Textbook of Diabetes and Pregnancy

SERIES IN MATERNAL–FETAL MEDICINE

Available

Of related interest

Textbook of Diabetes and Pregnancy

Second Edition

Edited by

Moshe Hod MD
Professor (Clinical) of Obstetrics and Gynecology
Director, Division of Maternal Fetal Medicine
Helen Schneider Hospital for Women
Rabin Medical Center
Sackler Faculty of Medicine, Tel-Aviv University
Petah-Tiqva
Israel

Lois Jovanovic MD
Clinical Professor of Medicine, University of Southern California
Keck School of Medicine
Adjunct Professor of Biomolecular Science and Engineering
University of California-Santa Barbara
CEO and Chief Scientific Officer
Sansum Diabetes Research Institute, Santa Barbara, CA
USA

Gian Carlo Di Renzo MD PhD
Professor and Chairman
Department of Obstetrics and Gynecology
Director
Centre of Perinatal and Reproductive Medicine, University Hospital
Perugia
Italy

Alberto de Leiva MD PhD MHE
Professor of Medicine and Director
Department of Endocrinology, Diabetes and Nutrition
Principal Investigator
EDUAB-CIBER BBN (ISCIII)
Hospital de la Santa Creu i Sant Pau, Universitat Autònoma
Barcelona
Spain

Oded Langer MD PhD
Babcock Professor and Chairman,
Department of Obstetrics and Gynecology
St. Luke's-Roosevelt Hospital Center
University Hospital for Columbia University
New York, NY
USA

informa
healthcare

First edition published in the United Kingdom in 2003

Second edition published in the United Kingdom in 2008 by Informa Healthcare, Telephone House, 69-77 Paul Street, London EC2A 4LQ. Informa Healthcare is a trading division of Informa UK Ltd. Registered Office: 37/41 Mortimer Street, London W1T 3JH. Registered in England and Wales number 1072954.

Tel: +44 (0)20 7017 5000
Fax: +44 (0)20 7017 6699
Website: www.informahealthcare.com

A CIP record for this book is available from the British Library.

Library of Congress Cataloging-in-Publication Data
Data available on application

ISBN-10: 0 415 42620 0
ISBN-13: 978 0 415 42620 6

Distributed in North and South America by
Taylor & Francis
6000 Broken Sound Parkway, NW, (Suite 300)
Boca Raton, FL 33487, USA

Within Continental USA
Tel: 1 (800) 272 7737; Fax: 1 (800) 374 3401
Outside Continental USA
Tel: (561) 994 0555; Fax: (561) 361 6018
Email: orders@crcpress.com

Distributed in the rest of the world by
Thomson Publishing Services
Cheriton House
North Way
Andover, Hampshire SP10 5BE, UK
Tel: +44 (0)1264 332424
Email: tps.tandfsalesorder@thomson.com

Composition by Cepha Imaging Pvt Ltd., Bangalore, India
Printed and bound in India by Replika Press Pvt. Ltd

To the most important people in my life

My wife Zipi, my sons Roy, Elad, and Yotam and my parents Esther and Michael
For their tolerance, patience and love – they made it all possible

Contents

Contributors

Salvatore Alberico, MD Obstetrical & Gynecologic Pathology, IRCCS Burlo Garofolo, Trieste, Italy

Emily Albertson, MD Sansum Diabetes Research Institute, Santa Barbara, CA, USA

Zarko Alfirevic, MD PhD FRCOG Professor of Fetal–Maternal Medicine, Liverpool Women's Hospital, Liverpool, UK

Yossef Bahagon Clalit Health Services, Hebrew University–Hadassah Medical School, Jerusalem, Israel

Madhuri S. Balaji, MB, FRSH Consultant Diabetologist, Dr V. Seshiah Diabetes Care & Research Institute, Chennai, India

V. Balaji, MD Consultant Diabetologist, Dr V. Seshiah Diabetes Care & Research Institute, Chennai, India

Jacob Bar, MD Division of Maternal Fetal Medicine, Helen Schneider Hospital for Women, Rabin Medical Center, Sackler Faculty of Medicine, Tel-Aviv University, Petah-Tiqva, Israel

Avi Ben-Haroush, MD Infertility & IVF Unit, Helen Schneider Hospital for Women, Rabin Medical Center, Sackler Faculty of Medicine, Tel-Aviv University, Petah-Tiqva, Israel

Noa Bischitz, BSc Laboratory of Teratology, Hebrew University–Hadassah Medical School & Israeli Ministry of Health, Jerusalem, Israel

Isaac Blickstein, MD Kaplan Medical Center, Rehovot and Hadassah–Hebrew University School of Medicine, Jerusalem, Israel

Paolo Bogatti, MD Obstetrical & Gynecologic Pathology, IRCCS Burlo Garofolo, Trieste, Italy

Bartolomé Bonet, MD PhD Head of the Department of Pediatrics and Neonatology, Fundacion Hospital Alcorcon, Madrid, Spain

Michael Brandle, MD MS Division of Endocrinology and Diabetes, Kantonsspital, St. Gallen, Switzerland

Eulàlia Brugués, MSc Head, Information Technology, Diabem Foundation, Barcelona, Spain

Lluis Cabero-Roura, PhD BD FRCOG AIAPM Professor & Chairman, Hospital Maternal–Infantil Vall d'Hebron, Barcelona, Spain

Maria Goya Canino, MD Hospital Maternal–Infantil Vall d'Hebron, Barcelona, Spain

Patrick M. Catalano, MD Case Western Reserve University at Metrohealth Medical Center, Cleveland, OH, USA

Rony Chen, MD Division of Maternal Fetal Medicine, Helen Schneider Hospital for Women, Rabin Medical Center, Sackler Faculty of Medicine, Tel-Aviv University, Petah-Tiqva, Israel

Frank A. Chervenak, MD New York Presbyterian Hospital, Weill Medical College of Cornell University, New York, NY, USA

Graziano Clerici, MD Centre for Perinatal & Reproductive Medicine, University of Perugia, Italy

Ohad Cohen, MD Institute of Endocrinology, Ch. Sheba Medical Center, Tel Hashomer, & Sackler School of Medicine, Tel Aviv University, Israel

Rosa Corcoy, MD PhD Consultant Physician, Hospital de la Santa Creu i Sant Pau, Assistant Professor, Universitat Autònoma, Barcelona, Spain & Centro de Investigaciòn Biomédica del Area de Bioingenieria, Biomateriales y Nanotecnologia, Instituto de Salud Carlos III

Antonio Cutuli, MD Centre for Perinatal & Reproductive Medicine, University of Perugia, Italy

Dana Dabelea, MD PhD Associate Professor, University of Colorado, Denver, CO, USA

M.G. Dalfrà Surgical Sciences Chair of Metabolic Disease, University of Padua, Italy

Kevin J. Dalton, DFMS LLM PhD FRCOG FCLM Consultant in Obstetrics & Gynecology and in Legal Medicine, University of Cambridge, Addenbrooke's Hospital, Cambridge, UK

Peter Damm, MD DMSc Centre for the Pregnant Woman with Diabetes, University Hospital of Copenhagen, Rigshospitalet, Denmark

Alberto de Leiva, MD PhD MHE Professor, Universitat Autònoma, Barcelona, Spain

Gernot Desoye, PhD Clinic of Obstetrics & Gynecology, Medical University of Graz, Austria

G. Di Cianni, Endocrinology and Metabolism Department, Section of Diabetes, University of Pisa, Italy

Gian Carlo Di Renzo, MD PhD Professor and Chairman, Department of Obstetrics and Gynecology, Director, Centre of Perinatal and Reproductive Medicine, University Hospital, Perugia, Italy

Tao Duan Shanghai Ist Maternity & Infant Hospital of Tongji University, Shanghai, China

Ulf J. Eriksson, MD PhD Professor, Uppsala University, Biomedical Center, Sweden

Inge M. Evers, MD University Hospitals, Utrecht, The Netherlands

Marco Orsini Federici University of Perugia, Italy

Dov Feldberg, MD Helen Schneider Hospital for Women, Rabin Medical Center, Sackler Faculty of Medicine, Tel-Aviv University, Petah-Tiqva, Israel

Benjamin Fisch, MD PhD Infertility Unit, Helen Schneider Hospital for Women, Rabin Medical Center, Sackler Faculty of Medicine, Tel-Aviv University, Petah-Tiqva, Israel

Mark Forbes Specialist Registrar, Diabetes Centre, Royal Devon & Exeter NHS Foundation Trust, Devon, UK

Pauline Green Consultant Obstetrician, Arrowe Park Hospital, Wirral, UK

David R. Hadden, MD FRCP Professor, Royal Maternity Hospital and Royal Victoria Hospital, Belfast, Northern Ireland, UK

Sylvie Hauguel-de Mouzon, PhD Professor of Reproductive Biology, Case Western Reserve University, Cleveland, OH, USA

John W. Hare, MD Senior Physician, Associate Clinical Professor of Medicine, Joslin Diabetes Center, Harvard Medical School, Boston, MA, USA

Linda Harnevo LifeOnKey Inc., Baltimore, MD, USA

Andrew T. Hattersley, DM FRCP FMedSci Professor of Molecular Medicine and Consultant Diabetologist, Peninsula Medical School, Exeter, UK

William W. Hay Jr., MD Professor of Pediatrics, University of Colorado, School of Medicine, Aurora, CO, USA

Yenon Hazan, MD Kaplan Medical Center, Rehovot and the Hadassah–Hebrew University School of Medicine, Jerusalem, Israel

William H. Herman, MD MPH Professor of Internal Medicine & Epidemiology, University of Michigan Medical Center, Ann Arbor, MI, USA

Emilio Herrera, PhD Professor and Chairman of Biochemistry, Faculties of Pharmacy & Medicine, Universidad San Pablo-CEU, Madrid, Spain

Michael Hirsch, Helen Schneider Hospital for Women, Rabin Medical Center, Sackler Faculty of Medicine, Tel-Aviv University, Petah-Tiqva, Israel

Moshe Hod, Professor (Clinical) of Obstetrics & Gynecology, Director, Division of Maternal Fetal Medicine, Helen Schneider Hospital for Women, Rabin Medical Center, Sackler Faculty of Medicine, Tel-Aviv University, Petah-Tiqva, Israel

Matías Uranga Imaz, MD Practice Works Chief UBA, Hospital Aleman & Hospital Fernandez, Buenos Aires, Argentina

Lois Jovanovic, MD CEO and Chief Scientific Officer, Sansum Diabetes Research Institute, Santa Barbara, CA, USA

Bari Kaplan, MD Helen Schneider Hospital for Women, Rabin Medical Center, Sackler Faculty of Medicine, Tel-Aviv University, Petah-Tiqva, Israel

Yoo Lee Kim, MD College of Medicine, Pochon CHA University, Seoul, Korea

John L. Kitzmiller, MD Good Samaritan Hospital, San Jose, & Sansum Medical Research Institute, Santa Barbara, CA, USA

Siri L. Kjos, MD Professor and Chief, Division of Women's Health, Obstetrics and Gynecology, University of Southern California Keck School of Medicine, Los Angeles, CA, USA

Eli Kupperman Sansum Diabetes Research Institute, Santa Barbara, CA, USA

Nieli Langer, PhD Associate Professor, Graduate School Division of Human Services, College of New Rochelle, New Rochelle, NY, USA

Oded Langer, MD PhD Babcock Professor and Chairman, Department of Obstetrics and Gynecology, St. Luke's-Roosevelt Hospital Center, University Hospital for Columbia University, New York, NY, USA

A. Lapolla, MD Surgical Sciences Chair of Metabolic Disease, University of Padua, Italy

Jeannet Lauenborg Centre for the Pregnant Women with Diabetes, Rigshospitalet, Copenhagen University Hospital, Denmark

C. Lencioni, Endocrinology and Metabolism Department, Section of Diabetes, University of Pisa, Italy

Nino Loia, MD Department of Ophthalmology, Rabin Medical Center, Petah Tiqva, Sackler Faculty of Medicine, Tel Aviv University, Israel

Roberto Luzietti, MD PhD Centre of Perinatal & Reproductive Medicine, University of Perugia, Italy

Karel Marsal, MD Consultant, University Hospital Lund, Sweden

Reuven Mashiach, MD Ultrasound Unit, Helen Schneider Hospital for Women, Rabin Medical Center, Sackler Faculty of Medicine, Tel-Aviv University, Petah-Tiqva, Israel

Massimo Massi-Benedetti, MD Chair of the School of Podology, University of Perugia, Italy

Gianpaolo Maso, MD Obstetrical & Gynecologic Pathology, IRCCS Burlo Garofolo, Trieste, Italy

Elisabeth R. Mathiesen, MD DMSc Chief Physician & Assistant Professor, Centre for the Pregnant Woman with Diabetes, University Hospital of Copenhagen, Rigshospitalet, Denmark

Maria Jose Mattioli, MD Hospital Fernandez, Buenos Aires, Argentina

Dídac Mauricio, MD PhD Director, Department of Endocrinology, University Hospital Arnao de Vilanova, Lleida, Spain

Laurence B. McCullough, PhD Center for Medical Ethics and Health Policy, Baylor College of Medicine, Houston, TX, USA

Israel Meizner, MD Head, Ultrasound Unit, Helen Schneider Hospital for Women, Rabin Medical Center, Sackler Faculty of Medicine, Tel-Aviv University, Petah-Tiqva, Israel

Nir Melamed, MD MSc Division of Maternal Fetal Medicine, Helen Schneider Hospital for Women, Rabin Medical Center, Sackler Faculty of Medicine, Tel-Aviv University, Petah-Tiqva, Israel

Giorgio Mello, MD SOD di Medicina Perinatale, Careggi University Hospital, Florence, Italy

Paul Merlob, MD Department of Neonatology, Helen Schneider Hospital for Women, Rabin Medical Center, Sackler Faculty of Medicine, Tel-Aviv University, Petah-Tiqva, Israel

Jorge H. Mestman, MD Professor of Medicine and Obstetrics & Gynecology, Keck School of Medicine, Los Angeles, CA, USA

Boyd E. Metzger, MD Tom D Spies Professor, Northwestern University, Feinberg School of Medicine, Chicago, IL, USA

Lars Mølsted-Pedersen, MD DMSc Centre for the Pregnant Woman with Diabetes, University Hospital of Copenhagen, Rigshospitalet, Denmark

Jeremy Oats, MD Clinical Director of Women's Services, Adjunct Professor, School of Public Health, La Trobe University, Carlton, Victoria, Australia

Yasue Omori, MD Director of Diabetes Center, Ebina General Hospital & Emeritus Professor of Tokyo Women's Medical University, Japan

Asher Ornoy, MD Laboratory of Teratology, Hebrew University–Hadassah Medical School & Israeli Ministry of Health, Jerusalem, Israel

Galia Oron Division of Maternal Fetal Medicine, Helen Schneider Hospital for Women, Rabin Medical Center, Sackler Faculty of Medicine, Tel-Aviv University, Petah-Tiqva, Israel

Henar Ortega, PhD Faculties of Pharmacy & Medicine, Universidad San Pablo-CEU, Madrid, Spain

Elena Parretti, MD PhD Firenze Nuovo Ospedale San Giovanni di Dio UO, Ginecologia e Ostetricia, Florence, Italy

Tamar Perri, MD Division of Maternal Fetal Medicine, Helen Schneider Hospital for Women, Rabin Medical Center, Sackler Faculty of Medicine, Tel-Aviv University, Petah-Tiqva, Israel

David J. Pettitt, MD Senior Scientist, Sansum Diabetes Research Institute, Santa Barbara, CA, USA

Dina Pfeifer Medical School, University of Zagreb, Croatia

Maria Rosaria Raspollini, MD PhD University of Florence School of Medicine, Florence, Italy

Drucilla J. Roberts, MD Massachusetts General Hospital & Harvard Medical School, Boston, MA, USA

Karl G. Rosén, MD PhD Plymouth Postgraduate Medical School, University of Plymouth, UK, & Neoventa Medical, Gothenburg, Sweden

David A. Sacks, MD Director, Maternal–Fetal Medicine, Kaiser Foundation Hospital, Bellflower & Clinical Professor Keck School of Medicine, University of Southern California, Los Angeles, CA, USA

Isabel Sánchez-Vera Department of Pediatrics and Neonatology, Fundacion Hospital Alcorcon, Madrid, Spain

V. Seshiah, MD DSc Chairman, Dr V. Seshiah Diabetes Care & Research Institute, Chennai, India

Eleazar Shafrir, PhD M Med Sci Professor of Biochemistry, Emeritus, Hadassah University, Kiryat Hadassah, Jerusalem, Israel

David Simmons, MA MBBS MRCP FRACP MD Waikato Clinical School, University of Auckland, Hamilton, New Zealand, and School of Rural Health, University of Melbourne, Victoria, Australia

Kinneret Tenenbaum-Gavish Division of Maternal Fetal Medicine, Helen Schneider Hospital for Women, Rabin Medical Center, Sackler Faculty of Medicine, Tel-Aviv University, Petah-Tiqva, Israel

Marta Viana, PhD Universidad San Pablo-CEU, Boadilla del Monte, Spain

Gerard H.A. Visser, MD PhD Professor of Obstetrics, University Medical Centre, Utrecht, The Netherlands

Liliana S. Voto, MD PhD Chairperson, Maternal & Childhood Department, Full Professor in Obstetrics, School of Medicine, Buenos Aires, University and Barceló School of Medicine, Argentina

Parri Wentzel, PhD Uppsala University, Biomedical Center, Sweden

Uri Wiesenfeld, MD Obstetrical & Gynecologic Pathology, IRCCS Burlo Garofolo, Trieste, Italy

Yariv Yogev, MD Division of Maternal Fetal Medicine, Helen Schneider Hospital for Women, Rabin Medical Center, Sackler Faculty of Medicine, Tel-Aviv University, Petah-Tiqva, Israel

Howard Zisser, MD Sansum Diabetes Research Institute, Santa Barbara, CA, USA

Foreword

The first edition of the *Textbook of Diabetes and Pregnancy*, edited by M. Hod and colleagues, was published five years ago. At that time, I mused about the uncertainty that yet another textbook on a well-established topic of clinical activity and research would be successful. The record of widespread circulation of the text speaks for itself, encouraging the preparation of the second edition that is now a reality.

There is a long history of collegiality among leaders in the field of diabetes and pregnancy. Reflecting this, the editor, M. Hod, is from Israel and he assembled a team of co-editors from three additional countries, the USA, Italy, and Spain. The more than 60 additional authors that contributed to the first edition were from equally diverse backgrounds, fields of expertise, and institutional and national affiliations. Likewise, the content of the volume was comprehensive and provided great depth in coverage of the field.

My assessment of the second edition is that it offers more of the same with improvements. The same group of editors has expanded the topics that were covered initially while retaining the excellent focus of the first edition. More than 100 authors have contributed to the 64 chapters of this edition. The Table of Contents now lists 5 chapters that deal with special issues that diabetes or gestational diabetes present in specific regions of the world, or in countries where rapid increases in chronic diseases (obesity, diabetes, cardiovascular disease) are occurring. In recognition of the challenges that attaining and sustaining "normalization" of glycemic control present in the management of Type 1 diabetes, and in anticipation of the availability of tools to address those challenges, chapters have been added that focus on the use of insulin pumps, the potential use of an "artificial pancreas" for treatment of diabetes during pregnancy, and the major impact of hypoglycemia. New chapters have also been added on key topics that are emerging, or projected to be of importance in the near future, e.g., genetics, infertility, electronic collection, management and application of health information.

In my opinion, the prospects are excellent for continued success with the second edition because of the forward-looking approach that Professor Hod and co-editors have adopted. I am confident that the second edition of Hod's *Textbook of Diabetes and Pregnancy* will continue to be a major resource for clinicians and investigators in the field of diabetes and pregnancy.

Boyd E. Metzger MD

Preface

The field of diabetes and pregnancy has come of age. From the conception of the terminology 'gestational diabetes' and 'diabetes in pregnancy' to the creation of an entire subspecialty, this textbook documents the 'gestation' of the field. Now we have even subdivided the field and have created subspecialists in gestational diabetes, and pregestational or diabetes in pregnancy, Type 1 and Type 2. In fact we have created our own internal debating groups as to the correct terminology for each type of diabetes and its impact on pregnancy and the pregnancy's impact on the type of diabetes. It is a great honor to be on the team of editors who have sought out the most creative and progressive of scientists, and learned from them the latest techniques and opinions as to the optimal management of all types of diabetes in pregnancy.

This textbook not only documents the past 80 years of progress in the field of diabetes and pregnancy, but also presents the most up-to-date tools, techniques and management protocols to ensure the optimal outcome of pregnancies complicated by diabetes. In addition, the areas that remain controversial are discussed in detail to enable the reader to come to an opinion while waiting for the evidence to validate many of the expert opinions presented in this book. A scan of the table of contents shows that every area in the field of diabetes and pregnancy has been covered. After a retrospective and historical perspective this textbook covers both gestational diabetes and the Type 1 and Type 2 diabetic woman who becomes pregnant. There are four chapters devoted to the history written by giants in the field who have had the opportunity to sit at the feet of the pioneers in our field: the great Drs Priscilla White, Norbert Freinkel, John O'Sullivan and Jørgen Pedersen. The authors of each of the subsequent chapters are world renowned. Thus if there is not the highest level of evidence-based literature to substantiate an opinion, the expert presents the data upon which a decision can be made about optimal care.

The most controversial topic today in the field of diabetes and pregnancy is in the area of screening and diagnosis. Here the evidence to date is presented and the justification for a multi-national, multi-center clinical trial to elucidate the optimal methods for screening and diagnosis are presented. In addition, the pure physiology of normal metabolism in pregnancy and the pathophysiology of diabetes in pregnancy are discussed in detail. These chapters set the stage for deriving the optimal therapy for the pregnant diabetic women and creating the algorithms that most closely mimic the normal physiology and metabolism of pregnancy.

The chapters devoted to malformations, placental pathology and defects of growth and development of the fetus are the strongest discussions to date in our understanding of diabetic fetopathy and teratogenesis. Based on this literature the reader will be motivated to learn the difficult protocols to achieve and maintain normoglycemia before, during and in-between all pregnancies complicated by diabetes.

The *Textbook of Diabetes and Pregnancy* also includes the latest theories and literature on the immunology of Type 1 diabetes and gives us hope that the near future holds the answers to prevention of this disease. Perhaps the solutions to the enigma may lead us to a cure of Type 1 diabetes. However, until there is a cure for diabetes, we must continually take on the burden of astutely diagnosing diabetes and treating all pregnant women who are at risk of an untoward outcome of pregnancy. Understanding and diagnosing all the metabolic abnormalities associated with pregnancy and providing the best management protocols to ensure a normal outcome of pregnancy is the objective. This textbook not only fulfills this objective, but also provides the answers for the clinician to help her/him to deliver optimal care of all pregnancies complicated by diabetes while we wait for the cure.

Only five years passed since we published the first edition of the textbook and it is most interesting to observe the changes that have occurred in the interval. A substantial amount of new evidence-based information was accumulated during these years on new technologies, devices, and new pharmacological treatment modalities, all aimed to improve maternal and fetal outcome in diabetic pregnancy. We added some 14 new chapters in this edition that broaden all aspects of our knowledge of physiology, pathophysiology, follow up and management of the mother and her offspring.

Thanks to the expertise and understanding of our collaborators, our editorial process has been stimulating and rewarding. To all of them our sincerest and deepest gratitude.

Moshe Hod
Lois Jovanovic
Gian Carlo Di Renzo
Alberto de Leiva
Oded Langer

Abbreviations

AA	arachidonic acid; *also*, autoantibody
AACC	American Association of Clinical Chemists
ACE	angiotensin-converting enzyme
ACE-I	angiotensin-converting enzyme inhibitors
acetyl CoA	acetyl coenzyme A
ACOG	American College of Obstetricians and Gynecologists
ACTH	adrenocorticotropic hormone
AD	abdominal diameter
ADA	American Diabetes Association
ADHD	attention deficit hyperactivity disorder
ADIPS	Australasian Diabetes in Pregnancy Society
AGA	appropriate or average for gestational age
AGC	antenatal glucocorticosteroids
AGE	advanced glycation endproducts
AHIMA	American Health Information Management Association
AMA	antimicrosomal antibodies
ATP	adenosine triphosphate
AUGC	areas under the glucose curve
BDecf	base deficit in extracellular fluid
bFGF	basic fibroblast growth factor
BMD	bone mineral densities
BMI	body mass index
BP	blood pressure
BPD	biparietal diameter
BPI	brachial plexus injury
CAD	caspase-activated-deoxyribonuclease; *also*, coronary artery disease
CDSS	clinical decision support systems
CEA	cost-effectiveness analyses
CEMACH	Confidential Enquiry into Maternal and Child Health (*in UK*)
CETP	cholesteryl ester transfer protein
CHD	coronary heart disease
CHO	total grams of carbohydrate in the meal
CI	confidence interval
CIR	carbohydrate-to-insulin ratio
CM	congenital malformations
CNS	central nervous system
CRBP	cytoplasmatic retinoid binding proteins
CRL	crown–rump length measurement
CRP	C-reactive protein
CSII	continuous subcutaneous insulin infusion
CT	computed tomography
CTG	cardiotocography
DAG	diacylglycerol
DCCT	Diabetes Control and Complications Trial
DHES	dehydroepianosterone sulfate

DIEPS	Diabetes in Early Pregnancy Study
DIPAP	Diabetes in Pregnancy Awareness and Prevention
DKA	diabetic ketoacidosis
DM	diabetes mellitus
DM-1	Type 1 diabetes mellitus
DM-2	Type 2 diabetes mellitus
DME	diabetic macular edema
DMPA	depo-medroxyprogesterone acetate
DPC	Diabetes in Pregnancy Center at Northwestern University, USA
DPP	Diabetes Prevention Program
DPSG	Diabetic Pregnancy Study Group
DRS	Diabetic Retinopathy Study
DSM-IV	Diagnostic and Statistical Manual-IV
DZ	dizygotic
ECG	electrocardiogram
ED	erectile dysfunction
EE	equine estrogen
EFA	essential fatty acid
EFM	electronic fetal monitoring
EFW	estimated fetal weight
EGF	endothelial growth factors
EHR	electronic health record
EPO	erythropoietin
ESIMS	electrospray ionization mass spectrometry
ETDRS	Early Treatment of Diabetic Retinopathy Study
ETSI	European Telecommunications Standards Institute
FABP	fatty acid binding protein
FAD	flavin adenine dinucleotide
FBS	fetal blood sampling
FDA	Food and Drug Administration (*in the USA*)
FDR	first degree relative
FDRs-DM1	first degree relatives of patients with DM-1
FECG	fetal ECG
FFA	free fatty acid
FFM	free fat mass
FGF-4	fibroblast growth factor-4 protein
FGF	fetal growth factor
FHR	fetal heart rate
FI	finger identification
FPG	fasting plasma glucose
FR	folate receptor
FSH	follicle-stimulating hormone
FT$_4$I	free thyroxine index
GABA	gamma amino butyric acid
GAPDH	glyceraldehyde-3-phosphate dehydrogenase
GCT	glucose challenge test

GDM	gestational diabetes mellitus	LH	luteinizing hormone
GH	growth hormone	LMC	lead maternity carer
GLUT1	glucose transporter	LMWA	low molecular weight antioxidant
GnRH	gonadotropin-releasing hormone	LPL	lipoprotein lipase
GSIS	glucose stimulated fetal insulin secretion	LTS	localization of tactile stimuli
GUR	glucose utilization rate	MA	microalbuminuria
HAPO	Hyperglycemia and Adverse Pregnancy Outcome study	MAP	mitogen activated protein
		MBG	mean blood glucose
HbAlc	glycosylated hemoglobin	MFP	manual form perception
HCG	human chorionic gonadotropin	MFPR	multifetal pregnancy reduction
HCS	human chorionic somatomam- motropin (*previously referred to as* human placental lactogen, HPL)	MGH	mild gestational hyperglycemia
		MM	methimazole
		MMR	maternal mortality ratio
HDL	high density lipoproteins	MNT	medical nutrition therapy
HERS	Heart and Estrogen/Progestin Replacement Study	MODY	mature onset diabetes of the young
		MPA	medroxyprogesterone acetate
HG	hyperemesis gravidarum	MPHWS	multi purpose health workers
HGF	hepatocyte growth factor	MRI	magnetic resonance imaging
HIT	health information technology	MSAFP	maternal serum alpha-feto-protein
HL	hepatic lipase	MZ	monozygotic
HLA	histocompatibility leukocytic antigen; *also*, human leukocyte antigen	NADH	nicotinamide adenine dinucleotide
		NEFA	non-esterified fatty acid
		NGT	normal glucose tolerance
HPL	human placental lactogen	NICU	neonatal intensive care unit
HPLC	high-performance liquid chromatography	NIDD	non-insulin-dependent diabetes mellitus
HRT	hormone replacement therapy	NIH	National Institutes of Health (*in USA*)
HVR	hypervariable region	NO	nitric oxide
ICM	inner cell mass	NOS	NO synthase
IDDM	insulin-dependent diabetes mellitus	NPDR	non-proliferative diabetic retinopathy
IFCC	International Federation of Clinical Chemistry	NTD	neural tube defects
		NZSSD	New Zealand Society for the Study of Diabetes
IFG	impaired fasting glucose	$1,25\text{-OH}_2\text{D}$	1,25-dihydroxyvitamin D
IFIH1	interferon-induced helicase region	25-OH D	25-hydroxyvitamin D
IGF	insulin-like growth factor	OAV	one abnormal OGTT value
IGF-I (or IGF-1)	insulin-like growth factor I	OBSQID OB	Stetrical Quality Indicators and Data
IGF-II (or IGF-2)	insulin-like growth factor II		
IGF-BPI	IGF binding protein I	PAD	perinatal aggregated data
IGFR	IGF receptor family	PAI	plasminogen activator inhibitor
IgG	immunoglobulin	PBSP	prognostically bad signs during pregnancy
IGT	impaired glucose tolerance		
IL-6	interleukin-6	PC-1	glycoprotein-1
IR	insulin receptor	PCC	preconception care
IRMA	intraretinal microaneurysm	PCO	polycystic ovary
IRS	insulin receptor substrate	PCOS	polycystic ovary syndrome
ISF	insulin sensitivity factors	PDR	proliferative diabetic retinopathy
ISO	International Standards Organization	PEDF	pigment-epithelium-derived factor
IT	information technology	PET	pre-eclampsia toxemia
IUD	intrauterine device	PG	plasma glucose; *also*, prostaglandin
IUGR	intrauterine growth restriction	PGDM	pre-gestational diabetes mellitus
IVF	*in vitro* fertilization	PGE2	prostaglandin E2
IVGTT	intravenous glucose tolerance tests	PGF	placental growth factor
KAP	knowledge, attitude and practice	PHR	personal health record
LADA	latent autoimmune diabetes of adulthood	PI	phosphatidylinositol
		PID	pelvic inflammatory disease
LBM	lean body mass	PIH	pregnancy-induced hypertension
LCPUFA	long-chain polyunsaturated fatty acid	PKC	protein kinase C
LDL	low density lipoprotein	PMNL	polymorphonuclear leucocytes
LGA	large for gestational age		

PNM	perinatal mortality	T$_4$	thyroxine
PPG	postprandial plasma glucose	TBG	thyroxine-binding globulin
PPV	positive predictive value	TDD	total daily insulin dose
PTCA	percutaneous transluminal coronary balloon angioplasty	TG	triglyceride
		TK	tyrosine kinase
PTU	propylthiouracil	TNF-α	tumor necrosis factor-alfa
PUFA	polyunsaturated fatty acids	TOBEC	total body electrical conductivity
RAIU	radioactive iodine uptake	TPO	thyroid peroxidase antibodies
RBF	retinal blood flow	THHG	transient hyperthyroidism of hyperemesis gravidarum
RBP	retinol binding protein		
RCT	randomized controlled trial	TTP-α	alfa-tocopherol transfer protein
RDS	respiratory distress syndrome	UKPDS	United Kingdom Prospective Diabetes Study
REM	rapid eye movement sleep		
ROS	reactive oxygen species	VBAC	vaginal birth after Cesarean
SAP-35	surfactant associated protein 35	VEGF	vascular endothelial growth factor
SCBU	special care baby unit	VH	vitreous hemorrhage
SHS	Strong Heart Study	VLDL	very low density lipoproteins
SOD	superoxide dismutase	VNTR	variable number tandem repeat
T$_3$	triiodothyronine		

1 History of diabetic pregnancy

David R. Hadden

Introduction

One hundred years ago the medical literature on diabetic pregnancy was very limited. Pregnancy itself was no less frequent, but the outcome was affected by so many other major problems that the influence of a medical disorder of a chronic nature was both unrecognized and disregarded. Diabetes mellitus was also less prevalent, due both to demographic differences in the age of the population and to epidemiological factors – mainly the absence of any effective treatment so that young people with diabetes had a life expectancy of only a few years. The diagnosis of diabetes depended on the demonstration of sugar in the urine and the well-known symptoms of thirst, polyuria and weight loss, but there was no accurate measurement to assess severity, and the distinction between what are now known as Type 1 and Type 2 diabetes was only anecdotal. There was no documentation of the specific long-term complications of hyperglycemia in the eyes, nerves, heart, kidneys or blood vessels.

Early history of diabetes

Diabetes was well recognized as a medical disorder more than 2000 years ago, and some well-known references are worth quoting. The ancient Egyptian Ebers papyrus, dating to 1500 BC, records abnormal polyuria; the Greek father of medicine, Hippocrates (466–377 BC), mentioned 'making water too often' and Aristotle also referred to 'wasting of the body.' Aretaeus of Cappodocia (AD 30–90) in Asia Minor (now Turkey) is credited with first using the name diabetes, which is Greek for a siphon, meaning water passing through the body: 'diabetes is a wasting of the flesh and limbs into urine – the nature of the disease is chronic, but the patient is short lived ... thirst unquenchable, the mouth parched and the body dry ...'. The famous Arabian physician Avicenna (AD 980–1027) recorded further important observations that maintained and extended the previous Greek knowledge through what became known in Europe as the Dark Ages: he described the irregular appetite, mental exhaustion, loss of sexual function, carbuncles and other complications. There are also references to diabetes in ancient Hindu texts (AD 500) as a 'disease of the rich, brought about by gluttony or over-indulgence in flour and sugar,' and in early Chinese and Japanese writings 'the urine of diabetics was very large in amount and so sweet that it attracted dogs.'[1,2]

After the European Renaissance the first physician to rediscover and record the sweetness of the urine in diabetes was Thomas Willis in London (1679), 'The diabetes or pissing evil ... in our age given to good fellowship and guzzling down of unalloyed wine,' and Mathew Dobson 100 years later in Liverpool first demonstrated chemically the presence of sugar in the urine of diabetic patients. The demonstration by Oscar Minkowski (1889) that removal of the pancreas in a dog unexpectedly resulted in uncontrolled polyuria – the urine sugar attracted flies in the laboratory to the puddles on the floor – was the significant observation that eventually led to the extraction of insulin from the pancreatic islets in Toronto in 1922.[3] The story of the discovery of insulin is a remarkable record of disappointment: it was almost discovered in 1906 by Zuelzer in Berlin, and then in 1912 by Scott in Chicago, but was actually extracted by Paulesco in Romania in 1920. However, the world recognizes the story of the Toronto group – including Banting, Best, Collip and Macleod – as the definitive discovery and in 1923 the Nobel Prize for medicine and physiology was awarded to two of them, Frederick Banting and JJR Macleod.[4]

Until then the only effective treatment for diabetes had been dietary, and it was well known that restriction of food would ameliorate the symptoms. John Rollo had demonstrated this with his patient Captain Meredith in the army in Ireland in 1797, who obeyed his doctor's advice, documented the reduction in urine volume and subsequent weight loss, and even extracted sugar from the urine by evaporation. The dietary approach was carried to its logical extreme by the over-enthusiastic approach of FM Allen in New York (1919), whose starvation therapy often temporarily returned the blood glucose to normal, but only succeeded in extending life for a year or so in the severe juvenile cases, all of whom became skeletally thin. Dr Elliott Joslin is remembered as the Boston physician who bridged the period immediately before insulin's discovery and the exciting clinical demonstration of its effectiveness in the following decade.[5] In London, Dr Robin Laurence, diabetic himself, on dietary therapy only in his early twenties, recorded how his life was saved in 1923 by a telegram from his doctor in King's College Hospital, 'I've got insulin, and it works – come back quick': he survived for many years and became the leading diabetes specialist in England.[6]

These two doctors, Joslin in Boston and Laurence in London, became the leaders of the revolution which would take place in both the opportunity for and the outcome of pregnancy in diabetic women.

Pregnancy and diabetes before the discovery of insulin

A full historical review of fertility and of the outcome of pregnancy in different parts of the world is beyond the scope of this chapter, but there are a number of aspects that are of particular relevance to the story of diabetes. Medical history, in particular, is constrained by publication bias, and there is much more available data regarding Europe and North America than in other parts of the world. The geographical and ethnic differences in the distribution, development and management of diabetes in different places at different times would be of great interest to review, but as the data are patchy and both diabetic and obstetric treatments often poorly defined, it may be that: 'History followed different courses for different peoples, because of differences among peoples' environments, not because of biological differences among peoples themselves.'[7] There are certainly both environmental and genetic reasons for the differing prevalence and incidence of diabetes in different countries, as much as for the different outcomes of pregnancy, but the international historical study of these factors is still in its infancy.

The collection of vital statistics first became available at varying times in the developed Western countries. The Scandinavian countries were first (Sweden 1749, Denmark 1801), England and Wales followed (1838) and then Russia (1867); although the process was initiated in the USA in 1880 it was not complete until 1933.[8] Fertility rates have varied as much as death rates and migration in different countries, so that population dynamics will have a considerable effect on reported statistics for a single condition such as diabetes in pregnancy. The classical Malthusian checks on death rate – disease, famine and war – and the effects of celibacy and restraint on birth rate, will have more effect on the overall outcome statistics of pregnancy in diabetic mothers than the diabetes itself. The general fertility rate for England and Wales was about 130 live births per 1000 women between the ages of 15 and 44 in 1840, but is now only half

that rate. At present the total fertility rate (average number of children born per woman) varies from 2.1 in western Europe to 6.7 in West Africa.[9] However, there is no doubt that untreated diabetes must have been virtually incompatible with successful pregnancy before about 1850. In 1856 Blott in Paris wrote that 'True diabetes was inconsistent with conception,' and certainly the then short life expectancy of a young woman with what we now call Type 1 diabetes before the discovery of insulin would support that statement. Recent speculation on the possible nutritional causes of the present-day epidemic of Type 2 diabetes in older patients means that any data on diabetes successfully treated by diet only (which was probably Type 2, rather than Type 1) is of considerable theoretical interest, but it is perhaps important that these cases were not often reported in the literature and may well have been missed due to not even testing the urine for sugar.

In the pre-insulin days, and for some time after, death of the mother during or soon after pregnancy from uncontrolled diabetes was the major risk. But maternal mortality was high for many reasons unrelated to diabetes, and retrospective analysis of data from England and Wales between 1850 and 1937 shows that poor interventional obstetric care with increased risk of puerperal sepsis was more important than social or economic deprivation.[10] The maternal mortality rates for Scandinavian countries were much lower, and it is now clear that this was due to better overall obstetric management in the prevention of sepsis; in the USA maternal mortality between 1921 and 1924 was 6.8 per 1000 births, in England and Wales 3.9 per 1000 births and in the Netherlands only 2.5 per 1000 births.[8] These differences at national level have been widely discussed, but must be borne in mind when considering the isolated effect of maternal diabetes over those years.

Overall perinatal mortality (death of the fetus after 28 weeks or within 7 days of delivery) has shown a more consistent fall over the same period of time in all Western countries. Most of the decline was in postneonatal mortality related to rising standards of living and nutrition, but also to improved public health measures – broadly speaking, the predominant form of infant mortality in Western countries was postneonatal in the nineteenth century and neonatal in the twentieth. There was no close link between neonatal and maternal mortality, but there were very considerable differences in each of these measures between countries at the time of discovery of insulin (Table 1.1). The overall infant mortality

Table 1.1 Overall maternal mortality and infant and neonatal mortality for selected countries at the time of discovery of insulin (from Loudon[8])

Country	Maternal deaths, 1921–1924, per 1000 births	Infant deaths, 1924, per 1000 births	Neonatal deaths, 1924, per 1000 births
The Netherlands	2.5	67.3	18.6
Japan	3.3	166.4	67.5
England/Wales	3.9	75.1	33.1
Australia	4.5	57.1	29.8
USA	6.8	70.8	38.6

rates in Scandinavian countries were persistently lower than in England and Wales, or Belgium, between 1920 and 1965, although all countries show a steady exponential decline.[8] As perinatal mortality is now used as a main comparator for the outcome of diabetic pregnancy, it is important to bear these long-standing historical trends in mind.

Congenital malformations are also an important comparator for obstetric results but the recognition of a possible link with maternal diabetes is much more recent: anecdotal accounts in small series in the 1940s were not supported until the report by the UK Medical Research Council in 1955[11] and the larger series from Copenhagen in 1964.[12] Historical records on the frequency of congenital malformations are very incomplete and it was not until the International Clearinghouse for Birth Defects began to operate after 1974 that any baseline data on the prevalence of congenital malformations became possible.[13] It is still difficult to compare results for specifically identified diabetic pregnancies with overall national malformation rates where the collection of cases is much less detailed.[14] Other obstetric complications such as pre-eclampsia appear today to be more common in diabetic pregnancy but it is difficult to trace this possible inter-relationship back to the days before organized antenatal care. Some of the cases where maternal death occurred in a diabetic pregnancy may have been due to eclampsia rather than diabetic coma.

Gestational diabetes

The concept of gestational diabetes, actually meaning hyperglycemia due to the pregnancy itself but in practice defined as 'carbohydrate intolerance of varying severity with onset or first recognition during pregnancy,' is also recent.[15] In the very first recorded case Bennewitz, in 1823, considered that the diabetes was actually a symptom of the pregnancy, and as the symptoms and the glycosuria disappeared after at least two successive pregnancies he had some evidence to support his views.[16] That lesser degrees of maternal hyperglycemia were also a risk to pregnancy outcome dates back to studies in the 1940s in the USA[17,18] and Scotland,[19] which showed increased perinatal mortality some years before the recognition of clinical diabetes mellitus. This led to the term prediabetes in pregnancy, and to poorly defined concepts of temporary and latent diabetes. The first prospective study of carbohydrate metabolism in pregnancy was established in Boston in 1954, using a 50 g, 1 h screening test, which has subsequently been widely adopted in the USA.[20] O'Sullivan[21] first used the name 'gestational diabetes' in 1961, following the term metagestational diabetes used by Dr JP Hoet in 1954 after his early studies in Louvain, Belgium.[22] At that time the US emphasis was on establishing criteria for the 100 g oral glucose tolerance test in pregnancy as an index of the subsequent risk of the mother developing established diabetes, and the well-known O'Sullivan criteria were derived on this basis.[23] At about the same time, Mestman in southern California, began to identify the very considerably increased perinatal mortality associated with abnormal oral glucose tolerance in the obstetric population of Los Angeles County Hospital, which then comprised > 60% Latino mothers with the rest African–American and

only a few Caucasian.[24] Subsequent studies in many parts of the world have extended the recognition of what has now become, in some places, an epidemic of hyperglycemia in pregnancy. Jorgen Pedersen also used the term gestational diabetes in his monograph in 1967, but preferred to so classify a mother only after delivery, when he had demonstrated that her abnormal glucose tolerance in pregnancy had actually returned to normal postpartum; this rigorous definition has proved too difficult to achieve in practice.[25,26] The true definition of hyperglycemia in pregnancy judged by the internationally acceptable 75 g oral glucose tolerance test awaits the results of the large Hyperglycemia and Adverse Pregnancy Outcome (HAPO) study.[27] The enthusiasm of the team at Northwestern University, Chicago, led by Norbert Freinkel and subsequently by Boyd Metzger has ensured that the concept of gestational diabetes is now firmly imprinted on the obstetric mind, as well as having established a major place as an epidemiological tool to study not only the immediate outcome of pregnancy but also the long-term effects on both mother and baby of the relatively short phase of hyperglycemia during the latter part of the pregnancy.

Important early publications

The historical development of understanding in obstetric, metabolic and pediatric disciplines over the past 100 years is perhaps best illustrated by several more extensive quotations and commentaries on seminal papers from the early literature.

HG Bennewitz. Diabetes mellitus – a symptom of pregnancy. MD Thesis, University of Berlin, 1824. [Translated from Latin][28]

This is the first reference to diabetes in pregnancy. Although the patient was young the clearly described onset of her symptoms during the pregnancy would now classify this as gestational diabetes. Is it possible that she only survived because she was a milder case who responded to diet, while all the more severe Type 1 diabetic patients died?

Henry Gottlieb Bennewitz publicly defended his thesis for the degree of Doctor of Medicine at the University of Berlin on 24 June 1824 (Figure 1.1). It is a simple case report and review of the literature on the causes and treatments of diabetes known at that time. His Greek derivation of the word diabetes and his one-line definition of the symptoms are unchanged today:

> Urine differing in quality and quantity from the normal ... accompanied by unquenchable thirst and eventual wasting.

Before giving the case history, he summarized his belief that the diabetic condition was in some way a symptom of the pregnancy, or due to the pregnancy. He noted that:

> Other disorders ... began to break out as the pregnancy matured ... the little fires which had hidden beneath the smouldering deceiving ashes broke forth and devoured again the woman's condition in the most wretched manner.

DE
DIABETE MELLITO,
GRAVIDITATIS SYMPTOMATE.

DISSERTATIO
INAUGURALIS MEDICA
QUAM
GRATIOSI MEDICORUM ORDINIS
CONSENSU ATQUE AUCTORITATE
IN
UNIVERSITATE LITTERARIA BEROLINENSI
PRO SUMMIS
IN MEDICINA ET CHIRURGIA HONORIBUS
RITE OBTINENDIS
DIE XXIV. M. IUNII A. MDCCCXXIV
H. L. Q. S.
PALAM DEFENDET
AUCTOR
HENR. GOTTL. BENNEWITZ
BEROLINENSIS.

OPPONENTIBUS:
W. DE MOELLER, MED. ET CHIR. DDR.
A. TIETZEL, MED. ET CHIR. DDR.
O. ZIMMERMANN, MED. ET CHIR. DDR.

BEROLINI,
TYPIS IOANNIS FRIDERICI STARCKII.

DIABETES MELLITUS: A SYMPTOM OF
PREGNANCY

An inaugural dissertation in medicine in which
its author
Heinrich Gottleib Bennewitz
of Berlin
will defend publicly with the consent and on the
authority of the distinguished order of doctors in
the University of Letters of Berlin to obtain in
due order the highest honours in medicine and
surgery, on the 24th day of the month of June in
the year 1824.
HLQS.
The opponents being
W. de Moeller, Doctor of Medicine and Surgery
A. Tietzel, Doctor of Medicine and Surgery
O. Zimmermann, Doctor of Medicine and
Surgery

Berlin, at the press of Johann Friederich Starck

Figure 1.1   The title page of Dr Bennewitz's thesis De diabete mellito, graviditatis symptomate,[28] with translation into English.

He was convinced that:

> The disease appeared along with pregnancy, and at the very same time …; when pregnancy appeared, it appeared; while pregnancy lasted, it lasted; it terminated soon after the pregnancy.

He showed a degree of humility when he remarked that his patient must be something of a rare bird.

The case history commences on 13 November 1823, when Frederica Pape, aged 22, was admitted at 7 months in her fifth pregnancy to the Berlin Infirmary. The first three pregnancies appear to have been unremarkable, but in the fourth in 1822 she had an onset of thirst and polyuria which had resolved spontaneously after delivery. These symptoms returned at an unspecified time in her fifth pregnancy: she had

> a really unquenchable thirst – she consumed more than six Berlin measures of beer or spring water, although the quantity of urine greatly exceeded the amount of liquid consumed, and the urine itself smelt like stale beer. Her voice was weak, skin dry, face cold and she complained of a dragging pain in her back.

Treatment was more a matter of belief than of understanding, but apart from having withdrawn 360 mL of venous blood all at once (the equivalent of thirty-six 10 mL routine blood tests today) and taking a high-protein diet, probably deficient in vitamins, she must have benefitted from the rest and care. The measurement of 2 oz of sugar in 16 lb (224 oz) of urine, which is equivalent to about 1% glycosuria, was Bennewitz's only biochemical evidence of diabetes mellitus. From about 32 to

36 weeks the patient had a recurrent sore throat and increased abdominal distension such that twins were suspected. When examined on 28 December 1823 the cervix was dilating and the fetal head already partially descended. On 29 December she had an obstructed labor, and the child died intrapartum, probably due to delay in the second stage. Bennewitz remarks that the baby was of

> such robust and healthy character whom you would have thought Hercules had begotten.

The infant weighed 12 lb, a fact witnessed carefully. Postpartum, in spite of continued dieting, sweating and purging, and the application of eight leeches, the patient's strength improved daily, and sugar disappeared from her urine. 'With nature to preserve and treat her, we dismissed our patient cured' (Figure 1.2).

Unfortunately, there is no record of the woman's subsequent health, perhaps because Dr Bennewitz presented his thesis within 6 months and having been successful in obtaining his doctorate, dropped out of academic medicine. This pregnancy would certainly qualify as 'carbohydrate intolerance of varying severity with onset or first recognition during pregnancy,' which was the definition agreed for gestational diabetes at the first workshop–conference in Chicago in 1980.

JM Duncan. On puerperal diabetes. Trans Obstet Soc London 1882; 24: 256–85[29]

Matthews Duncan graduated in Aberdeen and became one of the leading obstetricians of his day (Figure 1.3). This compilation of cases from the literature, from anecdotal reports and

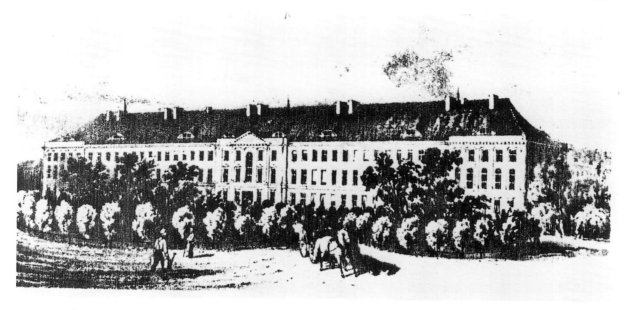

Figure 1.2   Die Charite in Berlin (1785–1800) from a lithograph by von C Koppen (from Murken AH, Vom Armenhospital zum Grossklinikum die Geschichte des Krankenhauses, Vom 18. Jahrhundert biszur Gegenwart Koln, Durmont, 1988, 39).

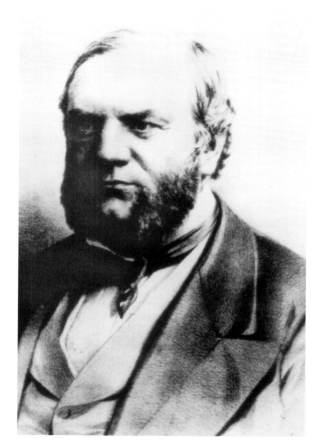

Figure 1.3   J Matthews Duncan MD: born in 1826, and educated in Aberdeen and Edinburgh. He studied obstetrics under Sir James Simpson and was closely involved in the discovery of chloroform. He moved to London in 1877 and had a large practice based at St Bartholomew's Hospital (courtesy of Dr DWM Pearson, Aberdeen).

from his own experience first identified the serious problem of diabetes to the obstetrical world. He recorded at least 22 pregnancies in 15 mothers between the ages of 21 and 38 (the data are confused in places): the mother survived the pregnancy for long enough to become pregnant again in nine instances, in five she died at the delivery and in six within a few months. The cause of maternal death was usually diabetic coma, although it is not possible to exclude eclampsia, and some must also have developed puerperal sepsis and one died from exacerbation of tuberculosis. Twelve of the 22 babies died, usually *in utero*, and they were usually of a large size: at least 10 survived and only three miscarriages are recorded: another 20 pregnancies seem to have occurred before the recorded cases, so some of these mothers must represent late-onset Type 2 or gestational diabetes, and these seemed to have a better prognosis for both mother and child.

So far as is known, all, with one exception, were multipara, the pregnancy of highest number being the tenth. They cannot be read without giving a strong impression of the great gravity of the complication, but they are not sufficiently numerous to justify any statistical argument based on the number of occurrences.

The histories further show that:

- Diabetes may come on during the pregnancy.
- Diabetes may occur only during pregnancy, being absent at other times.
- Diabetes may cease with the termination of the pregnancy, recurring some time afterwards.
- Pregnancy may occur during diabetes.

- Pregnancy and parturition may be apparently unaffected in its healthy progress by diabetes.
- Pregnancy is very liable to be interrupted in its course; and probably always by the death of the foetus.

JW Williams. The clinical significance of glycosuria in pregnant women. Am J Med Sci 1909; 137: 1–26[30]

Whitfield Williams was Professor of Obstetrics at the Johns Hopkins University and wrote the first major American textbook on obstetrics, which still survives today in the eighteenth edition. He was concerned that the demonstration of sugar in the urine in pregnancy would be overinterpreted. 'I know of no complication of pregnancy the significance of which is more variously interpreted than the presence of sugar in the urine of pregnant women.' Williams blamed Matthews Duncan for concluding that the detection of sugar in the urine constituted one of the most serious complications of pregnancy, as Duncan's views were accepted without question, although they were based on a small series of 22 pregnancies in 16 women collected from the then medical literature over 60 years, and his own small experience in Aberdeen. Williams presented six case reports to illustrate the various conditions in which sugar may be observed in the urine of pregnant women: simple lactosuria, transient glycosuria (two cases), alimentary glycosuria, recurrent glycosuria and mild diabetes. All resulted in a normal pregnancy outcome (although all the recorded birthweights were > 8 lb). He then analyzed the urinary records of 3000 consecutive patients in the obstetrical department of the Johns Hopkins Hospital, in 167 of whom sugar had been demonstrated by Fehling's solution. He concluded that 137 of these represented definite postpartum lactosuria, being recognized only during lactation, and that almost all the others who had been recognized in late pregnancy were similar. He was able accurately to distinguish glucose from lactose in a few cases and found only two of the 167 cases had definite glycosuria, and could thus be considered to have mild diabetes complicating pregnancy. This may be the first evidence of screening for gestational diabetes, suggesting a rather low prevalence in hospital practice in Baltimore, USA, nearly 100 years ago.

The major difficulty in the bedside measurement of reducing sugars by Fehling's test is no longer apparent, as all test strips now use a glucose oxidase system and recognize only glucosuria (lactosuria will still occur but no longer causes medical concern). Whitfield Williams then tabulated all reported cases (81) of diabetes complicating pregnancy from 1826 to 1907: he considered 15 cases to be doubtful, as glycosuria disappeared after delivery (including the famous patient first reported by Bennewitz in 1826, although he had not read the full case report in the original Latin). He calculated an overall immediate maternal mortality of 27%, with an additional 23% of mothers dying within the following 2 years. He concluded:

> Pregnancy may occur in diabetic women, or diabetes may become manifest during pregnancy; either is a serious complication, although the prognosis is not so alarming as is frequently stated.

EP Joslin. Pregnancy and diabetes mellitus. Boston Med Surg J 1915; 173: 841–9[31]

Joslin was the first internist to specialize in diabetes and wrote the first textbook on the subject. In 1915, 6 years before the discovery of insulin, he was able to describe seven personal cases of moderate or severe diabetes associated with pregnancy. He wished to take a more hopeful view, but admitted that little progress had been made. Of his seven cases, four were dead – one by suicide, one with uremic manifestations (? eclampsia), one of diabetic coma while under the care of a clairvoyant, and the fourth having survived one pregnancy with a healthy child died of pulmonary tuberculosis 2 months after losing her second child. But he was pleased that of the three remaining cases, one was in exceptionally good health, free from sugar and had a normal child, another in a tolerable condition having been pregnant three times but with only one child now living, and the remaining patient alive although severely ill with diabetes 6 years after confinement. He closed his paper with an optimistic comment: 'It is certainly true that with the improvements in the treatment of diabetic patients [he meant strict diet], diabetic women will be less likely to avoid pregnancy.'

E Brandstrup and H Okkels. Pregnancy complicated with diabetes. Acta Obstet Gynecol Scand 1938; 18: 136–63[32]

The immediate post-insulin period was marked by some euphoria by both patients and their doctors, but it took a long time for the very considerable fear of pregnancy to diminish, and to some extent that fear remains to the present day. A careful retrospective assessment of those early years of insulin at the Rikshospital in Copenhagen from 1926 to 1938 showed that although there had been no maternal deaths in 22 pregnancies in 19 diabetic women mostly treated with insulin (probably the more severe and often referred cases), the perinatal mortality was still 57%.[32] The 13 perinatal deaths included six stillbirths, two intrapartum deaths and five early neonatal deaths; of the 10 living children three were asphyxiated at birth, one weighed only 1500 g and one was 5250 g. Histological examination of the pancreas in two full-weight fetuses showed a pronounced increase in the size and number of the islets of Langerhans. Dr Brandstrup, who was in charge of these mothers' care during that time, set the scene for the future advances made by his successor Dr Jorgen Pedersen after World War II.

Brandstrup noted that most of his patients had been considered to be well adjusted with insulin treatment, but that they still had high levels of blood sugar for the greater part of the day. He had previously undertaken physiological studies in pregnant rabbits on the passage of carbohydrates across the placenta after intravenous injection, and had shown that while glucose and the pentoses passed across by a process of slow diffusion, the placental membrane was almost impermeable to disaccharides, including saccharose and lactose.[33] He described one patient treated in 1927, illustrated by a 24 h curve for blood sugar, who had been treated with two doses of insulin daily, felt well and was looked upon as treated

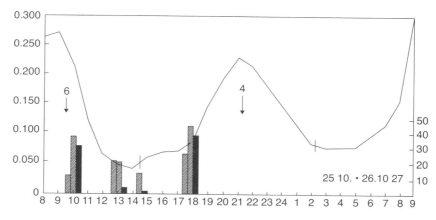

Figure 1.4   Blood sugar curve for a pregnant diabetic treated at the Rikshospital in Copenhagen in 1927, with two doses of insulin (6 units at 09.30 and 4 units at 21.00). Units are grams per cent blood sugar (0.100 g% = 100 mg/dl). Food intake is shown as histograms, with unidentified units on the right side (from Brandstrup and Okkels[32]).

adequately but he was unhappy with the level of control achieved (Figure 1.4).

The blood sugar is seen to keep at very high levels through a great part of the day. This feature is typical of the severe cases of diabetes under treatment with insulin, and it explains why the children are subject to intrauterine obesity through excessive supply of sugar also now in the epoch of insulin therapy. But these children are not only fat: they are large too. They present a condition of universal macrosomia … it seems probable that it is the maternal hyperglycemia alone that brings about the pathologic–anatomical changes in the child.

Conclusion

Further historical development of the management of diabetes in pregnancy will be considered in the next three chapters, which will focus on the work of Dr Jorgen Pedersen in Copenhagen, Dr Norbert Freinkel in Chicago and Dr Priscilla White in Boston. There is no doubt that had insulin not been discovered in 1922 then the present-day outlook for successful pregnancy in a diabetic mother would still remain very poor because of the continued maternal hyperglycemia, in spite of the enormous improvements in social, medical and obstetric care which has occurred in the intervening years.

REFERENCES

1. Peel J. A historical review of diabetes and pregnancy. Obstet Gynaecol Br Commun 1972; 79: 385–95.
2. Reece EA. The history of diabetes mellitus. In: Reece EA, Coustan DR, eds. Diabetes Mellitus in Pregnancy, 2nd edn. New York: Churchill Livingstone; 1995, pp. 1–10.
3. Banting FG, Best CH. The internal secretion of the pancreas. J Lab Clin Med 1922; 7: 256–71.
4. Bliss M. The Discovery of Insulin. Edinburgh: Paul Harris Publishing; 1983, pp. 20–58.
5. Joslin EP. Pregnancy and diabetes mellitus. Boston Med Surg J 1915; 173: 841–9.
6. Laurence RD, Oakley WG. Diabetic pregnancy. Q J Med 1942; 11: 45–54.
7. Diamond J. Guns, Germs and Steel: The Fates of Human Societies. New York: Norton & Co.; 1997, p. 25.
8. Loudon I. Death in Childbirth: An International Study of Maternal Care and Maternal Mortality 1800–1950. Oxford: Clarendon Press; 1992.
9. Chamberlain G. Birth rates. In: Turnbull A, Chamberlain G, eds. Obstetrics. Edinburgh: Churchill Livingstone; 1989, pp. 1105–10.
10. Turnbull A. Maternal mortality. In: Turnbull A, Chamberlain G, eds. Obstetrics. Edinburgh: Churchill Livingstone; 1989, pp. 1121–32.
11. Medical Research Council Conference on Diabetes and Pregnancy. The use of hormones in the management of pregnancy in diabetes. Lancet 1955; ii: 833–6.
12. Molsted-Pedersen L, Tygstrup I, Pederson J. Congenital malformations in newborn infants of diabetic women. Lancet 1964; i: 1124–6.
13. International Clearinghouse for Birth Defects Monitoring Systems. Congenital Malformations Worldwide. Amsterdam: Elsevier; 1991, pp. 1–8.
14. Kalter H. Of Diabetic Mothers and their Babies: An Examination of Maternal Diabetes on Offspring, Perinatal Development and Survival. Amsterdam: Harwood Academic Publishers; 2000, pp. 95–111.
15. Freinkel N. Of pregnancy and progeny. The Banting Lecture 1980. Diabetes 1980; 29: 1023–35.
16. Hadden DR. The development of diabetes and its relation to pregnancy: the long-term and short-term historical viewpoint. In: Sutherland HW, Stowers JM, Pearson DWM, eds. Carbohydrate Metabolism in Pregnancy and the Newborn II. London: Springer-Verlag; 1989, pp. 1–8.
17. Miller HC. The effect of the prediabetic state on the survival of the fetus and the birthweight of the newborn infant. N Engl J Med 1945; 233: 376–8.
18. Hurwitz D, Jensen D. Carbohydrate metabolism in normal pregnancy. N Engl J Med 1946; 234: 327–9.
19. Gilbert JAL, Dunlop DM. Diabetic fertility, maternal mortality and foetal loss rate. Br Med J 1949; i: 48–51.
20. Wilkerson HLC, Remein QR. Studies of abnormal carbohydrate metabolism in pregnancy. Diabetes 1957; 6: 324–9.
21. O'Sullivan JB. Gestational diabetes. Unsuspected, asymptomatic diabetes in pregnancy. N Engl J Med 1961; 264: 1082–5.
22. Hoet JP. Carbohydrate metabolism during pregnancy. Diabetes 1954; 3: 1–12.

23. O'Sullivan JB, Mahan C. Criteria for the oral glucose tolerance test in pregnancy. Diabetes 1964; 13: 278–85.

24. Mestman JH, Anderson GU, Barton P. Carbohydrate metabolism in pregnancy. Am J Obstet Gynecol 1971; 109: 41–5.

25. Pederson J. Diabetes og gravid: En introduktion. Ugeskr Laeger 1951; 113: 1771–7.

26. Pedersen J. The Pregnant Diabetic and her Newborn. Problems and management. Copenhagen: Munksgaard; 1967, p. 46.

27. HAPO Study Cooperative Research Group. The Hyperglycemia and Adverse Pregnancy Outcome (HAPO) study. Int J Gynecol Obstet 2002; 78: 69–77.

28. Bennewitz HG. De diabete mellito, gravidatatis symptomate. MD Thesis, University of Berlin, 1824. [Translated into English, deposited at the Wellcome Museum of the History of Medicine, Euston Road, London, 1987].

29. Duncan JM. On puerperal diabetes. Trans Obstet Soc London 1882; 24: 256–85.

30. Williams JW. The clinical signifcance of glycosuria in pregnant women. Am J Med Sci 1909; 137: 1–26.

31. Joslin EP. Pregnancy and diabetes mellitus. Boston Med Surg J 1915; 173: 841–9.

32. Brandstrup E, Okkels H. Pregnancy complicated with diabetes. Acta Obstet Gynecol Scand 1938; 18: 136–63.

33. Brandstrup E. On the passage of some substances from mother to fetus in the last part of pregnancy. Acta Obstet Gynecol Scand 1930; 10: 251–87.

2 The Priscilla White legacy

John W. Hare

Introduction

Priscilla White was a pure clinician who devoted her entire professional career to the treatment of diabetic patients. In particular, she had an interest in Type 1 diabetes in women and in youths. This interest led her to the treatment of diabetes in pregnancy, now a formal discipline which her life's work did much to create.

Priscilla White was born in 1900 and attended Radcliffe College (now merged with Harvard College). Since Harvard Medical School did not enroll women until just after World War II, she attended Tufts College Medical School. She was an intern at the Worcester (MA) Memorial Hospital because Boston hospitals did not accept women as house officers. She had worked as a medical student with Elliott Joslin, already well known in the field of diabetes, whose first textbook was published in 1916, six years before the availability of insulin. Elliott Joslin was greatly impressed with '… this early-rising, young medical student …' and invited her to join his staff in 1924. Legend has it that when she started her career at the Joslin Clinic she was given the task of treating young women with diabetes. Over time they grew up and began to have children, creating her lifelong interest in pregnancy. However, she wrote a chapter entitled Diabetes in Pregnancy in the 1928 edition of the Joslin-edited textbook *The Treatment of Diabetes Mellitus*.[1] This was too short a period for her young charges to have gone through puberty (often late in those days), married and conceived. Thus, her interest in pregnancy must have been manifest and acted upon from the very beginning.

Elliott Joslin was her mentor and a father figure until his death in 1962. Her association with him as a student came just at the exciting time when insulin became available, first given in Boston by Dr Joslin's assistant, Howard Root, in August 1922. It is hard to imagine what the times must have been like for those with diabetes and their doctors. Most diabetes diagnosed in the early twentieth century was symptomatic Type 1. Patients who survived were often severely cachectic as a result of both therapeutic design and pathophysiology. Their absence of fat precluded ketogenesis and thus allowed survival. In some way, the practice of diabetes in 1920 must have been like specializing in the treatment of HIV/AIDS today. Early insulin preparations – crude and cumbersome, consisting of 10 U/mL of crystalline insulin – required frequent and painful injections. It stopped the high proportion of deaths from ketoacidosis but permitted the subsequent expression of the vascular complications of diabetes with which there is now

so much concern. These points are relevant to the treatment of diabetes and pregnancy. Many women who became pregnant without the benefit of insulin treatment either died or lost the fetus because of ketoacidosis. Insulin therapy permitted an immediate and marked improvement in the survival of both mother and fetus. Over the next several decades it also permitted women with diabetes to survive and to develop vascular complications. The development of vascular complications, particularly microvascular, became the principal determinant of pregnancy outcomes. The significance of these complications was quickly perceived by Priscilla White and underlies the now famous White classification. Any subsequent or modern evaluation of diabetes and pregnancy must still adhere to this principle so perceptively noted by her.

An important dimension of White's character and personality was her ability to relate in the warmest way to her patients. She gave them enormous time and energy. A letter from a patient, quoted in a 1998 monograph by Donald M Barnett, MD (*Elliott P Joslin, MD: A Centennial Portrait*) is illustrative:

> Yes, I feel that I know Dr. White very well. I had first come to the Joslin Clinic in 1935 with newly discovered diabetes. … Dr. White's presence was such a help. Naturally she would chart and guide our medical therapy including the problematic Protamine Zinc Insulin in use at the time. She was endearingly optimistic and happy with each of us individually. She was a naturally beautiful woman and could easily engage in what I felt to be a genuine interest in fashion and feminine things that interest young women. I remember that Dr. White drove me from the Deaconess Hospital to the Faulkner Hospital in a terrible rainstorm as my due date neared.

White never married and had no children. Her great passion was her career and her small passion was her dogs. I have my own experiences with her love of dogs and her capacity for personal relationships. When I was a Junior Assistant Resident at the New England Deaconess Hospital in 1966, my first assignment was to Priscilla White's service. I would meet her early in the morning at the Boston Lying-in Hospital for rounds. Her secretary would afterwards drive us to the Joslin Clinic, where I would find my house officer's whites covered with dark daschund hairs. During this rotation, I told her a story about a boyhood birthday. Eight years later, when I joined the senior staff, she was near retirement and immediately recalled the story. That year was her fiftieth anniversary at the Joslin Clinic. Soon thereafter she began a gradual retirement and only occasionally appeared in our Pregnancy Clinic that she had begun over 50 years before. I subsequently inherited a number of her patients who expected me to give them as much time she did, and to write them a letter after each and every visit, something the time pressure of modern medicine no longer permitted.

White's mental acuity began to decline in the late 1970s and her remarkable mind failed her completely in the last years before her death in 1989. Her last paper, published in 1980, was co-authored with me and fittingly enough was her last revision of her world famous White classification. These revisions had been done from time to time over 30 years as data and experience dictated, e.g. adding class T for women who became pregnant after renal transplantation. The 1980 refinement removed gestational diabetes from the standard lettered taxonomy.

The early years

Priscilla White's first chapter in the Joslin-edited textbook *The Treatment of Diabetes Mellitus* appeared in 1928.[1] In it she reviewed the Joslin Clinic experience with 89 pregnancies. She made the then spectacular and hopeful statement that '... diabetes is no longer a contraindication to pregnancy.' To say such a thing makes clear that, for diabetic women before insulin, pregnancy was considered hopeless. Hope is the sentiment that has sustained thousands of diabetic women since, and permitted them to undergo the therapeutic demands and discomforts of pregnancy. This hope was made real and underpinned by the gathering of clinical evidence that documented the likelihood of a successful outcome. White's chapters were typical of those in early Joslin texts, and were largely, if not entirely, case reports and clinical series. In fact, much of her extensive bibliography is comprised of book chapters, clinical series and reviews reporting her collected experience as opposed to peer-reviewed publications of original research.

The dismal reproductive capacity of women in this era is easily inferred by reading White's somewhat optimistic statements in the obverse. For example, 'Insulin, it is true, has decreased the frequency of sterility among diabetic women, but the return to normalcy is slow,' meaning sterility had been and still remained a problem. In writing about success she said, 'Fourteen stillbirths, or 25 per cent, occurred among our 59 pregnancies coming to term.' She felt the 25% figure was an improvement because it represented a halving of the 50% risk for fetal death in the pre-insulin era. Sometimes the severity of the reality was obscure. A table summarized the outcomes of the 89 pregnancies: eight outcomes were unknown and four were 'undelivered.' I had to ask a colleague why this category was included, given all the other expected outcomes, such as stillbirths and miscarriage, were listed. It meant that the mother died. If not death in pregnancy, there was death thereafter. Another table in White's first chapter indicates that of 58 cases, 42 were still alive in June 1926, indicating an eventual mortality of 28% after pregnancy. Even more striking, 10 of the 16 women had developed their diabetes in 1922 or later, meaning that they died despite having short-term diabetes and

being insulin treated from the onset. One of the women had survived 23 years postpartum and another 15 years, i.e. they had diabetes in the pre-insulin era.

Some concepts now taken for granted began to emerge. For example, though gestational diabetes was not labeled as such, it was recognized: 'Pregnancy contracted during diabetes is less frequent than diabetes contracted during pregnancy.' The phenomenon of heightened insulin sensitivity postpartum was noted, though incorrectly ascribed to '... the passage of sugar from the blood to the breasts at lactation.' It was in this chapter that White made the prescient statement 'Controlled diabetes is essential to fetal welfare,' which has become the bedrock of modern management.

White was not the first to write about diabetes in pregnancy, but this chapter represents the beginning of a systematic clinical analysis of an astounding series of over 2200 cases (most of whom were insulin dependent) that made her famous, and allowed maternity for her patients and countless others all over the world.

Her chapter published in the sixth edition of the textbook edited by Joslin et al., *The Treatment of Diabetes Mellitus*, represents continued progress in understanding the natural history of diabetes in pregnancy and how to modify it.[2] She noted that the lack of fertility in diabetic women '... has been corrected in great measure in proportion to the extent of control of the disease.' White once again, to some degree by intuition and to some degree supported by data, hit the nail on the head by observing that '... the degree of hyperglycemia appears to be directly related to the frequency of spontaneous miscarriage or abortion.' She found that the abortion rate was 33% in controlled cases and only 2% in those well treated, which seems too low. All this was, of course, without benefit of anything more precise to assess control other than urine tests and occasional blood glucose levels done at the time of clinic visits.

However, one could not expect White to have understood all that is known today about the biology of diabetic pregnancy, and she did not. She admitted, 'The cause of overgrowth of the fetus of the diabetic is not known,' although she certainly recognized the problem. Fifty-six per cent of Joslin patients' infants had birthweights > 8 lb, compared with 9% of a control series [presumably 8 lb, or *c.* 3600 g, represented infants large for gestational age (LGA) or the ninetieth centile). She noted that 'The greatest growth of the embryo occurs in the last two months, at a time when the blood sugar is often normal,' which it surely was not. Another statement, now known to be wide off the mark, was 'Congenital defects are beyond our therapeutic control and are, we believe, related to a disease which is genetic in origin.' She later revised her opinion and in 1958 said that 'The 3 per cent mortality due to congenital anomalies can perhaps be lowered by avoiding such causes of anoxia as acidosis and hypoglycemia.'[3] This sentence attributing anomalies to metabolic changes presaged by 20 years the notion of hyper- and hypoglycemia as causes of malformations. These hypotheses could not be tested until self-blood-glucose monitoring and glycohemoglobin tests became available. She also felt that some malformations were '... due to chronic vascular insufficiency ...', but she was not alone in having to speculate as to the cause of fetal anomalies.

It is in the paper published in 1937 that White's most important contribution begins to germinate; namely that duration (and its relation to vascular disease) adversely affects outcome.[4] Although over a decade away from publishing her classification, one can see a hint of the concept emerging. She said that 'Long duration of diabetes decreases the number of living births,' but by long duration she meant > 1 year. In her discussion of toxemia (which must have included pregnancy-induced hypertension of all types) she noted that mothers over 30 years of age had a higher loss rate and more toxemia. Her most seriously erroneous construct is also mentioned here. She believed that toxemia, a major cause of fetal death, was caused by or related to hormonal imbalance. In particular, she believed prolan [human chorionic gonadotropin (hCG)] excess and estrin deficiency were related to toxemia. To support this thesis she cited both human and animal data derived from urine or bioassays which were immeasurably cruder than today's assays measured in picomoles. She said, 'Estrin therapy seems to be the logical method of treatment.' This belief would lead to the treatment of her pregnant women with sex steroids starting in 1938, and it was a therapy she refused to relinquish. Not until after her retirement was the practice stopped in 1975. The original basis for White's staunch belief in hormonal therapy was the paper published with Smith, Smith and Joslin in 1937.[4] The hypothesis was that prolan (hCG) was utilized in the placental production of estrogen, both by oxidation (early) and metabolism (late). She wrote: 'The damaged vascular tree of the diabetic may interfere with the blood supply to the uterus and placenta and with the normal production of its hormones.'[5] Her insistence on maternal sex steroid therapy is often overlooked in view of the more familiar linking of her name to her eponymous classification. When the White classification first appeared hormonal dysfunction was also a modality of classification, as well as the familiar alphabetized one based upon age, duration and complications. In fact, it occupied as much space in her discussion as did classes A–F. White firmly believed that this regimen improved fetal survival and increased the hormone doses from class A to class F. By the time her last chapter in *Joslin's Diabetes Mellitus* appeared in the 11th edition of this textbook in 1971,[6] hormonal therapy was no longer given in increasing doses by class. Class A (abnormal glucose tolerance, treated with diet alone) was excepted from treatment as it always had been.

In the 1980s, the Joslin Clinic formally surveyed the mothers known to have been treated with these hormones. No cases of gynecological cancer in their daughters or genitourinary abnormalities in their sons were reported other than cryptorchidism, which is common and may not have been related. However, anecdotal accounts of daughters having difficulty with habitual abortion and incompetent cervices have been received.

Finally, White also believed that diuretic therapy prevented hydramnios, edema and pre-eclampsia toxemia (PET), the latter having always been a major cause of fetal loss. Thus, at first encapsulated ammonium chloride, then injected mercurial diuretics and finally oral diuretics, thiazides in particular, were routinely used from the 1940s until 1975. Of course, diuretic therapy may have aggravated PET, the very condition it was meant to prevent.

The White classification

In 1949, White published the first version of the classification system which was to be the single most remembered thing about her work, and has been of immense clinical value to practitioners all over the world.[7] Part of the success of this classification was no doubt rooted in its rationale and utility, but part must have also been that the world leader in the field of diabetic pregnancy espoused it. She was almost precisely at the mid-point in her career and had been on the staff of the Joslin Clinic for 25 years. She was already well known and her eminence would have been helpful in facilitating its adoption. By way of historical perspective, in 1949 her great European clinical counterpart, Jørgen Pedersen, was just making his debut on the world stage of diabetes and pregnancy, and Norbert Freinkel had just received his medical degree.

Reading papers published by White only a year or two before the appearance of her classification so soon after is somewhat of a surprise. Although she had long recognized the importance of duration of diabetes as a risk factor for vascular disease, she did not particularly link it to pregnancy outcome and certainly not in a graded form, even shortly before 1949. In her 1946 chapter in the eighth edition of the book *The Treatment of Diabetes Mellitus*, edited by Joslin et al., she wrote about how quickly diabetes could cause vascular disease, noting that it was present in 70% of non-pregnant 20 year survivors of diabetes, i.e. not all patients with Type 1 diabetes lived 20 years.[8] By vascular disease she meant both macro- and microvascular, e.g. coronary heart disease and retinopathy. However, she did not discuss the implications of this observation for pregnant women. Despite the generally poor prognosis it is notable that only one maternal death had occurred in 271 pregnancies between January 1936 and March 1946. The one death was due to infectious hepatitis and occurred 8 weeks postpartum. Thus, the striking maternal mortality of the pre-insulin era was gone. Also of interest is her notation that congenital anomalies occurred in 12% of the infants as compared with 1.8% in the non-diabetic population, almost exactly what would be reported 35 years later when Joslin data were published which clearly and quantitatively linked periconceptual control to congenital anomalies by using first trimester glycohemoglobin levels.[9] In the patients studied in that paper, the overall anomaly rate was 12.9% and the non-diabetic rate in the USA was c. 2%.

In a 1947 paper entitled 'Pregnancy Complicating Diabetes of More Than Twenty Years Duration,' White rather tediously reviewed 10 cases, but stopped short of systematically linking duration and complications to outcome.[10] However, all the data that she collected and used in her classic 1949 paper[7] must have already been under review. Two years later the original classification appeared and had only six classes, though it was later to have as many as 10 (Box 2.1).

Another important point emerged in this paper.[7] White noted that 68% of stillbirths occurred after the 35th week of gestation. This was the rationale for early delivery of all patients, usually by Cesarean section. By 1953 the schema had been refined: class A was permitted to go to term, classes B and C were carried to 38 weeks, and classes D–F were delivered in the 35th week.[5] White reasoned that prematurity and atelectasis

---

Box 2.1   Priscilla White's first classification

Class A: Abnormal glucose tolerance test, treated with diet alone
Class B: Onset before the age of 20, duration < 10 years, no vascular disease
Class C: Onset between the ages of 10 and 19, duration 10–19 years or minimal vascular disease, including retinal arteriosclerosis or calcifications of lower extremity arteries*
Class D: Onset before the age of 10, duration > 20 years or retinitis, hypertension or albuminuria
Class E: Pelvic vascular calcification, iliac or uterine
Class F: All patients with nephritis (more than just albuminuria)

*Background retinopathy and lower extremity calcification were included in class D in later classifications.

(respiratory distress) were a lesser risk than stillbirth in the more severe classes.

The White classification underwent several revisions. In her 1971 chapter in *Joslin's Diabetes Mellitus*, which was her last, class E, pelvic vascular calcification, was no longer used.[6] This category had either been actively sought or incidentally diagnosed when X-ray pelvimetry was used. It was thought that pelvic or uterine arterial calcification caused feto-placental hypoxia and that this was important information. However, the recognition of the danger of X-rays to the fetus resulted in elimination of the category. Class G had been added some years before: this was a rather vague class and included 'multiple failures in pregnancy.' Class R had been added, and women with both retinopathy and renal disease were placed in a combined class termed class FR. Class H, women with coronary heart disease, and class T, women with prior renal transplantation, had yet to be added.

At the 1979 American Diabetes Association Symposium on Gestational Diabetes, the first of the series begun by Norbert Freinkel, the confusing issue of class A and gestational diabetes was raised. Implicit in raising the issue was the recognition that nearly everyone used the White classification. Class A was meant to include women treated with diet alone but was never synonymous with gestational diabetes; however, in common parlance it often came to be. The Joslin Clinic has traditionally had few patients with gestational diabetes, so the White classification never really needed to address the issue. At the Joslin Clinic women with gestational diabetes who required insulin were called gestational Bs as opposed to true Bs, meaning women with either pregestational diabetes or the onset of Type 1 diabetes in pregnancy. At the request of the symposium, I revised the classification and separated gestational diabetes from the traditional alphabetic list.[11] Priscilla White was invited to co-author the alteration with me in order to lend it credence, to which she readily agreed. As it turned out, this revision of the White classification was also her last publication (Box 2.2).

The basic soundness of White's clinical observations that duration and vascular disease were the major determinants of outcome became even clearer to me when I tried to revise the White classification for the 13th edition of *Joslin's Diabetes Mellitus* in 1994, in order to reflect most recent experience and to try to make it less confusing.[12] Class A had essentially disappeared; it did not include gestational diabetes and increasingly stringent standards of control meant that no one with pregestational diabetes went through pregnancy without insulin. Duration or onset in women with no complications

---

Box 2.2   Priscilla White's last classification

Gestational diabetes: Abnormal glucose tolerance test, euglycemia maintained by diet alone.
                             Diet alone insufficient, insulin required
Class A: Diet alone sufficient, any duration or onset age
Class B: Onset at the age of 20 or older, duration < 10 years
Class C: Onset between the ages of 10 and 19, or duration 10–19 years
Class D: Onset before the age of 10, duration > 20 years, background retinopathy or hypertension (not pre-eclampsia)
Class R: Proliferative retinopathy or vitreous hemorrhage
Class F: Nephropathy with > 500 mg/day proteinuria
Class RF: Criteria for both classes R and F coexist
Class H: Arteriosclerotic heart disease clinically evident
Class T: Prior renal transplantation

All classes following Class A require insulin therapy. Classes R, F, RF, H and T have no onset/duration criteria but usually occur in long-term diabetes. The development of a complication moves the patient to a lower class.

made no difference to outcome, so women in classes B and C, as well as those in uncomplicated class D, did not need to be separated. Classes E and G were obsolete. In my chapter, I ended up with three classifications! First, one specifically for gestational diabetes; second, the 1980 version of the White classification; and third, one just as cumbersome, which was based on the presence or absence of complications. Each category was identified by a specific complication rather than by using the more non-specific onset or duration. It did make sense to be specific about what the complication was, e.g. autonomic neuropathy or background retinopathy, and it did correlate with outcomes, but it was still cumbersome.

Most of the attention in diabetes complicating pregnancy today is not focused on Type 1 diabetes but the far more common gestational diabetes, and in particular on fetal outcome in gestational diabetes. (This is curious, because the standard O'Sullivan and Mahan diagnostic criteria,[13] since revised to reflect refinements in laboratory methodology, are based on a maternal, not fetal, outcome, the subsequent risk of developing diabetes.) I believe that there is an understandable difference in viewpoint between obstetricians who worry mainly about fetal outcome as opposed to physicians who have to treat the mothers for many years to come after delivery. I think it is for that reason, and because of the overwhelming predominance of Type 1 diabetes at the Joslin Clinic, that the White classification always took into account both maternal and fetal risk. For example, retinopathy (class R) poses no fetal risk but if aggravated by pregnancy it can cause maternal blindness.

The later years

By the mid-point in her career, Priscilla White was undeniably the doyenne of diabetic pregnancy. She continued to publish reviews and papers which extended and refined her experience. Jørgen Pedersen, who became well established as a student of and expert in diabetic pregnancy in the 1950s and 1960s, used her classification in a modified form. It was included in *The Pregnant Diabetic and Her Newborn*, his classic treatise published in 1967. Although he did adopt and modify White's classification, Pedersen also stated flatly that 'This department has never used hormone therapy.'[14] In fact, by this time few, if any, centers believed that estrogen and progesterone supplementation made any difference, and White was the only real advocate of its use. This became more of a bone of contention in the 1960s and 1970s, even within the Joslin Clinic.

White was an invited lecturer all over the world. She was asked to present her data on diabetes complicated by vascular disease at the International Federation of Gynecology and Obstetrics in Mexico City in 1976. However, she was troubled by thromboembolic venous disease and could not travel long distances. She asked me to present her paper for her. At the congress I met Jørgen Pedersen. He was interested in her data and, of course, knew her personally and inquired about her health. He also told me that he thought she should have discouraged her patients with renal disease from becoming pregnant, given the still poor prognosis for this subgroup. In retrospect, I see the differences in their viewpoints as reflecting his realism and her optimism. Patients with nephropathy clearly had the lowest expectation of success of any class, but she started her career when no one had much expectation of success. Having been an effector of triumph over adversity no doubt influenced her optimistic view.

Upon my return to Boston, I suggested that these data be published. She agreed and told me to go ahead. This resulted in a brief but remarkable summation of her experience entitled 'Pregnancy in Diabetes Complicated by Vascular Disease.'[15] Not only were 416 pregnancies with vascular disease (classes R, F, RF, E, H and T) presented but also summarized was a half century of her experience with over 2200 cases of diabetic pregnancy in which the fetal survival rates rose from only 54% at the beginning of her career to 94% by the end.

She was twice honored by the American Diabetes Association at its annual meeting. In 1960 she received the Banting Medal for Distinguished Scientific Achievement and delivered a lecture entitled Childhood Diabetes: Its Course and Influences on the Second and Third Generations. In 1978 she was the Outstanding Physician Clinician in Diabetes but this award, after her retirement, in reality recognized her as an Eminence grise.

It is of interest that her two contemporaries and colleagues at the Joslin Clinic, Howard Root and Alexander Marble, were both presidents of the American Diabetes Association. Howard Root became a Medical Director of the Clinic and a President of the Joslin Diabetes Center. Alexander Marble was a Research Director and President of the Joslin Diabetes Center. Priscilla White never achieved such high office within or without the Joslin Diabetes Center. She was made head of the Youth Division, created in the 1960s, which reflected her interest not only in pregnancy but also her long-term interest in the Joslin Camps for boys and girls. It may have been that this division was created, at least in part, to make up for her lack of a major title at the Joslin Diabetes Center. Root and Marble had academic appointments in medicine at Harvard; her appointment was in pediatrics at Tufts, her alma mater. She never sought a Harvard appointment because they would not admit her (or any other woman before 1945) to their medical school. To what degree her lack of official recognition, when compared to her peers Root and Marble, reflected intrinsic choices that led her down a different career path or extrinsic forces of latent sexism, or the interplay of both, is an open question.

Her legacies are direct and indirect. She can arguably be personally credited with creating the discipline of diabetes in pregnancy. Others were active in the field, but none were as single-mindedly devoted and as well known before 1950. Special interest groups for diabetic pregnancy now exist within multiple professional societies. Hundreds, if not thousands, of physicians and obstetricians have developed clinical and investigative interests in the field. There are thousands of direct legatees – her patients who became mothers and had children, grandchildren, and now great grandchildren – generations that would not have come into being had it not been for her. Also directly affected were residents and fellows who learned from her how to treat diabetic patients for the rest of their careers. Her indirect legatees are untold numbers of diabetic women all over the world whose doctors enabled them to bear children because she led the way.

REFERENCES

1. White P. Diabetes in pregnancy. In: Joslin EP, ed. The Treatment of Diabetes Mellitus, 4th edn. Philadelphia: Lea & Febiger; 1928, pp. 861–72.
2. White P. Pregnancy complicating diabetes. In: Joslin EP, Root HF, White P, Marble A, eds. The Treatment of Diabetes Mellitus, 6th edn. Philadelphia: Lea & Febiger; 1937, pp. 618–37.
3. White P. Pregnancy and diabetes. Diabetes 1958; 7: 494–5. [editorial]
4. Smith OW, Smith GvS, Joslin EP, White P. Prolan and estrin in the serum and urine of diabetic and nondiabetic women during pregnancy, with especial reference to pregnancy toxemia. Am J Obstet Gynecol 1937; 3: 365–79.
5. White P, Koshy P, Duckers J. The management of pregnancy complicating diabetes and of children of diabetic mothers. Med Clin N Am 1953; 37: 1481–96.
6. White P. Pregnancy and diabetes. In: Marble A, White P, Bradley RF, Krall LP, eds. Joslin's Diabetes Mellitus, 11th edn. Philadelphia: Lea & Febiger; 1971, pp. 581–98.
7. White P. Pregnancy complicating diabetes. Am J Med 1949; 5: 609–16.
8. White P. Pregnancy complicating diabetes. In: Joslin EP, Root HF, White P, et al., eds. The Treatment of Diabetes Mellitus, 8th edn. Philadelphia: Lea & Febiger; 1946 pp. 769–84.
9. Miller E, Hare JW, Cloherty J, et al. Elevated maternal hemoglobin A1c in early pregnancy and major congenital anomalies in infants of diabetic mothers. N Engl J Med 1981; 304: 1331–4.
10. White P. Pregnancy complicating diabetes of more than twenty years' duration. Med Clin N Am 1947; March: 395–405.
11. Hare JW, White P. Gestational diabetes and the White Classification. Diabetes Care 1980; 3: 394.
12. Hare JW. Diabetes and pregnancy. In: Kahn CR, Weir GC, eds. Joslin's Diabetes Mellitus, 13th edn. Philadelphia: Lea & Febiger; 1994, pp. 889–99.
13. O'Sullivan JM, Mahan CM. Criteria for the oral glucose tolerance test in pregnancy. Diabetes 1964; 13: 278–85.
14. Pedersen J. The Pregnant Diabetic and Her Newborn. Baltimore: Williams & Wilkins; 1967, pp. 112–18, 142.
15. Hare JW, White P. Pregnancy in diabetes complicated by vascular disease. Diabetes 1977; 26: 953–5.

3 The Pedersen legacy

Lars Mølsted-Pedersen

Introduction

As an introduction to this chapter it is appropriate to give a brief outline of the founder of the Copenhagen Centre for Pregnant Diabetics, my teacher, chief and during the years 1962–1978 also my personal good friend, the late Professor Jørgen Pedersen.

After his graduation as MD in 1938 he had a thorough training in Copenhagen hospitals and during his term as an assistant physician to HC Hagedorn at the Steno Memorial Hospital from 1943 to 1945 he became fascinated with the problems of diabetes and pregnancy. From 1945 to 1946 he held an appointment as registrar in the Obstetric Department, Rigshospital, University of Copenhagen, where, from 1946 to 1954, he worked as a voluntary consultant and from 1954 until his death in November 1978 as an appointed consultant for pregnant diabetics. Jørgen Pedersen was a very active teacher throughout his long career and from 1970 he held the chair of Professor of Internal Medicine at the University of Copenhagen.

As early as 1945, Jørgen Pedersen started his work on diabetes and pregnancy. He managed to build up a center for pregnant women with diabetes, a center which over the years has become well-known worldwide as The Copenhagen Centre for Pregnant Diabetics. His paramount aim was to diminish perinatal mortality through strict control of diabetes and special obstetric management. These efforts were widely successful, as the perinatal mortality during his leadership decreased from nearly 40 to 4%.

However, in connection with his clinical work a very comprehensive continuous research has been performed to elucidate the manifold and intricate pathogenetic problems around the diabetic mother and her conceptus. Some of the papers from the Copenhagen Centre are collected in three volumes from 1954, 1961 and 1966, and a fourth was sent out in January 1974 as a memorial volume by Pedersen's co-workers in honour of his 60th birthday.

A survey is given in Pederson's book *The Pregnant Diabetic and Her Newborn*, which was published in its first edition in 1967 and in a greatly revised second edition in 1977. This monograph not only deals with the treatment and prognosis of mother and child, but also with pathogenic, pathoanatomical, metabolic, endocrine and many other problems, largely based on investigations in the Copenhagen Centre.

A few characteristics of Jørgen Pedersen's working methods were: a repeated meticulous control to problems from varying aspects to confirm or weaken results; an ability to differentiate a large inhomogeneous material in groups to be individually evaluated; and a certain artistic ability to see new problems connected with the old ones, often linked with new discoveries and new techniques. These intellectual faculties combined with an unflagging perfectionism made him a highly admired leader of a multi-disciplinary research team.

It is well known that Jørgen Pedersen was one of the founders of the European Diabetic Pregnancy Study Group (DPSG). During its first 3 years he was a board member and from then until his death he was a highly esteemed and very active member of the group. In 1979, the board of the DPSG decided that a lecture in memory of Jørgen Pedersen should be given at the group's yearly meeting and since 1980 a Jørgen Pedersen memorial lecture has been given every year by a distinguished scientist within the field of diabetes and pregnancy.

Diabetes and pregnancy: 1940–1980

In 1946 it was decided, with Professor Brandstrup at the Rigshospital, University of Copenhagen, to centralize the management and study of diabetes and pregnancy to the Obstetrical Department of Professor Brandstrup, who previously had interest in the problems involved.[1,2]

The first study from the Copenhagen Centre was designed to find possible characteristics of the course of diabetes during pregnancy, to contribute to a quantitative elucidation of the incidence of alterations occurring and to set up rules for the supervision of pregnant diabetics.[3] Two typical periods in diabetic alterations took place, reaching a peak at about the second to third month and at about the seventh month. During the former period, an improvement in tolerance, lasting for an average of 2–3 months, was commonly observed. The manifestation of this improvement was insulin coma, or other insulin reactions, or an improvement in the degree of compensation. During the latter period there is often a decreased tolerance, manifesting itself as a diabetic precoma, acute acidosis or a necessity for raising the insulin dosage. The duration of this reduction in tolerance averaged 2 months.[3]

A treatment policy was described as follows:[3,4] referral to a diabetes center as early as possible in pregnancy; outpatient control every 2–3 weeks until the fifth gestational month and weekly thereafter. About 8 weeks before calculated term the patient was hospitalized for prophylactic purposes and remained as an inpatient until delivery, which was usually induced *c*. 3 weeks before term. This applied to uncomplicated cases. On the whole, the patients were hospitalized in the presence of any complications that failed to yield immediately to ambulatory measures. Perinatal mortality fell from *c*. 40 to 25% in the period from 1946 to 1952 and for the group with long-term control perinatal mortality was as low as 12%. However, in the period from 1956 to 1965 the total perinatal mortality was still as high as 18.5% and the focus was now on the high incidence of severe congenital malformations (CM), a subject which was still under debate in the 1950s and 1960s. In a paper from 1964, Mølsted-Pedersen et al.[5] showed in a convincing way that the incidence of severe CM was significantly higher in newborns of diabetic mothers and, furthermore, that fatal and multiple CM were five times higher in this group, and there was a significant correlation to the severity of the maternal diabetes. Based on these results, it was proposed that CM in infants of diabetic mothers were due in particular to the presence of maternal vascular complications with an insufficient blood supply to the uterus and placenta.

During the 1970s this view was changed in favor of the metabolic hypothesis, i.e. incomplete metabolic compensation at nidation and during the first trimester might be important. In a study from the late 1970s, a series comprising 949 newborn infants of diabetic mothers were treated at the Copenhagen Centre during pregnancy and delivery in the period from 1966 to 1977. The malformation rate was 8.2%.[6] By analyzing the series it was found that the rate of CM in White classes B–F was significantly reduced from 14.1 to 7.4% in infants whose mothers preconceptionally attended two hospitals which specialized in the treatment and ambulatory control of diabetes. The observation demonstrated the importance of procuring constant care for diabetic women outside pregnancy in order to decrease the malformation rate.

During the first half of the 1980s the rate of severe CM decreased significantly at the Copenhagen Centre. The explanation for this significant decline is not a simple one and the cause may be non-specific, but some points of possible relevance were reported.[7] Firstly, from *c*. 1980, diabetologists in Denmark had intensified their treatment of diabetics, especially that of the young. Secondly, in 1976 an outpatient clinic for instructions in contraception and planning for future pregnancies in diabetic women was organized at the Copenhagen Centre. A few years after the opening of this clinic a significant increase – from 35 to 70% – in the frequency of planned pregnancies was seen. Thirdly, some induced abortions were performed due to elevated levels of alpha-fetoprotein (ultrasound examination verified severe neural tube defects) and in a few diabetic women from classes D and F who had poorly regulated diabetic metabolism during conception and during the first gestational weeks, and moreover whose fetuses had a significant ultrasound-verified growth delay in early pregnancy, thereby having a significantly increased risk of severe CM (see below).[8]

The impact of preconceptional care has been strongly underlined by the Copenhagen Centre's later clinical experience (Table 3.1).[9] In unplanned pregnancies in Type 1 diabetic women, the rate of pregnancy complications and preterm deliveries are doubled compared to insulin-dependent diabetes mellitus (IDDM) women who preconceptionally planned their pregnancy. Furthermore, the incidence of severe CM and the perinatal mortality were markedly increased in the unplanned group.

In his thesis from 1952, Jørgen Pedersen[10] mentioned the hyperglycemia (maternal) – hyperinsulinism (fetal) hypothesis, but at that time direct measurements of plasma insulin were not possible. In the second edition of his book *The Pregnant Diabetic and Her Newborn*,[11] the hypothesis ran as follows: maternal hyperglycemia results in fetal hyperglycemia and, hence, in hypertrophy of fetal islet tissue with insulin hypersecretion. The hyperinsulinism in the presence of more than adequate supplies of glucose, abruptly eliminated at birth, explains several of the characteristic features observed in the offspring. Over the years the theory, its consequences and explanatory powers have been intensively discussed, especially in papers from the Copenhagen Centre.[12–15] The results of many pathoanatomical, clinical, physiological and biochemical investigations have adducted a nearly common agreement of the theory, which is now, more than 20 years after Pedersen's death, simply called the Pedersen theory.

White's[16] widely used classification of pregnant diabetes is based on factors present in the mother before pregnancy, particularly with regard to the severity of her diabetes and vascular complications. This classification indicates groups of pregnant women with a different basic fetal mortality risk and a different proneness to complications, and hence fetal mortality. However, a more individual prognosis was required.

In order to improve the possibilities of predicting the outcome of pregnancies in diabetics, a consecutive series of

Table 3.1   Major clinical differences in planned and unplanned pregnancies in pregestational Type 1 diabetic women – Copenhagen Series 1989–1992

	Pregnancies		
	Planned (%) (*n* = 133)	Unplanned (%) (*n* = 67)	*P*-value
Pregnancy complications	27.0	52.0	< 0.001
Preterm delivery (< 37 completed weeks)	19.0	39.0	< 0.005
Major congenital malformations	1.5	11.9	< 0.010
Perinatal mortality	0.8	5.9	< 0.100

304 pregnancies from the Copenhagen Centre in the 5-year period from 1959 to 1963 was analyzed. Patients with a poor prognosis were divided into four groups: pregnant women who developed (1) hyperpyretic pyelitis, (2) precoma or severe acidosis, (3) toxaemia or (4) could be designated as 'neglectors.'[17] These four groups are designated as PBSP (prognostically bad signs during pregnancy) and concern complications which become evident during the actual pregnancy. Although the classification may not be perfect, the inherent concept of the White classification, i.e. that the chance of a successful pregnancy is not the same for all pregnant diabetics, is fundamentally correct.[18] The simultaneous combined use of the two complementary classifications is recommended until more precise classifications are available.

Diabetes and pregnancy: 1980–present

In 1976 the Copenhagen Centre started to perform consecutively an ultrasound examination in the first trimester in all diabetic pregnancies to confirm the gestational age. Quite unexpectedly, it was observed that some fetuses in early diabetic pregnancy were smaller by ultrasound measurements than expected from the menstrual history and the term early growth delay was used to describe this phenomenon.[19] When assessing gestational age from a crown–rump length (CRL) measurement, the 95% confidence interval (CI) is +4–5 days. Therefore, significant early growth delay defines an ultrasound age that is at least 6 days less than the menstrual age.[20] There is a significant association between early growth delay and the quality of the diabetes regulation as assessed from the HbA1c concentration.[21] Correspondingly, there has been a significant decrease in the average early growth delay over the past 20 years, from 5.5 to 2.0 days, which is ascribed to the efforts made to improve diabetes regulation around the time of conception and during early pregnancy.

In 1981, it was reported that significant early growth delay predicted an increased risk of CM.[8] To examine whether this was still so, the series was divided at 1980, so that 1976–1979 roughly corresponds to an earlier report. The alarming high rate of malformations in the delay group (18%) fortunately has decreased (4%), and although early growth still may involve a higher risk of malformation the difference does not reach statistical significance. Again, it is believed that this is a result of an improved diabetes regulation around conception and in early pregnancy.

When looking at severe CM, spontaneous abortions and successful outcomes in the whole series of 376 pregnancies (Table 3.2), it is obvious that the too-small fetuses not only had a higher rate of CM [10 of 110 (9.1%) versus 6 of 266 (2.3%)] but also a higher rate of spontaneous abortions [6 of 110 (5.5%) versus 1 of 266 (0.4%)]. The chance of a successful outcome of pregnancy, i.e. delivery of a live, non-malformed baby, was significantly lower in the delay group [93 of 110 (85%) versus 252 of 266 (94%)]. These highly significant differences show that the early growth delay is a real phenomenon and not a result of inaccurate estimation of ovulation.[22]

In order to study postnatal development, the infants of the Copehagen Centre's 1981 report, together with a group of control infants, underwent a pediatric follow-up examination at the age of 4 years. The Denver Development Screening Test showed that the infants in the diabetes group had a slightly poorer psychomotor development than the control infants; only 83% had a normal score as opposed to 88% in the control group.[23] When the diabetes group was divided according to early growth delay, it appeared that only 69% of infants in the delay group had a normal score, thereby differing significantly from the non-delay infants (88%), who performed remarkably similarly to the control infants. In other words, in this series it was the delay infants alone that were responsible for the poorer performance in the diabetic group.

Summary on early growth delay

Some fetuses in early diabetic pregnancy are smaller than normal, i.e. exhibiting early growth delay. This is related to the quality of the diabetes regulation and gives a marked increase in the risk of fetal malformations, and predicts a poorer psychomotor development. A first trimester ultrasound study is essential and patient management should be guided by the ultrasound age.

Since the foundation of the Diabetes Centre at the Obstetric Department of the Rigshospital, 13 theses for the DMSc degree at the University of Copenhagen have been

Table 3.2 Analyses of early growth delay in 376 singleton pregnancies in Type 1 diabetic mothers – Copenhagen Series 1976–1995

	Delay	No delay
Included in the study	110	266
Spontaneous abortions < 16 weeks	6	1
Spontaneous abortions > 16 weeks	0	3
Induced abortions and intrauterine Fetal death	0	8
Delivery of live infant	104	254
Severe malformation	10	3
Trisomi 21	1	0
Successful outcome*	93 (85%)	251 (94%)

*P = 0.0053 (Fisher's exact probability test).

published, all of them dealing with the topic diabetes and pregnancy in every possible way. In 1977, the Diabetes Centre obtained its own laboratory, where it was possible to carry out hormone assays, glucose tolerance tests, etc.

The interest and activity in the field of gestational diabetes mellitus (GDM) has increased since the foundation of the centre and within the following two decades four DMSc theses dealing with GDM have been published. The most well known, and one often quoted in the medical literature, was written by the internist diabetologist Claus Kuhl: 'Serum insulin and plasma glucagon in human pregnancy – on the pathogenesis of gestational diabetes.'[24] After the death of Jørgen Pedersen, Claus Kuhl was appointed consultant for pregnant diabetics at the Copenhagen Centre for the next decade.

Another important work on GDM was done by the present leader of the Diabetes Centre, Peter Damm.[25] His DMSc was entitled 'Gestational diabetes mellitus and subsequent development of overt diabetes mellitus – a clinical, metabolic and epidemiological study.' He investigated the prognosis of women with previous GDM with respect to subsequent development of diabetes and also the identification of predictive factors for the development of overt diabetes in these women. He also evaluated insulin sensitivity in glucose-tolerant non-obese women with previous GDM and controls. A decreased insulin sensitivity due to a decreased non-oxidative glucose metabolism in skeletal muscle was found in women with previous GDM. The same group of previous GDM women had

a relatively reduced insulin secretion evaluated by IVGTT (intravenous glucose tolerance test). A longitudinal study of 91 GDM women showed a relatively reduced insulin secretion to oral glucose in pregnancy, postpartum, and 5–11 years later.

Damm's study showed that even non-obese glucose-tolerant women with previous GDM are charaterized by the metabolic profile of Type 2 diabetics, i.e. insulin resistance and impaired insulin secretion. Hence, the combination of this finding together with the significantly increased risk for development of diabetes indicates that all women with previous GDM should have a regular assessment of their glucose tolerance in the years after pregnancy.

Finally, it should be mentioned that the rigid outline for treatment of the pregnant diabetics described in one of the first publications from the Copenhagen Centre has been changed since the mid-1980s. The treatment is now much more individualized and, in uncomplicated diabetic pregnancies, all contact with the pregnant women takes place in the outpatient clinic and a planned delivery happens, on average, in gestational week 39.

The Copenhagen Centre for Pregnant Diabetics is still functioning well, with its own laboratory and a staff of obstetricians (led by Peter Damm) and diabetologists (led by Elisabeth Mathiesen) collaborating with the well-known neonatal department in Rigshospital. Several research projects are in progress with young research fellows working well with the Pedersen legacy.

REFERENCES

1. Brandstrup E, Okkels H. Pregnancy complicated with diabetes. Acta Obstet Gyncol Scand 1938; 18: 136–41.
2. Okkels H, Brandstrup E. Studies on the thyroid gland X. Pancreas, hypophysis and thyroid in children of diabetic mothers. Acta Pathol Microbiol Scand 1938; 15: 245–68.
3. Pedersen J. Course of diabetes during pregnancy. Acta Endocr 1952; 9: 342–64.
4. Pedersen J, Brandstrup E. Foetal mortality in pregnant diabetics. Lancet 1956; 1: 607–11.
5. Mølsted-Pedersen L, Tygstrup I, Pedersen J. Congenital malformation in newborn infants of diabetic women. Lancet 1964; 1: 1124–7.
6. Pedersen J, Mølsted-Pedersen L. Congenital malformations: the possible role of diabetes care outside pregnancy. In: Ciba Foundation Symposium 63. Amsterdam: Excerpta Medica; 1979, pp. 265–71.
7. Mølsted-Pedersen L. Significant decrease in severe congenital malformations and perinatal mortality in newborns of diabetic mothers. Paper presented at The Scandinavian Society for the Study of Diabetes, Copenhagen, Denmark, 25 May 1986.
8. Pedersen JF, Mølsted-Pedersen L. Early fetal growth delay detected by ultrasound marks increased risk of congenital malformation in diabetic pregnancy. Br Med J 1981; 283: 269–71.
9. Mølsted-Pedersen L, Damm P. How to organize care for pregnant diabetic patients. In: Mogensen CE, Standl E, eds. Concepts for the Ideal Diabetes Clinic. Berlin: deGruyter; 1993, pp. 199–214.
10. Pedersen J. Diabetes and Pregnancy – Blood Sugar of Newborn Infants. Copenhagen: Danish Science Press Ltd; 1952. [thesis]
11. Pedersen J. The Pregnant Diabetic and Her Newborn, 2nd edn. Munksgaard: Copenhagen, and Williams & Wilkins: Baltimore; 1977, p. 211.
12. Pedersen J, Osler M. Hyerglycemia as the cause of charactristic features of the foetus of newborns of diabetic mothers. Danish Med Bull 1961; 8: 78–82.
13. Pedersen J, Mølsted-Pedersen L. The hyperglycemia– hyperinsulinism theory and the weight of the newborn baby. In: Rodrigues RR,

Wallance-Owen J, eds. Diabetes. Amsterdam: Excerpta Medica; 1971, 678–82.
14. Mølsted-Pedersen L. Studies on carbohydrate metabolism in newborn infants of diabetic mothers. University of Copenhagen, 1974. [thesis]
15. Pedersen J. Fetal macrosomia. In: Sutherland HV, Stowers JM, eds. Carbohydrate Metabolism in Pregnancy and the Newborn. Edinburgh: Churchill Livngstone; 1975, pp. 127–39.
16. White P. Pregnancy and diabetes, medical aspects. Med Clin N Am 1965; 49: 1015–21.
17. Pedersen J, Mølsted-Pedersen L. Prognosis of the outcome of pregnancies in diabetics. A new classification. Acta Endocrinol 1965; 50: 70–7.
18. Pedersen J, Mølsted-Pedersen L, Andersen B. Assessors of fetal perinatal mortality in diabetic pregnancy. Analysis of 1332 pregnancies in the Copenhagen Series, 1946–1972. Diabetes 1974; 23: 302–6.
19. Pedersen JF, Mølsted-Pedersen L. Early growth retardation in diabetic pregnancy. Br Med J 1979; 1: 18–19.
20. Pedersen JF. Ultrasound studies on fetal crown–rump length in early normal and diabetic pregnancy. Danish Med Bull 1986; 33: 296–304.
21. Pedersen JF, Mølsted-Pedersen L, Mortensen HB. Fetal growth delay and maternal hemoglobin A1C in early diabetic pregnancy. Obstet Gynecol 1984; 64: 351–2.
22. Pedersen JF. Early fetal growth delay in diabetic pregnancy. Paper presented at the FIGO congress, Copenhagen, Denmark, 1997.
23. Petersen MB, Pedersen SA, Greisen G, et al. Early growth delay in diabetic pregnancy: relation to psychomotor development at age 4. Br Med J 1988; 26: 598–600.
24. Kuhl C. Serum insulin and plasma glucagon in human pregnancy – on the pathogenesis of gestational diabetes. University of Copenhagen, 1978. [thesis]
25. Damm P. Gestational diabetes mellitus and subsequent development of overt diabetes mellitus – a clinical, metabolic and epidemiological study. University of Copenhagen, 1998. [thesis]

4 The Freinkel legacy

Boyd E. Metzger

Introduction

Professor Norbert (Norbie) Freinkel (Figure 4.1) was a renowned scholar, investigator and teacher. Although it is now nearly two decades since his sudden, untimely death, Norbie's influence on the field of pregnancy and diabetes remains profound. What accounts for this enduring legacy? Norbie was a brilliant, intense, dedicated and insightful investigator. He was a gifted and prolific writer and used language with great skill and flair. Norbert Freinkel was a member of prestigious academic societies including the American Society of Clinical Investigation and the Association of American Professors and held important professional leadership positions, including the presidency of both the Endocrine Society and the American Diabetes Association.

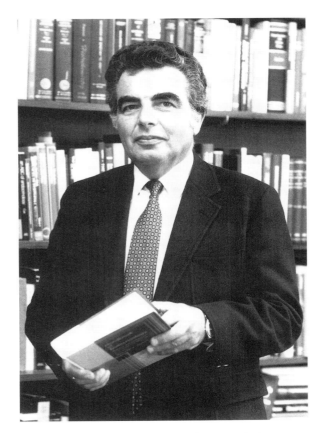

Figure 4.1 Norbert (Norbie) Freinkel.

However, in my estimation, an enduring legacy is built more on people that have benefitted from exposure to a stimulating research and intellectual environment and on the concepts that have been promoted, than on affiliations with prestigious organizations and recognition in 'high places.' Strong evidence of this is seen in the way that Norbert Freinkel's influence continues to be felt in the broad areas of nutrition and metabolism during pregnancy. In the short treatise that follows, I have summarized my perspective on some of the people and concepts that best convey the life and legacy of Norbert Freinkel. This perspective can be compared and contrasted with one that was provided 2 years after Norbie's death.[1]

Northwestern University's Diabetes in Pregnancy Center: Vehicle of the legacy

After making major, pioneering contributions to the understanding of thyroid hormone metabolism[2–4] and to other areas of endocrinology early in his career, in the mid 1960s Norbert Freinkel turned his interests and talents to the study of intermediary metabolism in normal and diabetic pregnancy.[4–7] By the early 1907s, he had established a Diabetes in Pregnancy Center (DPC) at Northwestern University and had attracted research collaborations globally. Over the next two decades, a virtual 'who's who' of the world's leading established and future investigators of intermediary metabolism in normal and diabetic pregnancy (basic and clinical) could be compiled from those that spent time as visiting scientists at the Northwestern University DPC. Several sources of objective support for this contention are cited below.

Following Norbie's sudden, untimely death,[8] the American Diabetes Association established the Norbert Freinkel Lecture through the support and encouragement of many colleagues, friends and patients. The Freinkel Lectureship is held under the auspices of the Diabetes in Pregnancy Council. On a triennial basis, it is integrated into the program of the International Diabetes Federation Congress. A review of the names of the Freinkel Lecturers chosen to date and the topics chosen for their lectures (Table 4.1) provides a vignette of the Freinkel legacy.

The Diabetic Pregnancy Study Group (DPSG), an affiliate of the European Association for the Study of Diabetes, held its first meeting in 1969. Norbie, then on a sabbatical leave at Cambridge University, was invited to be the 'keynote' speaker

Table 4.1   Norbert Freinkel Lectures

Lecturer	Year	Title of lecture
John Bell	1991-IDF	Genetic Susceptibility to IDDM
Lars Mølsted-Pedersen	1992	Management of Chronic Hypertension in the Pregnant Diabetic Woman
Boyd Metzger	1993	Diabetes Begets Diabetes: The Last Tenet of the Freinkel Hypothesis
John O'Sullivan	1994	The Birth of Gestational Diabetes
Ulf Eriksson	1995	Intracellular Mediators of Diabetic Embryopathy: Is There a Common Pathway?
John Kitzmiller	1996	Pregnancy Planning and Care for Women with Chronic Diabetic Complications
Donald Coustan	1997-IDF	Gestational Diabetes: 33 Years Without Consensus
David Pettitt	1998	Long-Term Impact on the Offspring: The Pima Experience
Thomas Buchanan	1999	Fetal and Maternal Risks in GDM: Sorting Wheat from Chaff
Patrick Catalano	2000-IDF	Insulin Resistance in Pregnancy and Gestational Diabetes: Implications for Mother and Fetus
Lois Jovanovic	2001	Glucose Mediated Macrosomia: The Over-Fed Fetus and the Future
Jorge Mestman	2002	History of Diabetes and Pregnancy: Lessons from the Past
Oded Langer	2003-IDF	The Diabetes In Pregnancy Dilemma: Leading Change With Proven Solutions
F Andre Van Assche	2004	The Fetal Origin of Adult Diseases
Steven Gabbe	2005	Gestational Diabetes Mellitus – What Have We Learned in 30 Years?
David Hadden	2006-IDF	Prediabetes and the Big Baby

at that inaugural DPSG event. The annual Jörgen Pedersen Lecture that was established by the DPSG in 1980 honors individuals who have made major contributions to the field. Norbie was an early Jörgen Pedersen Lecturer and the depth of his impact on diabetes and pregnancy is reflected in the fact that 9 of the 24 lecturers that were named between 1980 and 2006 have had ties to Norbie through collaboration or by time spent at the Northwestern University DPC. Another measure of his lasting legacy is illustrated by the fact that in the year 2006, more than 20% of the 61 members and honorary members of the DPSG have this kind of linkage with Norbert Freinkel.

The last illustration of the enduring human dimensions of the Freinkel legacy is proved through the composition of the editorship and authorship of this text. The lead editor and one or more of the contributing authors to 40% of the chapters in the book have associations with Norbie (first or second generation) by way of their collaboration with or training at the Northwestern University DPC.

Freinkel concepts of metabolic regulation in pregnancy

Beginning with his earliest studies of metabolic changes during pregnancy, Norbert Freinkel directed his interests to the mutual interplay between mother and fetus. He regarded these changes as adaptations to facilitate optimal development of the fetus. Norbie had the unparalleled ability to synthesize diverse observations into cohesive concepts with clinical application. Some examples are summarized briefly in the following paragraphs.

'Accelerated starvation'

In Freinkel's laboratory and others, it was demonstrated that the transition from a basal or overnight fasting metabolic status to the pattern that is characteristic of the 'prolonged fasted state or starvation' is exaggerated during pregnancy.[7] Since the exaggerated changes differed in both temporal and absolute dimensions, Norbie characterized this pattern as 'accelerated starvation.'[9] A number of clinical and epidemiological studies suggest that greater than normal levels of ketonemia/ketonuria during pregnancy may have adverse effects on fetal development and subsequently, adverse neurological consequences.[10–12] Thus, it is common clinical practice to avoid dietary manipulations during pregnancy that might enhance ketogenesis such as marked restriction of calorie or carbohydrate intake. However, since the demonstration of 'accelerated starvation' was initially documented in animal models and in women that were subjected to prolonged starvation prior to having termination of pregnancy in early or mid gestation, the relevance of 'accelerated starvation' to the clinical management of normal, healthy pregnancies was uncertain until the report entitled '"Accelerated starvation" and the skipped breakfast in late normal pregnancy'[13] was published from the Northwestern University DPC. As noted in Figure 4.2, this study illustrated that even the common practice of delaying or skipping breakfast until lunchtime is sufficient to provoke early metabolic changes (fall in concentration of plasma glucose and increases in FFA and β-hydroxybutyrate), that if continued for a relatively short interval, could result in the full metabolic profile of accelerated starvation.

'Facilitated anabolism'

The metabolic changes that can be observed during the disposition of food intake are numerous. Many aspects of a characteristic diurnal metabolic profile of pregnancy were described in reports from the Northwestern group. The mediation of the these changes and the implications for normal pregnancy as well as the states of altered nutrition or metabolism (obesity, diabetes, malnutrition) are not fully defined and continue to be of great interest to investigators. Norbie interpreted the perturbations that were observed in normal

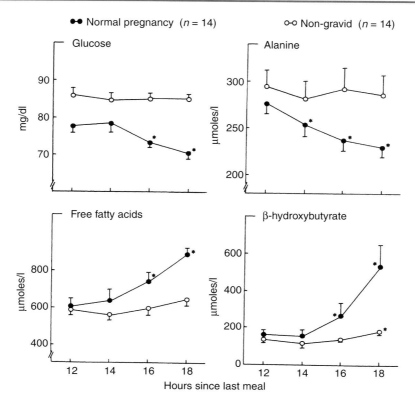

Figure 4.2   Changes in plasma concentration of glucose, alanine, free fatty acids, and β-hydroxybutyrate in non-pregnant and pregnant women between 12 h fast and 18 h fast during the third trimester. (Adapted from Fig. 1, reference 13.)

pregnancy as adaptations to assure an adequate delivery of nutrients to the fetus and coined the phrase 'facilitated anabolism'[14] to convey the aggregate changes. In his view, the insulin resistance of pregnancy plays a key role in bringing about the changes in carbohydrate, lipid and amino acid metabolism that 'facilitate anabolism.' Thus, during an OGTT in normal pregnant women, net area under the glucose curve (AUGC) was found to correlate with the overnight fasting concentration of free fatty acids (FFA) (Figure 4.3), and the decline in FFA after a glucose load was delayed despite the increasing glucose and insulin concentrations.[14] Though the postulated mechanisms differ from those originally proposed by Randle and others, the role of FFA metabolism as a concomitant and potentially mediating factor in insulin resistance is presently receiving renewed attention.[15] In the studies mentioned above, correlations were also found between triglycerides and AUGC and between basal and stimulated insulin and AUGC. The strong inter-relationships between glycemia, aminoacidemia, lipids and insulin sensitivity and secretion must be considered in trying to interpret correlations between triglycerides and birthweight or fetal body composition or between birthweight and maternal insulin sensitivity during and outside of pregnancy.[16]

Metabolic change as 'teratogens'

In the late 1970s and early 1980s, Freinkel and his group extended their focus beyond the factors that mediate insulin

secretion in the fetus, insulin-dependent fetal growth and other manifestations of third trimester fetal hyperinsulinism to consider the consequences of an altered intrauterine metabolic environment throughout gestation. Describing pregnancy as 'a tissue culture experience'[17] put this concept into sharp relief and Norbert Freinkel's 1980 Banting Lecture[18] was a masterful blend of an overview and integration of previous work in concert with a prescient grasp of the life-long implications of exposure to the intrauterine environment of diabetes mellitus. He illustrated clearly (Figure 4.4) that the consequences of metabolic disturbances at various times during gestation are different and that the implications of altered metabolism in GDM and in pre-existing diabetes are also different.

Through work in his laboratory at the DPC,[19–21] as well as through the subsequent and still ongoing work of those initially trained in embryo culture techniques at Northwestern, Norbert Freinkel was the driving force in demonstrating that at specific, finite times during gestation, the metabolic changes of diabetes, and metabolic changes that can occur through other mechanisms can be primary factors in teratogenesis. The capacity to define precisely the time and nature of specific metabolic insults led to the realization that the metabolic insults of DM on fetal development are probably multi-factorial and that recovery from the metabolic perturbation lags behind simple rectification of the altered concentration of metabolites. Though the specific mechanisms and molecular mediators that lead to dysmorphogenesis are not yet clear, these insights have stimulated efforts

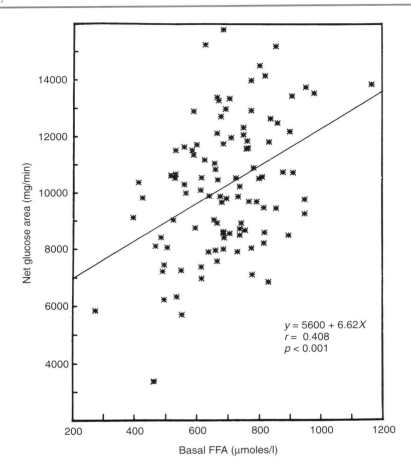

Figure 4.3   The relationship between the glycemic response to a 100 g glucose load during pregnancy and fasting FFA concentration. Regression equation was derived to relate fasting FFA at the time of glucose ingestion to the integrated changes in plasma glucose ('net glucose area') during the subsequent 3 h. Subjects were normal women at weeks 30–40 of pregnancy. (Adapted from Fig. 2, reference 14.)

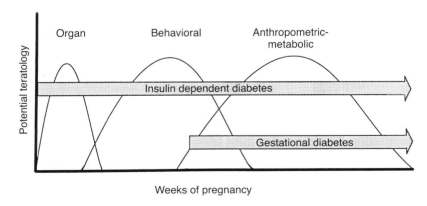

Figure 4.4   Potential long-range effects upon the fetus of chronic alterations in concentrations of maternal fuels during pregnancy. Fuel-mediated teratogenesis as the basis for long-range anatomic and functional changes. (Reproduced with permission from Fig. 12, reference 18.)

to establish optimal metabolic control before conception. Such efforts are highly successful when they are achieved though good control of DM before pregnancy is far from universal.[22]

Long-term consequences of intrauterine exposures

Testing the hypotheses that the consequences of alterations in intrauterine metabolic insult are conditioned by the time in gestation that the exposure occurred and that important outcomes may have latency before appearing much later in development required a long-term perspective. At the Northwestern University DPC, that was implemented through an NIH-funded 'Prospective, long term follow-up study of offspring of diabetic mothers' that has continued for more than two decades. It was initiated between 1978 and 1983 and focused on neurobehavioral development, adipose tissue development and obesity and β-cell function and glucose homeostasis. However, the majority of the studies that confirmed the initial hypotheses that lifelong functions of these tissues are vulnerable to intrauterine insult were not concluded until after Norbie's sudden, untimely death. For the purpose of this report, the commentary has been limited to several reports of Silverman and co-workers.[23–26] These indicate that risks of both obesity and altered glucose homeostasis (impaired glucose tolerance and Type 2 diabetes) in late childhood and adolescence are increased by exposure to the intrauterine environment of DM in mid and/or late gestation. The mechanisms by which adipose tissue development and glucose homeostasis are influenced in later life in offspring of diabetic mothers continue to be studied intensively. However, in the Northwestern DPC study, the risks were strongly associated with markers of fetal hyperinsulinism (primarily amniotic fluid insulin concentration measured at the time of third trimester amniocentesis).

Concurrently, the epidemiological studies in the Pima Indian population of Arizona by Pettitt and co-workers have provided very complementary findings.[27–29] However, in this population with the world's highest prevalence of Type 2 DM, direct information about fetal or neonatal insulin secretion is not available and large size at birth has served as the marker for infants that have been exposed to the intrauterine environment of diabetes mellitus.

The data from the Northwestern University DPC, from the Pima study, and from others, along with supporting evidence with animal models, provide convincing evidence that 'diabetes begets diabetes' through the intrauterine environment and is contributing significantly to the epidemic of Type 2 DM in adolescents and young adults, including a rising prevalence of gestational diabetes mellitus.[30] It remains to be determined if the vicious cycle can be effectively interrupted by more

timely diagnosis and effective therapy of diabetes antedating pregnancy (preexisting diabetes) and of GDM.

The Freinkel legacy and the future

This brief overview provides clear evidence that the legacy of Norbert Freinkel is being strongly sustained nearly two decades after his death. How this legacy will help shape the future directions of research and stimulate new clinical approaches is uncertain. However, the trail will not be difficult to follow. One area that will continue to reflect Norbie's concepts is future developments in GDM. Norbert Freinkel initiated and chaired the first two International Workshop Conferences on GDM. The third was in an early stage of planning at his death. Studies of GDM were initiated in the Northwestern University DPC for two reasons. The first objective was to learn more about the pathogenesis of GDM and progression to DM among women in this high-risk population. Women with previous GDM have been used successfully in efforts to develop pharmacologic and lifestyle strategies to prevent or delay the onset of Type 2 DM among high-risk subjects. Secondly, GDM was looked upon, as a good model to determine how much alteration of nutrient metabolism was required to have adverse effects on the offspring. The Hyperglycemia and Averse Pregnancy Outcome (HAPO) study[31] should soon provide an answer to that dilemma and foster the adoption of criteria for GDM that are based on the level of glycemia that is associated with clinically significant risk.

Acknowledgments

I had the extraordinary opportunity to know Norbie Freinkel as a friend and close professional mentor, advisor and colleague for more than 22 years. Now, nearly two decades have elapsed since his death and early reviews of his legacy. In this short report, I have concentrated on the extraordinary impact that Norbie's work and vision continue to exert on clinical and research aspects of pregnancy complicated by diabetes mellitus. I am convinced that in future decades, we still will be harvesting the rewards of that vision. In the course of this review, I alluded to the work of many others that I did not cite by specific literature reference. This was done to maintain the focus on the specific contributions of Norbert Freinkel and for the sake of brevity.

Work that was cited from the Northwestern University DPC received support from Research Grants DK 10699, HD 19070, HD 62903, HD/DK 34243; GCRC Grant RR48; and the Training Grant DK 07169.

REFERENCES

1. Metzger BE. The legacy of Norbert Freinkel: Maternal metabolism and its impact on the offspring, from embryo to adult. Diabetes in pregnancy. Norbert Freinkel memorial issue. Israel J Med Sci 1991; 27: 425–31.

2. Ingbar SH, Freinkel N, Hoeprich PD, Tthens FW. The concentration and significance of the butanol-extractable I[131] of serum in patients with diverse states of thyroidal function. J Clin Invest 1954; 33: 388–99.

3. Ingbar SH, Freinkel N. Simultaneous estimation of rates of thyroxine degradation and peripheral metabolism of thyroxine. J Clin Invest 1955; 34: 808–19.

4. Dowling JT, Freinkel N, Ingbar SH. Thyroxine-binding by sera of pregnant women, new-born infants and women with spontaneous abortion. J Clin Invest 1956; 35: 1263–76.

5. Goodner CJ, Freinkel N. Carbohydrate metabolism in pregnancy: the turnover of I^{131} insulin in the pregnant rat. Endocrinology 1960; 67: 862–72.

6. Bleicher SJ, O'Sullivan JB, Freinkel N. Carbohydrate metabolism in pregnancy. V. The interrelations of glucose, insulin and free fatty acids in late pregnancy and post partum. N Engl J Med 1964; 271: 866–72.

7. Herrera E, Knopp RH, Freinkel N. Carbohydrate metabolism in pregnancy. VI. Plasma fuels, insulin liver composition, gluconeogenesis and nitrogen metabolism during late gestation in the fed and fasted rat. J Clin Invest 1969; 48: 2260–72.

8. Obituary, Norbert Freinkel. Diabetes 1990; vol. 39.

9. Freinkel N. Effects of the conceptus on maternal metabolism during pregnancy. In: BS Leibel, GA Wrenshall, eds. On the Nature and Treatment of Diabetes. Amsterdam: Excerpta Medica Foundation; 1965, pp. 679–91.

10. Churchill JA, Berendes HW, Nemore J. Neuropsychological deficits in children of diabetic mothers. Am J Obstet Gynecol 1969; 105: 257–68.

11. Stebbens JA, Baker GL, Kitchell M. Outcome at ages 1, 3 and 5 years of children born to diabetic women. Am J Obstet Gynecol 1977; 127: 408–13.

12. Rizzo T, Metzger BE, Burns WJ, Burns KC. Correlations between antepartum maternal metabolism and child intelligence. N Engl J Med 1991; 325: 911–16.

13. Metzger BE, Ravnikar V, Vileisis RA, Freinkel N. "Accelerated starvation" and the skipped breakfast in late normal pregnancy. Lancet 1982; 1: 588–92.

14. Freinkel N, Metzger BE, Nitzan M, et al. Facilitated anabolism in late pregnancy: some novel maternal compensations for accelerated starvation. In: Proceedings of the VIII Congress of the International Diabetes Federation, Brussels, Belgium, July 1973. Excerpta Medica International Congress Series, No. 312. Amsterdam: Excerpta Medica; 1974, pp. 474–88.

15. Boden G. Role of free fatty acids in the pathogenesis of insulin resistance and NIDDM. Diabetes 1997; 46: 3–10.

16. Catalano PM, Thomas AJ, Huston L, Fung CM. Effect of maternal metabolism on fetal growth and body composition. Diabetes Care 1998; 21(suppl. 2): 85B–90B.

17. Freinkel N, Metzger BE. Pregnancy as a tissue culture experience: the critical implications of maternal metabolism for fetal development. In: Pregnancy Metabolism, Diabetes and the Fetus, Ciba Foundation Symposium 63. Amsterdam: Excerpta Medica; 1979, pp. 3–28.

18. Freinkel N. The Banting Lecture 1980. Of pregnancy and progeny. Diabetes 1980; 29: 1023–35.

19. Freinkel N, Lewis NJ, Akazawa S, Roth SI, Gorman L. The honeybee syndrome: implications of the teratogenicity of mannose in rat-embryo culture. N Engl J Med 1984; 310: 223–30.

20. Eriksson UJ, Lewis NJ, Freinkel N. Growth retardation during early organogenesis in embryos of experimentally diabetic rats. Diabetes 1984; 33: 281–4.

21. Freinkel N, Cockroft DL, Lewis NJ, et al. The 1986 McCollum Award Lecture. Fuel-mediated teratogenesis during early organogenesis: the effects of increased concentrations of glucose, ketones, or sommatomedin inhibitor during rat embryo culture. Am J Clin Nutr 1986; 44: 986–95.

22. Metzger BE, Buchanan TA. From research to practice. Diabetes and birth defects: insights from the 1980s, prevention in the 1990s. Conclusions. Diabetes Spectrum 1990; 3: 181–4.

23. Metzger BE, Silverman B, Freinkel N, et al. Amniotic fluid insulin concentration as a predictor of obesity. Arch Dis Child 1990; 65: 1050–2.

24. Silverman BL, Landsberg L, Metzger BE. Fetal hyperinsulinism in offspring of diabetic mothers: association with the subsequent development of childhood obesity. In: Williams CL, Kimm SYS, eds. Prevention and Treatment of Childhood Obesity, vol. 699. New York: American Academy of Sciences; 1993, pp. 36–45.

25. Silverman BL, Metzger BE, Cho NH, Loeb CA. Impaired glucose tolerance in adolescent offspring of diabetic mothers: relationship to fetal hyperinsulinism. Diabetes Care 1995; 18: 611–7.

26. Silverman BL, Rizzo TA, Cho NH, Metzger BE. Long-term effects of the intrauterine environment. Diabetes Care 1998; 21(suppl. 2): 142–9.

27. Pettitt DJ, Baird HR, Aleck KA. Excessive obesity in offspring of Pima Indian women with diabetes during pregnancy. N Engl J Med 1983; 308: 242–5.

28. Pettitt DJ, Aleck KA, Baird HR, et al. Congenital susceptibility to NIDDM: role of intrauterine environment. Diabetes 1988; 37: 622–8.

29. Dabelea D, Pettitt DJ, Hanson RL, et al. Birth weight, type 2 diabetes, and insulin resistance in pima indian children and young adults. Diabetes Care 1999; 22: 944–50.

30. Ferrera A, Kahn HS, Quesenberry CP, Riley C, Hedderson MM. An increase in the incidence of gestational diabetes mellitus: Northern California 1991–2000. Obstet Gynecol 2004; 103: 526–33.

31. HAPO Study Cooperative Research Group. The Hyperglycemia and Adverse Pregnancy Outcome (HAPO) Study. Int J Gynecol Obstet 2002; 78: 69–77.

5 Metabolism in normal pregnancy

Emilio Herrera and Henar Ortega

Introduction

During pregnancy, the mother adapts her metabolism to ensure the continuous supply of nutrients to the fetus in order to sustain its exponential growth. Among those nutrients crossing the placenta, glucose is quantitatively the most important, followed by amino acids. Although lipids cross the placenta in much lower proportion than the other nutrients, maternal lipid metabolism is consistently and intensely affected during pregnancy in order to satisfy maternal and fetal needs. Fetal growth and development also depend on other essential nutrients, like vitamins. The metabolism of certain vitamins is therefore affected during pregnancy to ensure their proper availability to the fetus. The purpose of this chapter is to review the main changes in carbohydrate, amino acids, lipid and vitamin metabolism that take place throughout pregnancy under normal conditions.

Carbohydrate metabolism

Glucose is the primary energy source of fetoplacental tissues. During early pregnancy, basal plasma glucose and insulin levels and hepatic gluconeogenesis are unchanged.[1] However, during late pregnancy, the mother develops hypoglycemia, which is specially manifest under fasting conditions, when the rate of gluconeogenesis from different substrates is enhanced.[2,3] The use of different substrates for such increased gluconeogenesis is variable: the conversion of glycerol to glucose rather than other more classical gluconeogenetic substrates like pyruvate or alanine is specially intense.[4] The development of maternal hypoglycemia despite the enhanced gluconeogenesis and the reduced consumption of glucose by maternal tissues, due to her insulin-resistant condition, is the result of the high rate of placental transfer of glucose, which is greater than that of any other substrate (Figure 5.1).[5] This preponderance of placental transfer of glucose over other metabolites has been demonstrated in different species. It is carried out by facilitated diffusion according to concentration-dependent kinetics and thanks to the presence of a high number of glucose transporters, particularly GLUT1.[6] The fetus does not synthesize glucose but uses it as its main oxidative substrate. This causes fetal glycemia to be normally lower than that of its mother,

allowing a positive maternal–fetal glucose gradient, which facilitates its placental transfer.

Protein and amino acid metabolism

The accretion of protein is essential for fetal growth and must be sustained by the active transfer of amino acids from maternal circulation. There is no evidence that pregnant women store protein during early pregnancy, when fetal needs are scarce. Therefore, the increased requirements of late pregnancy must be met by metabolic adjustments that enhance both dietary protein utilization and nitrogen retention in

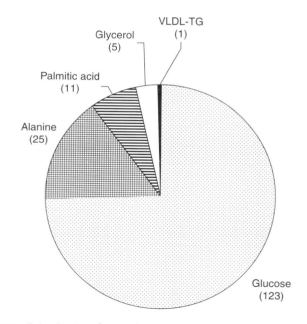

Figure 5.1 In situ placental transfer of D-glucose, L-alanine, palmitic acid, glycerol and VLDL-triacylglycerols (VLDL-TG) in 20-day pregnant rats. Placental transfer was measured by the infusion of ^{14}C-labeled substrates through the left uterine artery for 20 min and making the proper correction of data for specific activity dilution and uterine blood flow. Data are expressed as percentual value of all the studied substrates, numbers between breakers indicate the mean absolute value of the transfer for each substrate, expressed as nmol/min/g fetal body weight. Other details in reference 5.

order to satisfy fetal demands. Protein metabolism changes gradually throughout gestation, so that nitrogen conservation for fetal growth achieves full potential during the last quarter of pregnancy.[7] Nitrogen balance studies showed that the rate of maternal nitrogen retention between 20 and 40 weeks of gestation was greater than the predicted need,[8] leading to the proposal that the mother gains additional protein in her own tissues. The increased nitrogen retention in late pregnancy is due to a reduction in urinary nitrogen excretion as a consequence of decreased urea synthesis.[7] In late pregnancy, nitrogen balance is improved, allowing a more efficient use of dietary proteins.[9]

Although these alterations in protein metabolism during late pregnancy favor nitrogen conservation, pregnancy is associated with hypoaminoacidemia, which is specially evident during fasting, is present at early gestation, and persists throughout pregnancy.[10,11] Since insulin infusion in non-pregnant adults decreases both plasma amino acid levels and protein breakdown, it is proposed that the decrease in plasma amino acid levels found during normal pregnancy is not associated with the pregnancy insulin resistant condition. Thus, maternal hypoaminoacidemia reflects enhanced placental amino acid uptake. Additionally, maternal oxidation of branched-chain amino acids decreases in late pregnancy, increasing their availability for transfer to the fetus.[12]

Contrary to glucose, the concentration of most amino acids in fetal plasma is higher than that found in the mother, because placental transfer of amino acids is carried out by an active process, using selective transporters and metabolic energy.[13] This capacity to concentrate amino acids in the fetal side against the gradient versus maternal levels is clearly seen in the fed and 24 h fasted rat. As shown in Figure 5.2, under fed conditions, maternal plasma total amino acid levels are similar in 20 day pregnant rats and sex- and age-matched virgin animals, whereas the levels in fetal plasma are already higher than in the mother. However, after fasting, the decline of plasma amino acids in the late pregnant rat is greater than

that seen in virgin animals, whereas fetal plasma total amino acid concentration remains the same as when fed. Thus, under fasting, the fetal/maternal total amino acid ratio becomes even higher than when fed, showing the efficiency of the placenta in transfering amino acids against the gradient. A multiplicity of factors affects the overall placental amino acid delivery rates, including the activity and location of the amino acid transporter systems, changes in placental surface area, uteroplacental blood flow and maternal concentrations of amino acids,[13] all of which change as gestation advances and are dependent on maternal health conditions.[14]

Lipid metabolism

Accumulation of fat depots in maternal tissues and maternal hyperlipidemia are characteristic features during normal pregnancy. Besides, although lipids cross the placenta with difficulty, essential fatty acids (EFA) and long-chain polyunsaturated fatty acids (LCPUFA) are needed for fetal growth and development and must arrive from maternal circulation. Thus, throughout pregnancy there are major changes in lipid metabolism.

Adipose tissue metabolism

Fat accumulation takes place during the first two-thirds of gestation[15,16] and represents most of the increase in maternal structures that take place during pregnancy.[17] It is the result of both hyperphagia and enhanced lipid synthesis, and is driven by the enhanced adipose tissue insulin responsiveness that occurs during early pregnancy.[18]

Increments of maternal fat depots stop during the third trimester of gestation as a consequence of two changes: (1) a decrease in lipoprotein lipase (LPL) activity,[19] which mainly corresponds to that present in adipose tissue[20] and causes a decline in the hydrolysis and tissue uptake of triacylglycerols

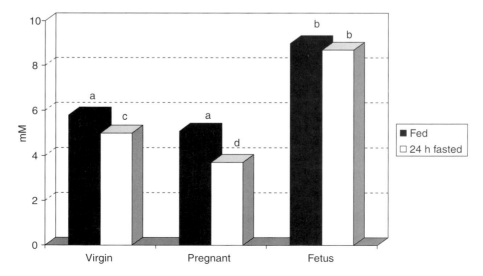

Figure 5.2   Plasma concentration of total amino acids in fed and 24 h fasted virgin and 20-day pregnant rats and their fetuses. Letters above each bar correspond to the statistical comparison between the groups: different letters indicate statistical differences (P < 0.05).

circulating in triacylglycerol-rich lipoproteins (chylomicrons and very low density lipoproteins, VLDL); and (2) an increased adipose tissue lipolytic activity, which is specially manifest under fasting conditions.[21,22]

The placental transfer of the products of adipose tissue lipolysis released into the circulation, non-esterified fatty acids (NEFA) and glycerol, is quantitatively low,[23] and therefore their main destiny is maternal liver. In liver, NEFA are converted into acyl-CoA, and glycerol into glycerol-3-phosphate, which are partially re-esterified for the synthesis of triacylglycerols. These are released back into the circulation in the form of VLDL, as maternal liver production is enhanced. In addition, whereas glycerol is also used as a preferential substrate for gluconeogenesis, NEFA are used for β-oxidation, leading to energy production and ketone body synthesis. These pathways are markedly increased under fasting conditions in late pregnancy.[3,24] Ketone bodies easily cross the placenta.[25] Although not synthesized by the fetus, in fetal circulation, they reach the same concentration as in the mother.[26] Different to what occurs in adults, ketone bodies can be used by the fetus not only as energetic fuels but as substrates for brain lipids.[27,28]

Thus, as shown in Figure 5.3, both the mother and the fetus benefit from the enhanced adipose tissue lipolytic activity during late pregnancy, and very especially during the fasting periods. The preferential conversion of glycerol to glucose allows the preservation of other gluconeogenic substrates like alanine and other amino acids for their transfer to the fetus. The active production of ketone bodies from fatty acids by fasting maternal liver, besides their transfer to the fetus, allows their use by certain maternal tissues such as skeletal muscle as alternative fuels. This production also saves glucose for its use by maternal tissues like the nervous system, which depends on glucose, as well as for its placental transfer.

Although pregnancy hormones may contribute to some of these changes, it is thought that the insulin-resistant condition of late pregnancy is the main factor contributing to the increased adipose tissue lipolytic activity and hepatic VLDL production, as well as the increased gluconeogenesis and ketogenesis under fasting conditions.

Hyperlipidemia

Hyperlipidemia normally develops during the last third of gestation and mainly corresponds to increases in triacylglycerols, with smaller rises in phospholipids and cholesterol.[17,19] Besides an increase in VLDL levels as a result of their enhanced liver production and decreased removal from circulation as a consequence of reduced adipose tissue LPL activity, the increase in plasma triacylglycerols corresponds to their proportional enrichment in both LDL and HDL,[19] lipoproteins that are normally poor in triacylglycerols. Such changes in the maternal lipoprotein profile and composition are the result of the simultaneous action of several factors, which are schematically summarized in Figure 5.4: (1) enhanced arrival of the adipose tissue lipolytic products, NEFA and glycerol, to the liver, which facilitates the hepatic synthesis of triacylglycerols and their subsequent release into the circulation as VLDL; (2) decreased removal of VLDL from circulation as a consequence of the reduced adipose tissue LPL activity; (3) increase in cholesteryl ester transfer protein (CETP) activity that takes place at mid-gestation,[29] facilitating the exchange of cholesterol by triacylglycerols from LDL and HDL with VLDL; and (4) intense decrease in hepatic lipase (HL)[19] which decreases the conversion of buoyant HDL$_{2b}$ triacylglycerol-rich particles, into small triacylglycerol-poor and cholesterol-rich particles (HDL$_3$), allowing the accumulation of the former.[19]

Besides the insulin-resistant condition, which enhances adipose tissue lipolytic activity and decreases its LPL activity,[30] the increase in plasma estrogen concentrations during gestation also contributes to maternal hypertriglyceridemia,

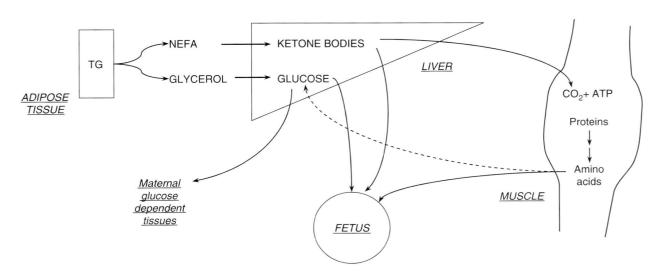

Figure 5.3 Schematic representation of maternal response to starvation during late pregnancy. Enhanced adipose tissue lipolysis increases the availability of glycerol in the liver, where it is used as preferential substrate for gluconeogenesis, and of non-esterified fatty acids (NEFA) for ketogenesis. Throughout this mechanism, the mother, besides producing glucose for the fetus and her own needs, preserves other gluconeogenic substrates, such as amino acids (mainly, alanine), and ensures their availability to the fetus.

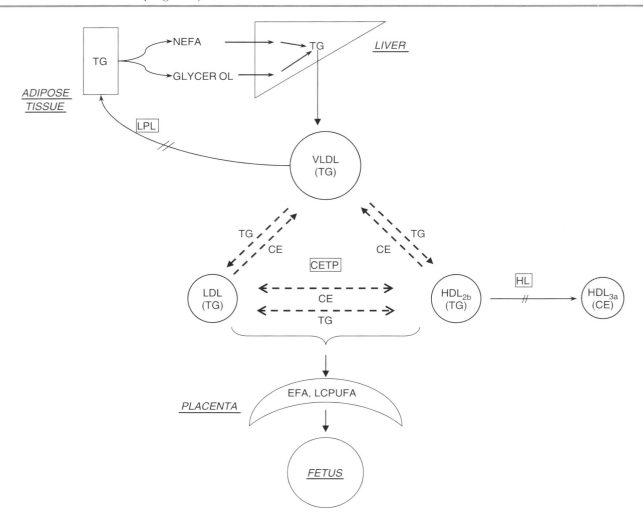

Figure 5.4   Schematic representation of the relationship of adipose tissue lipolytic activity with lipoprotein metabolism during late pregnancy, and its role as a source of essential- (EFA) and long-chain polyunsaturated fatty acids (LCPUFA) for the fetus. CE = cholesterol esters; CETP= cholesterol ester transfer protein; HDL = high density lipoproteins; LDL = low density lipoproteins; VLDL = very low density lipoproteins; LPL = lipoprotein lipase; HL = hepatic lipase.

since it enhances hepatic VLDL production[31] and decreases HL expression and activity.[32]

Benefits of maternal hypertriglyceridemia to the fetus and newborn

Although maternal triacylglycerols do not directly cross the placenta,[23] we think that there are several ways by which the fetus and newborn may benefit from maternal hypertriglyceridemia, as follows.

Use of triacylglycerols as metabolic fuels

Although adult liver does not normally express LPL activity, studies in the rat have shown that under fasting conditions during late pregnancy, there is an increment in liver LPL activity.[33] This liver LPL seems to be the result of the wash-out of LPL from extra-hepatic tissues carried out by the remnants of the triacylglycerol-rich lipoproteins. In this way, under fasting conditions, the maternal liver switches from an exporter organ to an importer of plasma triacylglycerols, which may be used

as substrates for ketogenesis. This allows the exaggerated increase in plasma ketone bodies, which, as commented above, save glucose in maternal tissues as well as cross the placental barrier and are directly metabolized by the fetus.

Placental transfer of polyunsaturated fatty acids (PUFA)

Essential fatty acids (EFA) and LCPUFA from either maternal diet or endogenous interconversion are mainly transported in their esterified form in maternal plasma lipoproteins rather than as NEFA.[34] The placenta expresses receptors for all the major plasma lipoproteins. It has different lipolytic activities, including LPL, phospholipase A_2 and an intracellular lipase and it also expresses fatty acid-binding proteins (for a review see Herrera et al.[35]). Thus, esterified PUFA in maternal plasma lipoproteins are taken up either intact through the placenta receptors or only their constituent fatty acids after hydrolysis. Within the placenta, fatty acids are re-esterified to be latterly hydrolyzed and, in their free form, finally diffuse to fetal plasma. This process, together with the direct transfer of NEFA and the intrinsic placental fatty acid metabolism, determines the actual rate of the selective placental fatty acid transfer, which is essential for fetal development.

Contribution to milk synthesis in preparation for lactation

Around parturition, there is a rapid increase in mammary gland LPL activity,[36] which, together with the low LPL activity in adipose tissue,[20] drive circulating triacylglycerols to the mammary gland. Through this mechanism there is a rapid disappearance of maternal hypertriglyceridemia,[19] and EFA and LCPUFA from maternal circulation are taken up by mammary gland for milk synthesis to become available to the suckling newborn, contributing to its normal development.

Vitamin metabolism in pregnancy

Adequate maternal micronutrient and vitamin status is especially critical during pregnancy and lactation. Several micronutrient deficiencies (like iron, iodine, zinc) are well established as contributors to abnormal prenatal development and/or pregnancy outcome. But less well-recognized for their importance are deficiencies of vitamins. Evidence is accumulating that maternal antioxidant status is important to prevent abnormal pregnancy outcomes. In lactation, the maternal status of several of these vitamins affects their concentration in breast milk. The main cause of multiple vitamin deficiencies is a poor quality diet, even though gene polymorphism can also impair vitamin absorption or alter their metabolism, and cause vitamin deficiency. In some diets high in unrefined grains and legumes, the amount of nutrients consumed may be adequate, but dietary constituents, such as phytanes and polyphenols, can also limit their absorption.

We summarize here the main changes in the metabolism of the vitamins during pregnancy which have the highest implications in fetal growth and development.

Hydrophilic vitamins

Folic acid

Folates act in different one-carbon transfer reactions, including purine and thymidylate biosynthesis, amino acid metabolism and formate oxidation. Purine and thymidylate biosynthesis is a fundamental requisite event underlying DNA and RNA synthesis. Thus, it is obvious that these folate-dependent reactions are essential for fetal growth and development and for maternal well-being.

Pregnancy is associated with an increased folate demand and, in some cases, leads to overt folate deficiency. The increase in folate requirement during pregnancy is due to the growth of the fetus and uteroplacental organs. Circulating folate concentrations decline in pregnant women who are not supplemented with folic acid.[37] Possible causes for the declines in blood folate include increased folate demand for the fetus, increased folate catabolism, increased folate clearance and excretion, decreased folate absorption, hormonal influence on folate metabolism as a physiological response to pregnancy and low folate intake.[38,39]

Whatever the reasons for the decline, it is essential that plasma folate be kept above a critical level (>7.0 nmol/L) because plasma maternal folate is the main determinant of transplacental folate delivery to the fetus. There is a strong positive association between maternal plasma, cord plasma and placental folate concentrations, suggesting that transplacental folate delivery depends on maternal plasma folate concentrations. In placental perfusion studies, it has been found that 5-methyltetrahydrofolate (the main form of folate in plasma) is extensively and rapidly bound in the placenta but transferred to the fetus in low amounts at a slow rate.[40] The placental folate receptor (FR) favors the binding of 5-methyltetrahydrofolate and can transfer folate against a concentration gradient; hence, the fetal perfusate is about 3-fold that of the maternal perfusate. The transfer of 5-methyltetrahydrofolate from the maternal to the fetal perfusate is not saturable in a range well above typical physiologic concentrations.[41] The placenta is rich in FR and is one of the tissues that express the α-isoform of FR (FR-α) in abundance. FR-α is a membrane-bound glycosylphosphatidylinositol-linked glycoprotein and the primary form of FR in the epithelial cells. The importance of FR-α in placental folate transfer is inferred from the fact that an FR-α knockout mouse is embryo-lethal.[42] Maternal folate status should be kept adequate to maintain plasma folate above a certain concentration for placental transfer.

Studies conducted in recent years led to recognition that supplementing with folic acid reduced the prevalence of folate deficiency in pregnancy and prevented pregnancy-related disorders. Data from these studies suggest that 200–300 μg folic acid per day is needed in addition to dietary folate to maintain normal folate status and to prevent folate deficiency during this time.[43,44]

Vitamin C

In addition to the prevention of scurvy, vitamin C has numerous other functions and is a co-factor for several enzyme systems. For humans, vitamin C is an essential vitamin, with an important antioxidant function. As antioxidant defense systems are important to protect tissues and cells from damage caused by oxidative stress, an imbalance between increased oxidative stress and decreased antioxidant defenses impairs fetal growth.[45] Thus, pregnant women utilize a defense mechanism, composed of antioxidant enzymes and nutrients including vitamin C, against oxidative stress and free-radical damage. It is believed that ascorbic acid, through conversion to dehydroascorbic acid, crosses the placenta to enter fetal circulation. Once dehydroascorbic acid is present in the fetal circulation, it is reduced back into ascorbic acid and is maintained in high concentrations on the fetal side of the placenta.[46] Maternal serum vitamin C levels during the second trimester of gestation are correlated with birthweight and length in full-term babies.[47]

Lipophilic vitamins

Because lipophilic vitamins are fat soluble, they share several common mechanisms with other lipidic substances concerning their metabolism and transfer to the offspring. Although lipophilic vitamins are essential during intrauterine and early postnatal life, little is known about their placental transfer during pregnancy and mammary gland uptake during lactation.

Vitamin D

Vitamin D metabolites have numerous potential physiological and pharmacological actions, but their principal physiological function is maintaining serum calcium and phosphorus concentrations in a range that supports cellular processes, neuromuscular function and bone mineralization. In humans, vitamin D (cholecalciferol or vitamin D_3) can be synthesized endogenously from 7-dehydrocholesterol in the epidermis of the skin after exposure to ultraviolet B radiation, or can come from dietary sources. Vitamin D_3 is then transported to the liver and hydroxylated to the inactive but biologically abundant 25-hydroxyvitamin D (25-OH D), which is the major circulating form of vitamin D. The active metabolite of vitamin D_3 is 1,25-dihydroxyvitamin D (1,25-$(OH)_2$ D), which is formed after further hydroxylation in the kidney. This active metabolite of vitamin D increases the efficiency of intestinal calcium absorption, decreases renal calcium excretion and, in conjunction with the parathyroid hormone (PTH), mobilizes calcium from bone.

Significant changes in maternal vitamin D and calcium metabolism occur during pregnancy to provide the calcium needed for fetal bone mineral accretion. Fetal $1,25(OH)_2D_3$ levels are low, whereas maternal levels are strikingly elevated during pregnancy before rapidly returning to normal after parturition.[48] This increase in maternal $1,25(OH)_2D_3$ levels appears to be caused by increased production rather than decreased clearance, but the precise source of the increased $1,25(OH)_2D_3$ synthesis has yet to be fully defined. There is evidence of 1α-hydroxylase activity in the placenta and deciduas, suggesting that these tissues might also contribute to $1,25(OH)_2D_3$ levels.[49] The placenta is a possible site of $1,25(OH)_2D_3$ production, independent of the maternal and fetal kidneys. The presence of a specific vitamin D receptor in placenta and deciduas has also been well documented, underlining the potential for autocrine or paracrine effects of $1,25(OH)_2D_3$ within these tissues.[50] The precise function of the $1,25(OH)_2D_3$ produced by placenta has yet to be fully defined. $1,25(OH)_2D_3$ passes through the placenta barrier bidirectionally to sustain the active transport of calcium across the placenta during late gestation, although current data suggest that the production of $1,25(OH)_2D_3$ by placenta may be less crucial to the maintenance of maternal and fetal calcium homeostasis than originally thought.[51] The fetus has developed several ways to either induce tolerance or escape from the maternal immune system, and it has been proposed that placental produced $1,25(OH)_2D_3$, acting in concert with other mechanisms, may play a key role in maintaining pregnancy by suppression of the maternal immune system.[52]

Approximately 25–30 g of calcium are transferred to the fetal skeleton by the end of pregnancy, most during the last trimester. It has been estimated that the fetus accumulates up to 250 mg/dL calcium during the third trimester. The three possible calcium sources that may supply the mother with the necessary calcium to support fetal growth include increased intestinal absorption from the diet, increased renal conservation, and increased bone mobilization.[53]

To date, there is no evidence to indicate a beneficial effect of vitamin D intake during pregnancy above amounts routinely required to prevent vitamin D deficiency among non-pregnant women.

Vitamin A

Vitamin A exists in several forms in animal tissues: retinol, retinal, retinoic acid and retinyl esters, mainly as retinyl palmitate. All forms of vitamin A are hydrophobic compounds that are highly unstable in the presence of O_2. A diet deficient in either retinol or in the provitamin A carotenoids that can be metabolized to retinol results in impaired growth, night blindness and ultimately, xerophthalmia and blindness. We now know that there are two metabolites of vitamin A, retinoic acid and retinal, which are responsible for growth and development by regulating gene expression, whereas retinal and its isomers are responsible for the visual function of vitamin A. The potential adverse effect of poor vitamin A status on pregnancy outcomes was demonstrated in an intervention study in a region of Nepal with endemic vitamin A deficiency: supplementation of these women with the recommended daily intake of vitamin A reduced maternal mortality by 40%, and supplementation with β-carotene reduced mortality by 49%. The apparent cause of the reduced mortality risk was a decreased susceptibility to infection.[54] Another advantage of vitamin A supplementation of pregnant women is that it can increase hemoglobin concentrations.[55]

During pregnancy, maternal plasma retinol concentrations fall as gestation advances (Figure 5.5),[56] and this effect reflects the increasing demands of the rapidly growing maternal and fetus tissues. Fetal retinol supply is essential, as retinoids are involved in growth and cellular differentiation of the fetus. Even though retinol is the only form of vitamin A that supports reproduction in full, all-*trans* retinoic acid appears to be the most important form for proper embryonic development. Vitamin A plays an essential role in the development of organs such as the lungs, heart, and skeleton; retinoic acid also enables the setting up of the vascular and nervous system, and is involved as a morphogenic agent during embryonic development.[57,58] Both cytoplasmatic and nuclear classes of retinoid binding proteins (CRBP, CRABP and RAR, RXR) are expressed early in development and are proposed to control the concentration of retinoic acid and the transcription activity of retinoid responsive genes, respectively. RAR regulate many developmental control genes, including homeobox genes and growth factor genes. Multiple fetal anomalies occur in vitamin A-deficient, as well as in RAR-deficient knockout mice, but an excess of vitamin A also induces the same type of abnormality: the importance of the abnormality depends on the period of gestation and the duration of the excessive or deficient supply.

The transfer of vitamin A from mother to fetus is carefully regulated in such a way that it allows vitamin A levels in the fetus to remain unaffected by alterations in maternal vitamin A status, except in conditions of deficiency or excess.[59] The placenta's vitamin A content increases in the last trimester of

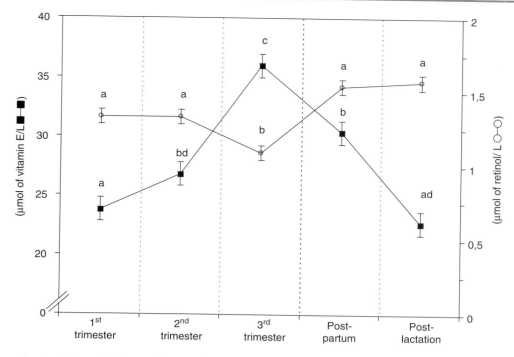

Figure 5.5   Plasma levels of vitamin E (α- and γ-tocopherol) and vitamin A (retinol) at different trimesters of pregnancy, 6–8 days postpartum and at postlactation in healthy women. Data are expressed as means ± SEM. Statistical comparisons are shown by the letters above the points. Different letters for the corresponding vitamin between the groups indicate statistical significance ($P < 0.05$).

pregnancy thanks to the supply of vitamin A from maternal stores (i.e. liver).[60] The amount of retinol provided to the fetus usually remains constant until maternal stores are almost totally depleted. Perfusion studies show that retinol is taken up and concentrated in the placenta, but the exact mechanism of transfer remains unknown. Although the retinol binding protein (RBP) seems to be involved,[61] it might be dispensable for retinol transfer,[62] because homozygous RBP-null mutant mice are viable and fertile. Studies in rats showed that in early gestation, maternal RBP is transported across the placenta and delivers retinol, whereas in late gestation, a different mechanism appears to be operating because fetal liver is capable of synthesizing RBP.[63] *In vivo* studies show that maternal RBP does not cross the placental membrane barrier in the last trimester of gestation and cannot enter fetal circulation.[64] In humans, serum apo-RBP (retinol-free) concentration appears to be elevated during pregnancy, suggesting that pregnancy may alter the affinity of RBP for retinol or induce the binding of the vitamin to other uncharacterized proteins.[65] Other forms of vitamin A, such as retinyl esters and retinoic acid, can also be taken up at the placental barrier.

Although under normal conditions there are no significant correlations between maternal and cord plasma concentrations of retinol or carotenoids, some authors report a weak but statistically significant correlation when the concentration of retinol in cord and maternal plasma are low.[66] Published studies in humans show that maternal subclinical vitamin A deficiency is related to neonatal subclinical vitamin A deficiency and to low birth weight,[66,67] and a high percentage of preterm neonates have marginal values of vitamin A (<0.35μmol/L).

The situation with vitamin A in early lactation is peculiar. Because of the limited transplacental transfer, infant liver stores of vitamin A at birth are small even in well-nourished populations, so newborns are greatly dependent on dietary intake of this vitamin to establish proper tissue stores, maintain rapid growth, and develop their immune system. Colostrum contains higher vitamin A concentration than milk, and has an important role to play in providing initial protection against vitamin A deficiency to the newborn.[68] The timing of colostrum ingestion seems to play a role in the efficiency of intestinal vitamin absorption: thus colostrum feeding on the day of birth is important for the establishment of absorptive mechanism allowing intestinal transport of fat-soluble vitamins. Further, breast milk is a good source of vitamin A and clinical vitamin A deficiency is rare in breast-fed infants during their first year of life.

Debate surrounds the use of retinol supplements during pregnancy. The use of retinol supplements in well-nourished mothers does not affect fetus concentrations. High doses of retinol are teratogenic, and in some countries pregnant women are advised to avoid retinol-containing supplements.[69] However, this advice may lead to vitamin A deficiency.[70] Serum retinol is a relatively insensitive indicator of body vitamin A status: only 1% of the body's reserves circulate in the plasma, and homeostatic mechanisms control concentrations via retinol binding protein concentrations.

Vitamin E

Dietary vitamin E is present as tocopherol, mainly α- and γ-tocopherol, and tocopheryl esters. As for retinyl esters, tocopheryl esters are hydrolyzed into tocopherol within the intestinal lumen by pancreatic esterase as well as by intestinal enzymes. The uptake of tocopherol by enterocytes appears to occur by passive diffusion, and the efficiency of the absorption is largely dependent on the quantity and type of fat present in the diet, even though β- and δ-tocopherol are poorly absorbed. Tocopherol is not re-esterified during the absorption process, which does not require any cellular transfer protein, and within the enterocyte, is incorporated to the chylomicrons and transported from the intestine to the lymphatic pathway to reach the bloodstream.

Plasma levels of vitamin E significantly increased from the first trimester of gestation and reached a maximum in the third trimester of gestation.[56,71,72] Different to vitamin A, there is no specific protein carrier protein in the serum to transport vitamin E, which circulates in its alcohol form in serum lipoproteins. Thus, changes in plasma α-tocopherol levels during pregnancy parallel maternal hyperlipidemia (see above), and are also accompanied by the increase of lipid peroxides. However, γ-tocopherol reaches a maximum concentration in maternal plasma at mid-gestation. The reason for this different concentration pattern between α- and γ-tocopherol during pregnancy is unknown, but could be related to differences in their tissue uptake and intracellular metabolism.

α-Tocopherol concentration in the plasma of human fetuses is lower than in their mothers, but rises towards the end of pregnancy. Since α-tocopherol is carried in plasma associated to the different lipoproteins, its uptake and handling by the placenta is similar to that of the other lipoprotein lipophilic components (see above in this chapter). Besides, the placenta expresses α-tocopherol transfer protein (α-TTP) and similar to the role of this protein in liver, it may actively contribute to the specific transfer of α-tocopherol to the fetus.[73,74]

Despite the existence of these processes, efforts to investigate the actual kinetics of the transfer of vitamin E by isolated human placental systems have found that although it is specific for natural RRR-α-tocopherol rather than any other form of vitamin E, its rate is very low, only 10% of passively transferred L-glucose. This justifies the consistent finding of much lower α-tocopherol levels in fetal plasma and red blood cells than in maternal ones, indicating an insufficient vitamin E supply for the fetus throughout gestation.

During lactation, vitamin E intake through milk is the way of supplying the newborn with an essential defense against oxygen toxicity and of stimulating the development of its immune system. A good supply of vitamin E to the offspring is therefore particularly critical in this period. The increase in vitamin E content in body tissues of the offspring following birth is attributed to the ingestion of colostrums and milk, emphasizing the limited placental vitamin E transfer and the importance of milk consumption. Colostrum contains higher vitamin E concentration than milk,[75] which may imply an active uptake by the mammary gland in compensation for the limited placental transport. A decline in maternal circulating vitamin E concentration is noticed at the end of gestation or in early lactation; this decrease may be the consequence of a considerable amount of α-tocopherol present in colostrum. The mechanism of transfer from blood into milk is not completely understood. Perhaps the transfer of vitamin E into milk occurs through a protein-mediated transport: the presence of an α-TTP like mechanism in the mammary gland cannot be excluded, nor can the presence of an SR-BI receptor in the mammary gland, which could be involved in the uptake of α-tocopherol from HDL. Further, the high concentration of vitamin E found in colostrum compared with mature milk might be due to an increase in activity of the mammary LDL receptors and thus, to an important uptake of LDL by the mammary gland around parturition. LPL also seems to influence in modulating the mammary gland uptake of α-tocopherol.[76] Contrary to the placental transfer, which remains low even with increased maternal serum levels, the transfer through colostrum and milk can be increased via higher vitamin E ingestion by the mother.

It is important to note that tocopherol is able to affect the metabolism of vitamin A in several tissues and may play a role in tissue retinol homeostasis. It has been shown to modulate the levels of retinol and total vitamin A in tissues such as the liver, kidney and intestine. *In vitro*, tocopherol exerts an inhibiting or stimulating action (depending on the tissue) on retinyl palmitate hydrolysis.

Summary

Maternal metabolic adaptations during pregnancy are mainly directed to maintaining a continuous availability of substrates to warrant fetal growth. Glucose, used as a primary energy source of fetoplacental tissues, is quantitatively the most important substrate crossing the placenta. During late pregnancy the mother develops hypoglycemia as a result of the high rate of placental transfer, despite of enhanced gluconeogenesis and reduced consumption of glucose. Amino acids cross the placenta against the gradient thanks to an active process. Fetal growth is sustained by the transfer of amino acids from maternal circulation. Protein metabolism changes gradually throughout gestation, and although during late pregnancy there is increased nitrogen retention, the mother develops hypoaminoacidemia, which is specially evident during fasting. Fat depot accumulation and maternal hyperlipidemia are characteristic features of pregnancy. Maternal adipose tissue lipolytic activity is increased and the main destination of released non-esterified fatty acids (NEFA) and glycerol is the liver, where they are used for the synthesis of triacylglycerols. Alternatively, in the case of glycerol, it is also used as a gluconeogenetic substrate and, in the case of NEFA, oxidized for ketogenesis. Major changes also occur in vitamin metabolism. Vitamin A and E are the most affected. Maternal plasma retinol falls as gestation advances, whereas vitamin E levels increase parallel to the increase in plasma lipids. Transplacental transfer of these vitamins is limited, but both the fetus and the newborn need them. They are taken up by mammary gland and their high content in colostrum seems to play an important role in the extrauterine adaptations of the suckling newborn.

Acknowledgments

Results reported in this chapter were obtained with grants from the Universidad San Pablo-CEU (19/03) and Ministerio de Educación y Ciencia of Spain (SAF2004-05998) and the Commission of the European Communities specific Research and Technological Development programme 'Quality of Life and Management of Living Resources' (QLK1-2001-00138; PeriLip). The authors thank Mis Linda Hamalainen for her editorial help.

REFERENCES

1. Catalano PM, Tyzbir ED, Wolfe RR, et al. Longitudinal changes in basal hepatic glucose production and suppression during insulin infusion in normal pregnant women. Am J Obstet Gynecol 1992; 167: 913–9.

2. Kalhan S, Rossi K, Gruca L, Burkett E, O'Brien A. Glucose turnover and gluconeogenesis in human pregnancy. J Clin Invest 1997; 100: 1775–81.

3. Herrera E, Knopp RH, Freinkel N. Carbohydrate metabolism in pregnancy. VI. Plasma fuels, insulin, liver composition, gluconeogenesis and nitrogen metabolism during gestation in the fed and fasted rat. J Clin Invest 1969; 48: 2260–72.

4. Herrera E. Metabolic adaptations in pregnancy and their implications for the availability of substrates to the fetus. Eur J Clin Nutr 2000; 54(suppl. 1): S47–S51.

5. Herrera E, Amusquivar E. Lipid metabolism in the fetus and the newborn. Diabetes Metab Res Rev 2000; 16: 202–10.

6. Jansson T, Wennergren M, Illsley NP. Glucose transporter protein expression in human placenta throughout gestation and in intrauterine growth retardation. J Clin Endocrinol Metab 1993; 77: 1554–62.

7. King JC. Physiology of pregnancy and nutrient metabolism. Am J Clin Nutr 2001; 71(suppl.): 1218S–25S.

8. Calloway DH. Nitrogen balance during pregnancy. In: Winick M, ed. Nutrition and Fetal Development. Philadelphia: Wiley & Sons; 1974, pp. 79–94.

9. Mojtahedi M, de Groot LCPGM, Boekholt HA, van Raaij JMA. Nitrogen balance of healthy Dutch women before and during pregnancy. Am J Clin Nutr 2002; 75: 1078–83.

10. Metzger BE, Unger RH, Freinkel N. Carbohydrate metabolism in pregnancy.XIV. Relationships between circulating glucagon, insulin, glucose and amino acids in response to a "mixed meal" in late pregnancy. Metabolism 1977; 26: 151–6.

11. Schoengold DM, DeFiore RH, Parlett RC. Free amino acids in plasma throughout pregnancy. Am J Obstet Gynecol 1978; 131: 490–9.

12. Fitch WL, King JC. Plasma amino acid, glucose, and insulin responses to moderate-protein and high-protein test meals in pregnant, nonpregnant, and gestational diabetic women. Am J Clin Nutr 1987; 46: 243–9.

13. Regnault TRH, De Vrijer B, Battaglia FC. Transport and metabolism of amino acids in placenta. Endocrine 2002; 19: 23–41.

14. Herrera E. Metabolic changes in diabetic pregnancy. In: Djelmis J, Desoye G, Ivanisevic M, eds. Diabetology of Pregnancy. Basel: Karger; 2005: 34–45.

15. Villar J, Cogswell M, Kestler E, et al. Effect of fat and fat-free mass deposition during pregnancy on birth weight. Am J Obstet Gynecol 1992; 167: 1344–52.

16. Lopez Luna P, Maier I, Herrera E. Carcass and tissue fat content in the pregnant rat. Biol Neonate 1991; 60: 29–38.

17. Herrera E, Lasunción MA, Gomez Coronado D, et al. Role of lipoprotein lipase activity on lipoprotein metabolism and the fate of circulating triacylglycerides in pregnancy. Am J Obstet Gynecol 1988; 158: 1575–83.

18. Ramos MP, Crespo-Solans MD, Del Campo S, Cacho J, Herrera E. Fat accumulation in the rat during early pregnancy is modulated by enhanced insulin responsiveness. Am J Physiol Endocrinol Metab 2003; 285: E318–28.

19. Álvarez JJ, Montelongo A, Iglesias A, Lasunción MA, Herrera E. Longitudinal study of lipoprotein profile, high density lipoprotein subclass, and postheparin lipases during gestation in women. J Lipid Res 1996; 37: 299–308.

20. Martín-Hidalgo A, Holm C, Belfrage P, Scott J, Herrera E. Lipoprotein lipase and hormone sensitive lipase activity and mRNA in rat adipose tissue during pregnancy. Am J Physiol 1994; 266: E930–5.

21. Williams C, Coltart TM. Adipose tissue metabolism in pregnancy: the lipolytic effect of human placental lactogen. Br J Obstet Gynaecol 1978; 85: 43–6.

22. Knopp RH, Herrera E, Freinkel N. Carbohydrate metabolism in pregnancy. VIII. Metabolism of adipose tissue isolated from fed and fasted pregnant rats during late gestation. J Clin Invest 1970; 49: 1438–46.

23. Herrera E, Lasunción MA. Maternal-fetal transfer of lipid metabolites. In: Polin RA, Fox WW, Abman SH, eds. Fetal and Neonatal Physiology. Philadelphia: Saunders; 2004, pp. 375–88.

24. Zorzano A, Lasunción MA, Herrera E. Role of the availability of substrates on hepatic and renal gluconeogenesis in the fasted late pregnant rat. Metabolism 1986; 35: 297–303.

25. Alonso de la Torre SR, Serrano MA, Medina JM. Carrier-mediated β-D-hydroxybutyrate transport in brush-border membrane vesicles from rat placenta. Pediatr Res 1992; 32: 317–23.

26. Herrera E, Gomez Coronado D, Lasunción MA. Lipid metabolism in pregnancy. Biol Neonate 1987; 51: 70–7.

27. Page MA, Williamson DH. Enzymes of ketone-body utilisation in human brain. Lancet 1971; 2: 66–9.

28. Shambaugh GE, Koehler RR, Yokoo H. Fetal fuels III: ketone utilization by fetal hepatocyte. Am J Physiol 1978; 235: E330–7.

29. Iglesias A, Montelongo A, Herrera E, Lasunción MA. Changes in cholesteryl ester transfer protein activity during normal gestation and postpartum. Clin Biochem 1994; 27: 63–8.

30. Ramos P, Herrera E. Reversion of insulin resistance in the rat during late pregnancy by 72-h glucose infusion. Am J Physiol Endocrinol Metab 1995; 269: E858–63.

31. Knopp RH, Bonet B, Lasunción MA, Montelongo A, Herrera E. Lipoprotein metabolism in pregnancy. In: Herrera E, Knopp RH, eds. Perinatal Biochemistry. Boca Raton: CRC Press; 2006, pp. 19–51.

32. Brinton EA. Oral estrogen replacement therapy in postmenopausal women selectively raises levels and production rates of lipoprotein A-I and lowers hepatic lipase activity without lowering the fractional catabolic rate. Arterioscler Thromb Vasc Biol 1996; 16: 431–40.

33. López-Luna P, Olea J, Herrera E. Effect of starvation on lipoprotein lipase activity in different tissues during gestation in the rat. Biochim Biophys Acta 1994; 1215: 275–9.

34. Herrera E. Lipid metabolism in pregnancy and its consequences in the fetus and newborn. Endocrine 2002; 19: 43–55.

35. Herrera E, Amusquivar E, López-Soldado I, Ortega H. Maternal lipid metabolism and placental lipid transfer. Horm Res 2006; 65 (suppl. 3): 58–63.

36. Ramirez I, Llobera M, Herrera E. Circulating triacylglycerols, lipoproteins, and tissue lipoprotein lipase activities in rat mothers and offspring during the perinatal period: effect of postmaturity. Metabolism 1983; 32: 333–41.

37. Cikot RJ, Steegers-Theunissen RP, Thomas CM, et al. Longitudinal vitamin and homocysteine levels in normal pregnancy. Br J Nutr 2001; 85: 49–58.

38. Caudill MA, Gregory JF, Hutson AD, Bailey LB. Folate catabolism in pregnant and nonpregnant women with controlled folate intakes. J Nutr 1998; 128: 204–8.

39. Higgins JR, Quinlivan EP, McPartlin J, et al. The relationship between increased folate catabolism and the increased requirement for folate in pregnancy. Br J Obstet Gynaecol 2000; 107: 1149–54.

40. Henderson GI, Perez T, Schenker S, Mackins J, Antony AC. Maternal-to-fetal transfer of 5-methyltetrahydrofolate by the perfused human placental cotyledon: evidence for a concentrative role by placental folate receptors in fetal folate delivery. J Lab Clin Med 1995; 126: 184–203.

41. Bisseling TM, Steegers EA, van den Heuvel JJ, et al. Placental folate transport and binding are not impaired in pregnancies complicated by fetal growth restriction. Placenta 2004; 25: 588–93.

42. Piedrahita JA, Oetama B, Bennett GD, et al. Mice lacking the folic acid-binding protein Folbp1 are defective in early embryonic development. Nat Genet 1999; 23: 228–32.

43. Rayburn WF, Stanley JR, Garrett ME. Periconceptional folate intake and neural tube defects. J Am Coll Nutr 1996; 15: 121–5.

44. Swain RA, St Clair L. The role of folic acid in deficiency states and prevention of disease. J Fam Pract 1997; 44: 138–44.

45. Myatt L, Eis AL, Brockman DE, et al. Differential localization of superoxide dismutase isoforms in placental villous tissue of normotensive, pre-eclamptic, and intrauterine growth-restricted pregnancies. J Histochem Cytochem 1997; 45: 1433–8.

46. Guajardo L, Beharry KD, Modanlou HD, Aranda JV. Ascorbic acid concentrations in umbilical cord veins and arteries of preterm and term newborns. Biol Neonate 1995; 68: 1–9.

47. Lee BE, Hong YC, Lee KH, et al. Influence of maternal serum levels of vitamins C and E during the second trimester on birth weight and length. Eur J Clin Nutr 2004; 58: 1365–71.

48. Kovacs CS, Kronenberg HM. Maternal-fetal calcium and bone metabolism during pregnancy, puerperium, and lactation. Endocrine Rev 1997; 18: 832–72.

49. Gray TK, Lowe W, Lester GE. Vitamin D and pregnancy: the maternal-fetal metabolism of vitamin D. Endocr Rev 1981; 2: 264–74.

50. Henry HL, Norman AW. Vitamin D: metabolism and biological actions. Annu Rev Nutr 1984; 4: 493–520.

51. Kovacs CS, Woodland ML, Fudge NJ, Friel JK. The vitamin D receptor is not required for fetal mineral homeostasis or for the regulation of placental calcium transfer in mice. Am J Physiol Endocrinol Metab 2005; 289: E133–44.

52. Evans KN, Bulmer JN, Kilby MD, Hewison M. Vitamin D and placental-decidual function. J Soc Gynecol Invest 2004; 11: 263–71.

53. Ritchie LD, Fung EB, Halloran BP, et al. A longitudinal study of calcium homeostasis during human pregnancy and lactation and after resumption of menses. Am J Clin Nutr 1998; 67: 693–6.

54. West Jr. KP, Katz J, Khatry SK, et al. Double blind, cluster randomised trial of low dose supplementation with vitamin A or beta carotene on mortality related to pregnancy in Nepal. The NNIPS-2 Study Group. BMJ 1999; 318: 570–5.

55. Tanumihardjo SA, Permaesih D, Muhilal. Vitamin A status and hemoglobin concentrations are improved in Indonesian children with vitamin A and deworming interventions. Eur J Clin Nutr 2004; 58: 1223–30.

56. Herrera E, Ortega H, Alvino G, et al. Relationship between plasma fatty acid profile and antioxidant vitamins during normal pregnancy. Eur J Clin Nutr 2004; 58: 1231–8.

57. Zachman RD. Role of vitamin A in lung development. J Nutr 1995; 125(6, suppl.): 1634S–8S.

58. Rohwedel J, Guan K, Wobus AM. Induction of cellular differentiation by retinoic acid in vitro. Cells Tissues Organs 1999; 165: 190–202.

59. Underwood BA. Maternal vitamin A status and its importance in infancy and early childhood. Am J Clin Nutr 1994; 59(2, suppl.): S517–24.

60. Ismadi SD, Olson JA. Dynamics of the fetal distribution and transfer of Vitamin A between rat fetuses and their mother. Int J Vit Nutr Res 1982; 52: 112–9.

61. Sivaprasadarao A, Boudjelal M, Findlay JB. Solubilization and purification of the retinol-binding protein receptor from human placental membranes. Biochem J 1994; 302(pt 1): 245–51.

62. Dancis J, Levitz M, Katz J, et al. Transfer and metabolism of retinol by the perfused human placenta. Pediatr Res 1992; 32: 195–9.

63. Takahashi YI, Smith JE, Goodman DS. Vitamin A and retinol-binding protein metabolism during fetal development in the rat. Am J Physiol 1977; 233: E263–72.

64. Quadro L, Hamberger L, Gottesman ME, et al. Transplacental delivery of retinoid: the role of retinol-binding protein and lipoprotein retinyl ester. Am J Physiol Endocrinol Metab 2004; 286: E844–51.

65. Sapin V, Alexandre MC, Chaib S, et al. Effect of vitamin A status at the end of term pregnancy on the saturation of retinol binding protein with retinol. Am J Clin Nutr 2000; 71: 537–43.

66. Gazala E, Sarov B, Hershkovitz E, et al. Retinol concentration in maternal and cord serum: its relation to birth weight in healthy mother-infant pairs. Early Hum Dev 2003; 71: 19–28.

67. Ghebremeskel K, Burns L, Burden TJ, et al. Vitamin A and related essential nutrients in cord blood: relationships with anthropometric measurements at birth. Early Hum Dev 1994; 39: 177–88.

68. Schweigert FJ, Bathe K, Chen F, Buscher U, Dudenhausen JW. Effect of the stage of lactation in humans on carotenoid levels in milk, blood plasma and plasma lipoprotein fractions. Eur J Nutr 2004; 43: 39–44.

69. Keusch GT. Vitamin A supplements: too good not to be true. N Engl J Med 1990; 323: 985–6.

70. Sanders TA. Vitamin A and pregnancy. Lancet 1990; 336: 1375.

71. González-Corbella MJ, Lopez-Sabater MC, Castellote-Bargallo AI, Campoy-Folgoso C, Rivero-Urgell M. Influence of caesarean delivery and maternal factors on fat-soluble vitamins in blood from cord and neonates. Early Hum Dev 1998; 53: S121–34.

72. Vriese SR, Dhont M, Christophe AB. Oxidative stability of low density lipoproteins and vitamin E levels increase in maternal blood during normal pregnancy. Lipids 2001; 36: 361–6.

73. Jishage K, Arita M, Igarashi K, et al. Alpha-tocopherol transfer protein is important for the normal development of placental labyrinthine trophoblasts in mice. J Biol Chem 2001; 276: 1669–72.

74. de Kaempf-Rotzoll DE, Horiguchi M, Hashiguchi K, et al. Human Placental trophoblast cells express alpha-tocopherol transfer protein. Placenta 2003; 24: 439–44.

75. Barbas C, Herrera E. Lipid composition and vitamin E content in human colostrum and mature milk. J Physiol Biochem 1998; 54: 167–73.

76. Martinez S, Barbas C, Herrera E. Uptake of alpha-tocopherol by the mammary gland but not by white adipose tissue is dependent on lipoprotein lipase activity around parturition and during lactation in the rat. Metabolism 2002; 51: 1444–51.

6 Intermediary metabolism in pregnancies complicated by gestational diabetes

Bartolomé Bonet, Marta Viana and Isabel Sánchez-Vera

Changes in intermediary metabolism during pregnancy

As has been shown in previous chapters, throughout pregnancy there are major changes in intermediary metabolism, changes that will facilitate the fetal needs of energy and precursors for fetal and placental growth, as well as for placental hormone synthesis. From a metabolic point of view, during gestation there are two different periods. In the first half of pregnancy, during the embryo development period, there are maternal changes that lead to storage of energy and nutrients.[1–3] The stored reserves will be used in the second half of pregnancy to facilitate rapid fetal and placental growth. During the first half of pregnancy, there is increased appetite and normal or increased insulin sensitivity. These changes will facilitate glucose and lipid uptake by adipose tissue, increasing the lipid stores.[1–3] In fact, during the first half of pregnancy, most women show an increase in adipose tissue mass.[4] Nevertheless, as pregnancy advances, and the fetal–placental unit is rapidly growing, a marked shift in the metabolic pathways is observed. This period is characterized by a state of insulin resistance, decreasing the uptake of glucose by the maternal tissues sensitive to insulin, mainly the white adipose tissue and muscle (Figure 6.1B). Such a condition facilitates the supply of glucose toward the fetus, where the daily glucose requirement is very high (30–50 g of glucose/day).[5] During this period of gestation, because of the high fetal glucose requirements and despite increased glucose production[6] and insulin resistance[1–3] after moderate periods of fasting, there is a trend toward lower maternal plasma glucose concentration. A blunted glucose curve is observed in normal pregnancies after an oral glucose tolerance test or a regular meal.[7,8] During the post-prandial period, such a curve will allow higher and prolonged plasma levels of glucose and therefore, a higher glucose supply to the fetus, as the glucose supply to the fetus is via passive glucose diffusion and therefore, concentration dependent.[9] This type of curve is thought to be secondary to the insulin resistance observed during the second half of gestation and not because of beta-cell dysfunction.

Plasma lipid changes during pregnancy

During gestation there are also relevant changes in lipid metabolism (Figure 6.1B), changes most marked in the second half of pregnancy, when both the plasma triglycerides and cholesterol reach the highest levels.[1,2,10,11] The high plasma levels of triglycerides seem to be secondary to both an increased hepatic synthesis of VLDL-TG, as well as a decreased lipoprotein lipase (LPL) activity in the adipose tissue in late gestation.[10,11] These changes are due to some of the hormonal changes observed during pregnancy. The increased production of VLDL-TG is secondary to the elevation of estradiol that takes place during gestation, as increased levels of estradiol stimulate the hepatic synthesis of triglycerides.[12,13] Both the placental lactogen (hPL), which reaches its maximum concentration by the end of pregnancy, and the insulin resistance that increases adipose tissue lipolysis, lead to an abundant supply of fatty acids to the liver.[14,15] The lower levels of adiponectin observed as pregnancy advances[16,17] may also play a role in the increased hepatic synthesis of triglycerides, as under this condition, in the liver there is a decrease in beta-oxidation[18] and therefore, the fatty acids are derived towards re-esterification and synthesis of triglycerides. The high plasma levels of triglycerides are used as a source of energy for the maternal tissues, sparing glucose for the fetus and the maternal organs that only use glucose as a source of energy. In addition, they are used by the placenta, where lipoprotein lipase is present[19] and therefore able to hydrolyze the VLDL-TG, releasing fatty acids, which are taken up by placental cells.[19] In fact, some studies show a positive relationship between maternal plasma triglycerides and birthweight.[20,21]

The elevation of the plasma levels of cholesterol, mainly from LDL,[1,2,10,11] will facilitate the substrate for the elevated synthesis of steroid hormones that takes place during pregnancy. By the end of pregnancy, plasma levels of estradiol are almost a thousand times higher than in non-pregnant women, while progesterone is ten times higher.[22] Cholesterol is also a source of precursors for the high synthesis of cell membranes that takes place in the fast-growing fetus.

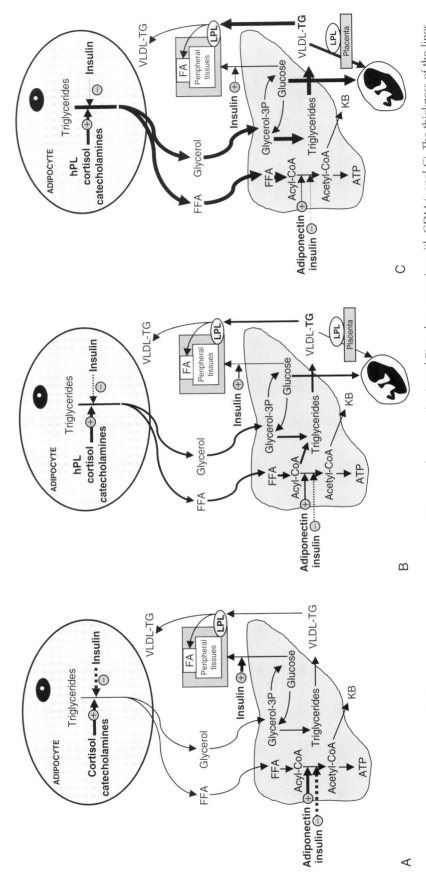

Figure 6.1   Intermediary metabolism in non-pregnant women (panel A), normal pregnancies (panel B) and pregnancies with GDM (panel C). The thickness of the lines relates the degree of stimulation (solid lines) or inhibition (dash lines) of either the metabolic pathway or the hormonal effects. TG: triglycerides; KB: ketone bodies; FFA: free fatty acids; FA: fatty acids; hPL: placental lactogen; LPL: lipoprotein lipase.

As occurs in carbohydrates and lipid metabolism, there are changes in protein metabolism throughout pregnancy. These changes develop gradually during gestation. By the end of pregnancy, when fetal growth is maximal, nitrogen retention is four times higher than in early pregnancy,[23] suggesting that amino acids are conserved for tissue synthesis. Nevertheless, the sum of total plasma amino acids declines by 15–25%, reflecting the enhanced uptake of amino acids by the placenta,[24] where there is an energy dependent active transport,[24,25] leading to a higher concentration of amino acids in fetal plasma. Such a mechanism facilitates the supply of amino acids for the rapid protein accretion that takes place in the fetus by the end of pregnancy.

Mechanisms of pregnancy-induced insulin resistance

The mechanisms involved in pregnancy-induced insulin resistance, although not fully understood, seem to be related to different factors. Firstly, in pregnant rats there is increased degradation of insulin by the placenta,[26] therefore insulin removal is accelerated. A similar phenomenon may occur in human pregnancies. Secondly, and probably most important, during the second half of gestation, there are several hormonal and metabolic alterations that facilitate the development of insulin resistance. Among them, there is the hypertriglyceridemia and the high plasma levels of non-esterified fatty acids, secondary to increased plasma levels of placental lactogen and increased lipolysis,[14,15] which lead to an increased cell metabolism of fatty acids, causing in turn, to an intracellular increase in the levels of NADH and ATP. This intracellular condition lowers the glucokinase activity and the cell ability to phosphorylate glucose, decreasing the cell uptake of this substance. Increased plasma levels of TNF-alfa have also been linked to insulin resistance.[27,28] The mechanism involved is probably related to a decrease in the insulin receptors. The high plasma levels of progesterone found during the second half of pregnancy also play a role in pregnancy-induced insulin resistance.[29] Adiponectin has been proposed as playing a role in the development of pregnancy-induced insulin resistance, as lower levels of adiponectin have been linked to a higher risk of developing gestational diabetes.[16,17] Nevertheless, the mechanism is not well understood. Adiponectin decreases as pregnancy advances and with increased adipose tissue mass, a condition also linked to the development of insulin resistance.

Mechanisms leading to the development of gestational diabetes

The mechanisms leading to the development of gestational diabetes mellitus (GDM) have not been fully defined but are probably related to both an exacerbation of the beta-cell dysfunction in subjects genetically predisposed to beta-cell alterations, which favors the development of GDM. In that sense, GDM will act like a Type 2 DM. In the present chapter we do not take into account situations where diabetes, although diagnosed during pregnancy, is secondary to auto-inmune processes or to the diagnosis of mature onset diabetes of the young (MODY) during pregnancy. Regarding the beta-cell dysfunction, several mechanisms could be involved in this process. High progesterone levels may play a relevant role.[30,31] Recently, in models of knock-out mice,[31] it has been shown that the lack of progesterone receptors is associated with a higher insulin secretion by beta-cells. Therefore the high levels of progesterone that develop during pregnancy may damage these cells. The hyperlipidemia observed during pregnancy may also decrease the capability of beta-cells to secrete insulin.[32,33] Although fatty acids may induce insulin secretion,[34] under certain circumstances, prolonged high levels of fatty acids may damage the beta-cell, decreasing insulin secretion. In fact, in an experimental animal model during pregnancy, a decrease in plasma free fatty acids and triglycerides increases insulin secretion after an oral glucose tolerance test.[35]

The higher food intake that develops during early pregnancy may lead to beta-cell hyperplasia. In certain genetically predisposed subjects, this higher supply of glucose and fatty acids to the beta-cell may increase the cell metabolism, leading to increased beta-cell apoptosis and cell death.[36,37] Such a phenomenon would compromise the capability of the beta-cells to secrete enough insulin in a period of high insulin requirements, because of the insulin resistance, and therefore, to the development of GDM. Further research is needed for a better understanding of the beta-cell dysfunction observed in GDM, in order to develop methods to improve this function and decrease the incidence of GDM.

Because the insulin resistance that takes place in the second half of pregnancy plays a key role in the development of gestational diabetes, any condition susceptible to exacerbating this resistance may play a role in the development of GDM. Higher plasma levels of triglycerides and NEFA and lower plasma levels of adiponectin have been associated with higher insulin resistance and therefore to a higher risk of developing GDM. Obesity also increases insulin resistance.[38,39] Added to the pregnancy-induced insulin resistance, it makes obese pregnant women more prone to the development of GDM.

Glucose alterations in gestational diabetes mellitus

Independent of the mechanisms involved, in GDM, there is a relative lack of insulin during a period of time with high insulin needs to compensate the insulin resistance that develops in the third trimester of pregnancy. When gestational diabetes develops, in the maternal tissues, where glucose uptake is insulin-dependent, this is further decreased and hyperglycemia develops. Because the materno-placenta–fetal transfer of glucose is concentration-dependent[9] under conditions of maternal hyperglycemia and placental normal function, there is increased placental transfer of glucose (Figure 6.1C), fetal hyperglycemia develops and secondary to this alteration, hyperinsulinism. As insulin is one of the main growth factors during fetal life,[40] this hyperinsulinemia leads to macrosomia and to the complications secondary to the delivery of a large baby, mainly both maternal perineal damage and birth trauma, including shoulder dystocia, Erbs palsy, etc. The hyperinsulinism remains in the newborn period and increases the risk of hypoglycemia, once the umbilical supply of glucose is suddenly arrested after delivery. Because of this process, the newborn will need frequent monitorization of blood glucose, early feeds and occasionally may require the intravenous administration of glucose. Hypoglycemia in the newborn, if not corrected, may lead to brain damage.[41] Fetal macrosomia also increases the risk of obesity, Type 2 diabetes mellitus and cardiovascular diseases later on in life.[42,43]

Lipid alterations in gestational diabetes mellitus

In gestational diabetes, as occurs in other conditions of insulin resistance and beta-cell dysfunction, there is an increase in plasma levels of triglycerides and cholesterol. This effect should be added to the physiological hyperlypidemia induced by pregnancy (Figure 6.1C).[10,11] Therefore, women with GDM have higher plasma levels of triglycerides and cholesterol than found in normal pregnancies (Figure 6.2).[44,45] The hyper-triglyceridemia found in gestational diabetes may also play a role in the fetal macrosomia observed in these pregnancies, as several authors have shown a positive correlation between the plasma levels of triglycerides and birthweight.[20,21]

Increased plasma levels of both triglycerides and cholesterol have been associated to structural alterations in LDL.[46,47] High triglycerides make LDL particles small and more dense.

Such particles are more susceptible to oxidation. Nevertheless, as pregnancy advances, the maternal milieu changes and conditions that both increase as well as decrease LDL susceptibility to oxidation are present. Higher levels of triglycerides and cholesterol are pro-oxidant,[48,49] but this effect may be blunted by higher levels of vitamin E and estradiol,[22] two powerful anti-oxidants whose levels are increased in pregnancy.[22] In fact, our group and others have shown that in normal pregnancies, as pregnancy advances, despite increased plasma levels of triglycerides and cholesterol, LDL susceptibility to oxidation decreases,[22,50] phenomenon that is partially explained by the high levels of estradiol observed at the end of pregnancy. Nevertheless, under conditions of exacerbated dys-lipidemia, the pro-oxidant effects may lead to increased LDL oxidation and to the consequences associated with this process. An increased LDL oxidation may have relevant consequences for the placenta as well as for the fetus. In a cell culture model of human placental trophoblasts and macrophages, LDL oxidation is cytotoxic.[51] If this process occured during pregnancy, it could damage the placenta. If such damage were extensive, the placental capability to transfer nutrients and oxygen to the fetus might be decreased, compromising fetal growth. In fact, our group has shown a correlation between LDL susceptibility to oxidation and birthweight,[22] suggesting that conditions where LDL oxidation is increased, fetal growth may be compromised. Furthermore, when oxidized LDL is taken up by human trophoblasts, through scavenger receptors and not by the LDL receptor, despite increasing the intracellular concentration of cholesterol, progesterone secretion is decreased (Figure 6.3).[52] These data suggest that the metabolism of cholesterol from oxidized LDL does not follow the physiological pathways required for hormonal synthesis. Therefore, under circumstances of increased LDL oxidation, there may be a lack of cholesterol for the placenta, decreasing the placental synthesis of steroidal hormones as well as the transfer of cholesterol to the fetus. As occurs in other conditions, increased LDL oxidation may also lead to vascular dysfunction,[53–55] decreasing the vascular blood flow and the nutrient transfer to the fetus. Therefore, increased LDL oxidation could affect the transfer of nutrients and oxygen to the fetus through different mechanisms, either damaging the placenta or decreasing the placental blood flow.

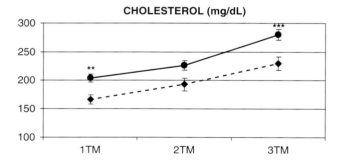

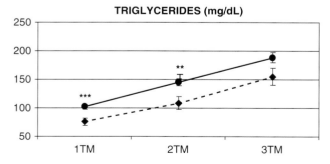

Figure 6.2 Changes in plasma levels of cholesterol and triglycerides throughout pregnancy in normal (dashed line) and pregnancies complicated with GDM (solid line). *Differences between control and GDM group. **$P < 0.01$; ***$P < 0.001$. (Data from Bonet, Viana, and Sánchez-Vera, unpublished results.)

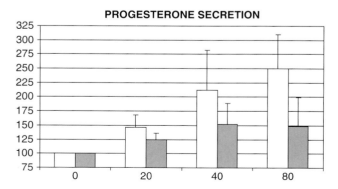

Figure 6.3 Progesterone secretion in trophoblast incubated with increasing concentrations of normal LDL (white bars) or oxidized LDL (black bars) (for details see Bonet et al.[52])

Finally, conditions of increased plasma levels of cholesterol and triglycerides have been linked to increased fatty streaks in the fetal arteries.[56,57] As a consequence, children from GDM pregnancies may have a higher incidence of these alterations than newborns from normal pregnancies. Further studies are needed to demonstrate if stillborns from GDM pregnancies also have increased incidence of fatty streaks in their arteries.

To sum up, in gestational diabetes, there is a combination of factors that may affect the nutrient supply to the fetus. Under certain conditions, increased supply of glucose and triglycerides towards the fetus may lead to increased fetal growth and macrosomia (Figure 6.3). Nevertheless, under certain conditions, the dyslipedemia found in gestational diabetes may lead to increased LDL oxidation to placental damage, and vascular dysfunction, leading to decreased transfer of nutrients towards the fetus and to intrauterine growth retardation (Figure 6.4). At the present time, most efforts are directed toward blood glucose normalization, and little attention has been paid to the dyslipedemia and to the LDL oxidation associated with this process. Further studies are needed to obtain a better understanding of the role of dyslipidemia in the maternal and fetal complications associated with gestational diabetes. There is a clear need of studies to determine which pregnancies with lipid alterations show compromised fetal growth.

Amino acid alterations in pregnancies complicated by gestational diabetes

In GDM there is an increase in a number of essential and nonessential amino acids in umbilical venous and arterial concentration,[58] compared to the values found in normal pregnancies. The higher plasma levels of fetal amino acids do not seem to be related to a higher concentration in maternal plasma, as only ornithine has been shown to increase in plasma from pregnant women with GDM.[58] More recently, studies analyzing maternal protein and amino acid metabolism by stable isotope methodologies did not find significant differences in either treated[59] or untreated GDM[60,61] compared to normal pregnancies. However, the elevation observed in the plasma amino acid concentration in umbilical, but not in maternal circulation, suggests that placental amino acid exchange and/or feto/placental metabolism is altered in GDM.[58]

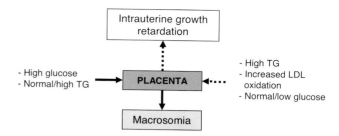

Figure 6.4 Potential mechanisms affecting fetal growth in pregnancies complicated by GDM. Solid lines show a stimulus in fetal growth and dash lines show a decrease in fetal growth.

Studies *in vitro* show that among the different amino acid transporters, the expression of system A, which mediates the transfer of neutral amino acids such as alanine, serine, and glutamine, is increased in diabetic pregnancies.[62,63] This, in turn, could increase the uptake and delivery of neutral amino acids into the fetus. However, it does not seem to be the primary cause of accelerated fetal growth. Other transporters such as the specific system for leucine (system L), have also been shown to be increased in microvillous plasma membranes isolated from GDM pregnancies with large babies for their gestational age.[62,63] Nevertheless, other authors did not find an increased activity of these transporters.[64] It is remarkable that leucine has been proven to be an effective stimulus for fetal insulin secretion in human pancreas studied *in vitro*.[65] *In vivo* studies applying stable isotope techniques have provided evidence to suggest that leucine, taken up across the microvillous plasma membranes, is rapidly transferred to the fetus, contributing to the accelerated fetal growth in these patients.[62,63] More studies are needed for a further clarification of the role of amino acid metabolic alterations associated with GDM.

Acknowledgments

Results reported in this chapter were obtained with grants from Universidad San Pablo-CEU (14/01) and from the Fondo de Investigación Sanitarias (Ministerio de Sanidad y Consumo) (00/0304 and 02/1731). The authors thank Miss Linda Hamalainen for her editorial help and to Amalia Quintanar for her technical assistance.

REFERENCES

1. Knopp RH, Montes A, Childs M, Li JR, Mabuchi H. Metabolic adjustments in normal and diabetic pregnancy. Clin Obstet Gynecol 1981; 24: 21–49.
2. Knopp RH, Bonet B, Zhu XD. Lipid Metabolism in pregnancy. In: Cowett RM, ed. Principles of Perinatal–Neonatal Metabolism. New York: Springer; 1998, pp. 221–58.
3. Catalana PM, Tyzbir ED, Wolfe RR, et al. Longitudinal changes in basal hepatic glucose production and suppression during insulin infusion in normal pregnant woman. Am J Obstet Gynecol 1992; 167: 913–9.
4. Hytten RE, Thomson AM, Taggart N. Total body water in normal pregnancy. Obstet Gynaecol Br Commun 1966; 73: 553–61.
5. Hay WW. Glucose metabolism in the fetal–placental unit. In: Cowett RM, ed. Principles of Perinatal–Neonatal Metabolism. New York: Springer 1998, pp. 337–67.
6. Kalhan S, Rossi K, Gruca L, Burkett E, O'Brien A. Glucose turnover and gluconeogenesis in human pregnancy. J Clin Invest 1997; 100: 1775–81.
7. Spelleacy WN, Goetz FC. Plasma insulin in normal late pregnancy. N Engl J Med 1963; 268: 988–91.
8. Bleicher SJ, O'Sullivan JB, Freinkel N. Carbohydrate metabolism in pregnancy. V. The interrelations of glucose, insulin, and free fatty acids in late pregnancy and postpartum. N Engl J Med 1964; 271: 866–72.
9. Hay WW. Placental nutrient metabolism and transport. In: Herrera E, Knopp RH, eds. Perinatal Biochemistry. Boca Raton, FL: CRC Press; 1992, pp. 93–130.
10. Knopp RH, Bonet B, Lasunción MA, Montelongo A, Herrera E. Lipoprotein metabolism in pregnancy. In: Herrera E, Knopp RH, eds. Perinatal Biochemistry. Boca Raton, FL: CRC Press; 1992, pp. 19–51.
11. Knopp RH, Montes A, Warth MR. Carbohydrate and lipid metabolism in normal pregnancy. In: Laboratory Indices of Nutritional Status in Pregnancy, Food and Nutrition Boards. Washington, DC: National Academy of Sciences; 1978, p. 35.

12. Knopp RH, Zhu XD, Bonet B. Effects of estrogens on lipoprotein metabolism and cardiovascular disease in women. Atherosclerosis 1994; 110: S83–S91.

13. Sacks FM. Gerhard M, Walsh BW. Sex hormones, lipoproteins, and vascular reactivity. Curr Opin Lipidol 1995: 6: 161–6.

14. Desoye G, Schweditsch O, Pfeiffer KP, Zechner R, Kostner GM. Correlation of homonones with lipid and lipoprotein levels during normal pregnancy and postpartum. J Clin Endocrinol Metab 1987: 64: 704–12.

15. Grumbach MM, Kaplan SL, Abramo CL, Bell JJ, Conte FA. Plasma free fatty acid response to the administration of chorionic "growth hormone prolactin". J Clin Endocrinol Metab 1966; 26: 478–82.

16. Retnakaran R, Hanley AJG, Raif N, et al. Reduced adiponectin concentration in women with gestational diabetes. Diabetes Care 2004; 27: 799–800.

17. Worda C, Leipold H, Gruber C, et al. Decreased plasma adiponectin concentrations in women with gestational diabetes mellitus. Am J Obstet Gynecol 2004; 191: 2120–4.

18. Kershaw EE, Flier JS. Adipose tissue as an endocrine organ. J Clin Endocrinol Metab 2004; 89: 2548–56.

19. Bonet B, Brunzell JD, Gown AM, Knopp RH. Metabolism of very-low density lipoprotein triglyceride by human placental cells: the role of the lipoprotein lipase. Metabolism 1992; 41: 596–603.

20. Knopp RH, Magee MS, Walden CE, Bonet B, Benedetti TJ. Prediction of infant birthweight by gestational diabetes screening test: importance of plasma triglyceride. Diabetes Care 1992; 15: 1605–13.

21. DiCianni G, Miccoli R, Volpe L, et al. Maternal triglyceride levels and newborn weight in pregnant women with normal glucose tolerance. Diabet Med 2005; 22: 21–5.

22. Sánchez-Vera I, Bonet B, Viana M, Quintanar A. López-Salva A. Increased low-density lipoprotein susceptibility to oxidation in pregnancies and fetal growth restriction. Obstet Gynecol 2005; 106, 345–51.

23. King JC. Physiology of pregnancy and nutrient metabolism. Am J Clin Nutr 2000; 71: 1218S–25S.

24. Phelps RL, Metzger BE, Freinkel N. Carbohydrate metabolism in pregnancy. XVII. Diurnal profiles of plasma glucose, insulin, free fatty acids, triglycerides, cholesterol, and individual amino acids in late normal pregnancy. Am J Obstet Gynecol 1981; 140: 730–6.

25. Cariappa R, Heath-Monning E, Smith CH. Isoforms of amino acid transporters in placental syncytiotrophoblast: plasma membrane localization and potential role in maternal/fetal transport. Placenta 2003; 24: 713–26.

26. Goodner CJ, Freinkel N. Carbohydrate metabolism in pregnancy: The degradation of insulin by extracts of maternal and fetal structures in the pregnant rat. Endocrinology 1959; 65: 957–67.

27. Kirwan JP, Hauguel-De Mouzon S, Lepercq J, et al. TNF-alpha is a predictor of insulin resistance in human pregnancy. Diabetes 2002; 51: 2207–13.

28. Hotamisligil GS, Murray DL, Choy LN, Spiegelman BM. Tumor necrosis factor alpha inhibits signaling from the insulin receptor. Proc Natl Acad Sci 1994; 91: 4854–8.

29. Kalchoff RK. Metabolic effects of pregesterone. Am J Obstet Gynecol 1982; 142: 735–8.

30. Branisteanu DD, Mathieu C. Progesterone in gestational diabetes mellitus: guilty or not guilty? Trends Endocrinol Metab 2003; 14: 54–5.

31. Picard F, Wanatabe M, Schoonjans K, et al. Progesterone receptor knockout mice have an improved glucose homeotasis secondary to beta-cell proliferation. Proc Natl Acad Sci USA 2002; 99: 15644–8.

32. Kasuga M. Insulin resistance and pancreatic beta-cell failure. J Clin Invest 2006; 116: 1756–60.

33. McGarry DJ, Dobbins RL. Fatty acids, lipotoxicity and insulin secretion. Diabetologia 1999; 42: 128–38.

34. Rojo-Martinez G, Esteva I, Ruiz de Aldana MS, et al. Dietary fatty acids and insulin secretion: a population-based study. Eur J Clin Nutr 2006; 60: 1195–200.

35. Sanchez-Vera I, Bonet B, Viana M, Herrera E, Indart A. Effect of acipimox on plasma lipids and glucose/insulin in pregnant rats. Int J Exp Diab Res 2002; 3: 233–9.

36. Prentki M, Nolan CJ. Islet Beta-cell failure in type 2 diabetes. J Clin Invest 2006; 116: 1802–12.

37. Kasuga M. Insulin resistance and pancreatic beta cell failure. J Clin Invest 2006; 116: 1756–60.

38. Kanh BB, Flier JS. Obesity and insulin resistance. J Clin Invest 2000; 106: 473–81.

39. King JC. Maternal obesity, metabolism and pregnancy outcomes. Annu Rev Nutr 2006; 26: 271–91.

40. Osler M, Pederson J. The body composition of newborn infants of diabetic mothers. Pediatrics 1960; 26: 985–92.

41. Chase HP, Marlow RA, Dabiere CS, Welch NN. Hypoglycemia and brain development. Pediatrics 1973; 52: 513–20.

42. Boney CM, Verma A, Tucker R, Vohr BR. Metabolic syndrome in childhood: Association with birth weight, maternal obesity and gestational diabetes mellitus. Pediatrics 2005; 115: 290–6.

43. McCance D, Pettit D, Hanson R, et al. Birth weight and non-insulin dependent diabetes: thrifty genotype, thrifty phenotype or surviving baby genotype? BMJ 1994; 308: 942–5.

44. Knopp RH, Chapman M, Bergelin R, et al. Relatioships of lipoprotein lipids to mild fasting hyperglycemia and diabetes in pregnancy. Diabetes Care 1980; 3: 416–20.

45. Hollingsworth DR, Grundy SM. Pregnancy-associated hypertriglyceridemia in normal and diabetic women. Differences in insulin-dependent, non-insulin-dependent, and gestational diabetes. Diabetes 1982; 31: 1092–7.

46. Silliman K, Shore V, Forte TM. Hypertriglyceridemia during late pregnancy is associated with the formation of small dense low-density lipoproteins and the presence of large buoyant high-density lipoproteins. Metabolism 1994; 43: 1035–41.

47. Sattar N, Greer IA, Louden J, et al. Lipoprotein subfraction changes in normal pregnancy: threshold effect of plasma triglyceride on appearance of small, dense low density lipoprotein. J Clin Endocrinol Metab 1997; 82: 2483–91.

48. Cominacini L, Pastorino AM, Garbin U, et al. The susceptibility of low-density lipoprotein to in vitro oxidative is increased in hypercholesterolemic patients. Nutrition 1994; 10: 564–6.

49. Liu ML, Ylitalo K, Vakkilainen J, et al. Susceptibility of LDL to oxidation in vitro and antioxidant capacity in familial combined hyperlipidemia: comparison of patients with different lipid phenotypes. Ann Med 2002; 34: 48–54.

50. De Vriese SR, Shont M, Christophe AB. Oxidative stability of low density lipoproteins and vitamin E levels increase in maternal blood during normal pregnancy. Lipids 2001; 36: 361–6.

51. Bonet B, Hauge-Gillenwater H, Zhu XD, Knopp RH. LDL oxidation and human placental trophoblast and macrophage cytotoxicity. PSEBM 1998; 217: 203–11.

52. Bonet B, Chait A, Gown AM, Knopp RH. Metabolism of modified LDL by cultured human placental cells. Atherosclerosis 1995; 112: 125–36.

53. Tanner FC, Noll G, Boulanger CM, Lüsscher TF. Oxidized low density lipoproteins inhibit relaxations of porcine coronary arteries: Role of scavenger receptor and endothelium-derived nitric oxide. Circulation 1991; 83: 2012–20.

54. Vergnani L. Effect of native and oxidized low-density lipoprotein on endothelial nitric oxide and superoxide production. Circulation 2000; 101: 1261–6.

55. Boulanger CM, Tanner FC, Dea MI, et al. Oxidized LDL induce mRNA expression and release of endothelin from human and porcine endothelium. Circ Res 1992; 70: 1191–7.

56. Napoli C, D'Armiento FP, Mancini FP, et al. Fatty streak formation occurs in human fetal aortas and is greatly enhanced by maternal hypercholesterolemia: intimal accumulation of LDL and its oxidation precede monocyte recruitment into early atherosclerotic lesions. J Clin Invest 1997; 100: 2680–90.

57. Napoli C, Glass CK, Witztum JL, et al. Influence of maternal hypercholesterolaemia during pregnancy on progression of early atheroesclerotic lesions in childhood: fate of early lesions in children (FELIC) study. Lancet 1999; 354: 1324–41.

58. Cetin I, Nobile de Santis MS, Tarico E, et al. Maternal and fetal amino acid concentrations in normal pregnancies and pregnancies with gestational diabetes mellitas. Am J Obstet Gynecol 2005; 192: 610–7.

59. Zimmer DM, Golichowski AM, Karn CA, et al. Glucose and amino acid turnover in untreated gestational diabetes. Diabetes Care 1996; 19: 591–6.

60. Butte NF, Hsu HW, Thotathuchery M, et al. Protein metabolism in insulin-treated gestational diabetes. Diabetes Care 1999; 22: 806–11.

61. Hod M, Lapidot A. Dynamic parameters of maternal amino acid metabolism and fetal growth. Isr J Med Sci 1996; 32: 530–6.

62. Jansson T, Ekstrand Y, Björn C, Wennergren M, Powell TL. Alterations in the activity of placental amino acid transporters in pregnancies complicated by diabetes. Diabetes 2002; 51: 2214–9.

63. Jansson T, Powell TL. Human placental transport in altered fetal growth: Does the placenta function as a nutrient sensor? A Review. Placenta 2006; 27(suppl. A): S91–7.

64. Kuruvilla AG, D'Souza SW, Glazier JD, Mahendran D, Maresh MJ. Altered activity of the system A amino acid transporter in microvillous membrane vesicles from placentas of macrosomic babies born to diabetic women. J Clin Invest 1994; 94: 689–95.

65. Milner RDG, Ashworth MA, Barson AJ. Insulin release from human foetal pancreas in response to glucose, leucine and arginine. J Endocrinol 1972; 52: 497–505.

7 Histopathology of placenta

Drucilla J. Roberts and Maria Rosaria Raspollini

Introduction

In 1892, Ballantyne wrote:

A diseased foetus without his placenta is an imperfect specimen, and a description of a foetal malady, unless accompanied by a notice of the placental condition, is incomplete. Deductions drawn from such a case cannot be considered as conclusive, for in the missing placenta or cord may have existed the cause of the disease and death. During intrauterine life the foetus, the membranes, the cord and the placenta form an organic whole, and disease of any part must react upon and affect the others.[1]

Indeed, a careful examination of the placenta contributes to the determination of the causes which underline fetal growth alterations, demise or neonatal conditions. The correlation between placenta histopathology and clinical data may allow the understanding of the sequence of pathologic events and getting information for the management of the neonate or future pregnancies.

At term, the human placenta is a focal, disk-like thickening of the membranous sac that is achieved by splitting the membranes into two separate sheets, the chorionic plate and the basal plate. Both sheets enclose the intervillous space, as cover and bottom. The intervillous space is perfused with maternal blood, which circulates, without its own vessel wall, directly around the trophoblastic surface of the placental villi. The human placenta is hemochorial in structure. The villi form from a complex tree-like projection of the chorionic plate into the intervillous space (Figure 7.1). The villous surface is surrounded by trophoblast and a core composed of a stroma that supports fetal vessels connected to the fetal circulation system via the chorionic plate and the umbilical cord. At the placental margin, the intervillous space is obliterated so that the chorionic plate and the basal plate fuse each other and thus form the chorion leave.[2]

Placental specimens are not routinely sent for pathological examination. Nevertheless, indications of placenta referral are many and include: fetal conditions requiring admission to neonatal intensive care unit, maternal diseases or disorders specific or complicated by pregnancy, with potential consequences to the neonate, such as maternal diabetes. In any case, the placenta should be grossly examined after the fetus is delivered, in order to identify any visible pathology. This macroscopic analysis should include measurement of the length and insertion site of the umbilical cord, the number of cord vessels, the state and the color of the fetal surface and fetal membranes, the maternal surface looking for abnormalities and/or the presence or absence of retroplacental clot, the color and the consistency of the villous tissue and the presence of chorionic plate lesions. Any abnormal findings at this point should necessitate a complete pathologic examination regardless of the clinical history.[3]

Pathophysiology of placenta alterations in diabetes

Maternal diabetes mellitus complicates pregnancy with combinations of growth-promoting and growth-restricting forces which may alter the normal growth trajectories of both the fetus and placenta. Diabetes may affect the maternal intrauterine environment by altering uteroplacental vascular function via the mediators of oxidative stress and inflammation. In an environment of abnormal metabolism, the placenta, which is the sole source of oxygen and nutrients for the fetus, affects the development of fetus.

At the earliest stage of pregnancy, the ovarian production of steroids allows the development of normal endometrial

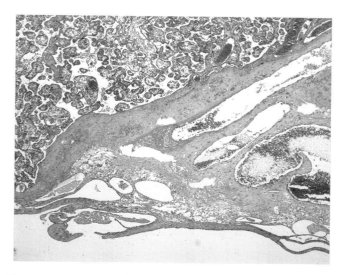

Figure 7.1 Hematoxylin–eosin section of normal placenta at term showing villi which form a complex tree-like projection of the chorionic plate into the intervillous space.

receptivity,[4] and insulin has been shown to modulate ovarian steroidogenesis.[5] Human pregnancy is associated with hyperinsulinemia and a progressive decline in insulin sensitivity.[6] Women with gestational diabetes mellitus appear to have abnormalities both in insulin secretion[7] and pronounced insulin resistance,[8] compared to women with normal glucose tolerance during pregnancy. Endothelial dysfunctions of decidual capillary network associated with insulin resistance include decreased vasodilation, increased leukocyte-endothelial cell adhesion and vascular permeability.[9,10] The primary mechanisms that contribute to these endothelial dysfunctions in diabetes appears to involve the activation of protein kinase C (PK-C) pathways and increased oxidative stress. Diabetes, as a pro-inflammatory state, has a negative effect on implantation, in a similar way to the contraceptive effect of intrauterine devices via induction of local inflammation.[11]

Within 2 weeks of pregnancy, the gestational sac is engaged with the maternal decidua. What follows is a necessary conversion of uterine spiral arteries: the media and elastica are loosened, and the endothelium is supported by connective tissue fibers. During this time, the conceptus develops in a low oxygen tension environment.[12] In diabetic pregnancies, increased oxidative stress to the cell, and/or the activation of protein kinase pathways (particularly PK-C and mitogen-activated PK) may create the basis for early damage in vessels formation of the placenta. In addition, the response of the fetal–placental vasculature to vasoconstrictor and vasodilator agents is significantly attenuated when compared to responses in nondiabetic placentas. Consequently, in cases of modified vascular responses, the diabetic placenta may not be able to adequately respond to demands for altered blood flow, resulting in fetal compromise.[13]

A physiologic state of insulin resistance is required during pregnancy to preferentially direct maternal nutrients towards the feto-placental unit, allowing adequate growth of the fetus. Type 1 diabetes during pregnancy is associated with dysregulation of glucose and oxygen metabolic pathways, both of which affect placental villous growth and function. Alteration of placental development may contribute to the associated increased risk of complications of pregnancy associated with diabetes such as pre-eclampsia, macrosomia, or fetal growth restriction, and to the state of relative fetal hypoxia. Different degree of changes in the syncytiotrophoblast, cytotrophoblast, trophoblastic basement membrane, and fetal vessels have been described, and have been attributed to the glycemic status.

Gross examination

The presence of chronic placental anomalies indicative of chronic insult (small or large placenta size, infarcts or hemorrhages, anomalies of insertion and defects of the cord, variations of placental shape, loss of transparency or increases of thickening of membranes, etc.) may already be diagnosed or suspected by gross macroscopic evaluation.

Generally, human placentas are round or oval, but other shapes are not uncommon. Anomalies of the placenta shape or multilobated placenta may develop from abnormal fetal genes (expressed in the placenta), abnormal maternal environment (such as the presence of submucosal leiomyomas or uterine scar), abnormal fetal–maternal interaction or early uteroplacental vascular compromise.[2] Sometimes, the anomalies of shape can be associated with unprotected membranous fetal vessels (such as vasa previa). The placental weight, which is evaluated after removing cord, membranes and maternal blood clots, is about 450–550 g at term pregnancy. The placental weight is related, other than to gestational age, to the weight of the fetus and to fetal gender. The fetal/placental weight ratio should be ~6–7 at term. Moreover, placental weight over the 95th or less than the 5th centiles for gestational age is often a sign of chronic insult. Maternal diabetes is a condition that can be associated with large placentas (more than 90 centiles), although the differential diagnosis largely include: fetal hydrops, congenital syphilis, villous edema, or Beckwith–Wiedemann syndrome.[14] Large placentas, however, should raise the suspicion for a maternal diabetic state.

The macroscopic analysis of the chorionic plate (fetal surface) should include evaluation of the chorionic vessels. Macroscopic features of dilated and/or discolored vessels suggest fresh thrombosis, while tan–white or yellow fibrosed vessels are indicative for an older thrombus. The rare finding of thrombosis of chorionic vessels is more common in maternal diabetes, but can also be seen in other pathological conditions such as thrombophilic states, fetal chromosomal disorders, vascular anomalies accompanied by local trauma or stasis (for example, true knots of the umbilical cord, velamentous cord insertion or umbilical cord entanglement),[15] toxic agents to fetal vessels, and some viral infections.[3]

The observation of the maternal surface of the placenta should demonstrate the normal mosaic of 20–40 cotyledons. This mosaic can be absent in pathologic conditions, such as vascular pathologies which may cause extensive fibrin deposition. The maternal surface may include the presence of adherent fresh blood clots, if recent, or old firm dry clots dissecting the placental parenchyma. These are findings related to placental abruption. The features, however, are also observed in placenta from patients carrying thrombophilic traits, maternal pre-eclampsia, or hypertension.

At term, the cut surface of placenta is red and spongy. A dark red color suggests congestion of capillaries, or choriangiosis that may be associated with maternal diabetes (see below). Placenta thickness is usually between 1.5 and 3 cm. A greater thickness is observed in diabetic placentas.

Cord and fetal membranes

The length of the cord at term is between 40 and 70 cm and the diameter is usually between 1 and 3 cm. A short or excessively long cord is related to an increased risk for fetal damage. Marginal cord insertion or velamentous cord insertion, which probably are due to disturbed implantation, may be also associated with fetal or neonatal damage. Histopathologic features such as thrombosis of vessels or the observation of a single artery should be already suspected by a macroscopic analysis of cord vessels. This sign may be indicative of vascular pathology, fetal malformations, and also presence of diabetes.

Fetal membranes and fetal surface of chorionic plate are normally clean and transparent making the color look blue on the chorionic plate and pink on the free membranes. A diffuse yellow/white–opaque feature is a feature seen with infiltration of granulocytes, lymphocytes and other inflammatory cells of acute chorioamnionitis, which may be also present in diabetic placentas. The brown color of the membranes may suggest hemosiderin deposition, while a green color may be present in the cases of meconium staining.[16] Combinations of pathologies are common, often the best description of membrane color is 'normal' or 'abnormal.'

Microscopic evaluation

Placental pathology in pregnancies complicated by maternal diabetes relates to the different aspects of the maternal disease. Although some findings are thought to be related to the direct effect of insulin on the placenta, most are due to associated maternal pathologies, especially hypertension. This makes the study of placental effects of hyperinsulinemia (in insulin resistance) and hyperglycemia difficult as most diabetic pregnancies

have other confounding variables, especially hypertension. What is known is often anecdotal or based on series of maternal diabetic pregnancies in which these confounding variables are either ignored or an attempt has been to ferret them out.

We do know that insulin does not cross the placenta into the fetal circulation but there is sufficient evidence that there are insulin receptors on trophoblast that can be up- or down-regulated according to maternal glucose status. The insulin effects of maternal diabetes, therefore, are indirect and are related directly to its effect on the placenta. Maternal glucose freely reaches the fetal circulation and the resulting fetal hyperglycemia has well described effects on the developing conceptus and are known for decades.[17] The placental findings in maternal diabetes are related with the glucose level and its control and have been well described in many different studies.[2,18–20]

Two of the most well documented effects of maternal diabetes in pregnancy include increased villous vasculature (chorangiosis),[21–27] and placental villous immaturity.[26,28–31] The increased villous vascularity (chorangiosis) may be a response to the relative hypoxemia due to the immaturity of the villi (characterized by centrally placed villous capillaries

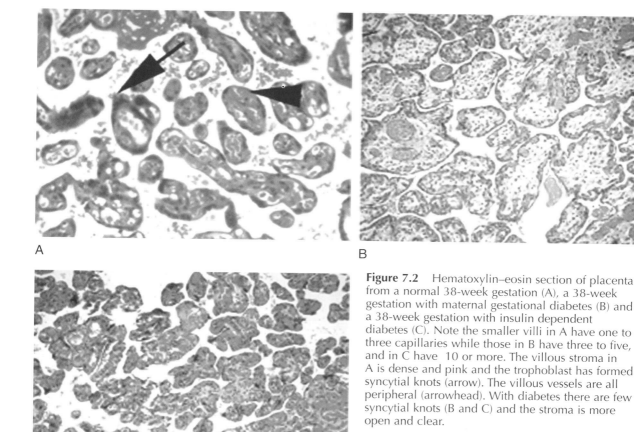

A

B

C

Figure 7.2 Hematoxylin–eosin section of placenta from a normal 38-week gestation (A), a 38-week gestation with maternal gestational diabetes (B) and a 38-week gestation with insulin dependent diabetes (C). Note the smaller villi in A have one to three capillaries while those in B have three to five, and in C have 10 or more. The villous stroma in A is dense and pink and the trophoblast has formed syncytial knots (arrow). The villous vessels are all peripheral (arrowhead). With diabetes there are few syncytial knots (B and C) and the stroma is more open and clear.

resulting in a greater distance for oxygen and nutrients to pass from maternal to fetal circulation).[32] Neither of these histopathologic findings are specific nor are they easily defined. In general, the non-hypertensive diabetic placenta has fewer syncytial knots, fewer vasculosyncytial membranes, larger villi, central villous vessels, and increased vessels per villous compared to placenta from diabetic pregnancies complicated by hypertension (Figure 7.2). Poor glucose control will exacerbate these findings and result in placentomegaly and macrosomia. The functional significance of these features is decreased oxygen and nutrient supply, due to the long diffusion distance from maternal to fetal vascular spaces. The pathology is not dramatic but distinctive and common. Given this as the baseline for diabetic placental pathology, complicating pathologies in the mother are added on.

Probably the most significant associated disease in diabetic mothers is hypertension/pre-eclampsia. Hypertension, whether pregnancy related (pre-eclampsia or pregnancy induced hypertension) or essential (therefore existing before pregnancy), can cause vascular damage to the uterus and results in poor blood flow to the placenta. The resulting uteroplacental insufficiency causes placental ischemia. The gross pathologic correlate of chronic significant uteroplacental insufficiency is stunted placental growth leaving a small organ (weighing below the 10th centile) and accelerated villous branching (hypermaturity)[33] (Figure 7.3). In addition, ischemic placentas often infarct or suffer abruption, chronic or acute (Figure 7.3). There is nothing specific or different about the histopathology of diabetic–hypertensive placentas as compared with hypertensive placentas alone.

An unusual finding that also observed in diabetic placentas is given by the infiltration of the membranes, chorionic plate, and umbilical cord by mature lymphocytes, plasma cells, and histiocytes, the so-called chronic chorioamnionitis.[34,35] Contrary to the acute pathology, chronic chorioamnionitis, which in approximately 80% of the cases is associated with villitis of unknown etiology, cannot be appreciated on gross examination.[36] Chronic chorioamnionitis may be due to infectious agents, but other causative mechanisms have been suggested, such as an imbalance of the systemic inflammatory milieu associated with insulin resistance in gestational diabetes mellitus.[37]

Pregnancy complicated by diabetes also has an increased risk for fungal placentitis.[38–44] This rare complication usually does not have significant sequelae for the fetus, but rarely can

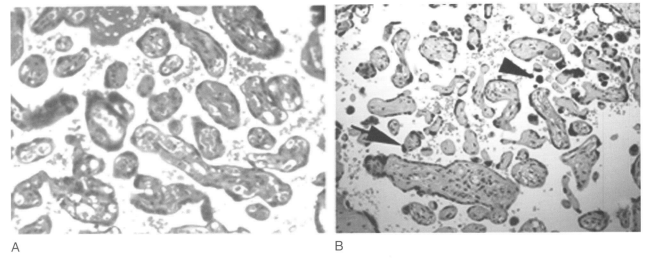

A

B

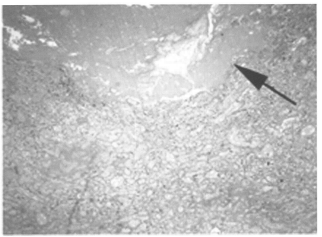

C

Figure 7.3 Section of a normal 38-week gestation (A), a 38-week gestation complicated with maternal insulin dependent diabetes mellitus and chronic hypertension (B and C) (hematoxylin–eosin). In B the villi are widely separated due to premature branching and the villi have fewer capillaries and larger and more numerous syncytial knots (arrow and arrowhead). C shows a chronic abruption with the retroplacental hematoma (arrow) with an indented and infracted parenchyma.

have catastrophic effects, including overwhelming sepsis.[45,46] The pathology is characteristic and includes a brisk funisitis (umbilical cord vasculitis) with peripheral umbilical cord abscesses (Figure 7.4).[42] The presence of invasive hyphae within the Wharton's jelly of the umbilical cord is thought to represent an increased risk for disseminated disease in the fetus/neonate, but in our experience most cases of even deeply invasive hyphae are benign (D. Roberts, unpublished data). The umbilical vasculitis and the presence of abscesses may be in association with acute chorioamnionitis. The abscesses typically have easily identifiable hyphae either superficially or invasive into Wharton's jelly and do not need special stains to be visualized. In the absence of hyphae visible by hematoxylin–eosin staining, fungal specific staining (silver stain) should be used. Abscesses on the surface of the umbilical cord are, nearly always, due to Candida although they can also be rarely seen with group B β-hemolytic Streptococcal infections.

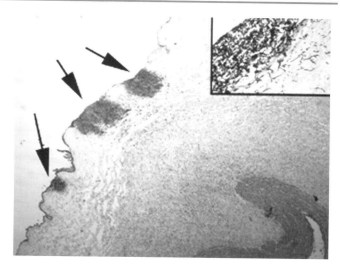

Figure 7.4 Hematoxylin–eosin section of an umbilical cord showing peripheral abscesses (arrow) which contain maternal white blood cells and abundant candidal forms (insert with silver stain).

Conclusions

The placenta in uncomplicated maternal diabetes is heavy, large, somewhat immature, and chorangiotic. The extent of placental findings is related to maternal insulin and glucose levels. Sometimes, maternal diabetes is associated with hypertension. Hypertension, *per se*, can cause vascular damage to the uterus and results in an impairment of blood flow to the placenta causing reduced placental growth and villous hypermaturity. There is nothing specific or different about the histopathology of diabetic and hypertensive placentas as compared with hypertensive placentas alone. In addition, pregnancies complicated by diabetes may have an increased risk for villitis, chorioamnionitis and funisitis. Probably, the interaction of genetic and environmental factors may explain this increased risk: recent data support the role of cytokines and immune response in the pathogenetic mechanisms underlying the effect of glucose intolerance in diabetes mellitus.

REFERENCES

1. Ballantyne JW. The Disease and Deformities of the Foetus, Vol. I. Edinburgh: Oliver and Boyd; 1892.
2. Benirschke K, Kaufman P, Baergen RN. The Pathology of the Human Placenta. Heidelberg: Springer-Verlag; 2006.
3. Roberts DJ, Oliva E. Clinical significance of placental examination in perinatal medicine. J Matern Fetal Neonat Med 2006; 19: 255–64.
4. Dominguez F, Avila S, Cervero A, et al. A combined approach for gene discovery identifies insulin-like growth factor-binding protein-related protein 1 as a new gene implicated in human endometrial receptivity. J Clin Endocrinol Metab 2003; 88: 1849–57.
5. Willis D, Mason H, Gilling-Smith C, et al. Modulation by insulin of follicle-stimulating hormone and luteinizing hormone actions in human granulosa cells of normal and polycystic ovaries. J Clin Endocrinol Metab 1996; 81: 302–9.
6. Fridman JE, Ishizuka T, Shao J, et al. Impaired glucose transport and insulin receptor tyrosyne phosphorylation in skeletal muscle from obese women with gestational diabetes. Diabetes 1999; 48: 1807–14.
7. Buchanan TA, Metzger BE, Freinkel N, et al. Insulin sensitivity and beta cell responsiveness to glucose during late pregnancy in lean and moderately obese women with normal glucose tolerance or mild gestational diabetes. Am J Obstet Gynecol 1990; 162: 1008–14.
8. Kautzky-Willer A, Prager R, Waldhausl W, et al. Pronounced insulin resistance and inadequate β-cell secretion characterize lean gestational diabetes during and after pregnancy. Diabetes Care 1997; 20: 1717–23.
9. Feener EP, King GL. Endothelial dysfunction in diabetes mellitus: role in cardiovascular disease. Heart Fail Monit 2001; 1: 74–82.
10. De Vriese AS, Verbeuren TJ, Van de Vorde J, et al. Endothelial dysfunction in diabetes. Br J Pharmacol 2000; 130: 963–74.
11. Ortiz ME, Croxatto HB, Bardin CW. Mechanisms of action of intrauterine devices. Obstet Gynecol Surv 1996; 51: S42–S51.

12. Jauniaux E, Burton GJ. Villous histomorphometry and placental bed biopsy investigation in type I diabetic pregnancies. Placenta 2006; 27: 468–74.
13. Myatt L, Kossenjans W, Sahay R et al. Oxidative stress causes vascular dysfunction in the placenta. J Matern Fetal Med 2000; 9: 79–82.
14. Torfs CP, van den Berg B, Oechsli FW, et al. Prenatal and perinatal factors in the etiology of cerebral palsy. J Pediatr 1990; 116: 615–9.
15. Redline RW. Clinical and pathological umbilical cord abnormalities in fetal thrombotic vasculopathy. Hum Pathol 2004; 35: 1494–8.
16. Miller PW, Coen RW, Benirschke K. Dating the time interval from meconium passage to birth. Obstet Gynecol 1985; 66: 459–62.
17. Driscoll S. Pathology of pregnancy complicated by diabetes mellitus. Med Clin North Am 1965; 49.
18. Haust MD. Maternal diabete mellitus-effects on the fetus and placenta. In: Naeye RL, Kissane JM, Kaufman N, eds. Perinatal Diseases. Baltimore: Williams & Wilkins; 1981, pp. 201–85.
19. Singer DB. The placenta in pregnancies complicated by diabetes mellitus. Perspect Pediatr Pathol 1984; 8, 199–212.
20. Fox H. The Pathology of the Placenta. W.B. Saunders Co.; 1997.
21. Asmussen I. Vascular morphology in diabetic placentas. Contrib Gynecol Obstet 1982; 9: 76–85.
22. Altshuler G. Chorangiosis. An important placental sign of neonatal morbidity and mortality. Arch Pathol Lab Med 1984; 108: 71–4.
23. Ogino S, Redline RW. Villous capillary lesions of the placenta: distinctions between chorangioma, chorangiomatosis, and chorangiosis. Hum Pathol 2000; 31: 945–54.
24. De La Ossa MM, Cabello-Inchausti B, Robinson MJ. Placental chorangiosis. Arch Pathol Lab Med 2001; 125: 1258.
25. Schwartz DA. Chorangiosis and its precursors: underdiagnosed placental indicators of chronic fetal hypoxia. Obstet Gynecol Surv 2001; 56: 523–5.

26. Evers IM, Nikkels PG, Sikkema JM, et al. Placental pathology in women with type 1 diabetes and in a control group with normal and large-for-gestational-age infants. Placenta 2003; 24: 819–25.

27. Gupta R, Nigam S, Arora P, et al. Clinico-pathological profile of 12 cases of chorangiosis. Arch Gynecol Obstet 2006; 274: 50–3.

28. Haust MD. Maternal diabetes mellitus – effects on the fetus and placenta. Monogr Pathol 1981; 22: 201–85.

29. Singer DB, Liu CT, Widness JA, et al. Placental morphometric studies in diabetic pregnancies. Placenta Suppl 1981; 3: 193–202.

30. Stoz F, Schuhmann RA, and Haas B. Morphohistometric investigations in placentas of gestational diabetes. J Perinat Med 1988; 16: 205–9.

31. Younes B, Baez-Giangreco A, al-Nuaim L, et al. Basement membrane thickening in the placentae from diabetic women. Pathol Int 1996; 46: 100–4.

32. Kingdom J, Huppertz B, Seaward G, et al. Development of the placental villous tree and its consequences for fetal growth. Eur J Obstet Gynecol Reprod Biol 2000; 92: 35–43.

33. Redline RW, Boyd T, Campbell V, et al. Maternal vascular underperfusion: nosology and reproducibility of placental reaction patterns. Pediatr Dev Pathol 2004; 7: 237–49.

34. Salafia CM, Silberman L. Placental pathology and abnormal fetal heart rate patterns in gestational diabetes. Pediatr Pathol 1989; 9: 513–20.

35. Jacques SM, Qureshi F. Chronic chorioamnionitis: a clinicopathological and immunohistochemical study. Hum Pathol 1998; 29: 1457–61.

36. Baerger RN. Manual of Bernirshke and Kaufmann's Pathology of the Human Placenta. New York: Springer; 2005.

37. Richardson A, Fulton C, Catlow D, et al. Cytokine profiles in pregnant women with gestational diabetes mellitus. Am J Obstet Gynecol 2006; 195: S163.

38. Delprado WJ, Baird PJ, Russell P. Placental candidiasis: report of three cases with a review of the literature. Pathology 1982; 14: 191–5.

39. Schwartz DA, Reef S. Candida albicans placentitis and funisitis: early diagnosis of congenital candidemia by histopathologic examination of umbilical cord vessels. Pediatr Infect Dis J 1990; 9: 661–5.

40. Reed BD. Risk factors for Candida vulvovaginitis. Obstet Gynecol Surv 1992; 47: 551–60.

41. Mazziotti F, Arena V, Lo Mastro F, et al. Diabetes and pregnancy: prophylaxis of genital infections. Ann Ist Super Sanita 1997; 33: 343–5.

42. Qureshi F, Jacques SM, Bendon RW, et al. Candida funisitis: A clinicopathologic study of 32 cases. Pediatr Dev Pathol 1998; 1: 118–24.

43. Kelekci S, Kelekci H, Cetin M, et al. Glucose tolerance in pregnant women with vaginal candidiasis. Ann Saudi Med 2004; 24: 350–3.

44. Grigoriou O, Baka S, Makrakis E, et al. Prevalence of clinical vaginal candidiasis in a university hospital and possible risk factors. Eur J Obstet Gynecol Reprod Biol 2006; 126: 121–5.

45. Gerberding KM, Eisenhut CC., Engle WA, et al. Congenital candida pneumonia and sepsis: a case report and review of the literature. J Perinatol 1989; 9: 159–61.

46. Levy I, Shalit I, Birk E, et al. Candida endocarditis in neonates: report of five cases and review of the literature. Mycoses 2006; 49: 43–8.

8 The placenta in diabetic pregnancy: Placental transfer of nutrients

Gernot Desoye, Eleazar Shafrir and Sylvie Hauguel-de Mouzon

Introduction

The placenta is a tissue of limited life span that serves an impressive array of diverse functions: selective forward transport of nutrients and gases to the fetus and reverse transport of metabolic waste products from the fetus to the maternal circulation; energy metabolism mainly to support various placental activities; metabolic modification of maternal nutrients destined for the fetus; synthesis of hormones, certain proteins and other molecules related to its function in gestation; maintenance of an immunologic barrier; transfer of heat and detoxification of xenobiotics. In fulfilling its pleiotropic functions the placenta serves as a substitute for fetal organs as long as these have not reached their full maturity, thereby sustaining and protecting fetal development. From these functions it becomes clear that the placenta should not be considered as a molecular sieve and transport vehicle only; it has many functions, which might affect both maternal and fetal metabolism as well as growth of the fetus. Inter-relation between fetal and placental growth has been repeatedly emphasized.

In general, the placenta is the organ accounting for the transfer of almost all nutrients and gases between mother and fetus and for the back-transfer of waste products from the fetus into the placenta and then further into the mother. In addition, extracellular pathways do exist. For example, some solutes including proteins may cross the amnion from the maternal circulation and then be ingested by fetal swallowing of amniotic fluid. However, the bulk of material being transferred between mother and fetus must all pass through the placenta.[1,2]

Upon reviewing the literature no clear-cut picture on the effects of gestational diabetes mellitus (GDM) on the placenta emerges, likely because of the variety of confounding factors that need to be controlled for in comprehensive studies, such as severity of disease, modality of treatment and quality of glycemic control. Critical for placental development and function and their potential alterations by maternal diabetes is also the duration of departures from normoglycemia. Hence, the time point of detection of GDM and subsequent institution of treatment appears important. The earlier in gestation this occurs the lesser the influence on placental development and function, and ultimately, on fetal growth and metabolism.

The extent of nutrient transfers from mother to fetus, and, hence, of fetal supply, is determined by a number of factors (Box 8.1). Below these will be considered separately and the influence of GDM discussed. We will focus on human pregnancy. Aspects of the placenta of animal pregnancy in diabetes will be covered in another chapter in this book.[3]

Maternal–fetal concentration gradients

Glucose

The human fetus is almost totally dependent on maternal glucose passing through the placenta,[4] since its own glucose production is minimal. From the arterio-venous concentration differences in the uterine and umbilical circulation it may be concluded that the human placenta takes up glucose from the maternal circulation and releases most of it into the fetal umbilical circulation.[5] A maternal–fetal glucose concentration gradient is normally observed at term.[6] Earlier in gestation, however, plasma glucose levels in the fetus may be equal to,[7] or even higher than those in the mother.[8,9] This is not consistently seen,[10] and apart from some exceptions, there exists a maternal–fetal concentration gradient throughout gestation in all species studied so far.

Fetal glucose utilization amounts to 38–43 μmol/kg at a maternal glucose level of 100 mg/dL.[4,11] This value will be higher in the presence of fetal hyperinsulinism. Because trans-placental passage of glucose among other factors is

---

Box 8.1 Factors that determine nutrient flux across the placenta

- Maternal–fetal concentration gradient
- Materal blood flow
- Placental structure and morphology
- Placental metabolism
- Placental transport activity
- Umbilical blood flow

directly proportional to the maternal–fetal glucose gradient[12,13] fetal hyperinsulinism will result in a lowering of fetal glucose levels with ensuing increase in trans-placental glucose flux in order to maintain fetal euglycemia. This notion is supported by the apparent independence of fetal glucose from fetal insulin levels.[14]

In well-controlled GDM women maternal glucose levels are slightly but not significantly elevated.[6] The umbilical cord glucose levels are elevated as compared to normal control subjects. However, the venous–arterial concentration difference is unchanged.[15]

Amino acids

Among the maternal plasma proteins, only IgG and albumin are able to be transported to the fetus in significant amounts.[16] Therefore, maternal amino acids provide by far the major source of nitrogen for both the placenta and the fetus. Total amino acid concentrations are higher in fetal plasma than in the maternal circulation.[17] The concentrations of most amino acids in the placenta exceed those in the maternal and fetal circulation, probably due to a high content in the syncytiotrophoblast. High amino acid concentrations are generally associated with a high rate of protein synthesis and are characteristic of rapidly growing tissues.

In human pregnancies complicated by gestational diabetes the concentrations of some amino acids (methionine, isoleucine, leucine, phenyalalanine, alanine and proline) are selectively increased in the fetal circulation with no apparent change in the maternal circulation.[18] This strongly suggests an altered amino acid metabolism in placenta, fetus or both or a change in maternal-to-fetal amino acid transfer.

Lipids and fatty acids

At delivery of a normal pregnancy the concentrations of cholesterol, triglycerides, total free fatty acids and lipid soluble vitamins is higher in the maternal than umbilical circulation.[19] However, individual fatty acids in the total plasma compartments such as total saturated fatty acids and arachidonic acid are selectively enriched in the umbilical cord blood.

In GDM the mothers have unchanged arachidonic acid and docosahexaenoic acid levels,[20] whereas the concentrations of both fatty acids are lower in their offspring than in normal pregnancies.[21]

GDM does not significantly alter maternal cholesterol levels, but maternal as well as fetal hypertriglyceridemia particularly in the VLDL and HDL fraction has been a well known feature of GDM.[22–25]

Utero-placental and feto-placental blood flow

Utero-placental and placental–umbilical blood flow determine the delivery to and removal from the area of exchange, i.e. syncytiotrophoblast and endothelium. A direct relationship between blood flow in the maternal and fetal placental circulation and extent of transfer is clearly established for flow-limited transport such as that of oxygen or carbon dioxide.

However, such a relation exists also for carrier-mediated transport as was clearly shown for glucose.[26] Therefore, uteroplacental and feto-placental blood flows are major determinants of overall maternal–fetal exchange. Absence of innervations strongly suggests that the vascular tone in the feto-placental circulation is regulated by local changes in autacoid or nitric oxide production. The details of this complex regulatory system are far from being understood, but it likely involves, locally produced vasoconstrictor and vasodilator components such as eicosanoids, endothelins and nitric oxide.

Invasion of cytotrophoblasts into maternal decidua and, subsequently, into spiral arteries results in their remodelling into low resistance vessels. Any impairment in this process may lead to a reduced flow of maternal blood into the intervillous space.

Diabetes is associated with modest modifications of vascular resistance in the uterine artery. There is a small increase in uterine artery vascular resistance in Type 1 diabetes[27] which is likely to reflect pre-gestational vasculopathy.[28] It has been proposed that some of these alterations originate from inadequate opening of the spiral arteries by a too shallow invasion of the cytotrophoblast, although there is no direct experimental evidence to support this hypothesis.

In GDM there is a positive correlation between uterine artery vascular impedance (resistance) and birthweight.[29] The relationship does not seem to be correlated with maternal glucose values, suggesting that hyperglycemia *per se* is not a causative factor.[30] This is also supported by the observation that acute hyperglycemia during pregnancy does not affect blood flow velocimetry characteristics in the umbilical or uterine arteries.[31] Therefore, flow-regulated increased placental transfer of nutrients may not be a mechanism underlying fetal macrosomia in diabetes if it occurs at all.

There is increasing evidence that oxidative stress arising from increased placental mitochondrial activity and production of reactive oxygen species (ROS), nitric oxide, carbon monoxide, and peroxynitrite is a general underlying mechanism of altered placental function and vascular reactivity.[32] This may even generate nitrative stress which can lead to covalent modification and hence altered activity of proteins. These are mechanisms likely to contribute to general fetal endothelial dysfunction in diabetes.[33]

Placental structure and morphology

The placenta is a complex organ made up of a variety of tissues that theoretically can contribute to transplacental transfer. All materials destined for transfer to the fetus must first be taken up by the microvillous membrane of the syncytiotrophoblast, the tissue which is in direct contact with maternal blood in the intervillous space. Once within the syncytium the molecules are either sequestered for modification (lipids) or metabolized for placental purposes (glucose), or they leave the syncytiotrophoblast by passing the basal syncytiotrophoblast membrane. The total surface area of the syncytiotrophoblast fronting to the maternal circulation and of the fetal-placental capillaries fronting to the fetal blood is 12 m^2. About 90% of the syncytiotrophoblastic surface are covered with microvilli that enlarge the surface area by 7-fold. About 5–10% of the syncytiotrophoblast surface area is made up by the epithelial plates. These are a specialized area, which accounts for most, if not all, transfer to the fetus. In these areas, the syncytiotrophoblast is very thin, devoid of cytoplasmic organelles and the basal laminas of the trophoblast and the endothelium of the feto-placental vessels are fused. Thus, no stromal tissue separates syncytiotrophoblast and endothelium. This architecture allows for a short 'diffusion distance' between the maternal and fetal bloodstream that at the end of gestation is about 3–5 μm in length.[34]

Diabetes is associated with major modifications of the structure and organization of the placenta leading to a variety of pathologies referred to as global placental dysfunction (reviewed in references 35–37). The surface area is particularly increased in the periphery of the villous tree. The diffusion distance between the maternal and fetal systemic circulations is increased due to a thickening of the trophoblastic basement membrane with higher amounts of collagen, predominantly Type IV.[38] Some collagens, e.g. Types IV, V and VI, contain a higher proportion of carbohydrates and it may be conceived that this is due to non-enzymatic glycation and mimics a situation of accelerated aging. The higher proportion of hyaluronic acid subfractions and heparan sulfate also contributes to increase the total glycosaminoglycan content of the villous connective tissue.[39] The sum of these morphological modifications modifies trophoblast barrier function particularly transplacental transfer mechanisms compared to normal pregnancy. For example, fetal hypoxia is one consequence of trophoblast basement-membrane thickening and may stimulate placental synthesis of angiogenic factors such as fetal growth factor (FGF), vascular endothelial growth factors (VEGF) and placental growth factor (PGF)-1.[40]

In Type 1 diabetes as well as in GDM, the villous stroma is slightly edematous with an over-representation of Hofbauer cells which are the placental resident macrophages.[41] The increased number of Hofbauer cells may contribute to a higher release of placental cytokines (leptin, TNF-alpha, interleukins) in the local environment and subsequently modify placental metabolic or endocrine functions.[42] Maternal diabetes is also associated with enlargement of the capillary surface area[43] with capillary proliferation and penetration of small newly formed vessels penetrating into the trophoblast.[44,45] The resulting hyper-vascularization and the increase in the surface area of exchange facilitate oxygen diffusion across the placenta to compensate for the impaired maternal–fetal transfer of diffusion-limited substances. Down-regulation in the surface expression of tight and adherens junctional molecules (occludin, zonula occludens protein-1) also participates in disrupting normal endothelial barrier function and angiogenesis.[46]

Classically, the occurrence of placentomegaly as a result of an increase in parenchymal tissue cellularity, is reflected by higher DNA content in pre-gestational and to a lesser degree in GDM.[47] Placentomegaly is closely correlated with fetal macrosomia confirming the close correlation of placental weight with that of the offspring.[48,49] Both tend to normalize with the quality of glycemic control achieved during pregnancy. Lower fetal insulin concentrations which results from better maternal glucose control may potentially limit the mitogenic effect of insulin in placental cells.[50] Another classic feature of the placentae in diabetic pregnancies is the higher content of glycogen, triglycerides and phospholipids than in normal pregnancies[6,51] indicative of increased nutrient storage capability.

Carrier-mediated transport

Glucose

The human fetus is almost totally dependent on maternal glucose passing through the placenta, since its own gluconeogenetic activity is minimal.[52] The key position of glucose for fetal maldevelopment in diabetes has prompted detailed studies into the molecular and regulatory mechanisms of maternal–fetal glucose transport and on their alterations in diabetes. The enormous amount of data on placental glucose transfer in pregnancy with diabetes may not be surprising given that glucose is the major energy substrate of the feto-placental tissue, accounting for almost 80% of oxidative needs at term.[53] In addition, myriads of studies have addressed the mechanisms for increased glucose availability over the last three decades. This was an essential component of the effort to obtain good glycemic control to limit maternal and fetal complications.

In most situations transplacental glucose transport in the maternal-to-fetal direction follows a downhill gradient involving GLUT1 as the predominant glucose transporter isoform. The recently cloned glucose transporter GLUT8 is also ubiquitously expressed in the term placenta with lower expression levels in diabetes, but its role in placental glucose utilization is elusive.[54] The high affinity isoform GLUT3[55] and the insulin-regulatable isoforms GLUT4[56] and GLUT12[57] have also been identified in the human placenta, but their location on endothelial cells and in the placental stroma, respectively, makes their direct contribution to maternal-to-fetal glucose transport unlikely. Rather they are involved in glucose back-transfer from the fetus into the placenta and uptake into cells surrounding the placental endothelium.

Maternal-to-fetal glucose transport involves GLUT1 on the trophoblast, where it is located on the microvillous and on the basal membrane, facing the maternal and fetal circulation, respectively. The transport system has a high capacity with saturation reached at glucose levels >20 mmol/L.[11] This system allows for a rapid transfer from the maternal to the fetal circulation.

Similar to other tissues trophoblast GLUT1 is regulated by ambient glucose levels, i.e. it is up-regulated under hypoglycemic and down-regulated under hyperglycemic conditions, respectively. Loss of functional GLUT 1 on the trophoblast surface is accounted for by lower GLUT1 transcript levels and, hence, translation[58] as well as by a hyperglycemia-induced translocation of GLUT1 from the surface to intracellular sites.[59] Kinetic studies demonstrated that the loss of GLUT1 at the cell surface alters glucose uptake only at concentrations close to or above 15 mmol/L,[58] a concentration that is not reached in diabetic patients that are controlled. This GLUT1 response to hyperglycemia must be acquired during gestation, because it is absent in the first trimester trophoblast.[60]

At this stage of gestation ketone bodies[61] and insulin[60] appear to reduce or increase GLUT1 levels, respectively.

At term of gestation Type-1 diabetes is associated with an increased expression of GLUT1 at the basement membrane, but not at the microvillous membrane, of the syncytiotrophoblast, whereas in gestational diabetes no such changes were observed regardless of offspring weight.[62–64] Total placental levels of GLUT1, GLUT3 and GLUT4 are unchanged in diabetes[65] suggesting that the protein content of these transporters is not modified although this awaits experimental confirmation.

Since transfer is determined by composite parameters such as maternal–fetal concentration gradient, blood flow, surface area of exchange and diffusion distance, placental metabolism as well as number and intrinsic activity of transporters, alterations in transporter levels alone will not predict *in vivo* changes. In gestational diabetes maternal–fetal glucose transport as measured by placental perfusion was reduced when the mothers were treated with diet alone,[66] whereas when they received insulin transport was higher as compared to the diet-treated group, but not different from non-diabetic controls.[67] However, at a pathological glucose concentration of 8 mmol/L no significant changes in maternal–fetal glucose transport were noted, when total placental weight was also taken into account (Figure 8.1).[66,67] It appears as if the potential changes at the molecular level of transporters are counterbalanced by morphological changes such as increased area of exchange and basement membrane thickening resulting in increased diffusion distance.

These results clearly demonstrate that the placenta does not contribute to any increase in transplacental glucose flux in gestational diabetes. This conclusion is also corroborated by the lack of change in the venous-arterial difference for glucose in the umbilical circulation in gestational diabetes.[15]

Since placental cells have such a high capacity for maternal–fetal glucose transfer it is not surprising that molecular changes

at the level of glucose transporters levels, if any, have no effect on transfer of glucose at physiological or pathophysiological glucose concentrations. This implies that transplacental glucose transfer is primarily limited by flow and, there is experimental evidence supporting that both utero-placental and umbilical blood flow affect glucose transfer.[26] Overall, the strongest determinant for glucose flux across the placenta is the maternal–fetal concentration gradient with some contribution by blood flow changes.

The high affinity glucose transporter GLUT3 is located on the feto-placental vessels and the insulin-regulatable transporters GLUT4 and GLUT12 in the placental stroma, i.e. a portion of the placenta that is more exposed to fetal rather than maternal blood. The functional significance of these transporters is unclear, but the placenta may have developed mechanisms to take up glucose from the fetal circulation. In fact glucose is also transported back from the fetus into the placenta[68] and the backflux is even increased in diabetes.[21] These transporters may extract glucose from the fetal circulation into the endothelial cells, where glucose may then be stored as glycogen. The endothelium is also richly endowed with glycogenin, the protein precursor for glycogen synthesis and glycogen is deposited predominantly around feto-placental vessels.[69,70] Therefore, the glycogen increments found in diabetes[6,51,69] may result from an increased glucose uptake from the feto-placental circulation. This would explain why the placenta in diabetes stores more glycogen than in non-diabetic pregnancies, although glycogen synthesis in the trophoblast is not stimulated by insulin or hyperglycemia.[71] Whether fetal insulin by activating GLUT4 or GLUT12 stimulates glucose uptake into the endothelium and, subsequently, also glycogen synthesis is unknown, but a net effect of fetal insulin on glycogen levels in the placenta was found[72] with little increase in fetal liver glycogen. The accumulated placental and fetal glycogen may then be broken down in case of fetal emergency demands

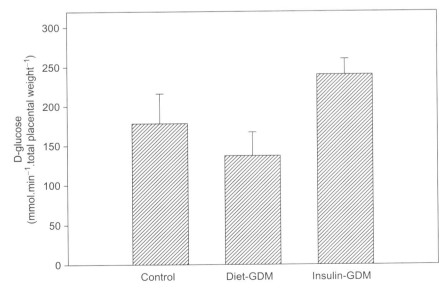

Figure 8.1   Comparison of total maternal–fetal D-glucose transfer (mean ± SEM) across the placenta at 8 mmol/L external D-glucose in normal, diet-treated and insulin-treated gestational diabetic (GDM) pregnancies. Adapted from Osmond et al.[67]

such as prolonged labor. Because of the low levels of glucose-6-phosphatase,[73] lactate will then be the outflowing product. Collectively, these data suggest that the placenta may serve as a buffer for excess fetal glucose, at least at term of gestation. Consequently, it can be envisioned that an overflow of this buffer, i.e. when the storage capacity is exhausted, may result in permanent fetal hyperglycemia and hyperinsulinemia.[74]

Amino acids

Amino acid uptake into cells generally occurs by a system of transporter molecules. These transporters show selective preference for certain amino acids although there is considerable overlap of specificity. Individual classes of transport systems were identified for neutral, cationic and anionic amino acids, respectively. Maternal amino acids provide by far the major source of nitrogen for the feto-placental tissues and, thus, are taken up by both the placenta and the fetus. The transport systems in the human term placenta resemble those described for various other tissues and cells.[75] Uptake of amino acids from the maternal and fetal circulation suggests the presence of specific transporters on both surfaces of the placenta. Maternal- and fetal-facing plasma membranes contain both common and distinct (systems ASC and t) systems for amino acid transport. To the best of our knowledge there is no available information on the spatial arrangement of amino acid transporters on the microvillous and basal syncytiotrophoblast membranes. Moreover, transport and transport systems in non-trophoblast cells of the placenta have not been characterized so far. Although the endothelium may not impose any limitation to placental-to-fetal amino acid transport, it may be involved in transport in the reverse direction i.e. from fetus to placenta and/or from placenta to mother.

The concentration of many amino acids is higher in the placenta as compared to the levels in the maternal or fetal circulation. A clear-cut explanation for this apparent discrepancy is still missing, but metabolism of amino acids by the placenta in general, or by the syncytiotrophoblast in particular, may influence transfer.[76] For example, one must assume passive diffusion of the amino acids along a concentration gradient for the Na+-independent systems.

Pyrimidine and purine synthesis are essential to build DNA blocks that rapid fetal growth requires. They are provided through glutamine/glutamate and asparagine/aspartate[16,77,78] cycles which involves back and forward transfer from fetus to placenta.

Despite the relative paucity of data, there is a general agreement that the ability to maintain normal serum levels of several amino acids is impaired in fetuses of diabetic mothers. However, a clear understanding of whether the transfer of a given amino acid will be increased or decreased relative to the type of diabetes has yet to be gained. In rodent models of experimental diabetes with various severity such as pregnant rats rendered diabetic by streptozotocin injection, fetal concentration of most amino acids is decreased in face of unchanged maternal-to-fetal ratio.[79,80] This also holds true for non-protein amino acid such as taurine and gamma amino butyric acid (GABA) which act as neurotransmitters to regulate fetal insulin secretion.[81] By contrast, an increased leucine turnover

which may modify its availability for placental uptake has been documented in insulin treated GDM women.[82] The concentrations of several essential amino acids and alanine were increased whereas glutamate was decreased in umbilical artery and vein in pregnancy with GDM.[18] The discrepancy between human and animal data cannot be currently explained although it should be underlined that maternal glucose homeostasis was clearly different. Whether or not the *in vivo* observations have molecular basis has not been yet established. An increase in system A and leucine has been observed in syncytiotrophoblast plasma membrane vesicles of non-insulin-dependent gestational diabetic mothers compared to normal (Figure 8.2),[83] whereas system L appeared unaffected.[84] However, this was not confirmed using dual perfusion of isolated cotyledons, a method that preserves the integrity of placental cell structure.[84–86] By contrast, the number of system A transporters per mg membrane protein was selectively reduced in diabetic pregnancies associated with fetal macrosomia.[84] Hence, different experimental models may lead to different results. These suggest there is not yet agreement whether maternal diabetes *per se* has an impact on placental amino acid transporters and require caution in generalizing inferences to the *in vivo* situation.

Lipids and fatty acids

At birth about 12–15% of the fetal body mass is fat, and about half of that fat is derived from maternal sources passing across the placenta over the whole period of gestation. The remainder may be due to the lipogenic activity of the fetal liver and other tissues. For most fatty acids a maternal–fetal concentration gradient exists and, hence, free fatty acids may traverse the placenta by simple diffusion, but the major proportion will bind to fatty acid transfer proteins on the microvillous membrane. In the syncytiotrophoblast cytoplasm the free fatty acids will bind to fatty acid binding proteins. These will serve as 'transporters' for the fatty acids enabling them to traverse the cytoplasm for immediate release into the fetal circulation. However, an intermediate esterification of free fatty acids to triglycerides within the placenta may also occur. This will then allow storage of triglycerides in the form of lipid droplets surrounded by droplet-associated proteins such as adipophilin and perilipin. These proteins are a prerequisite for recruitment of intracellular lipases. Subsequent lipolysis is required before the fatty acids can then be released into the fetal circulation.

Additional sources of fetal lipids are lipoprotein-borne triglycerides, phospholipids and cholesterol. The lipoproteins have to bind to their receptors, which can all be found at the syncytiotrophoblast surface. The binding of very low density (VLDL) and high density (HDL) lipoproteins to their receptors i.e., the VLDL receptor[87] and the major HDL receptor SR-BI,[88] is mediated by lipases, which also have a bridging function in addition to releasing fatty acids from the triglycerides and phospholipids. SR-BI not only binds HDL but mediates the selective uptake of HDL-cholesterol esters. Low density lipoproteins (LDL) bind to LDL receptors and will be internalized into the syncytiotrophoblast cytoplasm by receptor mediated endocytosis. In the cytoplasm cholesterol

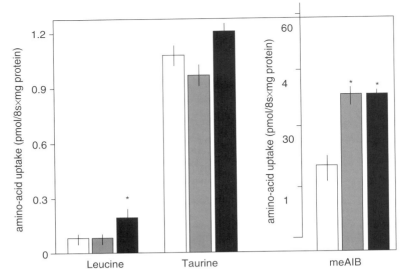

Figure 8.2   Carrier-mediated uptake of amino acids into microvillous plasma membrane vesicles of human term placenta. Leucine transported by system L is representative of essential amino acids. Taurine is representative of non-essential amino acids and MeAIB (methyl-α-isoaminobutyric acid) is representative of neutral amino acids such as alanine which are transported by sytem A. Data are means ± SE for 13 controls, non-macrosomic neonates (open bars), eight Type-1 diabetics with macrosomic neonates (full gray bars) and four GDM with macrosomic neonates (full black bars). *$P < 0.05$ versus controls. Adapted from Kalhan.[82]

esters may also be stored in the lipid droplets. A proportion of the cholesterol esters will be metabolized to serve as precursor for placental biosynthesis of steroid hormones. The mechanisms of further transfer from within the syncytiotrophoblast cytoplasm into the fetal circulation remain elusive, but will likely involve efflux transporters of the ABC family as well as SR-BI. Similar to triglycerides, phospholipids are hydrolyzed into their constituents predominantly by endothelial lipase, which can also be found on the syncytiotrophoblast surface, prior to their storage within the placenta. Placental storage capacity, however, is limited and does not prevent excessive flow of lipids to the fetus in a condition of maternal lipid excess, such as occurs in diabetes.

Diabetes is associated with well-known alterations in the level and composition of maternal lipids. Particularly, Type-1 diabetes in pregnancy is characterized by elevation of maternal plasma free fatty acids and triglycerides, as a result of loss of restraint on fatty acid mobilization from adipose tissue. The elevated lipid concentration may promote the transfer of free fatty acids and triglycerides across the placenta by increasing the maternal–fetal concentration gradient and by making other diabetes-related alterations that facilitate placental fat accumulation. Also in non-diabetic women concentrations of the free fatty acids myristate, palmitate, stearate and linoleate in maternal venous blood and umbilical vein blood are correlated.[89]

Among the fatty acid binding proteins (FABP) expressed in the placenta only the liver-type FABP is increased in diabetes whereas the heart-isoform is unchanged. The liver-type FABP has a preference for n-3 fatty acids such as α-linolenic acid, eicospentaenoic acid and docosahexaenoic acid, whereas the heart-type preferentially binds n-6 fatty acids such as linolenic acid and arachidonic acid. The uptake of arachidonate into the perfused human term placenta in Type-I diabetes is increased but changes in the FABPs are unlikely to account for this. Arachidonic acid is preferentially incorporated into triglycerides rather than into phospholipids of placental tissue and fetal effluent. Thus transfer and distribution among lipid classes of arachidonic acid are altered in Type-1 diabetic pregnancies.[90] The linoleate content, among others, in placental tissues is higher, while 20:5 n-3, 22:6 n-3 levels, and the ratios of 20:4 n-6/18:2 n-6 and 22:6 n-3/18:3 n-3 were reduced in diabetic pregnancies.[91] Therefore, a proportion of the arachidonic acid increments stored in the placenta in diabetes may also be derived by conversion of linoleate into arachidonic acid by elongation and desaturation reactions that occur in the human placenta.

The release of arachidonic acid, DHA and other 20-carbon PUFAs from cellular phospholipids is the rate-limiting step in the generation of lipid mediators of inflammation. This process involves the action of one or more phospholipases such as PLA$_2$. The expression of secretory PLA$_2$G$_2$ and G$_5$ is up-regulated in placenta of women with GDM having obese neonates whereas that of PLA$_2$G$_6$ was unchanged.[42] This may be a mechanism through which three to six times more arachidonate is converted to eicosanoids in a diabetic pregnancy than in a normal placenta. In addition, the transfer of eicosanoids into the opposing circulation was doubled in placentae from Type-I diabetics compared to normal placentae (Figure 8.3). The predominant direction of eicosanoid transfer in both groups of placentae was from the fetus into the maternal circulation. The relative amount of eicosanoids produced was also altered in placentae from Type-I diabetic pregnancies leading a lower ratio of prostacyclin I$_2$ to thromboxane A$_2$. This accounts for the imbalance in eicosanoid production, which is a strong contributing factor to placental vasoconstriction in diabetic pregnancies.[92]

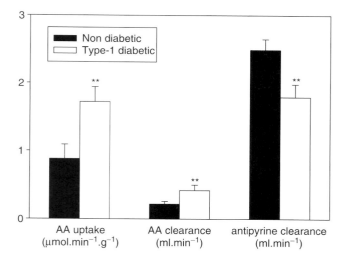

Figure 8.3 Uptake and clearance (means ± SD) into the fetal circulation of arachidonic acid (AA) in total placentas from normal and Type-1 diabetic pregnancies are increased, whereas clearance of the highly diffusible antipyrine is reduced. **$P < 0.01$ versus normal. Adapted from Kuhn et al.[92]

In addition, the concentration of placental products of PLA_2 hydrolysis such as DHA is positively correlated with placental weight. Collectively, these data indicate that qualitative as well as quantitative modifications of placental lipid content are associated with alterations of fetal growth in pregnancy with diabetes.

Nucleosides

Nucleosides such as adenosine or thymidine are rapidly taken up by cells. The characteristics of transport are consistent with facilitated diffusion, i.e. transport along a downhill concentration gradient by carrier-mediated transport mechanisms. Transport has a broad specificity including both purine and pyrimidine nucleosides. In the human placenta these transporters have been identified at the microvillous and basal membrane of the syncytiotrophoblast. Distinct from other tissues such as kidney and intestine the transporter is sodium independent. Transporters for adenosine are also present on the endothelium of placental vessels and the umbilical cord. At present it is questionable if maternal nucleosides will reach the fetal circulation. When thymidine and adenosine were used in perfusion studies they were extensively degraded.[93] Rather the nucleosides and in particular adenosine may serve local purposes in the regulation of the vascular tone.

In diabetes the transporters on the endothelium of the umbilical cord are down-regulated,[94] but not those on the trophoblast.[95] Because umbilical cord endothelial cells do not contribute to overall passage of nucleosides one can expect that the fetus in a diabetic pregnancy is supplied with sufficient nucleosides to ensure adequate formation of nucleotides as building block for RNA and DNA. The GDM-associated changes in nucleoside uptake into umbilical endothelial cells more likely result in an altered local regulation of the vascular tone by modifying the adenosine/L-arginine/nitric oxide pathway.[96]

Insulin and hypoglycemic compounds

The passage of plasma proteins across the human placental barrier in humans is a highly selective process. It cannot be predicted on a simple way based on physical properties, i.e. protein binding, lipid solubility or molecular weight. In diabetic pregnancy, the safe use of insulin, insulin analogs and oral hypoglycemic agents relies on the absence of transfer from maternal to fetal circulation. It has been known for years that free maternal insulin does not cross the materno-fetal barrier either in early or late pregnancy.[97–99] In addition, the absence of significant transfer of insulin lispro[100] makes insulins the primary therapeutic choices for treatment of pregnant women with diabetes. However, insulin-binding antibodies have been detected in newborn infants whose diabetic mothers received insulin therapy. This is due to increased titer of antibodies in insulin-treated mothers and, the higher the antibody titer of the mother the greater is the total insulin in the fetal circulation.[101] The question whether such exposure would have biological action in the fetus and participate to macrosomia has been raised. The poor correlation between the concentration of insulin antibody complexes in fetal plasma and birthweight argues against a major role of insulin therapy to enhance fetal growth.[102–104] However, none of these studies has addressed the relationship between the antibody titer and change in the ratio of lean/fat mass in the fetus.

Ex vivo perfusions of human placenta using radioactive antipyrine as a reference to assess for barrier integrity and perfusion constants is the 'gold standard' to quantify the passage of a substance from maternal into the fetal circulation.[105] It has been used to characterize the transplacental passage of several classes of anti-diabetic agents. Thiazolidinediones (rosiglitazone, pioglitazone), insulin sensitizers of the PPAR-gamma agonist family, as well as alpha-glucosidase inhibitors (acarbose) and biguanines (metformim) are oral hypoglycemic agents, which readily cross the placental barrier.[106] By contrast, glyburide a widely used sulfonylurea does not cross the placenta and is not metabolized by the placenta tissue at a significant extent.[107] Glipizide, another sulfonylurea, however, induced some changes in the placenta *in vitro*.[108] Agents with incretin effects such as the gut-derived peptide glucagons like peptide-1 GLP-1 have been recently developed as glucose dependent insulinotropic compounds. Exenatide, a synthetic exendin-4 which belongs to this class of molecules, shows negligible passage across the human placenta suggesting that maternal use of this peptide will result in negligible exposure to the fetus.[109]

Conclusion

In maternal diabetes mellitus the human placenta undergoes a number of changes. The extent of these predominantly depends on the quality of maternal glycemic control of mother and hence fetal glycemia. Structural changes are found mostly in the fetal aspect of the placenta. Maternal–fetal glucose transport across the placenta appears unchanged in diabetes. An increased flux will mainly be the result of a steeper concentration gradient between the maternal and fetal circulations. A reduced feto-placental blood flow may counteract to excessive fetal supply with glucose. Increased glucose storage in the placenta as glycogen may also contribute to some fetal protection although within small margins.

No clear-cut changes have been identified in the transport of amino acids, but studies using the perfusion system are pending. The mechanisms accounting for lipid transport across the placenta are far from being understood. Alterations in fatty acid uptake, metabolism and transport are known, but no information is available for more complex lipids such as triglycerides, phospholipids and lipoprotein–cholesterol.

REFERENCES

1. Desoye G, Shafrir E. Placental metabolism and its regulation in health and diabetes. Mol Aspects Med 1994; 15: 505–682.
2. Desoye G, Shafrir E. The human placenta in diabetic pregnancy. Diabetes Rev 1996; 4: 70–89.
3. Shafrir E, Desoye G. Pregnancy in diabetic animals. In: Hod M, Jovanovic L, DiRenzo GC, DeLeiva A, Langer O, eds. Textbook of Diabetes and Pregnancy. London: Martin Dunitz; 2007.
4. Kalhan SC, D'Angelo LJ, Savin SM, Adam PA. Glucose production in pregnant women at term gestation. Sources of glucose for human fetus. J Clin Invest 1979; 63: 388–94.
5. Metzger BE, Rodeck C, Freinkel N, Price J, Young M. Transplacental arteriovenous gradients for glucose, insulin, glucagon and placental lactogen during normoglycaemia in human pregnancy at term. Placenta 1985; 6: 347–54.
6. Desoye G, Hofmann HH, Weiss PA. Insulin binding to trophoblast plasma membranes and placental glycogen content in well-controlled gestational diabetic women treated with diet or insulin, in well-controlled overt diabetic patients and in healthy control subjects. Diabetologia 1992; 35: 45–55.
7. Aynsley-Green A, Soltesz G, Jenkins PA, Mackenzie IZ. The metabolic and endocrine milieu of the human fetus at 18–21 weeks of gestation. II. Blood glucose, lactate, pyruvate and ketone body concentrations. Biol Neonate 1985; 47: 19–25.
8. Bozzetti P, Ferrari MM, Marconi AM, et al. The relationship of maternal and fetal glucose concentrations in the human from midgestation until term. Metabolism 1988; 37: 358–63.
9. Nicolini U, Hubinont C, Santolaya J, et al. Maternal-fetal glucose gradient in normal pregnancies and in pregnancies complicated by alloimmunization and fetal growth retardation. Am J Obstet Gynecol 1989; 161: 924–7.
10. Forestier F, Daffos F, Rainaut M, Bruneau M, Trivin F. Blood chemistry of normal human fetuses at midtrimester of pregnancy. Pediatr Res 1987; 21: 579–83.
11. Hauguel S, Desmaizieres V, Challier JC. Glucose uptake, utilization, and transfer by the human placenta as functions of maternal glucose concentration. Pediatr Res 1986; 20: 269–73.
12. Stembera ZK, Hodr J. The relationship between the blood levels of glucose, lactic acid and pyruvic acid in the mother and in both umbilical vessels of the healthy fetus. Biol Neonat 1966; 10: 227–38.
13. Stembera ZK, Hodr J. Mutual relationships between the levels of glucose, pyruvic acid and lactic acid in the blood of the mother and of both umbilical vessels in hypoxic fetuses. Biol Neonat 1966; 10: 303–15.
14. Paterson P, Page D, Taft P, Phillips L, Wood C. Study of fetal and maternal insulin levels during labour. J Obstet Gynaecol Br Commun 1968; 75: 917–21.
15. Radaelli T, Taricco E, Rossi G, et al. Oxygenation, acid-base balance and glucose levels in fetuses from gestational diabetic pregnancies. J Soc Gynecol Invest 2005; 12(2, suppl.): 221A.
16. Dancis J, Schneider H. Physiology of the placenta. In: Falkner F, Tanner JM, eds. Human Gowth, Vol. 1. New York: Plenum Press; 1986, pp. 221–44.
17. Yudilevich DL, Sweiry JH. Transport of amino acids in the placenta. Biochem Biophys Acta 1985; 822: 169–201.
18. Cetin I, de Santis MS, Taricco E, et al. Maternal and fetal amino acid concentrations in normal pregnancies and in pregnancies with gestational diabetes mellitus. Am J Obstet Gynecol 2005; 192: 610–7.
19. Herrera E, Ortega H, Alvino G, et al. Relationship between plasma fatty acid profile and antioxidant vitamins during normal pregnancy. Eur J Clin Nutr 2004; 58: 1231–8.
20. Thomas BA, Ghebremeskel K, Lowy C, Offley-Shore B, Crawford MA. Plasma fatty acids of neonates born to mothers with and without gestational diabetes. Prostaglandins Leukot Essent Fatty Acids 2005; 72: 335–41.
21. Thomas CR, Eriksson GL, Eriksson UJ. Effects of maternal diabetes on placental transfer of glucose in rats. Diabetes 1990; 39: 276–82.
22. Hollingsworth DR, Grundy SM. Pregnancy-associated hypertriglyceridemia in normal and diabetic women. Differences in insulin-dependent, non-insulin-dependent, and gestational diabetes. Diabetes 1982; 31: 1092–7.
23. Couch SC, Philipson EH, Bendel RB, et al. Elevated lipoprotein lipids and gestational hormones in women with diet-treated gestational diabetes mellitus compared to healthy pregnant controls. J Diabetes Complications 1998; 12: 1–9.
24. Couch SC, Philipson EH, Bendel RB, Wijendran V, Lammi-Keefe CJ. Maternal and cord plasma lipid and lipoprotein concentrations in women with and without gestational diabetes mellitus. Predictors of birth weight? J Reprod Med 1998; 43: 816–22.
25. Merzouk H, Madani S, Prost J, et al. Changes in serum lipid and lipoprotein concentrations and compositions at birth and after 1 month of life in macrosomic infants of insulin-dependent diabetic mothers. Eur J Pediatr 1999; 158: 750–6.
26. Illsley NP, Hall S, Stacey TE. The modulation of glucose transfer across the human placenta by intervillous flow rates: an in vitro perfusion study. Trophoblast Res 1987; 2: 535-44.
27. Zimmermann P, Kujansuu E, Tuimala R. Doppler flow velocimetry of the uterine and uteroplacental circulation in pregnancies complicated by insulin-dependent diabetes mellitus. J Perinat Med 1994; 22: 137–47.
28. Pietryga M, Brazert J, Wender-Ozegowska E, et al. Abnormal uterine Doppler is related to vasculopathy in pregestational diabetes mellitus. Circulation 2005; 112: 2496–500.
29. Pietryga M, Brazert J, Wender-Ozegowska E, Dubiel M, Gudmundsson S. Placental Doppler velocimetry in gestational diabetes mellitus. J Perinat Med 2006; 34: 108–10.
30. Reece EA, Hagay Z, Assimakopoulos E, et al. Diabetes mellitus in pregnancy and the assessment of umbilical artery waveforms using pulsed Doppler ultrasonography. J Ultrasound Med 1994; 13: 73–80.
31. Yogev Y, Ben-Haroush A, Chen R, et al. Doppler sonographic characteristics of umbilical and uterine arteries during oral glucose tolerance testing in healthy pregnant women. J Clin Ultrasound 2003; 31: 461–4.
32. Myatt L. Placental adaptive responses and fetal programming. J Physiol 2006; 572(pt 1): 25–30.
33. Farias M, San Martin R, Puebla C, et al. Nitric oxide reduces adenosine transporter ENT1 gene (SLC29A1) promoter activity in human fetal endothelium from gestational diabetes. J Cell Physiol 2006; 208: 451–60.
34. Benirschke K, Kaufmann P, Baergen R. Pathology of the Human Placenta, 5th edn. New York: Springer.
35. Teasdale F. Gestational changes in the functional structure of the human placenta in relation to fetal growth: a morphometric study. Am J Obstet Gynecol 1980; 137: 560–8.
36. Teasdale F. Histomorphometry of the placenta of the diabetic women: class A diabetes mellitus. Placenta 1981; 2: 241–51.
37. Teasdale F, Jean-Jacques G. Morphometry of the microvillous membrane of the human placenta in maternal diabetes mellitus. Placenta 1986; 7: 81–8.
38. Leushner JR, Tevaarwerk GJ, Clarson CL, et al. Analysis of the collagens of diabetic placental villi. Cell Mol Biol 1986; 32: 27–35.
39. Wasserman L, Shlesinger H, Abramovici A, Goldman JA, Allalouf D. Glycosaminoglycan patterns in diabetic and toxemic term placentas. Am J Obstet Gynecol 1980; 138(7, pt 1): 769–73.

40. Arany E, Hill DJ. Fibroblast growth factor-2 and fibroblast growth factor receptor-1 mRNA expression and peptide localization in placentae from normal and diabetic pregnancies. Placenta 1998; 19: 133–42.

41. Sutton LN, Mason DY, Redman CW. Isolation and characterization of human fetal macrophages from placenta. Clin Exp Immunol 1989; 78: 437–43.

42. Varastehpour A, Radaelli T, Minium J, et al. Activation of phospholipase A2 is associated with generation of placental lipid signals and fetal obesity. J Clin Endocrinol Metab 2006; 91: 248–55.

43. Mayhew TM, Sorensen FB, Klebe JG, Jackson MR. Growth and maturation of villi in placentae from well-controlled diabetic women. Placenta 1994; 15: 57–65.

44. Asmussen I. Vascular morphology in diabetic placentas. Contrib Gynecol Obstet 1982; 9: 76–85.

45. Sherer DM, Salafia CM, Minior VK, et al. Placental basal plate myometrial fibers: clinical correlations of abnormally deep trophoblast invasion. Obstet Gynecol 1996; 87: 444–9.

46. Babawale MO, Lovat S, Mayhew TM, et al. Effects of gestational diabetes on junctional adhesion molecules in human term placental vasculature. Diabetologia 2000; 43: 1185–96.

47. Winick M, Noble A. Cellular growth in human placenta. II. Diabetes mellitus. J Pediatr 1967; 71: 216–9.

48. Clarson C, Tevaarwerk GJ, Harding PG, Chance GW, Haust MD. Placental weight in diabetic pregnancies. Placenta 1989; 10: 275–81.

49. Taricco E, Radaelli T, Nobile de Santis MS, Cetin I. Foetal and placental weights in relation to maternal characteristics in gestational diabetes. Placenta 2003; 24: 343–7.

50. Boileau P, Cauzac M, Pereira MA, Girard J, Hauguel-De Mouzon S. Dissociation between insulin-mediated signaling pathways and biological effects in placental cells: role of protein kinase B and MAPK phosphorylation. Endocrinology 2001; 142: 3974–9.

51. Diamant YZ, Metzger BE, Freinkel N, Shafrir E. Placental lipid and glycogen content in human and experimental diabetes mellitus. Am J Obstet Gynecol 1982; 144: 5–11.

52. Kalhan S, Parimi P. Gluconeogenesis in the fetus and neonate. Semin Perinatol 2000; 24: 94–106.

53. Battaglia FC, Meschia G. Principal substrates of fetal metabolism. Physiol Rev 1978; 58: 499–527.

54. Gorovits N, Cui L, Busik JV, et al. Regulation of hepatic GLUT8 expression in normal and diabetic models. Endocrinology 2003; 144: 1703–11.

55. Hauguel-de Mouzon S, Challier JC, Kacemi A, et al. The GLUT3 glucose transporter isoform is differentially expressed within human placental cell types. J Clin Endocrinol Metab 1997; 82: 2689–94.

56. Xing AY, Challier JC, Lepercq J, et al. Unexpected expression of glucose transporter 4 in villous stromal cells of human placenta. J Clin Endocrinol Metab 1998; 83: 4097–101.

57. Gude NM, Stevenson JL, Rogers S, et al. GLUT12 expression in human placenta in first trimester and term. Placenta 2003; 24: 566–70.

58. Hahn T, Barth S, Weiss U, Mosgoeller W, Desoye G. Sustained hyperglycemia in vitro down-regulates the GLUT1 glucose transport system of cultured human term placental trophoblast: a mechanism to protect fetal development? FASEB J 1998; 12: 1221–31.

59. Hahn T, Hahn D, Blaschitz A, et al. Hyperglycaemia-induced subcellular redistribution of GLUT1 glucose transporters in cultured human term placental trophoblast cells. Diabetologia 2000; 43: 173–80.

60. Gordon MC, Zimmerman PD, Landon MB, Gabbe SG, Kniss DA. Insulin and glucose modulate glucose transporter messenger ribonucleic acid expression and glucose uptake in trophoblasts isolated from first-trimester chorionic villi. Am J Obstet Gynecol 1995; 173: 1089–97.

61. Shubert PJ, Gordon MC, Landon MB, Gabbe SG, Kniss DA. Ketoacids attenuate glucose uptake in human trophoblasts isolated from first-trimester chorionic villi. Am J Obstet Gynecol 1996; 175: 56–62.

62. Gaither K, Quraishi AN, Illsley NP. Diabetes alters the expression and activity of the human placental GLUT1 glucose transporter. J Clin Endocrinol Metab 1999; 84: 695–701.

63. Jansson T, Ekstrand Y, Wennergren M, Powell TL. Placental glucose transport in gestational diabetes mellitus. Am J Obstet Gynecol 2001; 184: 111–6.

64. Jansson T, Lambert GW. Effect of intrauterine growth restriction on blood pressure, glucose tolerance and sympathetic nervous system activity in the rat at 3–4 months of age. J Hypertens 1999; 17: 1239–48.

65. Sciullo E, Cardellini G, Baroni MG, et al. Glucose transporter (Glut1, Glut3) mRNA in human placenta of diabetic and non-diabetic pregnancies. Early Pregnancy 1997; 3: 172–82.

66. Osmond DT, Nolan CJ, King RG, Brennecke SP, Gude NM. Effects of gestational diabetes on human placental glucose uptake, transfer, and utilisation. Diabetologia 2000; 43: 576–82.

67. Osmond DT, King RG, Brennecke SP, Gude NM. Placental glucose transport and utilisation is altered at term in insulin-treated, gestational-diabetic patients. Diabetologia 2001; 44: 1133–9.

68. Schneider H, Reiber W, Sager R, Malek A. Asymmetrical transport of glucose across the in vitro perfused human placenta. Placenta 2003; 24: 27–33.

69. Robb SA, Hytten FE. Placental glycogen. Br J Obstet Gynaecol 1976; 83: 43–53.

70. Jones CJ, Desoye G. Glycogen distribution in the capillaries of the placental villus in normal, overt and gestational diabetic pregnancy. Placenta 1993; 14: 505–17.

71. Schmon B, Hartmann M, Jones CJ, Desoye G. Insulin and glucose do not affect the glycogen content in isolated and cultured trophoblast cells of human term placenta. J Clin Endocrinol Metab 1991; 73: 888–93.

72. Goltzsch W, Bittner R, Bohme HJ, Hofmann E. Effect of prenatal insulin and glucagon injection on the glycogen content of rat placenta and fetal liver. Biomed Biochem Acta 1987; 46: 619–22.

73. Barash V, Riskin A, Shafrir E, Waddell ID, Burchell A. Kinetic and immunologic evidence for the absence of glucose-6-phosphatase in early human chorionic villi and term placenta. Biochem Biophys Acta 1991; 1073: 161–7.

74. Desoye G, Korgun ET, Ghaffari-Tabrizi N, Hahn T. Is fetal macrosomia in adequately controlled diabetic women the result of a placental defect? A hypothesis. J Matern Fetal Neonatal Med 2002; 11: 258–61.

75. Christensen HN. Role of amino acid transport and countertransport in nutrition and metabolism. Physiol Rev 1990; 70: 43–77.

76. Carroll MJ, Young M. The relationship between placental protein synthesis and transfer of amino acids. Biochem J 1983; 210: 99–105.

77. Schneider H, Mohlen KH, Challier JC, Dancis J. Transfer of glutamic acid across the human placenta perfused in vitro. Br J Obstet Gynaecol 1979; 86: 299–306.

78. Schneider H, Mohlen KH, Dancis J. Transfer of amino acids across the in vitro perfused human placenta. Pediatr Res 1979; 13(4, pt 1): 236–40.

79. Aerts L, Van Bree R, Feytons V, Rombauts W, Van Assche FA. Plasma amino acids in diabetic pregnant rats and in their fetal and adult offspring. Biol Neonate 1989; 56: 31–9.

80. Copeland Jr AD, Hendrich CE, Porterfield SP. Distribution of free amino acids in streptozotocin-induced diabetic pregnant rats, their placentae and fetuses. Horm Metab Res 1990; 22: 65–70.

81. Aerts L, Van Assche FA. Low taurine, gamma-aminobutyric acid and carnosine levels in plasma of diabetic pregnant rats: consequences for the offspring. J Perinat Med 2001; 29: 81–4.

82. Kalhan SC. Protein and nitrogen metabolism in gestational diabetes. Diabetes Care 1998; 21(suppl. 2): B75–8.

83. Jansson T, Ekstrand Y, Bjorn C, Wennergren M, Powell TL. Alterations in the activity of placental amino acid transporters in pregnancies complicated by diabetes. Diabetes 2002; 51: 2214–9.

84. Kuruvilla AG, D'Souza SW, Glazier JD, et al. Altered activity of the system A amino acid transporter in microvillous membrane vesicles from placentas of macrosomic babies born to diabetic women. J Clin Invest 1994; 94: 689–95.

85. Nandakumaran M, Al-Saleh E, Al-Shammari M, Harouny AK. Effect of hyperglycaemic load on maternal-foetal transport of L-leucine in perfused human placental lobule: in vitro study. Acta Diabetol 2005; 42: 16–22.

86. Nandakumaran M, Al-Shammari M, Al-Saleh E. Maternal–fetal transport kinetics of L-leucine in vitro in gestational diabetic pregnancies. Diabetes Metab 2004; 30: 367–74.

87. Wittmaack FM, Gafvels ME, Bronner M, et al. Localization and regulation of the human very low density lipoprotein/apolipoprotein-E receptor: trophoblast expression predicts a role for the receptor in placental lipid transport. Endocrinology 1995; 136: 340–8.

88. Wadsack C, Hammer A, Levak-Frank S, et al. Selective cholesteryl ester uptake from high density lipoprotein by human first trimester and term villous trophoblast cells. Placenta 2003; 24: 131–43.

89. Hendrickse W, Stammers JP, Hull D. The transfer of free fatty acids across the human placenta. Br J Obstet Gynaecol 1985; 92: 945–52.

90. Kuhn DC, Crawford MA, Stuart MJ, Botti JJ, Demers LM. Alterations in transfer and lipid distribution of arachidonic acid in placentas of diabetic pregnancies. Diabetes 1990; 39: 914–8.

91. Lakin V, Haggarty P, Abramovich DR, et al. Dietary intake and tissue concentration of fatty acids in omnivore, vegetarian and diabetic

pregnancy. Prostaglandins Leukot Essent Fatty Acids 1998; 59: 209–20.

92. Kuhn DC, Botti JJ, Cherouny PH, Demers LM. Eicosanoid production and transfer in the placenta of the diabetic pregnancy. Prostaglandins 1990; 40: 205–15.

93. Dancis J, Lee J, Mendoza S, Liebes L. Nucleoside transport by perfused human placenta. Placenta 1993; 14: 547–54.

94. Sobrevia L, Jarvis SM, Yudilevich DL. Adenosine transport in cultured human umbilical vein endothelial cells is reduced in diabetes. Am J Physiol 1994; 267(1, pt 1): C39–C47.

95. Osses N, Sobrevia L, Cordova C, Jarvis SM, Yudilevich DL. Transport and metabolism of adenosine in diabetic human placenta. Reprod Fertil Dev 1995; 7: 1499–503.

96. San Martin R, Sobrevia L. Gestational diabetes and the adenosine/L-arginine/nitric oxide (ALANO) pathway in human umbilical vein endothelium. Placenta 2006; 27: 1–10.

97. Adam PA, Teramo K, Raiha N, Gitlin D, Schwartz R. Human fetal insulin metabolismearly in gestation. Response to acutelevation of the fetal glucose concentration and placental tranfer of human insulin-I-131. Diabetes 1969; 18: 409–16.

98. Buse MG, Roberts WJ, Buse J. The role of the human placenta in the transfer and metabolism of insulin. J Clin Invest 1962; 41: 29–41.

99. Kalhan SC, Schwartz R, Adam PA. Placental barrier to human insulin-I125 in insulin-dependent diabetic mothers. J Clin Endocrinol Metab 1975; 40: 139–42.

100. Boskovic R, Feig DS, Derewlany L, et al. Transfer of insulin lispro across the human placenta: in vitro perfusion studies. Diabetes Care 2003; 26: 1390–4.

101. Bauman WA, Yalow RS. Insulin as a lethal weapon. J Forensic Sci 1981; 26: 594–8.

102. Jovanovic LG, Mills JL, Peterson CM. Anti-insulin antibody titers do not influence control or insulin requirements in early pregnancy. Diabetes Care 1984; 7: 68–71.

103. Lindsay RS, Ziegler AG, Hamilton BA, et al. Type 1 diabetes-related antibodies in the fetal circulation: prevalence and influence on cord insulin and birth weight in offspring of mothers with type 1 diabetes. J Clin Endocrinol Metab 2004; 89: 3436–9.

104. Menon RK, Cohen RM, Sperling MA, et al. Transplacental passage of insulin in pregnant women with insulin-dependent diabetes mellitus. Its role in fetal macrosomia. N Engl J Med 1990; 323: 309–15.

105. Challier JC, D'Athis P, Guerre-Millo M, Nandakumaran M. Flow-dependent transfer of antipyrine in the human placenta in vitro. Reprod Nutr Dev 1983; 23: 41–50.

106. Nanovskaya TN, Nekhayeva IA, Patrikeeva SL, Hankins GD, Ahmed MS. Transfer of metformin across the dually perfused human placental lobule. Am J Obstet Gynecol 2006; 195: 1081–5.

107. Elliott BD, Langer O, Schenker S, Johnson RF. Insignificant transfer of glyburide occurs across the human placenta. Am J Obstet Gynecol 1991; 165(4, pt 1): 807–12.

108. Desoye G, Barnea ER, Shurz-Swirsky R. Increase in insulin binding and inhibition of the decrease in the phospholipid content of human term placental homogenates in culture by the sulfonylurea glipizide. Biochem Pharmacol 1993; 46: 1585–90.

109. Hiles RA, Bawdon RE, Petrella EM. Ex vivo human placental transfer of the peptides pramlintide and exenatide (synthetic exendin-4). Hum Exp Toxicol 2003; 22: 623–8.

9 Nutrient delivery and metabolism in the fetus

William W. Hay Jr.

Introduction

Fetuses of diabetic mothers have markedly different growth rates and develop considerably different body compositions. Fetuses of poorly controlled diabetics who have wide swings in meal-associated plasma concentrations of glucose and fatty acids tend to be macrosomic, with large amounts of subcutaneous adipose tissue. In contrast, severely diabetic pregnant women, particularly those with vascular disorders and hypertension, frequently produce smaller placentas that transfer fewer nutrients to the fetus; their fetuses tend to be growth restricted and relatively devoid of body fat. To appreciate how such disparate patterns of growth can occur, it is important to understand the basic aspects of nutrient transport to the fetus and nutrient regulation of fetal metabolism and growth. In the following discussion, data from a variety of animal models, principally sheep, are used to augment and support the more limited information from humans.

Nutrients for the fetus

The principal metabolic nutrients in the fetus are glucose and amino acids. Glucose (including its metabolic product lactate) serves as the principal energy substrate in the fetus for maintenance of basal metabolism, energy storage in glycogen and adipose tissue, and energy requirements of protein synthesis and growth. Amino acids, while primarily providing the structural basis for protein synthesis and growth, also serve as oxidative substrates for energy production, especially when glucose is deficient. Fatty acids also are taken up by the fetus, where they are primarily used for structural components of membranes and for growth of adipose tissue. In humans, fatty acid oxidation occurs readily after birth, even in preterm infants, indicating that the lack of marked fatty acid oxidation in the fetus is primarily due to the ready supply and oxidation of glucose, lactate, and amino acids. Hormonal regulation of metabolic substrate utilization and growth in the fetus and the effects in the fetus of insulin and the insulin-like growth factors (IGFs) are important but secondary to the supply of nutrient substrates.[1-3]

Role of the placenta in nutrient transfer to the fetus

In mammals, the major determinant of intrauterine growth is the placental nutrient supply, which occurs primarily by diffusion and transporter mediated transport. In turn, these processes depend upon the size, morphology, blood supply, and transporter abundance of the placenta and on synthesis and metabolism of nutrients and hormones by the uteroplacental tissues.[4] The placenta contains membrane transporter proteins for glucose, lactate and fatty acids that facilitate their diffusional transport to the fetus by concentration gradients. The placenta also actively concentrates and then transfers amino acids to the fetal plasma, processes aided by the unique positioning of specific amino acid transporter proteins and systems on the maternal-facing and fetal-facing trophoblast membranes. The placenta also consumes nutrient substrates at a very high metabolic rate, producing part of the transplacental nutrient substrate gradient for glucose and fatty acids, as well as specific metabolic products of glucose, lipid, and amino acid metabolism that then provide a unique nutrient milieu in the fetal plasma.

Most of the increase in placental nutrient transfer capacity over gestation comes from increased placental growth, primarily of membrane surface area. Placental growth and development (size, morphology, and membrane transporter abundance) are regulated by imprinted paternally derived genes, such as the placental-specific Igf2–H19 gene complex.[5] Activity of these imprinted genes varies according to genetic supply; thus, a larger paternal Igf2 gene allele supply vs. maternal would lead to a larger placenta and the potential for a larger fetus. Activity also is affected by epigenetic modification, thereby allowing for considerable environmental influence over gene expression; for example, DNA methylation would tend to limit placental-specific Igf-2 gene activity and produce smaller placentas and potentially IUGR fetuses. Placental–fetal metabolic interaction, in which certain substrates transported directly to the fetus by the placenta are then metabolized into products for both fetal and, in turn, placental metabolism also provides a unique fetal nutrient metabolic milieu and tissue/organ-specific metabolic pathways.[1-3]

Table 9.1   Estimated human fetal nutrient substrate balance in late gestation

	Carbon (g/kg/day)	Calories (kcal/kg/day)
Requirement		
Accretion in carcass: non-fat (human)	3.2	32
Accretion in carcass: fat (human)	3.5	33
Excretion as CO_2	4.4	0
Excretion as urea	0.2	2
Excretion as glutamate	0.3	2
Heat (measured as O_2 consumption)	0.0	50
Total	11.6	119
Uptake		
Amino acids	3.9	45
Glucose	3.7	26
Lactate	1.7	21
Fatty Acids	1.1–2.2	17–34
Total	10.4–11.5	109–126

Adapted from (1) Hay and Regnault,[3] (2) Battaglia and Meschia,[6] and (3) Sparks et al.[7]

Nutrient supply and fetal metabolic rate

Estimates of carbon supply to the fetus are compared with requirements for energy production and storage in Table 9.1.[3,6,7] The fraction of fetal glucose utilization that actually produces CO_2 is only c. 0.5–0.6[4,8] (Table 9.2). Thus, carbon substrates other than glucose (lactate and amino acids, primarily) are required to meet the oxidative requirements imposed by the rate of fetal oxygen consumption.

At markedly reduced rates of glucose supply to the fetus, fetal glucose utilization rates decrease proportionally.[8,9] Under such short-term conditions (hours to days), fetal oxygen consumption remains at near normal rates, indicating active reciprocal oxidation of other substrates, such as glucose released from glycogen, lactate, amino acids, and, less important quantitatively, fatty acids and ketoacids. Over longer periods of reduced glucose supply (>2 weeks), fetal oxygen consumption tends to decrease by up to 25–30%. Because the rate of fetal growth decreases at the same time and to the same extent, the reduction in fetal oxygen consumption with prolonged nutrient deficiency probably represents the oxidative requirements of the decreased protein synthetic rate and metabolic requirements of growth.

Similar to nutrient deprivation, excess delivery of nutrients to the fetus, such as with maternal diabetes and hyperglycemia or experimental glucose infusion into the fetus or mother, decreases amino acid oxidation, but has little effect on fetal metabolic rate. A maximal increase of c. 15% in fetal oxygen consumption has been observed in fetal sheep infused directly with glucose. The balance of excess glucose consumption under these conditions maximizes glycogen stores and, in those fetuses that can produce abundant fat such as the human, augments the growth of adipose tissue. There is little evidence that excess amino acid supply enhances the growth of fetal lean body mass or linear growth. Thus, fetuses of diabetic mothers tend primarily to be macrosomic (i.e. obese).

Fetal carbohydrate supply and metabolism

The rate of glucose transfer from maternal to fetal plasma and the net rate of fetal glucose uptake are directly related to the maternal glucose concentration (Figure 9.1a).[10] Fetal growth rate, glycogen deposition, and fat production and storage in adipose tissue also are directly related to fetal glucose supply and uptake. Thus, it is not surprising that fetuses of hyperglycemic, diabetic mothers tend to contain more hepatic and muscle glycogen and body fat than do fetuses of more normally glycemic mothers, whether they are diabetic or not.

Table 9.2   Fetal carbon substrate oxidation in relation to fetal oxygen consumption (VO_2)*

Substrate	Oxidation fraction	Carbon for oxidation (mmol/min/kg)	Fraction of fetal VO_2
Glucose	0.55	0.09	0.29
Lactate	0.72	0.14	0.50
Amino acids	0.30	0.03	0.09
Total			0.88

*Estimates derived from data in fetal sheep in late gestation. (From (1) Battaglia and Meschia,[6] (2) Hay et al.,[8] and (3) Hay and Meznarich.[10])

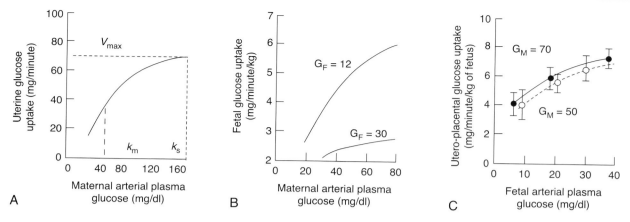

Figure 9.1   (a) Schematic representation of effect of maternal glucose concentration on uterine glucose uptake, based on experiments in which glucose was infused into pregnant sheep after an overnight fast to produce a large variety of maternal arterial blood glucose concentrations. Fick principle measurements were then made of net uterine glucose uptake rates versus the maternal arterial blood glucose concentration which shows saturation kinetics with an approximate K_m value in the physiological range of maternal glucose concentration (about 50–60 mg/dL). (Adapted from data in Hay and Meznarich.[10]) (b) Fetal glucose uptake (net transfer of glucose from placenta to fetal circulation) plotted against maternal arterial glucose concentration showing a saturable dependence of fetal glucose uptake on maternal glucose concentration. In addition, this relationship is left-shifted as fetal glucose concentration is decreased, showing that as fetal glucose concentration is decreased relative to that of the mother, which increases the maternal–fetal glucose concentration gradient, placental-to-fetal glucose transfer increases. (Adapted from data in Hay et al.[11]) (c) Net rate of uteroplacental glucose consumption in sheep, expressed per kilogram of fetus, plotted against fetal arterial plasma glucose. Solid line: values measured while maternal arterial plasma glucose was clamped at about 70 mg/dL. Dotted line: values measured while maternal arterial plasma glucose was clamped at about 50 mg/dL. These data show that although maternal glucose concentration determines glucose entry into the uteroplacenta and fetus, actual uteroplacental glucose consumption is regulated largely by the fetal glucose concentration. (Adapted from data in Hay et al.[11] Reproduced from Hay.[12])

In contrast to the direct relationship between maternal glucose concentration and uterine and fetal glucose uptake rates, the partition of uterine glucose uptake into fetal and uteroplacental glucose uptakes is separately regulated by fetal glucose concentration (Figure 9.1a).[10–12] A relatively higher fetal glucose concentration will diminish placental-to-fetal glucose transfer in favor of placental glucose consumption, while a relatively lower fetal glucose concentration will limit placental glucose consumption and enhance transfer of glucose into the fetal plasma. The concentration of glucose in the fetal plasma declines relative to that in the maternal plasma over the second half of gestation. This increases the transplacental glucose concentration gradient in later gestation, providing a greater driving force to supply glucose for the increasing glucose requirements of the growing fetus.[13] The decrease in fetal glucose concentration over the second half of gestation represents an absolute increase in glucose clearance. At least three principal mechanisms are responsible for this increase in glucose clearance: the size, cellularity, and glucose metabolic rate of the brain increases relative to other fetal tissues and organs; there is progressive development of fetal insulin secretion by the expanding mass of pancreatic islets and beta cells; finally, there is increased growth of insulin-sensitive tissues, primarily skeletal muscle, but also the heart and adipose tissue.

Fetal carbohydrate supply also includes lactate production in the placenta, which then is transported directionally into the fetus[2,6,14] by the monocarboxylate transporters MCT1 and MCT4. Placental production of lactate from glucose is probably more important than the concentration of these transporters in determining the amount of lactate transported to the fetus.[15]

Placental glucose transport

Glucose transporters

Placental glucose uptake and transfer are mediated by Na^+-dependent transport systems on both the maternal-facing microvillous and fetal-facing basal plasma membranes of the syncytiotrophoblast.[14] GLUT1 and GLUT3 are the predominant molecular isoforms of glucose transporters (GLUTs) in the placenta.[16–19] GLUT8 also has been found in the ovine placenta, and its abundance is reduced in placentas with intrauterine growth restriction, indicating that it also might have a quantitatively important functional role in placental glucose transport.[20] GLUT1 is localized in both microvillous and basal plasma membranes of the syncytiotrophoblast, as well as endothelial cells and the amnion. These locations provide transplacental regulation of glucose transport from maternal to fetal plasma, as well as the reverse when the fetus independently becomes hyperglycemic relative to the mother (e.g. experimental infusion of glucose or conditions of stress in the fetus when fetal glucose production develops). Expression of the higher affinity GLUT3 isoform in the human placenta is controversial and its participation in glucose uptake and transport has not been confirmed, although in the sheep placenta, cytochalasian binding assays indicate that GLUT3 might account for as much as 40% of glucose uptake by the end of gestation.[19] GLUT 3 also is confined primarily to the microvillous membranes of the syncytiotrophoblast where it logically might confer directionality of glucose flux across the trophoblast to the fetus, or at least ensure trophoblast glucose uptake when maternal and fetal glucose concentrations are reduced, as it has a greater affinity for glucose than GLUT1.[21] Despite considerable study, the regulation of placental glucose transporter expression and activity remain poorly defined.[22–24] Placental GLUT1 is acutely up regulated by hypoxia and hyperglycemia, while acute hypoglycemia leads to down regulation. Chronic changes in glycemia, both hyper- and hypoglycemia, generally are associated with diminished expression.[22] Thus maternal hyperglycemia causes a time-dependent decline in the entire placental glucose transporter pool (GLUT-1 and GLUT-3). In contrast, maternal hypoglycemia decreases GLUT-1 but not GLUT-3, resulting in a relatively increased GLUT-3 contribution to the placental glucose transporter pool, which could maintain glucose delivery to the placenta relative to the fetus when maternal glucose is low.[3] *In vitro* studies indicate that changes in GLUT concentrations are related to transport capacity, but this has not been demonstrated *in vivo*, except in experiments in which the transporters were competitively blocked by pharmacologic inhibitors;[19] such studies, however, did not discriminate among reductions of the different transporters to indicate their relative quantitative contributions to glucose uptake and transport.

Kinetics of glucose uptake and transport by the placenta

Although the effect of the maternal glucose concentration on net placental-to-fetal glucose transfer demonstrates saturation kinetics,[10] this relationship does not necessarily define the quantitative characteristics of placental-to-fetal glucose transport capacity, because as maternal glucose concentration and placental glucose transport are increased, both fetal glucose concentration and fetal glucose utilization rates increase. Other studies in which glucose was infused directly into the fetus have shown degrees of increase (slope) and saturation of fetal glucose utilization rates occurring at about the same fetal glucose concentrations as determined by maternal glucose infusions.[25] Thus, the maternal glucose infusion approach reflects fetal glucose consumption kinetics as well as those of placental-to-fetal glucose transfer. To address this experimental problem, different studies have used glucose clamp procedures to regulate the maternal-to-fetal glucose concentration gradient at different maternal and fetal glucose concentrations.[11] As shown in Figure 9.1b, placental-to-fetal glucose transfer is sensitive to a change in fetal glucose concentration, regardless of the maternal glucose level.[11,12]

Thus, at almost any maternal glucose concentration utero-placental glucose consumption is directly related to the fetal glucose concentration (Figure 9.1c). These observations imply that the fetal side of the utero-placenta is markedly more permeable to glucose than the maternal side. They also indicate that changes in the fetal glucose concentration have a strong influence on placental glucose flux and metabolism. The importance of this regulation of placental-to-fetal glucose transfer and net utero-placental glucose consumption by fetal glucose concentration is highlighted by observations in

chronically hypoglycemic pregnant sheep in which fetal glucogenesis develops,[9] thereby contributing glucose molecules to the fetal glucose pool and sustaining fetal glucose utilization at near-normal rates. As a result, the placental-to-fetal glucose concentration gradient and the placental-to-fetal glucose transfer rate are relatively reduced; under these circumstances, uteroplacental glucose consumption is maintained at near-normal rates for the level of maternal glycemia. Thus, fetal glucose production can compensate for reduced maternal glucose supply and sustain placental as well as fetal glucose utilization requirements.

Several other placental factors may affect placental glucose transport, including placental surface area, thickness of the various cell and tissue layers between the maternal and fetal plasma, rates of uterine and umbilical blood flow, and the placental glucose consumption rate. The effect of changes of placental thickness on glucose transport has not been studied, but there appears to be a direct relation between the maternal-to-fetal arterial glucose gradient and the amount of intervening placental and vascular tissue layers. Whether such tissue layers increase the gradient by glucose consumption or by imposing a barrier to transport, or both, is not known.

Gestational changes in placental glucose transfer

Placental glucose transport increases markedly over gestation. In sheep, the increase in transport capacity accounts for *c.* 60% of the increase in placental glucose transport, with an increase in the transplacental glucose concentration gradient accounting for the remaining 40%.[13] This increased transport capacity most likely reflects the growth of the surface area of the trophoblast and increased numbers of glucose transporters.[19,22,26] It has not been determined if increased trophoblast membrane glucose transporter concentrations occur as well.

Fetal glucose uptake and utilization

Glucose utilization rate in near-term fetal sheep averages *c.* 5–7 mg/min/kg.[27] This value is similar to those measured in term human newborn infants using stable isotope tracer methodology,[28] and is about half the value that occurs at mid-gestation in fetal sheep[9] when fetal growth, protein turnover, and fractional synthetic rates also are about twice those closer to term. The high correlation between fetal glucose utilization and growth rates indicates that glucose probably serves a major role as the energy supply for the protein synthesis required for growth. Indeed, fetal growth restriction is directly related to glucose deprivation.[29] Table 9.3 presents estimated utilization rates of glucose in several fetal organs and the remaining carcass of fetal sheep in late gestation. All organs are dependent on the plasma glucose concentration for their specific rate of glucose uptake, while skeletal muscle, heart, and liver develop insulin sensitivity in later gestation. It still is not known to what extent basal insulin concentration affects glucose uptake by specific organs and tissues in the fetus. An acute decrease in the fetal plasma insulin concentration (studies in fetal sheep), however, such as by somatostatin infusion,

Table 9.3   Metabolic rates in the fetus that account for glucose utilization (based on data in fetal sheep and estimates for human fetuses for brain)

	Glucose utilization rate (mg/min/kg fetus)	Percent of total
Whole fetus (sheep, measured)	5.0	100
Whole fetus (human, estimated)	6.0–8.0	100
Brain (sheep, measured)	0.8	16
Brain (human, estimated)	4.0	50–67
Heart (sheep, measured)	0.65	13
Lungs (sheep, estimated)	0.1	2
Liver (sheep, measured)	0.1	2
Red blood cells (human, estimated)	0.1	2
Gut (sheep, estimated)	??	??
Carcass/skeletal muscle (estimated, sheep)	3.25	65
Total of organs accounted for		
Sheep	5.0	100
Human	8.2	103–137

*Adapted from (1) Hay and Regnault,[3] (2) Battaglia and Meschia,[6] and (3) Sparks et al.[7]

does not affect measurements of fetal glucose utilization rate. These procedures do, though, lead to an increase in fetal glucose concentration. Thus, the basal plasma insulin concentration in the fetus appears to regulate glucose production but not utilization; the latter is more under the control of the plasma glucose concentration.

Fetal glucose transporters

GLUT1 is found throughout the fetal tissues and on all endothelial cells, and probably accounts for the majority of basal tissue glucose uptake from the fetal plasma. GLUT4 is found in the heart, adipose tissue, and skeletal muscle. In the fetal sheep, the GLUT1 protein concentration is up-regulated by hypoglycemia and hypoinsulinemia in skeletal muscle and adipose tissue, while there is no change in the brain.[30] In contrast, hyperglycemia appears to down-regulate GLUT1 protein concentrations in most tissues. Insulin-responsive GLUT4 protein is up-regulated by hypoglycemia, but in response to hyperglycemia it is initially up-regulated and then down-regulated to normal or less than normal levels in skeletal muscle and adipose tissue.[31,32] Acute hyperinsulinemia increases the whole fetal glucose utilization rate, principally in the heart and skeletal muscle,[14] and decreases the fetal plasma glucose concentration,[8] but it has been difficult to demonstrate in which organs this increased glucose utilization rate takes place. Hyperinsulinemia also appears to have acute effects on increasing protein concentrations for both GLUT1 and GLUT4.[31,32] Different studies among species, tissues studied, gestational ages, and conditions of glycemia and insulinemia show considerable variability and complexity of changes in glucose transporter concentrations during fetal life.[33]

Kinetics of the glucose utilization rate in the fetus

The principal actions of insulin in the human fetus are to increase protein anabolism and, by increasing cellular glucose uptake, to promote lipid formation and deposition in adipose tissue. In this situation, substrate supply (amino acids, glucose, fatty acids and triglycerides, and glycerol) is probably as or more important than insulin itself. The capacity for glucose utilization in the human fetus can only be estimated from measurements in prematurely born infants or in animal models such as the sheep. In preterm humans, doubling or even tripling of glucose utilization rate (GUR) from basal is possible.[34] GUR in fetal sheep follows Michaelis–Menten kinetics,[8] and is relatively limited to a doubling of basal GUR. This capacity is variable, however, as increased entry of glucose into the fetal plasma from the placenta increases fetal glucose concentration and insulin secretion, which, in turn, augments fetal glucose utilization, thus limiting further increases in the fetal glucose concentration. Glucose and insulin clamp experiments in fetal sheep, in which glucose or insulin or both are infused until GUR reaches maximal rates, have shown that plasma glucose and insulin concentrations act independently (i.e. additively) to increase glucose utilization and oxidation.[8] Despite wide changes in glucose utilization, the relative proportion of glucose oxidized during short-term 3–4-h studies (c. 55%) does not change significantly over the entire range of glucose utilized. Furthermore, because rates of oxygen consumption and thus the fetal metabolic rate do not vary significantly, if at all, under these circumstances, oxidation of other carbon substrates, such as amino acids and lactate, must increase in compensation. Indeed, sustained hypoglycemia in fetal sheep leads to a near doubling of the rate of leucine oxidation relative to the rate of leucine disposal from the plasma.[35]

In contrast to the acute effect of increased fetal plasma insulin concentrations to increase fetal glucose utilization and decrease fetal plasma glucose concentrations, an acute decrease of fetal plasma insulin concentration, for example, with somatostatin infusion, does not appear to affect the fetal glucose concentration or rate of glucose utilization.[36] It is possible that the decrease in insulin concentration allows fetal glucose production to develop under these conditions, which would limit glucose transfer to the fetus from the placenta, preventing a measurable increase in fetal glucose concentration. A chronic decrease of fetal plasma insulin concentration, however, either by pancreatectomy or injection of streptozotocin (a drug that leads to destruction of the pancreatic beta cells) into the fetus,[37,38] results in an increased fetal plasma glucose concentration. As discussed above, fetal hyperglycemia decreases placental to fetal glucose transfer. Chronic hyperglycemia in fetal sheep also is associated with decreased peripheral tissue insulin sensitivity and glucose utilization capacity[39] (and with decreased GLUT1 and GLUT4 transporter concentrations in skeletal muscle, liver, and adipose tissue, as discussed above[30–32]), as well as the potential release of insulin's normal inhibition of hepatic glucose production.

As a result of chronic fetal glucose deprivation, from whatever cause, fetal growth rate diminishes. Fetal insulin concentration is reduced in such hypoglycemic, glucose-deprivation conditions, and placental-to-fetal glucose transfer is secondarily reduced as a result of the compensatory development of fetal glucose production and relative increase in fetal glucose concentration. These results indicate that one growth-regulating effect of insulin in the fetus is its capacity to enhance glucose utilization, in addition to its independent and direct effects to stimulate protein synthesis via the classical insulin signal transduction cascade and inhibit protein breakdown. Examples of metabolic effects of increased glucose supply to the fetus are shown in Box 9.1.[14]

Fetal insulin secretion

Glucose-stimulated fetal insulin secretion (measured as an acute increase in fetal plasma insulin concentration) increases more than five-fold during the second half of gestation in fetal sheep.[40] Similar results appear to occur in human fetuses, derived from studies of human fetal islets *in vitro* and insulin secretion in preterm infants.[41] Fetal insulin secretion also can be modified by the degree, duration, and pattern of changes in the fetal plasma glucose concentration. Experiments in fetal sheep,[42] for example, have shown that sustained, marked, relatively constant hyperglycemia actually decreases both basal

and glucose stimulated fetal insulin secretion (GSIS); responsiveness to amino acids such as arginine also is diminished. In contrast, glucose-stimulated insulin secretion is augmented in most gestational diabetic women; in these cases, there is a strong tendency to develop increasingly exaggerated, meal-associated hyperglycemia in late gestation.[43] Similar results have been found in fetal sheep whose mothers received intermittent, pulsatile boluses of glucose intravenously.[44] Thus, a principal cause of enhanced fetal insulin secretion is variability in the magnitude and the intermittent nature of fetal glucose concentration, with pulsatile fetal hyperglycemia producing the largest increase in GSIS.

Fatty acids also stimulate fetal insulin secretion; their concentrations are increased in pregnant diabetics and in their fetuses in late gestation, perhaps contributing to augmented fetal insulin secretion.[43] Acute and chronic hypoglycemia, and probably hypoaminocidemia as well, diminish fetal insulin secretion.[36] Responsible mechanisms are not known, although presumably glucose activates insulin gene response elements, and both glucose and amino acids are necessary to develop mechanisms that regulate insulin secretion from the pancreatic beta cell.

In contrast to such variable hyperglycemic conditions that generally augment insulin secretion, sustained hypoglycemia usually diminishes fetal insulin secretion. For example, in fetal sheep in late gestation, fetal hypoglycemia produced by insulin infusion into the mother, produces normal to increased fetal pancreatic islet insulin content, but reduced fetal GSIS. Because these islets have normal glucose metabolism, ATP-activated potassium channel activity, and calcium entry through voltage-dependent calcium channels, the defective insulin secretion appears to be localized to insulin trafficking and/or exocytosis from the beta cell.[45] Recent studies in rats and sheep indicate that low protein diets in the mother, fetal amino acid deficiency, and intrauterine fetal growth restriction decrease fetal insulin secretion by decreased growth of the endocrine pancreas.[46,47] Vascular deficiency (decreased angiogenesis) is common in all of these islets in IUGR fetuses.[47] In addition, in IUGR fetal sheep caused by fetal nutrient

---

Box 9.1   Fetal responses to increased glucose supply

Acute: mild–moderate
- hyperglycemia
- increased insulin production, secretion, and hyperinsulinemia
- increased glucose utilization and oxygen consumption
- mild arterial hypoxemia
- increased placental lactate production, and fetal lactate uptake and utilization

Acute: severe
- increased fetal oxygen consumption, arterial hypoxemia and metabolic acidosis
- decreased placental perfusion leading to fetal demise

Chronic
- decreased insulin secretion and/or synthesis if hyperglycemia is marked and constant
- increased insulin secretion and/or synthesis if hyperglycemia is variable
- increased ratio of placental glucose consumption to placental glucose transfer increased erythropoietin production

(Adapted from Hay Jr WW. Nutrition and development of the fetus: carbohydrates and lipid metabolism. In: Walker WA, Watkins JB, eds. Nutrition in Pediatrics (Basic Science and Clinical Applications), 2nd edn. Neuilly-sur-Seine, France: Decker Europe; 1996, pp. 364–78.)

restriction from placental insufficiency, pancreatic beta cell replication is inhibited by cell cycle arrest of mitosis; islets are smaller and although they secrete insulin at normal to increased rates relative to their insulin content, they simply have less insulin because they contain fewer beta cells.[48] Other studies in rats have found that uteroplacental insufficiency induces oxidative stress and marked mitochondrial dysfunction in the fetal beta cell.[49] ATP production is impaired and continues to deteriorate with age. The activities of complexes I and III of the electron transport chain progressively decline in IUGR islets in these animals, followed by mitochondrial DNA point mutations that accumulate with age and are associated with decreased mtDNA content and reduced expression of mitochondrial-encoded genes. Mitochondrial dysfunction results in impaired insulin secretion. These results demonstrate that IUGR can induce mitochondrial dysfunction in the fetal beta cell leading to increased production of reactive oxygen species (ROS), which in turn damage mtDNA. A self-reinforcing cycle of progressive deterioration in mitochondrial function then could lead to a corresponding decline in beta cell function, finally reaching a threshold in mitochondrial dysfunction and ROS production that could lead to diabetes mellitus.

In all of these fetal conditions of under nutrition and metabolic insult, a final common pathway might be earlier and more frequent onset of later life diabetes based on decreased pancreatic capacity for growth and insulin production that began in fetal life, representing a fetal origin of an adult disease.[50]

Effect of other hormones on fetal glucose metabolism

Fetal thyroid hormone indirectly enhances fetal glucose utilization by increasing the fetal metabolic rate (oxygen consumption).[51] Changes in fetal plasma cortisol concentrations during late gestation have little effect on fetal glucose concentrations or on the rates of glucose utilization.[52] However, fetal plasma cortisol concentrations do increase in very late gestation, at which time cortisol-dependent increases in fetal hepatic glycogenolytic and gluconeogenic enzyme activities develop. These may enhance the glucogenic capacity of the fetus, thereby contributing to the endogenous glucose production observed in normal fetuses just before term and at the time of delivery.[53] Glucagon and circulating catecholamines (adrenal epinephrine and spillover norepinephrine from peripheral nerve endings) are normally present in modest concentrations in the fetal plasma, but they do stimulate fetal glucogenesis when infused into the fetus. Catecholamines promote glucose production at physiological levels,[54] but glucagon must reach relatively high concentrations in the fetal plasma to do this.[55]

Insulin, IGF and other growth factors

Acute changes in fetal plasma IGF-I concentrations appear to have little or no effect on fetal glucose kinetics.[56] Glucose does, however, act at the transcriptional level to regulate the production and plasma concentrations of both IGF-I and IGF-II.[57]

Plasma insulin also independently promotes IGF-I synthesis.[57,58] These observations indicate that the intracellular supply and/or concentration of glucose can regulate fetal IGF-I production. In turn, increased plasma IGF-I concentrations can inhibit protein breakdown,[58] as does insulin,[59] although this effect of IGF-I occurs primarily at higher glucose concentrations. Thus, both insulin and IGF-I indirectly enhance the capacity for glucose to promote fetal nitrogen balance and growth. In fetal sheep, an acute increase in the fetal insulin concentration activates proteins in the mitogen activated protein (MAP) kinase cascade but glucose does not, indicating that insulin might have independent and direct effects on stimulating protein synthesis, cell growth, and cell replication.[60] Similarly, acutely increased insulin concentrations in fetal sheep promote amino acid utilization and net nitrogen balance.[61] Such effects are probably short-lived, in that chronic infusions of insulin do not increase growth of lean tissues very much; instead, they contribute more to enhancing lipid production and storage in adipose tissue. Interestingly, insulin and amino acids act independently of glucose to promote amino acid synthesis into protein, in that reductions of glucose supply, utilization, and oxidation in the presence of increased insulin and amino acid concentrations do not alter amino acid oxidation, leaving their combined effect primarily on producing net protein balance.[62]

Fetal glucose carbon contribution to glycogen formation

Many fetal tissues, including the placenta, as well as the brain, liver, lung, heart, and skeletal muscle, produce glycogen over the second half of gestation.[63] Liver glycogen content increases with gestational age (Figure 9.2) and is the most important store of glycogen for systemic glucose needs, because only the liver contains sufficient glucose-6-phosphatase for release of glucose into the circulation. Skeletal muscle glycogen content increases during late gestation, whereas lung glycogen content decreases with loss of glycogen-containing alveolar epithelium, development of type II pneumocytes and onset of surfactant production.[64] Cardiac glycogen concentrations decrease with gestation as cellular hypertrophy develops. Despite this decrease, the cardiac glycogen content is essential for postnatal cardiac energy supply and cellular function; in fact, deficits of cardiac glycogen are associated with shortened survival time during periods of anoxia.[65] In this regard, it is important to note that fetal heart GLUT4 abundance increases in late gestation in IUGR fetuses relative to normally growing fetuses,[66] perhaps thereby maintaining its glucose uptake capacity and glycogen synthesis and storage despite the low circulating glucose concentrations that are characteristic of IUGR fetuses. Fetal glycogen synthetic rates vary from low, steady rates of accumulation in species with relatively long gestations, such as the human and sheep, to exceptionally high rates in species such as the rat that have relatively short gestations. In larger, more slow-growing fetuses (e.g. sheep, monkey, human), glycogen synthesis by the liver accounts for only a small (< 10%) portion of fetal glucose utilization.[67]

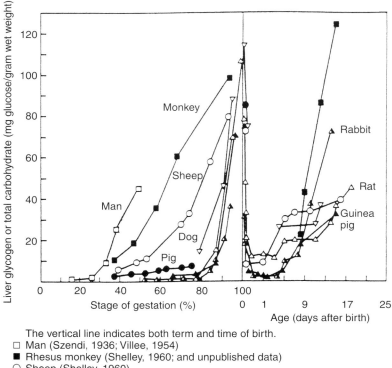

The vertical line indicates both term and time of birth.
- □ Man (Szendi, 1936; Villee, 1954)
- ■ Rhesus monkey (Shelley, 1960; and unpublished data)
- ○ Sheep (Shelley, 1960)
- ● Pig (Mendel & Leavenworth, 1907; McCance & Widdowson, 1959)
- ▽ Dog (Demant, 1887; Schlossmann, 1938)
- △ Rat (Stuart & higgins, 1935; Martinek & Mikulas, 1954; Jacquot, 1955; Stafford & weatherall, 1960)
- ▲ Rabbit (Szendi, 1936; Jost & Jacquot, 1955; Shelley, unpublished)
- ▲ Guinea-pig (Aron, 1922; Shelley, unpublished)

Figure 9.2 Liver glycogen in various species before and after birth. Hepatic glycogen content in several species is shown to increase with gestational age, decrease precipitously during the immediate postnatal period, and increase again with a normal neonatal diet. (From Shelly.[63])

Fetal glucogenesis

Tracer studies in humans[68] and sheep[10] have shown that when glucose tracer is infused into the mother the specific activity or enrichment ratio of tracer (labeled) glucose to non-labeled glucose in the fetal plasma is the same as in the maternal plasma. This demonstrates that the only source of glucose in the fetus is from the maternal plasma, otherwise, new glucose production into the fetal plasma from either the fetus itself or from the placenta would dilute the tracer glucose coming from the mother along with unlabeled glucose, thus lowering the fetal enrichment ratio. Furthermore, studies in fetal sheep have shown that the net uptake of glucose by the fetus from the placenta invariably is equal to the fetal glucose utilization rate, independently measured with glucose tracers.[69] Thus, there is no evidence for fetal glucose production under normal conditions. Also, there is little if any fetal glucogenesis under the conditions of short-term (1–4 h) changes in maternal and fetal glucose concentrations, the placental-to-fetal glucose transfer, and fetal glucose utilization rates. Measurable rates of fetal glucose production only develop significantly after prolonged periods (several days) of decreased fetal glucose supply, and sustained fetal hypoglycemia and hypoinsulinemia. The capacity of the fetus to make new glucose molecules from non-glucose substrates (e.g. lactate, amino acids, and glycerol)

varies considerably among species. In nearly all cases this appears to be a late gestational development, augmented by cortisol activation of phosphoenolpyruvate carboxykinase, the rate-limiting step for gluconeogenesis, and glucose-6-phosphatase, the enzyme necessary for release of glucose from the liver into the circulation.[70]

Fetal lipid metabolism

Placental lipid metabolism and fetal lipid supply

The amount and type of fatty acid or complex lipid transported by the placenta varies among species. Lipid transport varies according to the transport capacity of the placenta; it is greatest in the hemochorial placenta of the human, guinea pig and rabbit, and least in the epitheliochorial placenta of the ruminant and the endotheliochorial placenta of the carnivores.[71] There are many lipid substances in the plasma that are transported across the placenta that are essential for placental and fetal development, even if they do not contribute to nutritional or energy metabolism. Also, brown fat is common to all fetuses; it is essential for postnatal thermogenesis, even if the neonate is not 'fat' with white adipose tissue. Furthermore, many lipid substances entering the fetus are qualitatively different from those taken up by the uterus and utero-placenta, implying active placental metabolism of individual lipid substances. More complex pathways include lipoprotein dissociation by placental lipoprotein lipase activity, triglyceride uptake and metabolism (including metabolic pathways of oxidation, chain-lengthening, synthesis, and interconversions), and release into the fetal plasma as free fatty acids (FFA) or lipoproteins.[72] FFA uptake by the placenta and transfer to the fetus increase over gestation in response to a gestational increase in placental lipoprotein lipase activity, which appears to be increased by glucose and insulin.[73] Placental expression of the fatty acid transporter binding protein L-FAB also is increased in diabetic pregnancies.[74] Together, these changes perhaps contribute significantly to the greater lipid transport to the fetus and resultant macroscomia in gestational diabetics. A schema of placental lipid uptake, metabolism, transport and metabolic interaction with the fetus is shown in Figure 9.3.[2,72]

The fetal impact of maternal plasma FFA and lipid concentrations is reflected in the fetal lipid content and adipose tissue development. Fatter human fetuses develop in pregnant women who have higher plasma concentrations of fatty acids and other lipids, particularly among women with diabetes during pregnancy. In humans, umbilical venous–arterial fatty acid concentration differences in cord blood samples show that the net flux of non-esterified fatty acids into the fetus from the maternal circulation can account for the fetal requirement of fatty acids during the end of pregnancy.[75] Other estimates that are based on fetal lipid accumulation, as well as *in vitro* transfer experiments, estimate that as much as 50% of fetal fatty acid requirements are transferred across the human placenta.[14,75] Overall, therefore, it appears that there is a relatively direct relationship between the permeability of the placenta to lipids, especially fatty acids, and the adiposity

of the fetus at term. Human fetuses develop the most fat (15–18% of body weight at term), laboratory guinea pigs are second at *c.* 12%, laboratory rabbits third at *c.* 7%, and the sheep, because there appears to practically no fatty acid transfer except for essential fatty acids across the ovine placenta, only *c.* 3% (Figure 9.4).[3,7,14,71]

Fetal lipid metabolism

Physiological changes that develop in the fetus in late gestation and increase nutrient utilization, such as the increase in plasma insulin concentration, act to enhance net maternal-to-fetal fatty acid and lipid transport by increasing fatty acid utilization in the fetus (largely to develop adipose tissue).[7] Increased utilization of fatty acids by fetal tissues lowers fetal plasma fatty acid concentrations relative to those in the maternal plasma and increases the maternal-to-fetal fatty acid concentration gradients. For example, human maternal venous blood concentrations of fatty acids are directly related to the umbilical artery FFA concentrations and the umbilical vein-artery concentration differences of FFA.[75] In guinea pig placentas perfused *in vitro*, lowering the fatty acid concentrations in the fetal side perfusate relative to that in the maternal side perfusate independently increases fatty acid transfer across the placenta.[76]

Placental amino acid uptake and transport to the fetus

Growth of placental amino acid transport capacity

As pregnancy advances, the increasing protein synthetic and nitrogen balance demands of the growing fetus are met by an appropriate increase in placental amino acid transport. This enhanced transport is facilitated by increases in placental

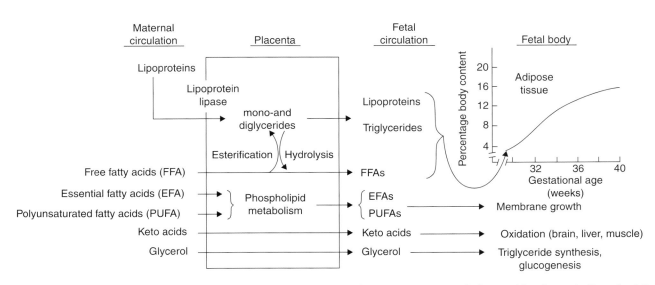

Figure 9.3 Schematic of placental–fetal inter-relationships in humans for various aspects of placental lipid metabolism, fetal lipid uptake and metabolism, and fetal lipogenesis into adipose tissue. (Adapted from (1) Hay Jr WW. Nutrition and development of the fetus: carbohydrates and lipid metabolism. In: Walker WA, Watkins JB, eds. Nutrition in Pediatrics (Basic Science and Clinical Applications), 2nd edn. Neuilly-sur-Seine, France: Decker Europe; 1996, pp. 364–78; and (2) Hay.[2])

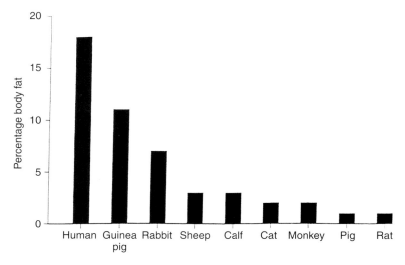

Figure 9.4   Fetal fat content at term as a percent of fetal body weight among species. (Adapted from (1) Hay Jr WW. Nutrition and development of the fetus: carbohydrates and lipid metabolism. In: Walker WA, Watkins JB, eds. Nutrition in Pediatrics (Basic Science and Clinical Applications), 2nd edn. Neuilly-sur-Seine, France: Decker Europe; 1996, pp. 364–78, 1996; (2) Hay,[2] (3) Battaglia and Meschia,[6] and (4) Sparks et al.[7])

perfusion, trophoblast membrane exchange area, transporter concentrations in the trophoblast membranes, and alterations in trophoblast membrane potential differences.[77] Because of the dominant effect of active transport of amino acids, modest variations within the normal range of uterine and umbilical (total placental) blood flow do not affect amino acid uptake by the placenta or transport to the fetus.[78] Some amino acid transport systems also increase their transport activity over gestation.[78–82] Changes in amino acid transporter concentration and transport capacity also are environmentally regulated; for example, placental System A activity and related amino acid transport are down-regulated in pregnant rats fed a low protein diet, perhaps contributing to the well characterized fetal growth restriction in such conditions.[83] Similarly, placental insufficiency in pregnant sheep exposed to high environmental temperatures appears related to early gestational increases in placental IGF-II and IGFBP-4, possibly thereby promoting angiogenesis but limiting exchange surface area.[84] Vectoral transport of amino acids from maternal to fetal plasma is further aided by adding transporter activity at the microvillous maternal-facing membrane that increases placental amino acid uptake, and by adding transporter activity at the basal fetal-facing membrane that facilitates transport of amino acids into the fetal plasma.

Fetal amino acid uptake

Amino acids are actively concentrated in the trophoblast intracellular matrix by Na^+/K^+-adenosine triphosphate-(ATP)ase- and H^+-dependent transporter proteins at the maternal-facing microvillous membrane of the trophoblast and then transported into the fetal plasma producing fetal–maternal plasma concentration ratios ranging from 1.0 to >5.0.[77,85] This active transport process is decreased by hypoxia and hypoglycemia *in vivo*.[86,87] *In vivo* studies also show that many amino acids are directly transported across

the placenta according to their concentration in maternal plasma, while *in vitro* studies produce opposite results, showing for example that low amino acid concentrations in incubation medium of primary cultures of trophoblast vesicles increases transport, indicating that synthesis of the transporters is in part responsible for their functional state.[88] Peptide uptake also has been observed. For example, protein molecules as small as albumin and as large as gamma-globulin pass from maternal to fetal plasma by pinocytosis with increasing efficiency as gestational age progresses.[89] This additional amount of protein probably provides little nutritional value, as shown by studies in the fetal lamb in which total amino nitrogen uptake is not different from the total amino nitrogen uptake in the form of amino acids.[90] Additional studies in sheep show that net total fetal amino acid uptake can account for up to 30–40% of the combined carbon requirements for oxidative metabolism and deposition in fetal protein, glycogen and fat, as well as providing 100% of the fetal nitrogen requirements.[90,91] The placenta and fetus also interact in a variety of ways to ensure amino acid supply to a large and complex set of vital developmental, metabolic and signaling processes that are unique to fetal growth and development (Figure 9.5).[3] In gestational diabetics in particular, there is increasing evidence that up-regulation of nutrient transport capacity in the placenta contributes significantly to nutrient supply to and growth of the fetus. Recent studies *in vivo* provide evidence for increased delivery of amino acids to the fetus in gestational diabetes (GDM) even when metabolic control is strict. Studies *in vitro* demonstrate an up-regulation of placental transport systems for certain amino acids in GDM associated with fetal overgrowth. GDM is also characterized by changes in placental gene expression, including up-regulation of inflammatory mediators and leptin. In Type 1 diabetes with fetal overgrowth the *in vitro* activity of placental transporters for glucose and certain amino acids as well as placental lipoprotein lipase is increased. Furthermore, both clinical observations in Type 1 diabetic

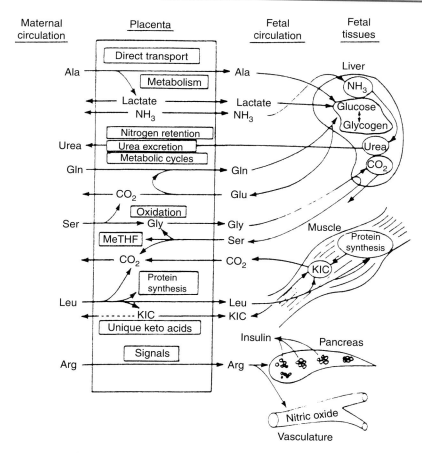

Figure 9.5 Schematic representation of a variety of placental–fetal metabolic interactions with respect to amino acid uptake by the placenta, metabolism in the trophoblast cells, direct transfer to the fetus, signaling of fetal vascular and metabolic processes, and utilization in fetal tissues. Ala = alanine; Gln = glutamine; Glu = glutamate; Ser = serine; Gly = glycine; Leu = leucine; KIC = α-ketoisocaproic acid; Arg = arginine; MeTHF = methyl-tetrahydrofolate; NH_3 = ammonia. (Adapted from (1) Hay,[2] and (2) Hay Jr WW. Fetal requirements and placental transfer of nitrogenous compounds. In: Polin RA, Fox WW, eds. Fetal and Neonatal Physiology. Philadelphia: WB Saunders; 1991, pp. 431–42.)

pregnancies and preliminary animal experimental studies suggest that even brief periods of metabolic perturbation early in pregnancy may affect placental growth and transport function for the remainder of pregnancy, thereby contributing to fetal overgrowth.[92]

Fetal amino acid metabolism

Fetal amino acid oxidation

Evidence for a relatively high rate of fetal oxidation of amino acids comes from three observations: amino acids are taken up by the fetus in excess of their rate of deposition in fetal protein;[90] fetal urea production rates are quite high;[93] fetal infusions of carbon-labeled amino acids have produced fetal production and excretion of labeled carbon dioxide.[94] The urea production rate in fetal sheep can account for 25% of fetal nitrogen uptake in amino acids. This magnitude of urea production also can account for up to *c*. 2% of total fetal carbon uptake and representing *c*. 6% of fetal carbon uptake in amino acids.[95] Such fetal urea production rates are large, exceeding neonatal and adult weight-specific rates, indicating

relatively rapid protein turnover and oxidation in the fetus.[95] Oxidation rates have been calculated for leucine (*c*. 25% of utilization), lysine (*c*. 10% of utilization) and glycine (*c*. 13% of utilization). These studies also demonstrate that the fetal oxidation–disposal rate ratio is directly related to the excess umbilical uptake of these amino acids above that required for protein accretion and to the plasma concentration of the amino acid.[90,96]

Fetal protein synthesis and turnover

The net umbilical uptake rates of several non-essential amino acids are less than their total rate of utilization, emphasizing the need for a relatively high rate of fetal amino acid production.[93] Protein synthetic rates also are quite high. Fractional protein synthetic rate (k_S) and fractional growth rate (k_G) in fetal sheep have been compared using two tracers, ^{14}C-leucine and ^{14}C-lysine, at different gestational ages (Figure 9.6).[96,97] The higher protein synthetic rate in the mid-gestation fetus is proportional to the higher metabolic rate and glucose utilization rate at that stage of gestation. Thus, protein synthesis relative to the amount of oxygen consumed

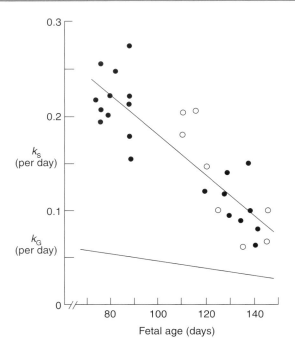

Figure 9.6 Fractional rate of protein synthesis (K_S) over gestation in fetal sheep studied with leucine (H) and lysine (O) radioactive tracers compared with the fractional rate of growth (K_G) in the lower portion of the figure (—). (Adapted from (1) Battaglia and Meschia,[6] (2) Meier et al.,[96] and (3) Kennaugh et al.[97])

decrease in the whole-body k_G.[99] Many anabolic endocrine–paracrine factors, such as insulin, pituitary, and placental growth hormone, placental lactogen, IGFs, and epidermal growth factors increase in late gestation. A direct relationship with such growth factors cannot be made, however, since most studies indicate an increasing concentration or secretion of these substances over gestation.[100] Simultaneous increases in binding proteins and changes in receptor density and binding capacity also develop that interact with and regulate the action of the various growth factors, thereby modulating their direct effects on promoting protein synthesis and cell growth.

Fetal skeletal muscle amino acid metabolism

Skeletal muscle in the fetal sheep takes up both essential and non-essential amino acids from the circulation,[101] reflecting the relatively high rate of protein synthesis and nitrogen accretion of the fetus. Under hyperinsulinemic conditions, in which glucose and amino acids are also infused to maintain normal concentrations, net uptake of most amino acids by skeletal muscle increases, reflecting reduced rates of proteolysis more than increased rates of protein synthesis. Protein synthesis is more strongly regulated by the plasma concentration of amino acids than by insulin alone. IGF-I acts similarly to insulin. Glucose utilization also increases the net protein balance, perhaps simply by substituting its carbon for that of amino acids in the tricarboxylic acid cycle, indicating that a positive energy balance and the provision of amino acids allow insulin (and IGF-1) to promote nitrogen accretion most effectively.[102,103]

Acknowledgments

Preparation of this manuscript was supported in part by research grants HD42815, HD28794 and DK52138 (WW Hay, PI) from the National Institutes of Health.

is quite constant from mid-gestation until term.[98] The reduction in the protein synthetic rate over gestation also is related to the changing proportion of body mass contributed by the major organs. For example, the body-weight-specific mass of skeletal muscle, which has a relatively lower k_S, increases more than other organs in late gestation, which would contribute to a

REFERENCES

1. Hay Jr WW. Energy and substrate requirements of the placenta and fetus. Proc Nutr Soc 1991; 50: 321–36.
2. Hay Jr WW. Metabolic interrelationships of placenta and fetus. Placenta 1995; 16: 19–30.
3. Hay Jr WW, Regnault TRH. Fetal requirements and placental transfer of nitrogenous compounds. In: Polin RA, Fox WW, Abman SH, eds. Fetal and Neonatal Physiology, 3rd edn. Philadelphia: WB Saunders; 2003, pp. 509–27.
4. Fowden AL, Ward JW, Wooding FPB, et al. Programming placental nutrient transport capacity. J Physiol 572; 1: 5–15.
5. Fowden AL, Sibley C, Reik W, Constancia M. Imprinted genes, placental development and fetal growth. Horm Res 2006; 65 (suppl. 3): 50–8.
6. Battaglia FC, Meschia G. An Introduction to Fetal Physiology. Orlando: Academic Press; 1986.
7. Sparks JW, Girard J, Battaglia FC. An estimate of the caloric requirements of the human fetus. Biol Neonate 1980; 38: 113–9.
8. Hay Jr WW, DiGiacomo JE, Meznarich HK, et al. Effects of glucose and insulin on fetal glucose oxidation and oxygen consumption. Am J Physiol 1989; 256: E704–13.
9. DiGiacomo JE, Hay Jr WW. Fetal glucose metabolism and oxygen consumption during sustained maternal and fetal hypoglycemia. Metabolism 1990; 39: 193–202.
10. Hay Jr WW, Meznarich HK. Effect of maternal glucose concentration on uteroplacental glucose consumption and transfer in pregnant sheep. Proc Soc Exp Biol Med 1988; 190: 63–9.
11. Hay Jr WW, Molina RD, DiGiacomo JE, et al. Model of placental glucose consumption and transfer. Am J Physiol 1990; 258: R569–77.
12. Hay Jr WW. Placental function. In: Gluckman PD, Heymann MA, eds. Scientific Basis of Pediatric and Perinatal Medicine, 2nd edn. London: Edward Arnold; 1996, pp. 213–27.
13. Molina RD, Meschia G, Battaglia FC, et al. Maturation of placental glucose transfer capacity in the ovine pregnancy. Am J Physiol 1991; 261: R697–R704.
14. Hay Jr WW. Nutrition and development of the fetus: carbohydrate and lipid metabolism. In: Walker WA, Watkins JB, Duggan CP, eds. Nutrition in Pediatrics (Basic Science and Clinical Applications), 3rd edn, Hamilton, Ontario: BC Decker; 2003, pp. 449–70.
15. Settle P, Sibley CP, Doughty IM, et al. Placental lactate transporter activity and expression in intrauterine growth restriction. J Soc Gynecol Investig 2006; 13: 357–63.
16. Jansson T, Wennergren M, Illsley MP. Glucose transporter protein expression in human placenta throughout gestation and in intrauterine growth retardation. J Clin Endocrinol Metab 1993; 77: 1554–62.
17. Hahn T, Hartmann M, Blaschitz A, et al. Localisation of the high affinity glucose transporter protein GLUT1 in the placenta of human,

marmoset monkey (Callithrix jacchus) and rat at different developmental stages. Cell Tiss Res 1995; 280: 49–57.

18. Wolf HG, Desoye G. Immunohistochemical localization of glucose transporters and insulin receptors in human fetal membranes at term. Histochemistry 1993; 100: 379–85.

19. Ehrhardt RA, Bell AW. Developmental increases in glucose transporter concentration in the sheep placenta. Am J Physiol 1997; 273: R1132–41.

20. Limesand SW, Regnault TRH, Hay Jr WW. Characterization of glucose transporter 8 (GLUT8) in the ovine placenta of normal and growth restricted fetuses. Placenta 2004; 25: 70–7.

21. Wooding FBP, Fowden AL, Bell AW, et al. Localisation of glucose transport in the ruminant placenta: implications for sequential use of transporter isoforms. Placenta 2005; 26: 626–40.

22. Das UG, Schroeder RE, Hay Jr WW, Devaskar SU. Time dependent regulation of rodent and ovine placental glucose transporter (Glut 1) protein. Am J Physiol 1998; 274: R339–47.

23. Das UG, He J, Ehrhardt RA, Hay Jr WW, Devaskar SU. Time-dependent physiological regulation of the ovine placental GLUT-3 glucose transporter protein. Am J Physiol 2000; 279: R2252–61.

24. Aldoretta PW, Carver TD, Hay Jr WW. Ovine uteroplacental glucose and oxygen metabolism in relation to chronic changes in maternal and fetal glucose concentrations. Placenta 1994; 15: 753–64.

25. Hay Jr WW, Meznarich HK, DiGiacomo JE, et al. Effects of insulin and glucose concentrations on glucose utilization in fetal sheep. Pediatr Res 1988; 23: 281–7.

26. Reid GJ, Flozak AS, Simmons RA. Increased expression of glucose transporter protein-1 (GLUT-1) in the growth retarded placenta. J Soc Gynecol Invest 1995; 2: 193.

27. Hay Jr WW, Sparks JW, Wilkening RB, et al. Fetal glucose uptake and utilization as functions of maternal glucose concentration. Am J Physiol 1984; 246: E237–42.

28. Sunehag AL, Haymond MW, Schanler RJ, Reeds PJ, Bier DM. Gluconeogenesis in very low birth weight infants receiving total parenteral nutrition. Diabetes 1999; 48: 791–800.

29. Carver TD, Quick Jr AN, Teng CC, et al. Leucine metabolism in chronically hypoglycemic, hypoinsulinemic growth restricted fetal sheep. Am J Physiol 1997; 272: E107–17.

30. Das UG, Schroeder RE, Hay Jr WW, Devaskar SU. Time-dependent and tissue-specific effects of circulating glucose on fetal ovine glucose transporters. Am J Physiol 1999; 276: R809–17.

31. Anderson MS, He J, Flowers-Ziegler J, et al. Effects of selective hyperglycemia and hyperinsulinemia on glucose transporters in fetal ovine skeletal muscle. Am J Physiol 2001; 50: R1256–63.

32. Anderson MS, Ziegler JA, Das UG, et al. Glucose transporter protein responses to selective hyperglycemia or hyperinsulinemia in fetal sheep. Am J Physiol 2001; 281: R1545–52.

33. Klip A, Tsakiridis T, Marette A, et al. Regulation of expression of glucose transporters by glucose: a review of studies in vivo and in cell cultures. FASEB J 1994; 8: 43–53.

34. Zarlengo KM, Battaglia FC, Fennessey P, Hay Jr WW. Relationship between glucose utilization rate and glucose concentration in preterm infants. Biol Neonate 1986; 49: 181–9.

35. van Veen LCP, Teng C, Hay Jr WW, et al. Leucine disposal and oxidation rates in the fetal lamb. Metabolism 1987; 36: 48–53.

36. DiGiacomo JE, Hay Jr WW. Effect of hypoinsulinemia and hyperglycemia on fetal glucose utilization and oxidation. Am J Physiol 1990; 259: E506–12.

37. Hay Jr WW, Meznarich HK, Fowden AL. Effect of streptozotocin of rates of ovine fetal glucose utilization, oxidation and production in the sheep fetus. Metabolism 1988; 38: 30–7.

38. Fowden AL, Hay Jr WW. The effects of pancreatectomy on the rates of glucose utilization, oxidation and production in the sheep fetus. Q J Exp Physiol 1988; 73: 973–84.

39. Aldoretta PW, Hay Jr WW. Chronic hyperglycemia induces insulin resistance and glucose intolerance in fetal sheep. Pediatr Res 2001; 49: 307A.

40. Aldoretta PW, Gresores A, Carver TD, Hay Jr WW. Maturation of glucose-stimulated insulin secretion. Biol Neonate 1998; 73: 375–86.

41. Van Assche FA, Hoet JJ, Jack PMB. Endocrine pancreas of the pregnant mother, fetus, and newborn. In: Beard RW, Nathanielsz PW, eds. Fetal Physiology and Medicine, 2nd edn. New York: Dekker; 1984, pp. 127–52.

42. Carver TD, Anderson SM, Aldoretta PW, et al. Glucose suppression of insulin secretion in chronically hyperglycemic fetal sheep. Pediatr Res 1995; 38: 754–62.

43. Catalano P, Buchanan TA. Metabolic changes during normal and diabetic pregnancies. In: Reece EA, Coustan DR, Gabbe SG, eds.

Diabetes in Women, 3rd edn. Philadelphia: Lippincott Williams & Wilkins; 2004, pp. 129–46.

44. Carver TD, Anderson SM, Aldoretta PW, et al. Effect of low-level plus marked 'pulsatile' hyperglycemia on insulin secretion in fetal sheep. Am J Physiol 1996; 271: E865–71.

45. Rozance PJ, Limesand SW, Hay Jr, WW. Decreased nutrient stimulated insulin secretion in chronically hypoglycemic late gestation fetal sheep is due to an intrinsic islet defect. Am J Physiol Endo Metab 2006; 291: E404–11.

46. Fowden AL, Hill DJ. Intrauterine programming of the endocrine pancreas. Br Med Bull 2001; 60: 123–42.

47. Dahri S, Reusen B, Remacle C, Hoet JJ. Nutritional influences on pancreatic development – potential links with non-insulin-dependent diabetes. Proc Nutr Soc 1995; 54: 345–56.

48. Limesand SW, Rozance PJ, Zerbe G, Hutton JC, Hay Jr WW. Attenuated insulin release and storage in fetal sheep pancreatic islets with intrauterine growth restriction. Endocrinology 2006; 147: 1488–97.

49. Simmons RA, Suponitsky-Kroyter I, Selak MA. Progressive accumulation of mitochondrial DNA mutations and decline in mitochondrial function lead to beta-cell failure, J Biol Chem 2005; 280: 28785–91.

50. Barker DJ. Adult consequences of fetal growth restriction. Clin Obstet Gynecol 2006; 49: 270–83.

51. Fowden AL, Silver MA. The effects of thyroid hormones on oxygen and glucose metabolism in the sheep fetus during late gestation. J Physiol 1995; 482: 203–13.

52. Fowden Al, Mundy L, Silver M. Developmental regulation of glucogenesis in the sheep fetus during late gestation. J Physiol 1998; 508: 937–47.

53. Fowden AL, Comline RS, Silver M. The effects of cortisol on the concentration of glycogen in different tissues in the chronically catheterized fetal pig. Q J Exp Physiol 1985; 70: 23–32.

54. Padbury JF, Ludlow JK, Ervin MG, et al. Thresholds for physiological effects of plasma catecholamines in fetal sheep. Am J Physiol 1992; 252: E530–7.

55. Devaskar SU, Ganguli S, Styer D, et al. Glucagon and glucose dynamics in sheep: evidence for glucagon resistance in fetus. Am J Physiol 1984; 246: E256–65.

56. Liechty EA, Boyle DW, Moorehead H, et al. Effects of circulating IGF-I on glucose and amino acid kinetics in the ovine fetus. Am J Physiol 1996; 271: E177–85.

57. Oliver MH, Harding JE, Breier BH, et al. Glucose but not mixed amino acid infusion regulates plasma insulin-like growth factor-I concentrations in fetal sheep. Pediatr Res 1993; 34: 62–5.

58. Han VKM, Fowden Al. Paracrine regulation of fetal growth. In: Ward RHT, Smith SK, Donnai D, eds. Early Fetal Growth and Development. London: RCOG Press; 1994, pp. 275–91.

59. Liechty EA, Boyle DA, Moorehead H, et al. Effect of hyperinsulinemia on ovine fetal leucine kinetics during prolonged maternal fasting. Am J Physiol 1992; 263: E696–702.

60. Stephens E, Thureen PJ, Goalstone ML, et al. Fetal hyperinsulinemia increases farnesylation of p21 Ras in fetal tissues. Am J Physiol 2001; 281: E217–23.

61. Thureen PJ, Scheer B, Anderson SM, Hay Jr WW. Effect of hyperinsulinemia on amino acid utilization in the ovine fetus. Am J Physiol 2000; 279: E1294–304.

62. Brown LD, Hay Jr WW. Effect of hyperinsulinemia on amino acid utilization and oxidation independent of glucose metabolism in the ovine fetus. Am J Physiol Endo Metab 2006; E1333–40.

63. Shelley HJ. Glycogen reserves and their changes at birth and in anoxia. Br Med Bull 1961; 17: 137–43.

64. Shellhase E, Kuroki Y, Emrie PA, et al. Expression of pulmonary surfactant apoproteins in the developing rat lung. Clin Res 1989; 37: 208A.

65. Mott JC. The ability of young mammals to withstand total oxygen lack. Br Med Bull 1961; 17: 144–8.

66. Barry JS, Davidsen ML, Limesand SW, et al. Developmental changes in ovine myocardial glucose transporters and insulin signaling during hyperthermia-induced intrauterine fetal growth restriction. Exp Biol Med 2006; 231: 566–75.

67. Sparks JW. Augmentation of glucose supply. Semin Perinatol 1979; 3: 141–55.

68. Marconi A, Cetin E, Davoli A, et al. An evaluation of fetal glucogenesis in intrauterine growth retarded pregnancies: steady state fetal and maternal enrichments of plasma glucose at cordocentesis. Metabolism 1993; 42: 860–4.

69. DiGiacomo JE, Hay Jr WW. Regulation of placental glucose transfer and consumption by fetal glucose production. Pediatr Res 1989; 25: 429–34.

70. Fowden AL. The endocrine regulation of fetal metabolism and growth. In: Gluckman PD, Johnston BM, Nathanielsz PW, eds. Advances in Fetal Physiology: Reviews in Honor of GC Liggins. Ithaca: Perinatology Press; 1989, pp. 229–43.

71. Widdowson EM. Growth and composition of the human fetus and newborn. In: Assali NS, ed. Biology of Gestation, Vol. 2. New York: Academic Press; 1968, pp. 1–48.

72. Coleman RA. Placental metabolism and transport of lipid. Fed Proc 1986; 45: 2519–23.

73. Magnusson-Olsson AL, Hamark B, Ericsson A, et al. Gestational and hormonal regulation of human placental lipoprotein lipase. J Lipid Res 2006; 47(11): 2551–61 (22 August, E-pub ahead of print).

74. Magnusson AI, Watterman IJ, Wennergren M, et al. Triglyceride hydrolase activities and expression of fatty acid binding proteins in the human placenta in pregnancies complicated by intrauterine growth restriction and diabetes. J Clin Endocrinol Metab 2004; 89: 4607–14.

75. Elphick MC, Hull D, Sanders RR. Concentrations of free fatty acids in maternal and umbilical cord blood during elective cesarean section. Br J Obstet Gynaecol 1976; 83: 539–44.

76. Hendrickse W, Stammers JP, Hull D. The transfer of free fatty acids across the human placenta. Br J Obstet Gynaecol 1985; 92: 945–53.

77. Thomas CR, Lowy C. Placental transfer of free fatty acids: factors affecting transfer across the guinea pig placenta. J Dev Physiol 1983; 5: 323–32.

78. Regnault TRH, de Vrijer B, Battaglia FC. Transport and metabolism of amino acids in placenta. Endocrine 2002; 19: 23–41.

79. Ayuk PT, Sibley C, Donnai P, et al. Development and polarization of cationic amino acid transporters and regulators in the human placenta. Am J Physiol 2000; 278: c1162–71.

80. Mahendran D, Byrne S, Donnai P, et al. Na$^+$ Transport, H$^+$ concentration gradient dissipation, and system A amino acid transporter activity in purified microvillous plasma membrane isolated from first-trimester human placenta: comparison with the term microvillous membrane. Am J Obstet Gynecol 1994; 171: 1534–40.

81. Novak DA, Beveridge MJ, Malandro M, Seo J. Ontogeny of amino acid transport system A in rat placenta. Placenta 1996; 17: 643–51.

82. Malandro MS, Beveridge MJ, Kilberg MS, Novak DA. Ontogeny of cationic amino acid transport systems in rat placenta. Am J Physiol 1994; 267: C804–11.

83. Jansson N, Pettersson J, Haafiz A, et al. Down-regulation of placental transport of amino acids precedes the development of intrauterine growth restriction in rats fed a low protein diet. J Physiol 2006; 1: 576(pt3): 935–46 (17 August, E-pub ahead of print).

84. de Vrijer B, Davidsen ML, Wilkening RB, et al. Altered placental and fetal expression of IGFs and IGF-binding proteins associated with intrauterine growth restriction in fetal sheep during early and mid-pregnancy. Pediatr Res 2006; 60(5): 507–12 (11 Sept, E-pub ahead of print.)

85. Smith CH, Moe AJ, Ganapathy V, et al. Nutrient transport pathways across the epithelium of the placenta. Annu Rev Nutr 1992; 12: 183–206.

86. Milley JR. Uptake of exogenous substrates during hypoxia in fetal lambs. Am J Physiol 1988; 254: E572–74.

87. Milley JR. Exogenous substrate uptake by fetal lambs during reduced glucose delivery. Am J Physiol 1993; 264(2, pt 1): E250–6.

88. Smith CH. Incubation techniques and investigation of placental transport mechanisms in vitro. Placenta 1981; 2: 163–8.

89. Dancis J, Lind J, Oratz M, et al. Placental transfer of proteins in human gestation. Am J Obstet Gynecol 1961; 82: 167–71.

90. Lemons JA, Adcock 3rd EW, Jones Jr MD, et al. Umbilical uptake of amino acids in the unstressed fetal lamb. J Clin Invest 1976; 58: 1428–34.

91. Marconi AM, Battaglia FC, Meschia G, et al. A comparison of amino acid arteriovenous differences across the liver, hindlimb and placenta in the fetal lamb. Am J Physiol 1989; 257: E909–15.

92. Jansson T, Cetin I, Powell TL, et al. Placental transport and metabolism in fetal overgrowth – a workshop report. Placenta 2006; 27(suppl. A), Trophoblast Research 20: S109–13.

93. Gresham EL, James EJ, Raye JR, et al. Production and excretion of urea by the fetal lamb. Pediatrics 1972; 50: 372–9.

94. van Veen LCP, Teng C, Hay Jr WW, et al. Leucine disposal and oxidation rates in the fetal lamb. Metabolism 1987; 36: 48–53.

95. Battaglia FC, Meschia G. Fetal nutrition. Annu Rev Nutr 1988; 8: 43–61.

96. Meier PR, Peterson RG, Bonds DR, et al. Rates of protein synthesis and turnover in fetal life. Am J Physiol 1981; 240: E320–4.

97. Kennaugh JM, Bell AW, Teng C, et al. Ontogenetic changes in the rates of protein synthesis and leucine oxidation during fetal life. Pediatr Res 1987; 22: 688–92.

98. Bell AW, Kennaugh JM, Battaglia FC, et al. Uptake of amino acids and ammonia at mid-gestation by the fetal lamb. Q J Exp Physiol 1989; 74: 635–43.

99. Waterlow JL, Garlick PJ, Millward DJ. Protein Turnover in Mammalian Tissues and in the Whole Body. Amsterdam: Elsevier/North-Holland Biomedical Press; 1978.

100. Milner RDG, Hill DJ. Interaction between endocrine and paracrine peptides in prenatal growth control. Eur J Pediatr 1987; 146: 113.

101. Wilkening RB, Boyle DW, Teng C, et al. Amino acid uptake by fetal ovine hindlimb under normal and euglycemic hyperinsulinemic states. Am J Physiol 1994; 266: E72–8.

102. Liechty EA, Boyle DW, Moorehead H, et al. Increased fetal glucose concentration decreases ovine fetal leucine oxidation independent of insulin. Am J Physiol 1993; 265: E617–23.

103. Liechty EA, Lemons JA. Changes in ovine fetal hindlimb amino acid metabolism during maternal fasting. Am J Physiol 1984; 246: E430.

10 Pathogenesis of gestational diabetes mellitus

Yariv Yogev, Avi Ben-Haroush and Moshe Hod

Introduction

Gestational diabetes mellitus (GDM) is characterized by carbohydrate intolerance of variable severity, with onset or first recognition during pregnancy. This definition applies whether or not there is a need for insulin and whether or not it disappears after the pregnancy. It does not apply to gravid patients with previously diagnosed diabetes.[1] A detailed discussion of glucose regulation in pregnancy is beyond the scope of this paper. However, two points are important for the discussion that follows. First, pregnancy is normally attended by progressive insulin resistance that begins near mid-pregnancy and progresses through the third trimester to levels that approximate the insulin resistance seen in individuals with Type 2 diabetes. The insulin resistance appears to result from a combination of increased maternal adiposity and the insulin-desensitizing effects of hormonal products of the placenta. The fact that insulin resistance rapidly abates following delivery suggests that the major contributors to this state of resistance are placental hormones. The second point is that pancreatic beta cells normally increase their insulin secretion to compensate for the insulin resistance of pregnancy. As a result, changes in circulating glucose levels over the course of pregnancy are quite small compared with the large changes in insulin sensitivity. Robust plasticity of beta-cell function in the face of progressive insulin resistance is the hallmark of normal glucose regulation during pregnancy.

Although pregnancy is a carbohydrate-intolerant state, only a small proportion of pregnant women (3–5%) develop GDM. As pregnancy advances, the increasing tissue resistance to insulin creates a demand for more insulin. In the great majority of women, insulin requirements are readily met, so the balance between insulin resistance and insulin supply is maintained. However, if resistance becomes dominant due to impaired insulin secretion, hyperglycemia develops. In the majority of such cases, it develops in the last half of pregnancy, with insulin resistance increasing progressively until delivery, when, in most cases, it rapidly disappears.

Controversy still exists about the screening and diagnosis of GDM. In the majority of cases, carbohydrate intolerance is asymptomatic and can be detected only by routine screening challenge tests. A detailed discussion of variations in the diagnostic criteria is beyond the scope of this chapter, but the main issue is that the diagnosis of GDM is based on the screening of a large number of apparently healthy young women.

As in Type 1 diabetes mellitus, GDM is associated with both insulin resistance and impaired insulin secretion.[2–4] The two disorders also share the same risk factors, have a corresponding prevalence within a given population and have the same genetic susceptibility; therefore, they are assumed to be etiologically indistinct, with one preceding the other.

In this chapter, the development of insulin resistance during pregnancy, hormones and newly discovered factors associated with insulin resistance and secretion, the insulin-signaling system during normal and diabetic pregnancy, and metabolic predictors of diabetes will be discussed.

Insulin sensitivity and resistance in pregnancy

The majority of women with GDM appear to have beta-cell dysfunction that occurs on a background of chronic insulin resistance. As noted above, pregnancy normally induces quite marked insulin resistance. This physiological insulin resistance also occurs in women with GDM. However, it occurs on a background of chronic insulin resistance to which the insulin resistance of pregnancy is partially additive. As a result, pregnant women with GDM tend to have even greater insulin resistance than normal pregnant women.

The cellular mechanisms underlying insulin resistance in normal and diabetic pregnancy are still unknown. The measurement of fasting insulin concentrations and the calculation of fasting insulin:glucose ratios can provide a qualitative but not a quantitative estimation of insulin sensitivity. In non-pregnant patients, hyperinsulinemic–euglycemic clamps[5] and minimal-model analysis of intravenous glucose tolerance tests (IVGTT)[6,7] have been used to obtain quantitative data about insulin action. The IVGTT model provides data on the glucose infusion that is required to maintain euglycemia during constant insulin infusion. However, its use in pregnancy is limited owing to the change in the relationship between common measures of body size, such as total body weight and body surface area. Catalano et al.[8,9] were the first to conduct a prospective longitudinal study using the hyperinsulinemic–euglycemic clamp model in obese and non-obese gravid women with normal glucose tolerance tests. They found a 47% decrease in insulin sensitivity in obese gravid women and a 56% decrease in lean gravid women. Differences in whole-body insulin sensitivity tend to be small in the third trimester, owing to the marked effects of pregnancy itself on insulin resistance. Nonetheless, precise and direct measures of insulin sensitivity applied during the third trimester have identified, in women with GDM, exaggerated resistance to insulin's ability to stimulate glucose utilization.[9]

The development of resistance to the glucose-lowering effects of insulin is a normal phenomenon of pregnancy. In a pioneer study, Burt et al.[10] demonstrated that pregnant women experience fewer hypoglycemic events in response to insulin infusion than non-gravid women. Accordingly, later research found women with normal pregnancies had progressively exaggerated insulin responses to ingested glucose, together with a slightly decreased glucose tolerance.[11,12] Using the IVGTT model, Buchanan et al.[13] and Cousins et al.[14] demonstrated a significant (70%) reduction in insulin sensitivity during the second trimester of normal pregnancy, with a return to normal values shortly after delivery. Ryan et al.[2] were the first to report quantitative differences in insulin sensitivity between normal and diabetic pregnancies. Other researchers noted that insulin sensitivity was lower in patients with GDM than in patients with normal pregnancies at 12–14 weeks of gestation, before the point of maximal physiological insulin resistance; however, the difference was not statistically significant. By the third trimester, insulin resistance was similar in the two groups.[8,14]

Much effort has been invested to identify the tissues that contribute to the insulin resistance of pregnancy. Findings in animal models indicate a 40% reduction in insulin-mediated glucose utilization by skeletal muscle, and a similar effect in cardiac muscle and fat cells.[15,16]

It remains unclear whether hepatic insulin sensitivity is altered during gestation. Kalhan et al.[17] and Cowett et al.[18] noted no significant differences in basal glucose production in pregnant women at term compared to non-pregnant control subjects when the data were expressed per kilogram of body weight; however, expression of the data in relation to pre-gravid weight yielded an increase in hepatic glucose production in late pregnancy.[19] Furthermore, in hyperinsulinemic–euglycemic clamp studies, hepatic glucose production was significantly less suppressed in lean and obese patients with GDM than in the control group.[8,9]

Hormonal effect in normal and diabetic pregnancy

Reproductive hormones tend to increase during pregnancy, most of them contribute to insulin resistance and altered beta-cell function.

Estrogen and progesterone

In early pregnancy, both progesterone and estrogen rise but their effects on insulin activity are counterbalanced. Progesterone causes insulin resistance whereas estrogen is protective.[20]

An IVGTT test given to estrogen-treated rats showed a significant decrease in glucose concentrations and a 2-fold increase in insulin concentration;[21] the addition of progesterone was associated with a 70% increase in the insulin response to a glucose challenge test, but there were no alterations in glucose tolerance.[22] In cultured rat adipocyte tissue treated with estrogen, there was no effect on glucose transport, but maximum insulin binding was increased. However, progesterone decreased both maximum glucose transport and insulin binding.[20,21]

Gonzalez et al.[23] evaluated the role played by progesterone and/or 17β-estradiol on sensitivity to insulin action that took place during pregnancy. Ovariectomized rats were treated with different doses of progesterone and/or 17β-estradiol in order to simulate the plasma levels in normal pregnancy rats. A hyperinsulinemic–euglycemic clamp was used to measure insulin sensitivity. The results suggested that the absence of female steroid hormones leads to decreased insulin sensitivity. Thus, the rise in insulin sensitivity during early pregnancy, when plasma concentrations of 17β-estradiol and progesterone are low could be due to 17β-estradiol. However, during late pregnancy, when both plasma concentrations of 17β-estradiol and progesterone are high, the role of 17β-estradiol may serve to antagonize the effect of progesterone, diminishing insulin sensitivity.[23]

Cortisol

Cortisol levels increase as pregnancy advances and by the end of pregnancy concentrations are threefold higher than in the non-pregnant state.[24] Rizza et al.,[25] in a clamp study, demonstrated that under infusion of high amounts of cortisol, hepatic glucose production increased and insulin sensitivity decreased. Findings in a skeletal muscle model showed that an excess of glucocorticoid is characterized by decreased total tyrosine phosphorylation of the insulin receptor; therefore, it seems logical that glucocorticoid-induced insulin resistance is related to a postreceptor mechanism. In a study by Ahmed and Shalayel,[26] 30 pregnant women with GDM and 30 pregnant women with impaired glucose tolerance (IGT) were compared with 30 pregnant women with normal glucose tolerance. The GDM and IGT groups were found to have significantly higher levels of serum cortisol than the control group.

Prolactin

During pregnancy, maternal prolactin levels increase 7- to 10-fold. Gustafson et al.[27] reported that the basal insulin concentration and post-challenge glucose and insulin responses were greater in women with hyperprolactinemia than in healthy controls. These findings were supported by studies showing that the culture of pancreatic islet cells with prolactin induces an increase in insulin secretion.[28] Skouby et al.[29] investigated the relationship between the deterioration in glucose tolerance and plasma prolactin levels in patients with normal and diabetic pregnancies. Oral glucose tolerance tests (OGTT) were performed in late pregnancy and postpartum. In late pregnancy, the GDM group had significantly elevated fasting glucose levels compared to the controls and, after glucose challenge, their insulin responses were significantly diminished and the suppression of glucagon less pronounced.

These differences in glucose metabolism were markedly reduced in the early post-partum period. There was no difference in basal prolactin concentrations between the two groups at either time point. The prolactin levels were also not altered during the OGTT tolerance tests, and there was no correlation between the deterioration in glucose tolerance and the prolactin concentrations in either group. Thus, abnormal prolactin levels are not of pathophysiologic importance in the development of GDM.

Human placental lactogen

Human placental lactogen (hPL) levels rise at the beginning of the second trimester, causing a decrease in phosphorylation of insulin receptor substrate (IRS)-1 and profound insulin resistance.[20] Beck and Daughday[30] demonstrated that overnight infusion of hPL results in abnormal glucose tolerance, and increased insulin and glucose concentration in response to an oral glucose challenge. Accordingly, Brelje et al.[31] found that in islet cell culture, hPL directly stimulates insulin secretion. This may indicate that hPL directly regulates islet cell function and is probably the principal hormone responsible for the increase in islet function observed during normal pregnancy.[31]

Leptin

Leptin is a 16 kDa protein encoded by the ob/ob (obesity) gene secreted by adipocyte tissue. It can modulate energy expenditure by direct action on the hypothalamus. Fasting insulin and leptin concentrations correlate closely with body fat, making leptin a good marker of obesity and insulin resistance. As receptors to leptin are found in skeletal muscle, the liver, the pancreas, adipocyte tissue, the uterus and the placenta, it may be responsible for both peripheral and central insulin resistance. Reductions in leptin concentrations are caused by weight loss, fasting, and starvation; leptin concentrations are increased with weight gain and hyperinsulinemia.

In animal models, using hyperinsulinemic–euglycemic clamp studies, infusion of leptin was found to increase the glucose infusion rate.[32] Leptin levels are significantly higher in pregnancy than in the non-pregnant state, especially during the second and third trimesters[33–35] and this change in circulating leptin concentrations are generally consistent with changes in maternal fat stores and glucose metabolism. Results of studies by Laivuori et al.[36] suggest that pregnancy-associated increases in maternal plasma leptin may result from an up regulation of adipocyte leptin synthesis in the presence of increasing insulin resistance and hyperinsulinemia in the latter half of pregnancy. Investigators have also shown that leptin directly affects whole body insulin sensitivity by regulating the efficiency of insulin-mediated glucose metabolism by skeletal muscle[37] and by hepatic regulation of gluconeogenesis.[38] Leptin may also wield an acute inhibitory effect on insulin secretion.[39] Yamashita et al.[40] suggested that an alteration in leptin action might play a role in GDM and fetal overgrowth weight gain. They found that pregnant mice treated with leptin had markedly lower glucose levels than controls during glucose and insulin challenge tests. However, despite the reduced energy intake and improved glucose tolerance, fetal overgrowth was not reduced.

Results provide evidence that leptin administration during late gestation can reduce adiposity and improve glucose tolerance in the model of spontaneous GDM. These data suggest that alterations in placental leptin levels may contribute to the regulation of fetal growth independently of maternal glucose levels.

Kautzky-Willer et al.[41] measured plasma concentrations of leptin and beta-cell hormones during fasting and after an oral glucose load (OGTT of 75 g) in pregnant women with GDM and normal glucose tolerance at 28 weeks gestation, and in women who were not pregnant. Plasma leptin was higher in the women with GDM than in the women with normal glucose tolerance, and higher in both these groups than in the non-pregnant controls. No change in plasma leptin concentrations was induced by OGTT in any group. Basal insulin release was higher in women with GDM than in the women with normal glucose tolerance. The authors concluded that women with GDM and no change in plasma leptin on oral glucose loading have increased plasma leptin concentrations during and after pregnancy. Vitoratos et al.[42] investigated the changes in leptin levels and the relationship between leptin substance and insulin and glucose in pregnant women with GDM. Plasma leptin levels were measured in peripheral vein blood samples from healthy and diabetic women at 29 and 33 weeks gestation. Results showed a correlation of plasma leptin levels with fasting plasma insulin levels and plasma glucose levels measured 1 h after oral administration of 50 g of glucose. Serum leptin levels were significantly higher in the women with GDM than in the women with uncomplicated pregnancies. The GDM group also showed a significant, positive correlation of serum leptin levels with glycosylated hemoglobin levels, fasting serum insulin levels and plasma glucose levels measured 1 h after administration of 50 g of glucose. Thus, levels of leptin are elevated in women with GDM, and leptin metabolism depends on insulin levels and the severity of the diabetes. Wiznitzer et al.[43] reported that umbilical cord leptin concentration was an independent risk factor for fetal macrosomia in non-diabetic pregnant women.

Other factors affecting gestational diabetes mellitus

Tumor necrosis factor-alfa

Tumor necrosis factor-alfa (TNF-α) has been implicated in the pathogenesis of insulin resistance in Type 2 diabetes mellitus, but only limited data are available with regard to GDM. Coughlan et al.[44] investigated the effect of exogenous glucose on the release of TNF-α from placental and adipose tissue obtained from normal and diabetic pregnant women. They found significantly greater TNF-α release under conditions of high glucose concentrations in the GDM group. As TNF-α has been implicated in the regulation of glucose and lipid metabolism, and in insulin resistance, these data are consistent with the hypothesis that TNF-α is involved in the pathogenesis and/or progression of GDM.

Catalano et al.[45] reported that changes in insulin sensitivity from early to late pregnancy correlated with a gradual increase in TNF-α levels, which in turn correlated with the percentage change in body weight.

Adrenomedullin

Adrenomedullin is a newly discovered hypotensive peptide involved in the insulin regulatory system and it may play a rule in modifying diabetes in pregnancy. Di Iorio et al.[46] studied its correlation to GDM. Adrenomedullin concentrations were measured in maternal and fetal plasma, and in amniotic fluid in diabetic and non-diabetic pregnancies. Overall amniotic fluid concentration was higher in the pregnant diabetic women (Type 1 or GDM) but there was no between group difference in maternal and fetal plasma levels. These findings suggest that placental adrenomedullin production is up-regulated in diabetic pregnancy and that it may be important to prevent excessive vasoconstriction of placental vessels.

Adiponectin

Adiponectin is an adipose tissue hormone, which is a specific plasma protein that is secreted by adipocytes. It may facilitate the regulation of the glucose and lipid metabolism. Adiponectin decreases the hepatic glucose production and insulin resistance by up-regulating fatty acid oxidation.[47] Adiponectin also suppresses the secretion of TNF-α by adipose tissue, a factor that is known to contribute to insulin resistance.[48] Studies have shown that adiponectin serum levels were decreased in obese subjects[49] and patients with Type 2 diabetes.[50] In studies with rhesus monkeys, adiponectin plasma levels were significantly decreased with the progression of obesity and insulin resistance.[51] In all probability, adiponectin increases insulin sensitivity by enhancing the beta oxidation of free fatty acids and by decreasing the intracellular concentrations of triglycerides.[52,53] In patients with Type 2 diabetes, who have the same risk factors for GDM, i.e. obesity, maternal age, ethnic origin, and family history, lower serum levels of adiponectin were detected. In mice, the intravenous administration of adiponectin was associated with loss of weight and reduced plasma concentrations of fatty acids;[54] the proportion of total body fat mass was correlated negatively with adiponectin serum levels.[55] The data suggests that low plasma adiponectin concentration during even early pregnancy may be associated with subsequent development of GDM.[56–58] Levels of adiponectin have been assessed in fetal cord at delivery.[58] A cord blood adiponectin level was extremely high in comparison to serum levels in children and adults and was positively correlated to fetal birth weights. No correlation was found between cord adiponectin levels and maternal body mass index, cord leptin, or insulin levels. Cord adiponectin levels were significantly higher compared with maternal levels at birth and no correlation was found between cord and maternal adiponectin levels. There were no significant differences between adiponectin levels at birth and 4 days postpartum. These findings indicate that adiponectin in cord blood is derived from fetal and not from placental or maternal tissues. The high adiponectin levels in newborns compared with adults may be the result of deficient negative feedback on adiponectin production stemming from lack of adipocyte hypertrophy, low percentage of body fat, or a different distribution of fat storage in newborns. Adiponectin may emerge as a significant factor in carbohydrate-fat metabolism and in the development of insulin resistance during pregnancy. Data suggests that there are decreased adiponectin levels in women with GDM compared with healthy control subjects. This finding supports the concept of a common pathogenesis between Type 2 diabetes and GDM. Although adiponectin level appears to rise throughout pregnancy, its contribution to gestation remains unclear.

Pancreatic beta-cell function in normal pregnancy and gestational diabetes mellitus

Insulin is the main hormone controlling blood glucose concentration. Most commonly, assessment of beta-cell function is made by measuring the fasting insulin concentration or the response to glucose infusion. Fasting plasma insulin increases gradually during pregnancy – by the third trimester levels are 2-fold higher than before pregnancy. Patients with GDM have fasting insulin levels equal to or higher than those of women with non-diabetic pregnancies, with the highest levels occurring in obese women with GDM.

During normal pregnancy, oral and intravenous glucose tolerance deteriorates only slightly, despite the reduction in insulin sensitivity.[13] The main mechanism responsible for that phenomenon is a gradual increase in insulin secretion by the beta cells. Kual[12] reported a hyperbolic relationship between insulin sensitivity and beta-cell responsiveness to glucose in both pregnant and non-pregnant women, pointing to a role for the beta cells in pathological states such as GDM and demonstrating the magnitude of the change in insulin secretion that is necessary to maintain glucose tolerance. The mechanism responsible for increase insulin secretion during pregnancy is not well understood. A major contributing factor is the increase in the beta-cell mass, a combination of hyperplasia and hypertrophy.[59] The increased beta-cell mass can contribute to the increased fasting insulin concentration despite normal or lowered fasting glucose concentrations in late pregnancy, and the enhanced insulin response to glucose during pregnancy (2- to 3-fold above non-pregnant levels).

In GDM, the early insulin response to OGTT (15–30 min after glucose ingestion) is reduced compared to non-diabetic pregnant control women, suggesting a defect in the beta-cell response.[60] First-phase beta-cell responses to glucose infusion in GDM patients is also been reported to be reduced. GDM tends to milder in women with a normal beta-cell response and they are at relatively low risk for developing diabetes.[61]

Genetics, immunology and gestational diabetes mellitus

Some GDM patients manifest evidence for autoimmunity towards beta cells (insulin autoantibodies and anti-islet cell antibodies); however, the prevalence of such autoimmunity has been reported to be extremely low (< 10%).[62,63] Mutations in the glucokinase gene occur in no more than 5% of GDM patients.[64] The inheritance of GDM was studied in a group of 100 women with previous GDM.[65] The women were reinvestigated 11 years postpartum and 60% were found to have either IGT or Type 2 diabetes. An investigation of their parents showed that a substantial proportion had neither parent affected with IGT or Type 2 diabetes, which suggests a polygenic inheritance or environmental influence rather autosomal dominance inheritance with high penetration rates. In addition, animal studies have shown that prenatal exposure to a diabetic intrauterine milieu increases the risk of GDM.

Harder et al.[66] reported that the prevalence of Type 2 diabetes was significantly greater in mothers than in fathers of women with GDM, and there was also significant aggregation of Type 2 diabetes in the maternal–grandmaternal line compared to the paternal–grandpaternal line. Therefore, that may suggest that a history of Type 2 diabetes on the mother's side might be considered as a particular risk factor for GDM.

The possible genetic background of GDM remains unclear. In particular, its association with human leukocyte antigen (HLA) class II polymorphism has been poorly studied and the results are conflicting. In attempt to clarify these discrepancies, Vambergue et al.[67] reported that the distribution of HLA class II polymorphism was not significantly different between GDM and IGT samples, and there was no significant variation in DRB1*03 and DRB1*04 allele frequencies. These data provide further evidence that Type 1 or insulin-dependent diabetes mellitus (IDDM) HLA class II susceptibility alleles cannot serve as genetic markers for susceptibility to glucose intolerance during pregnancy.

Ober et al.[68] studied the restriction fragment length polymorphisms near 'candidate diabetogenic genes' in order to identify molecular markers for GDM genes. Genotypes for the insulin hypervariable region (HVR), insulin-like growth factor II (IGF2), insulin receptor (IR), and glucose transporter (GLUT1) were studied in GDM and control subjects. The results supported the hypothesis that GDM has heterogeneous phenotypic and genotypic features, and that the risk for GDM in black and Caucasian subjects is not related to obesity *per se* but to interactions between obesity and IR alleles. In Caucasian women, IR and IGF2 alleles interact to confer an additional risk for GDM. Thus, in some women, genes responsible for susceptibility to GDM may be similar to the genes conferring risk of Type 2 diabetes, whereas in others, novel genes may contribute to GDM.

Insulin signaling system in normal pregnancy and in gestational diabetes mellitus

The action of insulin is triggered when it binds to the insulin receptor (IR). The IR belongs to the IGF receptor (IGFR) family, which possesses an intrinsic tyrosine kinase (TK) activity. The receptor is composed of two alfa subunits, each linked to a beta subunit and to each other by disulfide bonds; only the beta subunit has enzymatic TK activity. When insulin binds to the receptor, the conformational change activates the beta-subunit and autophosphorylation begins. Thus, activation of the TK enzyme leads to increased tyrosine phosphorylation

of cellular substrates. IRS-1, a cytosolic protein, binds to the phosphorylated intracellular substrates, thereby transmitting the insulin signal downstream. The distribution of the IRS proteins tends to be tissue specific: IRS-2 is more copious in the liver and pancreas, whereas both IRS-1 and IRS-2 are widely expressed in skeletal muscle. Insulin stimulates the activation and binding of the lipid kinase enzyme, phosphatidylinositol (PI)-3-kinase, and its binding to IRS-1. The formation of PI is essential for insulin action on glucose transport. Knockout of the IRS-1 gene causes only a moderate increase in insulin resistance due to increased insulin secretion, but not overt diabetes. In women with GDM, the skeletal muscle contains lower levels of IRS-1 protein and significantly less insulin-stimulated IRS-1 tyrosine phosphorylation, while levels of the IRS-2 protein are increased. These findings suggest that the insulin resistance of GDM may be exerted through a decrease in the insulin resistance cascade at the level of the IRS proteins. The increased IRS-2 level may be a compensation for the reduced IRS-1 level.[69] Glucose uptake by cells is mediated by a family of membrane proteins, GLUT1–GLUT4, which have a significant sequence similarity. GLUT4 is the main insulin-sensitive glucose transport, expressed uniquely in skeletal and cardiac muscles and adipose tissue. Garvey et al.[70] reported that in rectus abdominis taken from lean and obese women with GDM, GLUT4 content was similar. In GDM, GLUT4 gene expression is normal in skeletal muscles. To the extent that these muscles are representative of the total muscle mass, insulin resistance in skeletal muscle may involve impaired GLUT4 function or translocation, but not its depletion, as observed in adipose tissue. Garvey et al.[71] demonstrated that the insulin-stimulated glucose transport in adipocyte tissue was reduced by 60% at term in women with GDM compared to non-diabetic pregnant women. Moreover, the GLUT4 content in adipocytes was profoundly depleted in 50% of the GDM group. The whole group exhibited a novel abnormality in GLUT4 subcellular distribution; accumulation of GLUT4 in membranes co-fractionating with plasma membranes and high-density microsomes in basal cells, and absence of translocation in response to insulin. These data suggest that abnormalities in cellular traffic or targeting relegate GLUT4 to a membrane compartment from which insulin cannot recruit transporters to the cell surface. This has important implications for skeletal muscle insulin resistance in GDM. The membrane protein plasma cell membrane glycoprotein-1 (PC-1) has been identified as an inhibitor of insulin receptor TK (IRTK) activity. Shao et al.[69] investigated IR function and PC-1 levels in muscle from three groups of obese subjects: women with GDM, pregnant women with normal glucose tolerance and non-pregnant control subjects. No significant differences were found in basal IR tyrosine phosphorylation or IRTK activity among the three groups. After maximal insulin stimulation, IRTK activity increased in all subjects, but was lower in women with GDM by 25 and 39% compared with pregnant and non-pregnant control subjects, respectively. Similarly, IR tyrosine phosphorylation was significantly decreased in the subjects with GDM compared to the other two groups. Treatment of the IR with alkaline phosphatase to dephosphorylate serine/threonine residues significantly increased insulin-stimulated IRTK activity in the pregnant control and GDM subjects, but the rates were still lower than in the non-pregnant controls. PC-1 content in muscle from GDM subjects was increased by 63% compared with pregnant control subjects and by 206% compared with non-pregnant control subjects. PC-1 content was negatively correlated with IR phosphorylation and IRTK. Increased PC-1 content in the pregnant control and GDM groups suggests an excessive phosphorylation of serine/threonine residues in muscle IR, both of which may contribute to the pregnancy-associated decrease in IRTK activity. In GDM, changes worsened, even when controlling for obesity. These post-receptor defects in insulin signaling may contribute to the pathogenesis of GDM and the increased risk for Type 2 diabetes later in life.

Receptor autophosphorylation has also been reported to be impaired in GDM subjects, a finding consistent with their increased insulin resistance.[70] In addition, overexpression of membrane plasma cell differentiation factor-1 (i.e. PC-1) may play a role in developing insulin resistance by inhibiting the TK activity of the IR.[71] In GDM patients, PC-1 levels were significantly higher in skeletal muscle compared to non-diabetic pregnant women.[72]

Summary

GDM is carbohydrate intolerance resulting in hyperglycemia of variable severity with onset or first recognition during pregnancy. The incidence of GDM is 0.15–15%, and it corresponds to the prevalence of Type 2 diabetes and IGT within a given population. The predominant pathogenic factor in GDM could be inadequate insulin secretion. It has been convincingly demonstrated that GDM occurs as a result of a combination of insulin resistance and decreased insulin secretion. The similar frequencies of HLA-DR2, -DR3 and -DR4 antigens in healthy pregnant women and women with GDM,

and the low prevalence of markers for autoimmune destruction of the beta cells in GDM, rule out the possibility that GDM has an autoimmune origin. Pregnancy is associated with profound hormonal changes that have a direct effect on carbohydrate tolerance. In early pregnancy, both progesterone and estrogen levels rise, but their action on insulin is counterbalanced, as progesterone causes insulin resistance and estrogen is protective. In the second trimester, hPL, cortisol and prolactin levels all rise, causing decreased phosphorylation of IRS-1 and profound insulin resistance. In most subjects, pancreatic insulin secretion rise to meet this need, but in those with underlying beta-cell defects, hyperglycemia ensues. In women with GDM, the insulin resistance of pregnancy is exaggerated, especially if fasting hyperglycemia is present, and is related to additional defective tyrosine phosphorylation of the insulin receptor beta-subunit. Recent research suggests that the postreceptor mechanisms that contribute to insulin resistance of pregnancy are multifactorial, but are exerted at the beta-subunit of the IR and at the level of IRS-1. The resistance to insulin-mediated glucose transport appears to be greater in skeletal muscle from GDM subjects than from pregnancy alone. There is also a modest but significant decrease in the maximal IR tyrosine phosphorylation in muscle from obese GDM subjects. Results also suggest that increased IR serine/threonine phosphorylation and PC-1 could underlie the insulin resistance of pregnancy and contribute to the pathogenesis of GDM.

Whether additional defects are exerted further downstream from IRS-1 remains to be investigated. GDM is a predictor of diabetes (mainly Type 2) later in life. The cumulative incidence of Type 2 diabetes is 50% at 5 years. GDM is also a predictor, or even an early manifestation, of the metabolic (insulin resistance) syndrome. GDM is a cardiovascular risk factor and affected patients should be screened to prevent late complications.

REFERENCES

1. Metzger BE, Coustan DR. Summary and recommendations of the Fourth International Workshop–Conference on Gestational Diabetes Mellitus. Diabetes Care 1998; 21: B161–7.
2. Ryan EA, O'Sullivan MJ, Skyler JS. Insulin action during pregnancy: studies with the euglycemic clamp technique. Diabetes 1985; 34: 380–9.
3. Catalano PM, Tyzbir ED, Wolfe RR, et al. Carbohydrate metabolism during pregnancy in control subjects and women with gestational diabetes. Am J Physiol 1993; 264: E60–7.
4. Kuhl C. Insulin secretion and insulin resistance in pregnancy and GDM: implications for diagnosis and management. Diabetes 1991; 40: 18–24.
5. DeFronzo RA, Tobin JD, Andres R. Glucose clamp technique: a method for quantifying insulin secretion and resistance. Am J Physiol 1979; 237: E241–3.
6. Bergman RN, Ider YZ, Bowden CR, Cobelli C. Quantitative estimation of insulin sensitivity. Am J Physiol 1979; 236: E667–77.
7. Bergman RN. The Lilly Lecture 1989. Toward a physiological understanding of glucose tolerance: minimal model approach. Diabetes 1989; 38: 1512–28.
8. Catalano PM, Tyzbir ED, Roman NM, et al. Longitudinal changes in insulin release and insulin resistance in nonobese pregnant women. Am J Obstet Gynecol 1991; 165: 1667–72.
9. Catalano PM, Huston L, Amini SB, Kalham SC. Longitudinal change in glucose metabolism during pregnancy in obese women with

normal glucose tolerance and gestational diabetes mellitus. Am J Obstet Gynecol 1999; 180: 903–16.
10. Burt RL. Peripheral utilization of glucose in pregnancy. Insulin tolerance. Obstet Gynecol 1956; 2: 558–664.
11. Spellacy WN, Goetz FC. Plasma insulin in normal late pregnancy. N Engl J Med 1963; 268: 988–91.
12. Kuhl C. Glucose metabolism during and after pregnancy in normal and gestational diabetic women. Acta Endocrinol 1975; 79: 709–19.
13. Buchanan TA, Metzger BE, Freinkel N, Bergman RN. Insulin sensitivity and B-cell responsiveness to glucose during late pregnancy in lean and moderately obese women with normal glucose tolerance or mild gestational diabetes. Am J Obstet Gynecol 1990; 162: 1008–14.
14. Cousins L, Rea C, Crawford M. Longitudinal characterization of insulin sensitivity and body fat in normal and gestational diabetic pregnancies [abstract]. Diabetes 1988; 37: 251A.
15. Hauguel S, Leturque A, Gilbert M, Girard J. Effects of pregnancy and fasting on muscle glucose utilization in the rabbit. Am J Obstet Gynecol 1988; 158: 1215–8.
16. Leturque A, Ferre P, Burnol AF, et al. Glucose utilization rates and insulin sensitivity in vivo in tissues of virgin and pregnant rats. Diabetes 1986; 35: 172–7.
17. Kalhan SC, D'Angelo LJ, Savin SM, Adan SM. Glucose production in pregnant women at term gestation: sources of glucose for the human fetus. J Clin Invest 1979; 63: 388–94.

18. Cowett RA, Susa JB, Kahn CB, et al. Glucose kinetics in non-diabetic and diabetic women during third trimester of pregnancy. Am J Obstet Gynecol 1983; 146: 773–80.

19. Catalano PM, Ishizika T, Friedman JE. Glucose metabolism in pregnancy. In: Principles of Perinatal Neonatal Metabolism, 2nd edn. New York: Springer-Verlag; 1998, pp. 183–206.

20. Ryan EA, Ennes L. Role of gestational hormones in the induction of insulin resistance. J Clin Endocrinol Metab 1988; 67: 341–7.

21. Costrini NV, Kalkhoff RK. Relative effect of pregnancy estradiol and progesterone on plasma insulin and pancreatic islet insulin secretion. J Clin Invest 1971; 50: 992–9.

22. Kalkhoff RK, Jacobson M, Lemper D. Progesterone, pregnancy and the augmented plasma insulin response. J Clin Endocrinol 1970; 31: 24–8.

23. Gonzalez C, Alonso A, Alvarez N, et al. Role of 17beta-estradiol and/or progesterone on insulin sensitivity in the rat: implications during pregnancy. J Endocrinol 2000; 166: 283–9.

24. Gibson M, Tulchinski D. The maternal adrenal. In: Tulchinski D, Ryan KJ, eds. Maternal–fetal Endocrinology. Philadelphia: WB Saunders; 1980, pp. 129–43.

25. Rizza RA, Mandarino LJ, Gerich JE. Cortisol induced insulin resistance in man: impaired suppression of glucose production and stimulation of glucose utilization due to a postreceptor defect of insulin action. Clin Endocrinol Metab 1982; 54: 131–8.

26. Ahmed SA, Shalayel MH. Role of cortisol in the deterioration of glucose tolerance in Sudanese pregnant women. East Afr Med J 1999; 76: 465–7.

27. Gustafson AB, Banasiak MF, Kalkhoff RK. Correlation of hyperprolactinemia with altered plasma insulin and glucose: similarity to effects of late human pregnancy. J Clin Endocrinol Metab 1980; 51: 242–6.

28. Sorenson RL, Brelje TC, Roth C. Effect of steroid and lactogenic hormones on islet of Langerhans: a new hypothesis for the role of pregnancy steroids in the adaptation of islets to pregnancy. Endocrinology 1993; 133: 2227–33.

29. Skouby SO, Kuhl C, Hornnes PJ, Andersen AN. Prolactin and glucose tolerance in normal and gestational diabetic pregnancy. Obstet Gynecol 1986; 67: 17–20.

30. Beck P, Daughday WH. Human placental lactogen: studies of its acute metabolic effects and disposition in normal man. J Clin Invest 1967; 46: 103–10.

31. Brelje TC, Scharp DW, Lacy PE, et al. Effect of homologous placental lactogens, prolactins, and growth hormones on islet B-cell division and insulin secretion in rat, mouse, and human islets: implication for placental lactogen regulation of islet function during pregnancy. Endocrinology 1993; 132: 879–87.

32. Sivitz WI, Walsh SA, Morgan DA, et al. Effect of leptin on insulin sensitivity in normal rats. J Clin Invest 1997; 138: 3395–401.

33. Henson MC, Swan KF, O'Neil JS. Expression of placental leptin and leptin receptor transcripts in early pregnancy and at term. Obstet Gynecol 1998; 92: 1020–8.

34. Masuzaki H, Ogawa Y, Sagawa N. Nonadipose tissue production of leptin: leptin as a novel placenta-derived hormone in humans. Nat Med 1997; 3: 1029–33.

35. Highman TJ, Friedman JE, Huston LP, et al. Longitudinal changes in maternal serum leptin concentrations body composition and resting metabolic rate in pregnancy. Am J Obstet Gynecol 1999; 178: 1010–15.

36. Laivuori H, Kaaja R, Koistinen H, et al. Leptin during and after preeclamptic or normal pregnancy: its relation to serum insulin and insulin sensitivity. Metabolism 2000; 49: 259–63.

37. Cohen B, Novick D, Rubinstein M. Modulation of insulin activities by leptin. Science 1996; 274: 1185–8.

38. Rossetti L, Massillon D, Barzilai N, et al. Short term effects of leptin on hepatic gluconeogenesis and in vivo insulin action. J Biol Chem 1997; 272: 27758–63.

39. Ceddia RB, Koistinen HA, Zierath JR, et al. Analysis of paradoxical observations on the association between leptin and insulin resistance. FASEB J 2002; 16: 1163–76.

40. Yamashita H, Shao J, Ishizuka T, et al. Leptin administration prevents spontaneous gestational diabetes in heterozygous Lepr (db/+) mice: effects on placental leptin and fetal growth. Endocrinology 2001; 142: 2888–97.

41. Kautzky-Willer A, Pacini G, Tura A, et al. Increased plasma leptin in gestational diabetes. Diabetologia 2001; 44: 164–72.

42. Vitoratos N, Salamalekis E, Kassanos D, et al. Maternal plasma leptin levels and their relationship to insulin and glucose in gestational-onset diabetes. Gynecol Obstet Invest 2001; 51: 17–21.

43. Wiznitzer A, Furman B, Zuili I, et al. Cord leptin level and fetal macrosomia. Obstet Gynecol 2000; 96: 707–13.

44. Coughlan MT, Oliva K, Georgiou HM, et al. Glucose-induced release of tumor necrosis factor-alpha from human placental and adipose tissues in gestational diabetes mellitus. Diabet Med 2001; 18: 921–7.

45. Catalano P, Highman T, Huston L, Friedman J. Relationship between reproductive hormones/TNF-a and longitudinal changes in insulin sensitivity during gestation. Diabetes 1996; 45: 175a.

46. Di Iorio R, Marinoni E, Urban G, et al. Fetomaternal adrenomedullin levels in diabetic pregnancy. Horm Metab Res 2001; 33: 486–90.

47. Chandran M, Phillips SA, Ciaraldi T, et al. Adiponectin: More than just another fat cell hormone? Diabetes Care 2003; 26: 2442–50.

48. Hotamisligil GS. The role of TNF- and TNG receptors in obesity and insulin resistance. J Intern Med 1999; 245: 621–5.

49. Arita Y, Kihara S, Ouchi N, et al. Paradoxical decrease of an adipose-specific protein, adiponectin, in obesity. Biochem Biophys Res Commun 1999; 257: 79–83.

50. Weyer C, Funahashi T, Tanaka S, et al. Hypoadiponectimia in obesity and type 2 diabetes: Close association with insulin resistance and hyperinsulinemia. J Clin Endocrinol Metab 2001; 86: 1930–5.

51. Hotta K, Funahashi T, Bodkin NL, et al. Circulating concentrations of the adipocyte protein adiponectin are decreased in parallel with reduced insulin sensitivity during the progression to type 2 diabetes in rhesus monkeys. Diabetes 2001; 50: 1126–33.

52. Hu E, Liang P, Spiegelman BM. AdipoQ is a novel adipose-specific gene dysregulated in obesity. J Biol Chem 1996; 271: 10697–703.

53. Yamauchi T, Kamon J, Waki H, et al. The fat derived hormone adiponectin reverses insulin resistance associated with both lipoatrophy and obesity. Nat Med 2001; 7: 941–6.

54. Kubota N, Terauchi Y, Yamauchi T, et al. Disruption of adiponectin causes insulin resistance and neointimal formation. J Biol Chem 2002; 277: 25863–6.

55. Yang WS, Lee WJ, Funahashi T. Weight reduction increases plasma levels of an adipose-derived anti-inflammatory protein, adiponectins. J Clin Endocrinol Metab 2001; 86: 3815–19.

56. Ranheim T, Haugen F, Staff AC, et al. Adiponectin is reduced in gestational diabetes mellitus in normal weight women. Acta Obstet Gynecol Scand 2004; 83: 341–7.

57. Worda C, Leipold H, Gruber C, et al. Decreased plasma adiponectins concentrations in women with gestational diabetes mellitus. Am J Obstet Gynecol. 2004; 191: 2120–4.

58. Williams MA, Qiu C, Muy-Rivera M, et al. Plasma adiponectins concentrations in early pregnancy and subsequent risk of gestational diabetes mellitus. J Clin Endocrinol Metab. 2004; 89: 2306–11.

59. Van Assche FA, Aerts L, De Prins F. A morphological study of the endocrine pancreas in human pregnancy. Br J Obstet Gynecol 1978; 85: 818–20.

60. Swinn RA, Warham NJ, Gregory R, et al. Excessive secretion of insulin precursors characterizes and predicts gestational diabetes. Diabetes 1995; 44: 911–15.

61. Kjos SL, Peters RK, Xiang A, et al. Predicting future diabetes in Latino women with gestational diabetes: utility of early postpartum glucose tolerance testing. Diabetes 1995; 44: 586–91.

62. Damm P, Kuhl C, Buschard K, et al. Prevalence and predictive value of women with islet cell antibodies and insulin autoantibodies in women with gestational diabetes. Diabet Med 1994; 11: 558–63.

63. Catalano PM, Tyzbir ED, Simms EAH. Incidence and significance of islet cell antibodies in women with previous gestational diabetes. Diabetes Care 1990; 113: 478–83.

64. Stoffel M, Bell KL, Blacburn CL, et al. Identification of glucokinase mutations in subjects with gestational diabetes mellitus. Diabetes 1993; 42: 937–40.

65. McLeallan JAS, Barrow BA, Levy JC, et al. Prevalence of diabetes mellitus and impaired glucose tolerance in parents of women with gestational diabetes. Diabetologia 1995; 38: 693–8.

66. Harder T, Franke K, Kohlhoff R, Plagemann A. Maternal and paternal family history of diabetes in women with gestational diabetes or insulin-dependent diabetes mellitus type I. Gynecol Obstet Invest 2001; 51: 160–4.

67. Vambergue A, Fajardy I, Bianchi F, et al. Gestational diabetes mellitus and HLA class II (-DQ, -DR) association: the Digest Study. Eur J Immunogenet 1997; 24: 385–94.

68. Ober C, Xiang KS, Thisted RA, et al. Increased risk for gestational diabetes mellitus associated with insulin receptor and insulin-like growth factor II restriction fragment length polymorphisms. Genet Epidemiol 1989; 5: 559–69.

69. Shao J, Catalano PM, Yamashita H, et al. Decreased insulin receptor tyrosine kinase activity and plasma cell membrane glycoprotein-1 overexpression in skeletal muscle from obese women with gestational diabetes mellitus (GDM): evidence for increased

serine/threonine phosphorylation in pregnancy and GDM. Diabetes 2000; 49: 603–10.

70. Garvey WT, Maianu L, Hancock JA, et al. Gene expression of GLUT4 in skeletal muscle from insulin-resistant patients with obesity, IGT, GDM, and NIDDM. Diabetes 1992; 41: 465–75.

71. Garvey WT, Maianu L, Zhu J-H, et al. Multiple defects in the adipocyte glucose transport system cause cellular insulin resistance in gestational diabetes. Diabetes 1993; 42: 1773–85.

72. Goldfine ID, Maddux BA, Youngrem JF, et al. Membrane glycoprotein PC-1 and insulin resistance. J Cell Biochem 1998; 182: 177–84.

11 Fetal growth in normal and diabetic pregnancies

Patrick M. Catalano

Maternal and paternal factors associated with fetal growth

The problem of maternal diabetes and the increased population risk of obesity is becoming a greater problem not only in the developed areas of the world but also in developing countries with large populations and high birth rates. Because the increased risk of diabetes and obesity is now becoming manifest in adolescents and even children as young as 2–5 years,[1] the concept of *in utero* fetal programming assumes even more importance. Fetal programming is the effect of the *in utero* environment on events which have a permanent effect the organism's physiology or metabolism. In this chapter we will review normal fetal growth, fetal growth in infants of women with diabetes and fetal growth in infants of obese women.

Based on the studies of Hytten, greater than two-thirds of fetal growth occurs in the third trimester, with the fetus increasing weight from approximately 1000 to 3400 g.[2] Multiple factors contribute to the variability in fetal growth. These include ethnic, geographic and socio-economic factors. In the early 1960s the WHO reported that birthweight in various Indian populations was affected by socio-economic status, with neonates of women in lower socio-economic classes having smaller offspring than their more affluent counterparts.[3] Relative to geographic issues, high altitude has long been recognized as a factor resulting in decreasing birthweights as compared with those infants born at sea level; the decrease in oxygen tension at higher altitudes being the most ready explanation for the decreased birthweight.[4] Lastly, differences in various ethnic groups accounts for much of the variation in birthweight with Asian and African women having lighter babies in comparison with their Caucasian counterparts.[4]

Within the aforementioned parameters, however, the maternal environment during pregnancy has profound affects on *in utero* fetal growth. There is a strong correlation between maternal height and weight and fetal growth. In general, the taller and heavier a woman is prior to conception, the more her infant will weigh at birth.[5] These correlations are more robust in nulliparous as compared with multiparous women.[6] Similarly, there are also significant increases in birthweight related to maternal weight gain during gestation.[6] The interaction of maternal pregravid weight and weight gain on fetal growth are interesting relative to the underlying physiology

of fetal growth. Based on the studies of Abrams and Laros,[7] lean or underweight women will need to have a significant increase in weight gain in pregnancy in order to have a normally grown fetus. In contrast, the overweight and/or obese women will more likely have a larger baby, even with little or no weight gain. Maternal parity also has an affect on fetal growth. Increasing parity results in an increase of approximately 100 g with each successive pregnancy.[8] The effect appears to plateau after the fifth pregnancy. This may be related to increased maternal weight retention after successive pregnancies but does not appear to be related to maternal age, once adjusted for other co-variables.

The issue of maternal nutrition and fetal growth has been addressed in many animal studies, mostly addressing the issue of fetal programming in growth restricted models, although more recent work has focused on the problem of maternal obesity and obesogenic diets. In the human, the studies of Barker have addressed the issue of fetal programming in the human intrauterine growth restricted (IUGR) model.[9] The Barker hypothesis notes that poor nutrition *in utero* leads to fetal adaptations that produce permanent changes in insulin and glucose metabolism. For example, intra-uterine growth restriction followed by increased availability of food and/or decreased activity result in dysregulation such as the metabolic syndrome.[10] Lucas et al., however, suggested that

> size in early life is related to health outcomes only after adjustment for current size, it is probably the change in size between these points rather than fetal biology that is implicated.[11]

For example, in the Early Bird Study[12] 300 British children were followed longitudinally. Insulin resistance was the same in children who had high birthweight and remained at an elevated birthweight centile through age 5 years, compared with those who had a lower birthweight but attained a similar centile at age 5. In fact, the IUGR model for the fetal programming hypothesis is more robust relative to aspects of the metabolic syndrome such as hypertension rather than obesity.[13] Unfortunately, the human studies addressing the issue of maternal under nutrition in pregnancy mostly relate to starvation conditions during wartime. The best documented of these are the Dutch famine studies of 1944–1945.[14]

Starvation conditions had specific dates of onset and, with liberation, specific dates on the relief of starvation conditions. Nutritional developments in early pregnancy followed by increased access to food in later pregnancy results in babies being heavier at birth as compared with babies born either before or after the famine. This may represent *in utero* catch-up growth. In contrast, if the famine occurred during late gestation, the babies weighed less and were thinner at birth, with no change in length. Nutritional supplementation can improve birthweight. Based on the Guatemalan studies, the type of supplementation, i.e. protein or carbohydrate, may not make a difference in the increase in birthweight, assuming minimal protein requirements are achieved.[15]

Relative to maternal factors, paternal anthropometric factors have limited impact on fetal growth. Morton reported that half siblings of with the mother as the common parent, the correlation of birthweight between the half siblings was $r = 0.58$. In contrast, the correlation of birthweights between half siblings where the father was the common parent was only $r = 0.19$.[16] Animal cross-breeding studies support these findings. Walton and Hammond cross-bred Shetland ponies with shire horses. The size of the foals was approximately the same size as the foals of the maternal pure breed.[17] Thus, maternal regulation was more important in determining intrauterine growth than paternal factors. Lastly, Klebanoff using a Danish population registry, reported that paternal birthweight, adult height and weight together explained approximately 3% of the variance in birthweight, compared with 9% for the corresponding maternal factors.[18] In summary maternal factors, most importantly maternal pregravid weight has the strongest correlation with birthweight.

Genetic factors associated with fetal growth

Approximately 25% of fetal growth is presumed related to genetic factors. The most obvious example is that the average male newborn weighs 150 g more at birth in comparison with females, adjusted for any potential covariables. In 1998, Hattersley et al.[19] reported on the various phenotypic permutations associated with the single gene mutations in the glucokinase gene (Figure 11.1). Glucokinase phosphorylates glucose to glucose-6-phosphate in the pancreas and liver. A heterozygous glucokinase mutation results in hyperglycemia, usually with a mildly elevated fasting glucose and abnormal oral glucose tolerance test. This is due to both a defect in the sensing of glucose by the beta cell, resulting in decreased insulin release, and to a lesser degree from reduced hepatic glycogen synthesis. If the heterozygous mutation is present in the fetus, then the altered glucose sensing by the fetal pancreas will result in a decrease in insulin secretion. Because in the fetus insulin is a primary stimulus for growth, any defect in fetal insulin secretion will result in decreased fetal growth and possible growth restriction. Hence, depending on the mother, fetus or both have this gene defect in the glucokinase gene, the phenotype of the infant can vary from IUGR, through normal fetal growth and on to macrosomia.

In contrast, genetic imprinting may result in the offspring having the phenotype of an infant of a GDM mother, but the mother has normal glucose tolerance. Genetic imprinting is defined as the expression of either a maternal or paternal gene, the parent of origin of which determines the expression

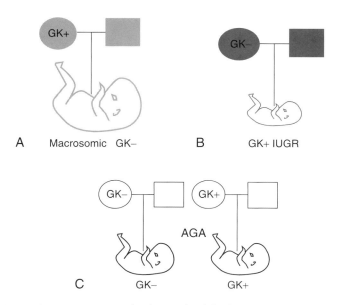

Figure 11.1   The glucokinse (GK) mutations: variation in fetal growth. If the heterozygous GK mutation in the mother and not the fetus (A), then the fetus is at risk for being macrosomic based on excess maternal nutrient availability (B) If only the fetus has the GK mutation, then the fetus is at risk for being intrauterine growth restricted (IUGR) because of the altered glucose sensing by the fetal pancreas, with resultant decreased fetal insulin secretion. (C) If the mother and the fetus either *both* have or do not have the GK mutation, then there is decreased risk of the fetus being macrosomic or IUGR. (Adapted from Hattersley et al.[19])

of a single allele of a gene. An example of genetic imprinting which results in the offspring having the phenotype of a GDM mother is the Beckwith–Wiedemann syndrome.[20] At birth these infants present with macrosomia, defined as an average birthweight of 4 kg with increased subcutaneous tissue and muscle mass. Other findings include neonatal polycythemia and hypoglycemia. The hypoglycemia may be related to increased IGF-2 expression, resulting in neonatal hyperinsulinemia. The most common situation is when the maternal copy of the gene (11p15.5) is inactivated. The only active copy of the gene is then the paternal copy. Hence, at birth the infant with Beckwith–Wiedemann syndrome may have the phenotype of an infant of a GDM mother based on macrosomia, hypoglycemia and polycythemia, whereas the mother may have completely normal glucose tolerance. The interaction of genes and the environment then have the potential to produce a myriad of phenotypes in the infant of the GDM mother, though fetal macrosomia still represents the most common phenotype.

Birthweight criteria for normal fetal growth

The criteria for normal fetal growth are population specific, based on issues reviewed earlier. Therefore most reports describe fetal growth in relationship to population percentiles, most usually less than 10th centile as SGA or small for gestational age, 10th to 90th centile as AGA or appropriate or average for gestational age and LGA for large for gestational age, i.e. birthweight greater than the 90th centile. These may be further delineated for gender and race. IUGR usually implies a neonate that is SGA and in addition has evidence of decreased intrauterine growth such as an increased head to abdominal ratio (asymmetric IUGR) or physiologically hypoglycemia at birth. At the other end of the birthweight spectrum, infants are often classified as macrosomic or overgrown if fetal weight is greater than 4000 g, although some define macrosomic if birthweight is greater than 4500 g. However, it has become apparent in the last 10 years that these criteria used to classify birthweight are not stable but rather represent a moving target.

In Canada and the United States there has been a significant decrease in term SGA neonates (11–27%) and increase in term LGA infants (5–24%) from 1985 to 1998. This increase has been observed in both Caucasians and African–Americans.[21] In Denmark, there has been a significant (16.7 to 20%) increase in macrosomic neonates defined as birthweight greater than 4000 g during the period from 1990 through 1999.[22] Similarly, in Sweden there has been a 23% increase in LGA newborns during the same period of time.[23] In our own population we have observed a mean 116 g increase in term birthweight from 1975 through 2004.[24] This increase in birthweight was observed not just at the 90th and 95th centiles but at the 5th and 10th centiles as well. Thus the increase in birthweight represents an entire population shift, not just an increase at the upper end of the birthweight scale. Although there were significant changes in the ethnic distribution of our population, the increase in birthweight over time remained once adjusted for as significant covariables. Lastly, when we performed a step-wise regression analysis, the 9.1 kg (20 pounds) increase in maternal weight we observed in our population at term from 1987 through 2004 had the strongest correlation with the observed increased birthweight.[24]

Body composition in the assessment of fetal growth

In an effort to improve our understanding of fetal growth we have elected to concentrate our studies on measures of body composition, i.e. fat and fat-free or lean body mass. The rationale for this approach stems as far back as 1923 from the work of Moulton, who described that the variability in weight within mammalian species was accounted for more by the fat mass rather than fat-free or lean body mass.[25] This concept was again examined by Sparks assessing body composition among 169 stillbirths. He described a relatively comparable accretion[26] of lean body mass in SGA, AGA and LGA fetuses, but considerable variation in the amounts of adipose tissue. The amount of fat in the SGA fetus was significantly less than the AGA fetus, which was less than that observed in the LGA fetus. Furthermore, relative to body composition, the human neonate is vastly different in comparison with other mammalian species. The term human fetus has the greatest percent body fat at birth (approximately 12–14%) in comparison with other common animal research models. For example, rodents have only approximately 1–3% body fat at birth. For these reasons, we have elected to assess fetal growth in our research protocols using measures of neonatal body composition. The methodologies we have employed in our studies include anthropometric, stable isotope and total body electrical conductivity (TOBEC). These methods have been described previously.[27–29]

The utility of using body composition in understanding fetal growth is exemplified by a previous study by our group evaluating the proportion of the variance in birthweight explained by body composition analysis of neonates, i.e. fat and fat-free mass. The mean birthweight of the population was 3553 ± 462 g and the mean percent body fat was 13.7 ± 4.2%. Fat free mass, which accounted for ~86% of mean birthweight accounted for 83% of the variance in birthweight. In contrast, body fat which accounted for only ~14% of birthweight, explained 46% of the variance in birthweight.[30] Measures of body composition can also help explain some of the variations in birthweight observed in a normal non-diabetic population. For example, it is well recognized that at term male neonates weigh on the average 150 g more than females. Based on studies by our group and others, male infants have greater fat-free mass but similar fat mass as compared with females.[31] Therefore although the percent body fat of females is greater than that of males, this is secondary to the decrease in fat-free mass rather than an increase in female fat mass. It is also well recognized that infants of women who smoke during pregnancy have neonates that are lighter (approximately 200 g) as compared to women who do not smoke and are at increased risk for being SGA. Lindsay et al. showed that the infants of women who smoked during pregnancy had significantly less fat-free mass (2799 ± 292 vs. 2965 ± 359 g, $P = 0.02$) but not

Table 11.1 Neonatal body composition and anthropometrics in infants of women with gestational diabetes (GDM) and normal glucose tolerance (NGT)*

	GDM (*n* = 195)	NGT (*n* = 220)	*P*-value
Weight (g)	3398 ± 550	3337 ± 549	0.26
Fat free mass (g)	2962 ± 405	2975 ± 408	0.74
Fat mass (g)	436 ± 206	362 ± 198	0.0002
Body fat (%)	12.4 ± 4.6	10.4 ± 4.6	0.0001
Tricep (mm)	4.7 ± 1.1	4.2 ± 1.0	0.0001
Subscapular (mm)	5.4 ± 1.4	4.6 ± 1.2	0.0001
Flank (mm)	4.2 ± 1.2	3.8 ± 1.0	0.0001
Thigh (mm)	6.0 ± 1.4	5.4 ± 1.5	0.0001
Abdomen (mm)	3.5 ± 0.9	3.0 ± 0.8	0.0001

*From Catalano et al.[33]

fat mass (343 ± 164 vs. 387 ± 216 g, *P* = 0.32). The decrease in fat-free mass was most apparent in the length on the long bones in the distal arms and legs.[32] In summary, neonatal body composition measures at term can assist in explaining some of the variation in birthweight observed in a normal population and provide a rationale for possible mechanisms.

Infants of women with gestational diabetes

There is an increased risk of fetal overgrowth or macrosomia in the infant of the women with gestational diabetes (GDM). The percentage of infants of women with GDM who fall within the normal birthweight centiles is often used as a positive outcome measure of glucose control and obstetrical management. We have recently published a series of studies comparing the body composition analysis of infants of women with normal glucose tolerance (NGT) and GDM within 48 hours of birth Table 11.1.[33] Although there was no significant difference in birthweight or fat-free mass between the groups, there was a significant increase in fat mass and percent body fat in the infants of the GDM mothers. The TOBEC body composition analyses were confirmed by the anthropometric/skinfold measures. These data were adjusted for potential confounding variables such as parity and gestational age without any significant change in results.

We further analyzed the data after stratification of the group into birthweight subsets, AGA[33] and LGA.[34] In Table 11.2, there are no significant differences in birthweights between the AGA infants of the GDM and NGT groups. However, there was again a significant increase in fat mass, percent body fat and skinfold measures in the infants of the GDM mothers as compared with the NGT. Interestingly, the fat-free mass in the infants of the GDM mothers was significantly less compared to the infants in the NGT group. The similar results were obtained when we limited the analysis to only LGA neonates (Table 11.3).[34] This relative increase in fat mass but not body weight may have obstetrical implications, such as the increased incidence of shoulder dystocia in GDM as compared with NGT neonates at similar birthweight categories. Based on these results, we conclude that birthweight alone may not be

Table 11.2 Neonatal body composition and anthropometrics in average for gestational age (AGA) infants of women with gestational diabetes (GDM) and normal glucose tolerance (NGT)*

	GDM (*n* = 132)	NGT (*n* = 175)	*P*-value
Weight (g)	3202 ± 357	3249 ± 372	0.27
Fat free mass (g)	2832 ± 286	2919 ± 287	0.008
Fat mass (g)	371 ± 163	329 ± 150	0.02
Body fat (%)	11.4 ± 4.6	9.9 ± 4.0	0.002
Tricep (mm)	4.5 ± 0.9	4.1 ± 0.8	0.0002
Subscapular (mm)	5.1 ± 1.1	4.5 ± 1.0	0.0001
Flank (mm)	4.0 ± 1.2	3.7 ± 0.8	0.007
Thigh (mm)	5.7 ± 1.2	5.2 ± 1.3	0.002
Abdomen (mm)	3.3 ± 0.9	3.0 ± 0.8	0.002

*From Catalano et al.[33]

Table 11.3 Neonatal body composition in large for gestational age (LGA) infants of women with gestational diabetes (GDM) and normal glucose tolerance (NGT)*

	GDM ($n = 50$)	NGT ($n = 52$)	*P*-value
Weight (g)	4060 ± 380	4120 ± 351	0.13
Fat free mass (g)	3400 ± 312	3564 ± 310	0.0009
Fat mass (g)	662 ± 163	563 ± 206	0.02
Body fat (%)	16.2 ± 3.3	13.5 ± 4.5	0.002

* From Durnwald et al.[34]

sensitive enough measure to recognize subtle difference in fetal growth in infants of GDM mothers.

Because many women with GDM are overweight or obese, we elected to perform a stepwise logistic regression analysis on the 220 infants of NGT and 195 term infants of GDM mothers previously described.[35] The results are given in Table 11.4. Not surprisingly, gestational age at term was the independent variable with the strongest correlation with both birthweight and fat-free mass. Maternal smoking had a negative correlation with both birthweight and fat-free mass and paternal weight had a weak correlation with only fat-free mass. In contrast, maternal pregravid BMI had the strongest correlation with fat mass ($r^2 = 0.066$) and percent body fat ($r^2 = 0.072$), therefore explaining approximately 7% of the variance in both fat mass and percent body fat. Although approximately 50% of the subjects had GDM, only 2% of the variance ($r^2 = 0.016$) in fat mass in this population was explained by a mother having GDM. Furthermore, Ehrenberg et al.[36] reported that the risk of having an LGA neonate was greatest for women with a history of diabetes (OR 4.4) when compared with maternal obesity (OR 1.6). However, there was 4-fold greater number of LGA babies born of obese women than women with diabetes because the relative prevalence of overweight/obesity to diabetes was 47 and 5%, respectively. Therefore, at least in our population, maternal obesity and not diabetes appears to be the more important factor contributing to the population's increase in mean birthweight.

Table 11.4 Stepwise regression analysis of factors relating to fetal growth and body composition in infants of women with gestational diabetes (n = 195) and normal glucose tolerance (n = 220)

Factor	r^2	Δr^2	P
Birthweight			
EGA	0.114	–	
Pregravid weight	0.162	0.048	
Weight gain	0.210	0.048	
Smoking (−)	0.227	0.017	
Parity	0.239	0.012	0.0001
Lean body mass			
EGA	0.122	–	
Smoking (−)	0.153	0.031	
Pregravid weight	0.179	0.026	
Weight gain	0.212	0.033	
Parity	0.225	0.013	
Maternal height	0.241	0.016	
Paternal weight	0.250	0.009	0.0001
Fat Mass			
Pregravid BMI	0.066	–	
EGA	0.136	0.070	
Weight gain	0.171	0.035	
Group (GDM)	0.187	0.016	0.0001
%Body Fat			
Pregravid BMI	0.072	–	
EGA	0.116	0.044	
Weight gain	0.147	0.031	
Group (GDM)	0.166	0.019	0.0001

Pregravid maternal obesity has the strongest correlation with neonatal measures of fat mass/% body fat in contrast to lean body mass.[35]

Table 11.5   Neonatal body composition and anthropometric measures of the lean/average and overweight/obese study groups*

Variable	Pregravid BMI < 25 kg/m² group	Pregravid BMI >25 kg/m² group	P-value
Birthweight (g)	3284 ± 534	3436 ± 567	0.051
Body composition (TOBEC)			
LBM (g)	2951 ± 406	3023 ± 410	0.22
Fat mass (g)	331 ± 179	406 ± 221	0.008
Body fat (%)	9.6 ± 4.3	11 ± 4.7	0.006
Skin folds (mm)			
Triceps	4.0 ± 0.9	4.4 ± 1.0	0.009
Subscapular	4.4 ± 1.2	4.9 ± 1.2	0.003
Flank	3.6 ± 0.9	4.0 ± 1.2	0.005
Thigh	5.2 ± 1.5	5.7 ± 1.4	0.058
Abdomen	2.9 ± 0.8	3.1 ± 1.0	0.099

*From Sewell et al.[37]

Infants of overweight and obese women

If infants of women with GDM have increased body fat rather than fat-free mass, what then is the difference if any in body composition between pregravid overweight/obese women as compared with lean or average weight women? Sewell et al. evaluated 76 singleton neonates of overweight/obese women and 144 neonates of lean/average women again using anthropometric and TOBEC measures of body composition.[37] None of these women had GDM. There were no significant differences in gestational age between the groups. Additionally, there were no significant differences in maternal age, parity, use of tobacco or obstetrical or maternal medical problems between the groups. However, 14% of the infants of the overweight/obese mothers had macrosomic infants (birthweight > 4 kg) as compared with only 5% in the neonates of the lean/average weight women ($P < 0.04$), while weight gain in the overweight/obese group was actually less (13.8 ± 7.5 vs. 15.2 ± 5.3 kg, $P < 0.001$) than in the lean/average weight women. The differences in neonatal body composition are depicted in Table 11.5. As was observed in the infants of GDM women, the infants of the overweight/obese women were significantly heavier because of an increase in fat mass (406 ± 221 vs. 331 ± 179 g, $P = 0.008$) and not fat-free mass (3023 ± 410 vs. 2951 ± 406 g, $P = 0.22$). In this study weight gain in overweight/obese women (BMI = 25) had the strongest correlation % body fat ($r^2 = 0.13$, $P = 002$), whereas weight gain was not significantly related to fat mass in the lean/average weight women. In summary, the increased birthweight observed in infants of obese women is similar to that observed in infants of women with GDM, i.e. an increase in fat mass rather than fat-free mass.

Since there is an independent affect of maternal pregravid weight and GDM on birthweight, Langer et al. reported that in women with pregravid obesity and well controlled GDM on diet alone, the odds of fetal macrosomia, defined as birthweight greater than 4000 g, was significantly increased (OR 2.12) as compared with those in women having a normal BMI. Similar results were found in lean and obese women with GDM, which was poorly controlled on diet or insulin. In contrast, well controlled GDM, whether lean or obese, as long as there managed with diet plus insulin, there was no significant increased risk of macrosomia with increasing pregravid BMI.[38] Hence, only in a well-controlled GDM patient on diet plus insulin was there no difference in the rate of fetal macrosomia in obese as compared to lean women. The effect of insulin on metabolites other than glucose may explain these observations.

Summary

There is a great variability in fetal growth in the human, based on both genetic and environmental factors. Although we cannot control our genes (with the possible exception of epigenetic phenomena), we may be able to affect fetal growth through alterations in the maternal environment. Based on these data, the maternal pregravid environment or factors in very early gestation may result in alterations in growth that have long term implications i.e. fetal programming. Much as the prevention of congenital anomalies in women with pregestational diabetes can be improved by tight glucose control prior to conception, so too may the more subtle effects of fuel mediated teratogenesis on fetal growth (as described by Freinkel),[39] be improved by preconceptual issues related to diet and weight regulation. Therefore a better understanding of the underlying genetic predispositions, physiology and mechanisms relating to maternal and feto-placental interactions as they relate to fetal growth are necessary.

REFERENCES

1. Ogden CL, Flegal KM, Carroll MD, et al. Prevalence and trends in overweight among U.S. children and adolescents. JAMA 2002; 288: 1728–32.
2. Hytten FD. Weight gain in pregnancy. In: Hytten FE, Chamberlain G, eds. Clinical Physiology in Obstetrics. Oxford: Blackwell Scientific Publications; 1991, pp. 173–203.
3. Lawrence W, Miller DG, Isaacs M, et al. Nutrition in pregnancy and lactation. Report of a WHO Expert Committee. WHO Expert Committee on Nutrition, Pregnancy and Lactation, 1965; 302: 1–54.
4. Ounsteid M, Ounsted C. On Fetal Growth Rate: Its Variations and Their Consequences. Clinics in Developmental Medicine, No. 46. Lavenham, Suffolk, UK: Lavenham Press; 1973.
5. Love EJ, Kinch RAH. Factors influencing the birth weight in normal pregnancy. Am J Obstet Gynecol 1965; 91: 342–9.
6. Humphreys RC. An analysis of the maternal and foetal weight factors in normal pregnancy. J Obstet Gynecol Br Emp 1954; 764–71.
7. Abrams BF, Laros RK. Prepregnancy weight, weight gain and birth weight. Am J Obstet Gynecol 1986; 4: 503–9.
8. Thompson AM, Billewicz WZ, Hytten FE. The assessment of fetal growth. J Obstet Gynecol 1968; 5: 903–16.
9. Barker DJP, ed. Fetal and Infant Origins of Adult Disease. Br Med J 1990; 301(6761): 1111.
10. Armitage JA, Khan IY, Taylor PD, et al. Developmental programming of the metabolic syndrome by maternal nutritional imbalance: How strong is the evidence from experimental animal models in mammals? J Physiol 2004; 561/2: 355–77.
11. Lucas A, Fentrell MS, Cule TJ. Fetal origins of adult disease – The hypothesis revisited. BMJ 1999; 319: 245–9.
12. Wilkin TJ, Metcalf BS, Murphy MJ, et al. The relative contribution of birth weight, weight change and current weight to insulin resistance in contemporary 5 year olds, the Early Bird Study. Diabetes 2002; 51: 3468–72.
13. Hypponen E, Power C, Davey-Smith G. Perinatal growth, BMI and risk of type 2 diabetes by early midlife. Diabetes Care 2003; 26: 2512–7.
14. Ravelli ACJ. Prenatal exposure to the Dutch famine and glucose tolerance and obesity at age 50. Thesis, University of Amsterdam, 1999, pp. 51–62.
15. Lechtig A, Habracht J-P, Delgado H, et al. Effect of food supplementation during pregnancy on birthweight. Pediatrics 1975; 56: 508–20.
16. Morton NE. The inheritance of human birth weight. Ann Hum Genetics 1955; 20: 125–34.
17. Walton A, Hammond S. Maternal effects on growth and conformation in Shire horse–Shetland pony crosses. Proc R Soc Lond B Biol Sci 1938; 125B: 311–35.
18. Klebanoff MA, Mednick BR, Schulsinger C, et al. Father's effect on infant birth weight. Am J Obstet Gynecol 1998; 178: 122–6.
19. Hattersley AT, Beards F, Ballantyne E, et al. Mutations in the glucokinase gene of the fetus result in reduced birth weight. Nature Genetics 1998; 19: 268–70.
20. Smith's Recognizable Patterns of Human Malformations, 5th edn. Philadelphia: WB Saunders; 1997, pp. 164–6.
21. Anath CV, Wen SW. Trends in fetal growth among singleton gestations in the United States and Canada, 1985 through 1998. Semin Perinatol 2002; 26: 260–7.
22. Surkan PJ, Hsieh C-C, Johansson A LU, Dickman PW, Cnattingius S. Reasons for increasing trends in large for gestational age births. Obstet Gynecol 2004 ; 104: 720–6.
23. Orskou J, Kesmodel U, Henrikson TB, Secker NJ. An increasing proportion of infants weigh more than 4000 grams at birth. Acta Obstet Gynecol Scand 2001; 80: 931–6.
24. Catalano PM. Management of obesity in pregnancy. Obstet Gynecol 2007; 109: 419–33.
25. Moulton CR. Age and chemical development in mammals. J Biol Chem 1923; 57: 79–97.
26. Sparks JW. Human intrauterine growth and nutrient accretion. Semin Perinatol 1984; 8: 74–93.
27. Fiorotto MC, Klish WJ. Total body electrical conductivity measurements in the neonate. Clin Perinatol 1991; 18: 611–27.
28. Catalano PM, Thomas AJ, Avallone DA, Amini SB. Anthropometric estimation of neonatal body composition. Am J Obstet Gynecol 1995; 173: 1176–81.
29. Fiorotto MC, Cochran WJ, Runk RC, Sheng J-P, Klish WJ. Total body electrical conductivity measurements: Effects of body composition and geometry. Am J Physiol 1987; 252: R798–800.
30. Catalano PM, Tyzbir ED, Allen SR, McBean JH, McAuliffe TL. Evaluation of fetal growth by estimation of body composition. Obstet Gynecol 1992; 79: 46–50.
31. Catalano PM, Drago NM, Amini SB. Factors affecting fetal growth and body composition. Am J Obstet Gynecol 1995; 172: 1459–63.
32. Lindsay CA, Thomas AJ, Catalano PM. The effect of smoking tobacco on neonatal body composition. Am J Obstet Gynecol 1997; 172: 1124–8.
33. Catalano PM, Thomas A, Huston-Presley L, Amini SB. Increased fetal adiposity: A very sensitive marker of abnormal in utero development. Am J Obstet Gynecol 2003; 189: 1698–704.
34. Durnwald C, Huston-Presley L, Amini S, Catalano P. Evaluation of body composition of large-for-gestational-age infants of women with gestational diabetes mellitus compared with women with normal glucose tolerance levels. Am J Obstet Gynecol 2004; 191: 804–8.
35. Catalano PM, Ehrenberg HM. The short- and long-term implications of maternal obesity on the mother and her offspring. Br J Obstet Gynecol 2006; 113: 1126–33.
36. Ehrenberg HM, Mercer BM, Catalano PM. The influence of obesity and diabetes on the prevalence of macrosomia. Am J Obstet Gynecol 2004; 191: 964–8.
37. Sewell M, Huston-Presley L, Super DM, et al. Increased neonatal fat mass and not lean body mass is associated with maternal obesity. Am J Obstet Gynecol 2006; 195: 1100–3.
38. Langer O, Yogev Y, Xenakis EMJ, Brustman L. Overweight and obese in gestational diabetes: The impact on pregnancy outcome. Am J Obstet Gynecol 2005; 192: 1368–76.
39. Freinkel N. Diabetic embryopathy and fuel-mediated organ teratogenesis: Lessons from animal models. Horm Metab Res 1988; 20: 463–75.

12 Pregnancy in diabetic animals

Eleazar Shafrir and Gernot Desoye

Introduction

It would be expected that pregnancy in many of the animal models of Type 1 or Type 2 diabetes would result in a typical overt diabetes or gestational diabetes mellitus (GDM). However, although this is true in cytotoxin-induced diabetes it is not in most genetically predetermined diabetes in animals. The lepr[db] mice, lepr[fa] rats and KK mice are infertile, and heterozygote siblings are used to obtain the homozygote individuals. Most studies of diabetes in pregnancy in animals have therefore been performed in cytotoxin-treated animals, predominantly rodents.

Streptozotocin-induced diabetes

Streptozotocin (STZ)-induced diabetes results from either intravenous or intraperitoneal (i.p.) injection of the toxin. Alloxan is also an effective diabetogenic agent but is now rarely used in pregnant animals. The mode of action of STZ and typical observations on the resulting diabetic derangements in various animal species have been extensively described in several reviews.[1–5] A wide range of animals may be used to elicit diabetes in pregnancy by STZ, including rabbits, pigs, sheep, and subhuman primates.[6–9]

However, the preferred and most often used experimental models are rodents because of their convenient maintenance, short length of pregnancy, multiparity (enabling studies on multiple fetuses and generations), and lack of special problems in termination of pregnancy and fetus recovery. The need for animal models for research of pathophysiology of diabetic pregnancy, a goal not fully attainable by study of human subjects, was underscored by Baird and Aerts.[10] Useful information on various animals suitable for perinatal metabolic research has been contributed by Susa.[11]

There is a marked difference in the effect of diabetes on the maternal, fetal and placental histopathology and metabolism depending on STZ dosage and time of injection. Rodents rendered diabetic before conception manifest hyperglycemia and hypoinsulinemia during organogenesis. As a result, they experience a high degree of fetal resorption and a high percentage of malformed fetuses.[12–16] Injection of STZ into rats in midgestation between days 5 and 14 of gestation, produces diabetes with a low percentage of fetal malformations, and provides the opportunity to follow the metabolic changes induced by maternal diabetes and to study those effects on the placenta and fetus.[17,18]

STZ injected into the mother does not affect the fetal pancreas. Although STZ crosses the placenta, its maternal half-life is of the order of minutes and the amount reaching the fetal circulation does not damage fetal beta cells, as investigated in rhesus monkeys.[19] Injection of STZ into rodents in the post-organogenesis phase, but before full pancreas development, also does not affect the function of the fetal pancreas, except of beta-cell degranulation secondary to the prevalent hyperglycemia.

Diabetes characteristics in pregnant STZ-induced diabetic rats

STZ-induced diabetes should serve mainly as a model for pregestational diabetes since the hyperglycemia and metabolic derangements are the result of beta-cell destruction, whereas GDM is characterized by insulin resistance and compensatory hyperinsulinemia with possible secondary lesion to beta cells as a result of the strain of oversecretion. Even moderate doses of STZ, which result in mild hyperglycemia, do not represent GDM, since the result is a limited insulin deficiency due to a reduced beta-cell mass.

Glucose and glycogen metabolism in STZ-induced diabetes

The decreased glucose uptake by muscles, the reduction in glucose transporter activity and concentration, and the increased hepatic glucose production in diabetes are well documented and discernible early. The hyperglycemia of diabetes is also a concentration-dependent factor causing increased deposition of glycogen in both rodent and human placentas (Figure 12.1).[20,21] It is remarkable that glycogen accumulation in the placenta occurs despite the maternal insulin deficiency, while the glycogen content in the typical insulin-sensitive maternal tissues (e.g. adipose tissue, muscle and liver) becomes reduced. Fetal liver glycogen content is increased most probably in response to the fetal hyperglycemia and consequent hyperinsulinemia. The responses

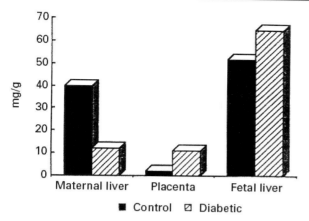

Figure 12.1   Glycogen content in the placenta and in maternal and fetal liver of control and streptozotocin (STZ)-induced diabetic rats on day 20 of gestation. Values are means of determinations in 20–26 rats at the mean level of plasma glucose of 6.0 and 24.5 mmol/L in control and diabetic rats, respectively. The insulinopenic STZ-induced diabetes caused a marked decrease in maternal hepatic glycogen content, whereas the placental glycogen content rose about 5-fold. Fetal liver glycogen also increased, but this was associated with intrafetal hyperinsulinemia. (Data adapted from Barash et al.[22])

of maternal insulin-sensitive tissues in insulinopenic diabetes are well known, entailing glycogen breakdown as regulated by the reciprocal activities of the enzymes glycogen synthase and glycogen phosphorylase. However, in the placenta these enzymes are not sensitive to insulin and the deposition of glycogen is positively correlated with the abundance of glucose.

This is accompanied by an increase in the intracellular concentration of glucose-6-phosphate,[22] a potent activator of the phosphorylated (inactive) form of glycogen synthase. Such a mechanism was shown to operate not only in diabetes but in normal pregnant animals rendered hyperglycemic by glucose infusion.[23] Thus, the placenta exhibits a mode of regulation of glycogen metabolism similar to other insulin-insensitive tissues, such as kidneys or intestine, which also accumulate glycogen in insulin-deficient diabetes in response to the augmented hyperglycemic gradient across the cells.[24–27]

Lipid metabolism and transport in STZ-induced diabetic rats

Hypoinsulinemic diabetes is known to result in fat release from adipose tissues, due to the weakened restraint of triglyceride (TG) lipolysis. In non-pregnant animals, this leads to increased hepatic fat oxidation and ketogenesis. However, in pregnant animals, additional tissues take up free fatty acids (FFA) released by lipolysis, namely the placenta and fetus. In STZ diabetic rats, a significant correlation was found between maternal levels of TG, placental TG and fetal TG, all of which were markedly elevated (Figure 12.2).[18] There was also a marked increase in TG and FFA in the fetal circulation. Fetal weight does not increase, probably due to the short duration of diabetic pregnancy insufficient for appreciable intrafetal fat accretion and also due to rather severe diabetes in these experiments.[18] In another report on diabetes in pigs, fetal obesity was observed.[28] Based on the pattern of distribution of the injected ^{14}C-fatty acid and [3]H₂O radioactivity, it was shown that the increment in fetal TG in STZ-induced diabetes

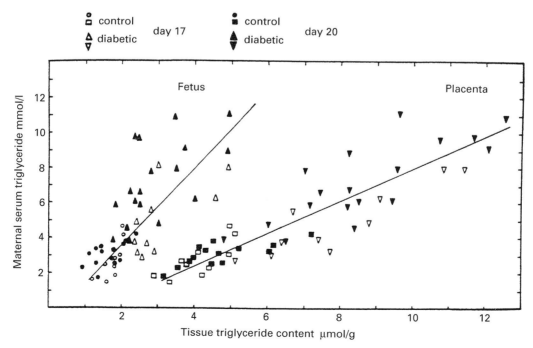

Figure 12.2   Relationship between the elevated triglyceride (TG) concentration in rat maternal circulation and the TG content in placentae and fetuses towards the end of gestation. Regression lines for placentae: $y = -1.1 + 0.9x$; $r = 0.88$; for fetuses: $y = -0.5 + 2.1x$; $r = 0.74$. Each point is a mean of TG values in five placentae and five fetuses from each of the 52 litters. (Reproduced from Shafrir and Khassis.[18])

is derived from the transfer of maternal TG and FFA rather than from increased *de novo* intrafetal lipogenesis.[18] The passage of lipids across the placenta involves an initial uptake of FFA and very-low-density-lipoprotein (VLDL)-borne TG from the circulation. The latter are lipolysed in the process of uptake in proximity to the tissue. The uptake of FFA does not represent a direct transfer to the fetus but a sequential process of intermediate re-esterification to TG and phospholipids within the placental cells, with subsequent lipolysis by an intracellular lipase and release to the fetal side.[29] The presence in the placenta of lipoprotein lipase-like activity was inferred from the change in the FFA:glycerol ratio during TG uptake (Table 12.1). In the face of an augmented maternal–fetal gradient of FFA and TG, there is an increased flow associated with a substantial amount of intracellular FFA. Thus, the transplacental passage in diabetes may also involve a diffusion of FFA along the membrane lipids of interfacial capillaries.[29]

The increased maternal–fetal transport of fat in STZ-induced diabetes was also demonstrated by an altered distribution of polyunsaturated fatty acids in maternal, placental, and fetal tissues near the time of delivery. These fatty acids must be of nutritional origin and therefore derived from the maternal circulation. A pronounced (60%) increase in the relative content of linoleate was recorded in the placental and fetal carcass TG, and as much as about 200% in the fetal liver.[30] This suggests that after placental transfer, the fetal liver is the primary recipient of fatty acid excess from the diabetic mother, but the fetal liver TG are then redistributed to other fetal tissues through the hepatic synthesis of VLDL.

Results similar to those in rodents have been obtained in diabetic pigs. Induction of diabetes in Yorkshire gilts during the third trimester of gestation resulted in a 2-fold increase in the carcass fat content in the progeny compared with controls injected with either saline or insulin[31] indicating a direct incorporation of maternal fatty acids into fetal adipocytes. Diabetes decreased the maternal lipogenesis while increasing the *de novo* fetal fat synthesis in pigs.[32]

Enzymes of metabolic pathways in diabetic pregnant animals

STZ-induced and Type 1 diabetes have, in general, far-reaching effects on the synthesis and activity of numerous rate-limiting enzymes in the pathways of carbohydrate, lipid and protein metabolism in both human and animal tissues. These enzymes respond to hormone alterations, which include insulin, glucocorticoids, triiodothyronine, and pregnancy-related hormones such as estrogen and progesterone. This involves both activity responses to changes in concentrations of metabolic effectors as well as translational or transcriptional influences at the DNA or mRNA level. To mention but a few, the regulatory enzymes of carbohydrate metabolism, glucokinase, hexokinase, pyruvate kinase, pyruvate dehydrogenase and glucose-6-phosphate dehydrogenase are severely reduced in the liver or adipose tissue, whereas those regulating gluconeogenesis, PEPCK and glucose-6-phosphatase, increase in activity and concentration. Similarly, lipogenic enzymes, e.g. acetyl coenzyme A (acetyl CoA) carboxylase, are markedly reduced in diabetes, both in concentration and in activity, whereas those responsible for TG lipolysis and FFA oxidation are enhanced. These changes have also been documented in pregnant diabetic animals, as exemplified in the STZ-induced diabetic rats[17] or alloxan-induced diabetic pigs.[32]

The placenta is an exception to these activity changes. The placental enzymes are constitutive, almost devoid of capacity to adapt in activity to diabetes or other hormonal and pathophysiological changes in the maternal organism.[17,33] Treatment of pregnant rats with different hormones or protracted fasting, which has a pronounced effect the activity of maternal hepatic and adipose tissue enzymes, is without appreciable effect on most placental enzymes in the rat[33,34] or rabbit.[35] Fetal liver enzymes do respond, although to a lesser extent than those in the maternal liver.[17,36] These observations suggest that, by maintaining the constancy of enzymatic function, the placenta confers metabolic stability to the fetus, thus shielding the fetus from hormonally induced fluctuations on the maternal side, and attenuating the possible variations in the metabolite flow and substrate availability to the fetus.

Table 12.1 Free fatty acid:glycerol ratio change during triglyceride (TG) uptake by the placenta and transfer to the fetus		
VLDL or tissue	**Ratio**
Injected VLDL*	1.23
Placenta	4.22
Fetal liver	5.43
Fetal carcass	5.88

*VLDL, very-low-density liproprotein. Doubly-labeled VLDL were prepared by the injection of ^{14}C-palmitate and ^{3}H-glycerol into rats followed by exsanguinations 20 min later and separation of the VLDL by ultracentrifugation. The isolated VLDL were injected into non-diabetic or STZ-induced diabetic rats (10 mg VLDL TG rat) on day 20 of gestation, and the ^{3}H:^{14}C ratio was measured after 2 h in the placenta, fetal liver and fetal carcass after extraction of lipids in chloroform:methanol 2:1. (Unpublished data of Shafrir, Barash, and Levy.)

Embryopathy in STZ-induced diabetic animals

One of the numerous problems confronted in overt diabetic pregnancy is fetal wastage together with a large percentage of congenital malformations, mainly in neural tissues and skeleton development. Cytotoxin-induced diabetic rodents are therefore preferred models for the study of fetal malformations. As mentioned before, a correlation exists between hyperglycemia in the organogenesis phase and the extent of malformations in the offspring of diabetic rodents.[16,37] Since hyperglycemia is the main culprit, apart from the study of malformations *in vivo*, normal or STZ-induced diabetic animals are often used as a source of embryos for *in vitro* studies after removal at various stages of gestation.[37–39]

As elegantly demonstrated by Strieleman et al.[40] and Hod et al.,[41,42] myoinositol is vital in preventing malformations. In cultured rat fetuses the teratogenicity of 400 mg/dL glucose was evident by a decrease in the concentration of inositol phosphates and in reduced DNA synthesis. The extent of neural and extraneural malformations rose about 10-fold. Addition of scylloinositol (a non-metabolizable isomer of inositol preventing its intracellular transport), at normal glucose concentrations, produced a decrease in cellular myoinositol and inositol phosphates, impaired growth with dysmorphogenesis, and malformations similar in extent to high glucose concentrations. Hod et al.[41,42] found that sorbinil (an inhibitor of aldose reductase) was ineffective in preventing malformations in cultured fetuses which amounted to > 50 versus 4% at normal glucose concentrations; however, the addition of 1.5 mg/mL of exogenous inositol substantially reduced the malformations.

Extensive investigations of the glucotoxicity of advanced glycation endproducts (AGE) and of the detrimental effect of oxidative radicals were performed by Erickson and associates, and are described in Chapter 24. It is worth emphasizing here that many of these studies were performed in cytotoxin-induced diabetic models or fetuses cultured in diabetic milleu. Zaken et al.[43] and Ornoy et al.[44] cultured 10.5-day-old normal fetuses in 'diabetic' serum containing 200 mg/dL glucose, 200 mg/dL β-hydroxybutyrate and 1 mg/dL acetoacetate. As determined by cyclic voltametry, a marked drop in natural, protective antioxidative components was noted, along with depletion of vitamins E and C. The malformations could, in large measure, be prevented by raising the antioxidant defences, using superoxide dismutase and resupplying vitamins E and C.

The particular contribution of the oxidative stress in the diabetic milieu is not only due to AGE but to the plethora of reducing equivalents emanating from high glucose metabolism.

The inflow of reduced nicotinamide adenine dinucleotide (NADH) to mitochondria is not only from the Krebs cycle metabolizing significant loads of glycolysis-derived products but also from the aldose reductase pathway. The mitochondrial electron transport system is overloaded, particularly at the flavin adenine dinucleotide (FAD)-dependent oxidase (flavoprotein) step, which results in extrusion of the reactive oxygen species as illustrated in Figure 12.3.

Neonatally STZ-administered rats (nSTZ)

Among the syndromes resembling mild Type 2 diabetes as a consequence of reduced beta-cell mass are rats which received neonatal STZ injection (nSTZ), either at the time of birth[45,46] or 2 days after birth.[46,47] It should be stressed, however, that these animals, although non-obese, do not represent a true Type 2 diabetes, but rather a model of limited insulin deficiency with little, if any, peripheral or hepatic insulin resistance.

The i.p. or intravenous injection of 90–100 mg/kg STZ into neonatal rats causes about 90% destruction of pancreatic beta cells with hyperglycemia that peaks 3–5 days thereafter. This acute diabetes is transient. Beta cells at the neonatal stage are endowed with a remarkable regeneration capacity, although up to 30% of mortality is also occurring. After 3–5 weeks, fasting plasma glucose and insulin levels return to normal, even though the regenerated cells are not completely normal and impairment in insulin secretion persists, as seen in the response to a glucose load. The inferior performance of the regenerated cells is further exposed by subjecting the young animals to stress. By 8 weeks and thereafter blood glucose is 150–180 mg/dL with impaired glucose tolerance (IGT)

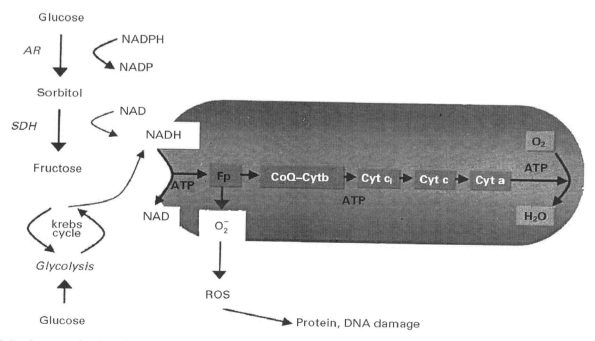

Figure 12.3   Sources of reduced nicotinamide adenine dinucleotide (NADH) flowing into the mitochondria, the Krebs tricarboxylic acid cycle and NADH derived from aldose reductase initiated dehydrogenation of glucose and the NAD-dependent conversion of sorbitol to fructose. In hyperglycemia, the flow of reducing equivalents is considerably increased, overloading the mitochondrial electron transport chain. The accumulation of reducing equivalents at the stage of flavin adenine dinucleotide (FAD) oxidase results in the production of reactive oxygen species with a detrimental effect on multiple feto-placental systems.

and a 50% decrease in pancreatic insulin content with mild hypoinsulinemia. As reviewed by Portha et al.,[48] the incompetence of the regenerated beta cells may be due to a reduced GLUT2 content limiting glucose entry and metabolism, and a decreased glucokinase affinity to glucose. More probably there is a reduced mitochondrial oxidation capacity of glucose-derived products, which is evident since leucine oxidation and insulinotropic action is similar to normal, i.e. acetyl CoA from leucine is metabolized without impediment. It has been suggested that the affected site is the FAD glycerol phosphate shuttle slowing the flow of reducing equivalence into the mitochondria. The activity of K^+ adenosine triphosphate (ATP) channels, the rate-limiting step in insulin secretion, may be also affected. The polarization of these channels allows Ca^{2+} entry into the cell, triggering the insulin secretion. However, no defect in K^+ ATP channels has been detected but their function may be slowed due to ATP deficiency.

One form of stress that exposes the latent diabetes in nSTZ rats is pregnancy. The basal plasma glucose concentration is elevated, both during the pregnancy and postpartum, and plasma insulin levels are reduced compared with those of normal pregnant rats. IGT was explicit during the response to a glucose load and persisted for 2 months postpartum. As demonstrated by Triadou et al.,[49] the secretion defect is particularly evident in the significantly decreased plasma insulin:glucose ratio during the pregnancy and postpartum (Table 12.2). Insufficient information is available on the pregnancy and malformations in the nSTZ model, and should be extensively explored because of the implication that the reduced or incompetent beta-cell mass may be an aggravating factor to human GDM. Complications in various tissues of the nSTZ rats have been reviewed by Schaffer and Mozaffari.[50]

It is of interest to mention the results of nSTZ injection into spontaneously hypertensive SHR rats. These insulin-resistant rats, which are used as a model of human essential hypertension, are prone to develop hypertensive cerebrocardiovascular disease with aging.[51] Diabetes was induced by i.p. injection of 75 mg STZ 2 days after birth and the animals were mated with untreated male SHR rats at 4–5 months of age.

Hyperglycemia of 20 mmol/L was evident during the pregnancy, with an elevated systolic blood pressure (213 vs. 192 mmHg) and albuminuria. The progeny was microsomic. nSTZ treatment of SHR rats decreased the lifespan of male offspring from about 18 to 15 months and raised the systolic blood pressure in correlation with their birthweight.[52,53] Such a model may be useful for the study of combined hypertension and diabetes.

Progeny of STZ-induced diabetic animals

With regard to the progeny of diabetic animals as models of insulin-deficient diabetes, it should be recalled that the intrauterine metabolic fuel milieu is untoward for the fetus. Fetal pancreatic beta cells are vulnerable to hyperglycemia and to changes in other metabolites. The inflicted injury persists after birth, resulting in mild, insulin-deficient diabetes and is propagated into successive generations.[54] STZ-induced diabetes was produced either by a low (30 mg/kg) or high (50 mg/kg) dose of STZ on day 1 of gestation, and created mild or severe maternal diabetes, respectively, resulting in a reduction in the maternal betacell content.[55,56] The characteristics of mild and severe STZ maternal diabetes, and its effect on the fetus, is shown in Table 12.3. Mildly diabetic mothers are moderately hypoinsulinemic and hyperglycemic, whereas severely diabetic mothers are insulin deficient, markedly hyperglycemic and hyperlipidemic, with low body weights.

In the fetal pancreas, beta-cell granulation starts at day 17 of gestation in non-diabetic rats, with a pronounced expansion in islet size, continuing up to the birth. In severely diabetic rats, hypertrophy of islets with poor granulation is observed on day 20 of gestation. The degranulated beta cells in the islets are evident but there is apparently no decrease in the beta-cell number.[56] The degranulation should be attributed to the secretory overtaxation of the newly organized endocrine pancreas, with granule depletion overtaking the usually rapid regranulation. This is striking on the day of birth in severely diabetic rats, showing, in addition to pronounced degranulation, disorganization of the rough endoplasmic reticulum,

Table 12.2   Pregnancy in normal and neonatal (nSTZ) streptozotocin injected rats

	Body weight (g)	Plasma glucose (mg/dL)	Plasma insulin (mU/L)	Insulin/glucose at 0–90 min
Neonatally STZ-treated rats				
Virgin	153 ± 3*	203 ± 5*	30 ± 3*	4 ± 1*
Pregnant (day 21)	281 ± 11*	128 ± 15*	52 ± 11	5 ± 1*
Postpartum (2 months)	265 ± 9	173 ± 5	47 ± 4	3 ± 1*
Normal rats				
Virgin	174 ± 3	156 ± 6	51 ± 7	19 ± 2
Pregnant (day 21)	330 ± 13	83 ± 3	45 ± 7	29 ± 4
Postpartum (2 months)	272 ± 5	145 ± 3	54 ± 5	10 ± 1

*Significant difference from corresponding control at $P < 0.05$. Data are means ± SE; $n = 7$–9 rats/group. The nSTZ rats were mated at 3–4 months and compared with control rats mated at 2.5–3 months. An i.v. glucose load (0.5 g/kg) was given during pregnancy and postpartum, and the integrated insulin increment was related to the glucose increment. (Adapted from Triadou et al.[50])

Table 12.3   Effect of severe and mild STZ diabetes on mothers and their progeny

	Non-diabetic	Mildly diabetic	Severely diabetic
Fetal weight (g)	2.0 ± 0.02	2.1 ± 0.05*	1.9 ± 0.02*
Fetal plasma glucose (mg/dL)	54 ± 2	69 ± 3*	317 ± 27*
Fetal plasma insulin (mU/L)	87 ± 7	103 ± 8*	45 ± 4*
Placental weight (g)	460 ± 20	462 ± 23	560 ± 31*
Placental glycogen (mg/g)	1.7 ± 0.1	1.6 ± 0.1	5.8 ± 0.3*
Offspring weight at 100 days (g)	209 ± 5	205 ± 3	186 ± 6*
Fasting plasma glucose (mg/dL)	91 ± 2	91 ± 1	94 ± 3
Plasma glucose at day 20 of gestation (mg/dL)	80 ± 3	110 ± 5*	98 ± 4*
Granulated beta cells in islets (%)	66 ± 2	50 ± 3	56 ± 2*

*Significant difference from control values at $P < 0.05$ at least. Data are means ± SE; n = 19–34 rats/groups. (Adapted from Aerts et al.[57] and Bihoreau et al.[58])

swelling of mitochondria and glycogen deposits. Insulin stores of the pancreas are correlated with morphological observations: at birth, the fetal insulin content is very low, compared with doubling of insulin stores in fetuses of non-diabetic rats at birth. The response to secretagogues is also concordant with the morphology and insulin content: fetal islets of mildly diabetic mothers are capable of response, whereas those of severely diabetic mothers have a minimal response, indicating a defective stimulus coupling.[57,58] Newborns of severely diabetic mothers exhibit microsomia (even if they are born about 1 day later than those of mildly diabetic mothers) in association with placentomegaly (Table 12.3). Newborns of mildly diabetic mothers are macrosomic, with a postnatal period of hypoglycemia followed by a mild hyperglycemia. At weaning after 1 month, these pups return to fasting normoglycemia, but they exhibit latent diabetes, as seen from the IGT with a low insulin:glucose ratio after a glucose load.

At about 3 months of age, the percentage of granulated cells in pancreatic islets is normal in the progeny of both mildly and severely diabetic mothers; however, the granules of the offspring of the severely diabetic mothers are pale,[54] suggesting insulin depletion. Fasting plasma glucose and insulin levels are normal, but even on slight stress, e.g. anesthesia, glucose and insulin become elevated. At 8 months of age, the situation worsens, basal hyperglycemia, IGT and resistance to insulin action increasing.[59] Half-maximal suppression of hepatic gluconeogenesis requires insulin concentration of about 50% higher than in controls.

The important aspect of the first generation of female offspring of diabetic mothers is their metabolic–endocrine reaction to pregnancy. They develop mild hyperglycemia and IGT during gestation, and their fetuses grow again in hyperglycemic fuel milieu, ensuing in derangements similar to those of the first generation fetuses. Islet hyperplasia and hypertrophy with beta-cell degranulation and hyperinsulinemia, with loss of insulin stores, are perpetuated in the subsequent female pregnant generations. The non-genetic consequence of the abnormal metabolic milieu gives credence to the concept that 'diabetes begets diabetes' by imprinting of alterations in metabolism in the fetus *in utero*, with a propensity to diabetes and

obesity in adult life.[60,61] The hyperglycemia may effect DNA mutagenesis of the reporter lacI transgene during embryonic development. In a transgenic mouse a 2-fold increase in mutation frequency of the IacI transgene was observed in fetuses developing in a hyperglycemic milieu.[62] This finding provides evidence for genotoxicity of the diabetic environment, suggested to be due to the effect of AGE, known for their mutagenicity.

It is worthy to note that similar changes in pancreatic function and characteristics of the offspring can be produced in non-diabetic rats by continuous glucose infusion during the last stage of pregnancy, strengthening the contention that the glycemia is mainly responsible for the persistent transgenerational GDM.[63,64] This was demonstrated by maintaining rats on protracted glucose infusion through indwelling catheters during the last third of gestation. Female offspring of the glucose-infused rats exhibited IGT when 3 months old that persisted during their pregnancy. The newborn second generation was hyperglycemic, hyperinsulinemic and macrosomic, quite similar to the second generation of rats born to STZ-induced diabetic mothers, and on adulthood became glucose intolerant with defective insulin secretion.

Mild gestational diabetes mellitus

A model much sought after is that of mild GDM that reverts to normal after delivery.[65] An attempt to provide such a model was made by transplanting STZ-induced diabetic female rats with isogeneic islets of Langerhans[66] and mating them with non-diabetic partners. The results were promising in that the hyperglycemia in dams transplanted with 700–1000 islets was moderate and no congenital anomalies were observed in the offspring.

Fetal hyperinsulinemia as a cause of macrosomia in pregnancy

Diabetes produces major changes in the hormonal and metabolic homeostasis in pregnancy that has divergent effects on maternal and feto-placental tissues. The hyperglycemia in cytotoxin-induced diabetes was considered to cause maternal tissue malfunction on the one hand and to induce the precocious commencement of fetal insulin secretion on the other. The profuse insulin secretion was assumed to promote fetal overgrowth by the excess of glucose, amino acids and other fuels.[67] The fetuses of STZ-induced diabetic rats were shown to have lower tissue DNA contents and DNA polymerase activities than those of normal or mildly diabetic mothers,[68] suggesting that the fetal tissue growth recedes as the severity of maternal diabetes increases. However, numerous observations underscore that the fetal macrosomia is insulin induced. In mild diabetes it comprises obesity as an important element, in addition to the selective organ overgrowth.

Fetal fat accretion may result from excessive de novo lipogenesis along with stimulated tissue growth during the fetal hyperinsulinemia, or from the excess of maternal lipids entering the fetal circulation because of the steep concentration gradient across the placenta in GDM (Figure 12.3). Fetal fat increment caused by the accelerated maternal transfer is dependent on maternal hypoinsulinemia or insulin resistance and is abetted by the concomitant fetal hyperinsulinemmia. Szabo and Szabo[69] and Skryten et al.[70] were among the first to suggest that the diabetes-augmented lipid gradient across the placenta contributes to fetal obesity. As mentioned above, in more recent studies the extent of endogenous fatty acid synthesis was measured by ^{3}H incorporation, whereas the transfer of maternal fat was monitored with a ^{14}C-labeled fatty acid.[18] In STZ-induced diabetic rats, the endogenous lipogenesis was substantial but was not higher than that in non-diabetic pregnant controls. In contrast, there was a marked increment in the ^{14}C-labeled, maternally derived fat in placental and fetal tissues during the last third of gestation. Thus, both the maternal contribution and the intrafetal fat synthesis appear to contribute to the fetal macrosomia, particularly in mild maternal diabetes, similar to the factors promoting adipose tissue hypertrophy in human gestation.[71]

In rats, the effect of hyperinsulinemia on fetal growth has been investigated by direct intrafetal insulin injection. Rat fetuses receiving 5 U of long-acting insulin on day 18 of gestation had their plasma insulin elevated for 24 h, with the body mass of fetuses exceeding that of saline-injected controls. At birth, the weight of insulin-injected fetuses rose significantly from 5.5 to 5.9 g.[72] Fetal hyperinsulinemia enhanced the hepatic and carcass fatty acid synthesis.[73]

Fetal hyperinsulinemia, achieved by transuteral injections of insulin on day 19 of gestation, resulted in macrosomia at birth, and in net increases in protein and mRNA synthesis in the brain, heart and liver.[74] However, one should be aware that maternal, in contrast to fetal, hyperinsulinemia, produced by implantation of insulin minipumps on day 14 of gestation, produced the opposite result: i.e. it deprived the fetus of fuels, retarded fetal growth and hepatic glycogen deposition, and delayed the onset of hepatic gluconeogenesis in the newborn by suppressing the PEPCK activity.[75]

Perhaps the most impressive demonstration of the induction of macrosomia by direct intrafetal insulin infusion was made by Susa and colleagues[76–78] in pregnant rhesus monkeys. Insulin infusion for 19 days during the last third of gestation resulted in a 23% increase in fetal weight, accompanied by placentomegaly. Fetal organomegaly was selective, with heart and spleen weights increasing significantly. Skeletal growth, assessed by the crown–heel length and the head circumference, remained unchanged, as did the lung, kidney, adrenal and thymus weights (Table 12.4). The levels of insulin-like growth factors I and II rose only in monkeys infused with a high dose of insulin. Because the fetal overgrowth was so prominent, even at moderate hyperinsulinemia, it was clear that insulin was the predominant effector of macrosomia.

The activities of fetal hepatic enzymes concerned with glycolysis were not affected by the hyperinsulinemia; gluconeogenic enzymes were suppressed but lipogenic enzymes became enhanced, indicating an increased de novo fetal fat synthesis.[78] Additional evidence that diabetic macrosomia entails an enhanced cholesterol and lipoprotein metabolism has recently been provided.[79] Macrosomic pups of mildly hyperglycemic STZ pregnant rats had elevated plasma low-density lipoprotein (LDL) and high-density lipoprotein (HDL) cholesterol associated with increased lecithin–cholesterol acyl transferase activity compared with normal birthweight controls. There was no change in hepatic cholesterol content, but hepatic HMG-CoA reductase and cholesterol 7α-hydroxylase activities were higher in both macrosomic males and females. By 3 months, macrosomic rats had developed hypercholesterolemia with a rise in all lipoproteins. These findings demonstrate that macrosomia throughout adulthood is associated with accentuation of both cholesterol synthesis and metabolism.

Table 12.4   Chronic hyperinsulinemia in fetal rhesus monkeys

| Insulin infusion | Plasma insulin (mU/L) | Weight (g) | | | | |
		Fetus	Placenta	Liver	Kidney	Heart
None	28 ± 12	372 ± 54	92 ± 12	11 ± 3	2.7 ± 0.5	2.3 ± 0.6
5 U/day	340 ± 208	459 ± 53*	125 ± 40	14 ± 2	3.0 ± 0.8	3.0 ± 0.7*
19 U/day	3625 ± 1700	474 ± 48*	142 ± 51*	17 ± 4	3.4 ± 0.9	3.7 ± 0.9*

*Significant difference between control and insulin-infused fetuses at $P < 0.05$. Insulin was infused for 20 days at day 145 of gestation. Data are means ± SE. (Adapted from Susa et al.[77])

Pregnant animals with genetically determined Type 1 diabetes and their heterozygotes

BB rats

BB rats offer a good opportunity to study the interaction of genetics, autoimmunity, and environment in the outcome of pregnancy. The attractive features of this spontaneously diabetic animal occur at the *c.* 3 month long prediabetic period prior to the onset of insulin dependency. Because the female BB rat is fertile at *c.* 60 days of age, it is possible to achieve pregnancy in the prediabetic period and to study GDM in an autoimmune animal. Brownscheidle and colleagues[80,81] found a high rate of perinatal mortality, and neural tube and skeletal defects. Intensive treatment with insulin decreased perinatal mortality and reduced the incidence of malformation from *c.* 40 to *c.* 10%, close to the rate in non-diabetic animals. Verhaege et al.[82] found a marked degranulation of beta cells in the fetuses of diabetic BB rats, indicating pancreas overstimulation *in utero* similar to that previously described in fetuses of STZ-induced diabetic rats. Baird et al.[83] obtained a good pregnancy outcome in their diabetic BB/E rats by individually adjusting insulin dosage by monitoring weight and glucuria. They found that insulin requirements during pregnancy doubled in comparison with those of non-pregnant diabetic BB rats. There was no significant difference in the size of litters produced by non-diabetic and diabetic treated animals, but the number of pups weaned per litter was significantly lower in diabetic animals and their growth rate fell off from 15 days of age. Stopping the insulin treatment for any 2 days between 2 and 9 days of gestation resulted in loss of maternal weight and ketosis, higher rates of fetus resorption, lower fetal and higher placental weights, and reduced skeletal maturity.[84]

Because BB rats represent a model for the study of perinatal morbidity, microsomia and malformations, attention was directed to early fetal growth processes. Embryo development in BB rats depends on successful trophoblast invasion into the uterine endometrium and protection of the conceptus, which may be antigenic to the maternal immunocompetent cells. Lea et al.[85] measured trophoblast proliferation by ^{3}H-thymidine incorporation during incubation with 8.5 day decidual extracts. Decidual supernatants from diabetes-resistant BB/E rats or non-diabetic Wistar rats significantly reduced trophoblast outgrowth relative to non-pregnant rats, as expected.

However, decidual supernatants from diabetic BB/E rats did not inhibit the trophoblast cell growth. This finding suggests that BB rat decidual cells secrete a profile of trophoblast reactive factors different to those from non-diabetic rats, and that this increase in the number of trophoblast cells may be related to the subsequent fetal intrauterine growth retardation and congenital malformations.

NOD mice

Among mildly diabetic NOD mice, offspring born before the onset of ketonuria (between 26 and 52 weeks of age) tend to be macrosomic, with a mean increase of 31% in body weight. They show a selective nephromegaly and adiposity compared with non-diabetic controls, but no cardiomegaly (Table 12.5).[86] The macrosomic progeny have a highly elevated pancreatic insulin content but smaller litter sizes. Presence of malformations and subsequent glucose intolerance should be investigated in this model as well as in its heterozygotes.

In further studies with NOD mice, it was observed that the maternal hyperglycemia may not be the only causative factor of macrosomia.[87] High parity and age are also associated with increased birthweights. Mild hyperglycemia plays a major role when age, maternal size, duration of gestation and parity are controlled. Pregnant NOD mice that received pancreas transplants from neonatal donors were demonstrated to have lower plasma glucose and glycohemoglobin levels, and their offspring had lower birthweights. Thus, the increased maternal beta-cell mass effectively reduced the macrosomia in the offspring of prediabetic NOD mice.[88] Placental glucose transporters and hexokinase I were also investigated in diabetic NOD mice.[89] The protein concentrations of these glucose-uptake- and phosphorylation-determining entities were not down-regulated so as to protect the fetoplacental unit from the maternal hyperglycemia-induced alterations, e.g. placental overgrowth and glycogen accumulation, and fetal hyperglycemia and hyperinsulinemia.

Pregnant animals with genetically determined Type 2-like diabetes

As mentioned before, animals with Type 2-like diabetic syndromes are generally infertile. This appears to be related to insulin resistance impairing the mediobasal hypothalamus–pituitary system, resulting in decreased gonadotropin release.[90,91]

Table 12.5	Macrosomia in the offspring of young, mildly diabetic NOD mice prior to the onset of insulin dependency				
	Maternal glucose (mg/dL)	Fetal weight (g)	Heart weight (mg/g)	Kidney weight (mg/g)	Pancreas insulin (mg/g)
Control	145 ± 8	1.4 ± 0.1	12 ± 1.7	9.6 ± 1.3	0.7 ± 0.0
Mildly diabetic	187 ± 5*	1.8 ± 0.1*	9.0 ± 2.3	10.4 ± 2.3	1.3 ± 0.2*

Significant difference at $P < 0.05$ at least for 14–19 mice. (Adapted from Formby et al.[87])

Breeding of these animals in most cases involves mating heterozygotes, among whom GDM is often detected.

C57 BIKS leprdb+ heterozygotes

These mice are highly attractive for the study of GDM. Only a few experimental protocols have been carried out with these animals,[92] but the information gained suggests that they may represent an excellent experimental approach. Heterozygous leprdb+ mice have a significant glucose intolerance and elevated glycohemoglobin levels during pregnancy, compared with pregnant homozygous non-diabetic siblings. There was no difference in litter size, whereas the mean weight of pups of heterozygous mice was significantly higher, with 19% of them > 95th percentile of the weight of pups from non-diabetic mice. The GDM in leprdb+ was extensively reviewed by Shao and Friedman.[93] They found that leprdb+ mice do not develop any diabetic symptoms in the non-pregnant state and have normal body weights, and plasma glucose and fasting insulin levels are similar to those in wild-type mice. During the early stages of pregnancy (days 1–15) there is no IGT, but from day 16 > 98% of leprdb+ mice have significantly higher glucose levels at 30 minutes and 1 h during i.p. glucose tolerance testing. At the end of day 19 of pregnancy, fasting plasma glucose levels are still in the normal range, despite IGT, and this finding is similar to most human GDM patients who may manifest insulin secretion adequate to compensate for the resistance. However, mice exhibit higher body weights and plasma insulin levels, and fetal macrosomia. After delivery all these parameters revert to normal.

The leprdb+ pregnant mice are extremely insulin resistant – they almost do not respond to injected insulin with a reduction of plasma glucose (Figure 12.4). Leprdb+ mice consume about 13% more food and gain more weight during pregnancy compared with their non-heterozygous siblings,

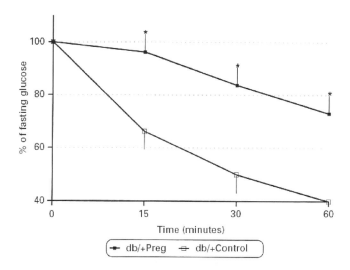

Figure 12.4 Response to exogenous insulin in pregnant leprdb mice compared with pregnant controls. At day 18 of gestation the mice were fasted for 6 h and then injected i.p. with 7.5 U/kg insulin. Glucose values are means + SE. *Significance $P < 0.02$ at least.

suggesting that the leptin receptor site is not fully recessive with regard to fat mass, and that heterozygosity at the leptin receptor may play a role in the susceptibility to environmental conditions favoring obesity and insulin resistance. IGT present despite significantly higher insulin levels, compared with normal pregnant or non-pregnant leprdb+ mice, and despite enhanced insulin synthesis and secretion in response to glucose, indicating insufficient compensation of hyperglycemia by insulin oversecretion. The wild-type pups from leprdb+ mothers return to normal body weights as adults, but +/+ female offspring in particular are more likely to become obese on a high-fat diet compared with the wild-type offspring of normal mothers. GLUT4 activity and translocation in GDM is reduced, but may be improved by transfection of the human GLUT4 gene.[94] Glucose-stimulated insulin secretion is increased and insulin receptor and its substrate (IRS)-1 activity reduced independent of food intake.

C57BL/6J mice

The non-obese, non-diabetic BL/6J mice, the genomic host of the ob/ob mutation, when placed on an affluent fat and sucrose-rich diet become hypertensive and insulin resistant with first-phase insulin release disappearing at 6 months of age.[95–97] Abnormalities, characterized by increased outflow from the sympathetic nervous system, deranged beta-cell function and adipocyte metabolism were found to be responsible for the resultant IGT and insulin-resistance syndrome. No hyperphagia or elevation in corticosterone levels was seen. Thus, inbred laboratory mice, without overt metabolic disturbance, were shown to be susceptible to nutritionally induced diabetes and obesity with marked hyperinsulinemia, hyperlipidemia and polygenic vulnerabilities. The C57/BL/6J mice retain their fertility after developing diabetes and are a potential model of GDM. Pregnancy produced significant hyperinsulinemia beyond the diet alone in BL/6J but not in control A/J mice. There were differences in the number and weight of pups per litter for either strain or diet groups. There was no fetal loss on a regular diet but a high rate of pup loss in the high-energy diet groups. There was no hyperglycemia, which was most probably compensated by hyperinsulinemia. Maternal mice returned to normal weights and glucose tolerances after birth, and there was no macrosomia in the progeny. These mice might be of interest for the study of GDM and pup loss elicited by high-energy diets.

Goto–Kakizaki rats

Apart from animals with spontaneous alterations leading to inappropriate hyperglycemia, a diabetic line was isolated by repeated breeding of normal animals. The selection was of individuals with minimal deviation from the mean response to a glucose load. This emphasizes the polygenic basis of diabetes within a 'normal' genetic mosaic. A GK diabetic line was obtained by breeding Wistar rats for > 35 generations in Japan, using a relative intolerance to a 2 g/kg glucose load as a selection index.[98] The GK rats are non-obese and non-hyperinsulinemic, their diabetes is inheritable but is stable with age. Insulin resistance is present and decreased hepatic insulin receptor numbers were noted with normal tyrosine

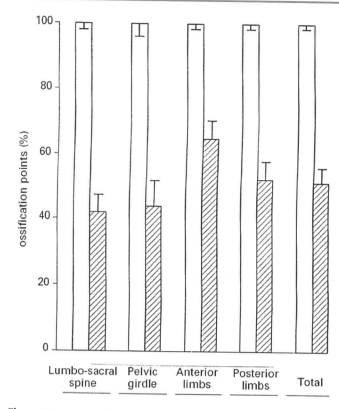

Figure 12.5 Number of ossification points in fetus as from Goto–Kakizaki (GK) rats (hatched bars) versus controls (open bars). Values are means + SE for 61 GK and 125 control fetuses expressed as a percentage of the control value. (From Malaisse-Laege et al.[99])

kinase (TK) activity per receptor. During pregnancy at 15–20 days gestation, GK rats had gained less weight than controls, though the number of fetuses in each litter was similar. The abortive fetal development averaged 40% compared with 6% in controls. A particular finding was the low number of ossification points in the lumbosacral spine, pelvic girdle, and anterior and posterior limbs (Figure 12.5).[99] These anomalies were not related to lower plasma insulin levels before or during the pregnancy and may be related to the impaired vitamin D metabolism in the GK rats.[100]

Nutrition-induced diabetes

When animals are fed a high carbohydrate diet, consisting mainly of fructose, they display features of Type 2 diabetes within a short time. Fasting hyperglycemia, hyperinsulinemia and hyper-lipidemia as well as insulin resistance develop.[101–103] Some of these features can be ameliorated by supplementing the diet with fish oil[104] or by troglitazone as a food admixture.[105] Although this has been known for a long time surprisingly little use has been made of this model in pregnancy. One additional effect of the diet is the development of hypertension. This was also found in pregnancy[106] suggesting that the fructose-induced diabetes may result in the development of sustained hypertension during pregnancy via the

insulin-resistance–hyperinsulinemia link. A similar model was developed on a high sucrose diet[107] but the effect of pregnancy on its metabolism is pending.

Psammomys obesus

The Israeli 'sand rat', *Psammomys obesus*, a desert gerbil, uses a predominantly vegetarian diet in its natural habitat. It has developed a high metabolic efficiency characteristic of a thrifty metabolism. When these animals are domesticated and fed a laboratory rodent diet, which is hypercaloric relative to their habitat staple, they develop hyperinsulinemia, hyperglycemia, and insulin resistance and beta-cell loss.[108,109] The latter is caused by overexpression of protein kinase Cε.[110,111] This animal serves as an excellent model for nutritionally induced Type 2 diabetes. When pregnant, *Psammomys* has similar pregnancy rates, but reduced litter size as compared with their counterparts kept on a low-energy diet.[112] Pregnancy duration is somewhat extended, but the offspring weighs less and had a shorter crown–rump length. In the postnatal period offspring neurodevelopment was delayed. After 4 weeks of life they develop diabetes.[111] This model may also be a valuable for studies into the effect of alterations in maternal lipid metabolism on malformations and fetal development. Accumulation of lipids and diacylglycerol (DAG) in the muscle has been noted in the insulin resistant *Psammomys*.[110,111] DAG is the causative lipid eliciting PKC overexpression, as illustrated in Figure 12.6. PKC phosphorylates serine residues on several components of the insulin signaling pathway inhibiting tyrosine phosphorylation and thus attenuating the downstream insulin signaling.

The intramyocellular accumulation of lipids in skeletal muscle is correlated with insulin resistance in human post GDM subjects,[113] indicating proneness to Type 2 diabetes. This is most probably due to PKC overexpression and results in reduced muscle glucose uptake by inducing insulin resistance. Zierath et al.[114] have shown that high-fat feeding impairs the recruitment of GLUT4 and produces a defect in the function of the phosphatidylinositol (PI)-3 kinase in muscle of lepr[db+] mice with GDM. It was found that serine phosphorylation of IRS-1 was associated with redistribution of PI-3 kinase to the beta subunit of the insulin receptor. This was suggested to result in the inhibition of the receptor tyrosine kinase activity and in the increase of the PKC expression in pregnancy that inhibits IRS serine phosphorylation. These data indicate that a new in-depth approach is needed to assess the insulin resistance in GDM at the molecular level of insulin signal transduction.

Conclusions

The choice of an animal model for the study of diabetes in pregnancy depends very much on the particular pathophysiological alteration exhibited by the animal and its relation to human diabetes, whether pre- or intragestational. It also depends on the specific interest of the investigator. Because of the complexity of human gestation and the variety of its complications, more than one model may be necessary for exploration, since the similarities between diabetic derangements in

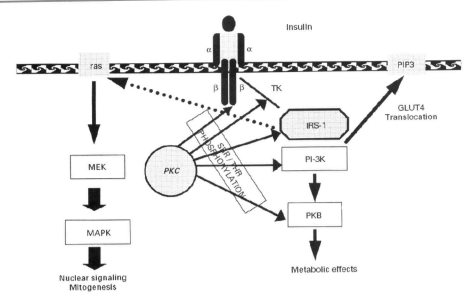

Figure 12.6 Principles of insulin signaling pathway inhibition by overexpression of protein kinase C (PKC) isoenzymes. The PKC activated serine phosphorylation affects the beta subunit of the insulin receptor (IR), the IR substrate (IRS), phosphatidylinositol (PI)-3 and PKB activities. The latter is responsible for activation of multiple metabolic systems. The mitogenic activity activated by insulin through MAP kinase is not affected by PKC.

certain animals and in the diabetic woman may be limited. The endocrine–metabolic aberrations and the histopathological lesions of diabetes in a given animal may either surpass or be constrained in relation to those encountered in human diabetes. Many new models, including a variety of mild and severe STZ-induced diabetes, are now available to fulfil the needs of this approach.

The use of STZ-generated diabetic pregnant animals was predominant until recently. These models represent the condition of absent or limited endogenous insulin presence. The proper approach to GDM is the use of models with normal or excessive endogenous insulin to compensate, or attempt to compensate, the salient insulin resistance of pregnancy. More models of this kind are becoming available, either from a genetic background or from nutritionally induced Type 2-like diabetes (some of them are described in this chapter). Investigators should increasingly turn to these models as well as developing further models of this kind in order to unravel

the various complications of insulin-resistant GDM and the associated macrosomia.

If malformations are of primary interest, one can use the preconceptionally induced STZ-induced diabetic animals or embryos cultured in a diabetic milieu, in which severe multiple malformations and fetal wastage are encountered. If malformations accompanying mild diabetes are the target, than the progeny of STZ-induced diabetic animals or neonatally STZ injected newborns should be selected. The nSTZ animals and the offspring of diabetic mothers are eminently suitable for the investigation of GDM with moderate insulin insufficiency. Effects on the fetal pancreas, particularly those governing beta-cell replication, are good research targets in these models. Much remains to be done on pancreas morphology and the possibility of stimulation of beta-cell replication *in vivo*.

However, insulin resistance most probably represents the main cause of GDM, with limitation of secretion appearing afterwards, unless there is a precondition affecting the

Table 12.6 Triglyceride (TG) levels in serum, liver and gastrocnemius muscle of control, mildly, and severely streptozotocin (STZ)-induced diabetic rats on day 20 of pregnancy

	Serum glucose (mmol/L)	Serum TG (mmol/L)	Liver TG (mg/g)	Muscle TG (mg/g)
Control	5.1 ± 0.3	2.4 ± 0.4	0.28 ± 0.3	0.040 ± 0.008
Mild diabetes	$11.5 \pm 0.7^*$	3.9 ± 0.6	$0.45 \pm 0.6^*$	$0.084 \pm 0.016^†$
Severe diabetes	$22.8 \pm 1.6^†$	$7.1 \pm 0.9^†$	$0.83 \pm 1.0^†$	$0.133 \pm 0.022^†$

*Significant difference between mild diabetic and control rats at $P < 0.05$ at least.
†Significant difference between mild and severe diabetic rats at $P < 0.02$ at least.
Values are means ± SE for 10 rats. (Unpublished data of E. Shafrir.)

efficiency of insulin secretion. Therefore, the emphasis should be placed on factors causing insulin resistance and insulin signaling malfunction in pregnancy, leading to macrosomia and fetal obesity, including the increased fetal lipogenesis in this condition. The heterozygote animals in a prediabetic stage introduce new facets of etiology of GDM on a range of backgrounds, spanning from pancreatic cell lability to peripheral and hepatic insulin resistance. Both hormonal alterations inducing insulin resistance in pregnancy and enhancing

muscle lipid deposition, which induces the accumulation of diacylglycerol and activation of PKC, should be actively explored together with possible effects on the insulin signaling pathway in pregnancy.

Another aspect, which should not be omitted, is the research possibly enabling the use of oral antidiabetic modalities, e.g. metformin or thiazolidinediones, to increase insulin sensitivity in pregnancy, counteracting hyperglycemia as the main culprit of pregnancy complications.

REFERENCES

1. Cooperstein SJ, Watkins D. Action of toxic drugs on islet cells. In: Cooperstein SJ, Watkins D, eds. The Islets of Langerhans. New York: Academic Press; 1981, pp. 387–425.
2. Shafrir E. Diabetes in animals. In: Porte Jr. D, Sherwin R, Baron A, eds. Diabetes Mellitus, 6th edn. New York: McGraw-Hill; 2003.
3. Okamoto H. The molecular basis of experimental diabetes. In: Okamoto H, ed. Molecular Biology of the Islets of Langerhans. Cambridge: Cambridge University Press; 1990, pp. 209–31.
4. Boquist L. Aspects of the diabetogenecity of alloxan and streptozotocin with special regard to a 'mitochondrial hypothesis.' In: Shafrir E, ed. Lessons from Animal Diabetes, Vol. 4. London: Smith-Gordin; 1992, pp. 1–16.
5. McNeill JH, ed. The Streptozotocin-induced Diabetic Rat. Section I. Experimental Models of Diabetes. Boca Raton: CRC Press; 1999.
6. Dickinson JE, Meyer BA, Chmielowiec S, Palmer SM. Streptozotocin induced diabetes mellitus in the pregnant ewe. Am J Obstet Gynecol 1991; 165: 1673–7.
7. Hay Jr WW, Meznarich HK. Use of fetal streptozotocin injection to determine the role of normal levels of fetal insulin in regulating uteroplacental and umbilical glucose exchange. Pediatr Res 1988; 24: 312–7.
8. Peterson CM, Jovanovic-Peterson L, Bevier W, Formby B. Animal models of diabetic pregnancy. Adv Diabetol 1992; 5(suppl. 1): 11–16.
9. Mintz DH, Chez RA, Hutchinson DL. Subhuman primate pregnancy complicated by streptozotocin induced diabetes mellitus. J Clin Invest 1972; 51: 837–47.
10. Baird JD, Aerts L. Research priorities in diabetic pregnancy today: the role of animal models. Biol Neonate 1987; 51: 119–27.
11. Susa JB. Methodology for the study of metabolism: animal models. In: Cowett R, ed. Principles of Perinatal–Neonatal Metabolism. New York: Springer-Verlag; 1991, 48–60.
12. Sybulski S, Maughan GB. Use of streptozotocin as diabetic agent in pregnant rats. Endocrinology 1974; 94: 1247–53.
13. Pitkin RM, Van Oren DE. Fetal effects of maternal streptozotin-diabetes. Endocrinology 1974; 94: 1247–53.
14. Golob EK, Rishi S, Becker KL, Moore C. Streptozotocin diabetes in pregnant and nonpregnant rats. Metabolism 1970; 19: 1014–9.
15. Prager R, Abramovici A, Liban E, Laron Z. Histopathological changes in the placenta of streptozotocin induced diabetes rats. Diabetologia 1974; 10: 89–91.
16. Eriksson UJ. Congenital malformations in animal models. Diabetes Res 1984; 1: 57–66.
17. Diamant YZ, Shafrir E. Placental enzymes of glycolysis, gluconeogenesis and lipogenesis in the diabetic rat and in starvation: comparison with maternal and fetal liver. Diabetologia 1978; 15: 481–591.
18. Shafrir E, Khassis S. Maternal–fetal transport versus new fat synthesis in the pregnant diabetic rat. Diabetologia 1982; 22: 111–7.
19. Reynolds WA, Chez RA, Bhuyan BK, Neil GL. Placental transfer of streptozotocin in the Rhesus monkey. Diabetes 1971; 23: 777–82.
20. Shafrir E, Barash V. Placental glycogen metabolism in diabetic pregnancy. Isr J Med Sci 1991; 27: 449–61.
21. Diamant YZ, Metzger BE, Freinkel N, Shafrir E. Placental lipid and glycogen content in human and experiment diabetes mellitus. Am J Obstet Gynecol 1982; 144: 5–11.
22. Barash V, Gutman A, Shafrir E. Mechanism of placental glycogen deposition in diabetes in the rat. Diabetologia 1983; 24: 63–8.
23. Barash V, Gimmon Z, Shafrir E. Placental glycogen accumulation and maternal-fed metabolic responses in hyperglycaemic non-diabetic rats. Diabetes Res 1986; 3: 97–101.
24. Sochor M, Baquer N, McLean P. Glucose overutilization in diabetes: evidence from studies on the changes in hexokinase, the pentose phosphate pathway, and glucuronate–xylulose pathway in rat kidney cortex in diabetes. Biochem Biophys Res Commun 1979; 86: 32–9.
25. Khandelwal RL, Zinman M, Knull HR. The effect of streptozotocin-induced diabetes on glycogen metabolism in rat kidney and its relationship to the liver system. Arch Biochem Biophys 1979; 197: 310–6.
26. Delaval E, Moreau E, Adriamanantsara S, Geloso JP. Renal glycogen content and hormonal control of enzymes involved in renal glycogen metablism. Pediatr Res 1983; 17: 766–9.
27. Anderson W, Jones AL. Biochemical and ultrastructural study of glycogen in jejunal mucosa of diabetic rats. Proc Soc Exp Biol Med 1984; 145: 268–72.
28. Ezekwe MO, Martin RJ. The effects of maternal alloxan diabetes on body composition, liver enzymes and metabolism and serum metabolites and hormones of fetal pigs. Hormone Metabolic Res 1980; 12: 136–9.
29. Shafrir E, Barash V. Placental function in maternal–fetal fat transport in diabetes. Biol Neonate 1987; 51: 102–12.
30. Goldstein R, Levy E, Shafrir E. Increased maternal–fetal transport of fat in diabetes assessed by polyunsaturated fatty acid content in fetal lipids. Biol Neonate 1985; 47: 343–49.
31. Kasser TR, Martin RJ, Allen CE. Effect of gestational alloxan diabetes and fasting on fetal lipogenesis and lipid deposition in pigs. Biol Neonate 1981; 40: 105–12.
32. Martin RJ, Makula A, Kasser TR. Placental metabolism and enzyme activities in diabetic pigs. Proc Soc Exp Biol Med 1980; 165: 39–43.
33. Shafrir E, Barash V, Zederman R, et al. Modulation of fetal and placental metabolic pathways in response to maternal thyroid and glucocorticoid hormone excess. Isr J Med Sci 1994; 30: 32–41.
34. Diamant YZ, Neuman S, Shafrir E. Effect of chorionic gonadotropin, triamcinolone, progesterone and estrogen on enzymes of placenta and liver in rats. Biochem Biophys Acta 1975; 385: 257–67.
35. Hauguel A, Leturque A, Gilbert M, et al. Glucose utilization by the placenta and fetal tissues in fed and fasted pregnant rabbits. Pediatr Res 1988; 23: 480–3.
36. Singh M, Feigelson M. Effects of maternal diabetes on the development of carbohydrate metabolizing enzymes in fetal rat liver. Arch Biochem Biophys 1981; 209: 655–67.
37. Styrud J, Thunberg L, Nybacka O, Eriksson UJ. Correlations between maternal metabolism and deranged development in the offspring of normal and diabetic rats. Pediatr Res 1995; 37: 343–53.
38. Chernicky CL, Redline RW, Tan HQ, et al. Expression of insulin-like growth factor-I and factor-II in conceptuses from normal and diabetic mice. Moles Reprod Dev 1994; 37: 382–90.
39. Sadler TW. Effects of maternal diabetes on early embryogenesis. I. The teratogenic potential of diabetic serum. Teratology 1980; 21: 339–47.
40. Strieleman J, Connors MA, Metzger BE. Phosphoinositide metabolism in the developing conceptus. Effects of hyperglycemia and scyllo-inositol on rat embryo culture. Diabetes 1992; 41: 989–97.
41. Hod M, Star S, Passonneau JV, et al. Effect of hyperglycemia on sorbitol and myo-inositol content of cultured rat conceptuses: failure of aldose reductase inhibitors to modify myo-inositol depletion and dysmorphogenesis. Biochem Biophys Res Commun 1986; 140: 974–80.
42. Hod M, Star S, Passonneau J, et al. Glucose-induced dysmorphogenesis in the cultured rat conceptus: prevention by supplementation with myo-inositol. Isr J Med Sci 1990; 26: 541–4.
43. Zaken V, Kohen R, Ornoy A. Vitamins C and E improve rat embryonic antioxidant defense mechanism in diabetic culture medium. Teratology 2001; 64: 33–44.

44. Ornoy A, Zaken V, Kohen R. Role of reactive oxygen species (ROS) in the diabetes-induced anomalies in rat embryos in vitro: reduction in antioxidant enzymes and low-molecular weight antioxidants (LMWA) may be the causative factor for increased anomalies. Teratology 1999; 60: 1–11.
45. Portha B, Picon L, Rosselin G. Chemical diabetes in the adult rat as the spontaneous evolution of neonatal diabetes. Diabetologia 1979; 17: 371–7.
46. Bonner-Weir S, Trent DF, Honey RN, Weir GC. Responses of neonatal rat islets to streptozotocin: limited B-cell regeneration and hyperglycemia. Diabetes 1981; 30: 64–9.
47. Bonner-Weir S, Leahy JL, Weir GC. Induced rat models of noninsulin-dependent diabetes. In: Renold AE, Shafrir E, eds. Lessons from Animal Diabetes, Vol. 2. London: Libby; 1988, pp. 295–300.
48. Portha B, Movassat J, Cousin-Tournel D, et al. Neonatally streptozotocin-induced (n-STZ) diabetic rats: a family of Type 2 diabetews models. In: Shefrir E, ed. Animal Models of Diabetes, 2nd edn. Francis & Thomas, CRC Press; Boca Raton; 2007.
49. Triadou N, Portha B, Picon L, Rosselin G. Experimental chemical diabetes and pregnancy in the rat: evolution of glucose tolerance and insulin response. Diabetes 1982; 31: 75–9.
50. Schaffer SW, Mozaffari M. The neonatal STZ model of diabetes in experimental models of diabetes. In: McNeill JH, ed. Experimental Models of Diabetes. Boca Raton: CRC Press; 1999, 231–56.
51. Iwase M, Wada M, Shinohara N, et al. Effect of maternal diabetes on longevity in offspring of spontaneously hypertensive rats. Gerontology 1995; 41: 181–6.
52. Wada M, Iwase M, Wakisaka M, et al. A new model of diabetic pregnancy with genetic hypertension: pregnancy in spontaneously hypertensive rats with neonatal streptozotocin-induced diabetes. Am J Obstet Gynecol 1995; 172: 626–30.
53. Iwase M, Wada M, Wakisaka M, et al. Effects of maternal diabetes on blood pressure and glucose tolerance in offspring of spontaneously hypertensive rats: relation to birth weight. Clin Sci 1995; 89: 255–60.
54. Aerts L, Holeman K, Van Assche FA. Maternal diabetes during pregnancy: consequences for the offspring. Diabetes Metabolic Rev 1990; 6: 147–67.
55. Van Assche FA, Gepts W, Aerts L. Immuno-cytochemical study of the endocrine pancreas in the rat during normal pregnancy and during experimental diabetic pregnancy. Diabetologia 1980; 18: 487–91.
56. Aerts L, Van Assche FA. Endocrine pancreas in the offspring of rats with experimentally induced diabetes. J Endocrinol 1981; 88: 81–8.
57. Bihoreau Mth, Ktorza A, Picon L. Gestational hyperglycemia and insulin release by the fetal rat pancreas in vitro: effect of amino acids and glyceraldehydes. Diabetologia 1986; 29: 434–9.
58. Aerts L, Holeman K, Van Assche FA. Impaired insulin response and action in offspring of severely diabetic rats. In: Shafrir E, ed. Lessons from Animal Diabetes, Vol. 3. London: Smith-Gordon; 1990, pp. 561–6.
59. Holemans K, Van Bree R, Verhaeghe J, et al. In vivo glucose utilization by individual tissues in virgin and pregnant offspring of severely diabetic rats. Diabetes 1993; 42: 530–6.
60. Gauguier D, Bihoreau MT, Ktorza A, et al. Inheritance of diabetes mellitus as consequence of gestational hyperglycemia in rats. Diabetes 1990; 39: 734–9.
61. Zhong S, Dunbar JC, Jen K-LC. Postnatal development in rat offspring delivered of dams with gestational hyperglycemia. Am J Obstet Gynecol 1994; 171: 753–63.
62. Lee At, Plump A, DeSimone C, et al. A role for DNA mutations in diabetes-associated teratogenesis in transgenic embryos. Diabetes 1995; 44: 20–4.
63. Bihoreau MT, Ktorza A, Kinebanyau MF, Picon L. Impaired glucose homeostasis in adult rats from hyperglycemic mothers. Diabetes 1986; 35: 979–84.
64. Ktorza A, Gauguier D, Bihoreau MT, et al. Long-term effects of gestational hyperglycemia: a non-genetic transmission of diabetes in the rat. Diabetologia 1988; 31: 510A.
65. Hellerstrom C, Swenne I, Eriksson UJ. Is there an animal model for gestational diabetes? Diabetes 1985; 34: 28–31.
66. Ryan EA, Tobin BW, Tang J, Finegood DT. A new model for the study of mild diabetes during pregnancy: syngeneic islet-transplanted STZ-induced diabetic rats. Diabetes 1993; 42: 316–23.
67. Freinkel N. Banting Lecutre 1980: Of pregnancy and progeny. Diabetes 1980; 29: 1023–35.
68. Kim YS, Jatoi I, Kim Y. Neonatal macrosomia in maternal diabetes. Diabetologia 1980; 18: 407–11.
69. Szabo AJ, Szabo O. Placental free fatty acid transfer and fetal adipose tissue development: an explanation of fetal adiposity in infants of diabetic mothers. Lancet 1974; 2: 498–9.
70. Skryten A, Johnson P, Samsioe G, Gustafson A. Studies in diabetic pregnancy I. Serum lipids. Acta Obstet Gynecol Scand 1976; 55: 211–5.
71. Enzi G, Inelmen EM, Caretta F, et al. Adipose tissue development 'in utero': relationships between some nutritional and hormonal factors and body fat mass enlargement in newborns. Diabetologia 1980; 18: 135–40.
72. Ogata ES, Collins Jr JW, Finley S. Insulin injection in the fetal rat: accelerated intrauterine growth and altered fetal and neonatal glucose homeostasis. Metabolism 1988; 37: 649–55.
73. Catlin EA, Cha C-JM, Oh W. Postnatal growth and fatty acid synthesis in overgrown rat pups induced by fetal hyperinsulinemia. Metabolism 1985; 34: 1110–4.
74. Johnson JD, Dunham T, Wogenrich FJ, et al. Fetal hyperinsulinemia and protein turnover in fetal rat tissues. Diabetes 1990; 39: 541–8.
75. Ogata ES, Paul RI, Finley SL. Limited maternal fuel availability due to hyperinsulinemia retards fetal growth and development in the rat. Pediatr Res 1987; 22: 432–7.
76. Susa JB, Neave C, Sehgal P, et al. Chronic hyperinsulinemia in the fetal rhesus monkey. Diabetes 1984; 33: 656–60.
77. Susa JB, Schwartz R. Effects of hyperinsulinemia in the primate fetus. Diabetes 1985; 34: 36–41.
78. McCormick KL, Susa JB, Widness JA, et al. Chronic hyperinsulinemia in the fetal rhesus monkey: effects on hepatic enzymes active in lipogenesis and carbohydrate metabolism. Diabetes 1979; 28: 1064–8.
79. Merzouk H, Madani S, Boualga A, et al. Age-related changes in cholesterol metabolism in macrosomic offspring of rats with streptozotocin-induced diabetes. J Lipid Res 2001; 42: 1152–9.
80. Brownscheidle CM, Davis DL. Diabetes in pregnancy: a preliminary study of the pancreas, placenta and malformations in the BB Wistar rat. Placenta 1989; 3(suppl): 203–16.
81. Brownscheidle CM, Wooten V, Mathieu MH, et al. The effects of maternal diabetes on fetal maturation and neonatal health. Metabolism 1983; 32: 148–55.
82. Verhaege J, Peeters TL, Vandeputte M, et al. Maternal and fetal endocrine pancreas in the spontaneously diabetic BB rat. Biol Neonate 1989; 55: 298–308.
83. Baird JD, Bone AJ, Eriksson UF. The BB rat: a model for insulin-dependent diabetic pregnancy. In: Renold AE, Shafrir E, eds. Lessons From Animal Diabetes, Vol. 2. London: Libby; 1988, pp. 412–7.
84. Eriksson UJ, Bone AJ, Turnbull DM, Baird JD. Timed interruption of insulin therapy in diabetic BB/E rat pregnancy: effect on maternal metabolism and fetal outcome. Acta Endocrinol 1989; 120: 800–10.
85. Lea RG, McCracken JE, Smith W, Baird JD. Disturbed development of the pre- implantation embryo in the insulin dependent BB/E rat. Diabetes 1996; 45: 1463–70.
86. Formby B, Schmid-Formby F, Jovanovic L, Peterson CM. The offspring of the female diabetic 'nonobese diabetic' (NOD) mouse are large for gestational ageand have elevated pancreatic insulin content: a new animal model of human diabetic pregnancy. Proc Soc Exp Biol Med 1987; 184: 291–4.
87. Bevier WC, Jovanovic-Peterson L, Formby B, Peterson CM. Maternal hyperglycemia is not the only cause of macrosomia: lessons learned from the nonobese diabetic mouse. Am J Perinatol 1994; 1: 51–6.
88. Chen H-M, Jovanovic-Peterson L, Desai TA, Peterson DM. Lessons learned from the non-obese diabetic mouse II: amelioration of pancreatic autoimmune isograft rejection during pregnancy. Am J Perinatol 1966; 13: 249–54.
89. Devaskar SU, Devaskar UP, Schroeder RE, et al. Expression of genes involved in placental glucose uptake and transport in the nonobese diabetic mouse pregnancy. Am J Obstet Gynecol 1994; 171: 1316–23.
90. Bestetti GE, Rossi GL. Effects of diabetes on functional and morphological complications in the hypothalamopituitary system of diabetic rodent models. A pathogenesis overview. In: Shafrir E, ed. Lessons from Animal Diabetes, Vol. 3. London: Smith Gordon; 1988, pp. 466–70.
91. Rossi GL, Bestetti GE. In vitro assessment of functional and morphological complications in the hypothalamopituitary system of diabetic rodent models. In: Shafrir E, ed. Lessons from Animal Diabetes, Vol. 3. London: Smith Gordon; 1988, pp. 471–4.
92. Kaufmann RC, Amankwah KS, Dunaway G, et al. An animal model of gestational diabetes. Am J Obstet Gynecol 1981; 141: 479–82.
93. Shao J, Friedman JE. Gestational diabetes and maternal insulin resistance in the C57BLKS/Jleprdb+ mouse – a unique model for understanding the impact on the fetus. In: Hansen B, Shafrir E, eds. Insulin Resistance and Insulin Resistance Syndrome. London: Taylor & Francis; 2002.

94. Ishizuka T, Klepcyk P, Liu S, et al. Effects of overexpression of human GLUT4 gene on maternal diabetes and fetal growth in spontaneous gestational diabetic C57BLKS/J Lepr (db/+) mice. Diabetes 1999; 48: 1061–9.

95. Livingston EG, Feinglos MN, Kuhn CM, et al. Hyperinsulinemia in the pregnant C57BL/6J mouse. Hormone Metabolic Res 1994; 26: 307.

96. Martin T, Collins S, Surwit RS. The C57BL/6J mouse as a model of insulin resistance and hypertension. In: Hansen B, Shafrir E, eds. Insulin Resistance and Insulin Resistance Syndrome. London: Taylor & Francis; 2002.

97. Petro AE, Surwit RS. The C57BL/6J mouse as a model of diet induced type 2 diabetes and obesity. In: Sima AAF, Shafrir E, eds. Animal Models of Diabetes. A Primer. London: Harwood Academic Press; 2000, pp. 337–50.

98. Ostenson CG. The Goto–Kakizaki rat. In: Shafrir E, ed. Animal Models of Diabetes, 2nd. edn. Taylor & Francis, CRC Press; 2007.

99. Malaisse-Lagae F, Vanhoutte C, Rypens F, et al. Anomalies of fetal development in GK rats. Acta Diabetol 1997; 34: 55–60.

100. Ishimura E, Nishizawa Y, Koyama H, et al. Impaired vitamin D metabolism and response in spontaneously diabetic GK rats. Miner Electrolyte Metab 1995; 21: 205–10.

101. Hwang IS, Ho H, Hoffman BB, Reaven GM. Fructose-induced insulin resistance and hypertension in rats. Hypertension 1987; 10: 512–6.

102. Zavaroni I, Sander S, Scott S, Reaven GM. Effect of fructose feeding on insulin secretion and insulin action in the rat. Metabolism 1980; 29: 970–3.

103. Luo J, Rizkalla SW, Lerer-Metzger M, et al. A fructose-rich diet decreases insulin-stimulated glucose incorporation into lipids but not glucose transport in adipocytes of normal and diabetic rats. J Nutr 1995; 125: 164–71.

104. Huang YJ, Fang VS, Juan CC, et al. Amelioration of insulin resistance and hypertension in a fructose-fed rat model with fish oil supplementation. Metabolism 1997; 46: 1252–8.

105. Lee MK, Miles PD, Khoursheed M, et al. Metabolic effects of troglitazone on fructose-induced insulin resistance in the rat. Diabetes 1994; 43: 1435–9.

106. Olatunji B, II, Nwachukwu D, Adegunloye BJ. Blood pressure and heart rate changes during pregnancy in fructose-fed Sprague–Dawley rats. Afr J Med Med Sci 2001; 30: 187–90.

107. Weksler-Zangen S, Yagil C, Zangen DH, et al. The newly inbred Cohen diabetic rat: a nonobese normolipidemic genetic model of diet induced type 2 diabetes expressing sex differences. Diabetes 2001; 50: 2521–9.

108. Shafrir E, Gutman A. Psammomys obesus of the Jerusalem colony: a model for nutritionally induced, non-insulin-dependent diabetes. J Basic Clin Physiol Pharmacol 1993; 4: 83–99.

109. Shafrir E, Ziv E. Cellular mechanism of nutritionally induced insulin resistance: the desert gerbil Psammomys obesus and other animals in which insulin resistance leads to detrimental outcome. J Basic Clin Physiol Pharmacol 1999; 9: 347–85.

110. Ikeda Y, Olsen GS, Ziv E, Hansen LL, Busch AK, Hansen BF, et al. Cellular mechanism of nutritionally induced insulin resistance in Psammomys obesus: overexpression of protein kinase Cepsilon in skeletal muscle precedes the onset of hyperinsulinemia and hyperglycemia. Diabetes 2001; 50: 584–92.

111. Shafrir E, Ziv E. Mosthaf L. Nutritionally induced insulin resistance and receptor defect leading to beta cell failure in animal models – human implications. Ann NY Acad Sci 1999; 892: 223–46.

112. Patlas N, Avgil M, Ziv E, Ornoy A, Shafrir E. Pregnancy outcome in the Psammomys obesus gerbil on low- and high-energy diets. Biol Neonate 2006; 90: 58–65.

113. Kautzky-Willer A, Krssak M, Winzer C, et al. Increased intramyocellular lipid concentration identifies impaired glucose metabolism in women with previous gestational diabetes. Diabetes 2003; 52: 244–51.

114. Zierath JR, Houseknecht KL, Goudi L, Kahn BB. High fat feeding impairs insulin stimulated GLUT4 recruitment via an early insulin-signaling effect. Diabetes 1997; 46: 215–23.

13 Immunology of gestational diabetes mellitus

Alberto de Leiva, Dídac Mauricio and Rosa Corcoy

Autoimmune gestational diabetes as a clinical entity

Pregnancy represents a distinct immunologic state; the fetus acts as an allograft to the mother, needing protection against potential rejection.[1,2] Humoral immunoreactivity does not change much during pregnancy, with the exception of lowered immunoglobulin G concentration at late phase, probably explained by placental transport.[3] Regarding cellular immunity, reduction,[4,5] elevation,[6] and no variation[7] in the number of different lymphocytic populations have been reported. The final effect of pregnancy on previously active autoimmune processes is controversial,[8,9] and multiple autoimmune disturbances may be manifested during pregnancy.[10]

In diabetic pregnancy, immunological abnormalities occurring in diabetes are superimposed on immunological changes of pregnancy, eventually influencing maternal and fetal outcomes.

DM-1 is considered an autoimmune disorder progressing toward the selective destruction of the beta cells. Subjects with DM-1 frequently display evidence of autoimmune disorders specific to other organs: thyroid, adrenal cortex, gastric mucosa, and antigliadin antibodies in childhood.

Gestational diabetes mellitus (GDM) is defined as an impairment of glucose tolerance first recognised at the index pregnancy.[11] For this category of women, an increased risk of progression to Type 2 diabetes mellitus (DM-2) has been repeatedly reported.[12–15] Nevertheless, a subset of women with GDM depicts one or several autoantibodies (AA) against various pancreatic islet cell autoantigens, typically detected in Type 1 diabetes (DM-1),[16] as well as in high risk subjects for the development of the disease, in particular, first degree relatives of patients with DM-1 (FDRs-DM1).[17] In Type 1A diabetes, a selective destruction of the insulin-producing cells occurred, mediated by T cells.

Autoimmune destruction of the beta cells is determined by multiple genetic susceptibility and modulated by undefined environmental factors. The autoimmune response may be detected for months or years before the clinical onset. Patients with Type 1 diabetes have an increased risk of other autoimmune disorders, including Graves disease, thyroiditis, Addison disease, celiac disease, and pernicious anemia. A minority of patients with Type 1 diabetes have no known

etiology and no evidence of autoimmunity (Type 1b diabetes; idiopathic Type 1 diabetes); most of these patients are of African or Asian origin. It is well known that autoimmunity against pancreatic islets may evolve in some instances as a highly aggressive process responsible of extreme insulinopenia, whereas in other occasions it leads to a slow and non-aggressive process, practically asymptomatic, recognized by humoral autoimmunity markers. During past years, islet autoantibodies have been demonstrated in the sera of a significant fraction (5–20%) of individuals with phenotypical characteristics of DM-2.[18–20] As a result, the term 'latent autoimmune diabetes of adulthood' (LADA) has been incorporated to define this new clinical variant of diabetes.[18–20]

Therefore, we define as autoimmune GDM a concrete subgroup of women depicting humoral autoimmune markers against pancreatic cells in association with glucose intolerance at pregnancy. Due to its potential high risk for progression to clinically overt insulinopenia, women with autoimmune GDM may be considered candidates for immune interventions.

Islet-cell autoantibodies

Islet cell autoantibodies include AA to islet cell cytoplasm (ICAs); to native insulin (IAAs); to glutamic acid decarboxylase (GAD65A);[21–23] and to two tyrosinephosphatases (insulinoma-associated antigens IA-2A and IA-2βA).[24,25] AA markers of immune destruction are present in 85–90% of newly onset Type 1 diabetes at the time that fasting hyperglycemia is first detected.[26]

The risk of developing DM-1 in first degree relatives (FDRs) of patients with the disease is about 5%, approximately 15-fold higher than the risk in the general population (1:250–300 lifetime risk). Screening FDRs can identify those at high risk for DM-1. Nevertheless, as many as 1–2% of healthy individuals display a single AA, and they are at low risk to develop DM-1.[27] Due to the low prevalence of DM-1 in the general population (c. 0.3%), the positive predictive value (PPV) of a single AA is low.[28] The presence of combined islet cell AA is associated with a risk of DM-1 up to >90%.[27,29] Only about 20% of subjects presenting with newly onset DM-1 express only a single autoantibody. Children and young adults carrying certain HLA-DR and/or DQB1 chains (*0602/*0603/*0301) are mostly protected from DM-1, but not from developing islet cell AA.[30] Screening of FDRs of patients with DM-1 or in the general population for islet cell AA is not recommended at present. Islet cell AA are usually measured in research protocols and clinical trials as surrogate end-points. It is important that AA should be measured only in accredited laboratories with an established quality-control program, and participation in a proficiency-testing protocol.

So far, no therapy has been recommended to prevent the clinical onset of DM-1 in islet cell AA positive individuals.[31]

Cytoplasmic islet cell autoantibodies in GDM

ICA were first described in 1974.[32] The investigated serum was incubated with a slide of human pancreas; the antigen–antibody interaction was visualized by fluorescence microscopy. Only the cytoplasm of endocrine cells depicted fluorescence, showing the non-specific character of the antibodies for the beta cells.

Circulating antibodies against the cytoplasm of islet cells (ICA) have been demonstrated in the great majority of individuals with DM-1 at the preclinical state and at the onset of clinically overt disease, and they persist in the circulation for various times. In pregnant women with DM-1 the reported frequencies of ICAs have been 11–62%.[33–35] ICAs are transferred by the placenta,[33] but their passage has not been associated with fetal/neonatal morbidity.

The presence of ICA in GDM was first reported by Steel et al.[36] with a frequency of 10%. Prevalence rates of 1–15% have been reported for ICA in GDM (Table 13.1).[14,36–49,52–57,59,63,64] These discordant results are probably explained by differences in investigated populations, methodology of assessing ICA, and dissimilar protocols of screening and diagnosing GDM.

Women with GDM positive for ICA, characteristically display low titers when compared with subjects with new-onset T1DM and FDR.[39,43,48,54,57,63] Our group has compared ICA titers in 38 ICA-positive women with GDM and 66 women with new-onset T1DM and results are displayed in Figure 13.1. However, in GDM, ICA persistance is higher in the long run.[56,65]

Insulin autoantibodies in GDM

The presence of IAA in the sera of DM-1 subjects before initiating insulin therapy was first reported by Palmer et al.[66] Later, IAA have been detected in 18–50% of newly diagnosed Type 1 diabetic patients.[67,68] Overall, 4–6% of FDRs are positive for IAA, a prevalence that is higher in young ICA

Table 13.1   Diabetes-related antibodies in women with gestational diabetes mellitus

First author, and reference	ICA prevalence (%)	IAA prevalence (%)	GADA prevalence (%)	IA2A prevalence (%)
Steel[36]	10			
Roma cohort[37,38]	5		3.6 †	
Freinkel[14]	7.5 #			
Stowers[39] *	12.5			
Catalano[40] *	1.6			
Bell[41]	2.8			
Stangenberg[42]	1.8			
Barcelona cohort[43–45]	12.4–14 #	1	1.5	0.2
Munich cohort[46,47]	8.5–11		9.5 #	6.2 #
Copenhagen cohort[48,49]	2.9 †	0 †	2.2 †	
Tuomilheto[50]			5.0	
Beischer[51] *			1.8	
Padova cohort[52,53]	2.8–2.9	1.5	1.4	0
Dozio[54]	10 †	3.0 †	0 †	0 †
Wittingham[55]	3		4	1
Panczel[56] *	14.7			
Kinalski[57] *	5.1 #		7.0 #	3.2 #
Mitchell[58]			6 #	
Bartha[59] *	0.98		10.8	
Kousta[60] *			4.0	
Weng[61] ◊			4.5 †	
Balaji[62]		41 #		
Bo[63]	6.5 #		4.1 #	
Jarvela[64]	12.5 #	5.9 #	4.7 #	1.0 †

For groups with several papers on the subject, the information has been summarized.
ICA, islet cell antibodies; IAA, insulin autoantibodies; GADA, glutamic-acid decarboxylase autoantibodies; IA2A, antibodies against IA2 protein (thyrosin-phosphatase).
*Measurements were performed at different times after delivery; † NS versus the control population; # $P < 0.05$ versus the control population; ◊ women had both GDM and a positive family history for diabetes mellitus. (Adapted from de Leiva et al.[83])

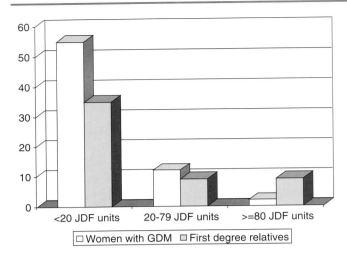

Figure 13.1   Titers of ICA in women with GDM and first degree relatives of Type 1 diabetic subjects with ICA positivity (Adapted from reference 81)

positive individuals. There are only a few reports on the prevalence of IAA in GDM, depicting rates of 0–6%.[44,48,52,54,64] Our group has measured IAA by the radiobinding assay described by Vardi.[69] We could observe that pregnancy itself does not influence IAA levels and that only 0.98% of non-selected women at diagnosis of GDM displayed IAA in their sera before initiation of treatment, frequency not different from that of a control group (0%, and lower than that reported in FDRs of subjects with DM-1 (4.7%) and in newly diagnosed Type 1 diabetic patients (16%).[70] Interestingly, the prevalence of IAA was higher in the group of ICA positive women with GDM than in the ICA negative group (11 vs. 0.7%).

Autoantibodies against glutamic acid decarboxylase and tyrosine phosphatase IA2 in GDM.

Baekkeskov et al.[71] identified the pancreatic islet beta-cell autoantigen of relative molecular mass 64k, as glutamic acid decarboxylase, a major target of AA associated with the development of DM-1. GAD is the biosynthesizing enzyme of the inhibitory neurotransmitter GABA (gamma-aminobutyric acid). Pancreatic beta cells and a subpopulation of central nervous system neurons express high levels of this enzyme. Most patients with a rare neurologic disease called stiff-man syndrome have autoantibodies to GABA-secreting neurons. The 64k antigen was found in beta cells as a hydrophilic soluble 65k form and a 64k hydrophobic form.[72]

In newly dignosed patients with DM-1, ICA positivity is depicted in 75–85% of cases, presence of GAD65A in about 60–70%, IA2A in 40%, and IA2βA in 20%. IAAs are positive in 90% of children who develop DM-1 before age 5, but in less than 40% of cases developing the disease after

the age of 12. At present, a panel of IAA, GAD, and IA2A/IA2βA is now available for screening purposes of autoimmune diabetes, possibly with ICAs used for confirmatory testing. It is likely that other islet cell antigens could lead to additional diagnostic and predictive tests for DM-1. The largest study on the prevalence of GAD65Ab in Type 2 diabetes is the United Kingdom Prospective Diabetes Study (UKPDS). Overall, 10% of patients tested positive for GAD65Ab, and the prevalence was inversely proportional to age.[73] This investigation also depicted that 84% of GAD-Ab+ patients 25–34 years old required insulin within 6 years in comparison with 34% of those older than 55 years. No patient with Type 2 diabetes was positive for IA-2Ab alone. GAD65Ab+ patients with Type 2 diabetes have lower fasting C-peptide levels and lower insulin response to orally administered glucose than do GAD65Ab patients, as well as fewer features of the metabolic syndrome, an indication of potential lower risk or cardiovascular events than average Type 2 diabetic subjects. An estimated 5–10% of patients with Type 2 diabetes have maturity-onset diabetes of youth, 10% may have LADA, and another 5–10% may have diabetes due to rare genetic disorders. Reported prevalences of GAD in women with GDM ranges from 0 to 10.8% (Table 13.1).[54,59] After the identification of IA2 as a target beta-cell antigen, several studies have shown a prevalence of IA2 antibodies in GDM between 0 and 6.2%.[45,47,53–55,57,64]

As for other DRA titers of GADA and IA2 in GDM have been also reported to be lower when compared to T12DM, autoimmune prediabetes and FDR.[55,63,74] GADA in women with GDM, have a distinct characteristic compared with FDR since they bind to fewer epitopes than the corresponding antibodies in FDR.[74]

Genetic markers in autoimmune GDM

Although genetic markers hold a most relevant promise for the future, they are of only limited clinical value in the evaluation and management of diabetic patients.

To screen for the genetic susceptibility for autoimmune-mediated Type 1A diabetes, HLA typing is most useful. The HLA complex on chromosome 6p21.3 is a major susceptibility locus, *IDDM1*. The HLA complex contains class I and II genes that code for several polypeptide chains. The class I genes are HLA-A, -B, and -C. The loci of class II genes are designated by three letters: the first, -D-, indicates the class, the second (-M,O, P, Q, R-) the family, and the third (-A or B-) the chain. Both classes of molecules are heterodimers: class I exhibits an alfa chain and β2-microglobulin; class II exhibits alfa and beta chains. The function of the HLA molecules is to present short peptides to T cells to initiate the immune response. Multiple genetic reports have demonstrated an association between various HLA alleles and autoimmune disorders. In caucasian DM-1 patients HLA-D genes contribute as much as 50% of the genetic susceptibility.[75]

HLA-DQ genes appear critical to the HLA-associated risk of DM-1A. In any individual four possible DQ dimers are encoded; positive risks for the disease are associated with alfa chains that have an arginine residue 52 and beta chains that lack an aspartic acid at residue 57. The highest genetic risk corresponds to those persons in whom all four HLA-DQ combinations meet this criterion (heterozygous for *HLA-DRB1*04-DQA1*0301-DQB1*0302 and DRB1*03-DqA1*0501-DQB1*0201*), with an absolute lifetime risk for DM 1A in the general population of 1:12. On the contrary, person who are protected are those with *DRB1*15-DQA1*0201-DQB1*0602 (Asp57+)* haplotypes.[76] People carrying out the *B1*0401 and 0405 subtypes of DRB1*04* are susceptible, whereas the **0403* and **0406* subtypes are protective.

So far, the genes of HLA complex have been most investigated genetic factors investigated in autoimmune GDM. The information obtained from various reports showed discordant results;[14,41,42,48,52,77–79] in these protocols, the number of investigated subjects was small, and the analyzed populations quite heterogeneous. Rubinstein et al. depicted a strong association between HLA DR3/DR4 and islet autoimmunity of women with GDM.[77] A similar observation was provided by Freinkel et al., showing a 2-fold increase in the frequency of DR3 and DR4 alleles in women with GDM.[14] Ferber et al.[79] investigated 184 German women with GDM; when compared with another group of 254 nondiabetic unrelated subjects, no elevation in the frequency of any HLA class allele was observed. Nevertheless, DR3 allele frequency was increased in GDM women with positivity to islet cell antibodies, particularly GADA ($P = 0.002$), as well as DR4 and DQB1*0302 ($P = 0.009$). Sixty percent islet antibody-positive women and 74% women who developed DM-1 after partum had a DR3/DR4 containing genotype. Combining the determination of susceptible HLA alleles (DR3, DR4) with islet autoantibody measurement increased the sensitivity of identifying GDM women developing postpartum DM-1 to 92%. Several reports could not found association between increased prevalence of class II alleles and the presence of humoral islet cell autoimmune markers in women with GDM.[42,52,78] Finally, Damm et al. showed a trend towards an increased frquency of DR3/DR4 and a decrease frequency of DR2 in women with GDM evolving to DM-1.[48]

Autoimmune GDM and the risk of developing postpartum DM-1

A main issue regarding autoimmune GDM is that of the potential increased risk for the development of DM-1 either at short term after partum or at longer follow-up. We can accept the proposal that the majority of women developing DM after GDM will evolve to DM-2;[12,14] nevertheless, a small but meaningful fraction will evolve to DM-1.

After delivery, the autoimmune process directed against beta cells may follow different pathways: (1) the restoration of normal glucose tolerance when pregnancy is over; (2) the appearance of DM-1 shortly after pregnancy; and (3) slow deterioration of the insulin secretory capacity due to the continuous progression of autoimmune destruction of the residual population of beta cells, resulting in a long subclinical period (LADA).

Already in the first study on ICA in GDM, three out of five ICA-positive gestational diabetic women developed classical DM-1A shortly after pregnancy.[36] Additional studies have

confirmed an increased risk of diabetes[43] or glucose intolerance[40] in these women. Positivity for either ICA or GADA increases the risk of T1DM at 2 years of follow-up, the risk increasing with the number of positive antibodies.[47,80] Some studies not showing an association between ICA[42] or GADA[61] with abnormal glucose tolerance at short term after delivery have a low statistical power. Overall, it is important to highlight that only two of the papers dealing with DRA and glucose tolerance after delivery performed statistical adjustment for other predictors.[42,47]

After describing ICA as being predictive of DM at the first assessment after delivery,[43] our team described an impairment of the acute insulin response to intravenous glucose in women with GDM with positivity for ICA and normal glucose tolerance after delivery, the response being superimposable to that of ICA-positive FDR.[81] Interestingly, a Finnish study on FDR of patients with LADA, demonstrated metabolic features similar to those described by us in women with GDM and positivity for ICA. These individuals, family members of LADA patients exhibited decreased insulin secretion, associated with increased risk genotypes.[82]

Most papers focusing on longer follow-up, describe also an increased risk of DM-1 in women with GDM and positivity for ICA.[48,49,56,64] GADA[49,51,64] and positivity for one or more islet cell antibodies,[49,80] with the risk increasing with the number of antibodies.[64] Not all authors describe a positive association between DRA positivity and DM at follow up, that in some cases,[39,53] but not in others[45,60] can be attributed to a low statistical power of the studies. For instance, in our population, despite the aforementioned association of ICA positivity with postpartum abnormal glucose tolerance, DRA positivity (ICA, GADA, IA2 alone or in any combination) were not predictive of diabetes mellitus at mid-term follow-up.[45] As in the case of short-term follow-up only some studies have adjusted for other predictors.[45,64,80]

Concluding remarks

Autoimmune GDM appears to be the result of the variable expression of autoimmunity against the beta cell, challenged by the higher functional demand associated with the insulin-resistant state of pregnancy. In this respect, autoimmune gestational diabetes can be considered a distinct clinical entity. There are different time-course patterns in the progression of autoimmune GDM: from the restoration of normal glucose tolerance when pregnancy is over (even with eventual disappearance of autoimmune markers), to the appearance of Type 1 diabetes shortly after partum, to an established state of glucose intolerance which may eventually progress, slowly, to a noninsulin dependent state, manifested as LADA. Furthermore, the course of the autoimmune destruction of the residual beta cell mass may be accelerated at any time-point resulting in a rapid-onset form of DM-1.

Women with autoimmune GDM must be regarded as a high-risk group for the development of DM-1 in any of its clinical forms. These women are candidates for immunomodulatory interventions to prevent diabetes after pregnancy.

Table 13.2   Abnormal glucose tolerance at follow-up in women with GDM and diabetes-related antibodies

First author, and reference	Follow-up	ICA	GADA	IA2A	Several DRA
Steel[36]	1 year	Predictive of T1DM			
Stowers[39]	Up to 22 years	Not predictive of the final state of glucose tolerance			
Catalano[40]	Up to 4 years	Predictive of IGT			
Stangenberg[42]	2–4 months	Not predictive of abnormal OGTT*			
Barcelona cohort[43,45]	Months/up to 11 years	Predictive of DM at short term			DRA positivity not predictive of DM, T1DM or T2DM at long term*
Copenhagen cohort[48,49]	Up to 11 years	Predictive of T1DM	Predictive of T1DM GADA at follow-up associated to T1DM and T2DM		
Beischer 1995[51]					
Munich cohort[47,80]	Up to 5 years/ up to 11 years	Predictive of T1DM*	Predictive of T1DM *	Not predictive of T1DM*	The risk of T1DM increases with the number of DRA*/
GAD and/or IA2 positivity predictive of DM at long term*					
Panczel[56]	Up to 14 years	Predictive of T1DM			
Kousta[60]	Up to 45 months		GADA at follow-up, not associated with differences in FBG or HOMA estimations of insulin secretion and sensitivity		
Weng[61]	1 year		No association with DM/IGT		
Padova cohort[53]	5 years				DRA positivity, borderline association to T1DM
Jarvela[64]	Up to 7 years	Predictive of T1DM*	Predictive of T1DM*	Not predictive of T1DM*	N of DRA predictive of T1DM*

For groups with several papers on the subject, information has been summarized.
*Adjusted for other predictors.
FBG: fasting blood glucose; HOMA: homeostasis model assessment; DM: diabetes mellitus; T1DM: Type 1 diabetes mellitus; IGT: impaired glucose tolerance.
There were no results for insulin autoantibodies (IAA).
(Adapted from de Leiva et al.[83])

REFERENCES

1. Gleicher N. Pregnancy and autoimmunity. Acta Haematol 1986; 76: 68–77.
2. Lewis JE, Coulam CB, Moore S. Immunologic mechanisms in the maternal-fetal relationship. Mayo Clin Proc 1986; 61: 655–65.
3. Mauroulis GB, Buckley RH, Younger GB. Serum immunoglobulin levels during normal pregnancy. Am J Obstet Gynecol 1971; 109: 971–6.
4. Galluzzo A, Giordano C, Bompiani GF. Cell-mediated immunity in diabetic pregnancy. In: Andreani D, Bompiani G, Di Mario U, Page Faulk W, Galluzzo A, eds. Immunobiology of Normal and Diabetic Pregnancy. Chichester: Wiley; 1990, pp. 273–81.
5. Bulmer R, Hancock W. Depletion of circulating T lymphocytes in pregnancy. Clin Exp Immunol 1977; 29: 302–7.
6. Clements PJ, Yu DTY, Levy J, Pearson CM. Human lymphocytes subpopulation: effects on pregnancy. Proc Soc Exp Biol Med 1976; 152: 664–72.
7. Dodson MG, Kerman RH, Lange CF, Stefani SS, O'Leary JA. T and B cells in pregnancy. Obstet Gynecol 1976; 49: 229–303.
8. Shonfeld Y, Schwarz RS. Immunologic and genetic factors in autoimmune diseases. N Engl J Med 1984; 311: 1019–29.
9. Giordano C. Immunobiology of normal and diabetic pregnancy. Immunol Today 1990; 11: 301–3.
10. Torry DS, McIntyre JA. The role of the antibody in pregnancy. In: Andreani D, Bompiani G, Di Mario U, Page Faulk W, Galluzo A, eds. Immunobiology of Normal and Diabetic Pregnancy. Chichester: Wiley; 1990, pp. 39–57.

11. Metzger BE, Coustan DM, and the Organizing Committee. Summary and recommendations of the Fourth International Workshop–Conference on Gestational Diabetes Mellitus. Diabetes Care 1998; 21(suppl. 2): B161–7.

12. Kjos SL, Buchanan TA. Gestational diabetes mellitus. N Engl J Med 1999; 341: 1749–56.

13. Buchanan TA, Metzger BE, Freinkel N, Bergman RN. Insulin sensitivity and B-cell responsiveness to glucose during late pregnancy in lean and moderately obese women with normal glucose tolerance or mild gestational diabetes. Am J Obstet Gynecol 1990; 162: 1008–14.

14. Freinkel N, Metzger BE, Phelps RL, et al. Gestational diabetes mellitus: heterogeneity of maternal age, weight, insulin secretion, HLA antigens, and islet cell antibodies and the impact of maternal metabolism on pancreatic B-cell and somatic development in the offspring. Diabetes 1985; 34(suppl. 2): 1–7.

15. Kim C, Newton KM, Knopp RH. Gestational diabetes and the incidence of type 2 diabetes: a systematic review. Diabetes Care 2002; 25: 1862–8.

16. Schranz DB, Lernmark A. Immunology in diabetes: an update. Diabetes Metab Rev 1998; 14: 3–29.

17. Palmer JP. Predicting IDDM: use of humoral immune markers. Diabetes Rev 1992; 1: 104–15.

18. Tuomi T, Groop LC, Zimmet PZ, et al. Antibodies to glutamic acid decarboxylase reveal latent autoimmune diabetes mellitus in adults with a non-insulin dependent onset of the disease. Diabetes 1993; 42: 359–62.

19. Turner R, Stratton I, Horton V, et al., for the UK Prospective Diabetes Study (UKPDS) Group: UKPDS 25. Autoantibodies to islet cytoplasm and glutamic acid decarboxylase for prediction of insulin requirement in type 2 diabetes. Lancet 1997; 350: 1288–93.

20. Zimmet PZ, Tuomi T, Mackay JR, et al. Latent autoimmune diabetes in adults (LADA): the role of antibodies to glutamic acid decarboxylase in diagnosis and prediction of insulin dependency. Diabet Med 1994; 11: 299–303.

21. Baekkeskov S, Aanstoot HJ, Christgau S, et al. Identification of the 64K autoantigen in insulin-dependent diabetes as the GABA-synthesizing enzyme glutamic acid decarboxylase Nature 1990; 347: 151–6. (Published erratum appears in Nature 1990; 347: 782.)

22. Kaufman DL, Erlander MG, Clare-Salzler M, et al. Autoimmunity to two forms of glutamate decarboxylase in insulin-dependent diabetes mellitus. J Clin Invest 1992; 89: 283–92.

23. Atkinson MA, Maclaren NK. Islet cell autoantigens in insulin dependent diabetes. J Clin Invest 1993; 92: 1608–16.

24. Lan MS, Wasserfall C, Maclaren NK, Notkins AL. IA-2, a transmembrane protein of the protein tyrosine phosphatase family, is a major autoantigen in insulin-dependent diabetes mellitus. Proc Natl Sci USA 1996; 93: 6367–70.

25. Lu J, Li Q, Xie H, et al. Identification of a second transmembrane protein tyrosine phosphatase, IA-2β, as an autoantigen in insulin-dependent diabetes mellitus: precursor of the 37-kDa tryptic fragment. Proc Natl Acad Sci USA 1996; 93: 2307–11.

26. American Diabetes Association. Report of the Expert Committee on the diagnosis and classification of diabetes mellitus. Diabetes care 1997; 20: 1183–201.

27. Maclaren N, Lan M, Coutant R, et al. Only multiple autoantibodies to islet cells (ICA), insulin, GAD65, IA-2 and IA-2β predict immune-mediated (type 1) diabetes in relatives. J Autoimmun 1999; 12: 279–87.

28. Harrison LC. Risk assessment, prediction and prevention of type 1 diabetes. Pediatr Diabetes 2001; 2: 71–82.

29. Verge CF, Gianani R, Kawasaki E, et al. Prediction of type I diabetes in first-degree relatives using a combination of insulin, GAD, and ICA512bdc/IA-2 autoantibodies. Diabetes 1996; 45: 926–33.

30. Schott M, Schatz D, Atkinson M, et al. GAD65 autoantibodies increase the predictability but not the sensitivity of islet cell and insulin autoantibodies for developing insulin dependent diabetes mellitus. J Autoimmun 1994; 7: 865–72.

31. Atkinson MA, Eisenbarth GS. Type 1 diabetes: new perspectives on disease pathogenesis and treatment. Lancet 2001; 358: 221–9.

32. Bottazo GF, Florin-Christensen A, Doniach D. Islet cell antibodies in diabetes mellitus with polyendocrine autoimmune deficiencies. Lancet 1974; ii: 1279–82.

33. Tingle AJ, Lim G, Wright VJ, Dimmick JE, Hunt JA. Transplacental passage of islet cell antibody in infants of diabetic mothers. Pediatr Res 1979; 13: 1323–5.

34. Falluca F, Di Mario U, Gargiulo P, et al. Humoral immunity in diabetic pregnancy: interrelationships with maternal/neonatal complications and maternal metabolic control. Diabet Metab 1985; 11: 387–95.

35. Mauricio D, Corcoy R, Codina M, et al. Frequency of islet-cell antibodies is not different in pregnant versus non-pregnant type 1 diabetic women [abstract]. Diabetes 1991; 40(suppl. 1): 277A.

36. Steel JM, Irvine WJ, Clarke BF. The significance of pancreatic islet cell antibody an abnormal glucose tolerance during pregnancy. J Clin Lab Immunol 1980; 4: 83–5.

37. Falluca F, Di Mario, Gargiulo P, et al. Humoral immunity in diabetic pregnancy: interrelationships with maternal/neonatal complications and maternal metabolic control. Diabet Metab 1985; 11: 387–95.

38. Fallucca F, Tiberti C, Torresi P, et al. Autoimmune markers of diabetes in diabetic pregnancy. Ann Ist Super Sanita 1997; 33: 425–8.

39. Stowers JM, Sutherland HW, Kerridge DF. Long-range implications for the mother. The Aberdeen experience. Diabetes 1985; 34(suppl. 2): 106–10.

40. Catalano PM, Tyzbir ED, Sims EAH. Incidence and significance of islet cell antibodies in women with previous gestational diabetes. Diabetes Care 1990; 13: 478–82.

41. Bell DSH, Barger BO, Go RCP, et al. Risk factors for gestational diabetes in black population. Diabetes Care 1990; 13(suppl. 4): 1196–201.

42. Stangenberg M, Agarwal N, Rahman F, et al. Frequency of HLA genes and islet cell antibodies (ICA) and result of postpartum oral glucose tolerance tests (OGTT) in Saudi Arabian women with abnormal OGTT during pregnancy. Diabetes Res 1990; 14: 9–13.

43. Mauricio D, Corcoy R, Codina M, et al. Islet cell antibodies identify a subset of gestational diabetic women with higher risk of developing diabetes mellitus shortly after pregnancy. Diabetes Nutr Metab 1992; 5: 237–41.

44. Mauricio D, Balsells M, Morales J, et al. Islet cell autoimmunity in women with gestational diabetes and risk of progression to insulin-dependent diabetes mellitus. Diabetes Metab Rev 1996; 12: 275–85.

45. Albareda M, Caballero A, Badell G, et al. Diabetes and abnormal glucose tolerante in women with previous gestational diabetes. Diabetes Care 2003; 26: 1199–205.

46. Ziegler AG, Hillebrand B, Rabl W, et al. On the appearance of islet associated autoimmunity in offspring of diabetic mothers: a prospective study from birth. Diabetologia 1993; 36: 402–8.

47. Füchtenbusch M, Ferber K, Standl E, Ziegler A-G, and participating centers. Prediction of type 1 diabetes postpartum in patients with gestational diabetes mellitus by combined islet cell autoantibody screening. A prospective multicenter study. Diabetes 1997; 46: 1459–67.

48. Damm P, Kühl C, Buschard K, et al. Prevalence and predictive value of islet cell antibodies and insulin antibodies in women with gestational diabetes. Diabet Med 1994; 11: 558–63.

49. Petersen JS, Dyrberg T, Damm P, et al. GAD65 autoantibodies in women with gestational or insulin dependent diabetes mellitus diagnosed during pregnancy. Diabetologia 1996; 39: 1329–33.

50. Tuomilehto J, Zimmet P, Mackay IR, et al. Antibodies to glutamic acid decarboxylase as predictors of insulin-dependent diabetes mellitus before clinical onset. Lancet 1994; 343: 1383–5.

51. Beischer NA, Wein P, Sheedy MT, et al. Prevalence of antibodies to glutamic acid decarboxylase in women who have had gestational diabetes. Am J Obstet Gynecol 1995; 173: 1563–9.

52. Lapolla A, Betterle C, Sanzari M, et al. An immunological and genetic study of patients with gestational diabetes mellitus. Acta Diabetol 1996; 33: 139–44.

53. Lapolla A, Fedele D, Pedini B, et al. Low frequency of autoantibodies to islet cell, glutamic acid decarboxylase and second-islet antigen in patients with gestational diabetes mellitus: A follow-up study. Ann NY Acad Sci 2002; 958: 263–6.

54. Dozio N, Beretta A, Belloni C, et al. Low prevalence of islet autoantibodies in patients with gestational diabetes mellitus. Diabetes Care 1997; 20: 81–3.

55. Wittingham S, Byron SL, Tuomilehto J, et al. Autoantibodies associated with presymptomatic insulin-dependent diabetes mellitus in women. Diabet Med 1997; 14: 678–85.

56. Panczel P, Kulley O, Luczay A, et al. Detection of antibodies against pancreatic islet cells in clinical practice. Orvosi Hetilap 1999; 140: 2695–701.

57. Kinalski M, Kretowski A, Telejko B, et al. Prevalence of ICA antibodies, anti-GAD and anti-IA2 in women with gestational diabetes treated with diet. Przegl Lek 1999; 56: 342–6.

58. Mitchell ML, Hermos RJ, Larson CA, Palomaki GE, Haddow JE. Prevalence of GAD autoantibodies in women with gestational diabetes. A retrospective analysis. Diabetes Care 2000; 23: 1705–6.

59. Bartha JL, Martínez del Fresno P, Comino-Delgado R. Postpartum metabolism and autoantibody markers in women with gestational diabetes mellitus diagnosed in early pregnancy. Am J Obstet Gynecol 2001; 184: 965–70.

60. Kousta E, Lawrence NJ, Anyakou V, Johnston DG, McCarthy MI. Prevalence and features of pancreatic islet cell autoimmunity in women with gestational diabetes from different ethnic groups. BJOG 2001; 108: 716–20.

61. Weng J, Ekelund M, Lehto M, et al. Screening for MODY mutations, GAD antibodies, and type 1-diabetes associated HLA genotypes in women with gestational diabetes mellitus. Diabetes Care 2002; 25: 68–71.

62. Balaji M, Shatauvere-Brameus A, Valaji V, Seshiah V, Sanjeevi CB. Women diagnosed with gestational diabetes mellitus do not carry antibodies against minor cell antigens. Ann NY Acad Sci 2002; 958: 281–4.

63. Bo S, Menato G, Pinach S, et al. Clinical characteristics and outcome of pregnancy in women with gestational hyperglycemia with and without antibodies to beta-cell antigens. Diabet Med 2003; 20: 64–8.

64. Järvela I, Juutinen J, Koskela P, et al. Gestational diabetes identifies women at risk for permanent Type 1 and Type 2 diabetes in fertile age. Predictive role of autoantibodies. Diabetes Care 2006; 29: 607–12.

65. Corcoy R, Albareda M, Ortiz A, et al. In women with GDM, glutamic acid decarboxylase and tyrosine phosphatase antibodies increase after delivery. Diabetologia 2000; 43(suppl. 1): A19.

66. Palmer JP, Asplin CH, Clemons P. Insulin antibodies in insulin dependent diabetics before insulin treatment. Science 1982; 222: 1337–9.

67. Karjalainen J, Salmena P, Ilonen J, Surcel HM, Knip M. A comparison of childhood and adult type I diabetes mellitus. N Engl J Med 1989; 320: 881–6.

68. Srikanta S, Richter AT, MacCulloch DK, et al. Autoimmunity to insulin, beta-cell dysfunction and development of insulin-dependent diabetes mellitus. Diabetes 1986; 36: 139–42.

69. Vardi P, Dib SA, Tuttleman M, et al. Competitive insulin antibody assay: prospective evaluation of subjects at high risk for development of type I diabetes mellitus. Diabetes 1987; 36: 1286–91.

70. Puig-Domingo M, Mauricio D, Morales J, et al. Proyecto de la Sociedad Española de Diabetes sobre prediabetes tipo 1. Av Diabetol 1992; 5(suppl. 2): 57–65.

71. Baekkeskov S, Aanstoot HJ, Christgau S, et al. Identification of the 64K autoantigen in insulin dependent diabetes as the GABA-synthesizing enzyme glutamic acid decarboxylase. Nature 1990; 347: 151–6.

72. Maclaren N, Lan M, Coutant R, et al. Only multiple autoantibodies to islet cells (ICA), insulin, GAD65, IA2 and IA2beta predict immune-mediated (type 1) diabetes in relatives. J Autoimmun 1999; 12: 279–87.

73. Turner R, Stratton I, Horton V, et al. UKPDS 25: Autoantibodies to islet-cell cytoplasm and glutamic acid decarboxylase for prediction of insulin requirement in type 2 diabetes. Lancet 1997; 350: 1288–93.

74. Füchtenbusch M, Bonifacio E, Lampasona V, Knopff, Ziegler AG: Immune responses to glutamic acid decarboxylase and insulin in patients with gestational diabetes. Clin Exp Immunol 2004; 135: 318–21.

75. Todd JA. Genetics of type 1 diabetes. Pathol Biol (Paris) 1997; 45: 219–27.

76. Redondo MJ, Kawasaki E, Mulgrew CL, et al. DR- and DQ-associated protection from type 1A diabetes: comparison of DRB1*1401 and DQA1*0102-DQB1*0602*. J Clin Endocrinol Metab 2000; 85: 3793–7.

77. Rubinstein P, Walker M, Krassner J, et al. HLA antigens and islet cell antibodies in gestational diabetes. Hum Immunol 1981; 3: 271–5.

78. Vambergue A, Fajardi I, Bianchi F, et al. Gestational diabetes mellitus and HLA class II (-DQ, -DR) association: the DIAGEST Study. Eur J Immunogenet 1997; 24: 385–94.

79. Ferber K, Keller E, Albert ED, Ziegler A-G. Predictive value of human leucocyte antigen Class II typing for the development of islet autoantibodies and insulin-dependent diabetes postpartum in women with gestational diabetes. J Clin Endocrinol Metab 1999; 84: 2342–8.

80. Löbnner K, Knopff A, Baumgarten A, et al. Predictors of postpartum diabetes in women with gestational diabetes mellitus. Diabetes 2006; 55: 792–7.

81. Mauricio D, Corcoy R, Codina M, et al. Islet cell antibodies and beta cell function in gestational diabetic women: comparison to first-degree relatives of Type 1 (insulin-dependent) diabetic subjects. Diabet Med 1995; 12: 1009–14.

82. Vauhkonen I, Niskanen L, Knip M, et al. Impaired insulin secretion in non-diabetic offspring of probands with latent autoimmune diabetes in adults. Diabetologia 2000; 43: 69–78.

83. de Leiva A, Mauricio D, Corcoy R. Diabetes related autoanti-bodies and gestational diabetes mellitus. Diabetes Care (in press).

14 Gestational diabetes: The consequences of not-treating

Oded Langer

The GDM controversy

Diabetes mellitus is one of the most common medical complications of pregnancy. Of all types of diabetes, gestational diabetes (GDM) accounts for approximately 90–95% of all cases of diabetes in pregnancy. GDM is defined as

> carbohydrate intolerance of variable severity with onset or first recognition during pregnancy. The definition is applicable regardless of whether insulin is used for treatment or the condition persists after pregnancy. It does not exclude the possibility that unrecognized glucose intolerance may have antedated the pregnancy.[1]

Since the late 1960s when O'Sullivan first suggested the term 'gestational diabetes', controversy has continuously surrounded this clinical entity even though it is associated with adverse pregnancy outcome, i.e. macrosomia, birth trauma, and neonatal hypoglycemia. Regardless of these serious results, opinions and anecdotes have been more prolific than research generated data on this issue. There is no consensus regarding diagnostic criteria, the utility of universal screening, or the association of gestational diabetes with perinatal morbidity and mortality. For example, Jarrett[2] concluded that GDM is 'a non-entity' whose only clinical association is with an increased maternal risk of subsequent diabetes.[1] The Scottish Intercollegiate Guidelines Network (SIGN) published a document regarding the management of diabetes in pregnancy in 2001. They reiterated that there is as yet no consensus on the definition, management or treatment of GDM, or the most appropriate strategies for screening, diagnosis and management of asymptomatic GDM. A document published in the United Kingdom in October 2003 from the National Institute for Clinical Excellence suggested that available evidence did not support routine screening for GDM. The Society of Obstetricians and Gynecologists of Canada[3] suggest in their guidelines that screening for GDM needs to target high risk women. They included obesity among the risk factors, using a cut-off BMI of 27 kg/m.[2] In a letter to the editor, Hunter and Milner[4] stated that 'gestational diabetes is a diagnosis still looking for a disease.'

According to these physicians, gestational diabetes is not convincingly associated with increased perinatal mortality or morbidity, and macrosomia *per se*, regardless of definition, is not a morbid condition.[3] Greene, in an editorial in the *New England Journal of Medicine* (2001) also questioned if GDM is a disease,[5] while in 2005 the same author in a different editorial in the same journal endorsed treatment for GDM. Beard and colleagues[6] in a review article concluded that gestational diabetes is a clinical entity associated with a significant incidence of diabetes in the later life of the mother and an increase in fetal and neonatal morbidity.

In the current era of evidence-based medicine, it is surprising that the opposing positions are not the result of data gleaned from authors' research but rather based upon opinions that lack evidence to support these opinions. In order to determine a research-based answer to this dilemma, it is time to cease the rhetoric and subdue the 'storm in a teacup.' Tolstoy may have summed it up best:

> I know that most men, including those at ease with problems of the greatest complexity, can seldom accept even the simplest and most obvious truth if it be such as would oblige them to admit the falsity of conclusions which they have delighted in explaining to colleagues, which they have proudly taught to others, and which they have woven, thread by thread, into the fabric of their lives.

In approaching this debate, three conditions need to be met in order to establish gestational diabetes as a clinical entity. To demonstrate:

1. Change from physiology to pathophysiology
2. Significant adverse outcome, i.e. maternal and/or fetal
3. That treatment improves adverse outcome

Change from physiology to pathophysiology

Identification of the primary metabolic disturbance in GDM would facilitate the development of interventions aimed at prevention as well as treatment. Gestational diabetes mellitus may provide the ideal model for investigating the primary defect which leads to the development of Type 2 diabetes.

Human pregnancy is an insulin-resistant condition. Although there is a 4- to 5-fold range of insulin resistance in the general population, there is a relatively uniform 40–50% increase (from the pregravid condition) in insulin resistance and increase in insulin secretion in obese patients of 60% in the first phase of secretion and 130% in the second phase.[7] These alterations in insulin have been previously ascribed to a variety of reproductive hormones such as human placental lactogen, cortisol, progesterone and estrogen.[8]

More recent data have implicated adypocyte/placental secreted factors such as cytokines, in particular tumor necrosis factor alfa (TNF-α) and leptin as active candidates in the alteration of insulin sensitivity in pregnancy. Adiponectin belongs to the family of adipocytokines which also includes leptin, TNF-α, resistin, interleukin-6 (IL-6), and others.[8,9] Adiponectin is associated with obesity, diabetes, cardiovascular disease and dyslipidemia.[10–12] From a metabolic standpoint, adiponectin produces an insulin-sensitizing effect on skeletal muscle, adipose tissue a and liver. It has been demonstrated that the level of adiponectins in class A2 and B gestational diabetes are associated with suppressed levels of adiponectins, similar to that found in other insulin-resistant states (Type 2 diabetes and obesity.)

Retnakaran et al.[13] reported that C-reactive protein (CRP) levels in late pregnancy relate to pregravid BMI and not to GDM *per se*. Assuming that the CRP concentrations in late gestation are a marker of insulin resistance, then a woman's pregravid BMI may be the strongest clinical indicator of the degree of her insulin resistance, even in late gestation. The lack of a relationship between CRP and GDM may reflect the wide variation of pregravid BMI to inflammation/insulin resistance rather than the relative uniform decreases observed during pregnancy.[14]

It has been shown that total oxidative and non-oxidative glucose metabolism is inversely related to increased visceral-to-subcutaneous fat ratio in obese women and to total fat content in lean women. Others have demonstrated decreased insulin sensitivity in subjects with a central pattern of fat distribution. Whatever the cause for increased insulin resistance

during pregnancy, in women who maintain normal glucose tolerance, it is offset by a 3- to 3.5-fold increase in insulin secretion.[17] The degree of insulin resistance during late gestation appears to be dependent primarily on pregravid maternal insulin resistance, which is quite variable, and secondarily on the 40–50% increases mediated through placental factors.

It is not too surprising that GDM develops in genetically susceptible women when they become pregnant. They probably have some degree of insulin resistance prior to pregnancy and normal pregnancy is associated with severe insulin resistance. Catalano et al.[15] found an approximate 21% decrease in insulin sensitivity occurring by 12–14 weeks of gestation and a 56% decrease in insulin sensitivity occurring by 34–36 weeks. Others have found similar results.[16–18]

In summary, gestational diabetes is characterized by pathogenesis deviating from the normal physiology of pregnancy which involves insulin resistance and decreased insulin secretion. Furthermore, similarity exists between the pathogenesis of GDM and Type 2 diabetes which are probably one disease at different stages on the spectrum of glucose intolerance.

Is there an associated increased adverse outcome in GDM?

The infants of GDM women are at an increased risk for stillbirth and aberrant fetal growth (macrosomia and growth restriction) as well as metabolic (e.g. hypoglycemia and hypocalcemia), hematological (e.g. bilirubinemia and polycythemia) and respiratory complications that increase neonatal intensive care unit admission rates and birth trauma (e.g. shoulder dystocia)[19,20] (Table 14.1).

Congenital anomalies and spontaneous abortions are not as serious complications in GDM as they are in pre-gestational diabetes. However, due to the relatively high rate of undiagnosed Type 2 (10%) diabetic women in the GDM population, there should be a concerted effort to rule out the presence of congenital malformations.

Fasting plasma glucose is accepted as the gold standard for severity of diabetes. This is true in Type 2 individuals and in GDM women. In an attempt to control for different GDM

Table 14.1 Selective neonatal outcomes between untreated and nondiabetic subjects

	Odd ratio	95% CI
LGA	3.28	2.53–4.60
Macrosomia	2.66	1.93–3.67
Ponderal index	1.91	1.46–2.50
Shoulder dystocia	4.07	1.63–10.16
Hypoglycemia	10.38	6.15–16.56
Polycythemia	10.88	6.16–19.18
Hyperbilirubinemia	3.87	2.64–5.67
Pulmonary complications	3.43	1.87–6.27
Cesarean section	1.88	1.45–2.43
NICU >24 h	4.11	2.37–7.10

Modified from Langer O. The Diabetes in Pregnancy Dilemma: Leading Changes with Simple Solutions, University Press of America, New York, 2006.

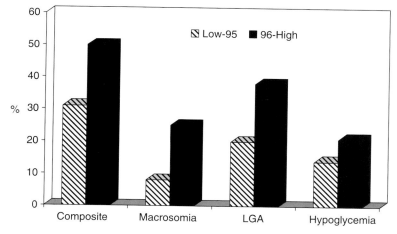

Figure 14.1   Outcome by fasting plasma severity for untreated GDM. (Modified from Langer O. The Diabetes in Pregnancy Dilemma: Leading Changes with Simple Solutions, University Press of America, New York, 2006.)

severity levels in the treated and untreated GDMs, we stratified the patients based on increases in fasting plasma glucose (10 mg increments) for each severity category. In the treated GDMs, there are similar rates of perinatal outcome for all fasting severity categories reiterating the importance of achieving targeted levels of glycemic control (Figure 14.1). In contrast, in the untreated GDMs, significant morbidity was found in each fasting plasma category of severity. In the untreated group, logistic regression revealed that fasting plasma glucose (severity of disease) had a significant independent impact when for every 10 mg increment there was an increased likelihood of adverse outcome (composite) by 15%; for each pound increase in obese patients, the likelihood of adverse outcome increase by 3%. For the treated GDMs, parity was found to have a 6% increment for every child and obesity and weight gain had a negligible effect although both were found to be statistically significant.

Neonatal complications

The adverse outcomes most commonly associated with GDM include increased perinatal mortality, macrosomia, shoulder dystocia, birth trauma, pre-eclampsia, Cesarean section, neonatal hypoglycemia, hypocalcemia, hyperbilirubinemia, and polycythemia. In addition, there are long-term effects

associated with GDM pregnancies such as an increased maternal risk of developing diabetes in the future and an increased risk of obesity and glucose intolerance in the offspring (Table 14.2).

Perinatal mortality

Perinatal mortality is the most significant perinatal outcome and early, albeit flawed studies, showed a 4-fold increase in perinatal mortality in women with GDM. These studies did not control for variables affecting perinatal mortality such as fetal malformations, maternal history of stillbirth, as well as advanced maternal age. Furthermore, all these studies probably included women with unrecognized pre-gestational diabetes, thus confounding the results. In addition, in most studies a labeling bias existed since a GDM diagnosis tends to enhance surveillance and interventions that may have a major impact on perinatal mortality. Some researchers have suggested that GDM has no or a negligible effect on mortality. This could be explained by two opposing views: GDM has no or a negligible effect on mortality; or, due to the overall decrease in perinatal mortality, excess fetal deaths due to unrecognized GDM could go unnoticed in smaller studies.

O'Sullivan and Mahan[21] first reported an association between GDM and perinatal death, documenting a 6.4% risk only in women with GDM who were older than 25 years of

Table 14.2   Intensified versus conventional management of GDM

	Conventional	Intensified	Control
Macrosomia (%)	13.6	7.01	8.1
Large for gestational age (%)	20.1	13.1	11.9
Metabolic complication (%)	13.3	3.1	2.9
Respiratory complication (%)	6.2	2.3	2.1
Shoulder dystocia (%)	1.4	0.4	8.7
Cesarean section (%)	22.0	15.0	14.0
n	1316	1145	4922

Modified from Langer O. The Diabetes in Pregnancy Dilemma: Leading Changes with Simple Solutions, University Press of America, New York, 2006.

age, and a relative risk of 4.3 over controls. Abell et al.[22] reported similar results in women with GDM with a 3.9% overall perinatal mortality rate. However, an analysis of 1016 GDM pregnancies from the author's institution documented an increased perinatal mortality rate (3.2%) only among those meeting the NDDG criteria for the diagnosis of GDM.[23] Schmidt et al.[24] evaluated the relation between the ADA and the WHO diagnostic criteria for GDM against pregnancy outcome. Of the 4977 women in the study, 2.6% had GDM by the ADA criteria and 7.2% by the WHO criteria. The perinatal death in the ADA group had an odds ratio of 3.10, 95% confidence interval 1.42–6.47. Similarly, the perinatal mortality by the WHO criteria had an odds ratio 1.59, 95% confidence interval 0.86–2.90 (not significant). Mondestin et al.[25] reported the results of a retrospective cohort study of U.S. data (1995–1997). These included 10 million nondiabetic gravids and 271,691 diabetic patients with fetal death rates of 4/1000 for the nondiabetic and 5.9/1000 for the diabetic patients. Fetal death rates increased when birthweight was >4250 g for nondiabetic and 4000 g for diabetic patients with a 2-fold increased rate in mortality in the diabetic group. The drawbacks of this study was the retrospective design and the lack of distinction between types of diabetes. However, it would be reasonable to assume that the majority of the diabetic patients were GDM which accounts for 90% of all diabetic pregnancies.

Clinicians must, therefore, consider the merits of establishing the diagnosis of GDM. Gestational diabetes, if untreated or not recognized, may be associated with an increased risk of intrauterine fetal death and commonly reported morbidities such as macrosomia, birth trauma, neonatal hypoglycemia, hyperbilirubinemia, hypoglycemia, and polycythemia. There is paucity of prospective data concerning some of these risks. However, it is generally agreed that women with GDM with significantly elevated fasting blood glucose levels appear to have an increased risk of intrauterine fetal death.

Macrosomia, shoulder dystocia and birth trauma

Being relatively common and easily documented, macrosomia is the perinatal outcome most investigators refer to when addressing GDM. Macrosomia is the primary outcome with relevant surrogate complications such as Cesarean section, shoulder dystocia and brachial plexus injury (BPI). The overall rate of macrosomia for the nondiabetic population is 7–9%.[26] In contrast, the incidence reported for macrosomia in GDM is management-dependent. When good glycemic control is not achieved, the incidence of macrosomia can be as high as 20–45%.[23] The macrosomic fetus is a result of diabetic fetopathy and is characterized by organomegaly.[27,28] Complications, directly and indirectly associated to fetal macrosomia are neonatal hypoglycemia, hypocalcemia, hyperbilirubinemia, and polycytemia; in addition to birth trauma, these are all the consequence of not treating or inadequate treatment of the disease.

Excessive fetal growth occurs in as many as 50% of pregnancies complicated by GDM. It was shown that the accelerated fetal growth is associated with the maternal glycemic profile. Infancy is a period of rapid adipose tissue accumulation and influences during fetal development are credible determinants of altered adiposity. The quantity of adipose

tissue as well as its distribution is a health/disease indicator. Previous methods for the assessment of body composition in infants have been indirect, i.e. skinfold measurement. This method was frequently used in 1990s but was unreliable in determining adiposity quantity or distribution. Adipose tissue magnetic resonance imaging is a direct, non-invasive fetus friendly serial of examinations. Adipose tissue deposits are quatified individually and totaled in order to provide an accurate measure of deposit-specific and total adiposity.[29] Assessing fetal/neonatal adiposity may enhance the understanding of the effect of differential factors on fetal growth. The variables associated with the accrual of fetal adipose tissue in late gestation are less well understood compared to birthweight and free fat mass.

Although fetal growth can be measured by birthweight, a more accurate way to characterize overgrowth is by estimation of body composition that includes lean body mass (LBM) and free fat mass (FM). Lean body mass is a metabolically active tissue and is relatively stable *in utero*. Free fat mass is more variable and sensitive to factors that affect fetal growth. Therefore, to more accurately characterize the diabetic fetopathy, measurements that can identify even minimal deviations from the norm are needed. Fat mass and lean body mass may provide the means.

Recent studies have shown conflicting results in the evaluation of infant body composition.[30,31] Catalano reported increased free fat mass in infants of GDM women, even when average weight for gestational age compared with infants of women with normal glucose tolerance.[30] Similarly, he demonstrated increased body fat in infants of GDM women requiring a Cesarean delivery compared with normal glucose tolerance despite similar birthweights. In contrast, we and Naeye[27,28] found an increase in lean body mass at the time of autopsy in overgrown infants of women with diabetes. In a study evaluating body composition of macrosomic infants of diabetic women, we demonstrated increased body fat and decreased lean body mass in infants of GDM women compared with normal glucose tolerance.[31]

Long-term effects of GDM

When addressing the issue of the long-term effects of GDM, one must differentiate between the long-term maternal effects and the prognosis for the offspring (Figures 14.2–14.4).

The mother

The increased risk of developing diabetes later in life for women with GDM is well known with the magnitude of the risk ranging from 20–80%.[32,33] In recent years, it was recognized that GDM women have up to 8-fold increased risk to develop metabolic syndrome. This syndrome is associated with a high rate of Type 2 diabetes and cardiovascular complications.

The neonate

Since Barker's primary epidemiologic studies in 1989[34,35] showing an inverse relationship between birthweight and mortality due to adult ischemic heart disease, it has become increasingly clear over the past decades that many fetal stresses

At Age 1 Year

LGA-GDM   AGA-GDM   LGA-NON-GDM AGA-NON-GDM

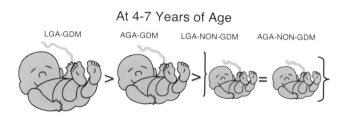

> ➤ LGA's of GDM mothers had a higher BMI, greater waist
> circumference and abdominal skinfold compared with all
> other study groups

> ➤ The mean 2-h postprandial glucose value for the 2nd and
> 3rd trimester correlated with waist circumference (r=0.28,
> P<0.04) and subscapular skin-fold (r=0.37,P<0.007)

Modified from Vohr, BR, Diabetes care, 1997;20,7:1066-72

Figure 14.2   Long term complications of the infant of the diabetic mother. Infant's age: 1 year. LGAs of GDM mothers had a higher BMI, greater waist circumference and abdominal skinfold compared with all other study groups. The mean 2-h post-prandial glucose value of the seond and third trimester correlated with waist circumference ($r = 0.28$, $P < 0.04$) and subscapular skinfold ($r = 0.37$, $P < 0.07$). (Modified from Vohr and McGarvey.[51])

may lead to fetal programming and the alteration of the normal developmental gene expression pattern. Research indicates that the child of the diabetic mother remains at increased risk for a variety of developmental disturbances: obesity,[36–39] impaired glucose tolerance or diabetes[40] and diminished neurobehavioral capacities.[41–47] Therefore, it would be reasonable to speculate that the process whereby a stimulus or insult (glucose toxicity and other metabolic fuels) acting at a critical period of development in early and during intrauterine life, may alter gene expression patterns for life.

Silverman et al. demonstrated that the growth of offspring of diabetic mothers is similar to nondiabetic populations after 12 months. However, after age 5, there was a rapid weight gain to a point at which at 8 years, almost half of the offspring of diabetic mothers had a weight at or above the 90th percentile. In addition, a slight upward trend in height was noted.[48] Pettitt et al. in the Pima Indian population demonstrated that by 5–9 years of age, both macrosomic and normal birthweight infants of GDM mothers are more obese than normal birthweight offspring of nondiabetic mothers.[49] Adiposity in

children is strongly correlated with childhood hypertension (both systolic and dystolic) and resembles the metabolic syndrome albeit at a younger age. Moreover, the presence of hypertension in LGA infants was suggested as a cause for this condition in children.[50] In another study, Vohr et al. reported that LGA infants of GDM mothers had higher BMI waist circumference and abdominal skin folds at one year compared to infants of nondiabetic mothers. The mean postprandial glucose value for the second and third trimester correlated with waist circumference ($r = 0.28$, $P < 0.04$) and subscapular skinfold ($r = 0.37$, $P < 0.007$). They concluded that macrosomic infants of GDM mothers have unique patterns of adiposity that are present at birth and persist at age 1 year.[51]

Cognitive development in children of diabetic mothers

Several studies evaluated the association between cognitive development and metabolic fuels in pre-existing and

At 4-7 Years of Age

LGA-GDM   AGA-GDM   LGA-NON-GDM   AGA-NON-GDM

> ➤ LGA infants of GDM mothers had a higher BMI,
> greater waist circumference and abdominal
> skinfold compared to AGA-GDM.

> ➤ No difference between non-GDM LGA and AGA.

Modified from Vohr et al, Diabetes care, 1999

Figure 14.3   Long-term complications of the infant of the diabetic mother. Infant's age: 4–7 years. (Modified from Vohr B et al. Diabetes Care 1999; 22(8): 128–91.)

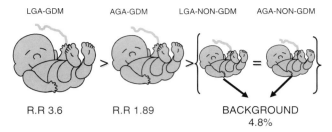

Figure 14.4   Long-term complications of the infant of the diabetic mother: metabolic syndrome at 11 years. (Modified from Boney CM et al. Pediatrics 2005; 115(3): e290–6.)

gestational diabetes. The research group at Northwestern University, Chicago, tested 73 pre-existing and 112 GDM infants for the relationship between maternal fasting plasma glucose and hemoglobin A_{1c} during the second and third trimesters on neonatal performance on the Brazelton Neonatal Behavioral Assessment scale. The Brazelton scale has gained wide asceptance as one of the premier instruments for integrative characterization of nervous system function in the newborn.[52] They found a significant correlation between glycemic control in three out of the four newborn behavioral dimensions on the scale. In each case, poor glycemic control was followed by a poor Brazelton rating of the neonate. The results were no different when gestational diabetic and pre-gestational diabetics were analyzed separately. Attribution of results to various prenatal events such as asphyxia, neonatal hypoglycemia or differences in socioeconomic status or ethnicity could not be made. Although the authors reported that their patients were well controlled, this statement is questionable since there was an approximate 30% rate of macrosomia (>4000 g), hypoglycemia and hyperbilirubinemia. On the other hand, this perinatal outcome demonstrated the long term complications one can anticipate when the level of glycemia remains uncontrolled.

Another study sponsored by the same group[53] evaluated the offspring of 95 pre-existing diabetic women and 101 GDM subjects. The children were assessed using the psychomotor development index of the Bayley Scales of Infant Development at 2 years of age and the Bruininks–Oseretsky Test of Motor Proficiency at ages 6, 8 and 9 years. They reported that the children's average scores on the Bruininks–Oseretsky test at ages 6–9 years correlated significantly with β-hydroxybutyrate in maternal second and third trimesters. There was also a borderline association between children's scores on the psychomotor development Index at age 2 and β-hydroxybutyrate. Similar findings were reported in another study.[54] Rizzo et al.[42] correlated measures of maternal glucose and lipid metabolism (fasting plasma glucose levels, hemoglobin A_{1c} levels, episodes of hypoglycemia, episodes of acetonuria, and plasma β-hydroxybutyrate and free fatty acid levels) with two measures of intellectual development in the offspring using the Bayley Scales of Infant Development for 2-year-olds and the Stanford–Binet Intelligence Scale for 3–5-year-olds expressed as an average of the three scores. The children's mental development index scores at the age of two correlated inversely with the mother's third-trimester plasma β-hydroxybutyrate levels; the average Stanford–Binet scores correlated inversely with third-trimester plasma β-hydroxybutyrate and free fatty acid levels.

Maternal diabetes during pregnancy may affect behavioral and intellectual development in the offspring. The associations between gestational ketonemia in the mother and a lower IQ in the child warrant continued efforts to avoid ketoacidosis and accelerated starvation in all pregnant women. Similar information was reported by Petersen et al. who suggested that first trimester intrauterine growth delay is associated with psychomotor deficit in the offspring at age 4–5. Presumably such delays are driven from mothers who were in poor glycemic control (elevated HbA_{1c}).[54] Sells et al. reported that late entry into treatment programs in pregnancy in pre-existing diabetic women resulted in lower scores on language measures and intellectual development of children through age 2 in comparison to women who maintained good control during pregnancy.[55] Finally, Stenninger et al. reported that children born to mothers with diabetes (probably GDM) who subsequently developed neonatal hypoglycemia, experienced long-term neurological dysfunction. The offspring evaluated at age 8 had more difficulties in validated screening tests for minimal brain dysfunction, were hyperactive, impulsive and easily distracted. On psychological assessment, they had a lower developmental score in comparison to the offspring of normoglycemic diabetic women and nondiabetic control patients.[56]

In summary, the existing evidence clearly suggests that there is adverse neurological and cognitive outcomes in addition to the possibility of early development of metabolic syndrome (hypertension, obesity and diabetes) when gestational diabetes is not treated or poorly managed. Of note, the adverse neonatal outcome is reported to be similar regardless of the type of diabetes. Finally, the maternal long-term implications for the future development of Type 2 diabetes should be included in the morbidity spectrum of this disease.

Clinical studies

There is paucity of information in the literature regarding outcome of pregnancy in untreated GDM. Ostlund et al.[57] studied 213 women prospectively who were identified with

IGT during pregnancy but remained undiagnosed and untreated. IGT was defined as fasting blood glucose level 121 mg/dL (<6.7 mmol/L) and 2-h blood glucose level 162–198 mg/dL (>9 and <11 mmol/L). They compared the untreated IGT to control and treated GDMs. The rate of macrosomia (>4000 g) was 33, 16, and 30%, and LGA 25, 4 and 25%, respectively. These findings demonstrate significant morbidity in the GDM and untreated groups. It also questions the efficacy of diabetic patient treatment. Similar findings were found relevant to metabolic complications, Erb's palsy, and neonatal intensive care admission. In their study, the obstetrician was not informed of the deviation in the glucose tolerance. They concluded that there is an increased independent association between Cesarean section rates, prematurity and LGA and macrosomic infants born to mothers with untreated IGT. The main problem in the Ostlund study is that the authors used a non-traditional definition for GDM which was a modification of the Lind definition.[58] It is not used in North America nor in the majority of European centers who follow the consensus agreement reached at the Fourth International Workshop on Gestational Diabetes.

Adams et al.[59] identified 16 cases of clinically unrecognized gestational diabetes diagnosed using the NDDG criteria and compared them to 64 nondiabetic controls. A third group consisted of 373 unmatched cases of GDM. The unrecognized group had 44% macrosomia, 44% LGA, 19% shoulder dystocia, 25% birth trauma and 13% metabolic or respiratory complications. The nondiabetic controls and the unmatched GDM group had rates of macrosomia 8 vs. 18%; LGA 5 vs. 13%; shoulder dystocia 3 vs. 4%; birth trauma 0 vs. 0.5%; metabolic/respiratory complications 0 vs. 10%, respectively. The study suggests that unrecognized GDM increases risks for neonatal complications such as LGA, macrosomia, shoulder dystocia, and birth trauma independent of maternal obesity and other confounding variables. Clinical recognition and dietary control of gestational diabetes are associated with a reduction in these perinatal morbid conditions. The limitation of this study is its small sample size; the results could have been affected by both alpha and beta errors.

Another series of studies was performed by the Toronto Tri-Hospital Gestational Diabetes Project.[60] In their first work, the investigators explored the function of the screening test. Their subsequent study addressed pregnancy outcomes for the 3637 subjects without a diagnosis of GDM whose caregivers were blinded to the OGTT results. There was a direct relationship between OGTT results and a number of adverse pregnancy outcomes including Cesarean delivery, neonatal macrosomia, and pre-eclampsia. When multivariate analysis was used to correct for the relative contribution of various other potential risk factors such as maternal obesity and age, the OGTT results continued to have a significant independent impact. For example, for every 18 mg/dL (1.0 mmol/L) increment in the 3-h OGTT value, the likelihood of Cesarean delivery rose by 10% even though the caregivers did not know the OGTT results. Similarly, for each 18 mg/dL (1.0 mmol/L) increase in the fasting plasma glucose level, the likelihood of macrosomia (birthweight ≥4000 g) increased by 100% even though the OGTT results were all in the presumed normal range.[61,62]

In another study, the OGTT results did not reach the NDDG threshold for GDM but did meet a lower set of thresholds that has been previously associated with increased morbidity.[63] In the untreated gestational diabetes group, the macrosomia rate of 29% was more than double the rates in the control and gestational diabetes mellitus groups (14 and 10%, respectively), while the Cesarean delivery rate was 30%, similar to the rate in the GDM subjects. In these untreated pregnancies, however, Cesarean delivery was significantly more likely when fetal macrosomia was present. These data demonstrate that the GDM treatment was apparently effective in reducing the rate of macrosomia, since undiagnosed and untreated women with mildly abnormal glucose tolerance manifested significantly increased fetal macrosomia.

Li et al.[64] randomly assigned 209 women into three groups based on the OGTT results. The first group, 'mild GDM' (n = 75) was based on NDDG criteria and remained untreated. The second group was GDM, diagnosed after a 75-g OGTT by WHO criteria and was treated. The third group consisted of normal, nondiabetic controls. The results showed a significantly higher rate of LGA, 29% in the untreated group (NDDG criteria), when compared to the nondiabetic control women. There was no significant difference in the rate of LGA between the treated GDM (WHO criteria) and the untreated group. This study again raises the issue that untreated GDM is associated with increased morbidity and questions the efficacy of glycemic control and the intervention in the treatment group. The relevance of this study is limited by the fact that the study group did not fulfill the diagnostic criteria for GDM. Thus, it is difficult to apply the results to the GDM population. In addition, neither the women nor their caregivers were blinded to the OGTT results thus allowing the women to initiate dietary and other lifestyle modifications that could have potentially affected glycemic control while leaving the caregivers exposed to a potential labeling bias. Increased morbidity in untreated GDM was demonstrated in several studies. The majority of these studies were retrospective, with small sample sizes, and the rate of metabolic and respiratory complications and neonatal intensive care admissions not reported.

Langer et al.[19] addressed many of the limitations posed by the above studies. Patients in the untreated group were recruited to the study after 37 weeks' gestation which in and of itself controls for lifestyle modifications such as diet that may influence pregnancy outcome. Additionally, patients and care providers were unaware of the GDM since the disease was diagnosed after week 37 which had left the fetus exposed to the glucose toxicity throughout pregnancy. Crowther et al.[20] randomly assigned women between 24 and 34 weeks of gestation to intervention and non-intervention groups to determine whether treatment of GDM reduced perinatal outcome. They also found that treatment reduced perinatal morbidity and may have also improved the women's health-related quality of life. The question remains how many of the undiagnosed GDMs were due to late development during pregnancy and how many were due to late identification. Even if some of the untreated cases were late onset of the disease, this will dilute the outcome results but will not be a confounding variable on the outcome. The diagnostic criteria used in the study are one of two accepted criteria and recommended in the last decade since it was supported by two international workshops on gestational diabetes which represent international consensus.[65,66]

The sample size in our and Crowther's studies were the largest, to date, of all previously published work. The power of the studies was sufficient to evaluate macrosomia, LGA, metabolic complications, respiratory complications, and neonatal intensive care admissions. Furthermore, by developing a composite outcome, Langer et al.[19] were able to evaluate the overall neonatal disease (morbidity) in addition to specific morbidity components. Finally, selection into the nondiabetic comparison group was designed to control for potential confounding variables. Two nondiabetic controls were matched to each untreated GDM case on the basis of the following characteristics: ethnicity, parity, gestational age at delivery (within one week), obesity, and number of prenatal visits. We found a 2- to 4-fold increased risk for large infants and shoulder dystocia; a 2- to 7-fold increased risk for metabolic and respiratory complications; a 4-fold increased risk for neonatal intensive care admissions; and, a 2-fold increased risk for Cesarean section.

Mild untreated hyperglycemia

The association between mild hyperglycemia (two or more abnormal values on the OGTT or patients with lower glucose thresholds) and adverse neonatal outcome has been a major concern for the past two decades especially for patients who could not reach the current 'gold standard' of the NDDG and the Fourth International Workshop on Gestational Diabetes. There are many cases of unrecognized and, therefore, untreated GDM and 'mild hyperglycemia.' With the current criteria for selective screening, some in the low risk group may include cases of unrecognized GDM. The cut-off point used in different centers (when screening is performed) varies from 130–140 mg/dL. However, it is well recognized that when using a glucose level of 140 mg/dL, approximately 10% of GDM cases will go undetected.[67] Women with one elevated value on the OGTT are not tagged by the current criteria as GDM. All suffer from glucose toxicity yet remain unrecognized GDM in most obstetric clinics. They are reinstated into the 'normal' population; we deliver them every day.

The scientific rationale for the use of two or more abnormal values is not based on evidence but rather on opinions. The explanation for those who support two abnormal values range from 'just because' to 'better reproducibility of the test.' However, data supporting these positions are lacking. If at all, the existing data suggests that one abnormal value has the same characteristics and predictive value as two or more values. The use of one abnormal value for diagnostic criteria of GDM is further supported by the fact that many obstetricians will use screening values of 180 mg/dL or greater as a single diagnosis for GDM and will treat based on this single result.

In 1987, we suggested, in a case control study, that women with one abnormal value on the OGTT results have a significantly increased risk for adverse pregnancy outcome when compared to nondiabetic and treated GDM women (two or more abnormal values on the OGTT).[68] In a follow-up

study, women with one abnormal value were randomized into treatment and non-treatment groups and compared to nondiabetic subjects. Again, the incidence of large infants was significantly higher in the untreated group. When patients were stratified into obese and non-obese for each study group (treated, untreated, and control), there was a significantly higher rate of large infants and metabolic complications in the untreated group. There was no significant difference in the rate of LGA between obese and non-obese patients.[69] In a third study, we compared the incidence of LGA infants in relation to the number of abnormal values on the OGTT. We found a similar rate of LGA infants when one, two, or three values were abnormal. This was especially true in patients with poor glycemic control.[70] Similar findings by Lindsay et al.[71] showed 18% LGA in his one-abnormal population. Neiger and Coustan[72] showed that women with one abnormal value even on the modified lower Coustan–Carpenter criteria when compared to the NDDG criteria when the OGTT was repeated after 4 weeks showed that about 33% had at least two abnormal values on the OGTT. This demonstrates the similarity between one or more abnormal values on the OGTT and the continuation of the disease during pregnancy.

Gruendhammer et al.[73] studied 152 women with 1 abnormal glucose value match controlled to 304 nondiabetic women with normal OGTT values. They found that women with only one abnormal OGTT value had increased risk in comparison to the control subjects. In another study[74] untreated one abnormal and GDM women had significantly higher abnormal glucose characterstics and an increased rate of adverse perinatal outcome in comparison to the control subjects. Another study evaluated the impact of pregnancy with different OGTT values. There was an LGA rate of 8.8% in the normal group; untreated one abnormal 19%; treated one abnormal 18.9%, and GDM 20%. The results demonstrate the increased morbidity with any abnormal value on the OGTT and that most likely the targeted levels of glycemic control were not achieved in treated patients.[75] Therefore, from mild to severe hyperglycemia defined as abnormal oral glucose tolerance test (one or more abnormal values), there are significantly higher rates of perinatal mortality and morbidity when these patients remain unrecognized and untreated.

Can treatment of GDM improve adverse outcome?

The potential for successful treatment of diabetes in pregnancy including GDM will determine pregnancy outcome. Thus, failure to achieve rate of successful outcome is not due to the questionable need for treatment but may suggest an inappropriate treatment approach. In a prospective quasi-randomized study[24] of 2461 GDM women we compared conventional ($n = 1316$) to intensified therapy ($n = 1145$). The two diabetic groups were compared to a nondiabetic control in a ratio of 2:1 selected in a randomized approach from our general population. The conventional therapy consisted of fasting plasma glucose and 2-h postprandial levels monitored on a weekly basis at clinic visits. In addition, patients were required to perform four times daily, visualized but not verified, self-monitoring of blood glucose. The women in the intensified group were selected per memory reflectance meter availability and instructed to test their blood glucose seven times daily with a memory reflectance meter to ascertain accurate and reliable blood glucose information. The study revealed, firstly, a significant adverse outcome for LGA and macrosomia, metabolic complications, respiratory complications, and shoulder dystocia rates when the conventional group was compared to the intensified therapy group. Secondly, there was a higher rate of neonatal intensive care unit admission and length of stay for the conventional group. Thirdly, with regards to maternal complications, no significant difference was found in the rates of pre-eclampsia, chronic hypertension or chorioamnionitis between the three study groups; the perinatal outcome variables also included Cesarean section rates. The above variables were all found to be comparable between the intensified and the nondiabetic controls. Fourthly, logistic regression to evaluate the net effect of potential contributing variables to the rate of macrosomia revealed that only mean blood glucose, gestational age at delivery, previous macrosomia, and previous GDM were significant, while obesity, parity, and ethnicity were non significant for the intensified group (Table 14.3). This study demonstrated that neonatal macrosomia is related to the level of blood glucose and that when this factor is controlled, the maternal size has minimal or no effect on fetal size in GDM women.

Persson et al.[76] assigned 202 women with GDM randomly to treatment with diet alone or diet plus insulin. A subgroup of the diet-treated group (14%) had insulin treatment added when prescribed limits for hyperglycemia were exceeded on the diet alone protocol. Frequencey of macrosomia was relatively low and did not differ in the two groups but was not specifically compared with such events in controls with normal carbohydrate metabolism. Thirty infants in the diet group and 40 infants in the insulin group showed one or more episodes of neonatal morbidity. The most common was neonatal hypoglycemia. It is also unclear if the data were analyzed with the intent to treat group. Drexel et al.[77] reported their efforts to prevent perinatal morbidity in GDM by tight metabolic control. Insulin therapy was initiated without a trial of diet alone if one or more values during the OGTT was >200 mg/dL. The therapeutic goals were capillary blood glucose concentration <130 mg/dL one hour after breakfast, absence of ketonuria, and weight gain ≤1 kg/month. When blood glucose concentration exceeded the acceptable range in diet-treated subjects, insulin treatment was added (lente, ≥12 U/day). Whereas insulin was used in most subjects, the frequency of macrosomia was no different in the intensely treated subjects with GDM (group 2) compared to the normal control group; the frequency of macrosomia in the group of GDM with limited treatment (group 3) was significantly higher than that in group 2. However, the frequency of unphysiological modes of delivery and of neonatal morbidity did not differ among the three groups of subjects. In addition, obesity, an important confounding variable in several of the studies cited, was not a common feature of these subjects. The protocol used in this study suggests earlier diagnosis and treatment of GDM than is customarily practiced in most centers.

Summary

Gestational diabetes in all severity levels (from one abnormal to maximum values) is associated with decreased insulin sensitivity and secretion. Furthermore, the majority of GDM women are prone to develop metabolic syndrome and Type 2 diabetes later in life.

All GDM severity levels will result in adverse neonatal outcome. Short-term neonatal complications include increased perinatal mortality, metabolic, respiratory, hematological complications, and neonatal trauma. Long-term neonatal implications include obesity, future diabetes and intellectual impairment and the early onset of metabolic syndrome.

Table 14.3   Perinatel outcome: Untreated and treated GDM

	Langer et al.[19]		Crowther et al.[20]	
	Untreated	**Treated**	**Untreated**	**Treated**
Macrosomia (%)	16.8	7.0	21	10
LGA (%)	29.4	10.7	22	13
Ponderal index (>2.85) (%)	21.7	13.8	—	—
NICU admission (%)	24.1	6.0	61	71
Metabolic complications (%)	29.0	10.0	14	16
Respiratory complications (%)	12.0	2.0	4.0	5.0
Shoulder dystocia (%)	2.5	0.9	3.0	1.0
Stillbirth (per 1000)	5.4	3.6	6.0	0.0
C/S (%)	23.7	23.2	32	31
n	555	1110	510	490

REFERENCES

1. Metzger BE, Coustan DR, and the Organizing Committee. Summary and recommendations of the 4th International Workshop Conference on gestational diabetes. Diabetes Care 1998; 21(suppl. 2): B161–7.20–22.
2. Jarrett RJ. Gestational diabetes: A non-entity? BMJ 1993; 306: 37–8.
3. Sermer M, Naylor CD, Farine D, et al. The Toronto Tri-Hospital Gestational Diabetes Project. A preliminary review. Diabetes Care 1998; 21: B33–B42.
4. Hunter DJS, Milner R. Gestational diabetes and birth trauma [letter]. Am J Obstet Gynecol 1985; 152: 918–9.
5. Greene MF. Oral hypoglycemic drugs for gestational diabetes [editorial]. New Engl J Med 2000; 343: 1178–9.
6. Beard RW, Hoet JJ. Is gestational diabetes a clinical entity? Diabetologia 1982; 4: 307–12.
7. Ryan E, Enns L. Role of gestational hormones in the induction of insulin resistance. J Clin Endocrinol Metab 1988; 67: 431–7.
8. Pittas AG, Joseph NA, Greenberg AS. Adipocytokines and insulin resistance. J Clin Endocrinol Metab 2004; 89: 447–52.
9. Hotta K, Funahashi T, Arita Y, et al. Plasma concentrations of a novel, adipose-specific protein, adiponectins, in type 2 diabetic patients. Arterioscler Thromb Vas Biol 2000; 20: 1595–9.
10. Matsubara M, Maruoka S, Katayose S. Decreased plasma adiponectins concentrations in women with dyslipidemia. J Clin Endocrinol Metab 2002; 87: 2764–9.
11. Yamauchi T, Kamon J, Waki H, et al. Globular adiponectins protected ob/ob mice from diabetes and ApoE-deficient mice from atherosclerosis. J Biol Chem 2003; 278: 2461–8.
12. Yamauchi T, Kamon J, Waki H, et al. The fat-derived hormone adiponectins reverses insulin resistance associated with both lipoatrophy and obesity. Nat Med 2001; 7: 941–6.
13. Retnakaran R, Hanley AJG, Raif N, et al. C-reactive protein and gestational diabetes: the central role of maternal obesity. J Clin Endocrinol Metab 2003; 88: 3507–12.
14. Catalano PM. Obesity and pregnancy – The propagation of a viscous cycle? [editorial]. J Clin End Metab 2003; 88: 3505–6.
15. Catalano PM, Tyzbir ED, Roman NM, et al. Longitudinal changes in insulin release and insulin resistance in non-obese pregnant women. Am J Obstet-Gynecol 1991; 165: 1667–72.
16. Buchanan TA, Xiang AH, Peters RK. Response of pancreatic β-cells to improved insulin sensitivity in women at high risk for type 2 diabetes. Diabetes 2000; 49: 782–8.
17. Xiang AH, Peters RK, Trigo E, et al. Multiple metabolic defects during late pregnancy in women at high risk for type 2 diabetes mellitus. Diabetes 1999; 48: 848–54.
18. Buchanan TA. Pancreatic β-cell defects in gestational diabetes: implications for the pathogenesis and prevention of type 2 diabetes [commentary]. J Clin Endocrinol Metab 2001; 86: 989–93.
19. Langer O, Yogev Y, Most O, Xenakis MJ. Gestational diabetes: The consequences of not treating. Am J Obstet Gynecol 2005; 192: 989–97.
20. Crowther CA, Hiller JE, Moss JR, et al. Effect of treatment of gestational diabetes mellitus on pregnancy outcomes. N Engl J Med 2005; 352: 2477–86.
21. O'Sullivan JB, Mahan CM, Charles D. Screening criteria for high-risk gestational diabetic patients. Am J Obstet Gynecol 1973; 116: 895.
22. Abell DA, Beischer NA, Wood C. Routine testing for gestational diabetes, pregnancy, hypoglycemia, and fetal growth retardation and results of treatment. J Perinat Med 1976; 4: 197–212.
23. Langer O, Rodriguez D, Xenakis EMJ, et al. Intensified versus conventional management of gestational diabetes. Am J Obstet Gynecol 1994; 170; 1036–47.
24. Schmidt MI, Duncan BB, Reichelt AJ, et al. Gestational diabetes mellitus diagnosed with a 2-h 75-g oral glucose tolerance test and adverse pregnancy outcomes. Diabetes Care 2001; 24: 1151–3.
25. Mondestin M, Ananth C, Smulian J, et al. Birth weight and fetal death in the United States: The effect of maternal diabetes during pregnancy. Am J Obstet Gynecol 2002; 187: 922–6.
26. ACOG. Practice Bulletin Clinical Management Guidelines: Fetal Macrosomia. Number 22, 2000.
27. Naeye RL. Infants of diabetic mothers: a quantitative, morphologic study. Pediatrics 1965; 35: 980–8.
28. Langer O, Kagan-Hallet K. Diabetic vs. non-diabetic infants: A quantitative morphological study. Proceedings of the 38th Annual Meeting of the Society for Gynecologic Investigation. San Antonio, Texas, 1992.
29. Uthaya S, Bell J, Modi N. Adipose tissue magnetic resonance imaging in the newborn. Hormone Research 2004; 62:(suppl. 3): 143–8.
30. Catalano PM, Thomas A, Huston-Presley L, et al. Increased fetal adiposity: a very sensitive marker of abnormal in-utero development. Am J Obstet Gynecol 2003; 189(6): 1698–704.
31. McFarland MB, Trylovich CG, Langer O. Anthropometric differences in macrosomic infants of diabetic and non-diabetic mothers. J Matern Fetal Med 1998; 7: 292–5.
32. Peters RK, Kjos SL, Xiang A, et al. Long-term diabetogenic effect of single pregnancy in women with previous gestational diabetes mellitus. Lancet 1996; 347: 227–30.
33. Kim C, Newton KM, Knopp RH. Gestational diabetes and the incidence of type 2 diabetes. Diabetes Care 2002; 25: 1862–8.
34. Barker D, Osmond C, Golding J, et al. Growth in utero, blood pressure in childhood and adult life, and mortality from cardiovascular disease. Br Med J 1989; 298: 564–7.
35. Barker DJ. In utero programming of cardiovascular disease. Theriogenology 2000; 53: 555–74.
36. Silverman B, Rizzo T, Green O, et al. Long-term prospective evaluation of offspring of diabetic mothers. Diabetes 1991; 40(suppl. 2): 121–5.
37. Pettitt DJ, Nelson RG, Saad MF, et al. Diabetes and obesity in the offspring of Pima Indian women with diabetes during pregnancy. Diabetes Care 1993; 16: 310–4.
38. Silverman BL, Rizzo TA, Cho NH, et al. Long-term effects of the intrauterine environment. The Northwestern University Diabetes in Pregnancy Center. Diabetes Care 1998; 21(suppl. 2): B142–9.
39. Dabelea D, Pettitt DJ. Intrauterine diabetic environment confers risks for type 2 diabetes mellitus and obesity in the offspring, in addition to genetic susceptibility. J Pediatr Endocrinol Metab 2001; 14: 1085–91.
40. Silverman B, Metzger B, Cho N, et al. Fetal hyperinsulinism and impaired glucose tolerance in adolescent offspring of diabetic mothers. Diabetes Care 1995; 18: 611–7.
41. Rizzo T, Freinkel N, Metzger B, et al. Correlations between antepartum maternal metabolism and newborn behavior. Am J Obstet Gynecol 1990; 163: 1458–64.
42. Rizzo T, Metzger B, Burns W, et al. Correlations between antepartum maternal metabolism and intelligence of offspring. N Engl J Med 1991; 325: 911–6.
43. Petersen MB, Pedersen S, Greisen G, et al. Early growth delay in diabetic pregnancy: relation to psychomotor development at age 4. BMJ 1988; 296: 598–600.
44. Visser G, Bekedam D, Mulder E, et al. Delayed emergence of fetal behavior in type 1 diabetic women. Early Hum Dev 1985; 12: 167–72.
45. Mulder E, Visser G, Bekedam D, et al. Emergence of behavioral states in fetuses of type 1 diabetic women. Early Hum Dev 1987; 15: 231–51.
46. Sells C, Robinson N, Brown Z, et al. Long-term developmental follow-up infants of diabetic mothers. J Pediatr 1994; 125: S9–S17.
47. Lincoln N, Faleiro R, Kelly C. Effect of Long-term glycemic control on cognitive function. Diabetes Care 1996; 19: 656–8.
48. Silverman B, Landsberg L, Metzger B. Fetal hyperinsulinism in offspring of diabetic mothers. Ann NY Acad Sci 1993; 699: 36–45.
49. Pettitt D, Knowler W, Bennett P, et al. Obesity in offspring of diabetic Pima Indian women despite normal birth weight. Diabetes Care 1987; 10: 76–80.
50. Vohr B, McGarvey S, Coll C. Effects of maternal gestational diabetes and adiposity on neonatal adiposity and blood pressure. Diabetes Care 1995; 18: 467–75.
51. Vohr B, McGarvey S. Growth patterns of large-for-gestational age and appropriate-for-gestational age infants of gestational diabetic mothers and control mothers at age 1 year. Diabetes Care 1997; 20: 1066–72.
52. Rizzo T, Dooley S, Metzger B, et al. Prenatal and perinatal influences on long-term psychomotor development in offspring of diabetic mothers. Am J Obstet Gynecol 1995; 173: 1753–8.
53. Rizzo T, Ogata E, Dooley S, et al. Perinatal complications and cognitive development in 2–5-year-old children of diabetic mothers. Am J Obstet Gynecol 1994; 171: 706–13.
54. Petersen M. Status at 4–5 years in 90 children and insulin-dependent diabetic mothers. In: Sutherland H, Stowers J, Pearson D, eds. Carbohydrate Metabolism in Pregnancy and the Newborn, IV. London: Springer-Verlag; 1989, pp. 353–61.
55. Sells C, Robinson N, Brown, et al. Long-term developmental follow-up infants of diabetic mothers. J Pediatr 1994; 125: S9–S17.
56. Stenninger E, Flink R, Eriksson B, et al. Long-term neurological dysfunction and neonatal hypoglycemia after diabetic pregnancy. Arch Dis Child Fetal Neonatal Ed 1998; 79: F174–9.

57. Ostlund I, Hanson U, Bjorklund A, et al. Maternal and fetal outcomes if gestational impaired glucose tolerance is not treated. Diabetes Care 2003; 26: 2107–11.

58. Lind T, Phillips PR. Influence of pregnancy on the 75-g OGTT: A prospective multicenter study. The Diabetic Pregnancy Study Group of the European Association for the Study of Diabetes. Diabetes 1991; 40(suppl. 2): 8–13.

59. Adams KM, Li H, Nelson RL, et al. Sequelae of unrecognized gestational diabetes. Am J Obstet Gynecol 1998; 178: 1321–32.

60. Sermer M, Naylor CD, Gare DJ, Kenshole AB, Ritchie JWK. For the Toronto Tri-Hospital Gestational Diabetes Investigators: Impact of increasing carbohydrate intolerance on maternal-fetal outcomes in 3,637 women without gestational diabetes. Am J Obstet Gynecol 1995; 173: 146–56.

61. Coustan DR. Management of gestational diabetes mellitus: A self-fulfilling prophecy? JAMA 1996; 275: 1199–200.

62. Coustan DR. Screening and testing for gestational diabetes mellitus. Obstet Gynecol Clin North Am 1996; 23: 125–36.

63. Magee MS, Walden CE, Benedetti TJ, et al. Influence of diagnostic criteria on the incidence of gestational diabetes and perinatal morbidity. JAMA 1993; 269: 609–15.

64. Li DF, Wong VC, O'Hoy KM, et al. Is treatment needed for mild impairment of glucose tolerance in pregnancy? A randomized controlled trial. Br J Obstet Gynaecol 1987; 94: 851–4.

65. Metzger BE, Coustan DR. Summary and Recommendations of the Fourth International Workshop Conference on Gestational Diabetes Mellitus. The Organizing Committee. Diabetes Care 1998; 21(suppl. 9): B161–7.

66. Summary and Recommendations of the Third International Workshop Conference on Gestational Diabetes. Diabetes 1991; 40(suppl. 2): 197–201.

67. Coustan DR, Nelson C, Carpenter MW, et al. Maternal age and screening for gestational diabetes: a population-based study. Obstet Gynecol 1989; 73: 557–61.

68. Langer O, Brustman L, Anyaegbunam A. The significance of one abnormal glucose tolerance test value on adverse outcome in pregnancy. Am J Obstet 1987; 157: 758–63.

69. Langer O, Anyaegbunam A, Brustman L, Divon M. Management of women with one abnormal oral glucose tolerance test value reduces adverse outcome in pregnancy. Am J Obstet Gynecol 1989; 161: 593–9.

70. Berkus MD, Langer O. Glucose tolerance test: Degree of glucose abnormality correlates with neonatal outcome. Obstet Gynecol 1993; 81: 344–8.

71. Lindsay MK, Graves W, Klein L. The relationship of one abnormal glucose tolerance test value and pregnancy complications. Obstet Gynecol 1989; 73: 103–6.

72. Neiger R, Coustan DR. The role of repeat glucose tolerance tests in the diagnosis of gestational diabetes. Am J Obstet Gynecol 1991; 165: 787–90.

73. Gruendhammer M, Brezinka C, Lechleitner M. The number of abnormal plasma glucose values in the oral glucose tolerance test and the feto-maternal outcome of pregnancy. J Obstet Gynecol Reprod Biol 2003; 108: 131–6.

74. Forest J, Masse J, Garrido-Russo M. Glucose tolerance test during pregnancy: The significance of one abnormal value. Clin Biochem 1994; 27: 200–4.

75. Bo S, Menato G, Gallo M, et al. Mild gestational hyperglycemia, the metabolic syndrome and adverse neonatal outcomes. Acta Obstet Gynecol Scand 2004; 83: 335–40.

76. Persson B, Strangenberg M, Hansson U, et al. Gestational diabetes mellitus (GDM): Comparative evaluation of two treatment regimes, diet versus insulin and diet. Diabetes 1985; 34 (suppl. 2): 101.

77. Drexel H, Bicher A, Sailer S, et al. Prevention of perinatal morbidity by tight metabolic control in gestational diabetes mellitus. Diabetes Care 1988; 11: 761–8.

15 Epidemiology of gestational diabetes mellitus

Avi Ben-Haroush, Yariv Yogev and Moshe Hod

Introduction

Gestational diabetes mellitus (GDM) is defined as carbohydrate intolerance that begins or is first recognized during pregnancy.[1] Although it is a well-known cause of pregnancy complications, its epidemiology has not been studied systematically.[2] One problem is the distinction of GDM, as currently defined, from pre-existing but un-diagnosed diabetes, so that the degree of clinical surveillance may have a major impact on the estimated prevalence of GDM in a given population. This is especially true in high-risk populations in which the onset of Type 2 DM occurs at an early age.[2] Furthermore, investigators use different screening programs and diagnostic criteria for GDM, making comparisons among studies difficult.

In this chapter the reported risk factors for GDM, differences in its racial distribution and evidence of a genetic or familial association will be discussed. The close relationship of GDM to polycystic ovary syndrome (PCOS), the question of the possibly greater risk of fetal malformations in GDM pregnancies and the effect of an abnormal glucose challenge screening test (GCT), by itself or together with an impaired glucose tolerance (IGT), on obstetric outcome will also be considered. The risk of hypertensive disorders in diabetic pregnancy and of future Type 2 DM will also be described.

Racial distribution of gestational diabetes mellitus

The prevalence of GDM varies in direct proportion to the prevalence of Type 2 DM in a given population or ethnic group.[1] The reported prevalence of GDM in the United States (US) ranges from 1 to 14%, with 2–5% being the most common rate.[3] In a study of the prevalence of diabetes and IGT in diverse populations in women between the ages of 20 and 39, the World Health Organization (WHO) Ad Hoc Diabetes Reporting Group[4] noted lower rates of diabetes (<1%) in Bantu (Tanzania), Chinese, rural Indian, Sri Lankan and some Pacific populations followed (1–3%) by Italian women, and white, black and Hispanic women in the US. Rural Fijian Indian and Aboriginal Australian women had a 7% prevalence; the highest rate was found in Pima/Papago and Nauruan Indians (14–22%). The prevalence of IGT was low (< 3%) in Chinese and Malays, and was >10% in black and Hispanic women in the US, urban Indian women in Tanzania, Pima and Nauruan Indians, and some other Pacific communities. The combined age-standardized prevalence of diabetes and IGT ranged from 0 to 36%, with >10% prevalence in one third of the populations, and >30% prevalence in Pima and Nauruan Indians. Importantly, in some populations more than half of the cases of diabetes were undiagnosed prior to the survey. IGT was mostly overlooked in routine clinical practice. Thus, a substantial proportion of abnormal glucose tolerance in pregnancy will be undetected without screening.

King[2] summarized the work of several research groups who had collected data on the prevalence of diabetes in pregnancy (Table 15.1). Their findings, together with the WHO study, show that for a given population and ethnicity, the risk of diabetes in pregnancy reflects the underlying frequency of Type 2 DM.

It remains unclear, however, if this marked racial and geographic variation represents true differences in the prevalence of GDM, because of the remarkably variable approaches used across different studies, including different methods of screening, different oral and intravenous glucose loads, and different diagnostic criteria. For example, Dooley et al.[5] demonstrated that race as well as maternal age and degree of obesity must be taken into account in comparing the prevalence of GDM in different populations. Their study included 3744 consecutive pregnant women who underwent universal screening. The population was 39.1% white, 37.7% black, 19.8% Hispanic and 3.4% Oriental/other. Black and Hispanic race, maternal age and percentage ideal body weight had a significant independent effect on the prevalence of GDM. The adjusted relative risk (RR) was higher in black [1.81, 95% confidence interval (CI) 1.13–2.89] and Hispanic (2.45, 95% CI 1.48–4.04) women than in white women. The degree of carbohydrate intolerance was similar across racial groups; nevertheless, when the 92 GDM patients under dietary control were analyzed separately, mean birthweight was found to be highest in the Hispanic women, and was lowest in the blacks and Orientals. Hence, race had a significant independent effect on birthweight, with maternal percentage ideal body weight a significant covariate. These findings are supported by a recent study showing that Asian woman were more likely to have GDM than Caucasian woman (31.7 vs. 14%, $P = 0.02$), despite their lower body mass index (BMI).[6]

Table 15.1 Prevalence of gestational diabetes mellitus as a percentage of all pregnancies

Population	Prevalence (%)
United States	
All ethnicities	4.0
Zuni Indian	14.3
California, US	
Chinese	7.3
Hispanic	4.2
African	1.7
Non-Hispanic white	1.6
Mexico	6.0
Melbourne, Australia	
Australian-born	4.3
Vietnam-born	7.8
Indian-born	15.0
African-born	9.4
Mediterranean-born	7.3
Arabian	7.2
Chinese	13.9
Northern European	5.2
Northern American	4.0
Illawarar, Australia	
All ethnicities	7.2
Asian	11.9
London, UK	
Caucasion	1.2
African	2.7
Asian	5.8
Scandiano, Italy	2.3
Israel	
Jewish	5.7
Bedouin	2.4
Karachi, Pakistan	3.5
South India	0.6
Pietermaritzburg, South Africa	
Predominantly Indian	3.8
Taipei, Taiwan	
Chinese	0.6
Hyogo, Japan	3.1

(From King,[2] with permission.)

Recently, Silva et al.[7] reported on ethnic differences in perinatal outcome of GDM. Neonates born to Native-Hawaiian/Pacific-Islander mothers and Filipino mothers had four and two times the prevalence of macrosomia, respectively, compared with neonates born to Japanese, Chinese, and Caucasian mothers. These differences persisted after adjustment for other statistically significant maternal and fetal characteristics. Ethnic differences were not observed for other neonatal or maternal complications associated with GDM, with the exception of neonatal hypoglycemia and hyperbilirubinemia. the authors concluded that this finding emphasizes the need to better understand ethnic-specific factors in GDM management and the importance of developing ethnic-tailored GDM interventions to address these disparities.

Risk factors for gestational diabetes mellitus

The traditional and most often reported risk factors for GDM are high maternal age, weight and parity, previous delivery of a macrosomic infant and a family history of diabetes. These and other reported risk factors are summarized in Table 15.2. It is of great importance that the clinician understand and use these characteristics, along with others, such as the racial and geographic attributed risk (discussed above), to improve screening programs and diagnostic accuracy, and perhaps to design better and more cost-effective selective screening and diagnostic tests.

Jang et al.[8] examined 3581 consecutive Korean women and found a 2.2% prevalence of GDM. The affected women were older, had higher prepregnancy weights, higher BMI, higher parities and higher frequencies of known diabetes in the family. The risk of diabetes was closely associated with previous obstetric outcome, such as congenital malformation, stillbirth, and macrosomia. The number of risk factors present in each individual increased the risk of diabetes, with the prevalence ranging from 0.6% in subjects without any risk factors to 33% in those with four or more. Thus, it is possible that selective screening may be cost-effective in situations where health resources are scarce and where total screening is impossible.[2]

Similar results were reported in a retrospective cohort study of 2574 pregnant women, which suggested that selective screening programs have a high true-positive yield.[8] An age of ≥ 30, a family history of diabetes, obesity (BMI ≥ 27) and previous fetal macrosomia were the most frequent risk factors. Just over half (54.2%) of the population presented with one or more risk factors. The positive predictive value (PPV) of screening increased with the number of risk factors, from 12% for the women with no risk factors to 40% for those with three or more risk factors.[9]

In another study, Jang et al.[10] demonstrated that in the racially homogeneous population of Seoul, Korea, besides pre-pregnancy BMI, age, weight gain and parental history of diabetes, short stature is an independent risk factor for GDM. Accordingly, Kousta et al.[11] reported that European and South Asian women with previous GDM were shorter than control women from the same ethnic groups, perhaps due to a common pathophysiological mechanism underlying GDM and the determination of final adult height. Others have reported similar results.[12]

In a large retrospective cohort study in Canada, Xiong et al.[13] evaluated 111,563 pregnancies and detected a 2.5% prevalence of GDM. The risk factors identified were age >35 years, obesity, history of prior neonatal death, and a prior Cesarean section. Interestingly, teenage mothers and women who drank alcohol were less likely to have GDM.

The risk factors mentioned above are mainly of maternal origin. However, cumulative knowledge about the long-term implications of exposure to the diabetic intrauterine environment (see Chapter 23) has led to the addition of the mother's fetal history to the risk factor list. Egeland et al.[14] investigated whether the mother's own characteristics at birth could predict her subsequent risk of GDM. Using linked generation

Table 15.2   Summary of reported risk factors for gestational diabetes mellitus

Risk factor	Author (reference)	Study and population	Results
MATERNAL FACTORS **Older age**			
	Jang et al.[7]	Universal screening with a 50-g glucose load at 24–28 weeks gestation of 3581 consecutive Korean women. At 1-h plasma glucose ≥ 130mg/dl, they underwent a 3-h 100-g OGTT. GDM prevalence was 2.2% (80 cases of GDM vs. 3432 normal controls)	Mean age of GDM and normal control groups, 31.7±4.0 and 28.9±3.3 years, respectively ($P < 0.001$)
	Jang et al.[9]	Same as above in 9005 pregnant women. GDM prevalence was 1.9% (173 GDM, 1735 IGT and 6955 normal controls)	Mean age of GDM and IGT groups versus normal controls, 31.1±4.2, 29.4±3.5, and 28.5±3.4 years, respectively ($P < 0.001$)
	Jimenez-Moleon et al.[8]	Retrospective cohort study on 2574 pregnant women	Among GDM patients 41.8% were older than 30 years of age, whereas 26.2% were younger than 25 years of age. The PPV of the screen for a single risk factor was 22.9 (95% CI 16.9–29.8)
	Xiong et al.[12]	Retrospective cohort study on 111,563 deliveries between 1991 and 1997 in 39 hospitals in Canada Average prevalence of GDM was 2.5% (2755 cases of GDM vs. 108,664 normal controls)	Age > 35 years in 22.4 and 10.3% of GDM and normal patients, respectively (adjusted OR = 2.34, 95% CI 2.13–2.58)
	Egeland et al.[13]	Medical Birth Registry of Norway study of all women born between 1967 and 1984 who gave birth between 1988 and 1998 ($n = 141{,}107$), excluding 2393 non-singleton pregnancies	GDM prevalence of 2.5%; age > 35
	Bo et al.[20]	126 pregnant women with GDM, 84 with IGT and 294 with normal glucose tolerance	Prevalence of GDM increased with age, from 1.5 per 1000 deliveries for women aged ≤ 20 to 4.2 for women aged ≥ 30 (OR = 2.8, 95% CI 1.9–4.3)
	Jolly et al.[80]	Retrospective analysis of 385,120 singleton pregnancies	Mean age of GDM, IGT and normoglycemic groups, 33.0±4.8, 33.0±4.9, and 31.8±4.4 years, respectively ($P = 0.02$)
	Lao et al.[81]	Prospective study of 97 GDM patients and 194 matched controls examined at the time of OGTT at 28–31 weeks gestation for serum ferritin, iron and transferrin concentrations. Managing obstetricians blinded to results	Pregnant women aged between 35 and 40 were at increased risk of GDM (OR = 2.63, 99% CI 2.40–2.89)
High parity			
	Jang et al.[7]	As described above	Mean parity of GDM and normal control groups, 0.6±0.9 and 0.4±0.5, respectively ($P < 0.05$)
	Jang et al.[9]	As described above	Parity ≥ 2 in 9.8% of GDM, 4.7% of IGT groups and 2.6% of controls ($P < 0.001$)
	Egeland et al.[13]	As described above	Age-adjusted OR (95% CI) for women with two, three, four or more deliveries compared with one delivery were 1.5 (1.2–1.9), 1.9 (1.4–2.5), and 3.3 (2.1–5.1), respectively
Pre-pregnancy weight			
	Jang et al.[7]	As described above	Mean weight of GDM and normal control groups, 56.4±9.2 and 51.6±6.4 kg, respectively ($P < 0.001$)
	Jang et al.[9]	As described above	Mean weight of GDM and IGT groups versus normal controls, 56.5±9.5, 52.4±7.2 and 51.6±6.4 kg, respectively ($P < 0.001$)
	Jimenez-Moleon et al.[8]	As described above	BMI > 27 in 12.3% of GDM patients. PPV of the screen for a single risk factor was 32.5 (95% CI 22.4–43.9)

Table 15.2   Summary of reported risk factors for gestational diabetes mellitus—(cont'd)

Risk factor Author (reference)	Study and population	Results
Pregnancy weight		
Xiong et al.[12]	As described above	Obesity ≥ 91kg detected in 15.8 and 7.3% of GDM and normal groups, respectively (adjusted OR = 2.40, 95% CI 2.06–2.98)
Pregnancy weight gain		
Jang et al.[9]	As described above	Mean weight gain of GDM, IGT and normal control groups, of 8.4±3.9, 8.3±3.3, and 8.1±8.1kg, respectively (NS)
Body mass index		
Jang et al.[7]	As described above	Only 1.3% of population was obese, but GDM prevalence increased significantly with increasing BMI. BMI ≥ 27 in 8.8% of GDM and 1.1% of control group (P < 0.001)
Jang et al.[9]	As described above	BMI ≥ 27.3 in 9.8% of GDM, 2.4% of IGT and 1.0% of controls (P < 0.001)
Bo et al.[20]	As described above	Mean BMI in GDM, IGT, and normoglycemic group, 25.4±5.3, 26.0±5.5, and 23.6±4.6, respectively (P = 0.002)
Kousta et al.[24]	91 previous GDM and 73 normoglycemic control women, a median (interquartile range) of 20 (11–36) and 29 (17–49) months postpartum, respectively	Women with previous GDM had higher BMI [26.4 (22.8–31.4) 31.4 vs. 23.8 (21.0–27.5), P = 0.002] and waist:hip ratio [0.82 (0.79–0.88) vs. 0.77 (0.73–0.81), P < 0.0001] than controls
Holte et al.[23]	34 women with GDM 3–5 years before the investigation and 36 controls with uncomplicated pregnancies, selected for similar age, parity and date of delivery	GDM patients had higher BMI than controls (25.2 vs. 22.2, P < 0.001)
Short stature		
Jang et al.[7]	As described above	Mean height of GDM and normal control groups, 158.1±4.8 and 159.7±4.2cm, respectively (P < 0.001)
Jang et al.[9]	As described above	≤ 157cm, the OR for GDM was two times greater compared to the ≥ 163cm group, even after controlling for age and BMI
Kousta et al.[10]	346 women with previous GDM and 470 controls with no previous history of GDM	European and South Asian women with previous GDM were shorter than control women from the same ethnic groups (European: 162.9±6.1 vs. 165.3±6.8 cm, P < 0.0001; South Asian: 155.2±5.4 vs. 158.2±6.3 cm, P = 0.003, adjusted for age)
Bo et al.[20]	As described above	GDM, IGT and normoglycemic groups had a mean height of 1.62±0.06, 1.61±0.006, and 1.63±0.07cm, respectively (P = 0.02)
Branchtein et al.[11]	5564 Brazilian women	Height < 150 cm associated with a 60% increase in the odds of GDM, independently of age, obesity, skin color, parity, family history, and previous GDM
Low birthweight		
Egeland et al.[13]	As described above	Birthweight < 2500 a risk factor for GDM with OR = 9.3, (95% CI 4.1–21.1, P < 0.001), as was weight for gestational age (centiles) < 10 with OR = 1.7, (95% CI 1.2–2.5)
α-thalassemia trait		
Lao and Ho[21]	Retrospective case–control study: 163 women with α-thalassemia trait compared to 163 controls matched for maternal age and parity, following each index case	GDM incidence higher in the study group (62.0 vs. 14.7%, P < 0.0001, OR = 11.74, 95% CI 6.37–21.63)
PCOS		
Holte et al.[23]	As described above	Compare with controls, GDM patients showed a higher prevalence of polycystic ovaries [14 of 34 (41%) vs. 1 of 36 (3%)]; greater clinical and biochemical evidence of hyperandrogenism and insulin resistance; and a higher prevalence of pregnancy-induced hypertension (50 vs. 15%; P < 0.05) during the index pregnancy; 15% developed overt diabetes

Continued

Table 15.2   Summary of reported risk factors for gestational diabetes mellitus—(cont'd)

Risk factor	Author (reference)	Study and population	Results
	Anttila et al.[25]	Retrospective comparative ultrasound study of ovaries in 31 women with GDM and 30 healthy controls matched for maternal age and BMI	14 women with GDM (44%) and two controls exhibited PCOS
	Kousta et al.[24]	As described above	Higher prevalence of PCOS in previous GDM group than controls [47 of 91 (52%) vs. 20 of 73 (27%), $P = 0.002$ overall, OR = 2.7, $P = 0.007$ by logistic regression allowing for ethnicity]
	Mikola et al.[26]	Retrospective study of 99 pregnancies in women with PCOS compared with an unselected control population	GDM developed in 20% of PCOS patients and 8.9% of controls ($P < 0.001$). BMI > 25 an important predictor of GDM (adjusted OR = 5.1; 95% CI 3.2–8.3), as is PCOS (adjusted OR = 1.9; 95% CI 1.0–3.5)
	Koivunen et al.[27]	33 women with a history of GDM and 48 controls	Higher prevalence of PCOS in GDM group (39.4% vs. 16.7%, $P = 0.03$); also higher serum cortisol, androgens and a greater area under the glucose curve
High intake of saturated fat			
	Bo et al.[20]	As described above	Only percentages of saturated fat (OR = 2.0, 95% CI 1.2–3.2) and polyunsaturated fat (OR = 0.85, 95%, CI 0.77–0.92) were associated with gestational hyperglycemia, after adjustment for age, gestational age and BMI
FAMILY HISTORY			
Familial history of diabetes			
	Jang et al.[7]	As described above	35% of GDM vs. 15.4% of normal controls ($P < 0.001$)
	Jang et al.[9]	As described above	30.1% of GDM, 17.6% of IGT and 13.2% of normal controls ($P < 0.001$)
	Jimenez- Moleon et al.[8]	As described above	14.8% of GDM patients. PPV of screen for a single risk factor = 25.9 (95% CI 16.8–36.9)
	Bo et al.[20]	As described above	41% of GDM, 33% of IGT and 28% of normal controls ($P = 0.04$)
	Holte et al.[23]	As described above	First-degree heredity of NIDD more prevalent in previous GDM than control group (24 vs. 6%, $P < 0.05$)
GDM in subject's mother			
	Egeland et al.[13]	As described above	GDM rate 30.6 (per 1000 women) in women whose mother had GDM versus 3.5 in controls (OR = 9.3, 95% CI 4.1–21.1)
PREVIOUS OBSTETRIC OUTCOME			
Congenital malformation			
	Jang et al.[7]	As described above	GDM in 20.7% of patients who had previous malformation versus 2.4% of patients who did not (OR = 22.5, 95% CI 7.15–70.96)
Stillbirth			
	Jang et al.[7]	As described above	GDM in 14.3% of patients who had previous stillbirth versus 2.6% of patients who did not (OR = 8.5, 95% CI 2.35–30.78)
	Xiong et al.[12]	As described above	Previous neonatal death in 1.3% of GDM group versus 0.6% of controls (adjusted OR = 2.09, 95% CI 1.06–1.34)
Macrosomia			
	Jang et al.[7]	As described above	GDM in 9.3% of patients who had previous macrosomia versus 2.5% of patients who did not (OR = 5.8, 95% CI 1.98–17.02)
	Jimenez-Moleon et al.[8]	As described above	OR = 5.8 in patients who had previous macrosomia – 4.9% of GDM patients. The PPV of the screen for a single risk factor was 37.5 (95% CI 21.1–56.3)
Cesarean section			
	Xiong et al.[12]	As described above	Previous CS in 14.8% of GDM group and 10.1% of controls (adjusted OR = 1.55, 95% CI 1.11–1.25)
Previous GDM			
	MacNeill et al.[44]	A retrospective longitudinal study including 651 women	Recurrence of GDM in 35.6% (95% CI 31.9–39.3%). Infant birthweight in the index pregnancy and maternal pre-pregnancy weight were predictive of recurrent GDM

Table 15.2   Summary of reported risk factors for gestational diabetes mellitus—(cont'd)

Risk factor	Author (reference)	Study and population	Results
	Major et al.[45]	78 patients with previous GDM	Recurrence rate 69%; more common with parity ≥1, BMI ≥30, GDM diagnosis at ≤ 24 weeks gestation, insulin requirement, weight gain of ≥ 7 kg (c. 15 pounds) and interval between pregnancies ≤ 24 months
	Spong et al.[46]	164 Hispanic patients with previous GDM	Recurrence rate 68%; more common with earlier diagnosis of GDM, requirement of insulin and hospital admissions in index pregnancy
	Foster-Powel and Cheung[79]	Retrospective review of 540 women	117 women had a subsequent pregnancy with recurrent GDM in 82 (70%). Risk factors were older age, race, BMI, and weight gain
PREGNANCY FACTORS			
High blood pressure in pregnancy			
	Ma and Lo[14]	Retrospective study of 84 pregnant women with normal and abnormal antenatal OGTT results who delivered in a 12-month period	MAP was increased from 28 weeks until delivery in gestational diabetics (n = 50) as compared with controls (n = 34). The OGTT fasting glucose value significantly correlated with MAP at 32 and 36 weeks gestation
Multiple pregnancy			
	Sivan et al.[29]	103 women with consecutive triplet pregnancies, compared to 85 women who elected to undergo fetal reduction to twins	Higher GDM rate in the triplet than the reduction group (22.3 vs. 5.8%)
	Schwartz et al.[30]	Total 29,644 deliveries, 429 twins	GDM increased in twin versus singleton deliveries (7.7 vs. 4.1%, P < 0.05)
	Hoskins[28]	3458 recorded twin live births. Calculated zygosity rate according to sex ratios	Estimated risk for DZ twin pregnancies relative to MZ pregnancies of 8.6 (95% CI 3.5–21.0)
	Wein et al.[31]	61,914 singleton and 798 twin pregnancies	GDM prevalence of 7.4% in twins vs. 5.6% in singletons (P = 0.025)
Increased iron stores			
	Lao et al.[81]	As described above	Log-transformed ferritin concentration was a significant determinant of OGTT 2-h glucose value
PROTECTIVE FACTORS			
Young age			
	Xiong et al.[12]	As described above	Age = 19 years in 2.6 and 8.5% of GDM and normal patients, respectively (adjusted OR = 0.35, 95% CI 0.27–0.44)
Alcohol use			
	Xiong et al.[12]	As described above	Alcohol use in 0.7 and 2.0% of GDM and normal patients, respectively (adjusted OR = 0.40, 95% CI 0.25–0.76)

BMI, Body mass index; CI, confidence interval; CS, Caesarean section; DZ, dizygotic; GDM, gestational diabetes mellitus; IGT, impaired glucose tolerance; MAP, mean arterial pressure; MZ, monozygotic; NIDDM, noninsulin-dependent diabetes mellitus; NS, non-significant; OGTT, oral glucose tolerance test; OR, odds ratio; PPV, positive predictive value.

data from the Medical Birth Registry of Norway for all women born between 1967 and 1984, who gave birth between 1988 and 1998, the authors identified 498 women aged < 32 years with GDM in one or more singleton pregnancies. They found that the women whose mothers had had diabetes during pregnancy were at increased risk of GDM themselves. Significant inverse trends in diabetes were noted in relation to birthweight, with an increased risk of GDM of 80, 60 and 40% in women whose birthweights were ≤ 2500, 2500–2999 and 3000–3499 g, respectively, compared with women in the 4000–4500 g group. Similar findings were observed for categories of weight for gestational age.

Is GDM a cause or an effect? A retrospective study from Hong Kong[15] in 84 normotensive women showed that progressive glucose intolerance throughout pregnancy is associated with an upward shift in blood pressure in the third trimester. Hence, it is possible that blood pressure changes below the diagnostic threshold for hypertensive disorders of pregnancy may help to identify women at increased risk of GDM.

The relationship between dietary fat and glucose metabolism has been recognized for many years. Epidemiological data in humans suggest that subjects with a higher fat intake are more prone to disturbances in glucose metabolism.[16] Several researchers have hypothesized that polyunsaturated fatty acid plays an essential role in the maintenance of energy balance and, through regulation of gene transcription, may improve insulin resistance.[17–19] A recent small study reported significantly lower cord vein erythrocyte phospholipid fatty acid concentrations in 13 women with GDM compared to 12 women with normal pregnancies.[20] Accordingly, Bo et al.[21] investigated the relationship between lifestyle habits and glucose abnormalities in 504 Caucasian women with and without conventional risk factors for GDM. They identified 126 women with GDM and 84 with IGT. These patients were older and shorter than the women with normal pregnancies, and had significantly higher prepregnancy BMI, higher rates of diabetes in first-degree relatives and higher intakes of saturated fat. In a multiple logistic regression model, all of these factors were associated with glucose abnormalities, after adjustment for gestational age. In the patients without conventional risk factors, only the percentages of saturated fats [odds ratio (OR) = 2.0, 95% CI 1.2–3.2) and polyunsaturated fats (OR = 0.85, 95% CI 0.77–0.92) were associated with gestational hyperglycemia, after adjustment for age, gestational age and BMI. Thus, the allegedly independent role of saturated fat in the development of gestational glucose abnormalities takes on greater importance in the absence of conventional risk factors. This suggests that glucose abnormalities could be prevented in some groups of women during pregnancy.

A possible expression of the still unknown genetic linkage in GDM was reported by Lao and Ho,[22] who detected GDM in 62% of 163 women with the α-thalassemia trait compared to 14.7% out of 163 controls matched for maternal age and parity.

Polycystic ovary syndrome and gestational diabetes mellitus

PCOS is a heterogeneous disorder affecting 5–10% of women of reproductive age. It is characterized by chronic anovulation with oligo-/amenorrhea, infertility, typical sonographic appearance of the ovaries, and clinical or biochemical hyperandrogenism. Insulin resistance is present in 40–50% of patients, especially in obese women.[23]

Holte et al.[24] reported a higher rate of ultrasonographic, clinical, and endocrine signs of PCOS in 34 women who had had GDM 3–5 years before, compared to 36 matched controls with uncomplicated pregnancies. Five of the women (15%) with previous GDM had developed manifest diabetes. The authors concluded that women with previous GDM and PCOS may form a distinct subgroup from women with normal ovaries and previous GDM, who may be more prone to develop features of insulin-resistance syndrome.

Many other researchers reported similar results. Kousta et al.[25] found a higher prevalence of PCOS in 91 women with previous GDM compared to 73 normoglycemic control women (52 vs. 27%, P = 0.002), and Anttila et al.[26] reported a 44% prevalence of PCOS in women with GDM, with no differences in BMI before pregnancy or in weight gain during pregnancy compared to controls. They suggested a screening program for GDM for these patients.

Mikola et al.[27] retrospectively evaluated 99 pregnancies in women with PCOS compared with an unselected control population. The average BMI and the nulliparity rate were higher in the PCOS group, as was the multiple pregnancy rate (9.1 vs. 1.1%). GDM developed in 20% of the patients with PCOS but only in 8.9% of the controls (P < 0.001). A BMI > 25 was the best predictor of GDM (adjusted OR = 5.1, 95% CI 3.2–8.3), and PCOS was an additional independent predictor (adjusted OR = 1.9, 95% CI 1.0–3.5).

Koivunen et al.[28] found that compared with 48 control women, 33 women with previous GDM more often had significantly abnormal oral glucose tolerance tests (OGTT), higher prevalences of polycystic ovaries (39.4 vs. 16.7%, P = 0.03), higher serum concentrations of cortisol, dehydroepiandrosterone and dehydroepiandrosterone sulfate, and a greater area under the glucose curve.

Multiple pregnancy and gestational diabetes mellitus

The number of fetuses in multifetal pregnancies is expected to influence the incidence of GDM owing to the increased placental mass and, thereby, the increase in diabetogenic hormones. However, the reports are somewhat conflicting, probably because of the heterogeneous populations studied.

In an interesting study of the prevalence of GDM in dizygotic (DZ) twin pregnancies with two placentae compared to monozygotic (MZ) twin pregnancies with one placenta, Hoskins[29] evaluated 3458 recorded twin deliveries and found that a higher proportion of different-sex compared with same-sex twin pregnancies were complicated by GDM (3.5 vs. 1.6%). The estimated risk for DZ twin pregnancies relative to MZ pregnancies was 8.6 (95% CI 3.5–21.0). The impact of fetal reduction on the incidence of GDM may support this theory. Sivan et al.[30] examined 188 consecutive triplet pregnancies of which 85 were reduced to twins. The rate of GDM was significantly higher in the triplet group than in the reduction group (22.3 vs. 5.8%).

Similar results were reported by Schwartz et al.[31] in a study of 29,644 deliveries. They found that GDM was significantly more frequent in the 429 twin deliveries (7.7 vs. 4.1%, P < 0.05). However, insulin requirements were not different, suggesting a minor clinical impact. Wein et al.[32] compared the prevalence of GDM between 61,914 singleton and 798 twin deliveries performed between 1971 and 1991. The difference was significant only for the earlier decade (5.6 vs. 7.4%, P = 0.025). However, in a follow-up program there was a trend toward a higher prevalence of overt diabetes in the women who had had a diabetic twin pregnancy (18.5%) compared to those who had had a diabetic singleton pregnancy (7.4%). Whether this represents a true increased risk for diabetes is unknown.

By contrast, using data derived from the Medical Birth Registry of Norway, Egeland and Irgens,[33] controlling for other risk factors such as advanced age, parity, maternal history of diabetes and the woman's own birthweight, found GDM in 6.6 per 1000 multiple pregnancies (n = 9271) and in 5.0 per 1000 singleton pregnancies (n = 640,700) (OR = 1.3, 95% CI 1.0–1.7, P = 0.03). However, analyses stratified by maternal age or parity yielded no elevated risk of GDM. Others have also failed to demonstrate a higher prevalence of GDM in multiple pregnancies.[34,35]

Genetic factors

Animal studies have shown that female fetuses exposed to a diabetic intrauterine milieu have an increased risk of subsequent GDM. In a family history study, Harder et al.[36] reported a significantly greater prevalence of diabetes (mainly Type 2 DM) in the mothers of women with GDM than in their fathers. A significant aggregation of Type 2 DM was also observed in the maternal–grandmaternal line compared to the paternal–grandpaternal line. However, in patients with IDDM there was no significant difference in the prevalence of any type of diabetes between mothers and fathers. Therefore, a history of Type 2 DM on the mother's side might be considered as a particular risk factor for GDM via 'intergenerative transmission' of Type 2 DM, which might be prevented by strict avoidance of GDM.

Dorner et al.[37] reported a significantly decreased familial diabetes aggregation on the maternal side in children with Type 1 DM born between 1974 and 1984 compared to those born between 1960 and 1973. This finding was explained by the improved prevention of hyperglycemia during pregnancy since 1974, and particularly of GDM in women with familial diabetes aggregation. These authors also noted a highly significant predominance of Type 2 DM in the great-grandmothers of individuals with infantile-onset diabetes compared to the paternal side. They suggested that GDM, which may represent a risk factor for diabetes transmission on the maternal side, is often followed by 'extra-gestational' Type 2 DM at a later age. Like Harder et al.,[36] these authors suggested that their findings were consistent with the suspected teratogenetic effect of GDM on diabetes susceptibility in the offspring, and that this was preventable by avoiding hyperglycemia in pregnant women and hyperinsulinism in fetuses.

Histocompatibility leukocytic antigen (HLA) studies are one way to establish a genetic linkage in certain diseases. In GDM, conflicting results have been reported. Kuhl[38] described similar frequencies of HLA DR2, DR3 and DR4 antigens in healthy pregnant women and women with GDM, and low prevalences of markers of autoimmune destruction of the beta cells in GDM pregnancies. Likewise, Vambergue et al.,[39] in a study of 95 women with GDM, 95 with IGT and 95 control pregnant women, found no significant difference in the distribution of HLA class II polymorphism among the groups. However, the GDM and IGT groups presented some particular HLA patterns, pointing to a genetic heterogeneity of glucose intolerance during pregnancy.

Lapolla et al.[40] evaluated 68 women with GDM and matched controls for the frequency of HLA A, B, C and DR antigens; the only significant differences were an increase in Cw7 and a decrease in A10 in the GDM group. Budowle et al.[41] reported that the Bf-F allele was found significantly less frequently in non-obese black women with GDM compared to controls, and suggested similar genetic associations in non-obese black women with GDM and with IDDM. Similarly, in another study, women with GDM who required insulin for glycemic control had a lower frequency of the Bf-F phenotype and a higher frequency of the Bf-f1 phenotype; they also had a lower frequency of the type 2 allele at the polymorphic locus adjacent to the insulin gene.[42]

Freinkel et al.[43] evaluated 199 women with GDM and 148 patients with normal pregnancies, and found that the HLA DR3 and DR4 antigens occurred significantly more often in black women with GDM. Ferber et al.,[44] in an analysis of 184 women with GDM, did not find an elevation in the frequency of any HLA class II alleles in GDM patients compared with nondiabetic unrelated subjects. However, the DR3 allele was noted significantly more frequently in 43 women with islet autoantibodies and in the 24 women who developed Type 1 DM postpartum. The cumulative risk of developing IDDM within 2 years after pregnancy in the GDM women with DR3 or DR4 was 22%, and in the women without these alleles was 7% ($P = 0.02$). The risk rose to 50% in the DR3- and DR4-positive women who had required insulin during pregnancy ($P = 0.006$). These results indicate that women with GDM who have islet autoantibodies at delivery or develop Type 1 DM postpartum have HLA alleles typical of late-onset Type 1 diabetes, and that both HLA typing and islet antibodies can predict the development of Type 1 DM postpartum.

Recurrence of gestational diabetes mellitus

MacNeill et al.[45] conducted a retrospective longitudinal study of 651 women who had had a diabetic pregnancy and at least one other thereafter. They found a 35.6% recurrence rate of GDM. Multivariate regression models showed that infant birthweight in the index pregnancy and maternal weight before the subsequent pregnancy were predictive of recurrent GDM.

Higher recurrence rates (69% of 78 patients) were reported by Major et al.[46] Recurrence was more common when the following variables were present in the index pregnancy: parity ≥ 1 (OR = 3.0), BMI ≥ 30 (OR = 3.6), GDM diagnosis ≤ 24 weeks gestation (OR = 20.4) and insulin requirement (OR = 2.3). A weight gain of = 7 kg (c. 15 pounds) (OR = 2.9) and an interval between pregnancies of ≤ 24 months (OR = 1.6) were also associated with a recurrence of GDM. Spong et al.[47] found a similarly high recurrence rate of 68% in 164 women with GDM. Risk factors for recurrence in this study were earlier diagnosis of GDM, insulin requirement and hospital admissions in the index pregnancy. Nohira et al.[48] evaluated the recurrence rate and risk factors of recurrent GDM. In 32 patients with GDM and 37 with one abnormal OGTT value (OAV) in their index pregnancies. The recurrence rate from index GDM and OAV were 65.6 and 40.5%. Age, BMI before pregnancy, an increased weight gain between pregnancies and a short interval between pregnancies were risk factors for recurrence from the initial GDM. An increased weight gain between pregnancies and a short interval between pregnancies were risk factors of development to GDM from the initial OAV. They concluded that the control of weight gain and interval between pregnancies could be important to reduce GDM recurrence.

Impaired glucose tolerance as a risk factor of adverse outcome

The cut-off level of glycemia beyond which the risk of an adverse outcome of pregnancy is increased is of major clinical importance in the management and initiation of therapy.

Nasrat et al.[49] examined pregnancy outcome in 212 women with IGT and 212 women with normal glucose tolerance. They found a higher mean age and higher parity in the IGT group. The babies in this group also had higher birthweights, lower levels of capillary blood glucose and higher hematocrit. Nevertheless, the proportion of babies with birthweights ≥ 2 standard deviations (SD) above the mean, neonatal capillary blood glucose < 28 mg/dL and hematocrit ≥ 65% was equal in the two groups. Therefore, the authors concluded that IGT does not lead to any adverse outcome. Similar findings were reported by Ramtoola et al.,[50] who failed to find an excess perinatal mortality in 267 pregnant women with IGT compared with a background population. The mean birthweight was significantly higher in the babies born to women with GDM and gestational IGT than in the background population, but not in the babies of women with pregestational diabetes. The incidence of macrosomia was highest in the GDM group and it was also significantly increased in the pregestational diabetes group, but not in the IGT group, even though the latter had the highest gestational age at delivery. Both hypoglycemia and hyperbilirubinemia were significantly more common in the infants of women with pregestational and gestational diabetes than in the infants of women with gestational IGT.

By contrast, Moses and Calvert[51] suggested that the clinically optimal level for glycemia during pregnancy should be as near to normal as possible. They studied the proportion of assisted deliveries and the proportion of infants admitted to special care in relation to the range of glucose tolerance, and found an association between glycemia and both outcomes. For assisted deliveries, risk increased only in the higher range (126–142 mg/dL), but for admission to special care there was a linear trend.

Conflicting results were also reported by others. Al-Shawaf et al.[52] found that women with gestational IGT were older and more obese, had higher parities and had heavier babies than pregnant women with normal screening plasma glucose. Roberts et al.[53] found no significant difference in the incidence of antenatal complications between mothers with normal glucose tolerance and IGT ($n = 135$ each). Although the IGT group had higher rate of induced labor and Cesarean section, there was no between-group difference in fetal outcome or neonatal morbidity. Tan and Yeo,[54] in a retrospective analysis of 944 women with IGT in pregnancy (8.6%) with 10,065 women with normal pregnancies, noted that even when maternal age and obesity were excluded, the IGT group had a significantly higher risk of labor induction (RR = 1.15); Cesarean section (RR: overall = 1.43, elective = 1.72, emergency = 1.31); Cesarean section for dystocia/no progress (RR = 1.60), macrosomia (RR = 1.69, 1.76 and 1.61 for birthweights = 97th, 95th and 90th percentiles, respectively) and shoulder dystocia (RR = 2.84). The risk of hypertensive disease (RR = 1.22) and Cesarean section for fetal distress/thick meconium-stained amniotic fluid (RR = 1.53) were also higher in the IGT group, but the differences were not statistically significant when maternal age and obesity were excluded. There was no significant difference in the rates of low Apgar scores at 1 and 5 min between the two groups.

It is possible that some of the adverse outcomes associated with excess maternal weight were in fact related to GDM. It is also possible that some of the complications attributed to GDM,

especially the milder form of IGT, were actually related to excess maternal weight. Jacobson and Cousins[55] reported that good glycemic control did not normalize birthweight percentiles and that maternal weight at delivery was the only significant predictor of birthweight percentile. Thus, IGT diagnosed for the first time in pregnancy might only be a feature of excess maternal weight but not in itself a pathological condition. The clinical significance of IGT has also been disputed.[48,56] Lao and Ho,[57] in a retrospective case–control study, examined the impacts of IGT on the outcome of singleton pregnancies in 128 Chinese women with a high BMI (> 26) and IGT, compared with 128 women with matched high BMI and normal OGTT results. The IGT group was older, with more previous pregnancies, higher incidences of previous GDM, and higher hemoglobin and fasting glucose concentrations. There were no differences in the prepregnancy weight, gestational weight gain or weight or BMI at delivery, and no difference in obstetric complications, mode of delivery, or gestational age or mean infant birthweight. However, the birthweight ratio (relative to mean birthweight for gestation), incidence of large-for-gestational-age (LGA) infants (birthweight > 90th percentile) and macrosomic infants (birthweight ≥ 4000 g), and events of treated neonatal jaundice were all significantly higher in the IGT group. Thus, some of the complications attributed to GDM are probably related to maternal obesity, but IGT could still affect infant birthweight despite dietary treatment that normalizes maternal gestational weight gain.

In another recent study of 2904 pregnant women the following outcomes measures increased significantly with increasing glucose values on the OGTT: shoulder dystocia, macrosomia, emergency Cesarean section, assisted delivery, hypertension, and induction of labor.[58] However, when corrections were made for other risk factors, hypertension and induction of labor were only marginally associated with glucose levels.

Aberg et al.[59] conducted a population-based study of maternal and neonatal characteristics and delivery complications in relation to findings for the 75-g, 2-h OGTT at 25–30 weeks gestation. The OGTT value was < 140 mg/dL in 4526 women, 140–162 mg/dL in 131 women and ≥ 162 mg/dL in 116 women with GDM. An additional 28 cases of GDM were identified, giving a prevalence of 1.2%. An increased rate of Cesarean section and infant macrosomia was observed in the group with a glucose tolerance of 140–162 mg/dL and in the GDM group. Advanced maternal age and a high BMI were found to be risk factors for increased OGTT values.

Abnormal glucose tolerance test as a risk factor for adverse pregnancy outcome

Is an abnormal GCT alone, without GDM, a risk factor for adverse pregnancy outcome? Using fetal weight and anthropometric characteristics as their parameters, Mello et al.[60] evaluated 1615 white women with singleton pregnancies who underwent universal screening for GDM in two periods of pregnancy. They divided the population into three groups according to the GCT results: (1) 172 patients with abnormal

GCT in both periods; (2) 391 patients with a normal GCT in the early period and an abnormal GCT in the late period; and (3) 1052 patients with a normal GCT in both periods (control group). The incidence of LGA infants was significantly higher in group 1 (40.7%) and group 2 (22.0%) than in the control group (8.3%), and significantly higher in group 1 than in group 2. The newborns of group 1 had higher birthweights than those of group 2 and the control group, and the newborns of the control group had significantly greater lengths and mean cranial circumferences. Group 1 babies had significantly lower ponderal indexes, thoracic circumferences and weight:length ratios than controls, and significantly larger cranial/thoracic circumferences.

Weijers et al.[61] defined mild gestational hyperglycemia (MGH) as a positive GCT in the presence of a negative OGTT. Of the 1022 consecutive women evaluated, 813 (79.6%) were healthy, 138 (13.5%) had MGH and 71 (6.9%) had GDM. There was a stepwise significant increase in mean fasting glucose and C-peptide levels among the three diagnostic groups. Maternal age, non-Caucasian ethnicity and pre-pregnancy BMI were all associated with GDM, whereas only maternal age and pre-pregnancy BMI were associated with MGH. Therefore, it appears that additional factors promoting the loss of beta-cell function distinguish MGH from GDM. One of these factors is ethnicity.

To determine the predictive value of a negative GCT in subsequent pregnancies, Nahum[62] studied 62 pregnancies of women who had given birth during the past 4 years for whom third-trimester 1-h, 50-g glucose screening test results were available for both pregnancies. He found that the GCT results were significantly correlated between the two pregnancies ($r = 0.49$, $P < 0.001$) and concluded that a negative GCT of < 140 mg/dL during pregnancy is strongly predictive of a negative screening result in a succeeding pregnancy within 4 years.

Are women with one elevated 3-h glucose tolerance test value at risk for adverse perinatal outcomes? In a recent retrospective cohort study[63] perinatal outcomes in women with one elevated glucose tolerance test value were compared with the outcomes in women who screened negative by GCT. Of 14,036 women who met the study criteria, women with one elevated glucose tolerance test value exhibited higher rates of Cesarean delivery (in nulliparous women only), pre-eclampsia, chorioamnionitis, birthweight > 4000 g and > 4500 g, and neonatal admission to the intensive care nursery as compared with women who screened negative ($P < 0.05$ for all).

Early gestational diabetes mellitus diagnosis as a risk factor

Early onset of GDM is a high-risk factor. Bartha et al.[64] found that among 3986 pregnant women, those with early-onset GDM ($n = 65$) were more likely to be hypertensive (18.46 vs. 5.88%, $P = 0.006$), have higher glycemic values and greater needs for insulin therapy (33.85 vs. 7.06%, $P < 0.001$) than those in whom diabetes developed later ($n = 170$). All cases of neonatal hypoglycemia ($n = 4$) and all perinatal deaths ($n = 3$) were in this group. The women with early GDM also had an increased risk of postpartum diabetes mellitus, whereas those

with late-onset GDM had a minimal risk.[65] The percentages of overt diabetes and abnormal glucose tolerance were significantly higher in the early pregnancy group ($n = 30$) than in the late-pregnancy group ($n = 72$) (26.7 vs. 1.4 and 40 vs. 5.56%, respectively).

Congenital malformations

Schaefer-Graf et al.,[66] in a review of 4180 pregnancies complicated by GDM ($n = 3764$) or Type 2 DM ($n = 416$), reported that the congenital anomalies in the offspring affected the same organ systems described in pregnancies complicated by Type 1 DM. The risk of anomalies rose with increasing hyperglycemia at diagnosis or presentation for care. However, most other reports had conflicting findings. Bartha et al.[64] failed to find an increase in major congenital malformations associated with GDM, as did Kalter[67] in a comprehensive review of the literature. An exception is the recent Swedish Health Registry study covering over 1.2 million births between 1987 and 1997.[68] The authors identified 3864 infants born to women with pre-existing diabetes and 8688 infants born to women with GDM. The total malformation rate in the first group was 9.5% and in the second group 5.7%, similar to the rate in the general population. However, the GDM group was characterized by an excess of certain malformations, suggesting that a subgroup of GDM are at increased risk of diabetic embryopathy, perhaps due to pre-existing but undetected Type 2 DM.

Martinez-Frias et al.[69] analyzed 19,577 consecutive infants with malformations of unknown cause and compared those born to mothers with GDM with those of nondiabetic mothers. Their findings indicated that GDM is a significant risk factor for holoprosencephaly, upper/lower spine/rib anomalies, and renal and urinary system anomalies. However, owing to the heterogeneous nature of GDM, which includes previously unrecognized and newly diagnosed Type 2 DM, they could not rule out the possibility that the teratogenic effect is related to latent Type 2 DM. Nevertheless, they concluded that pregnancies complicated by GDM should be considered at risk for congenital anomalies.

Recently, Virtanen et al.[70] evaluated the prevalence of maternal glucose metabolism disorders during pregnancy in newborn boys having normal testicular descent or congenital cryptorchidism. After adjustment for possible confounding factors, abnormal maternal glucose metabolism was significantly more common in the group of cryptorchid boys [diet-treated gestational diabetes, $P = 0.0001$; odds ratio, 3.98 (95% CI, 1.97–8.05); diet-treated gestational diabetes or only an abnormal result in oral glucose tolerance test, $P = 0.0016$; odds ratio, 2.44 (95% CI, 1.40–4.25)] when compared with boys with normal testicular descent.

By contrast, the relationship between GDM and the development of congenital malformations was examined in another population-based retrospective study using birth certificate data for all live-born children delivered between 1984 and 1991 in Washington State.[71] The prevalence of congenital malformations was 7.2, 2.8 and 2.1% among the offspring of mothers with established diabetes ($n = 8869$), GDM ($n = 1511$) and no diabetes ($n = 8934$), respectively.

That is, the rate of congenital malformations in the GDM group was only slightly higher than in the control group (OR = 1.3, 95% CI 1.0–1.6).

Hypertensive disorders

Pre-eclampsia and gestational hypertension are apparently more frequent in women with GDM. A large study by Xiong et al.[13] detected pre-eclampsia in 2.7% of 2755 patients with GDM compared with only 1.1% of 108,664 patients with normal pregnancies (adjusted OR = 1.3, 95% CI 1.20–1.41). Similar results were observed for gestational hypertension. Likewise, Dukler et al.[72] studied 380 primiparous women with pre-eclampsia and 385 primiparous control women for a total of 1207 and 1293 deliveries, respectively. When adjusted for confounding variables, GDM was strongly associated with the recurrence of pre-eclampsia in the second pregnancy (OR = 3.72, 95% CI 1.45–9.53).

Go et al.,[73] in an 11-year follow-up study of a cross-sectional sample of African–American women with a history of GDM (n = 289), reported one of the highest rates of microalbuminuria (MA) of all ethnic groups. The presence of MA was not associated with insulin resistance, but it was significantly and independently associated with glycosylated hemoglobin (HbAlc) levels and hypertension. Hence, hypertension and glucose intolerance influence MA through different mechanisms, and screening for MA should be considered in this patient population.

Conditions associated with increased insulin resistance, such as GDM, PCOS and obesity, may predispose patients to essential hypertension, hypertensive pregnancy, hyperinsulinemia, hyperlipidemia and high levels of plasminogen activator inhibitor-1, leptin, and tumor necrosis factor-alpha. These findings may also be associated with a possible increased risk of cardiovascular complications in these women.[74] Joffe et al.[75] provided further support for the role of insulin resistance in the pathogenesis of hypertensive disorders of pregnancy. In a prospective study of 4589 healthy nulliparous women, they found that the women with GDM had an increased relative risk of pre-eclampsia and all hypertensive disorders (RR = 1.67, 95% CI 0.92–3.05 and RR = 1.54, 95% CI 1.28–2.11, respectively). RR were not substantially reduced after further adjustment for race and BMI (OR = 1.41 and 1.48, respectively). Furthermore, even within the normal range, multivariate analysis demonstrated that the level of plasma glucose 1 h after a 50-g oral glucose challenge was an important predictor of pre-eclampsia.

Innes et al.[76] evaluated 54 normotensive women who developed hypertension in pregnancy and 51 controls with normotensive pregnancies, matched for parity. Mean post-load glucose levels and the total glucose area under the curve were significantly higher in the cases than in the controls, and were positively correlated with peak mean arterial pressure. After adjustment for potential confounders, 2-h post-load glucose levels remained strongly related to the risk for hypertension and to peak mean arterial blood pressure, as did the total glucose area under the curve. The cases were also more likely to have had one abnormal OGTT. Stratifying analyses by case severity (pre-eclampsia and gestational hypertension) yielded similar results. Among all subjects, more cases than controls were also diagnosed with GDM (31 vs. 12%, P = 0.008).

Risk of Type 2 diabetes

Women with GDM have a 17–63% risk of Type 2 DM within 5–16 years.[77] However, the risk varies according to different parameters. For example, Greenberg et al.,[78] in a study of 94 patients with GDM, reported that the most significant predictor of 6-weeks postpartum diabetes was insulin requirement, with RR = 17.28 (95% CI 2.46–134.42), followed by poor glycemic control, IGT and a GCT = 200 mg/dL. All of these factors probably represent the magnitude of the insulin resistance, which is the hallmark of future diabetes and of other vascular complications. Similarly, Bian et al.[79] reported a diagnosis of diabetes 5–10 years postpartum in 33.3% of patients with previous GDM (n = 45), but only 9.7% (n = 31) of these with IGT and 2.6% (n = 39) of normal controls. Two or more abnormal OGTT values during pregnancy, a blood glucose level exceeding the maximal values at 1 and 2 h after oral glucose loading, and high pregnancy BMI were all useful predictors of diabetes in later life. In a recent study of 227 women,[80] in an average of 5.8 years after the diagnosis of GDM, the majority of women still have chronic insulin resistance. One third has either IGT, IFG or Type 2 DM. Despite the above, only 37% of women with a history of GDM were screened for postpartum DM according to guidelines published by the American Diabetes Association.[81]

To determine if recurrent episodes of insulin resistance (i.e. another pregnancy) contribute to the decline in beta-cell function that leads to Type 2 DM in high-risk individuals, Peters et al.[82] investigated 666 Latino women with a history of GDM. Among the 87 (13%) who completed an additional pregnancy, the rate ratio of Type 2 DM increased to 3.34 (95% CI 1.80–6.19), compared with women without an additional pregnancy, after adjustment for other potential diabetes risk factors during the index pregnancy (antepartum oral glucose tolerance, high fasting glucose, gestational age at diagnosis of GDM) and during follow-up (postpartum BMI, glucose tolerance, weight change, breastfeeding and months of contraceptive use). Weight gain was also independently associated with an increased risk of Type 2 DM; the rate ratio was 1.95 (95% CI 1.63–2.33) for each 4.5 kg gained during follow-up after adjustment for the additional pregnancy and the other potential risk factors. These data show that a single pregnancy, independent of the well-known effect of weight gain, accelerates the development of Type 2 DM in women with a high prevalence of pancreatic beta-cell dysfunction.

What about milder, diet-controlled GDM? Damm[83] reported abnormal glucose tolerance in 34.4% of 241 women 2–11 years after a diabetic pregnancy (3.7% Type 1 DM, 13.7% Type 2 DM, 17% IGT), in contrast to a control group in which none of the women had diabetes and 5.3% had IGT. The independent risk factors for later development of diabetes were high fasting glucose levels at diagnosis of GDM, delivery > 3 weeks before term and abnormal OGTT

2 months postpartum. Low insulin secretion at diagnosis of GDM was also an independent risk factor. Even the non-obese glucose-tolerant women with previous GDM had a metabolic profile of Type 2 DM, i.e. insulin resistance and impaired insulin secretion. Thus, the first OGTT should probably be performed 2 months postpartum to identify the women who are already diabetic and the women at highest risk of later development of overt diabetes.[83] Similarly, Lauenborg et al.[84] reported that the prevalence of the metabolic syndrome was three times as high in women with prior diet-treated GDM, compared with age-matched control subjects. Interestingly, according to a recent study, both women with a history of GDM as well as their children are at greater risk of progressing to Type 2 DM.[85] Whether this effect is due to a genetic or an *in utero* influence has yet to be determined.

Summary

The 1997 WHO estimates of the prevalence of diabetes in adults showed an expected total rise of > 120% from 135 million in 1995 to 300 million in 2025.[2] These numbers also include GDM, and should alert physicians to the need to direct special attention to this population, especially in developing countries.

The data presented in this chapter indicate that the epidemiology of GDM is characterized by several features.

- Differences in screening programs and diagnostic criteria make it difficult to compare frequencies of GDM among various populations. Nevertheless, race has been proven to be an independent risk factor for GDM, which varies in prevalence in direct proportion to the prevalence of Type 2 DM in a given population or ethnic group.
- There are several identifiable predisposing factors for GDM (Table 15.2).
- In the absence of risk factors, the incidence of GDM is low. Therefore, some authors suggest that selective screening may be cost-effective, especially in view the forecasted rise in the burden of GDM.
- PCOS is an important risk factor for GDM, with special similarity in the existence of insulin resistance.
- The genetic diathesis is not well understood.
- The recurrence rate of GDM (35–80%) is influenced by parity, BMI, early diagnosis of GDM, insulin requirement, weight gain and by the interval between pregnancies.
- Pregnant women with IGT and an abnormal GCT may be at increased risk of an adverse outcome relative to woman with a normal glucose tolerance and a normal GCT.
- Women with an early diagnosis of GDM represent a high-risk subgroup, with an increased incidence of obstetric complications, recurrent GDM and development of Type 2 DM.
- Another subgroup of GDM is characterized by an increased risk of a diabetic embryopathy, perhaps due to pre-existing but undetected Type 2 DM. This should be considered in all patients with early diagnosis of GDM, accompanied by appropriate patient counseling.
- Hypertensive disorders in pregnancy and afterwards may be more prevalent in women with GDM. One possible mechanism is insulin resistance.
- Women with GDM are at increased risk of developing Type 2 DM, especially obese patients, those who were diagnosed before 24 weeks gestation and those who required insulin for glycemic control.

REFERENCES

1. American College of Obstetricians and Gynecologists: Gestational Diabetes. Practice Bulletin No. 30, September 2001.
2. King H. Epidemiology of glucose intolerance and gestational diabetes in women of childbearing age. Diabetes Care 1998; 21(suppl. 2): B9–B13.
3. Coustan DR. Gestational diabetes. Diabetes in America. In: National Institutes of Diabetes and Digestive and Kidney Diseases, 2nd edn. NIH Publication No 95-1468. Bethesda: NIDDK; 1995, pp. 703–17.
4. WHO Ad Hoc Diabetes Reporting Group. Diabetes and impaired glucose tolerance in women aged 20–39 years. World Health Stat 1992; 45: 321–7.
5. Dooley SL, Metzger BE, Cho NH. Influence of race on disease prevalence and perinatal outcome in a US population. Diabetes 1991; 40: 25–9.
6. Gunton JE, Hitchman R, McElduff A. Effects of ethnicity on glucose tolerance, insulin resistance and beta cell function in 223 women with an abnormal glucose challenge test during pregnancy. Aust N Z Obstet Gynaecol 2001; 41: 182–6.
7. Silva JK, Kaholokula JK, Ratner R, Mau M. Ethnic differences in perinatal outcome of gestational diabetes mellitus. Diabetes Care. 2006; 29: 2058–63.
8. Jang HC, Cho NH, Jung KB, et al. Screening for gestational diabetes mellitus in Korea. Int J Gynecol Obstet 1995; 51: 115–22.
9. Jimenez-Moleon JJ, Bueno-Cavanillas A, Luna-del-Castillo JD, et al. Predictive value of a screen for gestational diabetes mellitus: influence of associated risk factors. Acta Obstet Gynecol Scand 2000; 79: 991–8.
10. Jang HC, Min HK, Lee HK, Cho NH, Metzger BE. Short stature in Korean women: a contribution to the multifactorial predisposition to gestational diabetes mellitus. Diabetologia 1998; 41: 778–3.
11. Kousta E, Lawrence NJ, Penny A, et al. Women with a history of gestational diabetes of European and South Asian origin are shorter than women with normal glucose tolerance in pregnancy. Diabet Med 2000; 17: 792–7.
12. Branchtein L, Schmidt MI, Matos MC, et al. Short stature and gestational diabetes in Brazil. Brazilian Gestational Diabetes Study Group. Diabetologia 2000; 43: 848–51.
13. Xiong X, Saunders LD, Wang FL, Demianczuk NN. Gestational diabetes mellitus: prevalence, risk factors, maternal and infant outcomes. Int J Gynaecol Obstet 2001; 75: 221–8.
14. Egeland GM, Skjærven R, Irgens LM. Birth characteristics of women who develop gestational diabetes: population based study. Br Med J 2000; 321: 546–7.
15. Ma RM, Lao TT. Maternal mean arterial pressure and oral glucose tolerance test results. Relationship in normotensive women. J Reprod Med 2001; 46: 747–51.
16. Lichtenstein AH, Schwab US. Relationship of diatary fat to glucose metabolism. Atherosclerosis 2000; 150: 227–43.
17. Clarke SD. Polyunsaturated fatty acid regulation of gene transcription: A mechanism to improve energy balance and insulin resistance. Br J Nutr 2000; 83(suppl. 1): s59–s66.
18. Clarke SD. Polyunsaturated fatty acid regulation of gene transcription: A molecular mechanism to improve the metabolic syndrome. J Nutr 2001; 131: 1129–32.
19. Rustan AC, Nenseter MS, Drevon CA. Omega-3 and omega-6 fatty acids in the insulin resistance syndrome. Lipid and lipoprotein metabolism and atherosclerosis. Ann NY Acad Sci 1997; 827: 310–26.
20. Wijendran V, Bendel RB, Couch SC, et al. Fetal erythrocyte phospholipid polyunsaturated fatty acids are altered in pregnancy complicated with gestational diabetes mellitus. Lipids 2000; 35: 927–31.

21. Bo S, Menato G, Lezo A, et al. Dietary fat and gestational hypergly-caemia. Diabetologia 2001; 44: 972–8.
22. Lao TT, Ho LF. Alpha-thalassaemia trait and gestational diabetes mellitus in Hong Kong. Diabetologia 2001; 44: 966–71.
23. Franks S, Gilling-Smith C, Waston H. Insulin action in the normal and polycystic ovary. Metab Clin North Am 1999; 28: 361–78.
24. Holte J, Gennarelli G, Wide L, Lithell H, Berne C. High prevalence of polycystic ovaries and associated clinical, endocrine, and metabolic features in women with previous gestational diabetes mellitus. J Clin Endocrinol Metab 1998; 83: 1143–50.
25. Kousta E, Cela E, Lawrence N, et al. The prevalence of polycystic ovaries in women with a history of gestational diabetes. Clin Endocrinol (Oxf) 2000; 53: 501–7.
26. Anttila L, Karjala K, Penttila RA, Ruutiainen K, Ekblad U. Polycystic ovaries in women with gestational diabetes. Obstet Gynecol 1998; 92: 13–16.
27. Mikola M, Hiilesmaa V, Halttunen M, Suhonen L, Tiitinen A. Obstetric outcome in women with polycystic ovarian syndrome. Hum Reprod 2001; 16: 226–9.
28. Koivunen RM, Juutinen J, Vauhkonen I, et al. Metabolic and ste-roidogenic alterations related to increased frequency of polycystic ovaries in women with a history of gestational diabetes. J Clin Endocrinol Metab 2001; 86: 2591–9.
29. Hoskins RE. Zygosity as a risk factor for complications and outcomes of twin pregnancy. Acta Genet Med Gemellol 1995; 44: 11–23.
30. Sivan E, Maman E, Homko CJ, et al. Impact of fetal reduction on the incidence of gestational diabetes. Obstet Gynecol 2002; 99: 91–4.
31. Schwartz DB, Daoud Y, Zazula P, et al. Gestational diabetes mellitus: metabolic and blood glucose parameters in singleton versus twin pregnancies. Am J Obstet Gynecol 1999; 181: 912–14.
32. Wein P, Warwick MM, Beischer NA. Gestational diabetes in twin pregnancy: prevalence and long-term implications. Aust NZ J Obstet Gynaecol 1992; 32: 325–7.
33. Egeland GM, Irgens LM. Is a multiple birth pregnancy a risk factor for gestational diabetes? Am J Obstet Gynecol 2001; 185: 1275–6.
34. Fitzsimmons BP, Bebbington MW, Fluker MR. Perinatal and neonatal outcomes in multiple gestations: assisted reproduction versus spontaneous conception. Am J Obstet Gynecol 1998; 179: 1162–7.
35. Henderson CE, Scarpelli S, Larosa D, Divon MY. Assessing the risk of gestational diabetes in twin pregnancies. J Natl Med Assoc 1995; 87: 757–8.
36. Harder T, Franke K, Kohlhoff R, Plagemann A. Maternal and paternal family history of diabetes in women with gestational diabetes or insulin-dependent diabetes mellitus type I. Gynecol Obstet Invest 2001; 51: 160–4.
37. Dorner G, Plagemann A, Reinagel H. Familial diabetes aggregation in type 2 diabetics: gestational diabetes an apparent risk factor for increased diabetes susceptibility in the offspring. Exp Clin Endocrinol 1987; 89: 84–90.
38. Kuhl C. Etiology and pathogenesis of gestational diabetes. Diabetes Care 1998; 21(suppl. 2): B19–B26.
39. Vambergue A, Fajardy I, Bianchi F, et al. Gestational diabetes mellitus and HLA class II (-DQ, -DR) association: The Digest Study. Eur J Immunogenet 1997; 24: 385–94.
40. Lapolla A, Betterle C, Sanzari M, et al. An immunological and genetic study of patients with gestational diabetes mellitus. Acta Diabetol 1996; 33: 139–44.
41. Budowle B, Huddleston JF, Go RC, Barger BO, Acton RT. Association of HLA-linked factor B with gestational diabetes mellitus in black women. Am J Obstet Gynecol 1988; 159: 805–6.
42. Bell DS, Barger BO, Go RC, Goldenberg RL, Perkins LL. Risk factors for gestational diabetes in black population. Diabetes 1990; 13: 1196–201.
43. Freinkel N, Metzger BE, Phelps RL, et al. Gestational diabetes mellitus: a syndrome with phenotypic and genotypic heterogeneity. Horm Metab Res 1986; 18: 427–30.
44. Ferber KM, Keller E, Albert ED, Ziegler AG. Predictive value of human leukocyte antigen class II typing for the development of islet autoan-tibodies and insulin-dependent diabetes postpartum in women with gestational diabetes. J Clin Endocrinol Metab 1999; 84: 2342–8.
45. MacNeill S, Dodds L, Hamilton DC, Armson BA, Vanden Hof M. Rates and risk factors for recurrence of gestational diabetes. Diabetes Care 2001; 24: 659–62.
46. Major CA, deVeciana M, Weeks J, Morgan MA. Recurrence of gestational diabetes: Who is at risk? Am J Obstet Gynecol 1998; 179: 1038–42.
47. Spong CY, Guillermo L, Kuboshige J, Cabalum T. Recurrence of gestational diabetes mellitus: identification of risk factors. Am J Perinatol 1998; 15: 29–33.
48. Nohira T, Kim S, Nakai H, et al. Recurrence of gestational diabetes mellitus: rates and risk factors from initial GDM and one abnormal GTT value. Diabetes Res Clin Pract 2006; 71: 75–81.
49. Nasrat AA, Augnesen K, Abushal M, Shalhoub JT. The outcome of pregnancy following untreated impaired glucose intolerance. Int J Gynecol Obstet 1994; 47: 1–6.
50. Ramtoola S, Home P, Damry H, Husnoo A, Ah-Kion S. Gestational impaired glucose tolerance does not increase perinatal mortality in a developing country: cohort study. Br Med J 2001; 28: 1025–6.
51. Moses RG, Calvert D. Pregnancy outcomes in women without gestational diabetes mellitus related to the maternal glucose level. Diabetes Care 1995; 18: 1527–33.
52. Al-Shawaf T, Moghraby S, Akiel A. Does impaired glucose tolerance imply a risk in pregnancy? Br J Obstet Gynaecol 1998; 95: 1036–41.
53. Roberts RN, Moohan JM, Foo RL, et al. Fetal outcome in mothers with impaired glucose tolerance in pregnancy. Diabet Med 1993; 10: 438–43.
54. Tan YY, Yeo GS. Impaired glucose tolerance in pregnancy – is it of consequence? Aust NZ J Obstet Gynaecol 1996; 36: 248–55.
55. Jacobson JD, Cousins L. A population-based study of maternal and perinatal outcome in patients with gestational diabetes. Am J Obstet Gynecol 1989; 161: 981–6.
56. Li DFH, Wong VCW, O'Hoy KMKY. Is treatment needed for mild impairment of glucose tolerance in pregnancy? A randomized controlled trial. Br J Obstet Gynaecol 1987; 94: 851–4.
57. Lao TT, Ho LF. Impaired glucose tolerance and pregnancy outcome in Chinese women with high body mass index. Hum Reprod 2000; 8: 1826–9.
58. Jensen DM, Damm P, Sorensen B, et al. Clinical impact of mild carbohydrate intolerance in pregnancy: a study of 2904 nondiabetic Danish women with risk factors for gestational diabetes mellitus. Am J Obstet Gynecol 2001; 185: 413–9.
59. Aberg A, Rydhstroem H, Frid A. Impaired glucose tolerance associ-ated with adverse pregnancy outcome: a population-based study in southern Sweden. Am J Obstet Gynecol 2001; 184: 77–83.
60. Mello G, Parretti E, Mecacci F, et al. Anthropometric characteristics of full-term infants: effects of varying degrees of 'normal' glucose metabolism. J Perinat Med 1997; 25: 197–204.
61. Weijers RN, Bekedam DJ, Smulders YM. Determinants of mild gestational hyperglycemia and gestational diabetes mellitus in a large Dutch multiethnic cohort. Diabetes Care 2002; 25: 72–7.
62. Nahum GG. Correlation between 1-hour 50-gram glucose screening test values in successive pregnancies. Obstet Gynecol 2001; 97(suppl. 1): S39–S40.
63. McLaughlin GB, Cheng YW, Caughey AB. Women with one elevated 3-hour glucose tolerance test value: are they at risk for adverse perinatal outcomes? Am J Obstet Gynecol. 2006; 194: e16–9.
64. Bartha JL, Martinez-Del-Fresno P, Comino-Delgado R. Gestational diabetes mellitus diagnosed during early pregnancy. Am J Obstet Gynecol 2000; 182: 346–50.
65. Bartha JL, Martinez-del-Fresno P, Comino-Delgado R. Postpartum metabolism and autoantibody markers in women with gestational diabetes mellitus diagnosed in early pregnancy. Am J Obstet Gynecol 2001; 184: 965–70.
66. Schaefer-Graf UM, Buchanan TA, Songster G, Montoro M, Kjos SL. Patterns of congenital anomalies and relationship to initial maternal fasting glucose levels in pregnancies complicated by type 2 and gestational diabetes. Am J Obstet Gynecol 2000; 182: 313–20.
67. Kalter H. The non-teratogenicity of gestational diabetes. Paediatr Perinat Epidemiol 1998; 12: 456–8.
68. Aberg A, Westbom L, Kallen B. Congenital malformations among infants whose mothers had gestational diabetes or preexisting diabetes. Early Human Dev 2001; 61: 85–95.
69. Martinez-Frias ML, Bermejo E, Rodriguez-Pinilla E, Prieto L, Frias JL. Epidemiological analysis of outcomes of pregnancy in gestational diabetic mothers. Am J Med Genet 1998; 78: 140–5.
70. Virtanen HE, Tapananainen AE, Kaleva MM, et al. Mild gestational diabetes as a risk factor for congenital cryptorchidism. J Clin Endocrinol Metab. 2006; 91: 4862–5.
71. Janssen PA, Rothman I, Schwartz SM. Congenital malformations in newborns of women with established and gestational diabetes in Washington State, 1984–91. Paediatr Perinat Epidemiol 1996; 10: 52–63.
72. Dukler D, Porath A, Bashiri A, Erez O, Mazor M. Remote prognosis of primiparous women with preeclampsia. Eur J Obstet Gynecol Reprod Biol 2001; 96: 69–74.
73. Go RC, Desmond R, Roseman JM, et al. Prevalence and risk factors of microalbuminuria in a cohort of African–American women with gestational diabetes. Diabetes Care 2001; 24: 1764–9.

74. Solomon CG, Seely EW. Brief review: hypertension in pregnancy: a manifestation of the insulin resistance syndrome? Hypertension 2001; 37: 232–9.

75. Joffe GM, Esterlitz JR, Levine RJ, et al. The relationship between abnormal glucose tolerance and hypertensive disorders of pregnancy in healthy nulliparous women. Calcium for Preeclampsia Prevention (CPEP) Study Group. Am J Obstet Gynecol 1998; 179: 1032–7.

76. Innes KE, Wimsatt JH, McDuffie R. Relative glucose tolerance and subsequent development of hypertension in pregnancy. Obstet Gynecol 2001; 97: 905–10.

77. Kjos SL, Buchanan TA. Gestational diabetes mellitus. N Engl J Med 1999; 341: 1749–56.

78. Greenberg LR, Moore TR, Murphy H. Gestational diabetes mellitus: antenatal variables as predictors of postpartum glucose intolerance. Obstet and Gynecol 1995; 86: 96–101.

79. Bian X, Gao P, Xiong X, et al. Risk factors for development of diabetes mellitus in women with a history of gestational diabetes mellitus. Chin Med J (Engl) 2000; 113: 759–62.

80. Hunger-Dathe W, Mosebach N, Samann A, Wolf G, Muller UA. Prevalence of impaired glucose tolerance 6 years after gestational diabetes. Exp Clin Endocrinol Diabetes 2006; 114: 11–7.

81. Smirnakis KV, Chasan-Taber L, Wolf M, et al. Postpartum diabetes screening in women with a history of gestational diabetes. Obstet Gynecol. 2005; 106: 1297–303.

82. Peters RK, Kjos SL, Xiang A, Buchanan TA. Long-term diabetogenic effect of single pregnancy in women with previous gestational diabetes mellitus. Lancet 1996; 347: 227–30.

83. Damm P. Gestational diabetes mellitus and subsequent development of overt diabetes mellitus. Dan Med Bull 1998; 45: 495–509.

84. Lauenborg J, Mathiesen E, Hansen T, et al. The prevalence of the metabolic syndrome in a danish population of women with previous gestational diabetes mellitus is three-fold higher than in the general population. J Clin Endocrinol Metab 2005; 90: 4004–10.

85. Fletcher B, Gulanick M, Lamendola C. Risk factors for type 2 diabetes mellitus. J Cardiovasc Nurs 2002; 16: 17–23.

86. Foster-Powel KA, Cheung NW. Recurrence of gestational diabetes. Aust NZ J Obstet Gynaecol 1998; 38: 384–7.

87. Jolly M, Sebire N, Harris J, Robinson S, Regan L. The risks associated with pregnancy in woman aged 35 years or older. Hum Reprod 2000; 15: 2433–7.

88. Lao TT, Chan PL, Tam KF. Gestational diabetes mellitus in the last trimester – a feature of maternal iron excess? Diabet Med 2001; 18: 218–23.

16 Gestational diabetes in Latin America

Liliana S. Voto, Maria Jose Mattioli and Matías Uranga Imaz

Maternal mortality in Latin America and the Caribbean

The Latin American and Caribbean region, included among the developing countries, has severe deficiencies regarding their socio-economic situations, medical care, women's status, prenatal care, and maternal and perinatal morbidity and mortality.

According to the World Health Organization,[1] the estimated number of maternal deaths in 2000 for the world was 529,000. These deaths were almost equally divided between Africa (251,000) and Asia (253,000), with about 4% (22,000) occurring in Latin America and the Caribean, and less than 1% (2500) in the more developed regions of the world. In terms of the maternal mortality ratio (MMR), the world figure is estimated to be 400 per 100,000 live births. By region, the MMR was highest in Africa (830), followed by Asia (330), Oceania (240), Latin America and the Caribbean (190), and the developed countries (20).

According to the Latin-American & Caribbean Regional Office of UNICEF,[2] the risk of maternal mortality in the developed compared with the developing world in 1990 was 1:1800 versus 1:48, with an incidence of 1:140 for South America.

Although the rate of maternal mortality is apparently low, it has remained similar in the last decade. For example, in our country, Argentina, the MMR was 5.2 in 1990, 4.4 in 1995, 3.5 in 2000 and 4.0 in 2004, which shows it has been very difficult to lower it.[3]

The MMR in the region is 190/100,000 live births, with big differences between countries.[4] According to the last publication of UNICEF in 2005, while in Uruguay, Chile, Cuba, Santa Lucia, Argentina, Costa Rica and Brasil MMR is below 50/100,000, in Peru, Bolivia and Haiti MMR is over 150/100,000.

In Argentina, the last publication of the Ministry of Health[5] shows a MMR of 4.0 (MMR expressed by 10,000 live births). These figures refer to the whole country; however, different Argentine provinces show wide variations, ranging from a rate of 2.8 in Buenos Aires to 13.6 in the province of La Rioja and 13.1 in Jujuy.

In a systematic review recently published by Khan et al.,[6] hypertensive disorders were the first cause of death (25.7%, number of deaths: 777) in Latin America and the Caribbean.

Incidence and prevalence of diabetes in the region

Diabetes continues to be a major concern for public health in the Americas and, unfortunately, its prevalence is likely to increase in Latin America and the Caribbean countries due to the demographic changes these countries are experiencing.

According to King et al.,[7] the number of diabetic people in the Americas is expected to rise from 35 million in 2000 to 64 million in 2025, and the incidence of diabetes in Latin America will increase from 52% to about 62% (around 40 million people),[7] as a result of the aging process of the population and of increased sedentary habits and hypercaloric diets, both of which lead to obesity.

King et al. also found that the incidence of diabetes is higher in women than in men in both developed and developing countries; in the latter it usually affects middle-aged women rather than the elderly, as is the case in developed countries. The male/female ratio shows how risk factors such as diet, low physical activity and obesity are distributed differently between the two sexes, and therefore should be taken into consideration in public welfare decision-making.

Regrettably, epidemiological surveys on diabetes are not carried out on a regular, systematic basis in Latin American and Caribbean countries. The few that have been conducted in different countries 'differ in important methodological features such as selection of the study population, age, sampling method and diagnostic criteria, making comparative studies not very reliable.'[8]

According to the National Household Survey, the prevalence of diagnosed diabetes in Costa Rica in 1998 was 2.8 and 9.4% in the general population and in people aged 40 or older, respectively.[9]

Studies conducted in South America show that the prevalence of diabetes ranges from 6 to 9%, with the lowest rates among the Aymara Indians in Chile (only 1.5%). The prevalence rate among the Mapuche Indians in Chile has increased from 1.0% in 1985 to 4.1%, which may be accounted for by the assimilation of other societies' habits into their culture (such as lack of physical activity and a hypercaloric diet). This acculturation process may explain increasing rates in the rest of Latin America.

The prevalence of diabetes among people aged 35–64 was found to be higher than 10% in Mexico, Trinidad and Tobago and Bolivia, with the highest rate in Jamaica (15.6%). The rest of the countries showed moderate prevalence rates ranging from 3 to 10%, the lowest rates being found in La Plata, Argentina (3.0%). While diabetes prevalence rates were over 10% in men in Jamaica, Mexico and Chile, they were moderate in men from other countries. In women, rates were highest in Jamaica, Mexico, Trinidad and Tobago and Bolivia, moderate (3–9%) in Brazil, Colombia, Paraguay and Surinam, and lowest in Argentina (2.6%).

Frequency of diabetes mellitus in the region

The prevalence of gestational diabetes in Latin American and the Caribbean Region may range from 1 to 14% of pregnancies, depending on the population studied. Gestational diabetes mellitus (GDM) represents nearly 90% of all pregnancies complicated by diabetes.[10]

In a recent communication of the World Health Organization in 2005,[11] it was reported that the global frequency of diabetes in pregnancy in the region was 0.77%; while in Cuba it was 1.75%, the highest rate in Latin America, followed by Argentina with 1.39% (Table 16.1).

According to the Argentine Ministry of Health,[12] over a total number of pregnant women (100,556 patients) the prevalence of diabetes in pregnancy in 2005 was 0.8% ($n = 789$ patients) (Table 16.2).

Risk factors

Pedro B Landabure was a direct disciple of Bernardo Houssay. On 28 December 1954 he founded the Argentine Society of Diabetes, and presided over it during the period from 1955 to 1956. He pioneered investigations on diabetes mellitus (DM) in Argentina and Latin America and described the Landabure syndrome as consisting of:

- history of macrosomic neonates (newborns weighing >4000 g)

Table 16.1   Number of women with diabetes in pregnancy in Latin America and the Caribbean

Country	Number of women	Women with diabetes	
		Number	Percent
Argentina	10,294	143	1.39
Brazil	15,166	143	0.94
Cuba	12,642	221	1.75
Ecuador	12,414	18	0.14
Mexico	20,889	173	0.83
Nicaragua	5,636	6	0.11
Paraguay	3,414	15	0.44
Peru	16,041	23	0.14
Total	96,496	742	0.77

Table 16.2   Types of diabetes in pregnancy in Argentina during 2005

	Number of patients	Percent
Type 1 diabetes	129	16.3
Type 2 diabetes	86	10.9
Gestational diabetes	463	58.7
No date	111	14.1
Total	789	100

- maternal obesity (>10% maternal weight increase with respect to height and age); history of fetal congenital malformations
- habitual abortion
- prematurity
- low birthweight
- polihydramnios
- glycosuria in pregnancy
- perinatal mortality
- multiparity and maternal age >35 years.

In 1981 Pedersen[13] developed the prognostically bad signs of diabetic pregnancy, which disagree with the White classification in one category. Pederse's ill prognosis signs are:

- moderate to severe ketoacidosis
- gestational hypertension
- chronic pyelonephritis
- maternal negligence

Overweight and obesity play an important role not only because of their high frequency, but also because of their contribution to the development of GDM.[14] Universal GDM screening is more effective than that based on risk factors, detecting more cases, allowing for an earlier diagnosis and showing better perinatal results.[15]

Personal experience at the Juan A Fernandez Hospital

The Juan A Fernandez Hospital is a tertiary level, high-risk pregnancy referral center. Between 1994 and 2001, the Maternal Infant Department assisted 72 pregnant women with a diagnosis of DM; in 55% of the cases the women were between the ages of 19 and 34, and in 45% of the cases the women were >34 years of age. Seventeen percent of the patients had a history of perinatal mortality. Seven women (9.7%) lacked prenatal care. Gestational age at the first prenatal visit was >30 weeks in 22.2 % of the cases.

The most frequently associated maternal pathologies were urinary infection and hypertension. Hospitalization during gestation was required for 48.6% of the patients. Gestational age at delivery was >37 weeks in 74% of the population. Cesarean sections were performed in 51.3% of the cases. There were four intrauterine death. Neonates were vigorous at 1 and 5 min after birth in 88 and 93% of the cases, respectively.

High and low birthweights were observed in 18.16 vs. 15% of the newborns, respectively. Neonatal assessment detected an 18% incidence of preterm babies.

Six neonates required hospitalization in the neonatal intensive care unit (NICU). Five newborns presented with respiratory distress syndrome, mechanical ventilation was required in two cases. There was one neonatal death, giving an overall perinatal survival rate of 93%.

Conclusions

From this group's personal experience, it can be concluded that, despite late first prenatal visits, when pregnant women receive prenatal care before birth, perinatal results are acceptable.

However, the question remains as to how many diabetic patients never reach prenatal care, are never detected, or approach the hospital to deliver a dead or macrosomic fetus without a final diagnosis of the pathology that has led to this end.

These are the deficiencies of a developing country which lacks a continuous, efficient maternal–infant policy, in contrast to highly trained medical staff, who cannot achieve the desired reduction in maternal, fetal and neonatal morbidity and mortality. This not only affects the care of patients with DM; unknown numbers of young women die of hemorrhage and infections. This is a consequence of the absence of prenatal care, with patients reaching health centers at the last minute, some of which lack the facilities to make a fast diagnosis and provide timely treatment.

Argentine physicians are aware of risk factors and prevention of fetal malformations by achieving periconceptional glycemic control through preconception care.[16] However, at present this can only be applied to a minority of fertile age women from higher socioeconomic backgrounds who can comply with prenatal care guidelines. The aim is to make this case standard, fighting against hundreds of obstacles that hinder the way towards the preventive care of women's health.

REFERENCES

1. Maternal Mortality in 2000: Estimates developed by WHO, UNICEF and UNFPA. Department of Reproductive Health and Research, World Health Organization, Geneva, 2004.
2. UNICEF. Oficina Regional para América Latina y el Caribe. Mortalidad Materna. Estrategia para su reducción en América Latina y el Caribe. Análisis y recomendaciones para la región. Geneva: UNICEF; 1999.
3. Ministerio de Salud de la República Argentina. Indicadores básicos 2006. www.msal.gov.ar
4. UNICEF. Oficina Regional para América Latina y el Caribe. Los objetivos de desarrollo del milenio tienen que ver con la infancia. Avances y desafíos en América Latina y el Caribe, 2005. www.unicef.org
5. Ministerio de Salud de la República Argentina. Informe 2004 – Serie 5 N° 48/05.
6. Khan KS, Wojdyla D, Say L, et al. WHO analysis of causes of maternal death: a systematic review. Lancet 2006; 367: 1066–74.
7. King H, Aubert RE, Herman WH. Global burden of diabetes, 1995–2025. Diabetes Care 1998; 21: 1414–31.
8. Barceló A, Rajpathak S. Incidence and prevalence of diabetes mellitus in the Americas. Pan Am J Public Health 2001; 10.
9. Morice A, Roselló M, Arauz AG, et al. Diabetes mellitus in Costa Rica. Serie de Documentos Técnicos. San José: INCIENSA; 1999.
10. American Diabetes Association. Diagnosis and classification of diabetes mellitus. Diabetes Care 2006; 29: S43–48.
11. Villar J, Valladares E, Wojdyla D, et al., for the WHO 2005 Global Survey on Maternal and Perinatal Health Research Group. (Personal communication.)
12. Sistema Informático Perinatal. Min. Salud de la República Argentina – 2005.
13. Pedersen J. La diabética gestante y su recién nacido. (Editorial Salvat: Buenos Aires, 1981).
14. Etchegoyen GS, de Martín ER. Gestational diabetes. Determination of relative importante of risk factors. Medicina (Buenos Aires) 2001; 61: 235–8.
15. Griffin ME, Coffey M, Jonson H, et al. Universal vs. Risk factor-based screening for gestational diabetes mellitus: detection rates, gestational diagnosis and outcome. Diabetes Med 2000; 17: 26–32.
16. Ray JG, O'Brien TE, Chan WS. Preconception care and the risk of congenital anomalies in the offspring of women with diabetes mellitus: a meta-analysis. Q J Med 2001; 94: 435–44.

17 Diabetes and pregnancy in advancing nations: India

V. Seshiah, V. Balaji and Madhuri S. Balaji

Introduction

The prevalence of diabetes is increasing globally and India is no exception. WHO indicates an expected total rise from 135 million in 1995 to 300 million (120%) in 2025,[1] in the prevalence of diabetes in adults. These numbers include women with Gestational diabetes mellitus (GDM).[2] GDM is considered as a transient abnormality of glucose intolerance during pregnancy.[3] Women with GDM are at increased risk of diabetes in future as are their children and the following subsequent generations. This fact should alert physicians to the necessity of devoting special attention to this segment of the population especially in developing countries.[2]

Implications

The usual recommendation of lifestyle modifications or drug intervention for prevention of diabetes is likely to delay or postpone the development of overt diabetes in persons diagnosed with abnormal glucose tolerance. These measures essentially target only the post-primary prevention of diabetes whereas the aim should be primary prevention of diabetes by keeping genetically or otherwise susceptible individuals normoglycemic, apart from preventing them from developing Type 2 DM.[4] In this respect, women with GDM become the ideal group for primary prevention of diabetes.[5] The diagnosis of GDM offers a unique opportunity in identifying individuals who will benefit from early therapeutic intervention with diet and exercise, thus normalizing body weight to delay or even possibly prevent the onset of diabetes.

Awareness

The success of a project for preventing any disease en masse mainly depends on an awareness of the disease amongst a population. But the general population, especially of India, are not aware of the possibility of glucose intolerance occurring during pregnancy and its consequences.

Hence, a baseline study was undertaken by the present authors to assess the knowledge, attitude, and practice (KAP) in a sample population of the study area, namely, Chennai city.

The city is divided into 424 health subunits. Each subunit has a population in the range of 30,000 to 51,000. Health aspects of each unit are monitored by the Multi Purpose Health Workers (MPHWS). A pilot survey showed that a precoded questionnaire was over-estimating, due to the intelligent guesses made by the respondents, and hence it was decided to use an open-end questionnaire.

The findings of this KAP study showed lack of knowledge and awareness about GDM among the population. The percentage awareness was only 13.2% (95% CI, 12.6–13.9%), which was a disturbing observation. The authors have launched and are still continuing an intensive campaign to inform the public about GDM through cinema theatre slides, cable TV scrolls, visual aids in public transport, wall posters, stencils, wall paintings, handouts, and speaker van campaigns. A repeat KAP study was performed after 1 year to assess the effect of the ongoing awareness creation program. The awareness of GDM among the general population has increased to an appreciable level of 23.5% (95% CI, 22.6–24.4%).

Prevalence

The epidemiology of GDM is subject to various factors such as the population to be screened, the screening methods, the gestational weeks for screening and the glycemic criteria for diagnosis. Screening recommendations range from inclusion of all pregnant women (universal) to the exclusion of all other women except those with very specific risk factors (selective): e.g. age >25 years, obesity: BMI >30, ethnicity: Hispanic, Native American, Asian–American, African–American, family history: first degree relative, and previous GDM or large for gestational age infant.[6] Different ethnic groups when exposed to the same environmental setting, experienced a widely variable risk. Among ethnic groups in South Asian countries, Indian women have the highest frequency of GDM (15%), followed by Chinese (13.9%), Vietnam-born (7.8%) and Australian-born (4.3%).[7]

The frequency of diabetes in the child-bearing age group of women for a given population and ethnicity mirrors that of the underlying frequency of Type 2 DM in that population.[7] Among Indians, the prevalence of impaired glucose tolerance (IGT) in the age groups of 20–29 years and 30–39 years was

Table 17.1   Prevalence of gestational diabetes mellitus in different parts of India 2002

Author/investigator	Center	Number of pregnant women screened	Prevalence rate (%)
Balaji et al.	North Chennai, Tamil Nadu	891	16.2
Anjalakshi et al.	South Chennai, Tamil Nadu	1002	15
K. P. Paulose	Trivandrum, Kerala	750	15
Mary John	Ludhiana, Punjab	220	17.5
Prasanna Kumar	Bangalore, Karnataka	49	12
Shyam Mukundan	Alwaye, Kerala	200	21
Aruyerchelvan	Erode, Rural Tamil Nadu	562	18.8
TOTAL		3674	16.55

found to be 12.2 and 15.3%, respectively. No gender difference was seen in the prevalence of IGT.[8] It was observed in a national survey performed in 2002, the frequency of the occurrence of GDM was 16.55% by WHO criteria[9] which was closer to the prevalence of IGT in the child-bearing age group of women in India.[8] Parallel to the increased prevalence of diabetes and IGT in the general population, the frequency of GDM had also increased. The prevalence of GDM was 2% in 1982[10] (IGT, 2%[11]) which increased to 7.62% in 1991[12] (IGT, 8.2%[13]), and doubled to 16.55% in 2002[9] (IGT, 14.5%[8]). The prevalence data published[9] included pregnant women attending different health care providing centres spread in different parts of the country (Table 17.1).

This phenomenal increase in the prevalence of GDM prompted the authors to initiate a project on 'Diabetes in Pregnancy Awareness and Prevention (DIPAP)', funded by the World Diabetes Foundation and supported by the government of Tamil Nadu, India. To obtain community-based prevalence data under the DIPAP project, the author's group screened 4151 pregnant women (during 2004–2005) in an

urban area, taking Chennai city of Tamil Nadu, India, as the sampling population. GDM diagnosis was based on the WHO criteria of 2 h plasma glucose (PG) ≥140 mg/dL with 75 g OGTT. In this community-based study, the prevalence of GDM was 17.9%. The prevalence of GDM had increased from 16.55 to 17.9% in 2 years. This trend indicates that the anticipated projection of prevalence of GDM by 2012 would be closer to 30–35% (Figure 17.1). This project is also being carried out simultaneously in a rural area and the target population to be screened is 3600. So far, 2936 women have been screened and the prevalence of GDM is 10.4% in the rural area. With the available information, there is a definite divide between the rural and urban areas in the prevalence of GDM. The reason for this difference will be known only after the completion of the project, but the possible cause for the low prevalence may be due to the less mechanized, agriculture-based lifestyle in the rural area.

Geographical variations in the prevalence of GDM

Prevalence of GDM varies from one region to another in the same country. Though the overall prevalence of GDM in India was 16.55%, the frequency varied from 12 to 21% in different parts of the country.[9] A low prevalence of GDM was observed in the hilly areas of Jammu and Kashmir[14] (north India) 4.4%, Imphal[15] (north-east India) 2.2%, and in Yercaud[16] (south India) 3.5%. This low prevalence could be attributed to the lifestyle adapted by the people living in the hostile terrain. The prevalence of GDM in other developing countries also showed regional variations. In Mexico, the prevalence of GDM varied from 4.3 to 11% when screening was done in different parts of the country.[17] The rate of abnormal screening test results ranged from 8.0 to 20.7% for different regions of Poland.[18] Among Pan Arab countries, Saudi Arabia (12.5%) and Bahrain (13.5%) had the highest prevalence of GDM.[19,20] The frequency of GDM in Argentina was between 2 and 12% depending upon the population studied and geographical variations.[21]

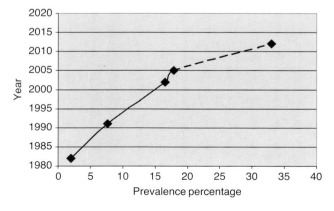

Figure 17.1   Anticipated projection of GDM prevalence in India.

Rationale for universal screening

Selective screening based on risk factors scored poorly in predicting GDM.[22] If selective screening is employed, it is likely that 16% of GDM women will go undetected.[23] Further selective screening recommended by ADA may be applicable for women belonging to the ethnic group with low prevalence of GDM. Whereas, among ethnic groups in South Asian countries, Indian women have the highest frequency of GDM necessitating universal screening.[24] The recognition of glucose intolerance during pregnancy is more relevant in the Indian context, as Indian women have 11-fold risk of developing GDM compared to Caucasians.[25]

Compared to selective screening, universal screening for GDM detects more cases and improves maternal and offspring prognosis.[26] Cost analysis of universal screening when compared with risk factor screening showed only a negligible difference.[22] Thus universal screening appears to be the most reliable and desired method for the detection of GDM.[22] For universal screening the test should be simple and cost effective. The two-step procedure of screening with the 50 g glucose challenge test (GCT) and then diagnosing GDM based on OGTT is not feasible in a country like India, because pregnant women may have to visit the antenatal clinic twice and at least three to five blood samples have to be drawn, which they resent. WHO recommendation serves both as a one-step screening and diagnostic procedure, and is easy to perform besides being economical.[27] WHO criteria of 2 h PG $\geq$ 140 mg/dL identifying a large number of cases may have a greater potential for prevention.[28] The WHO procedure for screening and diagnosis of GDM is being followed in the DIPAP project and the same has been recommended in the Indian Guidelines for Gestational Diabetes Mellitus.[29]

Gestational weeks for screening

The current recommendation is to perform screening test between 24 and 28 weeks of gestation, though there are reports that claim about 40–66% of women with GDM can be detected early during pregnancy.[30,31] Nahum et al. also suggest that the ideal period to screen for GDM is around 16 weeks of gestation and even earlier in high-risk groups with a history of fetal wastage.[32] The interim analysis based on the gestational weeks of the GDM women in the DIPAP project revealed that, 16.3% had glucose intolerance within 16 weeks, 23.1% between 17 and 23 weeks and remaining 60.6% more than 24 weeks of gestation.[33] These studies stress the need for screening for GDM during the early weeks of gestation. GDM diagnosis may not be missed by screening around 24–28 weeks of gestation, but a substantial number of pregnant women who develop GDM in the earlier weeks of pregnancy are likely to have delayed diagnosis and may not receive appropriate medical care. Further, early screening for glucose intolerance and care could avoid some diabetes-related complications in women with gestational diabetes.[34] To validate the above observation the present author's group screened 207 pregnant women attending their referral center for diabetes and pregnancy with a 75 g OGTT. Among them, 87 (42.03%) were

diagnosed with GDM. Women in whom GDM was detected between 0 and 23 weeks of gestation were classified as group 1 (54 (62.7%)) and beyond 24 weeks of gestation as group 2 (33 (37.93%)). All were treated and followed till confinement. In India, the normal birthweight varies between 2.5 and 3.5 kg.[35] There was no statistically significant difference ($P < 0.05$) between the birthweight of the neonates born to Normal glucose tolerance (NGT) women (3.28 ± 0.50 kg) and GDM women in group 1 (3.13 ± 0.55 kg). In group 2, the neonatal birthweight was 3.42 ± 0.58 kg which is the upper limit of the normal range in Indian new born babies. The observation of this study was that, by early detection of glucose intolerance during pregnancy and by giving adequate care to the antenatal women, a good fetal outcome can be achieved similar to that of NGT pregnant women.[36]

Yet another observation from the DIPAP project was that, out of 17.9% pregnant women diagnosed to have GDM, 12.7% of them were detected to have GDM in the first visit and the remaining 5.2% at subsequent visits. This finding stresses the fact that women with NGT in the first visit are to be advised to undergo glucose tolerance test in the subsequent visits.

Demographic findings in DIPAP project

The demographic details of the 4151 pregnant women screened in the DIPAP project are given below in Table 17.2.

The proportion of GDM increased with increasing age and BMI. There was a significant association between BMI and GDM ($P < 0.001$) but gravida did not show significant association ($P > 0.05$). The mean gestational weeks for all the women screened was 24.2 ± 7.74. The mean gestational weeks of screening GDM and NGT women was 25.5 ± 7.67 and 23.9 ± 7.73, respectively. The family history of DM was positive in 37.5% of GDM and in 24.5% of NGT women. The prevalence rates of GDM in the sedentary, moderate, and heavy activity group were 19.1, 17.8, and 12.9%, respectively.

Women whose blood pressure was $\geq$120 mmHg systolic or $\geq$80 mmHg diastolic were considered to have hypertension. The proportion of hypertension ($P < 0.0001$) was significantly higher in GDM (25.6%) compared to NGT women (18.8%). The odds ratio of developing hypertension

Table 17.2	Demographic details	
	GDM $n = 741$	**NGT $n = 3410$**
Age (years)	24.94 ± 3.81	23.38 ± 3.43
BMI (kg/m²)	23.33 ± 4.19	21.57 ± 3.87
Gravida	Primi: 352 (47.5%)	Primi: 1669 (48.9%)
	Multi: 389 (52.5%)	Multi: 1741 (51.1%)
Gestational weeks at screening	25.5 ± 7.67	23.9 ± 7.73
Positive family history of DM	278 (37.5%)	835 (24.5%)

was 1.489 (95% CI, 1.224–1.812). Women with a BP of ≥140/90 mmHg were advised methyldopa to control their hypertension.

The mean hemoglobin level of the NGT women was 10.30 ± 0.93 g% and that of the GDM was 10.36 ± 0.96 g%. There was no significant difference between the hemoglobin levels of GDM and NGT women.

Management

The goal in the management is to avoid both low birthweight and macrosomic babies, as they are prone to develop diabetes in adolescence and adult life.[37] In India, both under-nutrition and over-nutrition exist during pregnancy. There are two reported studies in India that relate size at birth to future risk of Type 2 DM. In Mysore, low birthweight did not increase the risk of diabetes but babies who were short and fat at birth (higher BMI) were at increased risk.[38] Fall et al. speculate that the rise in Type 2 DM in Indian urban populations would have been triggered by mild obesity in mothers, leading to glucose intolerance during pregnancy, macrosomic changes in the fetus, and insulin deficiency in adult life.[38] Yet another study attributes high prevalence of Type 2 DM and IGT in Indian people linked to poor fetal growth[39] which is at variance to the observation by Fall et al.

Medical nutrition therapy

The meal pattern should provide adequate calories and nutrients to meet the needs of pregnancy. The meal plan advised has to be simple, easy to achieve, understand, and follow. The MNT recommended is based on their routine dietary habits and glycemic excursions that occur with the meal. In a normal person, the peak of plasma glucose is higher after breakfast (due to the 'dawn phenomenon') than after lunch and dinner, and insulin secretion also matches the glycemic excursions that occur with these three meals.[40] Since GDM mothers have deficiency in first phase insulin secretion, the quantity of food at one time should also be less, to overcome this insulin deficiency, particularly after breakfast. To avoid the postprandial plasma glucose peaking with breakfast, the authors guide their women with GDM to distribute calorie consumption especially the breakfast into two portions 'split breakfast'. This implies splitting the usual breakfast into two halves and consuming these portions with a 2-h gap between them. By this, the undue peak in plasma glucose levels after ingestion of the total quantity of breakfast at one time is avoided. For example, if four slices of bread (applies to all type of breakfast menu) is taken for breakfast at 8 am, the postprandial peak plasma glucose is 140 mg: when the same quantity is divided into two equal portions, i.e. one portion (two slices of bread) at 8 am and the remaining two slices after 2–3 h, the postprandial peak plasma glucose falls by 20–30 mg.

Insulin therapy

The policy followed in India is to advise human insulin in women with GDM who failed to achieve fasting plasma glucose (FPG) of ≤90 mg/dL and 1.5 h post-meal plasma glucose level of ≤120 mg/dL with MNT. The aim is to maintain post-meal peak plasma glucose level of ≤120 mg/dL. A number of studies have established the benefits of maintaining the plasma glucose at this level.[41–43] Due to the pharmacokinetic action of human regular insulin, a considerable segment of pregnant women with GDM fail to achieve optimum glycemic control, mostly the postprandial plasma glucose. In them, the best option is to administer ultra short acting analogues, insulin lispro (Humalog) or insulin aspart (Novo rapid). Novo rapid is given freely in all the government institutions in the state of Tamil Nadu, India. These analogues improve the postprandial glucose control in pregnant women with Type 1, Type 2 DM and GDM, and are also safe and effective.[44–46]

Oral hypoglycemic agents

Glibenclamide

Glibenclamide (Glyburide) may be an alternative safe therapy for many GDM women who are hesitant to take insulin. This drug decreases insulin resistance and improves insulin secretion, the pathogenic factors in the causation of hyperglycemia in GDM.[47,48] Another advantage is that the human placental transfer of glibenclamide is negligible. Maternally administered glibenclamide in pharmacologic doses, and even doses greatly exceeding therapeutic levels, may not reach the fetus.[49] The landmark study by Langer et al. concluded that glyburide was as effective as insulin in maintaining desired glycemic levels and resulted in comparable outcome.[50] The author's group undertook a prospective study comparing insulin and glibenclamide in GDM. In this study, both glibenclamide and insulin treatment achieved equally good glycemic control and the perinatal outcome was not different.[51] The important observation of this study was that the mean dose of glibenclamide required at term was 1.45 ± 0.57 mg/day and mean insulin requirement at term was 21.7 ± 13.55 units/day to achieve the same glycemic level.[51] It is noteworthy that glibenclamide is very economical and cost effective compared to insulin, which is not only expensive but also inconvenient as it has to be taken parenterally. Ultimately, the therapy preference depends on the patient's choice and physician's decision.

Metformin

Women with polycystic ovary syndrome (PCOS) are advised metformin to induce ovulation. The drug is not withdrawn if a woman conceives while on metformin therapy and the maximum dose prescribed in the author's clinical practice is 1500 mg. If the plasma glucose is not under control with metformin, insulin is always added. No adverse pregnancy outcome with metformin therapy was observed. A preliminary study showed that metformin was safe in pregnant, glucose intolerant women either as an adjunct to insulin treatment or even as a monotherapy.[52] A prospective study found no adverse influence on the pregnancy outcome in PCOS women treated throughout pregnancy with metformin.[53]

Monitoring glycemic control

The continuous glucose monitoring has demonstrated that the time interval from meal to peak postprandial glucose level was approximately 90 min and was similar in all the evaluated types of diabetic pregnancies (insulin treated or diet only) and is not affected by the level of glycemic control. Moreover, no difference was obtained in postprandial glycemic profile between breakfast, lunch or dinner.[43] Hence the present policy in India, from August 2006, is to maintain FPG <90 mg/dL and 1.5 h post-meal plasma glucose <120 mg/dL during pregnancy.[29]

Target glycemic level

Increased birthweight of neonates occurred even when the mother's glucose tolerance was less than the glycemic criteria recommended by WHO (2-h PG >140 mg/dL) for diagnosis of GDM. Increasing carbohydrate intolerance in women without overt GDM was associated with graded increase in the incidence of macrosomia.[54] The author's group confirmed that the occurrence of macrosomia was continuum as the 2 h PG with 75 g OGTT increased from 120 mg/dL.[55] A similar outcome was also documented in the DIPAP community based study. The birthweight of the neonates born to 2315 pregnant women was available for analysis. Among these women 415 (17.5%) were GDM and of them 58 (13.9%) delivered big babies. The number of big babies in the NGT group was 147 and out of them 49 (33.3%) were born to mothers whose 2-h PG ≥120 mg/dL (75 g OGTT). Pregnant women who do not meet the diagnostic criteria of GDM but have 2-h PG ≥120 mg/dL (75 g OGTT) should not be ignored and this level needs cognizance. The study by Sunil Gupta et al. corroborates this finding.[56]

Pattern of delivery

In the rural areas, every pregnant woman in the village is visited by the village health nurse. A periodic antenatal checkup is done by the medical officers attached to the primary health centers which have the facility to conduct normal delivery. Women who may have difficulty in normal delivery are referred to the district headquarters hospital where a specialist obstetrician service is available.

In urban areas, pregnant women are taken care by the Multi Purpose health workers (MPHW). Centers run by the municipality or corporation in their area. These maternity centers have facilities for normal deliveries and Cesarean sections. High-risk pregnant women are referred to tertiary level maternity hospitals attached to teaching medical colleges.

The pattern of delivery in a district headquarters hospital, maternity centers of the corporation and teaching hospitals of Chennai, are given in the Table 17.3.

The Cesarean section rate was high in all these hospitals even in NGT women. This is due to the health policy of the government, which considers every pregnancy as high risk. Additionally, the preference of some parents to have only one child has resulted in a high rate of Cesarean sections. Another reason could be that some people in Indian society believe that a child has to be born at an auspicious time based on astrological prediction. If the natural delivery time of the child does not coincide with the prediction, then Cesarean section is resorted to. The total Cesarean section rates in the public, charitable and private hospitals were 20, 38, and 47% respectively.[57] The Cesarean rate in a maternity hospital increased from 1.9 to 16% within 10 years.[58] The perinatal mortality rate showed a significant reduction from 69 per 1000 to 36 per 1000, despite higher Cesarean rates.[58] The present trend in developing countries is for increased use of Cesarean section.[59]

Prevention

Screening for glucose intolerance during pregnancy is not done routinely and probably the undiagnosed glucose intolerance that has been occurring in the past has resulted in the increased prevalence of diabetes in India. This is likely to be true as GDM has a far-reaching consequence in predisposing their offspring to glucose intolerance. This observation was substantiated and documented in Pima Indians by Dabelea et al.[60] Children born in 1965 to women with GDM were followed up until 2000. By the time they reached 35 years, more than half of the group had diabetes.[60] Hence, as a policy to identify GDM and its consequences in the infant, a 75 g OGTT has been recommended to all women in the population during the third trimester of pregnancy.[60] Now it is obvious that taking care of women with GDM is the first step in the primary prevention of diabetes. To achieve this goal, the Diabetes In Pregnancy Study group India (DIPSI)

Table 17.3   Pattern of deliveries in public maternity centers and hospitals

Year and type of hospital	Total deliveries	Cesarean section
District headquarters hospital		
2004–2005	44,970	6018 (13.4%)
2005–2006	45,454	6681 (14.7%)
Maternity centers of the corporation		
2004–2005	16,495	1574 (9.5%)
2005–2006	16,516	2154 (13%)
Teaching medical college (tertiary-care hospitals)		
2004–2005	17,543	7646 (43.6%)
2005–2006	16,687	6722 (40.3%)

was formed in 2005. This study group has framed the guidelines to be followed in the management of GDM.[29] The Government of Tamil Nadu, India, has accepted these guidelines and promulgated an order by which screening for glucose intolerance during pregnancy has become mandatory.

The important aspect of diabetes and pregnancy is that the intrauterine millieu interieur, whether one of nutritional deprivation or one of nutritional plenty, results in changes in pancreatic development and peripheral response to insulin that may lead to adult-onset GDM and Type 2 DM.[61] Thus, timely action taken now in screening all pregnant women for glucose intolerance, achieving euglycemia in them and ensuring adequate nutrition may prevent in all probability, the vicious cycle of transmitting glucose intolerance from one generation to another.[62]

No single period in human development provides a greater potential than pregnancy for long range pay off via relatively short range period of enlightened metabolic manipulation. (Norbert Frienkel)

Conclusion

- GDM women are at increased risk of future diabetes as are their children and following generations.

- Prevalence of GDM varies from one region to another in the same country.
- Compared with selective screening, universal screening for GDM detects more cases and improves maternal and offspring prognosis.
- Asian Indian women are ethnically more prone to developing glucose intolerance compared to other ethnic groups.
- GDM based on 2-h 75 g OGTT defined by WHO predicts adverse pregnancy outcome and warrants treatment.
- A 2-h 75 g post-plasma glucose ≥140 mg/dL serves both as screening and diagnostic criteria besides being a simple and economical one-step procedure.
- Early screening for glucose intolerance and care could avoid some diabetes-related complications in women with gestational diabetes.
- Woman with NGT at the first visit are advised to undergo a glucose tolerance test during the subsequent visits.
- The meal pattern advised has to be simple, and easy to understand and follow.
- The goal is to maintain mean plasma glucose of 105 mg/dL.
- Occurrence of macrosomia was continuum as the 2-h PG increased from 120 mg/dL and this level needs cognizance.
- The present trend in the developing countries is for increased use of Cesarean section.
- Taking care of the women with gestational diabetes is envisaged as the first step in the primary prevention of diabetes.

REFERENCES

1. King H, Aubert RE, Herman WH. Global burden of diabetes, 1995–2025. Prevalence, numeric estimates and projections. Diabetes Care 1998; 21: 1414–31.
2. Ben Haroush A, Yogev Y, Hod M. Epidemiology of gestational diabetes mellitus. In: Hod M, Jovanovic L, Di Renzo GC, de Leiva A, Langer O, eds. Textbook of Diabetes and Pregnancy, 1st edn. London: Martin Dunitz, Taylor & Francis; 2003, pp. 64–89.
3. O'Sullivan JB. Gestational diabetes and its significance. In: Camerini-Davalos R, Cole HS, eds. Early Diabetes. New York: Academic Press; 1970, pp. 339–44.
4. Tuomilehto J. A paradigm shift is needed in the primary prevention of type 2 diabetes. In: Ganz M, ed. Prevention of type 2 diabetes. Chichester, UK: John Wiley; 2005. pp. 153–65.
5. Girling J, Dornhorst A. Pregnancy and diabetes mellitus. In: Pickup JC, Williams G, eds. Textbook of Diabetes, 3rd edn. Oxford, UK: Blackwell Publishing; 2003, pp. 65–66.
6. Mazze R. Epidemiology of Diabetes in Pregnancy. In: Langer O, ed. The Diabetes In Pregnancy Dilemma, Leading change with Proven Solutions. Maryland: University Press of America; 2006, pp. 13–22.
7. King H. Epidemiology of glucose intolerance and gestational diabetes in women of childbearing age. Diabetes Care. 1998; 21(suppl. 2): B9–B13.
8. Ramachandran A, Snehalatha C, Kapur A, et al., for the Diabetes Epidemiology Study Group in India (DESI). High prevalence of diabetes and impaired glucose tolerance in India: National Urban Diabetes Survey. Diabetologia 2001; 44: 1094–101.
9. Seshiah V, Balaji V, Balaji MS, et al. Gestational diabetes mellitus in India. J Assoc Physicians India 2004; 52: 707–11.
10. Agarwal S, Gupta AN. Gestational diabetes. J Assoc Physicians India 1982; 30: 203.
11. Ramachandran A, Jali MV, Mohan V, et al. High prevalence of diabetes in an urban population in south India. BMJ 1988; 297: 587–90.
12. Narendra J, Munichoodappa C. Prevalence of glucose intolerance during pregnancy. Int J Diab Dev Countries 1991; 11: 2–4.
13. Ramachandran A, Snehalatha C, Dharmaraj D, et al. Prevalence of glucose intolerance in Asian Indians. Diabetes Care 1992; 15: 1348–55.
14. Zargar AH, Sheikh MI, Bashir MI, et al. Prevalence of gestational diabetes mellitus in Kashmiri women from the Indian subcontinent. Diabetes Res Clin Pract 2004; 66: 139–45.
15. Dorendra Singh I, Bidhumukhi Devi Th, Ibeyaima Devi Kh, et al. Gestational Diabetes Mellitus among the Manipuri Women: The prevalence and the risk factors. Journal of Diabetes Association of India April–June 1999; 39: 15–18.
16. Uvaraj MG. Study of prevalence of abnormal glucose tolerance during pregnancy in the hamlets of Shervaroy hills. Diabetes 2007; 56(suppl 1): A 702.
17. Forsbach G, Vazquez-Lara J, Alvarez-y-Garcia C, et al. Diabetes and pregnancy in Mexico. Rev Invest Clin 1998; 50: 227–31.
18. Wojcikowski C, Krolikowska B, Konarzewska J, et al. The prevalence of gestational diabetes mellitus in Polish population. Givekol Pol 2002; 73: 811–6.
19. Ardawi MS, Nasrat HA, Jamal HS, et al. Screening for gestational diabetes mellitus in pregnant females. Saudi Med J 2000; 21: 155–60.
20. Al Mahroos S, Nagalla DS, Yousif W, et al. A population-based screening for gestational diabetes mellitus in non-diabetic women in Bahrain. Ann Saudi Med 2005; 25: 129–33.
21. Voto LS, Imaz MU, Margulies M. Gestational diabetes in developing countries. In: Hod M, Jovanovic L, Di Renzo GC, de Leiva A, Langer O, eds. Textbook of Diabetes and Pregnancy, 1st edn. London: Martin Dunitz, Taylor & Francis; 2003, pp. 183–190.
22. Shamsuddin K, Mahdy ZA, Siti Rafiaah I, et al. Risk factor screening for abnormal glucose tolerance in pregnancy. Diabet Med 2000; 17: 376–80.
23. Soonthornpun S, Soonthornpun K, Aksonteing J, al. A comparison between a 75g and a 100g oral glucose tolerance test in pregnant women. Int J Gynecol Obstet 2003; 81: 169–73.
24. Beischer NA, Oats JN, Henry OA, et al. Incidence and severity of gestational diabetes mellitus according to country of birth in women living in Australia. Diabetes 1991; 40(suppl. 2): 35–8.
25. Dornhost A, Paterson CM, Nicholls JS, et al. High prevalence of GDM in women from ethnic minority groups. Diabetic Med 1992; 9: 820–2.
26. Cosson E, Benchimol M, Carbillon L, et al. Universal rather than selective screening for gestational diabetes mellitus may improve fetal outcomes. Diabetes Metab 2006 Apr; 32(2):140–6.
27. Seshiah V, Balaji V, Balaji MS, et al. One step procedure for screening and diagnosis of gestational diabetes mellitus. J Obstet Gynecol Ind 2005; 55: 525–9.
28. Schmidt MI, Duncan BB, Reichelt AJ, et al. for the Brazilian Gestational Diabetes Study Group: Gestational diabetes mellitus

diagnosed with a 2-h 75-g oral glucose tolerance test and adverse pregnancy outcomes. Diabetes Care 2001; 24: 1151–5.

29. Seshiah V, Das AK, Balaji V, et al., and the Diabetes in Pregnancy Study Group. Gestational diabetes mellitus guidelines. J Assoc Physicians India 2006; 54: 622–8.

30. Meyer WJ, Carbone J, Gauthier DW, et al. Early gestational glucose screening and gestational diabetes. J Reprod Med 1996; 41: 675–9.

31. Super DM, Edelberg SC, Philipson EH, et al. Diagnosis of gestational diabetes in early pregnancy. Diabetes Care 1991; 14: 288–94.

32. Nahum GG, Wilson SB, Stanislaw H. Early pregnancy glucose screening for gestational diabetes mellitus. J Reprod Med 2002; 47: 656–62.

33. Seshiah V, Balaji V, Madhuri S, et al. Early screening for Gestational Diabetes. Diabetes 2006; 55(suppl. 1): A606.

34. Bartha JL, Martinez-Del-Fresno P, Comino-Delgado R. Early diagnosis of gestational diabetes mellitus and prevention of diabetes related complications. Eur J Obstet Gynecol Reprod Biol 2003; 109: 41–4.

35. Paul VK, Deorari AK, Singh M. Management of low birth weight babies. In: Parthasarathy A, Menon PSN, Nair MKC, et al., eds. IAP Textbook of Pediatrics, 2nd edn, New Delhi: Jaypee Brothers; 2002, p. 60.

36. Seshiah V, Alexander C, Balaji V, et al. Glycemic control from early weeks of gestation and pregnancy outcome. Diabetes 2006; 55(suppl 1): A 604.

37. Jovanovic L. American Diabetes Association's Fourth International Workshop – Conference on Gestational Diabetes Mellitus: Summary and Discussion. Diabetes Care 1998; 21(suppl. 2): B131–7.

38. Fall CH, Stein CE, Kumaran K, et al. Size at birth, maternal weight, and type 2 diabetes in South India. Diabet Med 1998; 15: 220–7.

39. Yajnik CS, Fall CH, Vaidya U, et al. Fetal growth and glucose and insulin metabolism in four year old Indian children. Diabet Med 1995; 12: 330–6.

40. Polonsky KS, Given BD, Van Cauter E. Twenty four hour profiles and pulsatile patterns of insulin secretion in normal and obese subjects. J Clin Invest 1988; 81: 442–8.

41. de Sereday MS, Damiano MM, Gonzalez CD, et al. Diagnostic criteria for gestational diabetes in relation to pregnancy outcome. J Diabetes Complications 2003; 17: 115–119.

42. Franks PW, Looker HC, Kobes S, et al. Gestational glucose tolerance and risk of type 2 diabetes in young Pima Indian offspring. Diabetes 2006; 55: 460–5.

43. Ben-Haroush A, Yogev Y, Chen R, et al. The post prandial glucose profile in the diabetic pregnancy. Am J Obstet Gynecol 2004; 191: 576–81.

44. Hermansen K, Colombo M, Storgaard H, et al. Improved postprandial glycemic control with biphasic human insulin in patients with Type 2 diabetes. Diabetes Care 2002; 25: 883–888.

45. Jovanovic L, Ilic S, Pettitt DJ, et al. Metabolic and immunologic effects of insulin lispro in gestational diabetes. Diabetes Care 1999; 22: 1422–7.

46. Balaji V, Madhuri S, Balaji, Seshiah V. Insulin Aspart – Safe During Pregnancy. Abstract volume of the 37th Annual Meeting of the Diabetes and Pregnancy Study Group, Myconos, Greece, September 2005.

47. Groop LC, Barzilai N, Ratheiser K, et al. Dose-dependent effects of glyburide on insulin secretion and glucose uptake in humans. Diabetes Care 1991; 14: 724–7.

48. Rossetti L, Giaccari A, DeFronzo RA. Glucose toxicity. Diabetes Care 1990; 13: 610–30.

49. Elliott BD, Langer O, Schenker S, et al. Insignificant transfer of glyburide occurs across the human placenta. Am J Obstet Gynecol 1991; 165(4, pt 1): 807–12.

50. Langer O, Cornway DL, Berkus MD, et al. A comparison of glyburide and insulin in GDM. N Engl J Med 2000; 343: 1134–8.

51. Anjalakshi C, Balaji V, Balaji MS, et al. A prospective study comparing insulin and glibenclamide in gestational diabetes mellitus in Asian Indian women. Diabetes Res Clin Pract 2006; 2007 June; 76(3):474–5.

52. Ramachandran A, Snehalatha C, Vijayalakshmi S, et al. Use of metformin in pregnancies with diabetes: A case series from India. J Assoc Physicians India 2005; 53: 157–8.

53. Glueck CJ, Goldenberg N, Pranikoff J, et al. Height, weight and motor–social development during the first 18 months of life in 126 infants born to 109 mothers with polycystic ovary syndrome who conceived on and continued metformin throughout pregnancy. Hum Reprod 2004; 19: 1323–30.

54. Sermer M, Naylor CD, Farine D, et al. The Toronto Tri Hospital Gestational diabetes project – A preliminary review. Diabetes Care 1998; 21(suppl. 2): B33–B42.

55. Balaji V, Balaji MS, Seshiah V, et al. Maternal glycemia and neonates birth weight in Asian Indian women. Diabetes Res Clin Pract 2006; 73: 223–4.

56. Gupta S. Gestational diabetes mellitus (GDM): Do we need to revise the standard criteria for diagnosis? Diabetes Res Clin Pract 2002; 56(suppl. 1): S45.

57. Sreevidya S, Sathiyasekaran BW. High Caesarean rates in Madras (India): a population-based cross sectional study. Br J Obstet Gynaecol 2003; 110: 106–11.

58. Mehta A, Apers L, Verstraelen H, et al. Trends in Cesarean section rates at a maternity hospital in Mumbai, India. J Health Popul Nutr 2001; 19: 306–12.

59. Onsrud L, Onsrud M. Increasing use of Cesarean section, even in developing countries. Tidsskr Nor Laegeforen 1996; 116: 67–71.

60. Dabelea D, Knowler WC, Pettitt DJ. Effect of diabetes in pregnancy and offspring: follow up research in the Pima Indians. J Matern Fetal Med 2000; 9: 83–8.

61. Savona-Ventura C, Chircop M. Birth weight influence on the subsequent development of gestational diabetes mellitus. Acta Diabetol 2003; 40: 101–4.

62. Aerts L, Van Assche FA. Intra-uterine transmission of disease. Placenta. 2003 Nov; 24(10): 905–11.

18 Diabetes and pregnancy in New Zealand

David Simmons and Jeremy Oats

Background

New Zealand is a developed nation with a land mass of 270,500 km^2 over two major islands (North Island and South Island). The population of 3,737,277 in 2001 included 2,868,009 of European descent (predominantly from the British Isles), 526,281 Maori (indigenous Polynesians who arrived mainly between 800 and 1200 AD), 231,801 Pacific peoples (mainly from Samoa, Tonga, Cook Islands, Niue and Tokelau Islands from the 1960s) and 237,459 Asians (who have arrived since the nineteenth century, but particularly in the 1990s).[1] The high prevalence of Type 2 diabetes among Maori was first reported in the early 1960s.[2] Subsequently, an increasing prevalence of diabetes among Tokelauan immigrants to New Zealand was found compared with those who remained in the islands.[3] The growth in numbers with diabetes across New Zealand Europeans, Maori and Pacific people became apparent from studies in South Auckland and data relating to complications (e.g. renal failure) in the 1990s.[4] Subsequent data has shown that this epidemic of diabetes is continuing unabated and now includes Asians.[5]

The mean age at diagnosis of diabetes is lower among Maori and Pacific people when compared with Europeans (41 vs. 45 vs. 50 years).[6] However, it is felt that the age at diagnosis is now dropping with increasing numbers of children and adolescents diagnosed with Type 2 diabetes (increasing in the Auckland adolescent diabetes clinic from 12.5% of incident cases 1997–1999 to 35.7% in 2000–2001).[7] Diabetes in pregnancy (particularly gestational diabetes (GDM) and Type 2 diabetes) is also increasing with over doubling of numbers in Auckland, although this is partly due to demographic and possibly screening trends.[8]

Organization of maternity services

New Zealand currently has a socialized healthcare system with no out-of-pocket expenses for public hospital and outpatient services, subsidised visits to primary care and subsidised medications. Care is funded through 21 District Health Boards with varying population sizes. In 1996, New Zealand introduced a lead maternity carer (LMC) system, whereby one health professional is chosen by the woman, with responsibility for assessment of her needs, planning care for mother and baby, and being responsible for ensuring provision of maternity services.[9] Payment by the government-funded health services is the same, independent of profession of the LMC. This system was associated with an increase in the number of self-employed midwives and a reduction in the number of private general practitioner and obstetrician deliveries. Women with diabetes in pregnancy are generally recommended to be referred to a local public diabetes in pregnancy specialist service, although distance and availability can be issues for some women. With referral, particularly if the women is insulin treated, lead care is transferred to specialist services.

The first specific Diabetes in Pregnancy Clinic in New Zealand was established at National Womens Hospital in the 1950s by Wilton Henley and an audit of the clinical work in 1968–1987 was published in 1990. During this period, the perinatal mortality rates fell from 6.7 to 0.5% among women with GDM and 15.2 to 2% among those with established diabetes.[10] A number of innovations were introduced in South Auckland, an area with a high proportion of Maori and Pacific people, after a diabetes in pregnancy clinic was established by Dr David Scott and Mr Bill Mercer in 1982. Dr David Scott was the first in New Zealand to introduce the 50 g polycose glucose challenge test as a screening test in 1983, and community-wide screening for GDM in 1984. The use of the insulin pump in diabetes in pregnancy was also first introduced to New Zealand through South Auckland in 1983. In Type 2 diabetes and GDM, the use of the insulin pump was associated with improvements in glycemic control within 1–4 weeks in 79% of women.[11] A further innovation was the introduction of a combined community and clinic Diabetes Midwifery Educator service in 1991 to combine the skills of the midwife and diabetes educator.[12] This innovation was associated with improvements in glycemia (laboratory 2-h postprandial glucose concentration 6.3 ± 1.3 to 5.7 ± 1.0 mmol/L, P <0.01) and an increase in the proportion starting insulin as an outpatient was increased (from 14 to 89%). The proportion receiving a postnatal oral glucose tolerance test remained low but increased from 10 to 29% (P <0.01).

National Womens Hospital is one of the two coordinating centres in Australia and New Zealand for the MiG study (Metformin in GDM), a randomized trial of metformin compared with insulin use in GDM. Trial results are due in 2007.

The study is partly based on their experience with the use of metformin in 214 Type 2 diabetes in pregnancy.[13] When compared with insulin treated women, those treated with metformin had similar rates of preeclampsia, perinatal loss, and neonatal morbidity.

Criteria for GDM in New Zealand and epidemiology of diabetes in pregnancy

New Zealand currently diagnoses GDM using a 75-g 2-h oral glucose tolerance test. Criteria for GDM are a fasting glucose of >5.5 mmol/L and/or 2-h glucose of >9.0 mmol/L. This is undertaken if there is a high risk of GDM early in pregnancy or after a 50 g glucose challenge test >7.8 mmol/L at 24–28 weeks gestation. These criteria are known as the Australasian Diabetes in Pregnancy Society (ADIPS) New Zealand criteria[14] or New Zealand Society for the Study of Diabetes (NZSSD) criteria.[15] They are more restrictive than the ADIPS Australia criteria (which uses a 2-h post-load level of >8.0 mmol/L): in a United Arab Emirates study,[16] approximately 26–46% fewer cases were diagnosed depending on gestation. While these diagnostic criteria are used throughout New Zealand,[17] there have been differences in perspectives on whether to screen all women for GDM or only those with risk factors. Although ADIPS recommends that all women be offered screening for GDM,[14] until 2006, the New Zealand College of Midwives recommended screening women with risk factors for GDM.[18] There are currently discussions being held about moving to an offer of screening for GDM to all pregnant women.

Penetration of screening has been an issue, making estimates of the prevalence of GDM difficult to make. The prevalence is thought to have increased based upon global trends, the extent of the National Womens Hospital increase in clinic numbers (NWH)[8] and the New Zealand population trends in obesity.[19] Obesity and weight gain are major issues among Maori and Pacific women. For example, cross-sectional data from 4,885 births in South Auckland in 1994[20] showed weight differences between European, Maori, and Pacific women aged <20 years and over 40 years of 6, 11, and 16 kg, respectively (Figure 18.1).

In South Auckland, with a high proportion of Maori and Pacific women, risk factor screening using American Diabetes Association criteria was estimated to have identified 97.9% of women as being at risk.[21] In this setting, development of GDM was also more likely to be associated with twin pregnancies in South Auckland.[22]

The only population based study of GDM screening in New Zealand, adjusting for penetration of screening, came from South Auckland.[20] This study, in the mid 1990s, used ADIPS criteria with prevalences of 3.3, 7.9, 8.1, and 5.5% for Europeans, Maori, Pacific, and Other women, respectively.[20] There were significant ethnic differences in screening (36.8, 47.3, 68.5, 50.0%, respectively), but comparable attendance at OGTT (72.6–81.8%). Among Europeans, there was no significant increase in screening with increasing numbers of risk factors. Recent data suggest that the penetration of screening is approximately 61% based upon the ratio between

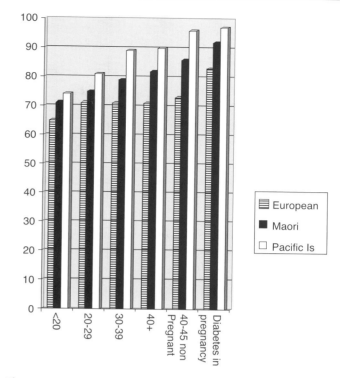

Figure 18.1 Weight at booking in South Auckland by age and ethnicity.

50 g glucose challenge tests and the number of births per annum (Unpublished, Ministry of Health, 2006). Penetration ranges between 20 and 89% depending on district.

No recent prevalence data for diabetes in pregnancy (pre-existing or gestational diabetes) exist. Women of child-bearing age in South Auckland had a prevalence of known diabetes up to 6.8% (Figure 18.2).[23]

Among New Zealand women with existing diabetes, 6% Europeans, 18% Maori, and 16% Pacific women were diagnosed during pregnancy.[6] Those with diabetes diagnosed in pregnancy are over three times more likely to default from both primary and specialist care compared with patients diagnosed in other ways.[24]

Management and outcomes of diabetes in pregnancy

Management guidelines now generally follow those published by ADIPS for either GDM[14] or pre-gestational diabetes.[25]

The importance of pre-conceptual care was audited in the early 1990s from the long-standing Canterbury (New Zealand) insulin-treated register.[26] This cohort includes predominantly European participants with Type 1 diabetes. With an 86% response, all women recognized the importance of good blood glucose control during pregnancy and 69% were using some form of contraception (combined oral contraceptive pill (35%), the progesterone-only pill (12%), condoms (24%), vasectomy (12%), and tubal ligation (12%)).

Outcomes at National Womens Hospital were particularly poor in women with Type 2 diabetes in pregnancy between

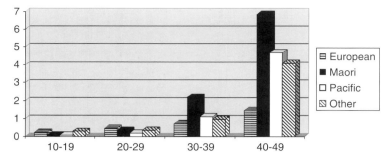

Figure 18.2   Prevalence of known diabetes among women of child-bearing age.

1985 and 1997. The cohort had high rates of perinatal mortality in Type 2 diabetes in pregnancy (46.1/1000), when compared with general rates (12.5/1000), Type 1 diabetes (12.5/1000) and GDM (8.9/1000).[27] Late fetal death (28 weeks gestation to term) was increased 7-fold, with intermediate fetal death (20–28 weeks gestation) and neonatal death increased 2.5-fold. Congenital malformations only accounted for 10% of the perinatal mortality. Those with Type 2 diabetes included women with GDM subsequently found to have diabetes post-natally. One confounding factor in these analyses was the high proportion of Pacific women who have higher rates of late fetal death in the background population.[28] Congenital anomalies were also studied in this cohort with 7.2% of women with Type 1 diabetes having major congenital anomalies, compared with 4.4% of women with known Type 2 diabetes, 4.6% in women with ongoing (Type 2) diabetes after GDM and 0.9% among other women with GDM.[29]

Admission rates to the Neonatal Intensive Care Unit after GDM and Type 2 diabetes in pregnancy at National Womens Hospital were 29 and 40%, respectively.[30] Those admitted had high rates of pre-term delivery (46%), emergency Cesarean section (40%), hypoglycemia (51%) and respiratory distress (40%).

GDM in New Zealand is associated with significant morbidity, partly due to the high proportion of women with likely undiagnosed diabetes, as well as the higher background rates of morbidity among non-European women.[31,32] An audit of all pregnancies complicated by GDM between 1991 and 1994 showed that, post-natally, permanent diabetes was present persisted in 4.3% Europeans, 21.4% Maori, 21.7% Pacific and 12.0% others and a further 4.3, 14.3, 26.7, and 12.0% had IGT or IFG respectively.[31] Ethnic differences were also shown for the age at which GDM was diagnosed (29 ± 5 vs. 31 ± 7 vs. 32 ± 5 vs. 30 ± 5 years), smoking rates (24.6, 63.2, 15.2, 2.4%), previous GDM rates (19.3, 34.2, 35.4, 16.7%) and gestation at booking (13 vs. 18 vs. 19 vs. 12 weeks) but not at referral to the diabetes in pregnancy service. Maori, Pacific and other patients had higher fasting glucose concentrations at diagnosis. Birthweight was higher among Pacific patients, whose babies were also more likely to have neonatal hypoglycemia <1.6 mmol/L. Neonatal hypoglycemia was related to fasting glucose at diagnosis, mean antenatal fingerprick glucose and a history of previous GDM. There were no ethnic differences in induction rates (34.2%), neonatal unit admission (27.1%), Cesarean section rates (16.7–22.4%) or insulin use (42.1–61.6%).

The determinants of birthweight among European, Maori, and Pacific women have been investigated in two studies. At National Women's Hospital between 1987 and 1989,[33] the birthweights of babies from women with GDM, pre-gestatational diabetes and control women were found to be related to pre-pregnancy body mass index, cigarette smoking, height, weight gain, and hypertension, but neither ethnicity nor fructosamine. In contrast, among women without GDM in South Auckland in 1994–1995,[34] large babies (4+ kg) were most common among Pacific people and less common among Maori (24.3, 8.9 vs. 18.8%) among Europeans. Birthweight increased significantly with maternal weight in all ethnic groups. Smoking and being Maori were independently associated with smaller babies (58.1% Maori women being smokers vs. <30% in the other ethnic groups). Across the groups, a 1-h 50-g glucose challenge test result 5.2–6.2 mmol/L was associated with 54% more large babies, and >6.3 mmol/L was associated with over double the number of large babies, this association was strongest with Pacific women.

Only one study of breastfeeding among women with diabetes in pregnancy has been undertaken in New Zealand.[35] Breastfeeding rates at discharge among women with GDM were 84.0% compared with 69.0% among women with Type 2 diabetes. The main influences on breastfeeding on discharge were breastfeeding as the initial feeding method, APGAR score, admission to baby unit and Cesarean section. There were no significant ethnic differences in breastfeeding rates.

Long-term outcomes

No prospective follow up study of women with past GDM has yet been published. A median 6-year follow-up of 14 women with diabetic nephropathy after pregnancy showed significant morbidity particularly progression to renal replacement therapy in 36%.[32]

Inter-generational effects of diabetes in pregnancy have been researched in a number of ways.

Possible ethnic differences in predisposition to Type 2 diabetes have been shown from studies of umbilical cord blood and neonatal anthropometry. The first study from 401 women showed that both Pacific and Maori babies had higher cord fructosamine concentrations than European babies.[36] However, Pacific Island babies were also heavier, and had higher cord insulin concentrations and subscapular skinfold thickness than European babies.[36] A subsequent study of 123 normal pregnancies showed that Polynesian babies had a higher cord insulin: C-peptide ratio than European women[37] in the setting of greater maternal obesity and marginally elevated (but 'normal') maternal glycemia. Umbilical cord insulin was associated with higher neonatal blood pressure:[38] the reasons for this remain unclear, although it may reflect associations underlying the metabolic syndrome.

Umbilical cord leptin concentration are also higher among Polynesians compared with Europeans and South Asians and those from pregnancies complicated by GDM and Type 2 diabetes.[39,40] There were no ethnic differences in cord SHBG, sex hormones, or IGF-I, although pregnancies complicated by diabetes are associated with higher IGF-I levels.[41] It was postulated that Polynesians and offspring of women with GDM have leptin resistance at birth, the latter possibly due to fuel-mediated teratogenesis affecting the adipo-insular axis.[42]

A 2 year 8 month follow-up of the babies from this study showed that the adiposity of the offspring was correlated with maternal pre-pregnancy weight and maternal serum triglyceride concentration but not ethnicity (except that South Asian children experienced faster weight gain than other ethnic groups).[43]

A household prevalence study of known diabetes among 55,518 residents found that those with Type 2 diabetes were more likely to have a diabetic mother than father (Europeans, 21.7 vs. 9.9%; Maori, 17.6 vs. 11.4%; Pacific Islands, 15.7 vs. 5.3%).[34] Adjusting for ethnicity, diabetic women with past diabetes in pregnancy were 2.05 times as likely to have diabetic offspring as women who had not had diabetes in pregnancy. However, a follow up study of twenty-seven 5–10-year-old offspring of women with Type 1 or Type 2 diabetes reported no influence of intra-uterine hyperglycaemia on alterations in glucose regulation, but did not adjust for ethnic differences in the proportions in the different groups.[44]

Conclusion

New Zealand is facing an growing number of women with diabetes in pregnancy as a result of demographic shifts, growing obesity and particularly the increasing numbers of non-European women developing GDM and Type 2 diabetes at a younger age. Research among New Zealand Asian women is sparse, but Maori and Pacific women experience poorer outcomes, partly as a result of longer (and often pre-gestational) fetal exposure to hyperglycemia and maternal obesity. Of greatest concern is the growing evidence that the offspring of these women are at high risk of future diabetes and obesity.

REFERENCES

1. 2001 New Zealand Census. www.stats.govt.nz [Accessed 26 September 2006].
2. Prior IAM. A health survey in a rural Maori community with particular emphasis on the cardiovascular, nutritional and metabolic findings. NZ Med J 1962; 61: 333.
3. Ostbye T, Welby TJ, Prior IAM, Salmond CE, Stokes YM. Type 2 (non-insulin-dependent) diabetes mellitus, migration and westernisation: The Tokelau Island Migrant study. Diabetologia 1989; 32: 585–90.
4. Simmons D. Diabetes and its complications in New Zealand: an epidemiological perspective. NZ Med J 2000; 113: 42–3.
5. Joshy G. Simmons D. Epidemiology of diabetes in New Zealand: revisit to a changing landscape. NZ Med J 2006; 119: U2003.
6. Simmons D, Gatland BA, Leakehe L, Fleming C. Ethnic differences in diabetes care in a multiethnic community in New Zealand. Diabetes Res Clin Pract 1996; 34(suppl.): S89–S93.
7. Hotu S, Carter B, Watson PD, Cutfield WS, Cundy T. Increasing prevalence of type 2 diabetes in adolescents. J Paediatr Child Health 2004; 40: 201–4.
8. National Women's Annual Clinical Report 2005. National Women's Health, Auckland District Health Board.
9. Ministry of Health. Health and Disability Services Act, Section 51. Ministry of Health, Wellington, New Zealand, 1993.
10. Roberts AB, Pattison NS. Pregnancy in women with diabetes mellitus, twenty years experience: 1968–1987. NZ Med J 1990; 103: 211–3.
11. Simmons D, Thompson CF, Conroy C, Scott DJ. Use of insulin pumps in pregnancies complicated by type 2 diabetes and gestational diabetes in a multiethnic community. Diabetes Care 2001; 24: 2078–82.
12. Simmons D, Conroy C, Scott DJ. Impact of a diabetes midwifery educator on the diabetes in pregnancy service at Middlemore Hospital. Prac Diab Int 2001; 18: 119–22.
13. Hughes RC, Rowan JA. Pregnancy in women with Type 2 diabetes: who takes metformin and what is the outcome? Diabet Med 2006; 23: 318–22.
14. Hoffman L, Nolan C, Wilson JD, Oats JJN, Simmons D. Gestational diabetes mellitus – management guidelines. The Australasian Diabetes in Pregnancy Society. Med J Aust 1998; 169: 93–7.
15. Colman PG, Thomas DW, Zimmet PZ, et al. New classification and criteria for diagnosis of diabetes mellitus. Position Statement from the Australian Diabetes Society, New Zealand Society for the Study of Diabetes, Royal College of Pathologists of Australasia and Australasian Association of Clinical Biochemists. Med J Aust 1999; 170: 375–8.
16. Agarwal MM, Dhatt GS, Punnose J, Koster G. Gestational diabetes: dilemma caused by multiple international diagnostic criteria. Diabet Med 2005; 22: 1731–6.
17. Cutchie W, Simmons D, Cheung NW. Comparison of international and New Zealand guidelines for the care of pregnant women with diabetes. Diabet Med 2006; 23: 460–8.
18. New Zealand College of Midwives. Gestational diabetes: NZCoM Consensus statement. Christchurch, New Zealand: NZCoM; 1996 (updated 2002).
19. Ministry of Health. Tracking the obesity epidemic – Public Health Intelligence Occasional Bulletin No 24. Wellington: MOH; 2004.
20. Yapa M, Simmons D. Screening for gestational diabetes mellitus in a multiethnic population in New Zealand. Diabetes Res Clin Pract 2000; 48: 217–23.
21. Simmons D. Gestational diabetes mellitus: growing consensus on management but not diagnosis. NZ Med J 1999; 112: 45–6.
22. Simmons D, Yapa M. Association between twin pregnancy and hyperglycemia in a multi-ethnic community in New Zealand. Diabetes Care 2002; 25: 934–5.
23. Simmons D, Harry T, Gatland B. Prevalence of known diabetes in different ethnic groups in inner urban South Auckland. NZ Med J 1999; 112: 316–9.
24. Simmons D, Fleming C. Prevalence and characteristics of diabetic patients with no ongoing care in South Auckland. Diabetes Care 2000; 23: 1791–3.
25. McElduff A, Cheung NW, McIntyre HD, et al. The Australasian Diabetes in Pregnancy Society consensus guidelines for the management of patients with type 1 and type 2 diabetes in relation to pregnancy. Med J Aust 2005; 183: 373–7.
26. Gibb D, Hockey S, Brown LJ, Lunt H. Attitudes and knowledge regarding contraception and prepregnancy counselling in insulin dependent diabetes. NZ Med J 1994; 107: 484–6.
27. Cundy T, Gamble G, Townend K, et al. Perinatal mortality in Type 2 diabetes mellitus. Diabet Med 2000; 17: 33–9.
28. Craig ED, Mantell CD, Ekeroma AJ, Stewart AW, Mitchell EA. Ethnicity and birth outcome: New Zealand trends 1980–2001.

Part 1. Introduction, methods, results and overview. Aust NZ J Obstet Gynaecol 2004; 44: 530–6.

29. Farrell T, Neale L, Cundy T. Congenital anomalies in the offspring of women with type 1, type 2 and gestational diabetes. Diabet Med 2002; 19: 322–6.

30. Watson D, Rowan J, Neale L, Battin MR. Admissions to neonatal intensive care unit following pregnancies complicated by gestational or type 2 diabetes. Aust NZ J Obstet Gynaecol 2003; 43: 429–32.

31. Simmons D, Thompson CF, Conroy C. Incidence and risk factors for neonatal hypoglycaemia among women with gestational diabetes mellitus in South Auckland. Diabet Med 2000; 17: 830–4.

32. Bagg W, Neale L, Henley P, MacPherson P, Cundy T. Long-term maternal outcome after pregnancy in women with diabetic nephropathy. 2003; 116: U566.

33. Cundy T, Gamble G, Manuel A, Townend K, Roberts A. Determinants of birth-weight in women with established and gestational diabetes. Aust NZ J Obstet Gynaecol 1993; 3: 249–54.

34. Simmons D. Relationship between maternal glycaemia and birthweight among glucose tolerant women from different ethnic groups in New Zealand. Diabet Med.

35. Simmons D, Conroy C, Thompson CF. In-hospital breast feeding rates among women with gestational diabetes and pregestational Type 2 diabetes in South Auckland. Diabet Med 2005; 22: 177–81.

36. Simmons D, Baker J, James A, Roberts A. Has the process causing noninsulin dependent diabetes start at birth? Evidence in neonates from a population with a high prevalence of diabetes. NZ Med J 1992; 105: 326–8.

37. Simmons D. Differences in umbilical cord insulin and birth weight in non-diabetic pregnancies of women from different ethnic groups in New Zealand. Diabetologia 1994; 37: 930–6.

38. Simmons D. Association between neonatal blood pressure and umbilical cord insulin concentration. Diabet Med 1997; 14: 196–9.

39. Simmons D, Breier BH. Fetal overnutrition in polynesian pregnancies and in gestational diabetes may lead to dysregulation of the adipoinsular axis in offspring. Diabetes Care 2002; 25: 1539–44.

40. Westgate JA, Lindsay RS, Beattie J, et al. Hyperinsulinemia in cord blood in mothers with type 2 diabetes and gestational diabetes in New Zealand. Diabetes Care 2006; 29: 1345–50.

41. Simmons D. Interrelation between umbilical cord serum sex hormones, sex hormone-binding globulin, insulin-like growth factor I, and insulin in neonates from normal pregnancies and pregnancies complicated by diabetes. J Clin Endocrinol Metab 1995; 80: 2217–21.

42. Robertson SP, Simmons D. Early childhood growth in ethnic groups predisposed to NIDDM: a prospective study. Diabetes Res Clin Pract 1998; 40: 137–43.

43. Simmons D, Gatland BA, Leakehe L, Fleming C. Frequency of diabetes in family members of probands with non-insulin-dependent diabetes mellitus. J Intern Med 1995; 237: 315–21.

44. Hunter WA, Cundy T, Rabone D, et al. Insulin sensitivity in the offspring of women with type 1 and type 2 diabetes. Diabetes Care 2004; 27: 1148–52.

19 Gestational diabetes in China

Tao Duan

Introduction

Gestational diabetes mellitus (GDM) was classified as an independent type of DM by WHO in 1979, but it was still a rare disease in China at that time and was not taught at medical schools. GDM was first listed as an independent chapter in Chinese textbooks of obstetrics and gynecology in 1980. Before then, very few papers were published about the disease.

The incidence of GDM in China

Descriptions of DM can be seen in ancient literatures from China, India, Egypt, Greece, and Rome, although it is not necessarily the same as the 'DM' we are talking about today. In the last two decades, the Chinese economy has developed rapidly, and the disease profile of Chinese people has changed greatly because of the new way of life. Diseases due to malnutrition and infection have been greatly reduced, while cancer and chronic diseases such as cardiovascular diseases and DM are now major health problems. According to data from 1996, the incidence of DM and impaired glucose tolerance in the Chinese population above 20 years of age were 3.2 and 4.8%, respectively, and is almost 10% in large cities such as Beijing and Shanghai. The incidence of DM increased dramatically from early 1980s to the mid 1990s, and the number of DM patients increased four to five times during that period, reaching 30–40 million. The total number of Chinese people with abnormal blood glucose is now about 100 million (Table 19.1).

In China, screening for GDM was first started in 1980. Prior to this time, the reported incidence was very low (0.24%). In the past 10 years, although screening has been carried out in most large Chinese cities, this is not the case for small cities and rural areas. China is such a big country, and the income, way of life, and food habits vary greatly. Additionally, the standards for screening and diagnosis of GDM are also different, so the reported incidence of GDM also varies greatly. There is no reported incidence of GDM for whole China, only the incidence for different regions. In Shanghai, the incidence of GDM is 2.88% (ADA), 3.86–5.33% for Beijing, 2.1% (WHO) and 3.8% (NDDG) for Tianjin.

The incidence of GDM is also different for the different ethnic groups in China; even in Asia, it varies from region to region. Although it is found that Chinese women are at high risk for GDM, the reported incidence of GDM is only 0.6% in Taiwan and 2.2% for South Korea; all values are lower than those for mainland China.

The pathogenesis and mechanism of GDM

In the last 5 years, many researches have been done to explore the pathogenesis and mechanism of GDM in China. Lao from Hong Kong reported that α-thalassemia, high hemoglobin, elevated blood–iron concentration in late pregnancy, and HBsAg carriers could increase the risk for GDM and so Chinese women are at high risk for GDM. Zhang from Beijing reported the close relationship between family history of DM, GDM, and GIGT, especially the strong relationship between DM of a mother and GDM of her daughter. Ying from Shanghai reported that the unsaturated fatty acid content in lipocyte membrane of GDM patients is lower than that of normal pregnant women, and the saturated fatty acid content in lipocyte membrane of GDM patients is higher than that of normal pregnant women. Li from Guangzhou analyzed the genotype of HLA-2DRB1 in GDM patients, and found that the frequency of HLA-2DRB1 34 is higher in patients of GDM and GIGT.

Table 19.1 Incidence of diabetes mellitus (DM) in the Chinese population

Year	DM (%)	Impaired glucose tolerance (%)
1980	1.00	–
1989	2.02	2.95
1994	2.51	3.20
1996	3.21	4.8
2002	4–5	–

Standards for screening and diagnosis of GDM

In the last decades, the incidence of GDM has been increasing gradually in China, but it varies from region to region. One of the main reasons for the difference is the standard of diagnosing GDM: everyone has his or her own reason to use ADA or NDDG or WHO standard. There are two different opinions regarding the standard of diagnosing GDM: one group of doctors insists on having only one official standard for the sake of convenience; the other group wishes to wait and compare the effectiveness of different standards, and to try to select the best for the Chinese population. Some doctors have even tried to suggest a real Chinese standard, because they think ADA, NDDG, and WHO standards are not based on the Chinese population. The newly formed Chinese GDM working group is now trying to set up a national standard for the screening and diagnosis of GDM in China.

In her study, Yang from Beijing suggested that the 3-h glucose test could be saved without affecting the final result of OGTT, and if an OGTT 2 h glucose >6.7 mmol/L is used as the cut-off value for GIGT, the incidence of GIGT will be increased greatly, so its feasibility as a cut-off value should be studied further. After careful study of the perinatal outcomes, Wu from Beijing suggested that the 50-g glucose screening test should be best done early in pregnancy, i.e. by 12–14 weeks, as well as later in pregnancy, i.e. by 28 weeks.

The effect of GDM on maternal complications and perinatal outcomes

Many researches have shown that if GDM is managed properly, the incidence of maternal and fetal complications could be reduced significantly. Yang from Beijing reported that, in their series of GDM patients, only the incidence of pre-eclampsia, macrosomia, and neonatal erythrocytosis were higher than those of euglycemic pregnant women. This might not be the case in small cities and rural areas where GDM screening is still not carried out; undetected GDM might lead to severe maternal, fetal, and neonatal complications. Diabetes is only diagnosed when maternal diabetic ketoacidosis or fetal death occurred. This scenario will not change until the importance of GDM is recognized by more obstetricians and there is universal screening for GDM throughout China, so that GDM patients are diagnosed and managed properly.

Management of GDM

The goal of managing GDM is to achieve euglycemia or almost euglycemia. If this could be done, the maternal and perinatal outcomes will be as good as that of the normal pregnant women. Just like in diabetes of nonpregnant women, the management of GDM includes nutritional management, exercise, and medical treatment; the importance of glucose monitoring can not be over-emphasized.

Nutritional management

Dietary control is very important not only for GDM patients, but also for normal pregnant women. The incidence of macrosomia is about 5–10% in most Chinese hospitals. If GDM is not detected and managed properly, the incidence of macrosomia could be as high as 50%. But if dietary control is carried out strictly, most patients do not need insulin therapy and the incidence of macrosomia could be greatly reduced. The ideal dietary control should provide the necessary nutrition to both mother and fetus, achieve well-controlled glucose levels, and avoid hypoglycemia and ketosis. The ideal body weight (IBW = height − 100) should be calculated first, and the daily calorie requirement is calculated according to the standard of 30–35 kcal/kg. The proportions of carbohydrate, protein, and fat are 40–50, 25–30, and 25–30%, respectively. In order to counter-balance the effects of day and night fluctuation of anti-insulin hormones of pregnant women, GDM patients are advised to have five meals a day. The proportion of calories should be divided reasonably, breakfast 10%, lunch 30%, dinner 30%, and 10% for three snacks. Vitamin E and unsaturated fatty acid are also recommended in the diet to against the possible teratogenic effect of free radicals caused by GDM.

The problem of clinical nutrition in China is that we do not have sufficient well-trained, qualified dietitians and dietary control can not be carried out as well as we wish. The average birthweight of Chinese newborn is around 3200–3400 g,which is much heavier than the average birthweight of Japanese newborns (3000 g).

Medical treatment

The most commonly used drug is recombinant human insulin.

Exercise

Proper exercise could help to control the glucose level of GDM patients, because it is believed that exercise could increase the sensitivity of peripheral tissues to insulin. Some Chinese hospitals already ask GDM patients to exercise, especially the upper limbs. Because most Chinese doctors and patients are somewhat conservative about exercise during pregnancy, there is still a long way to go before the value of exercise is widely accepted by GDM patients in China.

Follow-up of GDM after delivery

GDM patients are encouraged to breast feed their babies after delivery. Patients receiving insulin could benefit more from breast feeding because the dosage of insulin could be reduced after breast feeding. Breast-fed babies could also benefit as the incidence of Type 2 DM is lower in breast fed babies when they grow up. More and more Chinese doctors are becoming aware of the importance of breast feeding in GDM patients, the rate of breast feeding in GDM patients has been increasing steadily.

About 30% of GDM patients will still have persistent abnormal glucose tolerance after delivery and some will eventually develope Type 2 DM. So it is recommended that 75-g OGTT should be done 6–8 weeks after delivery or after breast feeding ceases. For women with a history of GDM, a low-dose oral contraceptive is not a contraindication.

A multicenter study to follow up the outcomes of GDM after delivery has just started in China, but it will be many years before the final results are available.

Shanghai model of managing diabetes during pregnancy

One general hospital in Shanghai has been selected as the referral center for diabetes (including GDM) during pregnancy for the whole Shanghai area. This center is also responsible for setting up guidelines, coordinating clinical trials, and collecting data. It is hoped that, by doing so, GDM can be studied and managed more efficiently.

Perspectives

GDM study group

The GDM study group of the Chinese Perinatal Society was established in April 2005, and the first meeting has been held. The group's aims are to:

- Disseminate knowledge of GDM throughout China and encourage more doctors to screen, diagnose, manage, and follow-up the disease
- Encourage more hospitals to become involved in the study and management of GDM
- Organize multicenter clinical trials and training concerning GDM
- Organize national meetings to discuss aspects of GDM
- Establish a network of cooperation about managing GDM

The e-mail address of the group is gdm2005_china@yahoo.com.cn, and a website will soon be established.

Clinical guideline

In the future, a clinical guideline about GDM will be written by the group. However, one guideline is not enough for China, because the medical conditions and levels of doctors in China are so 'heterogeneous'! In large Chinese cites, the average GDP per capita is around 8000–10,000 US dollars, while in poor western China, the average GDP per capita is only around 700–800 US dollars, which is almost the same level as in some African countries. Therefore, one clinical guideline is theoretically not acceptable for this scenario. One practical way of solving this problem is to have two versions of the clinical guidelines: the 'standard version' for big hospitals, and a 'basic version' for the other hospitals.

REFERENCES

1. Sun WJ, Gao XL. Meeting summary of 1st national congress of GDM. Chinese J Perinat Med 2005; 8: 324–5.
2. Lao ZX, Ma JM. GDM – The risk factors of Chinese women and long term effects. Chinese J Perinat Med 2005; 8: 321–3.
3. Yang HX. The epidemiology of GDM. Chinese J Gen Pract 2005; 4: 453–5.
4. Ying H, Wang DF, et al. The relationship between fatty acid composition of adipose cell membrane and insulin resistance. Curr Adv Obstet Gynecol 2004; 13: 8–10.
5. Ying H, Wang DF, et al. Effects of dietary fat on onset of gestational diabetes mellitus. Chinese J Obstet Gynecol 2006; 41: 729–31.
6. Shen YH, Chen X, et al. The descriptive analysis of the neonatal birth weight of 18 counties in the Jiangsu and Zhejiang provinces in China. Chinese J Perinat Med 2003; 6: 229–32.
7. Yang HX, Zhou SM. The clinical analysis of maternal and perinatal prognosis of GDM. Chinese J Obstet Gynecol 1993; 28: 139–41.

20 Diabetes and pregnancy in Japan

Yasue Omori

Introduction

The history of diabetes and pregnancy started in Europe and the USA after the discovery of insulin in 1921 and Japan followed about 30 years later. However, until the 1960s, Japan had very few diabetic young women and generally doctors advised them not to become pregnant. In those days, our medical schools taught students that diabetic patients should not become pregnant because of the high risks attached. If women became pregnant and the presence of diabetes was not diagnosed, it was considered possible that stillborn babies would result. Therefore, doctors strongly encouraged pregnant diabetic patients to abort their pregnancies.

However, during the mid 1960s clinical research into diabetes and pregnancy began in Japan. Since then, diabetic patients have been well informed by their doctors and the media that it is safe to become pregnant.

Young Japanese diabetics are mainly Type 2

As I have reported from time to time, Japanese diabetes is predominantly Type 2. This also applies to juvenile onset diabetes. Figure 20.1 shows the chronological change of pregnant diabetics treated by myself from the first delivery of diabetic pregnant women in Tokyo Women's Medical University from 1964 until my retirement in 1997.

This figure demonstrates two characteristics of pregnant diabetics. Firstly, there is a drastic increase of the number of diabetic pregnant women since the 1960s. Secondly, it indicates that the number of Type 2 diabetic pregnant women is greater than Type 1. In the Diabetes Center of Tokyo Women's Medical University (TWMU), Type 1 diabetic pregnant women constituted 32.3% of the total. This was made possible by the rigid supervision of the diabetologists for children of the hospital. However, generally, there is 95% Type 2 diabetic women and only 5% Type 1 throughout Japan.

Figure 20.2 shows the type of diabetes diagnosed before the age of 30 at the Diabetes Center of TWMU from 1960 to 2004.[1] A total number of 4063 patients were used for this data. There were 1746 Type 1 and 2317 Type 2 patients. It demonstrates the characteristics of Japanese young patients. The number of

Type 1 diabetic patients decrease until the age of 30, and the incidence of diabetes in girls is higher than boys.

Type 2 diabetic patients can be detected in children from as early as 1 year, and the number of patients increases as they grow older. Males are more affected than females. Laakso, from Finland, considered that the number of Type 2 diabetic patients increases from 30 years of age.[2]

The above findings clearly indicate that juvenile onset diabetes differs between ethnic groups. Research by Ogata et al. confirms the findings of the Asian group in The SEARCH for Diabetes in Youth.[3]

Incidence of deliveries from women with abnormal carbohydrate metabolism throughout Japan

In 1971, I started to survey the status of diabetes and pregnancy throughout Japan every 5 years. This research is still being carried out by appointed members of the Japanese Association of Diabetes and Pregnancy. The classification of the type of diabetes in the survey by questionnaire was difficult due to the lack of knowledge of the disease by the doctor respondents. Therefore, pregnant women with abnormal carbohydrate metabolism are included in Type 1, Type 2, and gestational diabetes in Table 20.1.

The incidences of deliveries from women with abnormal carbohydrate metabolism throughout Japan from 1996 to 2002 have increased from 0.55 to 0.87%.[4] The number of both GDM and prediabetic women are increasing year by year. Diagnosis of GDM was used as a diagnostic criterion in Japan.[5]

Special problems of Type 2 diabetic pregnant women based on a nationwide survey

In the first survey from 1971 to 1975, perinatal mortality was very high (10.8%), although the number of deliveries from pregnant diabetic women was very few.[6] Throughout Japan, diabetes control was not good, therefore the mortality rate,

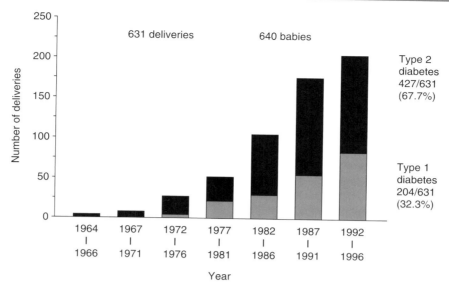

Figure 20.1 Chronological change of pregnant diabetics 1964.2-1996.12 Diabetes Center. Tokyo Women's Medical College.

including intrauterine death, was very high. However, 20 years later in the fifth survey conducted from1991to 1995, it had decreased to 2.2% (Figure 20.3). Moreover, in the sixth survey from 1996 to 2002, perinatal mortality rate improved to 0.7%.[4] This is believed to be a result of disseminating the information that normalizing blood glucose was important.

In contrast, the rate of congenital malformations has remained basically unchanged staying around 6% between the time of the first survey to the fifth survey. In the sixth survey, the congenital malformation rate from diabetic mothers whose type of diabetes could be determined was 5.2% in children from both Type 1 and Type 2 diabetic mothers.

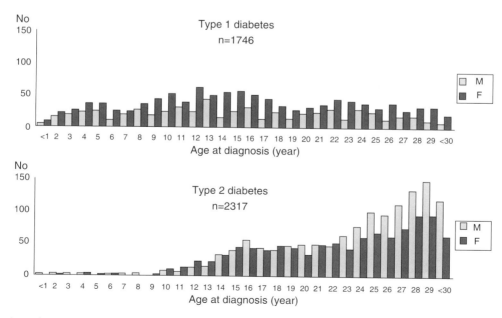

Figure 20.2 Number of patients with T1D and T2D diagnosed before the age of 30. Diabetes Center, TWMU, 1960–2004: Ogawa Y, Unchigata Y, et al., Diabetes Care 2007; 30(5) e30.

Table 20.1   The number of incidences of deliveries from women with abnormal carbohydrate metabolism throughout Japan 1996 – 2002

Year	Total No. of deliveries	Women with abnormal carb. metab.	Incidence
1996	100.213 (cases)	547 (cases)	0.55 (%)
1997	101.785	615	0.60
1998	107.066	698	0.65
1999	105.765	734	0.69
2000	110.728	822	0.74
2001	108.331	882	0.81
2002	106.539	936	0.87
Total	740.427	5.224	0.70

By Working group (M. Sanaka, N. Toyota et al.) of Japanese Association of Diabetes and Pregnancy.

There is a relationship between congenital malformation rate and HbA1c levels by 10 weeks of gestation.[4] When HbA1c levels are more than 8%, the congenital malformation rate increases greatly. Based on my experience in the Diabetes Center of TWMU the congenital malformation rate of children from pregnant diabetic women diagnosed during pregnancy was 12.7%.[7]

It had been reported that the formation of congenital abnormalities of children from diabetic mothers is complete until 7 weeks of gestation.[8]

Steel et al.[9] and Fuhrman et al.[10] reported that congenital malformations could be prevented by pre-pregnancy management. Despite insistence upon the importance of planned pregnancy, some pregnancies occur and diabetes remains undetected or, in the worst cases, patients with bad control are referred only after pregnancy.

The chronological changes in pre-pregnancy management in patients I have treated at the Diabetes Center of TWMU are shown in Figure 20.4. The rate of pre-pregnancy management was around 70% in Type 1 diabetics, and 40% in Type 2 diabetics and the rate has not changed since then.

Although a high rate of congenital malformations in newborns from diabetic mothers still exists and is still a big problem, nowadays, advances in medical treatment ensure that diabetic women never have to experience the grief of losing their unborn babies.

Through these data, special problems of Type 2 diabetic pregnant women were identified as:

* First diagnosis of diabetes at pregnancy: the diabetes is undiagnosed and untreated until pregnancy.

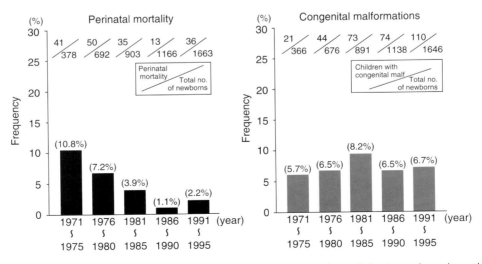

Figure 20.3   Perinatal mortality and Congenital malformations among newborns from diabetic mothers throughout Japan

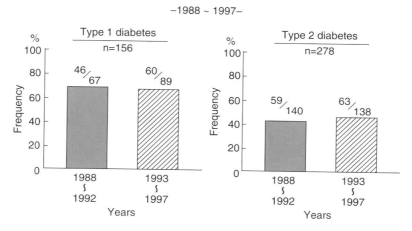

Figure 20.4   Comparison of Prepregnancy Management of Type 1 and Type 2 Diabetic Pregnant Women

- Diabetic pregnant women with microangiopathy: formation of diabetic complications takes a long time; even so, there are some pregnant women with retinopathy or nephropathy.
- Diabetic complications affect mother and fetus.
- The number of patients with GDM, including Type 2 diabetic women, is still increasing.

Diabetic retinopathy or nephropathy during pregnancy

According to my experiences at the Diabetes Center of TWMU, 12.7% of pregnant diabetic women diagnosed during pregnancy had simple retinopathy and 4.2% had proliferative retinopathy (Table 20.2).[7] Fortunately, treatment for retinopathy has advanced remarkably.

However, nephropathy continues to be a serious problem. I treated diabetic pregnant women with nephropathy at the Diabetes Center of TWMU from 1964 to 1996. There were 13 deliveries out of 631 and only 2.1% had nephropathy. Their incidence is not significantly different. Six (2.9%) were Type 1 and seven (1.6%) were Type 2 diabetics.

The clinical features of 13 patients were very severe. All had background or proliferative retinopathy and their HbA1c levels were almost all high when they were referred to our hospital. Their pregnancy could not continue to full term and birthweight of the newborn was low. Prognosis after delivery was very serious.

A comparison of incidences of diabetic pregnant women with nephropathy was made. During my 32 years at the

Table 20.2   Congenital malformations and diabetic retinopathy among GDM patients and pregnant diabetics diagnosed during pregnancy

	Diabetes Center, Tokyo women's Medical University			
	Cases	Congenital malformations 104 deliveries 105 babies	Simple retinopathy	Proliferative retinopathy
GDM	104/1571 (6.6%)	2/105 (1.9%)	0	0
		71 deliveries 71 babies		
Pregnant diabetic women diagnosed during pregnancy	71/1571 (4.5%)	9/71 (12.7%)	9/71 (12.7%)	3/71 (4.2%)

by Omori

Table 20.3 Incidence of diabetic pregnant women with nephropathy

	Diabetes Center, Tokyo Women's Medical Univ.		
	Feb. 1964 ~ Dec. 1996 over a 32-year period	Jan. 1997 ~ Dec. 2003 *Over a 7-Year period	
Type 1	6/204 (2.9%)	12/185 (6.5%)	
Type 2	7/427 (1.6%)	9/133 (6.8%)	
Total	13/631 deliv. (2.1%)	21/318 (6.6%)	

*Sanaka M. et. al., JDP 6 (1) 127 – 135, 2007.

Diabetes Center of TWMU only 2.1% of my patients had nephropathy. In contrast, a more recent study conducted by my colleagues for a period of 7 years from 1997 to 2003, showed that there was 6.6% of patients with nephropathy (Table 20.3).[11]

The following reasons may in one way or another have contributed to the increase of diabetic pregnant women with nephropathy: (1) their diabetes may have not been treated until pregnancy; or (2) treatment may have been discontinued sometimes; or (3) perhaps the patients had been treated by physicians who did not specialize in diabetes.

A clinical research related to nephropathy was performed by Yokoyama, one of my colleagues at the TWMU.[12] Cumulative incidences of diabetic nephropathy in early onset Type 1 and Type 2 diabetic patients is shown in Figure 20.5. He compared the incidence of diabetic nephropathy between Type 1 and Type 2 diabetics during four periods.

From 1965 to 1984, medical treatment for Type 1 diabetes became more advanced. Consequently, incidences of diabetic nephropathy in early onset Type 1 diabetic patients decreased. In contrast, with the same advanced medical treatment, incidences of diabetic nephropathy in early onset Type 2 diabetic patients has not changed, even in more recent years.

Based on the result of the study, we can speculate that Type 2 diabetes may be more prone to microangiopathy, and the development of nephropathy may be influenced by the lack of a diagnosis of the disease over a long time. Additionally, discontinuing treatment may also have contributed to the results of the study.

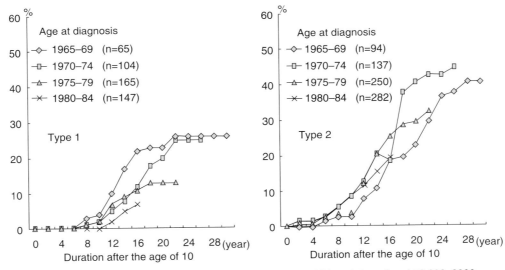

Yokoyama H, et al., Kidney International 58:302, 2000.

Figure 20.5 Cumulative incidence of diabetic nephropathy in early onset Type 1 and Type 2 diabetes patients

Differences between Type 1 and Type 2 diabetic pregnancies

I observed differences between Type 1 and Type 2 diabetic women and compared BMIs before pregnancy, family history, insulin requirement during pregnancy, weeks at delivery, neonatal birthweight, and neonatal complications.[13] I found no obvious differences. The following points should be noted in relation to treatment.

In Type 1 diabetic pregnant women:

- Duration from onset of disease to pregnancy is long. If disease control is poor, there are many cases with retinopathy or nephropathy.
- The requirement for insulin during pregnancy is greater than for nonpregnant women.
- Major malformation is predominant in congenital malformations.
- Fulminant-type diabetes which was discovered in Japan relates to pregnancy.[14]

In Type 2 diabetic pregnant women:

- The time of onset is unclear.
- Sometimes diabetes is detected at the first pregnancy, and there are pregnant women with retinopathy or nephropathy.
- GDM will develop to Type 2 diabetes.

Treatment for Type 1 and Type 2 diabetes in pregnant women is the same, although treatment of pregnant women with Type 2 diabetes is easier than Type 1. Insulin secretion in the Type 1 diabetic patients is non-existent, but some secretion remains in Type 2 diabetic patients.

Conclusion

In countries where Type 2 diabetes is dominant, even juvenile diabetics, detection of diabetes before pregnancy should be practised in order to prevent complications for a mother and fetus before and during pregnancy.

REFERENCES

1. Ogawa Y, Uchigata Y, Otani T, Iwamoto Y. Proportion of Diabetes type in early-onset diabetes in Japan. Diabetes Care 2007; 30: e30.
2. Laakso M, Pyorala K. Age of onset and type of diabetes. Diabetes Care 1085; 8: 114–7.
3. SEARCH for Diabetes in Youth Study Group: The burden of diabetes mellitus among US youth: SEARCH for Diabetes in Youth study. Pediatrics 2006; 118: 1510–8.
4. Sanaka M, Toyoda N, et al. Working group of Japanese Association of Diabetes and Pregnancy. Summary of national survey of glucose intolerance during pregnancy in Japan. J Japan Soc Diabetes Pregnancy 2005; 5: 37–41.
5. Sugawa T, Takagi S. Report of the Committee for Nutrition and Metabolism: the Japan Society of Gynecology and Obstetrics. A proposal of a guideline for the diagnosis of glucose intolerance particularly of gestational diabetes mellitus. J Japan Soc Gynecol Obstet 1984; 36: 2055–8.
6. Omori Y. Current Status of Diabetes and Pregnancy throughout Japan – 1971–1995. Diabetes Frontier 1999; 10(5), P664:671.
7. Omori Y. Classification of diabetic pregnancy. In: Hod M, Jovanovic L, Di Renzo GC, de Leiva A, O Langer O, eds. Textbook of Diabetes and Pregnancy. London: Martin Dunitz, Taylor & Francis; 2003, pp. 158–67.
8. Mills JL, Baker L, Gordman AS. Malformation in infants of diabetic mothers occur before the seventh gestational week. Implications for treatment. Diabetes 1979; 28: 292–3.
9. Steel JM, Johnstone FD, Smith AF, Duncan LJP. Five years experience of a "prepregnancy" clinic for insulin- dependent diabetics. Br Med J 1982; 285: 353–6.
10. Fuhrmann K, Reiher H, Semmler K, et al. Prevention of congenital malforations in infants of insulin-dependent diabetic mothers. Diabetes Care 1983; 6: 219–23.
11. Sanaka M, Minei S, Iwamoto Y. Occurrence of pregnancy for diabetics with nephropathy. J Japan Soc Diabetes Pregnancy 2006; 6: 127–35.
12. Yokoyama H, Okudaira M, Otani T, et al. Higher incidence of diabetic nephropathy in Type 2 than in Type 1 diabetes in early-onset diabetes in Japan. Kidney Int 2000; 58: 302–11.
13. Omori Y, Minei S, Tetsuo T, et al. Current status of pregnancy in diabetic women (A comparison of pregnancy in IDDM and NIDDM). DRCP 1994; 24(Suppl.): S273–8.
14. Shimizu I, Makino H, Imagawa A, et al. Clinical and immunogenetic characteristics of fulminant type 1 diabetes associated with pregnancy. J Clin Endocrinol Metab 2006; 91: 471–6.

21 Detection and diagnostic strategies for gestational diabetes mellitus

Boyd E. Metzger and Yoo Lee Kim

Introduction

Gestational diabetes mellitus (GDM) is one of the most common medical complications of pregnancy. The widely used definition of GDM ('carbohydrate intolerance of varying degrees of severity with onset or first recognition during pregnancy')[1] has been accepted for more than a quarter of a century. Nevertheless, for many years, there has been much debate and controversy about GDM with respect to: (1) its clinical significance and benefit of treatment; (2) optimal strategies for detection and diagnosis, and (3) appropriate treatment goals and methods. Publication of the results of a randomized clinical trial that compared standard treatment of GDM to no intervention and showed better outcomes with treatment[2] has reduced concerns about the benefit of identifying GDM. However, the polarization of opinion about the detection and diagnosis of GDM has not abated. In 2003, the U.S. Preventive Services Task Force concluded that: 'because of the lack of high-quality evidence concerning critical issues, we are unable to determine the extent to which screening has an important impact on maternal and neonatal health outcome' and recommended a randomized controlled trial to answer remaining questions.[3]

The Fourth International Workshop–Conference on GDM considered these issues in depth.[4] More 'flexible' positions were taken concerning screening and diagnostic criteria for GDM than had been recommended by the contributors to the previous workshop conferences.[5,6] For the first time, a strategy for potential 'exclusion from blood glucose testing' on the basis of below average risk for GDM, rather than performing blood glucose testing of all pregnant women was offered.[4] On the issue of diagnostic criteria, the Summary and Recommendations of the Fourth International Workshop Conference on GDM[4] stated "data presented at the conference indicated that the infants of women who meet these lower Carpenter–Coustan criteria are at similar risk for perinatal morbidity, including macrosomia, as those patients identified using the NDDG criteria."[1]

Thus, the Carpenter and Coustan criteria[7] were recommended for interpretation of the 100-g OGTT. In addition, criteria for interpretation of a 75-g 2-h OGTT were proposed, but not endorsed.[4] It was also acknowledged that the recommendation from the World Health Organization (WHO) that levels of glycemia during pregnancy should be interpreted according to the criteria used outside of pregnancy[8] has gained acceptance in some centers. This practice was likewise not endorsed.[4] The recommendations of the American Diabetes Association's 'Position Statement on Gestational Diabetes Mellitus'[9] closely parallel those of the Fourth International Workshop Conference.[4] The Fifth International Workshop Conference on GDM has endorsed the recommendations for screening and diagnosis of GDM[10] that were reached at the Fourth GDM Conference.[4]

The objective of this chapter is to assess the current status of issues regarding the detection and diagnosis of GDM. The positions taken at the Fourth International Workshop Conference on GDM serve as a point of reference. New approaches to detection and diagnosis of GDM that have been recommended in the interim have been summarized. Initial reports from the Hyperglycemia and Adverse Pregnancy Outcome Study[11,12] will become available during 2007. The primary goal of the HAPO study is to determine the degree of glucose intolerance short of diabetes that conveys a clinically important risk for adverse perinatal outcome. The data that have been collected in the HAPO study should permit the selection of 'outcome-based' criteria for the diagnosis of GDM. When translation of this information is implemented, strategies for detection and diagnosis of GDM may well be changed extensively from their current status. For the interim, the primary focus is on recent studies that have bearing on the problems of detection and diagnosis of GDM as currently defined, in conjunction with a less comprehensive review of historically important earlier reports.

Screening strategies

There is no debate about the longstanding observation that when overt diabetes mellitus (DM) occurs during pregnancy it is associated with adverse maternal and fetal outcomes.

Since early diabetes, especially Type 2 DM, is usually asymptomatic, virtually all care-givers are alert to the need to detect and treat overt diabetes. Therefore, they all engage in some form of a screening process. Indeed, it has been acknowledged that systematically taking a personal and family medical history represents a form of screening, or at least, an assessment of risk. Furthermore, though the presence of glucosuria is neither very sensitive, nor specific for the identification of diabetes during pregnancy, it remains a common practice to test urine for glucose and protein at each prenatal visit. The differences then, are not whether to screen for glucose intolerance during pregnancy, but rather, differences revolve about the following four questions: (1) what level or severity of glucose intolerance should be identified and treated; (2) how prevalent is the condition; (3) which patients require blood glucose testing in order to identify the individuals that need to be detected; and (4) are the sensitivity, specificity, and reproducibility of the screening procedure that is recommended adequate to serve the intended purpose? Some of these questions have remained controversial for more than three decades. In the meantime, the need to resolve the issues has become acute because the prevalence of GDM has increased substantially during the last decade.[13,14] In the sections that follow, we have attempted to provide an overview of the contemporary issues that relate to detection of GDM.

Use of high-risk characteristics as a screening tool

Historically, investigators and clinicians were aware of the serious adverse outcomes associated with maternal diabetes and instances of diabetes mellitus being present during pregnancy with its disappearance postpartum were documented many years before GDM became designated as a distinct entity.[15] These factors prompted some clinicians to begin testing for diabetes during pregnancy among women with a history of previous 'poor obstetric outcomes', those with severe obesity or with a strong family history of diabetes. After definitions of abnormal glucose tolerance in pregnancy were established, many continued to apply the strategy of limiting testing to such 'high-risk' subjects. On the other hand, in the 1950s, it was a common practice to use the measurement of blood glucose concentration 1-h after ingesting a 50-g glucose load as a screening test for glucose intolerance or diabetes mellitus in various populations. It was in this context that O'Sullivan and co-workers developed the 50-g glucose challenge test[16,17] in concert with the criteria that they proposed for interpretation of a 100-g OGTT during pregnancy.[16] In the original study, a sensitivity of c.80% was achieved with the proposed cutoff value of 130 mg/dL (venous whole blood). O'Sullivan's group[17] and others in years following[18–21] demonstrated much higher yields of GDM by performing the glucose challenge test (GCT) on all pregnant women rather than doing blood glucose testing only on those with high-risk characteristics. Furthermore, it was more cost-effective, since fewer diagnostic OGTTs were performed on the basis of a GCT than when high-risk characteristics are used to select women for a full diagnostic test. Nevertheless, selecting subjects for diagnostic tests on the basis of high-risk features remains popular, in part because it does not require blood glucose testing on two separate occasions.

Screening based on risk stratification

For many years, some experts have advised that 'risk assessment' for GDM should be conducted as part of the initial prenatal evaluation and that those considered 'high risk' on the basis of historical factors should undergo initial blood glucose testing early in pregnancy.[22] This strategy has also been suggested in the 'Summary and Recommendations' reports of the International Workshop Conferences on GDM. However, in practice, this point is commonly overlooked, resulting in a delay in the detection of GDM until after the 24–28 week window is reached, i.e. the standard or routine time for testing. Published reports from the Toronto Tri Hospital Study[23,24] and other data confirming a low prevalence of GDM among younger women[25] prompted the participants of the Fourth and Fifth International Workshop Conferences[4,10] and the ADA Expert Committee[9] to recommend a strategy for potential 'exclusion from blood glucose testing' on the basis of below-average risk for GDM (Box 21.1) rather than relying on the former strategy of testing only on the basis of perceived 'high-risk'. It is important to emphasize that *all* of the low-risk characteristics must be present for an individual to qualify for exclusion from blood glucose testing. As indicated in the Summary & Recommendations of the Fourth and Fifth GDM Workshop Conferences,[4,10] when blood glucose testing is required, either a one-step procedure (diagnostic test performed on all subjects) or a two-step procedure (initial screening test in all cases, with the diagnostic test reserved for those above a defined threshold value) is acceptable.

A number of groups have reported results of their efforts to apply the Fourth International Workshop Conference and American Diabetes Association endorsed guidelines for the identification of subjects to be excluded from blood glucose testing based on their low-risk characteristics.[4,9] Williams et al.[26] analyzed their screened population and those with a diagnosis of GDM using the NDDG criteria[1] that were also used in the Toronto Tri Hospital study.[23,24] They found that if the recommendations of the Fourth International Workshop Conference and the ADA[4,9] had been applied, few cases with GDM would have been missed (4%); however, most (c. 90%) would still have required blood glucose testing. Danilenko-Dixon et al.[27] did a retrospective analysis of 18,504 women that were universally screened for GDM with the 50-g GCT over an 11-year interval at the Mayo Clinic, Rochester, MN. They also found that use of the guidelines[4,9,10] would have failed to screen and detect only a small proportion (3%) of the women with GDM but would have required that 90.4% of the population receive the GCT. Corcoy et al.[28] determined the prevalence of low-risk characteristics in 917 women in the general population and among 1635 women with GDM at their hospital in Barcelona, Spain. Only 1.3% of GDM were classified as low risk; whereas the proportion of the general population with these characteristics was 7.0% ($P < 0.001$). Moses et al.[29] reported that lean Caucasian women, <25 years of age, had a prevalence of GDM that was 2.8%, compared to 6.3% overall, and suggested that the published guidelines for identifying pregnancies that could be excluded from blood

Box 21.1   Screening strategy for detecting gestational diabetes mellitus*

GDM risk assessment should be ascertained at the first prenatal visit

Low risk *Blood glucose testing not routinely required if all of the following characteristics are present*
- Member of an ethnic group with a low prevalence of GDM
- No known diabetes in first-degree relatives
- Age <25 years
- Weight normal at birth[†]
- Weight normal before pregnancy
- No history of abnormal glucose metabolism
- No history of poor obstetric outcome

Average risk [††]*Perform blood glucose testing at 24–28 weeks in the following*
- All subjects not classified as low risk or high risk
- Subjects initially designated high risk that did not have GDM at early testing

High risk *Perform blood glucose testing as soon as feasible after booking if one or more of the following characteristics are present*
- Severe obesity according to local standards
- Strong family history of Type 2 diabetes mellitus
- Previous history of GDM or glucose intolerance outside of pregnancy
- Glucosuria

If GDM is not diagnosed, blood glucose testing should be repeated at 24–28 weeks, or at any time a patient has symptoms or signs that are suggestive of hyperglycemia

*Based on Metzger and Coustan.[4]
[†]Based on Metzger et al.[10]
[††]Blood glucose testing by: (1) the two-step procedure: 50-g glucose challenge test (GCT) followed by a diagnostic oral glucose tolerance test (OGTT) in those meeting the threshold value in the GCT; or (2) a one-step procedure: diagnostic OGTT performed on all subjects.

glucose testing[4,9,10] require further study. It should be noted, however, that Moses et al. used criteria for the diagnosis of GDM that yield a much higher prevalence of GDM than is the case when the NDDG[1] or Carpenter–Coustan[7] criteria are applied. It must be emphasized that the strategy for identifying cases to be excluded from blood glucose testing has been formally tested only for the application of the NDDG diagnostic criteria.[1]

Some novel approaches to identifying subjects at low risk have been reported. Southwick and Wigton[30] found only 9.2% with a positive GCT and a prevalence of GDM of only 1.5% among young (<20 years of age) Hispanic women and they suggested that blood glucose testing of this subgroup of young pregnant women might not be warranted. Young et al.[31] looked at the prevalence of a positive GCT and of GDM in a group of 352 women that were seen for prenatal care with a second pregnancy after an interval of ≤4 years. All had a negative GCT (<7.8 mmol/L) during the index pregnancy, but <10% would have qualified for exclusion from blood glucose testing on the basis of low-risk characteristics. In the second pregnancy, 12 had a positive GCT but none met the NDDG diagnostic criteria for GDM[1] on the diagnostic OGTT. They concluded that women with a normal GCT in one pregnancy have a minimal risk of GDM in near future and could be excluded from blood glucose testing in a pregnancy occurring within the next 4 years.

Blood glucose screening tests: Two-step procedure

Glucose challenge test

The GCT, described briefly in the previous section, is the screening test most commonly used by those who employ a two-step procedure for GDM detection and diagnosis; however,

the test has limitations and many critics. It is relatively complex in that it involves administration of a specific glucose load and requires phlebotomy 60 min later. At threshold values that achieve the desired degree of sensitivity, the GCT has relatively low specificity. Furthermore, results are not highly reproducible. It is important to consider several factors in deciding whether or not to use the GCT. These include: (1) the proportion of screened subjects on which it is feasible to do the diagnostic test; (2) the diagnostic criteria that will be used in the interpretation of the OGTT; and (3) the desired levels of sensitivity and specificity.

Many variations of the 1-h GCT have been explored. Doing the GCT in the overnight fasting state or without controlling the interval since last eating has been compared in two studies with opposing conclusions being reached. No reasons for the difference are apparent.[32,33] Many investigators have proposed using cutoff values for a positive GCT other than the ≥7.8 mmol/L plasma glucose concentration that was extrapolated by the NDDG[1] from the original whole blood glucose cutoff value of >7.2 mmol/L originally used by O'Sullivan et al.[17] with different levels of sensitivity and specificity reported. There is also evidence that the cutoff values needed to obtain similar levels of sensitivity and specificity in the diagnosis of GDM differ when using the NDDG criteria or the Carpenter–Coustan diagnostic criteria.[34,35] Others have proposed that higher specificity can be achieved without loss of sensitivity by varying the value for a positive test according to the interval between the last intake of food and the time of the GCT.[24,25,36,37] Use of 50-g of glucose polymer[38] or of a quantity of jelly beans equivalent to 50-g of glucose[39] as test doses have been advocated as ways of improving the palatability of the test dose (less nausea or vomiting, factors that require the test to be repeated) while maintaining performance similar to that seen with the usual GCT procedure. Although some of these proposed alternatives are appealing, none of these modified GCT procedures has been used widely and none has consistently been found to be superior to the standard way of doing the GCT.

Analysis of samples collected at random times

Collecting blood samples for measurement of glucose concentrations without regard to time of day or interval since the last food intake (random sampling time) has also been advocated as a simpler and adequate method for blood glucose screening.[40] However, others have found this approach to be very insensitive for the detection of subjects with degrees of glucose intolerance short of overt diabetes mellitus.[41,42]

Fasting plasma glucose as a screening test

Many investigators have found a relatively strong correlation between the concentrations of fasting plasma glucose (FPG) and postprandial plasma glucose (PPG) in nonpregnant subjects with normal glucose metabolism, impaired glucose tolerance (IGT) or early Type 2 DM. For example, the association between FPG and PPG was used to select individuals at high risk for IGT as candidates for enrollment in the Diabetes Prevention Program (DPP). The DPP demonstrated that progression from IGT to diabetes could be prevented or delayed by lifestyle changes or the use of metformin.[43]

The concentration of FPG has also been examined as a means of detecting subjects at risk for GDM (Table 21.1).[44–48] Some investigators have reported an upper level for FPG that has high specificity for the diagnosis of GDM (≥90 %);[44,45,47,48] however, such values cannot be used as the sole marker for GDM since most cases have a FPG concentration below the putative threshold. Other investigators have attempted to identify a level of FPG that can specifically exclude individuals with GDM. In different studies, various 'cutoff values' have been recommended because a certain blood glucose level could exclude approximately one-third to one-half of the population from further testing beyond this 'simple test'.[44,47]

Significant limitations in most of these studies reduce the ability to extrapolate the findings to the obstetric population at large. First, in only two of the studies[46,47] were measurements of FPG and a diagnostic OGTT performed on an 'unselected' population of pregnant subjects. Population-based measurements are needed to verify that the defined upper level of FPG truly has acceptably high specificity for the presence of GDM. For example, it has been reported that women with normal carbohydrate metabolism who were severely obese failed to show a fall in FPG during pregnancy and actually tended to have a small increase.[49] That report does not contain the FPG values from the obese subjects; however, the inter quartile ranges given for the values in early pregnancy and the subsequent upward trend in values that was observed indicate that in the third trimester, values in excess of 5.8 mmol/L were present in some of the obese pregnant subjects with normal glucose tolerance. It is also important to establish that putative lower 'cutoff levels' truly have sufficient specificity to be used to exclude GDM in normal weight and lean pregnant

women. Finally, the usefulness of FPG as a 'screening tool' depends on the criteria used for the diagnosis of GDM. This is clearly illustrated in the report by Reichelt et al.[47] (Table 21.1). The optimal sensitivity/specificity relationship for the detections of diabetes mellitus during pregnancy (WHO criteria[8]) was found for a FPG ≥4.9 mmol/L; whereas, sensitivity for the detection of gestational impaired glucose tolerance (WHO criteria,[8]) was much lower. Instead, a value of 4.5 mmol/L was chosen as the 'lower limit' cutoff for excluding GDM or gestational IGT. This value had a sensitivity of 82% and negative predictive value of 97% and could be used to eliminate the need for a diagnostic OGTT in about half the population.

In the aggregate, the studies that are summarized in Table 21.1 do not make a convincing case that a single measurement of FPG can be cost-effectively substituted for the 1-h GCT as a screening test. In the largest, most complete study from Brazil,[47] the cutoff would have to be set at 4.5 mmol/L and 49% of the subjects would have to undergo an OGTT to ensure the detection of c. 81% of GDM cases. Finally, in the studies summarized in Table 21.1, the specific levels of FPG that have been suggested as high or low 'cutoff values' vary. This may be a function of true differences among populations. Alternatively, variation may result from different analytical methods or specific analytical instruments that were employed for the studies. Either option suggests that the choice of a specific FPG concentration to screen for subjects at increased or low risk for GDM may need validation for each center and population before this strategy is implemented.

Methodological and instrumentation issues

The comments about methodology and instruments above serve as an introduction to consideration of the potential utility of measuring the capillary blood glucose concentration with strip and meter technology to identify subjects that should have a diagnostic OGTT. During fasting, concentrations of glucose in capillary and venous blood are similar, but concentrations differ in the postprandial state, being higher in capillary than venous blood. Though whole blood is sampled for most analyses by strip–meter techniques, glucose is actually measured in a plasma ultrafiltrate with many of the techniques that are currently in use. However, the validity of a given method is ultimately established by the precision and accuracy of the measurements. Careful review of published data[50,51] indicated that a lack of precision would be an important issue for most systems. Thus, to maintain the desired sensitivity, thresholds for positive tests would have to be lowered to values that would reduce specificity and greatly increase the number of cases referred for OGTT. In addition, when precision and accuracy are deemed to be adequate, it remains essential to establish stability over time and to participate in a standardized external quality assurance scheme. Such schemes are not typically available for office-based procedures. Dillon et al.[52] have proposed an approach that combines meter based testing and laboratory measurements at the time of the GCT. They found that meter values of 6.1 or 8.6 mmol/L predicted plasma glucose values in the laboratory of <7.5 or >7.5 mmol/L (threshold for positive GCT) with 95% confidence. Thus, they could confidently discharge those with meter values <6.1mmol/L without waiting for laboratory analyses to be

Table 21.1   Fasting plasma glucose as a screening tool for the detection of GDM

Authors	Population studied	Diagnostic criteria	Assay method	Screening/diagnostic algorithm	Results				
					FPG (mm/L)	Sen. (%)	Spec. (%)	PPV (%)	NPV (%)
Agarwal et al.[44]	United Arab Emirate Selected by positive GCT Mean age: 30.2 ± 5.62 n = 368	Carpenter/ Coustan	Glucose oxidase	Prospective 50-g GCT: If (≥7.8), 100-g 3-h OGTT	4.4* 5.3†	97 79	28 91	38 80	95 90
Atilano et al.[45]	USA Selected by positive GCT 54% White; 19% Hispanic; 11% Asian; 8% Black; 8% other n = 512	NDDG	Not reported	Retrospective 50-g GCT: If (≥7.8), 100-g 3-h OGTT	FPG (mm/L) 5.8	20.2	99.7	95.8	81.4
Perucchini et al.[46]	Switzerland Unselected 63% White; 19% Asian; 6% African; 12% other Mean age: 28.4 ± 0.2 BMI 23.8 ± 0.2 n = 520	Carpenter/ Coustan	Hexokinase	Prospective All subjects had: 50-g GCT and 100-g 3-h OGTT	Threshold (mm/L) GCT: 7.8 FPG: 4.8	59 81	91 76		
Reichelt et al.[47]	Brazil Consecutive ≥20 years 45% White; 14% Black; 41% mixed Mean age 27.9 ± 5.5 BMI 26.1 ± 4.1 n = 5010	WHO Diabetes mellitus 2 h PG ≥11.1 Gestational IGT≥7.8; <11.1	Glucose oxidase	Prospective All subjects had 75-g 2-h OGTT	**Diabetes mellitus** FPG (mm/L) 4.9 **Gestational impaired glucose Tolerance** FPG (mm/L) 4.5*	88 / 81	78 / 54	1.3 / 12	100 / 97
Sacks et al.[48]	USA Selected by positive GCT n = 968	NDDG	Glucose oxidase	Retrospective 50-g GCT: If (≥7.8), 100-g 3-h OGTT	FPG (mm/L) 4.9 4.7 4.5	80 90 95	40 21 11		

*Value suggested as cutoff below which the prevalence rate of GDM is so low that the full diagnostic OGTT need not be done.

†Value suggested as cutoff with a sufficiently high specificity for the diagnosis of GDM so that the full diagnostic OGTT need not be done.

completed and could immediately schedule the diagnostic OGTT without confirming a result in the laboratory in those with meter values ≥8.6 mmol/L. For those with a meter value between 6.1 and 8.6 mmol/L the decision regarding further testing was deferred until the plasma glucose concentration was determined in the laboratory. Although this appears to be a workable approach, only clinical laboratory based and certified methods should be used for diagnostics tests.

Blood glucose screening tests: One-step procedure

Some investigators and clinicians favor using a one-step process, that is, performing a diagnostic test on all subjects that require blood glucose testing as defined by risk-assessment (Box 21.1). This approach may be cost-effective under two circumstances. First, if the diagnostic test that is used is not complicated to administer, e.g. a single sample drawn 2 h after a 75-g glucose load,[53] it approaches the standard GCT in simplicity. Secondly, in populations that have a very high prevalence of GDM (as is the situation among Pima women, other Native American groups and aboriginal populations), a high proportion will have a positive GCT and require the diagnostic OGTT. In this circumstance, it is cost-effective to administer the full diagnostic test to all subjects.

Diagnostic oral glucose tolerance test

Overview

As indicated in the introduction, there has been longstanding controversy about the optimal diagnostic test and criteria for interpretation of glucose tolerance tests in pregnancy. A brief overview may help to put some of the issues into perspective. In the original epidemiological study of OGTT in pregnancy by O'Sullivan and Mahan,[16] the objective was to devise a scheme that identified women at risk for diabetes mellitus outside of pregnancy sometime in the future. That objective was fulfilled in O'Sullivan's group's long-term follow-up of the original cohort of women[16,54] and it has been validated extensively in other populations.[55–60] Evidence that GDM may be associated with adverse perinatal events was found later.[17,61,62] O'Sullivan and Mahan's criteria for the interpretation of OGTTs in pregnancy were based on measurements of glucose concentration in whole blood.[16] Extrapolation of these values to approximate plasma glucose equivalent values has limitations and the need to do so has generated some of the controversy regarding diagnostic criteria for GDM. That issue has been covered in detail in other reports[1,4,7,9,10,63] and will not be addressed here.

For more than three decades, many other procedures and criteria for the diagnosis of gestational diabetes have been proposed and used. The scope of this chapter does not permit a comprehensive summary of this large body of work. In these reports, criteria for GDM have been derived from OGTTs that were performed in a variety of specific groups of subjects. In some instances, this was a population of pregnant women, in other cases criteria for GDM have been derived from studies in a general population of nonpregnant subjects. Prior to the HAPO study, no large studies have been completed in which

the primary objective was to specifically and independently determine associations between maternal glycemia and the risk of adverse pregnancy outcome. In a much smaller study, Gilmer and Beard reported values for area under the curve of a 2-h OGTT that could predict risk of neonatal hypoglycemia.[64]

Limitations

Many have concluded that the criteria for the diagnosis of GDM that are presently used fail to capture a significant proportion of the cases at risk for adverse outcomes. In fact, evidence has been reported to suggest that the relationship between maternal glycemia and macrosomia is a continuum.[65–67] As mentioned previously, the participants in the Fourth International Workshop Conference on GDM[4] reviewed available evidence and concluded that the infants of women who meet the lower Carpenter–Coustan[7] criteria for GDM are at similar risk for perinatal morbidity, including macrosomia, as those patients identified according to the NDDG criteria.[1] Some have reported higher than expected rates of complications and morbidity in cases with one-abnormal value on the diagnostic OGTT.[68,69] Others have reported an increase in adverse outcomes, in particular macrosomia, among GCT positive cases with nondiabetic or normal OGTT values by NDDG criteria[25,66,70,71] and among cases meeting the WHO criteria for IGT, or similar levels of glycemia.[72–74] Other investigators have failed to confirm the above findings or emphasize the potential role of confounding factors such as obesity, and continue to counsel against adopting more inclusive criteria for the diagnosis of GDM.[75–77] In concluding this part of the discussion, it is important to indicate that two issues are commonly overlooked when outcomes are compared among groups with GDM, lesser degrees of glucose intolerance or normal glucose metabolism. First, it is very likely that the treatment of GDM will have reduced the expected effects of hyperglycemia in that group. Secondly, it has been shown repeatedly that knowledge of glucose levels and/or the classification of glucose tolerance status may influence the decisions of healthcare providers.

Conclusions

Recommendations of the Fourth and Fifth International Workshop Conferences on GDM

As indicated in the introduction, the conclusions reached by the participants in the Fourth International Workshop Conference on GDM regarding screening and diagnosis[4] have served as a point of reference in the present review. The participants of the Fifth Workshop Conference[10] endorsed these conclusions. The role of risk assessment was summarized in detail previously and in Box 21.1. Threshold glucose concentrations for interpretation of both 100-g and 75-g OGTTs were recommended[4] and are presented in Tables 21.2 and 21.3, respectively. These recommendations have received both support and criticism (see above). At the time of the Fourth Workshop Conference, information on outcomes in pregnancies with GDM diagnosed with the criteria recommended for the 75-g OGTT were lacking. Some new OSC use of

Table 21.2   Diagnosis of GDM: 100-g oral glucose tolerance test*

Specimen	Concentration[†]	
	mg/dL	mmol/L
Fasting	95	5.3
One hour	180	10.0
Two hour	155	8.6
Three hour	140	7.8

*The test should be performed in the morning after an overnight fast of at least 8 h but not more than 14 h and after at least 3 days of unrestricted diet (≥ 150 g carbohydrate per day) and physical activity. The subject should remain seated and should not smoke throughout the test.
[†]The cutoff values are those proposed by Carpenter and Coustan[7] for extrapolation of the whole blood glucose values found by O'Sullivan and Mahan[16] to plasma or serum glucose concentrations. Two or more of the venous plasma concentrations must be met or exceeded for a positive diagnosis.

Table 21.3   Diagnosis of GDM: 75-g oral glucose tolerance test*

Specimen	Concentration[†]	
	mg/dL	mmol/L
Fasting	95	5.3
One hour	180	10.0
Two hour	155	8.6

*The test should be performed in the morning after an overnight fast of at least 8 h but not more than 14 h and after at least 3 days of unrestricted diet (≥ 150 gm carbohydrate per day) and physical activity. The subject should remain seated and should not smoke throughout the test.
[†]Cutoff values for the 75-g, 2-h oral glucose tolerance test in pregnancy are, of necessity, arbitrary. The lack of definitive data relating such test results to perinatal outcome made it difficult for the panel and the Organizing Committee of the Fourth International Workshop Conference on GDM to arrive at a consensus.[4]

these criteria and the WHO IGT criteria were not endorsed for clinical use until such data became available from studies of large numbers of subjects. Some additional information is now available for consideration. In the Brazil GDM project approximately 5000 pregnant women underwent a 75-g OGTT.[74] In that cohort, 2.4% met the ADA 75-g OGTT criteria for GDM.[9] However, a recent preliminary report suggests that more women meet the diagnostic threshold for GDM when challenged with 100 g of glucose than when they receive a 75-g test dose.[78]

Authors' recommendations

One consequence of applying lower glycemic thresholds in the interpretation of the OGTT is entirely predictable; namely, that the prevalence of GDM is higher when these criteria are used in any given population. In published studies, the magnitude of the difference is not constant from one population to another, but the relative change is substantial. Data from several studies that have been reported in the past few years[7,2,74–76] are summarized in Table 21.4. The choice of criteria has major implications for both the cost and complexity of prenatal care. The controversial issues that have been summarized in this report will continue until data such as those from the ongoing HAPO study[11,12] provide information from which criteria for the diagnosis of GDM that are based on the specific relationships between maternal glycemia and perinatal outcome can be formulated. After weighing all of these outstanding issues, we advise established programs to continue using one of the recommended screening/diagnostic strategies[1,4,8–10] for routine clinical care and we encourage ongoing collection of additional population-based data. We hope that our overview of the issues will be of assistance in making a choice for those establishing new programs, clinics or practices.

Table 21.4   Impact of diagnostic criteria on the prevalence of GDM

Authors	Population studied	Diagnostic criteria	Assay method	Screening/ Diagnostic algorithm	Prevalence	
Deerochanawong et al.[72]	Thailand Randomly selected n = 709	WHO IGT: 2-h PG ≥7.8 NDDG GDM	Glucose oxidase	Prospective All subjects had: 50-g GCT; if ≥7.8, 100-g OGTT	WHO GCT (+) NDDG	15.7% 11.7% 1.4%
Rust et al.[75]	USA Selected: positive GCT n = 434	NDDG Carpenter/Coustan (C/C) Sacks	Not reported	Retrospective 50-g GCT; if >7.8, 100-g 3-h OGTT	NDDG C/C Sacks	R Risk 1 1.5 1.7
Schmidt et al.[74]	Brazil Consecutive ≥ 20 years n = 4977	WHO[11] ADA 75-g[12]	Glucose oxidase	Prospective All subjects had 75-g OGTT	WHO ADA	7.2% 2.4%
Schwartz et al.[76]	USA Unselected n = 8857	NDDG Carpenter/Coustan (C/C)	Glucose oxidase	Retrospective 50-g GCT; if >7.8, 100-g 3-h OGTT	GCT (+) NDDG C/C	18.7% 3.2% 5.0%

ADA, American Diabetes Association; GCT, glucose challenge test; IGT, impaired glucose tolerance; NDDG, National Diabetes Data Group; OGTT, oral glucose tolerance test; PG, plasma glucose; WHO, World Health Organization.

REFERENCES

1. National Diabetes Data Group. Classification and diagnosis of diabetes mellitus and other categories of glucose intolerance. Diabetes 1979; 28: 1039–57.
2. Crowther CA, Hiller JE, Moss JR, et al., for the Australian Carbohydrate Intolerance Study in Pregnant Women (ACHOIS) Trial Group. Effect of treatment of gestational diabetes mellitus on pregnancy outcomes. N Engl J Med 2005; 352: 2477–86.
3. Brody SC, Harris R, Lohr K. Screening for gestational diabetes: a summary of the evidence for the U.S. Preventive Services Task Force. Obstet Gynecol 2003; 101: 380–92.
4. Metzger BE, Coustan DR, and The Organizing Committee. Summary and Recommendations of the Fourth International Workshop–Conference on Gestational Diabetes Mellitus. Diabetes Care 1998; 21(suppl. 2): 161–7.
5. Freinkel N. Summary and recommendations of the second International Workshop–Conference on Gestational Diabetes Mellitus. Diabetes 1985; 34(suppl. 2): 123–6.
6. Metzger BE, and the Organizing Committee. Summary and recommendations of the Third International Workshop–Conference on Gestational Diabetes Mellitus. Diabetes 1991; 40(suppl. 2): 197–201.
7. Carpenter MW, Coustan DR. Criteria for screening tests for gestational diabetes. Am J Obstet Gynecol 1982; 144: 763–73.
8. Alberti KGMM, Zimmet PZ, for the WHO Consultation. Definition, diagnosis and classification of diabetes mellitus and it complications. Part 1: Diagnosis and classification of diabetes mellitus. Provisional report of a WHO consultation. Diabet Med 1998; 15: 539–53.
9. American Diabetes Association. Gestational diabetes mellitus: a Position Statement. Diabetes Care 2004; 27(suppl. 1): S88–S90.
10. Metzger BE, Buchanan TA, Coustan DR, et al. Summary and recommendations of the 5th International Workshop–Conference on Gestational Diabetes Mellitus. Diabetes Care 2007; 30(suppl. 2): S251–S260.
11. HAPO Study Cooperative Research Group. The Hyperglycemia and Adverse Pregnancy Outcome (HAPO) Study. Int J Gynecol Obstet 2002; 78: 69–77.
12. Nesbitt GS, Smye M, Sheridan B, Lappin TRJ, Trimble ER, the HAPO Study Cooperative Research Group. Integration of local and central laboratory functions in a worldwide multicentre study: experience from the Hyperglycemia and Adverse Pregnancy Outcome (HAPO) Study. Clinical Trials 2006; 3: 397–407.
13. Ferrera A, Kahn HS, Quesenberry CP, Riley C, Hedderson MM. An increase in the incidence of gestational diabetes mellitus: Northern California 1991–2000. Obstet Gynecol 2004; 103: 526–33.
14. Dabelea D, Snell-Bergeon JK, Hartsfield CL, et al. Increasing prevalence of gestational diabetes mellitus (GDM) over time and by birth cohort. Diabetes Care 2005; 28: 579–84.
15. Hadden D. A historical perspective on gestational diabetes. Diabetes Care 1998; 21(suppl. 2): B3–B4.
16. O'Sullivan JB, Mahan CM. Criteria for the oral glucose tolerance test in pregnancy. Diabetes 1964; 13: 278–85.
17. O'Sullivan JB, Mahan CM, Charles D, Dandrow RV. Screening criteria for high-risk gestational diabetic patients. Am J Obstet Gynecol 1973; 116: 895–900.
18. Lavin JP. Screening of high-risk and general populations of gestational diabetes: clinical application and cost analysis. Diabetes 1985; 34(suppl. 2): 24–7.
19. Marquette GP, Klein VR, Niebyl JR. Efficacy of screening for gestational diabetes. Am J Perinatol 1985; 2: 7–9.
20. Coustan DR, Nelson C, Carpenter MW, et al. Maternal age and screening for gestational diabetes: a population based study. Obstet Gynecol 1989; 73: 557–61.
21. Griffin ME, Coffey M, Johnson H, et al. Universal vs. risk factor-based screening for gestational diabetes mellitus: detection rates, gestation at diagnosis and outcome. Diabet Med 2000; 17: 26–32.
22. Mestman JH, Anderson GV, Barton P. Carbohydrate metabolism in pregnancy. Am J Obstet Gynecol 1971; 109: 41–5.
23. Naylor CD, Sermer M, Chen E, Farine D. Selective screening for gestational diabetes mellitus. N Engl J Med 1997; 337: 1591–6.
24. Sermer M, Naylor CD, Farine D, et al., for the Toronto Tri-Hospital Gestational Diabetes Investigators: The Toronto Tri-Hospital Gestational Diabetes Project. Diabetes Care 1998; 21(suppl. 2): B33–B42.
25. Sacks DA, Abu-Fadil S, Karten GJ, Forsythe AB, Hackett JR. Screening for gestational diabetes with the one-hour 50-g glucose test. Obstet Gynecol 1987; 70: 89–93.
26. Williams CB, Iqbal S, Zawacki CM, et al. Effect of selective screening for gestational diabetes. Diabetes Care 1999; 22: 418–21.
27. Danilenko-Dixon DR, Winter JTV, Nelson RL, Ogburn PL. Universal versus selective gestational diabetes screening: Application of 1997 American Diabetes Association recommendations. Am J Obstet Gynecol 1999; 181: 798–802.
28. Corcoy R, Garcia-Patterson A, Pau E, et al. Is selective screening for gestational diabetes mellitus worthwhile everywhere? Acta Diabetol 2004; 41: 154–7.
29. Moses RG, Moses J, Davis WS. Gestational diabetes: Do lean young Caucasian women need to be tested? Diabetes Care 1998; 21: 1803–6.
30. Southwick RD, Wigton TR. Screening for gestational diabetes mellitus in adolescent Hispanic Americans. J Reproductive Med 2000; 45: 31–4.
31. Young C, Kuehl TJ, Sulak PJ, Allen SR. Gestational diabetes screening in subsequent pregnancies of previously healthy patients. Am J Obstet Gynecol 2000; 182: 1024–6.
32. Coustan DR, Widness JA, Carpenter MW, et al. Should the fifty-gram, one-hour plasma glucose screening test for gestational diabetes be administered in the fasting or fed state? Am J Obstet Gynecol 1986; 154: 1031–5.
33. Lewis GF, McNally C, Blackman JD, Polonsky KS, Barron WM. Prior feeding alters the response to the 50-g glucose challenge test in pregnancy. Diabetes Care 1993; 16: 1551–6.
34. Bonomo M, Gandini ML, Mastropasqua A, et al., for the Definition of Screening Methods for Gestational Diabetes Study Group of the Lombardy Section of the Italian Society of Diabetology. Which cutoff level should be used in screening for glucose intolerance in pregnancy? Am J Obstet Gynecol 1998; 179: 179–85.
35. Monteros AE, Parra A, Hidalgo R, Zambrana M. The after breakfast 50-g, 1-hour glucose challenge test in urban Mexican pregnant women: its sensitivity and specificity evaluated by three diagnostic criteria for gestational diabetes mellitus. Acta Obstet Gynecol Scand 1999; 78: 294–8.
36. Sermer M, Naylor CD, Gare DJ, et al. Impact of time since last meal on the gestational glucose challenge test. Am J Obstet Gynecol 1994; 171: 607–16.
37. Cetin M, Cetin A. Time-dependent gestational diabetes screening values. Int J Gynecol Obstet 1997; 56: 257–61.
38. Reece EA, Gabrielli S, Abdalla M, et al. Diagnosis of gestational diabetes by use of al glucose polymer. Am J Obstet Gynecol 1989; 160: 383–4.
39. Lamar ME, Kuehl TJ, Cooney AT, et al. Jelly bean as an alternative to a fifty-gram glucose beverage for gestational diabetes screening. Am J Obstet Gynecol 1999; 181: 1154–7.
40. Stangenberg M, Persson B, Nordlander E. Random capillary blood glucose and conventional selection criteria for glucose tolerance testing during pregnancy. Diabetes Res 1985; 2: 29–33.
41. Nasarat AA, Johnstone FD, Hasan SAM. Is random plasma glucose an efficient screening test of abnormal glucose tolerance in pregnancy? Br J Obstet Gynaecol 1988; 95: 855–60.
42. McElduff A, Goldring J, Gordon P, Wyndham L. A Direct comparison of the measurement of a random plasma glucose and a post-50 g glucose load glucose, in the detection of gestational diabetes. Aust NZ J Obstet Gynecol 1994; 34: 28–30.
43. Diabetes Prevention Research Group. Reduction in the incidence of type 2 diabetes with lifestyle intervention or Metformin. N Engl J Med 2002; 346: 393–403.
44. Agarwal MM, Hughest PF, Punnose J, Ezimokhai M. Fasting plasma glucose as screening test for gestational diabetes in a multi-ethnic, high-risk population. Diabet Med 2000; 17: 720–6.
45. Atilano LC, Parritz AL, Lieberman E, Cohen AP, Barbieri RL. Alternative methods of diagnosing gestational diabetes mellitus. Am J Obstet Gynecol 1999; 181: 1158–61.
46. Perucchini D, Fischer U, Spinas GA, et al. Using fasting plasma glucose concentrations to screen for gestational diabetes mellitus. BMJ 1999; 319: 812–5.
47. Reichelt AJ, Franco LJ, Spichler ER, et al. Fasting plasma glucose is a useful test for the detection of gestational diabetes. Diabetes Care 1998; 21: 1246–9.
48. Sacks DA, Greenspoon JS, Fotherington N. Could the fasting plasma glucose assay be used to screen for gestational diabetes? J Reprod Med 1992; 37: 907–9.
49. Mills JL, Jovanovic L, Knopp R, et al. Physiological reduction in fasting plasma glucose concentration in the first trimester of normal pregnancy: The diabetes in early pregnancy study. Metabolism 1998; 47: 1140–4.

50. Carr SR, Slocum J, Tefft L, Haydon B, Carpenter MW. Precision of office-based blood glucose meters in screening for gestational diabetes. Am J Obstet Gynecol 1995; 173: 1267–72.

51. Carr SR. Screening for gestational diabetes mellitus. A perspective in 1998. Diabetes Care 1998; 21(suppl. 2): B14–8.

52. Dillon AE, Menard MK, Rust P, Newman RB, Van Dorsten JP. Glucometer analysis of one-hour glucose challenge samples. Am J Obstet Gynecol 1997; 177: 1120–3.

53. Pettitt DJ, Knowler WC, Baird R, Bennett PH. Gestational diabetes: Infant and maternal complications of pregnancy in relation to third-trimester glucose tolerance in the Pima Indians. Diabetes Care 1980; 3: 458–64.

54. O'Sullivan JB. The interaction between pregnancy, diabetes, and long-term maternal outcome. In: Reece EA, Coustan DR, eds. Diabetes Mellitus in Pregnancy: Principles and Practice. New York: Churchill Livingstone; 1988, pp. 575–85.

55. Mestman JH, Anderson GV, Guadalupe V. Follow-up study of 360 subjects with abnormal carbohydrate metabolism during pregnancy. Obstet Gynecol 1972; 39: 421–5.

56. Grant PT, Oats JN, Beischer NA. The long-term follow-up of women with gestational diabetes. Aust NZ J Obstet Gynaecol 1986; 26: 17–22.

57. Dornhorst A, Bailey PC, Anyaoku V, et al. Abnormalities of glucose tolerance following gestational diabetes. Q J Med 1990; 77: 1219–28.

58. Damm P, Kühl C, Bertelsen A, Molsted-Pedersen L. Predictive factors for the development of diabetes in women with previous gestational diabetes mellitus. Am J Obstet Gynecol 1992; 167: 607–16.

59. Metzger BE, Cho NH, Roston SM, et al. Prepregnancy weight and antepartum insulin secretion predict glucose tolerance five years after gestational diabetes mellitus. Diabetes Care 1993; 16: 1598–605.

60. Kjos SL, Peters RK, Xiang A, et al. Predicting future diabetes in Latino women with gestational diabetes: Utility of early postpartum glucose tolerance testing. Diabetes 1995; 44: 586–91.

61. O'Sullivan JB, Charles D, Mahan CM, Dandrow RV. Gestational diabetes and perinatal mortality rate. Am J Obstet Gynecol 1973; 116: 901–4.

62. Gabbe SG, Mestman JH, Freeman RK, Anderson GV, Lowenstein RI. Management and outcome of class A diabetes mellitus. Am J Obstet Gynecol 1977; 127: 465–9.

63. Sacks DA, Abu-Fadil S, Greenspoon JS, Foftheringham N. Do the current standards for glucose tolerance testing in pregnancy represent a valid conversion of O'Sullivan's original criteria? Am J Obstet Gynecol 1989; 161: 638–41.

64. Gilmer MD, Beard RW, Brooke FM, Oakley NW. Carbohydrate metabolism in pregnancy. Part II. Relation between maternal glucose tolerance and glucose metabolism in the newborn. BMJ 1975; 3: 402–4.

65. Sacks DA, Greenspoon JS, Abu-Fadil S, et al. Toward universal criteria for gestational diabetes: the 75-gram glucose tolerance test in pregnancy. Am J Obstet Gynecol 1995; 172: 607–14.

66. Sermer M, Naylor CD, Gare DJ, et al., for the Toronto-Tri Hospital Gestational Diabetes Investigators. Impact of increasing glucose intolerance on maternal–fetal outcomes in 3637 women without gestational diabetes. Am J Obstet Gynecol 1995; 173: 146–56.

67. Jensen, DM, Damm P, Sorensen, B, et al. Clinical impact of mild carbohydrate intolerance in pregnancy: a study of 2904 nondiabetic Danish women with risk factors for gestational diabetes. Am J Obstet Gynecol 2001; 185: 413–9.

68. Berkus M, Langer O. Glucose tolerance test: Degree of glucose abnormality correlates with neonatal outcome. Obstet Gynecol 1993; 81: 344–8.

69. Lindsay MK, Graves W, Klein L. The relationship of one abnormal glucose tolerance test value and pregnancy complications. Obstet Gynecol 1989; 73: 103–6.

70. Leikin EL, Jenkins JH, Pomerantz GA, Klein L. Abnormal glucose screening tests in pregnancy a risk factor for fetal macrosomia. Obstet Gynecol 1987; 69: 570–3.

71. Bevier WC, Fischer R, Jovanovic L. Treatment of women with an abnormal glucose challenge test (but a normal oral glucose tolerance test) decreases the prevalence of macrosomia. Am J Perinatol 1999; 16: 269–75.

72. Deerochanawong C, Putiyanum C, Wongsuryrat M, Serirat S, Jinayon P. Comparison of National Diabetes Data Group and World Health Organization criteria for detecting gestational diabetes mellitus. Diabetologia 1996; 39: 1070–3.

73. Moses RG, Moses M, Russell KG, Schier GM. The 75-g glucose tolerance test in pregnancy. Diabetes Care 1998; 1807–11.

74. Schmidt MI, Duncan BB, Reichelt AJ, et al. Gestational diabetes mellitus diagnosed with a 2-h 75-g OGTT and adverse pregnancy outcomes. Diabetes Care 2001; 24: 1151–5.

75. Rust OA, Bofill JA, Andrew ME, et al. Lowering the threshold for the diagnosis of gestational diabetes. Am J Obstet Gynecol 1996; 175: 961–5.

76. Schwartz ML, Ray WN, Lubarsky SL. The diagnosis and classification of gestational diabetes mellitus: Is it time to change our tune ? Am J Obstet Gynecol 1999; 180: 1560–71.

77. Penninson EH, Egerman RS. Perinatal outcomes in gestational diabetes: A comparison of criteria for diagnosis. Am J Obstet Gynecol 2001; 184: 1118–21.

78. Mello G, Elena P, Ognibene A, et al. Lack of concordance between the 75-g and 100-g glucose load tests for the diagnosis of gestational diabetes mellitus. Clin Chem 2006; 52: 1679–84.

22 Diabetic embryopathy in the pre-implantation embryo

Asher Ornoy and Noa Bischitz

Introduction

Diabetes mellitus can cause, in addition to birth defects and/or intra-uterine death, decreased fertility in males and females. As maternal diabetes may affect embryonic development at different developmental stages, an important question relates to the stage at which the developing embryo may be affected. Does the first fault occur at the zygote, the morula, blastula or perhaps even earlier, at the oocyte phase?

This chapter will discuss the influence of maternal diabetes on the embryo at the pre-implantation and pre-organogenetic phase, i.e the first week post-fertilization in rodents and the first 2 weeks in man.

The pre-implantation period is a very initial process of pregnancy, when most women do not know that they are pregnant. This is one of the main reasons that make this process so difficult to investigate. Therefore, in order to understand these early events in diabetic pregnancies, most studies were carried out on diabetic animal models.

Maternal diabetes in rodents influences embryonic and fetal development in a very similar manner to that of humans.[1] Hence, most studies discussed in this chapter were carried out on diabetic rats and mice or in *in vitro* models. We will describe the effects of maternal diabetes starting from the ovum and gradually continuing to later pre-implantation stages, and then discuss proposed mechanisms of action.

Changes in oocytes

Most studies on the effects of maternal diabetes on early pregnancy focused on the zygote; only a few recent studies have started to examine the oocytes. In the developing oocyte, the surrounding granulosa cells support its growth and provide hormonal supplementation. There are several interactions between the oocyte and the granulosa cells such as paracrine signaling and gap junctional communication. These interactions are critical for the oocyte differentiation and growth.[2]

Chang et al.[3] suggested that maternal diabetes adversely affects pre-ovulatory oocyte maturation, oocyte development and granulosa cell apoptosis in mice. Their main hypothesis was how reduction in paracrine communication between the granulosa cells and the oocyte in diabetes causes a matura-

tional delay. Indeed, in chronic hypoinsulinemic and hyperglycemic mice (Akita diabetic mice) or in acutely hyperglycemic and hypoinsulinemic mice (induced by streptozotocin (STZ) injection) the pre-ovulatory follicles and oocytes were small with more apoptotic follicular cells in comparison to controls. In addition, there was a delay in meiotic maturation, up-regulation in the expression of cell-death signaling proteins and a decrease in the expression level of key gap junction proteins such as connexin-43 that are necessary for communication.

In conclusion, maternal diabetes, as evidenced from the studies in mice, may interrupt the normal communication of the oocyte and its surrounding cells, increase apoptosis thus leading to abnormal development of the oocyte. This might, if extrapolated to man, cause menstrual disturbances, different embryonic insults or very early miscarriage, as indeed found in diabetic women.[4]

The zygote and morula

The mechanism of the developmental delay of the zygote is not clear. Some studies investigated in rats the development of the zygote in STZ induced maternal diabetes or *in vivo*. Diabetes was induced in rats by ablation of the insulin secreting islets cells by STZ. These studies showed delay in early developmental progression of the zygotes and reduced implantation rates.[4] Other studies carried out on embryos recovered from NOD diabetic or nondiabetic mice 72 h after fertilization showed an increased percentage of embryos at the one-cell stage, as these embryos could not continue their normal dividing process.[5] When these embryos were further cultured in the presence of high concentrations of D-glucose, severe growth retardation was demonstrated. No impairment of growth was observed following culture in high concentrations of L-glucose. Similar results were obtained when two-cell stage mouse embryos were obtained from nondiabetic mice but cultured on culture media containing high concentrations of D-glucose.[6]

Other studies have examined substrate utilization in the developing mouse embryos. Many zygotes that were incubated in high concentrations of glucose or lactate, failed to progress to the two-cell stage.[6,7] Moreover, it is known that mouse embryos begin to utilize glucose for several synthetic processes at the eight-cell stage,[7] and therefore the stages of morula and early blastocysts are highly susceptible to high glucose concentrations.

It can be concluded that high glucose levels at the earliest developmental stages, starting from one to two cells, can influence the future embryonic development and might even stop cell division and growth.

The blastocyst

Leunda-Casi et al.[8] examined how high levels of glucose influence mouse blastocysts. Embryonic exposure to high levels of D-glucose for a short time impaired trophectoderm differentiation, and the outgrowth of the trophectoderm was increased. This effect was secondary to a deficiency in fibroblast growth factor-4 protein (FGF-4) in the inner cell mass. Addition of FGF-4 to the blastocysts pretreated with high glucose normalized trophoblastic growth. The authors conclude that FGF-4 is important in the normal differentiation of the trophoblast and that these observations could explain some of the morphological changes detected in the placentae of diabetic pregnancies.[8]

A comparison between blastocysts from STZ diabetic to normal rats indicated that the former contained a lower number of cell nuclei in the inner cell mass (ICM) on day 5 post-fertilization. The proportion of morulae versus blastocysts was also different from controls, as the diabetic animals had more embryos persisting in the morula stage in comparison to controls or to rats injected with sub-diabetogenic doses of STZ, and hence not diabetic.[9] Treatment of the diabetic rats with insulin during the pre-implantation period (days 1–6 of pregnancy), normalized embryonic growth and development.[10] These studies demonstrate that the embryonic damage is due to the diabetes and not to the possible action of STZ. In the same line, other studies have shown that STZ induced diabetic rats had a 15–20% decrease in the total cells number of the ICM, a 20–25% decrease in the implantation rate and a similar reduction in the number of blastocysts.[4] However, the implanted blastocysts seem to be normal, as their protein synthesis was similar to that of implanted blastocysts from nondiabetic animals.

In contrast to the reduction in the number of ICM cells, high glucose concentrations did not change the number of trophoblastic cells.[4] Hinck et al.[11] studied the differentiation of Rcho-1 rat trophoblastic cells into giant cells in a culture medium supplemented with different concentrations of glucose. High glucose concentrations increased the number of trophoblastic cells, their nuclei were smaller and contained more DNA compared to control cells. While the cells cultured in control culture media increased their progesterone secretion, addition of high glucose concentrations inhibited that increase. Apoptosis was not increased with the addition of glucose. These morphological and physiological changes (reduction in progesterone secretion) could interfere with implantation and may possibly explain the increased rate of early abortions in man.

In conclusion, high glucose increases apoptosis of the ICM and may cause embryonic death. Trophoblastic cells are not diminished in number; on the contrary, their number may even increase.

In vitro studies performed by us

Culture in 'diabetic' culture medium

We cultured pre-implantation mouse blastocysts for 72 h in RPMI medium with the addition of 10% fetal bovine serum, and found 20–24% of embryonic developmental arrest.[12] Addition of high concentrations of glucose, acetoacetate, β-hydroxybutyrate, glucagon and insulin were all embryotoxic, inducing a high percentage of embryonic death. However, while the concentrations of most substances were much higher than possibly found in diabetes, the embryotoxic glucose concentrations were only 300 mg %, concentrations often observed in diabetes. Moreover, a combination of β-hydroxybutyrate, acetoacetate and glucose, in relatively low concentrations, was more embryotoxic than each of the substances individually. In addition, 50% serum from STZ-induced diabetic rats added to the culture medium caused 53% of embryonic developmental arrest, while 20% and 50% of rat and human control serum did not reduce the number of normally developing embryos.

Culture in sera from diabetic pregnant women

In two sets of experiments we cultured mouse embryos on RPMI culture medium with 30 or 50% serum obtained from women with pre-gestational (PGD) Type 1, Type 2 or gestational diabetes (GD), in comparison to similar concentrations of serum from nondiabetic women.[12] The results are shown in Tables 22.1 and 22.2.

At first we cultured two- to four-cell mouse embryos for up to 72 h to the early blastocyst stage in 30% serum from pregnant women with PGD or with GD and found that a high proportion of these embryos stopped from further developing within 24–72 h of culture (Table 22.1). The developmental stage of the living embryos was also reduced, but this reduction was significant only after 72 h of culture (Table 22.1). When we cultured early blastocysts in 50% diabetic serum, about half of the blastocysts died within the first 48 h of culture, but from that stage, all living embryos had spread on the Petri dish and continued to develop normally. Hence, the developmental stages of the living embryos were not different from that of controls (Table 22.2). There was a negative correlation between the degree of diabetic control and the extent of damage to the embryos. The sera from women with good control had less deleterious effects on the zygotes, morulae or early blastocysts. Sera from women with GD were also less embryotoxic than sera from women with PGD.

These results imply that human diabetic serum may stop mouse morulae and/or early blastocysts from further development, and retard the development of living morulae. However, these sera do not retard the development of living

Table 22.1   Effects of 30% serum from diabetic pregnant women on the developmental stages of two- to four-cell stage mouse embryos cultured for 72 h. Results are given as number of living embryos and their developmental stage

Source of serum	Time		
	0 h	48 h	72 h
Control	2.0 ± 0.05 (195)	8.1 ± 1.0 (177)	10.5 ± 0.7 (173)
Type 1	2.2 ± 0.4 (170)	7.0 ± 0.7 (159)	8.9 ± 0.7* (128)*
Type 2	2.3 ± 0.4 (128)	7.6 ± 0.8 (101)	9.2 ± 0.8* (84)*
Geotational diabetes	2.1 ± 0.1 (215)	7.8 ± 1.2 (188)	9.3 ± 0.5* (160)

Values are mean ± SD (number of embryos).
*Significantly lower than control, $P < 0.05$.

late blastocysts, and do not interfere with their hatching. The developmental stage specificity of the hyperglycemia-induced injuries is apparently related to age-specific metabolic changes.

Summary

The observations in diabetic mice and rats show that maternal diabetes may damage early embryonic development. This might lead to early embryonic death and, if pertinent to the human situation, to very early miscarriage, even before pregnancy is clinically recognized. Whether such pre-implantation very early spontaneous abortions really occur in diabetic women is currently unknown.

Spontaneous abortions in diabetic women

If the data in animal models is relevant to man, it is expected that diabetic women will have an increased rate of early miscarriages. Indeed, most human studies observed increased rate of spontaneous abortions in women with PGD. For example, a retrospective sample of 164 pregnancies during 1956 to 1975 with 78 insulin-dependent diabetic women was examined in order to evaluate the risk of clinically recognizable spontaneous abortions in diabetic women in comparison to the normal population.[13] This study was done before the policy of meticulous control of diabetes in pregnancy. The risk of spontaneous abortions among the diabetic females was almost double compared to the nondiabetic women. Later retrospective studies from 1980 to 2000 showed lower differences in the rate of spontaneous abortions between the diabetic and the nondiabetic women. Jovanovic at el.[14] followed 389 diabetic and 429 nondiabetic pregnant women. They found that the mean pregnancy loss rates were 12% in diabetic and 13% in normal pregnancies. When they examined the glucose blood levels they found that both nondiabetic and diabetic women had high glucose levels. However, the level of hyperglycemia tolerated in the diabetic pregnancies before reaching the threshold of fetal sensitivity was higher than that in nondiabetic pregnancies, implying maternal, placental, or fetal defenses to the stress of hyperglycemia.

Table 22.2   Effects of 50% serum from diabetic pregnant women on the developmental stages of mouse blastocysts cultured for 72 h. Results are given as the number of living embryos and their developmental stage

Source of serum	Time		
	0 h	48 h	72 h
Control	7.8 ± 0.6 (105)	10.5 ± 0.7 (98)	11.7 ± 0.7 (97)
Type 1	7.6 ± 0.2 (144)	10.6 ± 0.7 (77)*	11.8 ± 0.1 (77)*
Type 2	7.4 ± 0.5 (132)	10.6 ± 0.7 (63)*	11.8 ± 0.2 (62)*
Gestational diabetes	7.9 ± 0.5 (183)	10.6 ± 0.4 (125)*	11.9 ± 0.0 (123)*

Values are mean ± SD (number of embryos).
*Significantly lower than control, $P < 0.05$.

It can be assumed that these significant differences are caused by the differences in the control of diabetes, and with improved glycemic control, the rate of spontaneous abortions is reduced. This is in accordance to the fact that serum from well treated diabetic women was less deleterious to mouse embryos in culture than serum from poorly controlled diabetic women.[15]

Possible mechanisms of action of diabetes on the early embryo

Several mechanisms were shown to play a role in diabetes-induced early embryopathy in animals. Elucidation of these mechanisms of action may help to understand the human situation. We will, therefore, discuss these mechanisms mainly based on experimental animal models.

Apoptosis

Hyperglycemia induced excessive cell death in the ICM of rat blastocysts, which was characterized mainly by nuclear fragmentation. It was shown that these cells contain a large amount of the clusterin transcripts, a gene associated with apoptosis. The over-expression of clusterin in blastocysts of STZ diabetic rats indicates that these embryos may be affected by subtle disruptions in the expression pattern of critical developmental genes.[16] Similar to the previous study, blastocysts from diabetic rats and mice showed increased nuclear chromatin degradation in the ICM cells.[17,18] These and other studies demonstrate that in pre-implantation embryogenesis, hyperglycemia triggers increased apoptosis, especially at the blastocyst stage. Maternal hyperglycemia caused a decrease in the expression of facilitative glucose transporter genes such as GLUT1, GLUT2, and GLUT3, which was associated with the reduction in glucose transport to the embryo and a decrease in intra-embryonic free glucose.[18] This mechanism acts as a signal for cell death which triggers p53 activity. The hyperglycemia-induced cell death signal increases the expression of the pro-apoptotic protein BAX, which is a member of the Bcl-2 family.[18] In addition, mRNA levels and protein expression of BAX were higher in blastocysts cultured in hyperglycemic culture medium or in blastocysts obtained from STZ-induced diabetic mice.[18] In rat blastocysts in culture, transcription of the Bcl-2 gene and the activity of the protein were also markedly increased in the presence of high glucose concentrations in the culture medium.[19] These events induced by hyperglycemia, lead to activation of caspases, to DNA fragmentation, and morphologic changes consistent with apoptosis. This cascade (Figure 22.1), connecting the expression of Bcl-2 and/or BAX with cell death signals involving p53, suggests that the hyperglycemia induces embryonic hypoglycemia due to the decrease in the glucose transport expression and induces the p53 apoptotic cascade.[18,19]

Of the different glucose transporters existing in the early embryo, GLUT8 was recently found to be one of the most important.[20] This transporter is regulated by insulin. During early differentiation of the mouse blastocyst there is a significant increase in glucose demand, and insulin causes GLUT8 to

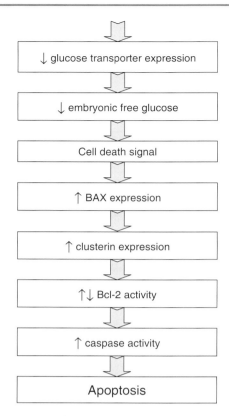

Figure 22.1 Hyperglycemia-induced apoptosis. (Modified from Keim et al.[21])

move to the plasma membrane, thus increasing the uptake of glucose, which is then converted to lactic acid. It is presumed that, similar to other glucose transporters, hyperglycemia decreases GLUT8 hence reducing the uptake of glucose by the ICM, inducing cell death.

Mouse blastocysts, genetically BAX deficient (BAX$^{-/-}$) obtained from diabetic dams, showed lower chromatin degradation and apoptosis than BAX-positive (BAX$^{+/+}$) embryos. Furthermore, the embryos from the BAX deficient diabetic mice had lower rates of malformations and resorption on day 14 of pregnancy.[18] These data propose that increased apoptosis in the blastocysts might indicate future increased early embryonic death or malformations, as observed in diabetic pregnancies.

The second apoptotic compound, Bcl-2, belongs to a family of proteins that operate in the effectors phase of apoptosis and may either promote or inhibit apoptosis. An increase in the expression of the anti-apoptotic Bcl-2 mRNA was observed in rat blastocysts which were cultured in 28 mM glucose for 24 h, compared to blastocysts incubated in 6 mM glucose.[19] When the Bcl-2 expression was inhibited, using antisense oligodeoxynucleotide, there was an increase of chromatin degradation in blastocysts incubated in high glucose concentrations. The addition of specific inhibitors to caspase-3 and caspase-activated-deoxyribonuclease (CAD) prevented the degradation of rat blastocysts.[19]

A third apoptotic compound, clusterin, a disulfide-linked heterodimeric protein associated with the clearance of cellular debris and apoptosis, was twice higher in embryos of diabetic rats than in control embryos.[17] When rat and mouse blastocysts were incubated with high glucose concentrations, there was an increase in BAX, in clusterin expression and nuclear chromatin degradation.[18,19]

It can be concluded that the significant loss of progenitor cells from the ICM makes the embryos more sensitive to later developmental deficiencies. Furthermore, it was reported that normal embryogenesis can occur only if sufficient number of functional ICM cells are available.[21] Increased apoptosis at this early stage of development may lead to spontaneous miscarriage or congenital malformations. Figure 22.1 summarizes the steps leading to diabetes-induced increased apoptosis.

Oxidative stress and antioxidants

Many studies implied that the causes of diabetic embryopathy may be secondary cellular damage from overproduction of reactive oxygen species (ROS) or/and decreased antioxidant defense mechanism in the embryonic cells.[15,22–24] The source of ROS is complex and non-specific. The main question is whether deranged oxidant antioxidant status can occur at this early stage of pre-implantation embryonic development. We found that serum from diabetic women can induce oxidative stress in the mouse blastocysts,[15] apparently in a way similar to that induced in post-implantation embryos.[22] This was evidenced by reduced concentrations of low molecular weight antioxidants (LMWA) such as glutathione and vitamins C and E. The pre-implantation mouse embryos cultured in serum from diabetic pregnant women had lower concentration of LMWA compared to embryos cultured in serum from nondiabetic women. It seems, therefore, that diabetic metabolic factors may induce embryotoxicity in pre-implantation embryos through derangement of the antioxidant defense mechanism. Leunda-Casi et al.[24] found that hyperglycemia may increase ROS generation, and this might be one of the reasons for increased cell apoptosis as evidenced in this study by the TUNEL technique. Similar findings were reported by others in mouse zygote and blastocysts.[25] One of the key mediators that was suggested as essence for apoptosis is hydrogen peroxide.[26] Violation of this balance by high glucose concentrations can cause massive cell damage, increase in apoptotic events and defective embryonic development. When there are high levels of glucose they need to be degraded, and the result is a high production of ketone bodies and an increase in the production of ROS.

Fertilization and embryonic development take place in an environment of low oxygen tension. Oxygen tension is gradually increasing with advanced gestation, once placentation is well established and maternal uterine arterioles are not obliterated by trophoblastic cells.[27,28] Oxidative stress also seems to play an important role in the early phases of embryonic development and hence antioxidants may play a significant role in preventing damage to the embryos.[13,22,26–28]

ROS mediate their action through many of the proinflammatory cytokines. They can influence the oocyte, sperm and embryos. During pregnancy, there are increased numbers of polymorphonuclear leucocytes (PMNL) which can cause superoxide ions increase. This oxidative stress may regulate the expression of cytokine receptors in the placenta, cytotrophoblastic cells, vascular endothelial cells, and smooth muscle cells. In addition, several studies have also demonstrated the significant role of free radicals in placental function. Oxidative damage to the trophoblastic cells early in pregnancy or to the placenta during the establishment of its maternal circulation, may also cause early pregnancy loss.[26–28]

Growth factors and cytokines

Cytokines and growth factors play an active role in the normal implantation process. They also have important roles in the pathogenesis of diabetes-induced organ damage, and those that interrupt the reproductive tract are able to cause pre-implantation embryopathy.[29–31] There are only few reports that refer to cytokines expression in the diabetic uterus. Insulin-like growth factor 2 (IGF-II) synthesis is down-regulated and, to the contrary, tumor necrosis factor-alfa (TNF-α) synthesis is up-regulated around the implantation sites in diabetic rat females.[32,33] Wuu et al.[34,35] showed a correlation between reduction in the concentrations of mRNA encoding IGF-II and embryonic growth retardation 2 days after initiation of implantation in C57B1/6J pregnant mice. However, later observations demonstrated that maternal diabetes did not affect the uterine IGF-I expression. Detection of TNF-α revealed over-expression in the mRNA as well as in the protein concentrations in the pre-implantation uterus of STZ-induced diabetic Wistar rats.[32] The majority of TNF-α protein synthesis was located in the epithelium lining the uterine lumen. Despite normalization of glycemia by addition of insulin to the diabetic animals, it did not prevent the overproduction of TNF-α in the uterus.[33] Incubation of rat and mouse uterine cells in different glucose concentrations induced stimulation of TNF-α secretion in uterine epithelial cells, apparently mediating the release of other cytokines, i.e. interleukin 1β from the subepithelial population of macrophages after their direct activation by hyperglycemia. There is evidence that high levels of TNF-α in utero can be harmful to the embryonic development at the implantation phase. Embryos exposed to high levels of TNF-α and surviving to term were significantly smaller than control embryos.[34–36] Mouse embryonic stem cells (ES) indicate that TNF-α inhibit cell proliferation in the ICM lineage and decreased their differentiation potential.[35] Further evidence for the hypothesis that TNF-α contributes to the harmful influence of maternal diabetes on pre-implantation development was found in blastocysts from Wistar rats. Culture medium was produced from normal and diabetic uterine cells; blastocysts of Wistar rats incubated in these media showed diminished growth in the diabetic medium, but improved significantly (not completely) by pre-treating the blastocysts with anti-sense oligonucleotide which blocked the embryonic TNF-α receptors.[36]

To conclude, there is increased secretion of TNF-α in diabetic rats and mice at the pre-implantation period which may harm the embryos, interfering with normal embryonic growth.

Metabolic factors

Glucose metabolism

The mouse blastocysts glucose supplement can be provided by the glucose transporters (i.e. GLUT1, GLUT8), by passive diffusion and by an active transport system.[20,37,38] In human and mouse blastocysts, the uptake of deoxyglucose is very active, and its concentrations in the mouse embryos were found to be 30 times higher than in the culture medium.[38] This transport was blocked by cytochalasin B but not by substances that usually block the active transport of glucose in the gut or kidney, emphasizing that this mechanism is unique to the early developing embryo.

Suppression of GLUT1 in preimplantation embryos by antisense GLUT1 is known to produce ICM apoptosis, in a way similar to high glucose concentrations. In addition, in the GLUT1 transporter deficient mouse the embryos and fetuses were found to exhibit the same damage and anomalies as observed in the offspring of diabetic animals,[39] further demonstrating the importance of glucose transport to normal early embryonic development.

Down-regulation of GLUT1 mRNA and protein expression in mouse trophoblasts and in human term placental trophoblasts[40–42] was observed after exposure to high glucose concentrations. It has therefore been suggested that the glucose transporter is regulated in the placenta by glucose, and that as a protective mechanism for the embryo, the transporter is being moved from the cell surface into an intracellular position, thus decreasing glucose uptake in hyperglycemia. This mechanism seems to protect the embryo from the toxic effects of high glucose concentrations.

Nitric oxide and prostaglandins

In the pre-implantation period, when the trophoblastic cells penetrate the decidua, there is an increase in vascular permeability and other inflammation-like changes. This increase in vascular permeability is related to vasoactive agents like nitric oxide (NO) and prostaglandins (PGs), as both are associated with increased vascular permeability, vasolidation and increased blood flow in the uterus. At the beginning of implantation in the rat uterus there is an increase in the NO synthase activity, synthesizing more NO and in the production of PGE, $PGF_{2\alpha}$ and PGI_2.[43,44] Moreover, when the synthesis of NO or PGs in the uterus is blocked, there is a decrease in the number of implanted rat embryos. During pre-implantation, there is an over-sensitivity to metabolic disturbances and the external environment can easily affect embryonic development. Novaro et al.[44] studied the uterine synthesis and temporal pattern of two vasoactive agents: NO and PGE, both modulating the implantation process in rats with noninsulin-dependent diabetes mellitus (NIDD) and found that the activity of NO synthase in the rat uterus and the production of prostaglandin E were increased in diabetes. In addition, the temporal profile of their activity was different from the control animals, and the number of implanted embryos was reduced. However, the implantation rate was not different between the diabetic and control animals.

While the NO increase was observed in different tissues, PGE production was located at the implantation sites and remained high after the implantation. The authors suggest that the increase of PGE synthesis in diabetic uterine tissue is a secondary effect. First there is an increase in the NO production, the NO regulates the synthesis of the PGs; together they have a positive influence on glucose metabolism and on the process of vasodilatation in the uterus. The rate and timing of the beginning of implantation are not altered by diabetes, but diabetes may damage the early blastocysts, reducing the number of embryos that are able to implant normally.[44]

Effects on male fertility

Studies suggest that sexual dysfunction is frequently associated with diabetes in men and in experimental animals.[45] Many of these problems result from diabetes-induced changes in the vascular system as well as in the peripheral and central nervous system that are related to changes in endocrine function.[46] Numerous studies have documented abnormalities in testicular function and spermatogenesis in diabetic animals.[47] In addition, studies demonstrated reduction in the activity of ATPases and phosphatases in the epidermis and in spermatozoa.[48] Impotence, infertility, and retrograde ejaculation have been described in diabetic men, but the etiology remains unclear. The reduction in the fertility of men with long standing diabetes, by affecting spermatogenesis, seems to be similar to the effects of diabetes on the ova.

Conclusions

As there is practically no data in man except for reduced fertility and increased spontaneous abortions in diabetics, most research was done on animal models. A direct extrapolation of these studies to man must be with great caution, as it may lead to wrong conclusions. In addition, in most *in vivo* animal studies, diabetes was induced by ablation of insulin production, and it is possible that some of the results stem from the technique of diabetes production. However, many of the results were obtained also *in vitro*, including studies on human diabetic serum that served as culture medium, strengthening the simulation to man. There is a need for human additional studies to verify the different proposed mechanisms of diabetic-induced early embryopathy.

Summary

Glucose blood levels can influence most processes related to oocyte maturation, fertilization, and early embryonic development. Good glycemic control in diabetic women even before pregnancy is diagnosed, can decrease or possibly prevent most of these effects that, if not prevented, may have long-term consequences on early and possibly late embryonic development.

REFERENCES

1. Polanco Ponce AC, Revilla Monsalve MC, Palomino Garibay MA, Islas Andrade S. Effect of maternal diabetes on human and rat fetal development. Gynecol Obstet Mex 2005; 73: 544–52.
2. Ackert CL, Gittens JE, O'Brien MJ, Eppig JJ, Kidder GM. Intercellular communication via connexin 43 gap junctions is required for ovarian folliculogenesis in the mouse. Dev Biol 2001; 233: 258–70.
3. Chang AS, Dale AN, Moley KH. Maternal diabetes adversely affects preovulatory oocyte maturation, development, and granulosa cell apoptosis. Endocrinology 2005; 146: 2445–53. E-pub 17 February 2005.
4. Pampfer S. Peri-implantation embryopathy induced by maternal diabetes. J Reprod Fertil 2000; 55(suppl.): 129–39.
5. Diamond MP, Moley KH, Pellicer A, Vaughn WK, DeCherney AH. Effects of streptozotocin- and alloxan-induced diabetes mellitus on mouse follicular and early embryo development. J Reprod Fertil 1989; 86: 1–10.
6. Moley KH, Vaughn WK, DeCherney AH, Diamond MP. Effect of diabetes mellitus on mouse pre-implantation embryo development. J Reprod Fertil 1991; 93: 325–32.
7. Biggers JD, Whittingham DG, Donahue RP. The pattern of energy metabolism in the mouse oocyte and zygote. Proc Natl Acad Sci USA 1967; 58: 560–7.
8. Leunda-Casi A, De Hertogh R, Pampfer S. Decreased expression of fibroblast growth factor-4 and associated dysregulation of trophoblast differentiation in mouse blastocysts exposed to high D-glucose in vitro. Diabetologia 2001; 44: 1318–25.
9. De Hertogh R, Vanderheyden I, Pampfer S, et al. Stimulatory and inhibitory effects of glucose and insulin on rat blastocysts development in vitro. Diabetes 1991; 40: 641–7.
10. De Hertogh R, Vanderheyden I, Pampfer S, Robin D, Delcourt J. Maternal insulin treatment improves pre-implantation embryo development in diabetic rats. Diabetologia 1992; 35: 406–8.
11. Hinck L, Thissen JP, Pampfer S, De Hertogh R. Effect of high concentrations of glucose on differentiation of rat trophoblast cells in vitro. Diabetologia 2003; 46: 276–83.
12. Ornoy A, Zusman I. Embryotoxic effects of diabetes on pre-implantation embryos. Isr J Med Sci 1991; 27: 487–92.
13. Greene MF. Spontaneous abortions and major malformations in women with diabetes mellitus. Semin Reprod Endocrinol 1999; 17: 127–36.
14. Jovanovic L, Knopp RH, Kim H, et al. Elevated pregnancy losses at high and low extremes of maternal glucose in early normal and diabetic pregnancy; evidence for a protective adaptation in diabetes. Diabetes Care 2005; 28: 1113–7.
15. Ornoy A, Kimyagarov D, Yeffee P, et al. Role of reactive species in diabetes-induced embryotoxicity; Studies on preimplantation mouse embryos cultured in serum from diabetic pregnant women. Isr J Med Sci 1996; 32: 1066–73.
16. Pampfer S, Vanderheyden I, McCracken JE, Vesela J, De Hertogh R. Increased cell death in rat blastocysts exposed to maternal diabetes in utero and to high glucose or tumor necrosis factor-α in vitro. Development 1997; 124: 4827–36.
17. Moley KH, Chi MM, Knudson CM, et al. Hyperglycemia induce apoptosis in pre-implantation embryos through cell death effector pathways. Nature Med 1998; 4: 1421–4.
18. Chi MM, Pingsterhouse J, Carayannopoulos M, et al. Decrease glucose transporter expression triggers Bax-dependent apoptosis in the murine blatocysts. J Biol Chem 2000; 275: 40252–7.
19. Pampfer S, Cordi S, Vanderheyden I, et al. Expression and role of Bcl-2 in rat blastocysts exposed to high D-glucose. Diabetes 2001; 50: 143–9.
20. Carayannopoulous MO, Maggie M, Chi MM, et al. Glut 8 is a glucose transporter responsible for insulin-stimulated glucose uptake in the blastocyst. Proc Natl Acad Sci USA 2000; 97: 7313–8.
21. Keim AL, Chi MY, Moley KH. Hyperglycemia-induced apoptotic cell death in the mouse blastocyst is dependent on expression of p53. Mol Reprod Dev 2001; 60: 214–24.
22. Zaken V, Kohen R, Ornoy A. Vitamins C and E improve rat embryonic antioxidant defense mechanism in diabetic culture medium. Teratology 2001; 64: 33–44.
23. Parchment RE. The implications of a unified theory of programmed cell death, polyamines, oxyradicals and histogenesis in the embryo. Int J Dev Biol 1993; 37: 75–83.
24. Leunda-Casi A, Genicot G, Donnay I, Pampfer S, De Hertogh R. Increased cell death in mouse blastocysts exposed to high D-glucose in vitro; implications of an oxidative stress and alterations in glucose metabolism. Diabetologia 2002; 45: 571–9.
25. Burton GJ, Hempstock J, Jauniaux E. Oxygen, early embryonic metabolism and free radical-mediated embryopathies. Reprod Biomed Online 2003; 6: 84–96.
26. Agarwal A, Gupta S, Sikka S. The role of free radicals and antioxidants in reproduction. Curr Opin Obstet Gynecol 2006; 18: 325–32.
27. Jauniaux E, Watson AL, Hempstock J, et al. Onset of maternal arterial blood flow and placental oxidative stress. A possible factor in human early pregnancy failure. Am J Pathol 2000; 157: 2111–22.
28. Jauniaux E, Hempstock J, Greenwold N, Burton GJ. Trophoblastic oxidative stress in relation to temporal and regional differences in maternal placental blood flow in normal and abnormal early pregnancies. Am J Pathol 2003; 162: 115–25.
29. Pankewycz OG, Guan JX, Benedict JF. Cytokines as mediators of autoimmune diabetes and diabetic complications. Endocr Rev 1995; 16: 164–76.
30. Chernicky CL, Redline RW, Tan HQ, et al. Expression of insulin-like growth factors I and II in conceptuses from normal and diabetic mice. Mol Reprod Dev 1994; 37: 382–90.
31. Banerjee S, Smallwood A, Moorhead J, et al. Placental expression of interferon-gamma (IFN-gamma) and its receptor IFN-gamma R2 fail to switch from early hypoxic to late normotensive development in preeclampsia. J Clin Endocrinol Metab 2005; 90: 944–52.
32. Pampfer S, Vanderheyden I, Wuu YD, et al. Possible role for TNF-alpha in early embryopathy associated with maternal diabetes in the rat. Diabetes 1995; 44: 531–6.
33. Pampfer S, Vanderheyden I, De Hertogh R. Increased synthesis of tumor necrosis factor-alpha in uterine explants from pregnant diabetic rats and in primary cultures of uterine cells in high glucose. Diabetes 1997; 46: 1214–24.
34. Wuu YD, Pampfer S, Becquet P, et al. Tumor necrosis factor alpha decreases the viability of mouse blastocysts in vitro and in vivo. Biol Reprod 1999; 60: 479–83.
35. Wuu YD, Pampfer S, Vanderheyden I, Lee KH, De Hertogh R. Impact of tumor necrosis factor alpha on mouse embryonic stem cells. Biol Reprod 1998; 58: 1416–24.
36. Pampfer S, Vanderheyden I, Vesela J, De Hertogh R Neutralization of tumor necrosis factor alpha (TNF alpha) action on cell proliferation in rat blastocysts by antisense oligodeoxyribonucleotides directed against TNF alpha p60 receptor. Biol Reprod 1995; 52: 1316–26.
37. Gardner DK, Leese HJ. The role of glucose and pyruvate transport in regulating nutrient utilization by preimplantation mouse embryos. Development 1988; 104: 423–9.
38. Chi MM, Manchester JK, Basuray R, et al. An unusual active hexose transport system in human and mouse preimplantation embryos. Proc Natl Acad Sci USA 1993; 90: 10023–5.
39. Heilig CW, Saunders T, Brosius FC, et al. Glucose transporter-1-deficient mice exhibit impaired development and deformities that are similar to diabetic embryopathy. Proc Natl Acad Sci USA 2003; 100: 613–8.
40. Ogura K, Sakata M, Yamaguchi M, Kurachi H, Murata Y. High concentration of glucose decreases glucose transporter-1 expression in mouse placenta in vitro and in vivo. J Endocrinol 1999; 160: 443–52.
41. Hahn T, Barth S, Weiss U, Mosgoeller W, Desoye G. Sustained hyperglycemia in vitro down-regulates the GLUT1 glucose transport system of cultured human term placental trophoblast; a mechanism to protect fetal development? FASEB J 1998; 12: 1221–31.
42. Hahn T, Hahn D, Blaschitz A, et al. Hyperglycemia-induced subcellular redistribution of GLUT1 glucose transporters in cultured human term placental trophoblast cells. Diabetologia 2000; 43: 173–80.
43. Kennedy TG. Evidence for a role for prostaglandins in the initiation of blastocyst implantation in the rat. Biol Reprod 1977; 16: 286–91.
44. Novaro V, Jawerbaum A, Faletti A, Gimeno MA, Gonzalez ET. Uterine nitric oxide and prostaglandin E during embryonic implantation in non-insulin-dependent diabetic rats. Reprod Fertil Dev 1998; 10: 217–23.

45. Amador A, Steger RW, Bartke A, et al. Pituitary and testicular function in spontaneously hypertensive rats. J Androl 1983; 4: 67–70.

46. Calvo JC, Baranao JL, Tesone M, Charreau EH. Hypothalamic-hypophyseal–gonadal axis in the streptozotocin-induced diabetic male rat. J Steroid Biochem 1984; 20: 769–72.

47. McVary KT, Rathnau CH, McKenna KE. Sexual dysfunction in the diabetic BB/WOR rat; a role of central neuropathy. Am J Physiol 1997; 272(1, pt 2): R259–67.

48. Kuhn-Velten N, Schermer R, Staib W. Effect of streptozotocin-induced hyperglycaemia on androgen-binding protein in rat testis and epididymis. Diabetologia 1984; 26: 300–3.

23 Congenital malformations in diabetic pregnancy: Prevalence and types

Paul Merlob

Introduction

The association between maternal diabetes mellitus and congenital malformations in newborns may well be causal; however, the teratogenic mechanism remains unclear.[1] The prevalence and the described type of malformations vary among different studies and a predictable malformation syndrome has not been identified.[1] This chapter discusses the prevalence and types of structural congenital malformations in infants of mothers with diabetes mellitus (IDM) or gestational diabetes (IGDM). Their etiology and pathogenesis are presented in two other chapters of this book.

Historical data

Many studies of small groups of infants (from 1930 to 1950), including malformed infants, were not conclusive. It was only after 1960 that large, controlled, population- or hospital-based studies of offspring of mothers with diabetes began to appear in the literature.

In 1964, Molsted-Pedersen et al.[2] studied 853 IDM born between 1926 and 1963 and weighing more than 1000 g. They noted a 6.4% rate of congenital malformations, compared to only 2.1% in a control group of 1212 infants born to nondiabetic mothers in the same hospital, but during 1958 and 1960. Further analysis revealed that the presence of maternal vascular complications was associated with a significantly greater risk of fatal, major (but not mild), and multiple malformations in the infants.

Two years later, Naeve[1] analyzed the frequency of congenital malformations in infants of 2592 diabetic mothers, 892 women known to have become diabetic 5 or more years after delivery, 1262 infants of women married to diabetic men and an equal number of infants of nondiabetic pregnancies. A significantly higher rate of congenital malformations was noted in the study group (13.1%) than in the control group (5.3%), with a relative risk of any malformation of 2.47. The frequency of malformations increased steadily with the severity of the maternal diabetes scaled by White's classification.

The largest review of malformations associated with diabetic pregnancy, performed by Kucera[3] in 1971, included the data available from the world literature between 1945 to 1965, covering 7101 infants born to diabetic mothers and a control group of more than 400,000 healthy infants derived from the registries of the World Health Organization. The prevalence of congenital malformations was 4.79% in the study population compared with 0.65% in the controls.[3] However, information regarding the criteria used for the diagnosis and management of diabetes, and for the diagnosis and classification of the malformations, was not consistently available.

The results of the Collaborative Perinatal Project, using data from hospitals throughout the United States, were reported in 1975.[4] A total of 567 overt diabetic pregnancies, 372 gestational diabetic pregnancies, and 47,408 nondiabetic pregnancies were analyzed. Congenital malformations were identified in a significantly higher proportion of infants of mothers with overt diabetes (17.1%) than in infants of nondiabetic mothers (8.4%). The infants of mothers with gestational diabetes had an 8.9% rate of malformations, almost equal to that of the control group.

In 1976, Soler et al.[5] studied 701 IDM born in Birmingham, UK, between 1950 and 1974, of whom 8.1% were found to have a congenital malformation compared to 1.7% in the control group. In the same year, Day and Insley,[6] in a study of 205 IDM born in the same area between 1969 and 1974, reported a malformation rate of 12%, compared to 6% in the control nondiabetic group.

After 1980, investigations in the field expanded worldwide. Although their specific figures differed considerably, in almost all of them, the prevalence rates were significantly higher in IDM than in the general newborn population. However, even the largest studies[7–11] comprised a relatively small absolute number of congenital malformations in offspring of women with pregestational insulin-dependent diabetes.[11]

Prevalence

The prevalence of congenital malformations has been evaluated predominantly in women with Type 1 diabetes (pregestational insulin-dependent diabetes), with rates ranging mainly from 4.1 to 17.1%. Despite improvements in obstetric care, with strict control of diabetes and good pregnancy surveillance, the rate of major malformations in infants of mothers with Type 1 diabetes remains two to three times that of the general population. Comparisons among the different studies are very difficult, if not impossible, for several reasons:

• The diagnostic classification of diabetes varies among and even within countries.
• Screening for the detection of diabetes has not been undertaken in the same manner and scale in all geographic regions.
• The timing and degree of preconception and postconception care differs.
• The diagnosis, definition, and classification of congenital malformations varies largely among studies.
• The methods used to detect fetal and neonatal malformations are different.
• Other confounding factors, such as maternal age, obesity, ethnicity, and uptake of folic acid, are rarely taken into account.

These confounding factors may explain the great variability in the reported prevalence rates of congenital malformations in Type 1 diabetic pregnancies and they should be taken into account when prevalence of malformations is studied.

It is important to emphasize that the demographic pattern of diabetes in pregnancy is changing: increasing numbers of young women are being diagnosed as having Type 1 diabetes, and the number of people diagnosed as having Type 2 diabetes is also increasing.[12,13]

With regard to gestational diabetes, several authors have reported an association with major malfomations and the same types of anomalies were found as in the offspring of women with pregestational Type 1 diabetes.[8,14–17] Although the risk is apparently lower, being that gestational diabetes accounts for approximately 90% of all cases of diabetes-complicated pregnancy,[18] the overall effect of this risk has important clinical and public health connotations.

In a fairly recent study, Sheffield et al.[10] found that women with pre-gestational diabetes or gestational diabetes plus fasting hyperglycemia had a 3- to 4-fold greater risk of congenital malformations in their offspring than the general population, whereas infants of women with mild gestational diabetes had malformation rates no different than the general nondiabetic population. Nevertheless, it is important to remember that gestational diabetes is a heterogenous disorder that includes previously unrecognized or newly diagnosed non-gestational diabetes mellitus.[8,16] These patients (with pre-existing but undetected Type 2 diabetes) represent a subgroup of IGDM with an increased risk for occurrence of congenital malformations.

Type 2 diabetes (associated with both increasing insulin resistance and abnormality of insulin secretion) is increasing explosively.[12,19] As in all diabetic pregnancies, infants born to mothers with Type 2 diabetes are also at increased risk of having congenital malformations.[15,19] The most common

malformations[19] were cardiac (53%) followed by musculo-skeletal (27%). These results are almost similar to rates previously identified in women with Type 1 diabetes.[19] The majority of malformations occurred in those with poor glycemic control who did not received pre-pregnancy care.[19,20]

The prevalence of congenital malformations in all types of maternal diabetes is in good relationship with:

• The severity of the maternal diabetes (White's class)
• The control of maternal diabetes (expressed by HbA1c)

An increased prevalence of malformations occurring in parallel with the severity and duration of the diabetes has been described.[21] For example, the frequency of major malformations among offspring has been reported to be 4.4% in White's classes B and C, 9.7% in class D, and 16.7% in class F, with an overall prevalence of 6.4% in all infants of diabetic mothers as compared with 2% in the general population.[21]

The same increase of prevalence of malformations was observed in relation to the HbA1c levels. For example, a frequency of 5.1% of malformations has been reported for a HbA1c of 7.0–8.5%, 22.9% for a level of 8.6–9.9% and 21.7% for a level of HbA1c above 10%.[22] Even a slightly raised of HbA1c during early pregnancy in women with Type 1 diabetes carries an increased risk for fetal malformations.[23]

Types of malformations

The congenital malformations of IDM and IGDM constitute a spectrum known as diabetic embryopathy (DE).[21,24] This spectrum implies errors of morphogenesis which appear between the third and the seventh week of embryonic development (end of blastogenesis and organogenesis).[25] Within this spectrum of DE, cardiac, skeletal, central nervous system (CNS), uro-genital, gastro-intestinal, facial and multiple malformations were repeatedly described (Table 23.1). Congenital malformations in IGDM and offspring of women with Type 2 diabetes affect the same organ systems that have been previously described in pregnancies with Type 1 diabetes.[15] The most commonly affected organ systems were cardiac (37.6%), musculo-skeletal (14.7%), CNS (9.8%), and multiple malformations (16%).[15]

It has been debated whether maternal diabetes exerts a non-specific teratogenic effect expressed in a universally increased risk of all congenital malformations or whether the disease should be regarded as a specific teratogen associated with a distinct pattern of congenital abnormalities.[11] The spectrum in DE is large and highly variable; however, most studies have reported an increase of specific malformations especially involving the heart, the skeleton (particularly sacral agenesis), the kidneys and CNS.[7] Regarding cardiac malformations, the strongest association with maternal diabetes was found in infants with defects of primary congenital cardiogenesis, whereas most abnormalities arising later in cardiac development were not associated with diabetes.[9] Others found a strong teratogenic effect on four specific types of malformations: renal agenesis, obstructive urinary tract, cardiac and multiple abnormalities, as opposed to an unspecific increased general risk of congenital malformations.[11]

Table 23.1   Congenital malformations in infants of diabetic mothers

Organ system	Malformations	
	Common	Rare, occasional
Cardiac	Corrected transposition Ventricular septal defect Coarctation Atrial septal defect Cardiomyopathy	Tetralogy of Fallot Hypoplastic left heart Single ventricle Double-outlet right ventricle Pulmonic stenosis Anomalous venous return
Skeletal	Sacral agenesis Vertebral and rib anomalies Limb reduction defects	Polydactyly Syndactyly Clinodactyly Clubfoot
CNS	Anencephaly Neural tube defects Microcephaly Hydrocephalus	Occipital encephalocele Holoprosencephaly Septo-optic dysplasia
Uro-genital	Hydronephrosis Renal agenesis Ureteral duplication Multicystic dysplasia Hypospadias	Hypoplastic genitalia Micropenis Ambiguous genitalia Megalo-urethera
Gastro-intestinal	Duodenal atresia Ano-rectal atresia Esophageal atresia	Malrotation Volvulus Omphalocele Gastroschisis Diaphragmatic hernia

Facial	Cleft lip
	Cleft palate
	Ears
	  microtia
	  anotia
	  atresia of canal ear
	  hairy ears
	  hearing loss
	Eyes
	  cataract
	  coloboma
	  optic nerve hypoplasia
		Choanal atresia
		Absent depressor anguli oris muscle
		Fused orbits

Others	Single umbilical artery	Laterality defects Tracheal stenosis Branchial arch anomalies

Cardiac malformations

Cardiac malformations are the most common congenital malformations of IDM, and they occur significantly more often in IDM than in infants of nondiabetic mothers.[7,21] Rowland et al.[26] reported a 4% prevalence of cardiac malformations in a series of 470 IDM, a 5-fold higher rate than in the general population (0.8%). Becerra et al.[7] found that infants of mothers with gestational diabetes who required insulin during the third trimester of pregnancy were 20.6 times more likely to have major cardiovascular malformations than infants of nondiabetic mothers. No such difference was noted in infants of mothers with gestational diabetes who did not require insulin.[7]

Loffredo et al.,[9] in a population-based case–control study of 4390 IDM and 3572 healthy infants, observed that pre-conceptional maternal diabetes was strongly associated with cardiovascular malformations of early embryonic origin (OR = 4.7) and cardiomyopathy (OR = 15.1), but not with obstructive and shunting defects (OR = 1.4). There was a strong association of cardiovisceral and cardiac chamber discordance, i.e. 'corrected' (levo-) transposition of the great arteries, but not with 'pure' transposition, i.e. intact ventricular septum or ventricular septal defect.[9] Among outflow tract anomalies, the risk was strongly associated with normally related great arteries (OR = 6.6) but not with simple transposition. These findings imply a specific effect of maternal diabetes on certain subtypes of cardiac malformations and may have important clinical and preventive implications.[9]

Skeletal malformations

Maternal diabetes has been associated with sacral agenesis, also termed sacral dysgenesis or caudal regression.[3] This is a complex malformation characterized by the absence or maldevelopment of the sacrum and coccyx, with or without hypoplastic femurs, dislocated hips, defects in tibias or fibulas, or other lower-limb malformations. Affected babies often have anomalies of other organ systems as well. Sacral agenesis occurs in about 0.2–0.5% of IDM, representing a 200- to 400-fold higher rate than in the general population.[5,21]

CNS malformations

Anencephaly is the most common CNS malformation associated with diabetic pregnancy, affecting 0.57% of IDM,[21] which is 3-fold higher than the rate in the general population (0.19%).[21] IDM also have a high prevalence of neural tube defects (1.95 vs. 0.2% in the general population).[27] One study of experimental diabetes induced after the period of organogenesis noted no effect on the CNS of the offspring.[21]

Uro-genital malformations

Kucera[3] was the first to report an increased rate of urological malformations in IDM. The most frequent renal malformations in IDM are renal agenesis, ureteral duplication, and hydronephrosis.[1,11,24] Hypospadias is the most frequent genital malformation in IDM and IGDM.[11,24]

Gastro-intestinal malformations

The abdominal malformations shown to occur with a higher prevalence in IDM include ano-rectal, duodenal, and lower-intestine atresia.[21,24] Malrotation, volvulus, and abdominal wall defects have also been described.

Facial malformations

Facial anomalies in IDM and IGDM have been described in only a small number of reports.[7,16,28–31] The most frequent were oro-facial clefts[7,16] and ear and eye abnormalities.[1,7,29] Interestingly, some studies reported an association of maternal diabetes with certain facio-skeletal syndromes, such as femoral–facial syndrome and oculoauriculovertebral polytopic field defect.[29–32] Therefore, IDM and IGDM should be carefully evaluated for facial malformations.[29–32]

Other anomalies

A single umbilical artery occurs in about 6.4% of IDM, a 5-fold higher rate than in the general population.[21] This mild malformation might be associated with other, major, structural anomalies.

Multiple malformations

Many studies found a strong association between pre-gestational maternal diabetes and multiple-system malformations (not defined as a syndrome) in the offspring.[4,11] For example, 27.5% of all malformed infants in the Collaborative Perinatal Project[4] had multiple anomalies. Aberg et al.[16] observed that 6% of their malformed IDM had more than one anomaly compared to 0.57% of the control group. They concluded that there is a clear-cut increase in the risk of multiple malformations in infants of mothers with pre-existing diabetes, but not of mothers with GDM.[16] In the infants with multiple malformations, the same organ systems were affected as in the whole group of IDM, with highest rates for cardiac malformations, atresias, clefts, limb reduction, and hypospadias.

Mild malformations

Studies on mild malformations in IDM and IGDM are relatively scarce,[33–35] and no randomized double-blind investigations have been performed to date. The results of the case–control studies are contradictory, with some showing significant differences but others not. No association was observed between the severity of the metabolic derangement (HbA1c) in the mother and the appearance of mild malformations in the offspring.[34,35] This was also true for White's class, duration of diabetes, maternal age, and cigarette smoking.[33]

Preconception care and reduced risk of congenital malformations

Many prospective controlled studies worldwide have demonstrated that strict metabolic control of maternal diabetes before conception and during pregnancy can prevent most neonatal complications, including congenital malformations.[36] Ray et al.[20] conducted a systematic review of all published studies on preconception care (PCC) (eight prospective and eight retrospective studies were included in the final analysis) involving a total of 1192 infants whose mothers had received PCC and 1459 infants of mothers who had not. The pooled rate of major malformations was lower in the infants of the PCC recipients (2.1%) than in non-recipients (6.5%), with a relative risk of 0.36. Interestingly, the risk of major malformations was lowest in the one study in which folic acid was administered periconceptionally.[37] The essential problem is that a substantial percentage of diabetic women do not attend PCC programs[20] and do not take prenatal folic acid and multivitamins, just as in the general population.[38] Greater efforts by the medical community are needed to promote education of the public, improve maternal access to PCC programs, and maximize the interventions associated with improved pregnancy outcome.[20]

Summary

Maternal diabetes mellitus (Types 1 and 2) and gestational diabetes with fasting hyperglycemia are associated with a 2- to

3-fold increase in the risk of congenital malformations in offspring compared with the general population. Although no specific malformation syndrome has been identified, cardiac, skeletal, CNS, and multiple malformations are the most frequently described. Up to 50% of all perinatal deaths of offspring of diabetic mothers are due to congenital malformations.[39] Congenital malformations also pose a seri-ous social and financial burden to both the individual family and society at large.[21] Therefore, the medical community must ensure that programs for preconception care are made available to diabetic mothers for strict control of their disease before conception and during pregnancy. This could prevent the occurrence of most neonatal complications, including congenital malformations.

REFERENCES

1. Naeve C. Congenital malformations in offspring of diabetics. Perspect Pediatr Pathol 1984; 8: 213–22.
2. Molsted-Pedersen L, Tygstrup I, Pedersen J. Congenital malformations in newborn infants of diabetic women: correlation with maternal diabetic vascular complications. Lancet 1964; I: 1124–6.
3. Kucera J. Rate and type of congenital anomalies among offspring of diabetic mothers. J Reprod Med 1971; 7: 61–70.
4. Chung CS, Myrianthopoulos NC. Factors affecting risk of congenital malformations, II: Effect of maternal diabetes. Birth Defects Orig Artic Ser 1975; 11: 23–38.
5. Soler NG, Walsh CH, Malins JM. Congenital malformations in infants of diabetic mothers. Q J Med 1976; 45: 303–13.
6. Day RE, Insley J. Maternal diabetes mellitus and congenital malformations: survey of 205 cases. Arch Dis Child 1976; 51: 935–8.
7. Becerra JE, Khoury MJ, Cordero JF, Erickson JD. Diabetes mellitus during pregnancy and the risks for specific birth defects: a population-based case-control study. Pediatrics 1990; 85: 1–9.
8. Martinez-Frias ML, Bermejo E, Rodriguez-Pinilla E, et al. Epidemiological analysis of outcomes of pregnancy in gestational diabetic mothers. Am J Med Genet 1998; 78: 140–5.
9. Loffredo CA, Wilson PD, Ferencz C. Maternal diabetes: an independent risk factor for major cardiovascular malformations with increased mortality of affected infants. Teratology 2001; 64: 98–106.
10. Sheffield JS, Butler-Koster EG, Casey BM, et al. Maternal diabetes mellitus and infant malformations. Obstet Gynecol 2002; 100: 925–30.
11. Nielsen GL, Norgard B, Puho E, et al. Risk of specific congenital abnormalities in offspring of women with diabetes. Diabet Med 2005; 22: 693–6.
12. MacIntosh MCM, Fleming KM, Bailey JA, et al. Perinatal mortality and congenital anomalies in babies of women with type 1 or type 2 diabetes in England, Wales and Northern Ireland: population-based study. Br Med J 2006; 333: 177–82.
13. Hotu S, Carter B, Watson PD, Cutfield WS, Cundy T. Increasing prevalence of type 2 diabetes in adolescents. J Paediatr Child Health 2004; 40: 201–4.
14. Kousseff BG. Gestational diabetes mellitus (class A): a human teratogen? Am J Med Genet 1999; 83: 402–8.
15. Shaefer-Graf UM, Buchanan TA, Xiang A, et al. Patterns of congenital anomalies and relationship to initial maternal fasting glucose levels in pregnancies complicated by type 2 and gestational diabetes. Am J Obstet Gynecol 2000; 182: 313–20.
16. Aberg A, Westbom L, Kallen B. Congenital malformations among infants whose mothers had gestational diabetes or preexisting diabetes. Early Hum Dev 2001; 61: 85–95.
17. Schaefer UM, Songster G, Xiang A, et al. Congenital malformations in offspring of women with hyperglycemia first detected during pregnancy. Am J Obstet Gynecol 1997; 177: 1165–71.
18. Xiong X, Saunders LD, Wang FL, Demianczuk NN. Gestational diabetes mellitus: prevalence, risk factors, maternal and infant outcomes. Int J Gynaecol Obstet 2001; 75: 221–8.
19. Dunne F, Brydon P, Smith K, Gee H. Pregnancy in women with type 2 diabetes: 12 years outcome data 1990–2002. Diabet Med 2003; 30: 734–8.
20. Ray JG, O'Brien TE, Chan WS. Preconception care and the risk of congenital anomalies in the offspring of women with diabetes mellitus: a meta-analysis, Q J Med 2001; 94: 435–44.
21. Albert-Reece A, Hobbins JC. Diabetic embryopathy: pathogenesis, prenatal diagnosis and prevention. Obstet Gynecol Survey 1986; 41: 325–35.
22. Miller E, Hare JW, Cloherty JP, et al. Elevated maternal hemoglobin A1c in early pregnancy and major congenital anomalies in infants of diabetic mothers. N Engl J Med 1981; 304: 1331–4.
23. Suhonen L, Hiilesmaa V, Teramo K. Glycaemic control during early pregnancy and fetal malformations in women with type 1 diabetes mellitus. Diabetologia 2000; 43: 79–82.
24. Merlob P, Reisner SH. Fetal effects from maternal diabetes, In: Buyse L, ed. Birth Defects Encyclopedia, 1st edn. Cambridge: Blackwell Scientific; 1990, pp. 700–2.
25. Mills JL, Baker L, Goldman AS. Malformations in infants of diabetic mothers occur before the seventh gestational week: implications for treatment. Diabetes 1978; 28: 292–3.
26. Rowland TW, Hubbell JP, Nadas AS. Congenital heart disease in infants of diabetic mothers. J Pediatr 1973; 83: 815–20.
27. Milunsky A, Alpert E, Kitzmiller JL, Younger MD, Neff RK. Prenatal diagnosis of neural tube defects. The importance of serum alpha-feto protein screening in diabetic pregnant women. Am J Obstet Gynecol 1982; 142: 1030–2.
28. Ramos-Arroyo MA, Rodriguez-Pinnila E, Cordero JP. Maternal diabetes: the risk of specific birth defects. Eur J Epidemiol 1992; 8: 503–8.
29. Lin HJ, Owens TR, Sinow RM, et al. Anomalous inferior and superior venae cavae with oculoauriculovertebral defect: review of Goldenhar complex and malformations of left-right asymmetry. Am J Med Genet 1998; 75: 88–94.
30. Ewart-Toland A, Yankowitz J, Winder A, et al. Oculoauriculovertebral abnormalities in children of diabetic mothers. Am J Med Genet 2000; 90: 303–9.
31. Spilson SV, Kim HJE, Chung KC. Association between maternal diabetes mellitus and newborn oral clefts. Ann Plast Surg 2001; 47: 477–81.
32. Wang R, Martinez-Frias ML, Graham JM. Infants of diabetic mothers are at increased risk for the oculo-auriculo-vertebral sequence: a case-based and case–control approach. J Pediatr 2002; 141: 611–7.
33. Rosenn B, Miodovnik M, St. John Dignan P, et al. Minor congenital malformations in infants of insulin-dependent diabetic women: association with poor glycemic control. Obstet Gynecol 1990; 76: 745–9.
34. Hod M, Merlob P, Friedman S, et al. Prevalence of minor congenital anomalies in newborns of diabetic mothers. Eur J Obstet Gynecol Reprod Biol 1992; 44: 111–6.
35. Simpson JL, Elias S, Martin AO, et al. Diabetes in pregnancy, Northwestern University Series (1977–1981), I, Prospective study of anomalies in offspring of mothers with diabetes mellitus. Am J Obstet Gynecol 1983; 146: 263–70.
36. Hod M, Merlob P. A meta-analysis of perinatal complications of maternal diabetes. Can they be prevented? Early Preg Biol Med 1996; 2: 15–7.
37. Kitzmiller JL, Gavin LA, Gin GD, et al. Pre-conception care of diabetes. Glycemic control prevents congenital anomalies. JAMA 1991; 265: 731–6.
38. Itikala PR, Ruuska SE, Oakley Jr. GP, Kloeblen-Tarver AS, Klein L. Periconceptional intake of folic acid among low-income women. JAMA 2000; 283: 3074.
39. Meyer BA, Palmer SM. Pregestational diabetes. Semin Perinatol 1990; 14: 12–23.

24 Post-implantation diabetic embryopathy

Ulf J. Eriksson and Parri Wentzel

Introduction

The mechanisms behind diabetes-induced embryonic dysmorphogenesis are still partly a question mark. Despite increased clinical efforts to improve glycemic control during diabetic pregnancy, the rate of congenital malformations remains increased in studies of diabetic gestation of Type 1,[1–4] Type 2,[4–7] and gestational diabetes mellitus (GDM).[5,8]

Both environmental factors and genetic predisposition seem to be of importance in diabetic embryopathy. Several teratological pathways have been suggested, often from clinical experience, and subsequently characterized in various experimental systems. The maternal teratogenic factors most often indicated are hyperglycemia[9–12] and ketonemia.[13–22] Major teratogenic processes in embryonic tissues so far identified include alterations of signaling systems such as metabolism of inositol,[23–28] sorbitol,[23,25,27,29,30] arachidonic acid/prostaglandins,[24,31,32] folic acid,[33,34] and reactive oxygen species,[35–38] as well as alterations in the activation of PKC isoforms.[39–42] The embryonic formation of glycated proteins,[43–45] and the maternal and fetal genotypes[46–50] are also suggested to influence the teratological events in diabetic pregnancy.

The growing knowledge in teratology has not yet generated any major alterations or added any new therapeutical agents to the clinical handling of diabetic pregnancy. The importance of maintaining normoglycemia and avoiding ketonemia are common knowledge; however, no systematic attempt to evaluate the potential of antioxidative treatment,[35] or to study the possible beneficial effects of administering folic acid[33] to pregnant diabetic women has been reported, as yet.

Inositol

High glucose concentration *in vitro* causes decreased levels of inositol in the embryo due to impaired uptake,[28] yielding an embryonic deficiency of inositol[23,27,51] concomitant with an increased rate of embryonic dysmorphogenesis. Supplementation of inositol to high glucose cultured embryos,[24–26] or dietary addition to diabetic pregnant rodents[52–55] diminishes both the inositol deficiency and the rate of embryonic maldevelopment. Furthermore, adding the inositol uptake inhibitor *scyllo*-inositol to the culture medium of rodent embryos

causes similar changes to the embryos, i.e. both inositol deficiency and embryonic maldevelopment.[39,51,56] In addition, similarly to the glucose-induced damage, both the inositol deficiency and the embryo maldevelopment caused by *scyllo*-inositol can be diminished by addition of inositol to the culture medium.[39,51,56] These findings identify inositol deficiency as a likely component of diabetic teratogenesis.[57]

However, addition of antioxidants diminish both glucose-induced and *scyllo*-inositol-induced embryonic dysmorphogenesis *in vitro*;[39,58] therefore the inositol deficiency appears to induce embryonic oxidative stress, which, in turn, causes embryonic maldevelopment.

The immediate effect of lowered inositol concentration would be decreased levels of the phosphoinositides (PI, PIP and PIP2) and their products in the embryonic tissue.[51] A lack of PIP2 would subsequently yield less IP3 and diacylglycerol, both of which are stimulators of protein kinase C (PKC) activity. A lowered PKC activity would exert a number of effects, including lowered activity of phospholipase A2, the key enzyme in the metabolism of triglycerides and phospholipids.[59] A decrease of phospholipase A2 activity would subsequently diminish the availability of free arachidonic acid, and thereby diminish the production and metabolism of prostaglandins, as discussed below.

Sorbitol

Exposure to a diabetic environment yields enhanced embryonic formation of sorbitol.[23,25,27,29,30] Several studies of aldose reductase inhibitors in pregnant diabetic animals have managed to lower the increased sorbitol levels, however, without diminishing the increased malformation rates.[23,25,60] Sorbitol accumulation, therefore, appears to be a side phenomenon of the teratogenic pathway.

Arachidonic acid/prostaglandins

Disturbed metabolism of arachidonic acid and prostaglandins has been found in previous studies of experimental diabetic pregnancy. Intraperitoneal injections of arachidonic acid to pregnant diabetic rats diminished the rate of neural tube damage,[61] as did enriching the diet of the pregnant diabetic rats with arachidonic acid.[54,62,63] Addition of arachidonic acid to the culture medium was shown to block the embryonic dysmorphogenesis elicited by high glucose concentration.[61,64,65] Addition of PGE$_2$ to the culture medium also blocks glucose-induced teratogenicity in vitro,[24,65] as well as maldevelopment of embryos cultured in diabetic serum.[66] Measurements of PGE$_2$ have indicated that this prostaglandin is decreased in embryos of diabetic rodents during neural tube closure,[67,68] in high glucose cultured embryos,[68] as well as in the yolk sac of embryos of diabetic women.[69]

Previous studies have shown, however, that the uptake of arachidonic acid by embryonic yolk sacs is increased in a hyperglycemic environment.[32] This finding would preclude an uptake deficiency of arachidonic acid in the conceptus of diabetic pregnancy, a result supported by the demonstration of unchanged concentration of arachidonic acid in membranes of high glucose cultured embryos in vitro.[70] Recent measurements in day-12 embryos indicate a decreased arachidonic acid concentration in offspring from diabetic rats.[55] A downregulation of the gene expression of COX-2, the inducible form of the COX enzyme, as well as a GSH-dependent enhancement of the conversion of the precursor PGH$_2$ to PGE$_2$ has also been demonstrated.[68] Thus, the PGE$_2$ concentration of day-10 embryos and membranes was decreased after exposure to high glucose in vitro or diabetes in vivo. In vitro addition of NAC to high glucose cultures restored the PGE$_2$ concentration.[68] Hyperglycemia/diabetes-induced downregulation of embryonic COX-2 gene expression may be an early event in diabetic embryopathy, leading to lowered PGE$_2$ levels and dysmorphogenesis, presumably because this pathway plays an important role in neural tube development. Antioxidant treatment does not prevent the decrease in COX-2 mRNA levels but restores PGE$_2$ concentrations, suggesting that diabetes-induced oxidative stress aggravates the loss of COX-2 activity. From these data, it may be concluded that decreased availability of arachidonic acid and the resulting decrease in several prostaglandins, in particular PGE$_2$, is likely to be involved in the teratogenicity of diabetic pregnancy.[63]

Other studies have shown that a diabetes-like environment increases isoprostane levels[68] and decreases embryonic PGE$_2$ concentration[67,68,71] in embryonic tissues. Isoprostanes, e.g. 8-epi-PGF$_{2\alpha}$, are prostaglandin-like compounds formed in situ from peroxidation of arachidonic acid by non-enzymatic, free radical-catalyzed reactions and they therefore serve as indicators of lipid peroxidation[72–74] with independent teratogenic activity.[75]

Folic acid

The risk of congenital malformations,[76,77] including neural tube defects (NTDs)[78] in diabetes pregnancy is 2- to 5-fold higher than in normal, nondiabetic pregnancy. Fortification of the US diet with folic acid in the late 1990s coincided with a reduced incidence of NTDs from 37.8 to 30.5 per 100,000 live births – appreciatively a 20% reduction (Figure 24.1).[79]

Rodent embryos were exposed to a diabetic environment in vivo and in vitro (high glucose embryo culture) and at the same time subjected to supplementation of folic acid.[33,34] The folic acid treatment increased folic acid concentration in the embryos and almost completely abolished the diabetes/glucose-induced dysmorphogenesis, i.e. both the growth retardation and somatic maldevelopment in the offspring.[33,34] In this context, the reports suggesting that folic acid may act as an antioxidant may offer an explanation for the findings of a marked antiteratogenic effect by folic acid on embryos exposed to a diabetic environment (Figure 24.2).

Reactive oxygen species

The notion that diabetes is associated with oxidative stress has been suggested by several authors.[80–84] Increased lipid peroxidation and generation of reactive oxygen species (ROS) were found in diabetic rats, measured as increased serum F2-isoprostane levels,[85] and increased electron spin clearance rate.[86] Cyclic voltammetric studies have also indicated increased levels of lipid peroxidation in diabetic rats,[87] and the F2-isoprostane 8-epi-PGF$_{2\alpha}$ is increased in embryos exposed to high glucose levels in vitro[68] and diabetes in vivo.[34]

The first indisputable evidence of an involvement of oxidative stress in the pathogenesis of diabetic embryopathy was the demonstration that treatment with antioxidative agents largely normalizes malformation rates in vitro,[20,35,36,88–90] and in vivo.[38,54,58,65,91–97] Furthermore, antioxidative treatment normalizes several of the markers of oxidative stress, such as serum F$_2$-isoprostane levels,[85] electron spin clearance rate,[86] and the concentration of embryonic isoprostane in vitro,[68] and in vivo.[34]

Adding scavenging enzymes, e.g. SOD, catalase or glutathione peroxidase, to the culture medium protects rat embryos from dysmorphogenesis induced by high glucose concentration in vitro.[35] Teratogenic concentrations of β-hydroxybutyrate or the branched chain amino acid analog β-ketoisocaproic acid can be blocked by addition of SOD to the culture medium,[36] and addition of SOD or NAC diminishes the dysmorphogenesis caused by diabetic serum.[58] In a study of the early development of cranial neural crest cells, it was shown that high glucose inhibited, and NAC normalized, the migration and proliferation of these cells, and that control cells of nonneural origin were not affected by either treatment.[98] Examination of litters of diabetic rats demonstrated lowered α-tocopherol (vitamin E) concentration in day-11 embryos and in the liver of day-20 fetuses.[94]

Analogously, dietary treatment with 5% vitamin E diminished the malformation rate in embryos of MD rats and largely normalized embryonic growth in vivo.[34] Thus, maternal diabetes increased the number of malformed embryos and, in particular, increased the proportion of embryos showing an open neural tube, whereas vitamin E treatment of the pregnant diabetic rats normalized both of these parameters. In embryos cultured in high glucose concentration, we noted increased isoprostane levels, and supplementation of folic acid to the culture medium decreased embryonic isoprostane concentration (Figure 24.3).[34]

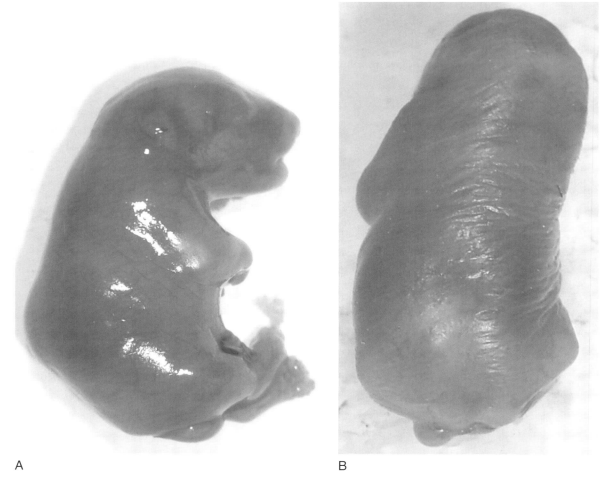

A   B

Figure 24.1   (A and B) A fetus of a manifestly diabetic rat showing a neural tube defect resembling a spina bifida in the lower left sacral region.

Embryonic neural tissue subjected to high glucose concentration show increased superoxide production, as measured in a Cartesian diver system.[99] One effect of increased intracellular ROS production would be inhibition of the

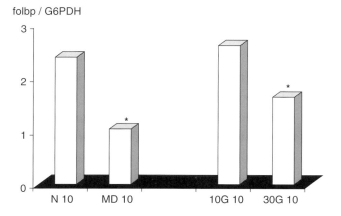

folbp / G6PDH

Figure 24.2   Expression of the folate transporter folbp in embryos of normal (N) and manifestly diabetic (MD) rats, and in embryos cultured in 10 or 30 mmol/L glucose (10G or 30G). The gene expression is normalized with that of the house-keeping gene G6PDH.

rate limiting enzyme of the glycolysis, Glyceraldehyde-3-phosphate dehydrogenase (GAPDH), since this enzyme has displayed sensitivity to ROS in several different conditions of oxidative stress.[100] This sensitivity resides in the thiol group of cysteine residue 149 in the active site of the enzyme.[101,102] Oxidation of the thiol group by NO or ROS leads to decreased enzyme activity,[103] and blocking of this process by antioxidants protects the activity of the enzyme.[104] In rat embryos subjected to a diabetic environment *in vivo* or *in vitro*, decreased GAPDH activity was found,[105] and addition of the antioxidant NAC prevented the decrease in activity.[105] In addition, when the enzyme was inhibited by iodoacetate, NAC addition also blocked the inhibition (Figure 24.4).[105]

Bovine endothelial cells have been shown to produce excess amount of superoxide in response to hyperglycemia.[106] Diminishing this overproduction of ROS via inhibition of the electron transport, by uncoupling oxidative phosphorylation, or by addition of SOD, blocked other markers of intracellular imbalance, such as sorbitol accumulation, activation of PKC, formation of advanced glycation end products, and NF-kB activation.[106]

Similar effects of ROS-mediated GAPDH inhibition have been found in embryos subjected to high glucose concentrations,

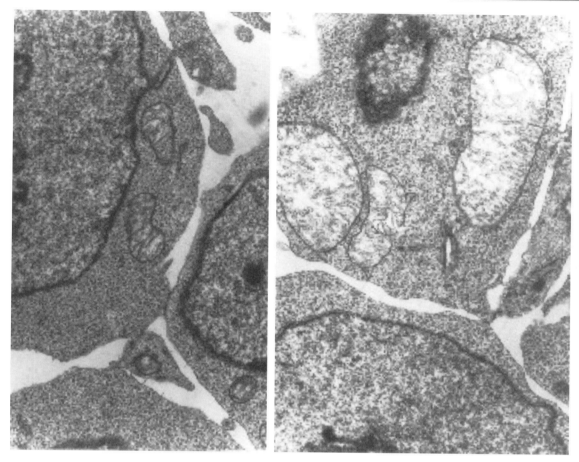

Figure 24.3   Neuroepithelium of embryos of normal (left) and manifestly diabetic (right) rat. Note the marked mitochondrial swelling in the latter cells.

i.e. sorbitol accumulation,[23,25,27,29,30] activation of (some isoforms of) PKC,[39-42] enhanced activity in the hexosamine shunt,[107] and increased formation of glycosylation intermediaries, such as deoxyglucosone.[44] Which of these ROS-mediated effects that will prove to be the major teratogenic pathway is under investigation (Figure 24.3).

High-amplitude mitochondrial swelling was demonstrated in embryonic neuroectoderm of embryos exposed to a diabetic environment,[108,109] a swelling diminished by antioxidative treatment of the mother,[110] implicating an embryonic ROS imbalance, with conceivable consequences for the rate of apoptosis in susceptible cell lineages in the embryo.[111,112] A diabetic milieu causes mitochondrial overproduction of ROS, which is suggested to give rise to apoptosis. The mitochondrion has an important role in the apoptotic machinery and previous studies have suggested that an altered apoptotic rate may affect the maldevelopment of embryos subjected to a diabetic milieu.[113,114] Combined supplementation of two compounds with antioxidative features (folic acid and vitamin E) to pregnant diabetic rats diminished diabetes-induced dysmorphogenesis and normalized apoptotic-associated protein levels.[115]

In addition, fetuses and embryos of diabetic rodents display increased rates of DNA damage,[116-118] another indication of enhanced ROS activity in the embryonic tissues.

The bulk of data implicates oxidative stress and ROS excess as an important component in the etiology of diabetic embryopathy. The data also suggest that long-term exposure to high glucose creates embryonic ROS excess either from increased ROS production,[99] or from diminished antioxidant defense capacity.[88,89,119] ROS excess may be small, restricted to particular cell populations,[120,121] and likely to vary with gestational time and nutritional status, making direct ROS determinations difficult.

Increasing ROS in embryos leads to malformations,[122,123] suggesting that ROS excess may also have a role in the teratogenic process(es) of phenytoin medication,[124,125] ethanol abuse,[120,121,126] and, recently, thalidomide administration.[127] Therefore, ROS excess may constitute a common element in a number of teratogenic situations, including diabetic pregnancy.[128]

Protein kinase C activity

PKC signaling is associated with apoptosis, especially the isoforms PKCδ[129] and PKCζ.[130] It has been suggested that PKCδ is involved in stabilizing p53 proteins[131] and is related to reactive oxygen species production,[132] both of which would ultimately lead to apoptotic cell death.

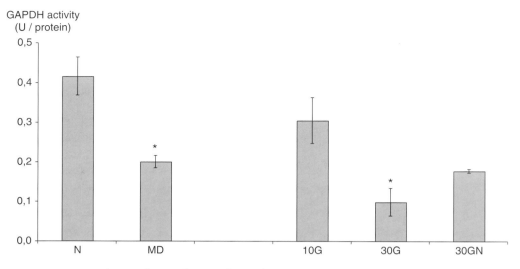

Figure 24.4   GAPDH activity in embryos of normal (N) and manifestly diabetic (MD) rats and in embryos cultured in 10 or 30 mmol/L glucose (10G or 30G), with or without addition of NAC (30GN).

In experimental diabetic pregnancy, altered activation of several PKC isoforms in the embryo was found to be associated with a hyperglycemic environment.[40,41] The addition of CHC and NAC to the culture medium with high glucose normalized the malformations in embryos cultured for 24 h, and addition of PKCδ and PKCζ-specific inhibitors to the culture medium with high glucose also normalized the malformations. PKCδ activity was higher in embryos cultured in medium with high glucose for 24 h when compared with embryos cultured in low glucose concentration. Supplementation of CHC and NAC to high glucose medium normalized PKCδ activity.[42]

These findings would implicate PKC activity changes in the diabetic embryopathy, however, since the previously discussed inositol deficiency is likely to decrease PKC activity, and blunt inhibition of PKC activity also causes embryonic developmental damage,[39,133] the exact relationships between maternal diabetes and embryonic PKC isoforms activity warrant further scientific attention.

Genetics of diabetic dysmorphogenesis

Despite similar teratological exposure, the effect of any teratogen, including maternal diabetes/hyperglycemia, varies between individuals. In addition to stochastic conditions, genetic predisposition determines the effect of each teratogen on a particular individual.[134,135]

Although predisposing genetic conditions for diabetes are clearly present in offspring of diabetic parents[136,137] as the offspring of a diabetic father has higher risk of developing the disease than the offspring of a diabetic mother,[138–142] it has been established that diabetic men do not have an increased risk of fathering malformed offspring.[143,144] This indicates that the genes predisposing to diabetes do not induce congenital malformations. In contrast, maternal diabetes has been suggested to be associated with Down's syndrome,[145–147] and

has also been suggested to predispose for optic nerve hypoplasia in female offspring.[148] A genetic element may be present in the etiology of diabetic embryopathy,[149] a notion supported by experimental data.[37,46,48-50,150,151]

It has been suggested that the absence of a specific malformation pattern for diabetic embryopathy signals the presence of several teratological factors and mechanisms in diabetic pregnancy.[152] Likewise, the number of different teratogenic agents identified would indicate that diabetic embryopathy is of complex etiology.[21,153,154]

We have previously found that both the maternal and fetal genome are involved in the etiology of the diabetes-induced (skeletal) malformations by comparing the incidence of malformations between different rat strains.[48] We could demonstrate that a specific variant of the catalase enzyme is present in rats that are malformation-prone (Cs-1a), whereas another variant of the catalase protein was present in rats that do not develop malformations in response to maternal diabetes (Cs-1b),[50] which can be demonstrated in the closely related U (malformation-prone) and H (malformation-resistant) Sprague–Dawley substrains that we have characterized.[48,155,156]

Thus, embryonic catalase activity was lower in embryos from normal U rats than in embryos from normal H rats, and that maternal diabetes augments this difference.[46] We sequenced catalase cDNA and the promotor region of the catalase gene in the U and H rat,[47] and found one nucleotide mutation in the 5'-UTR-region of the U rat cDNA and a heterozygocity in the U rat gene promoter. Therefore, the decreased catalase mRNA levels may result from different regulation of transcription (promotor), and the difference in the electrophoretic mobility in zymograms[50] may be a result of posttranslational modifications of the catalase protein (Figure 24.5). Using L4, an inbred U rat substrain with about 25% skeletal malformations when the mother is diabetic, and inbred Wistar Furth rats (no diabetes-inducible skeletal malformations), we performed a global gene linkage analysis of the skeletal malformations and found strong coupling to seven regions on chromosomes 4, 10, 14, 18, and 19, and

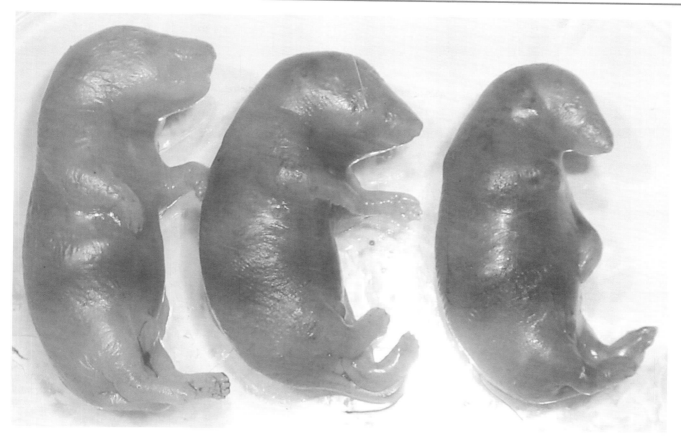

Figure 24.5   Fetuses of manifestly diabetic rats, displaying normal morphology (left), mild micrognathia (middle) and severe micrognathia (right).

a weaker coupling to the region of chromosome 3 where the catalase gene resides. The characterization of candidate gene and construction of congenic strains will be future work in this rat model of diabetic embryopathy.

There are several indications of a genetic element in the etiology and pathogenesis of the dysmorphogenesis in diabetic pregnancy. Thus, high glucose *in vitro* and diabetes *in vivo* alter the expression of the ECM genes B1-laminin and fibronectin in embryos.[157] These genes are also altered in placentae of diabetic rats, fibronectin is overexpressed and laminin is suppressed.[158] The expression of genes controlling the defense against oxidative stress also shows diabetes-induced alterations in expression, in a recent study embryos of diabetic rats demonstrated decreased expression of CuZnSOD, MnSOD, and Gpx-1 and Gpx-2 compared with embryos from normal rats (Wentzel et al. submitted).

The Pax-3 gene expression was found to be reduced in embryos of diabetic mice,[159,160] and this transcription factor may regulate the gene expression of the licensing factor cdc-46,[161] and a gene, Dep-1,[162] as well as p53,[163] all of which may be of importance for a correct neural tube closure. Null mutation of the Pax-3 gene yields the *Splotch* mouse displaying neural tube defects.[159,164] It has also been shown that the decreased Pax-3 expression in embryos of diabetic mice could be normalized by treatment of the mother with antioxidants,[165] thereby demonstrating a coupling between ROS excess and a teratologically important change in gene expression.

One conclusion from the genetic experimental efforts is that there are no universal gene identified to be responsible for enhanced (or decreased) susceptibility to diabetic embryopathy.

Conclusions and future directions

Diabetic embryopathy has a complex etiology and pathogenesis. The studies of etiologic factors in the pathogenesis of congenital malformations has revealed a complex process in which the diabetic state simultaneously induces alterations in a series of teratogenically capable pathways. These pathways are intertwined, and several of them seem to result in an imbalance of the ROS metabolism, yielding a ROS excess in teratogenically sensitive cell populations, an imbalance ultimately causing the congenital malformations. Blocking the ROS excess may be a valid way to diminish the disturbed development caused by the diabetic environment.

There is experimental evidence in favor of a major teratological role of ROS excess, however, there are no clinical studies, as yet, attempting to address the therapeutical potential of antioxidative treatment in pregnant diabetic women. Likewise, the possible advantage of folic acid supplementation in diabetic pregnancy has not been clinically evaluated.

Acknowledgments

The authors wish to gratefully acknowledge the support from The Swedish Research Council, The Family Ernfors Fund, The Novo Nordisk Foundation, and The Swedish Diabetes Association.

REFERENCES

1. Ray JG, O'Brien TE, Chan WS. Preconception care and the risk of congenital anomalies in the offspring of women with diabetes mellitus: a meta-analysis. Q J Med 2001; 94: 435–44.

2. Platt MJ, et al. St Vincent's Declaration 10 years on: outcomes of diabetic pregnancies. Diabet Med 2002; 19: 216–20.

3. Evers IM, de Valk HW, Visser GH. Risk of complications of pregnancy in women with type 1 diabetes: nationwide prospective study in the Netherlands. BMJ (Clin Res edn.) 2004; 328: 915–24.

4. Verheijen EC, Critchley JA, Whitelaw DC, Tuffnell DJ. Outcomes of pregnancies in women with pre-existing type 1 or type 2 diabetes, in an ethnically mixed population. Br J Obstet Gynaecol 2005; 112: 1500–3.

5. Schaefer-Graf UM, et al. Patterns of congenital anomalies and relationship to initial maternal fasting glucose levels in pregnancies complicated by type 2 and gestational diabetes. Am J Obstet Gynecol 2000; 182: 313–20.

6. Brydon P, et al. Pregnancy outcome in women with type 2 diabetes mellitus needs to be addressed. Int J Clin Pract 2000; 54: 418–9.

7. Dunne F, Brydon P, Smith K, Gee H. Pregnancy in women with Type 2 diabetes: 12 years outcome data 1990–2002. Diabet Med 2003; 20: 734–8.

8. Garcia-Patterson A, et al. In human gestational diabetes mellitus congenital malformations are related to pre-pregnancy body mass index and to severity of diabetes. Diabetologia 2004; 47: 509–14.

9. Cockroft DL, Coppola PT. Teratogenic effect of excess glucose on head-fold rat embryos in culture. Teratology 1977; 16: 141–6.

10. Sadler TW. Effects of maternal diabetes on early embryogenesis. II. Hyperglycemia-induced exencephaly. Teratology 1980; 21: 349–56.

11. Ellington SKL. In vivo and in vitro studies on the effects of maternal fasting during embryonic organogenesis in the rat. J Reprod Fertil 1980; 60: 383–8.

12. Moley K, Chi M, Manchester J, McDougal D, Lowry O. Alterations of intraembryonic metabolites in preimplantation mouse embryos exposed to elevated concentrations of glucose: a metabolic explanation for the developmental retardation seen in preimplantation embryos from diabetic animals. Biol Reprod 1996; 54: 1209–16.

13. Sadler TW, Horton WEJ. Effects of maternal diabetes on early embryogenesis: the role of insulin and insulin therapy. Diabetes 1983; 32: 1070–4.

14. Horton WEJ, Sadler TW. Effects of maternal diabetes on early embryogenesis. Alterations in morphogenesis produced by the ketone body β-hydroxybutyrate. Diabetes 1983; 32: 610–6.

15. Lewis NJ, Akazawa S, Freinkel N. Teratogenesis from beta-hydroxybutyrate during organogenesis in rat embryo organ culture and enhancement by subteratogenic glucose. Diabetes 1983; 32(suppl. 1): 11A.

16. Hunter ES, Sadler TW, Wynn RE. A potential mechanism of DL-beta-hydroxybutyrate-induced malformations in mouse embryos. Am J Physiol 1987; 253: E72–E80.

17. Shum L, Sadler TW. Embryonic catch-up growth after exposure to the ketone body D,L-beta-hydroxybutyrate in vitro. Teratology 1988; 38: 369–79.

18. Moore DCP, Stanisstree, M, Clarke CA. Morphological and physiological effects of beta-hydroxybutyrate on rat embryos grown in vitro at different stages. Teratology 1989; 40: 237–51.

19. Shum L, Sadler TW. Biochemical basis for D,L-beta-hydroxybutyrate-induced teratogenesis. Teratology 1990; 42: 553–6.

20. Ornoy A, Zaken V, Kohen R. Role of reactive oxygen species (ROS) in the diabetes-induced anomalies in rat embryos in vitro: reduction in antioxidant enzymes and low-molecular-weight antioxidants (LMWA) may be the causative factor for increased anomalies. Teratology 1999; 60: 376–86.

21. Buchanan TA, Denno KM, Sipos GF, Sadler TW. Diabetic teratogenesis. In vitro evidence for a multifactorial etiology with little contribution from glucose per se. Diabetes 1994; 43: 656–60.

22. Wentzel P, Eriksson UJ. Insulin treatment fails to abolish the teratogenic potential of serum from diabetic rats. Eur J Endocrinol 1996; 134: 459–66.

23. Hod M, Star S, Passonneau JV, Unterman TG, Freinkel N. Effect of hyperglycemia on sorbitol and myo-inositol content of cultured rat conceptus: failure of aldose reductase inhibitors to modify myo-inositol depletion and dysmorphogenesis. Biochem Biophys Res Commun 1986; 140: 974–80.

24. Baker L, Piddington R, Goldman A, Egler J, Moehring J. Myo-inositol and prostaglandins reverse the glucose inhibition of neural tube fusion in cultured mouse embryos. Diabetologia 1990; 33: 593–6.

25. Hashimoto M, et al. Effects of hyperglycaemia on sorbitol and myo-inositol contents of cultured embryos: treatment with aldose reductase inhibitor and myo-inositol supplementation. Diabetologia 1990; 33: 597–602.

26. Hod M, Star S, Passonneau J, Unterman TG, Freinkel N. Glucose-induced dysmorphogenesis in the cultured rat conceptus: prevention by supplementation with myo-inositol. Isr J Med Sci 1990; 26: 541–4.

27. Sussman I, Matschinsky FM. Diabetes affects sorbitol and myo-inositol levels of neuroectodermal tissue during embryogenesis in rat. Diabetes 1998; 37: 974–81.

28. Weigensberg MJ, Garcia-Palmer F-J, Freinkel N. Uptake of myo-inositol by early-somite rat conceptus. Transport kinetics and effects of hyperglycemia. Diabetes 1990; 39: 575–82.

29. Eriksson UJ, Naeser P, Brolin SE. Increased accumulation of sorbitol in offspring of manifest diabetic rats. Diabetes 1986; 35: 1356–63.

30. Eriksson UJ, Brolin SE, Naeser P. Influence of sorbitol accumulation on growth and development of embryos cultured in elevated levels of glucose and fructose. Diabetes Res 1989; 11: 27–32.

31. Pinter E, et al. Yolk sac failure in embryopathy due to hyperglycemia: ultrastructural analysis of yolk sac differentiation associated with embryopathy in rat conceptuses under hyperglycemic conditions. Teratology 1986; 33: 73–84.

32. Engström E, Haglund A, Eriksson UJ. Effects of maternal diabetes or in vitro hyperglycemia on uptake of palmitic and arachidonic acid by rat embryos. Pediatr Res 1991; 30: 150–3.

33. Wentzel P, Gareskog M, Eriksson UJ. Folic acid supplementation diminishes diabetes- and glucose-induced dysmorphogenesis in rat embryos in vivo and in vitro. Diabetes 2005; 54: 546–53.

34. Wentzel P, Eriksson UJ. A diabetes-like environment increases malformation rate and diminishes prostaglandin E(2) in rat embryos: reversal by administration of vitamin E and folic acid. Birth Defects Research. Part A. Clin Mol Teratol 2005; 73: 506–11.

35. Eriksson UJ, Borg LAH. Protection by free oxygen radical scavenging enzymes against glucose-induced embryonic malformations in vitro. Diabetologia 1991; 34: 325–31.

36. Eriksson UJ, Borg LAH. Diabetes and embryonic malformations. Role of substrate-induced free-oxygen radical production for dysmorphogenesis in cultured rat embryos. Diabetes 1993; 42: 411–9.

37. Hagay ZJ, et al. Prevention of diabetes-associated embryopathy by overexpression of the free radical scavenger copper zinc superoxide dismutase in transgenic mouse embryos. Am J Obstet Gynecol 1995; 173: 1036–41.

38. Eriksson UJ, Simán CM. Pregnant diabetic rats fed the antioxidant butylated hydroxytoluene show decreased occurrence of malformations in the offspring. Diabetes 1996; 45: 1497–502.

39. Wentzel P, Wentzel CR, Gareskog MB, Eriksson UJ. Induction of embryonic dysmorphogenesis by high glucose concentration, disturbed inositol metabolism, and inhibited protein kinase C activity. Teratology 2001; 63: 193–201.

40. Hiramatsu Y, et al. Diacylglycerol production and protein kinase C activity are increased in a mouse model of diabetic embryopathy. Diabetes 2002; 51: 2804–10.

41. Gareskog M, Wentzel P. Altered protein kinase C activation associated with rat embryonic dysmorphogenesis. Pediatr Res 2004; 56: 849–57.

42. Gareskog M, Wentzel P. N-Acetylcysteine and a-cyano-4-hydroxycinnamic acid alter protein kinase C (PKC)-δ and PKC-δ and diminish dysmorphogenesis in rat embryos cultured with high glucose in vitro. J Endocrinol 2007; 192: 207–14.

43. Wolff SP, Jiang ZY, Hunt JV. Protein glycation and oxidative stress in diabetes mellitus and ageing. Free Radic Biol Med 1991; 10: 339–52.

44. Eriksson UJ, Wentzel,P, Minhas HS, Thornalley PJ. Teratogenicity of 3-deoxyglucosone and diabetic embryopathy. Diabetes 1998; 47: 1960–6.

45. Thornalley PJ. Advanced glycation and the development of diabetic complications. Unifying the involvement of glucose, methylglyoxal and oxidative stress. Endocrinol Metab 1996; 3: 149–66.

46. Cederberg J, Eriksson UJ. Decreased catalase activity in malformation-prone embryos of diabetic rats. Teratology 1997; 56: 350–7.

47. Cederberg J, Galli J, Luthman H, Eriksson UJ. Increased mRNA levels of Mn-SOD and catalase in embryos of diabetic rats from a malformation-resistant strain. Diabetes 2000; 49: 101–7.

48. Eriksson UJ. Importance of genetic predisposition and maternal environment for the occurrence of congenital malformations in offspring of diabetic rats. Teratology 1988; 37: 365–74.

49. Otani H, Tanaka O, Tatewaki R, Naora H, Yoneyama T. Diabetic environment and genetic predisposition as causes of congenital malformations in NOD mouse embryos. Diabetes 1991; 40: 1245–50.

50. Eriksson UJ, den Bieman M, Prins JB, van Zutphen LFM. Differences in susceptibility for diabetes-induced malformations in separated rat colonies of common origin. In: 4th FELASA Symposium. Lyon, France: Fondation Marcel Mérieux; 1990, pp. 53–57.

51. Strieleman PJ, Connors MA, Metzger BE. Phosphoinositide metabolism in the developing conceptus. Effects of hyperglycemia and scyllo-inositol in rat embryo culture. Diabetes 1992; 41: 989–97.

52. Akashi M, et al. Effects of insulin and myo-inositol on embryo growth and development during early organogenesis in streptozocin-induced diabetic rats. Diabetes 1991; 40: 1574–9.

53. Reece EA, Khandelwal M, Wu YK, Borenstein M. Dietary intake of myo-inositol and neural tube defects in offspring of diabetic rats. Am J Obstet Gynecol 1997; 176: 536–9.

54. Reece AE, Wu YK. Prevention of diabetic embryopathy in offspring of diabetic rats with use of a cocktail of deficient substrates and an antioxidant. Am J Obstet Gynecol 1997; 176: 790–8.

55. Khandelwal M, Reece EA, Wu YK, Borenstein M. Dietary myo-inositol therapy in hyperglycemia-induced embryopathy. Teratology 1998; 57: 79–84.

56. Strieleman PJ, Metzger BE. Glucose and scyllo-inositol impair phosphoinositide hydrolysis in the 10.5-day cultured rat conceptus: a role in dysmorphogenesis? Teratology 1993; 48: 267–78.

57. Baker L, Piddington R. Diabetic embryopathy: a selective review of recent trends. J Diabetes Comp 1993; 7: 204–12.

58. Wentzel P, Thunberg L, Eriksson UJ. Teratogenic effect of diabetic serum is prevented by supplementation of superoxide dismutase and N-acetylcysteine in rat embryo culture. Diabetologia 1997; 40: 7–14.

59. Lapetina EG. Regulation of arachidonic acid production: role of phospholipases C and A2. Trends Pharmacol Sci 1982; 3: 115–8.

60. Eriksson UJ, Andersson A, Efendic S, Elde R, Hellerström C. Diabetes in pregnancy: effects on the fetal and newborn rat with particular regard to body weight, serum insulin concentration and pancreatic contents of insulin, glucagon and somatostatin. Acta Endocrinol (Kbh) 1980; 94: 354–64.

61. Goldman AS, et al. Hyperglycemia-induced teratogenesis is mediated by a functional deficiency of arachidonic acid. Proc Natl Acad Sci USA 1985; 82: 8227–31.

62. Reece EA, et al. Dietary polyunsaturated fatty acid prevents malformations in offspring of diabetic rats. Am J Obstet Gynecol 1996; 175: 818–23.

63. Wiznitzer A, Furman B, Mazor M, Reece EA. The role of prostanoids in the development of diabetic embryopathy. Semin Repro Endocrinol 1999; 17: 175–81.

64. Pinter E, et al. Arachidonic acid prevents hyperglycemia-associated yolk sac damage and embryopathy. Am J Obstet Gynecol 1986; 155: 691–702.

65. Wentzel P, Eriksson UJ. Antioxidants diminish developmental damage induced by high glucose and cyclooxygenase inhibitors in rat embryos in vitro. Diabetes 1998; 47: 677–84.

66. Goto MP, Goldman AS, Uhing MR. PGE2 prevents anomalies induced by hyperglycemia or diabetic serum in mouse embryos. Diabetes 1992; 41: 1644–50.

67. Piddington R, Joyce J, Dhanasekaran P, Baker L. Diabetes mellitus affects prostaglandin E2 levels in mouse embryos during neurulation. Diabetologia 1996; 39: 915–20.

68. Wentzel P, Welsh N, Eriksson UJ. Developmental damage, increased lipid peroxidation, diminished cyclooxygenase-2 gene expression, and lowered PGE2 levels in rat embryos exposed to a diabetic environment. Diabetes 1999; 48: 813–20.

69. Schoenfeld A, et al. Yolk sac concentration of prostaglandin E2 in diabetic pregnancy: further clues to the etiology of diabetic embryopathy. Prostaglandins 1995; 50: 121–6.

70. Pinter E, et al. Fatty acid content of yolk sac and embryo in hyperglycemia-induced embryopathy and effect of arachidonic acid supplementation. Am J Obstet Gynecol 1988; 159: 1484–90.

71. Jawerbaum A, et al. Diminished levels of prostaglandin E in type I diabetic oocyte-cumulus complexes. Influence of nitric oxide and superoxide dismutase. Reprod Fertil Dev 1999; 11: 105–10.

72. Morrow JD, Harris TM, Roberts 2nd LJ. Noncyclooxygenase oxidative formation of a series of novel prostaglandins: analytical ramifications for measurement of eicosanoids. Anal Biochem 1990; 184: 1–10.

73. Morrow JD, Awad JA, Boss HJ, Blair IA, Roberts II LJ. Non-cyclooxygenase-derived prostanoids (F2-isoprostanes) are formed in situ on phospholipids. Proc Natl Acad Sci USA 1992; 89: 10721–5.

74. Davi G, et al. In vivo formation of 8-iso-prostaglandin F2alpha and platelet activation in diabetes mellitus: effects of improved metabolic control and vitamin E supplementation. Circulation 1999; 99: 224–9.

75. Wentzel P, Eriksson UJ. 8-Iso-PGF(2alpha) administration generates dysmorphogenesis and increased lipid peroxidation in rat embryos in vitro. Teratology 2002; 66: 164–8.

76. Kucera J. Rate and type of congenital anomalies among offspring of diabetic women. J Reprod Med 1971; 7: 61–70.

77. Aberg A, Westbom L, Kallen B. Congenital malformations among infants whose mothers had gestational diabetes or preexisting diabetes. Early Human Dev 2001; 61: 85–95.

78. Martínez-Frias ML. Epidemiological analysis of outcomes of pregnancy in diabetic mothers: identification of the most characteristic and most frequent congenital anomalies. Am J Med Genet 1994; 5: 108–13.

79. Honein MA, Paulozzi LJ, Mathews TJ, Erickson JD, Wong LY. Impact of folic acid fortification of the US food supply on the occurrence of neural tube defects. J Am Med Assoc 2001; 285: 2981–6.

80. Oberley LW. Free radicals and diabetes. Free Radic Biol Med 1988; 5: 113–24.

81. Gillery P, Monboisse JC, Maquart FX, Borel JP. Does oxygen free radical increased formation explain long term complications of diabetes mellitus? Medic Hypotheses 1989; 29: 47–50.

82. Baynes JW. Role of oxidative stress in development of complications in diabetes. Diabetes 1991; 40: 405–12.

83. Schmidt AM, et al. Advanced glycation endproducts (AGEs) induce oxidant stress in the gingiva: a potential mechanism underlying accelerated periodontal disease associated with diabetes. J Periodontal Res 1996; 31: 508–15.

84. West IC. Radicals and oxidative stress in diabetes. Diabet Med 2000; 17: 171–80.

85. Palmer AM, et al. Dietary antioxidant supplementation reduces lipid peroxidation but impairs vascular function in small mesenteric arteries of the streptozotocin-diabetic rat. Diabetologia 1998; 41: 148–56.

86. Sano T, Umeda F, Hashimoto T, Nawata H, Utsumi H. Oxidative stress measurements by in vivo electron spin resonance spectroscopy in rats with streptozotocin-induced diabetes. Diabetologia 1998; 41: 1355–60.

87. Elangovan V, Shohami E, Gati I, Kohen R. Increased hepatic lipid soluble antioxidant capacity as compared to other organs of streptozotocin-induced diabetic rats: a cyclic voltammetry study. Free Radic Res 2000; 32: 125–34.

88. Trocino RA, et al. Significance of glutathione depletion and oxidative stress in early embryogenesis in glucose-induced rat embryo culture. Diabetes 1995; 44: 992–8.

89. Ishibashi M, et al. Oxygen-induced embryopathy and the significance of glutathione-dependent antioxidant system in the rat embryo during early organogenesis. Free Radic Biol Med 1997; 22: 447–54.

90. Zaken V, Kohen R, Ornoy A. Vitamins C and E improve rat embryonic antioxidant defense mechanism in diabetic culture medium. Teratology 2001; 64: 33–44.

91. Viana M, Herrera E, Bonet B. Teratogenic effects of diabetes mellitus in the rat. Prevention with vitamin E. Diabetologia 1996; 39: 1041–6.

92. Sivan E, et al. Dietary vitamin E prophylaxis and diabetic embryopathy: Morphologic and biochemical analysis. Am J Obstet Gynecol 1996; 175: 793–9.

93. Simán CM, Eriksson UJ. Vitamin C supplementation of the maternal diet reduces the rate of malformation in the offspring of diabetic rats. Diabetologia 1997; 40: 1416–24.

94. Simán CM, Eriksson UJ. Vitamin E decreases the occurrence of malformations in the offspring of diabetic rats. Diabetes 1997; 46: 1054–61.

95. Sakamaki H, et al. Significance of glutathione-dependent antioxidant system in diabetes-induced embryonic malformations. Diabetes 1999; 48: 1138–44.

96. Cederberg J, Siman CM, Eriksson UJ. Combined treatment with vitamin E and vitamin C decreases oxidative stress and improves fetal outcome in experimental diabetic pregnancy. Pediatr Res 2001; 49: 755–62.

97. Cederberg J, Eriksson UJ. Antioxidative treatment of pregnant diabetic rats diminishes embryonic dysmorphogenesis. Birth Defects Research. Part A. Clin Mol Teratol 2005; 73: 498–505.

98. Suzuki,N, Svensson K, Eriksson UJ. High glucose concentration inhibits migration of rat cranial neural crest cells in vitro. Diabetologia 1996; 39: 401–11.

99. Yang X, Borg LAH, Eriksson UJ. Altered metabolism and superoxide generation in neural tissue of rat embryos exposed to high glucose. Am J Physiol 1997; 272: E173–80.

100. Janero DR, Hreniuk D, Sharif HM. Hydroperoxide-induced oxidative stress impairs heart muscle cell carbohydrate metabolism. Am J Physiol 1994; 266: C179–88.

101. Rivera-Nieves J, Thompson WC, Levine RL, Moss J. Thiols mediate superoxide-dependent NADH modification of glyceraldehyde-3-phosphate dehydrogenase. J Biol Chem 1999; 274: 19525–31.

102. Ishii T, et al. Critical role of sulfenic acid formation of thiols in the inactivation of glyceraldehyde-3-phosphate dehydrogenase by nitric oxide. Biochem Pharmacol 1999; 58: 133–43.

103. Morgan PE, Dean RT, Davies MJ. Inhibition of glyceraldehyde-3-phosphate dehydrogenase by peptide and protein peroxides generated by singlet oxygen attack. Eur J Biochem FEBS 2002; 269: 1916–25.

104. McKenzie SM, Doe WF, Buffinton GD. 5-aminosalicylic acid prevents oxidant mediated damage of glyceraldehyde-3-phosphate dehydrogenase in colon epithelial cells. Gut 1999; 44: 180–5.

105. Wentzel P, Ejdesjo A, Eriksson UJ. Maternal diabetes in vivo and high glucose in vitro diminish GAPDH activity in rat embryos. Diabetes 2003; 52: 1222–8.

106. Nishikawa T, et al. Normalizing mitochondrial superoxide production blocks three pathways of hyperglycaemic damage. Nature 2000; 404: 787–90.

107. Horal M, Zhang Z, Stanton R, Virkamaki A, Loeken MR. Activation of the hexosamine pathway causes oxidative stress and abnormal embryo gene expression: involvement in diabetic teratogenesis. Birth Defects Research. Part A. Clin Mol Teratol 2004; 70: 519–27.

108. Horton WE, Sadler TW. Mitochondrial alterations in embryos exposed to beta-hydroxybutyrate in whole embryo culture. Anat Rec 1985; 213: 94–101.

109. Yang X, Borg LAH, Eriksson UJ. Altered mitochondrial morphology of rat embryos in diabetic pregnancy. Anat Rec 1995; 241: 255–67.

110. Yang X, Borg LAH, Simán CM, Eriksson UJ. Maternal antioxidant treatments prevent diabetes-induced alterations of mitochondrial morphology in rat embryos. Anat Rec 1998; 251: 303–15.

111. Forsberg H, Eriksson UJ, Welsh N. Apoptosis in embryos of diabetic rats. Pharmacol Toxicol 1998; 83: 104–11.

112. Gareskog M, Cederberg J, Eriksson UJ, Wentzel P. Maternal diabetes in vivo and high glucose concentration in vitro increases apoptosis in rat embryos. Repro Toxicol 2007; 23: 63–74.

113. Moley K, Chi M, Knudson C, Korsmeyer S, Mueckler M. Hyperglycemia induces apoptosis in pre-implantation embryos through cell death effector pathways. Nature Med 1998; 4: 1421–4.

114. Moley KH. Hyperglycemia and apoptosis: mechanisms for congenital malformations and pregnancy loss in diabetic women. Trends Endocrinol Metab 2001; 12: 78–82.

115. Gareskog M, Eriksson UJ, Wentzel P. Combined supplementation of folic acid and vitamin E diminishes diabetes-induced embryotoxicity in rats. Birth Defects Research. Part A. Clin Mol Teratol 2006; 76: 483–90.

116. Lee AT, Reis D, Eriksson UJ. Hyperglycemia induced embryonic dysmorphogenesis correlates with genomic DNA mutation frequency in vitro and in vivo. Diabetes 1999; 48: 371–6.

117. Lee AT, Plump A, DeSimone C, Cerami A, Bucala R. A role for DNA mutations in diabetes-associated teratogenesis in transgenic embryos. Diabetes 1995; 44: 20–4.

118. Viana M, Aruoma OI, Herrera E, Bonet B. Oxidative damage in pregnant diabetic rats and their embryos. Free Rad Biol Med 2000; 29: 1115–21.

119. Menegola E, Broccia ML, Prati M, Ricolfi R, Giavini E. Glutathione status in diabetes-induced embryopathies. Biol Neonate 1996; 69: 293–7.

120. Davis WL, et al. Ethanol induces the generation of reactive free radicals by neural crest cells in vitro. J Craniofac Genet Dev Biol 1990; 10: 277–93.

121. Chen SY, Sulik KK. Free radicals and ethanol-induced cytotoxicity in neural crest cells. Alcohol Clin Exp Res 1996; 20: 1071–6.

122. Jenkinson PC, Anderson D, Gangolli SD. Malformations induced in cultured rat embryos by enzymically generated active oxygen species. Teratog Carcinog Mutagen 1986; 6: 547–54.

123. Anderson D, Francis AJ. The modulating effects of antioxidants in rat embryos and Sertoli cells in culture. Basic Life Sci 1993; 61: 189–200.

124. Winn LM, Wells PG. Phenytoin-initiated DNA oxidation in murine embryo culture, and embryoprotection by the antioxidative enzymes superoxide dismutase and catalase: evidence for reactive oxygen species mediated DNA oxidation in the molecular mechanism of phenytoin teratogenecity. Mol Pharmacol 1995; 48: 112–20.

125. Winn LM, Wells PG. Maternal administration of superoxide dismutase and catalase in phenytoin teratogenicity. Free Rad Biol Med 1999; 26: 266–74.

126. Kotch LE, Chen S-E, Sulik KK. Ethanol-induced teratogenesis: free radical damage as a possible mechanism. Teratology 1995; 52: 128–36.

127. Parman T, Wiley MJ, Wells PG. Free radical-mediated oxidative DNA damage in the mechanism of thalidomide teratogenicity. Nature Med 1999; 5: 582–5.

128. Eriksson UJ. Oxidative DNA damage and embryo development. Letter Nature Med 1999; 5: 715.

129. Santiago-Walker AE, et al. Protein kinase C delta stimulates apoptosis by initiating G1 phase cell cycle progression and S phase arrest. J Biol Chem 2005; 280: 32107–14.

130. Leroy I, de Thonel A, Laurent G, Quillet-Mary A. Protein kinase C zeta associates with death inducing signaling complex and regulates Fas ligand-induced apoptosis. Cell Signal 2005; 17: 1149–57.

131. Lee SJ, Kim DC, Choi BH, Ha H, Kim KT. Regulation of p53 by activated protein kinase C-delta during nitric oxide-induced dopaminergic cell death. J Biol Chem 2006; 281: 2215–24.

132. Domenicotti C, et al. A novel role of protein kinase C-delta in cell signaling triggered by glutathione depletion. Biochem Pharmacol 2003; 66: 1521–6.

133. Ward KW, Rogers EH, Hunter ES. Dysmorphogenic effects of a specific protein kinase C inhibitor during neurulation. Reprod Toxicol 1998; 12: 525–34.

134. Kapron C, Trasler D. Genetic determinants of teratogen-induced abnormal development in mouse and rat embryos in vitro. Int J Dev Biol 1997; 41: 337–44.

135. Morrison K, et al. Susceptibility to spina bifida; an association study of five candidate genes. Ann Human Genet 1998; 62: 379–96.

136. Degnbol B, Green A. Diabetes mellitus among first and second-degree relatives of early onset diabetes. Ann Human Genet 1978; 42: 25–47.

137. Tillil H, Köbberling J. Age-corrected empirical genetic risk estimates for first degree relatives of IDDM patients. Diabetes 1982; 36: 93–9.

138. Warram JH, Krolewski AS, Gottlieb MS, Kahn CR. Differences in risk of insulin-dependent diabetes in offspring of diabetic mothers and diabetic fathers. New Engl J Med 1984; 311: 149–52.

139. Dahlquist G, et al. The Swedish childhood diabetes study – results from nine year case register and a one year case–referrent study indicating that type 1 (insulin-dependent) diabetes mellitus is associated with both type 2 (non-insulin-dependent) diabetes mellitus and autoimmune disorders. Diabetologia 1989; 32: 2–6.

140. McCarthy BJ, Dorman JS, Aston CE. Investigating genomic imprinting and susceptibility to insulin-dependent diabetes mellitus: an epidemiological approach. Genet Epidemiol 1991; 8: 177–86.

141. Pociot F, et al. A nationwide population-based study of the familial aggregation of insulin-dependent diabetes in Denmark. Diabetologia 1993; 36: 870–5.

142. Tuomilehto J, Podar T, Tuomilehto-Wolf E, Virtala E. Evidence for importance of gender and birth cohort for risk of IDDM in offspring of IDDM parents. Diabetologia 1995; 38: 975–82.

143. Comess LJ, Bennett PH, Burch TA, Miller M. Congenital anomalies and diabetes in the Pima Indians of Arizona. Diabetes 1969; 18: 471–7.

144. Chung CS, Myrianthopoulos NC. Factors affecting risks of congenital malformations. II. Effect of maternal diabetes on congenital malformations. Birth Defect 1975; 11: 23–38.

145. Stoll C, Alembik Y, Dott,B, Roth MP. Study of Down syndrome in 238,942 consecutive births. Ann Genetique (Paris) 1998; 41: 44–51.

146. Narchi H, Kulaylat N. High incidence of Down's syndrome in infants of diabetic mothers. Arch Dis Child 1997; 77: 242–4.

147. Pelz J, Kunze J. Down's syndrome in infants of diabetic mothers [letter; comment]. Arch Dis Child 1998; 79: 199–200.

148. Nelson M, Lessell S, Sadun AA. Optic nerve hypoplasia and maternal diabetes mellitus. Arch Neurol 1986; 43: 20–5.

149. Van Allen MI, Myhre S. New multiple congenital anomalies syndrome in a stillborn infant of consanguinous parents and a prediabetic pregnancy. Am J Med Genet 1991; 38: 523–8.

150. Endo A, Ingalls TH. Chromosomal anomalies in embryos of diabetic mice. Arch Environ Health 1968; 16: 316–25.

151. Yamamoto M, Endo A, Watanabe G, Ingalls TH. Chromosomal aneuploidies and polyploidies in embryos of diabetic mice. Arch Environ Health 1971; 22: 468–75.

152. Khoury MJ, Becerra JE, Cordero JF, Erickson JD. Clinical–epidemiologic assessment of pattern of birth defects associated with human teratogens: application to diabetic embryopathy. Pediatrics 1989; 84: 658–65.

153. Sadler TW, Hunter ES, Wynn RE, Phillips LS. Evidence for multifactorial origin of diabetes-induced embryopathies. Diabetes 1989; 38: 70–4.

154. Zusman I, Yaffe P, Raz I, Bar-On H, Ornoy A. Effects of human diabetic serum on the in vitro development of early somite rat embryos. Teratology 1989; 39: 85–92.

155. Eriksson UJ, Dahlstrom VE, Lithell HO. Diabetes in pregnancy: influence of genetic background and maternal diabetic state on the incidence of skeletal malformations in the fetal rat. Acta Endocrinol (Suppl) (Kbh) 1986; 277: 66–73.

156. Styrud J, Thunberg L, Nybacka O, Eriksson UJ. Correlations between maternal metabolism and deranged development in the offspring of normal and diabetic rats. Pediatr Res 1995; 37: 343–53.

157. Cagliero E, Forsberg H, Sala R, Lorenzi M, Eriksson UJ. Maternal diabetes induces increased expression of extracellular matrix components in rat embryos. Diabetes 1993; 42: 975–80.

158. Forsberg H, Wentzel P, Eriksson UJ. Maternal diabetes alters extracellular matrix protein concentrations in rat placentae. Am J Obstet Gynecol 1998; 179: 772–8.

159. Phelan SA, Ito M, Loeken MR. Neural tube defects in embryos of diabetic mice: role of the Pax-3 gene and apoptosis. Diabetes 1997; 46: 1189–97.

160. Fine EL, Horal M, Chang TI, Fortin G, Loeken MR. Evidence that elevated glucose causes altered gene expression, apoptosis, and neural tube defects in a mouse model of diabetic pregnancy. Diabetes 1999; 48: 2454–62.

161. Hill AL, Phelan SA, Loeken MR. Reduced expression of Pax-3 is associated with overexpression of cdc46 in the mouse embryo. Dev Genes Evol 1998; 208: 128–34.

162. Cai H, et al. Role of diacylglycerol-regulated protein kinase C isotypes in growth factor activation of the Raf-1 protein kinase. Mol Cell Biol 1997; 17: 732–41.

163. Pani L, Horal M, Loeken MR. Rescue of neural tube defects in Pax-3-deficient embryos by p53 loss of function: implications for Pax-3-dependent development and tumorigenesis. Genes Dev 2002; 16: 676–80.

164. Conway S, Henderson D, Copp A. Pax3 is required for cardiac neural crest migration in the mouse: evidence from the splotch (Sp2H) mutant. Development 1997; 124: 505–14.

165. Li R, Chase M, Jung SK, Smith PJ, Loeken MR. Hypoxic stress in diabetic pregnancy contributes to impaired embryo gene expression and defective development by inducing oxidative stress. Am J Physiol Endocrinol Metab 2005; 289: E591–9.

25 Management of gestational diabetes mellitus

Massimo Massi-Benedetti, Marco Orsini Federici and Gian Carlo Di Renzo

Diabetes and pregnancy

Global fetal and infant loss, perinatal mortality, neonatal mortality, and malformations rates are significantly greater if the mother is affected by diabetes than in the nondiabetic population.[1] Studies conducted by Casson et al.[2] confirm that among unselected populations of women with insulin dependent diabetes mellitus (IDDM), pregnancy loss remains significantly higher than in the normal population. The diagnosis of congenital anomalies is also more accurate in infants of diabetic mothers since they are more carefully looked for in respect to control infants and because of the more frequent autoptic evaluation due to the higher mortality rate.[3] Consolidated experiences clearly correlate fetal and maternal complications to the degree of metabolic control during pregnancy indicating without a doubt the need for an effective metabolic and obstetric management of women with different degrees of alteration of the glucose homeostasis during pregnancy.

Gestational diabetes mellitus

Diagnosis

Approximately 7% of all pregnancies are complicated by GDM, resulting in more than 200,000 cases annually. The prevalence may range from 1 to 14% of all pregnancies, depending on the population studied and the diagnostic tests adopted.[4]

Risk factors for GDM are well known and their presence allows the identification of three risk categories: (1) *high risk*, which is characterized by marked obesity, diabetes in first-degree relatives, history of glucose intolerance, previous infants with macrosomia, current glycosuria; (2) *average risk*, which includes women that fit neither in the low- nor high-risk categories; and (3) *low risk*, which includes women of the age <25 years, normal weight before pregnancy, member of an ethnic group with a low prevalence of GDM, with no known diabetes in first-degree relatives, and no history of abnormal glucose tolerance, nor of poor obstetric outcome.[5]

Risk assessment for GDM should be undertaken at the first prenatal visit. Women with clinical characteristics consistent with a high risk of GDM should undergo glucose testing as soon as feasible. A fasting plasma glucose level >126 mg/dL (7.0 mmol/L) or a casual plasma glucose >200 mg/dL (11.1 mmol/L) meets the threshold for the diagnosis of diabetes and if confirmed on a subsequent day rules out the need for any glucose challenge. In the absence of this degree of hyperglycemia, the screening for GDM in women with high-risk characteristics should be performed according to two different procedures: the one-step procedure and the two-step procedure. The one-step procedure consists of a diagnostic OGTT (oral glucose tolerance test) performed on all subjects, while the two-step procedure before a 50-g glucose challenge test (GCT) followed by a diagnostic OGTT in those meeting the threshold value in GCT (see Chapter 13).

Women at average risk should be evaluated at 24–28 weeks of gestation; even for this category of women both procedures are indicated and in the case of negative results test should be repeated later.

In cases where low-risk profile blood glucose testing has not been routinely required, a fasting plasma glucose measurement between 24 and 28 weeks of gestation has been considered sufficient.[5] However, in 1998 Carr[6] demonstrated that using the risk categories approach to define screening strategies, 44–53% of GDM was undiagnosed. The lack of universally accepted criteria for screening GDM could induce inappropriate procedures with consequent diagnostic bias as recently demonstrated in a national survey conducted in Italy on performances of GDM screening in different laboratories.[7] Considering the importance of adequately treating GDM to prevent maternal and fetal complications, a reliable and accurate diagnosis is essential; in this regard, the multinational HAPO Study might provide a definitive answer for the criteria to be used.[8]

Monitoring and therapy

Once the diagnosis of GDM has been confirmed, the woman should be closely monitored until the early postpartum period. The general goal of therapeutic interventions in GDM is to achieve and maintain blood glucose as near to normal as possible in order to reduce morbidity and mortality of the mother, the fetus, and the newborn.

In order to provide high-quality care a multidisciplinary team approach is essential, including a diabetologist, a nurse who specializes in diabetes, a dietician, obstetricians, the midwife, and the neonatologist.[9]

Strict metabolic surveillance is required, with reviews every 1–2 weeks directly or by phone contact[9] with the target to detect and prevent hyperglycemia.

Daily blood glucose self-monitoring (SMBG) appears to be superior to intermittent office monitoring of plasma glucose.[10] For women treated with insulin, various evidence indicates that postprandial monitoring is superior to pre-prandial monitoring. De Veciana et al.[11] showed that postprandial glucose measurements were significantly better for predicting a lower daily insulin dose, HbA1c level, birthweight, and a reduced risk for Cesarean section, large for gestational age, and neonatal hypoglycemia.

This evidence has been confirmed in a recent study[12] demonstrating that postprandial blood glucose monitoring may increase the percentage of women achieving good metabolic control and reduce the risk of pre-eclampsia, and neonatal triceps skinfold thickness.

Based on this consideration Gabbe et al. concluded that women with GDM should test blood glucose four times a day, measuring fasting and postprandial glucose after each main meal.[13] Postprandial blood glucose should be monitored either 1 or 2 h after a meal, even though 1 h should be preferred as it corresponds to the blood glucose postprandial peak in healthy pregnant women. Measuring 1 h postprandial blood glucose was found to be associated with a reduced risk of complications and delayed progression to insulin treatment with respect to 2-h evaluation, in a group of GDM women on medical nutrition therapy.[14]

Urine glucose monitoring is not useful in GDM as it does not allows for fine tuning of therapy and can be an unreliable indicator of metabolic control due to the changes of the renal glucose threshold occurring during pregnancy.

A novel and promising option for metabolic monitoring can be represented by the systems for continuous subcutaneous monitoring that have been demonstrated to be effective in optimizing treatment in diabetic pregnant women.[15] Data from continuous glucose monitoring studies in GDM women confirmed that 1 h is the most reliable time point for assessing postprandial control.[16]

HbA1c should be evaluated every 4–6 weeks[17] to assess the response to the applied therapeutic regime and the accuracy of SMBG. Considering the physiological reduction of HbA1c levels noted in nondiabetic pregnant mainly due to lower glycation rate[18] and increased erythrocytes volume,[19] the target HbA1c level during GDM should be as close as possible to 5%.[20]

Urine or capillary ketones should be evaluated every morning in the first trimester as it can be useful in detecting insufficient caloric or carbohydrates intake in women treated with restricted caloric intake.[21]

Follow-up at the diabetes clinic should be performed monthly until the 28th week of gestation, fortnightly until the 36th week and weekly until term.[22] Additional clinic visits should be programmed if needed. Maternal surveillance should include monitoring of blood pressure and of urinary protein excretion to detect hypertensive disorders. Special attention should be paid to the evaluation of the presence and the evolution of diabetes complications. A urine test, which should include a culture, should be done fortnightly, and serum creatinine, microalbuminuria, and proteinuria every trimester. Eyes must be examined at the first trimester and successively as the need arises. ECG should be evaluated at the first visit.

All women with GDM should receive nutritional counselling by a dietician. The first therapeutic step recommended is the individualization of medical nutrition therapy (MNT) depending on maternal weight and height. MNT should include the provision of adequate calories and nutrients to meet the needs of pregnancy and should be consistent with the target defined for maternal blood glucose. Non-caloric sweeteners may be used in moderation.[23]

The daily energy intake recommended for women with ideal weight in the normal range is 30 kcal/kg of the ideal weight; for obese women 20–25 kcal/kg of the ideal weight, and for underweight women is 40 kcal/kg of the ideal weight.

For obese women (BMI >30 kg/m^2), a 30–33% caloric restriction (to about 25 kcal/kg actual weight per day) has been shown to reduce hyperglycemia and plasma triglycerides with no increase in ketonuria.[24]

Meals should be constituted of 50–60% of carbohydrates (breakfast <45%, lunch 55%, and dinner 50%), 25–30% of lipids and 10–20% of proteins. The overall carbohydrates content should not be less than 175 g/day with the possible need of a late evening snack to reduce the risk of morning ketosis.[25] An effective MNT regime is crucial in GDM treatment allowing a reduction of risk of perinatal serious complication and of morning hyperketonemia that has been associated with increased risk of neonatal complications.[26]

Caloric intake should be modified if the woman practices physical activity. In case of moderate exercise lasting 30–60 min and a starting blood glucose of 100–160 mg/dL (5.5–8.8 mmol/L), an increased intake of 15 g of carbohydrates is suggested. If starting blood glucose is between 161 and 250 mg/dL (8.9–13.9 mmol/L) the carbohydrate intake is not to be changed. In presence of frank hyperglycemia (blood glucose >250 mg/dL (13.9 mmol/L), with ketonuria, exercise should not be performed until metabolic control has been normalized.[27]

The increase in weight during pregnancy should depend on the pre-gestational weight. Women with BMI <19.8 should have a weight increase of 12.5–18 kg; BMI between 19.5 and 25, a weight increase of 11.5–16 kg; and in the case of overweight, i.e. BMI >25, the weight increase should be 7–11.5 kg.[28] Insulin is the pharmacologic therapy that most consistently has been shown to reduce fetal morbidities when added to MNT.

The recent Australian Carbohydrates Intolerance Study (ACHOIS) demonstrated a relatively large population of GDM women for whom intensive treatment with either insulin or MNT or SMBG effectively reduces the incidence of perinatal complications.[29] Selection of pregnancies for insulin therapy can be based on the level of maternal glycemia with or without assessment of fetal growth characteristics. When maternal glucose levels are used, insulin therapy is recommended when MNT fails to maintain self-monitored glucose at the following levels: fasting blood glucose ≤105 mg/dL (5.8 mmol/L) or 1-h postprandial blood glucose ≤155 mg/dL

(8.6 mmol/L) or 2-h postprandial blood glucose ≤ 130 mg/dL (7.2 mmol/L).[25]

Measurement of the fetal abdominal circumference early in the third trimester can be considered another indicator to define the need to start insulin therapy. In 1998 Buchanan et al.[30] tested the utility of this approach to drive therapy choice. They proposed the following decisional cascade: diet therapy as the first approach with fasting blood glucose evaluation every 2 weeks. If fasting blood glucose is above 105 mg/dL (5.8 mmol/L), insulin should be started. If fasting blood glucose remains below this threshold until 29–33 weeks insulin should not be prescribed; thereafter fetal ultrasound could be used to define the need for insulin therapy (see Chapter 27). If the abdominal circumference is under the 70th percentile diet therapy alone should be continued. If abdominal circumference is above the 70th percentile insulin therapy should be started independently of the glycemic values.[30]

In order to achieve and maintain a good metabolic control a basal–bolus regime should be adopted. Human regular insulin or rapid acting insulin analogues can be used to control postprandial hyperglycemia. Different studies showed that rapid acting analogues are safe during pregnancy contemporary allowing better metabolic control and increased compliance with respect to human regular insulin.[31–34]

Basal insulinization can be provided either with NPH insulin or continuous subcutaneous insulin infusion which are effective in regulating inter-prandial periods.[35,36] Even if preliminary experiences in gestational diabetes are promising,[37,38] long-lasting insulin analogues are not actually recommended due to the lack of definitive data on their safety during pregnancy.

The generally suggested starting dose is 0.7 U/kg of body weight. The doses and timing of the insulin regimen, should be thereafter guided by SMBG with particular attention to the insulin adjustment in the second and third trimesters. In fact, from weeks 20 and 32 of gestation there is a physiological progressive increase in insulin requirement up to 50% of the initial dose.[39] Thus usually the average insulin dose is 0.8 U/kg in the second trimester, 0.9 U/kg in the third trimester and 1.0 U/kg at term.[40]

The most effective insulin regime for insulin therapy during pregnancy consists of four injections per day. In 1999, Nachum et al.[41] compared the twice daily insulin injection regimen versus four daily in a cohort of more than 400 pregnant women with diabetes. They showed that a regime of four daily insulin injections improved metabolic control and perinatal outcomes better than the twice daily injections; moreover, the intensified therapy did not increase the risk of hypoglycemia in the mothers.

A higher risk of hypoglycemia with intensified insulin therapy can be observed during the first trimester of gestation when there is an increase of passive diffusion of glucose across the placenta and an impaired counter-regulation response.

The continuous subcutaneous insulin infusion (CSII) therapy through the utilization of insulin pumps could represent an optimal means to improve metabolic control with a reduction of the risk of hypoglycemia in diabetic pregnant women. Several studies have shown a better or at least equal efficacy of the CSII in metabolic control than the optimized multiple daily injections regimen with a reduction of mild and severe hypoglycemic episodes, provided that correct criteria have been used for the selection of the candidates for CSII.[42,43]

Oral glucose-lowering agents have generally not been recommended during pregnancy due to their capability to cross the placenta inducing fetal abnormalities. Different studies with glyburide, a second generation sulfonylurea, showed its efficacy in controlling fasting and postprandial glucose levels during pregnancy with similar beneficial effects on pregnancy complications as insulin therapy.[44,45] Moreover Langer et al. demonstrated that glyburide did not significantly cross the placenta.[46] Thus, at present, various authors consider glyburide as a valid therapeutic option for GDM.[47,48]

Metformin is increasingly used for polycystic ovary syndrome (PCOS); preliminary experiences of PCOS women treated with metformin throughout the pregnancy did not demonstrate an increased risk of complications in children.[49,50]

Programs of moderate physical exercise have been shown to lower maternal fasting and postprandial glucose concentrations in women with GDM.[51] In fact, physical exercise can improve unsatisfactory metabolic control in a diabetic pregnant patient on diet therapy alone.

Controversial results are provided about the safety of exercise for the fetus. Some authors demonstrated an exercise-induced fetal bradycardia while others did not find cardiac effects in the fetus deriving from the mother's exercise.[52,53]

The same contrasting results were also shown with regard to uterine activity; some authors[54] found that it was increased by exercise, while other authors found that it was not affected by exercise.[55]

Physical exercise with utilization of upper body muscles was demonstrated to be safer than exercise that involves lower body muscles.[56] However, physical exercise that can increase blood pressure needs to be avoided because of the risk of pre-eclampsia in GDM.

Although the impact of exercise on neonatal complications awaits to be defined through rigorous clinical trials, the beneficial glucose-lowering effects warrants a recommendation that women without medical or obstetric contraindications be encouraged to start or continue a program of moderate exercise as a part of treatment for GDM. Jovanovic et al. suggested light exercise of at least 20 min per day three times per week.[57]

Increased surveillance for pregnancies at risk for fetal demise is appropriate, particularly when fasting glucose levels exceed 105 mg/dL (5.8 mmol/L) or the pregnancy progresses past term. The initiation, frequency, and specific techniques used to assess fetal well-being will depend on the cumulative risk the fetus bears from GDM and any other concomitant medical/obstetric condition. Assessment for asymmetric fetal growth by ultrasonography, particularly in the early third trimester, may aid in identifying fetuses that can benefit from maternal insulin therapy (see Chapters 27 and 30).

The timing of beginning and the frequency of fetal monitoring depend on the presence of complications of the pregnancy such as pre-eclampsia, hypertension, antepartum hemorrhage, and fetal growth retardation. The intensity and the type of monitoring should be dictated by the severity of the obstetric complication. Ultrasonography should be considered around the 24th week to detect abnormalities of fetal growth and signs of polyhydramnios.[11] Ultrasonography has also been proposed as a more accurate method of estimation of fetal weight. Unfortunately, the reported mean error ranges from 300 to 550 g (11.6 to 19.4 ounces) (see Chapter 30).[58]

Delivery

GDM is not an indication for delivery by Cesarean section nor for delivery before 38 completed weeks of gestation. The prolongation of the gestation beyond 38 weeks increases the risk of fetal macrosomia without reducing Cesarean section rates, so that delivery during the 38th week has been recommended unless obstetric considerations dictate otherwise.[11] Other authors suggest prolonging pregnancy till the due time in women treated with diet alone and presenting good metabolic control.[13]

Cesarean section should be considered in case of macrosomia to reduce the risk of dystocic delivery and the maternal consequences.[59] The main objectives during labor are to maintain normal glycemic values, adequate hydration and caloric intake.[60,61] If women are only on diet therapy, it is suggested that breakfast is avoided on the morning when the delivery is planned. During delivery an intravenous infusion of saline solution at a rate of 100–150 mL/h and regular glucose monitoring are advised.

In the case of women on insulin treatment it has to be considered that labor determines a reduction of insulin need and an increase of caloric necessity. The day before labor, women should follow their usual insulin and diet regimen with an injection of bedtime intermediate insulin adjusted to produce a satisfactory fasting blood glucose. On the morning of the delivery, women should not receive either breakfast or rapid acting insulin bolus. An intravenous insulin infusion of 1–2 units of short-acting insulin per hour together with a 5% glucose solution or a saline solution at 100–150 mL/h is recommended. Blood glucose should be evaluated every hour and the insulin infusion should be adjusted accordingly in order to obtain a glycemic target between 70 and 130 mg/dL (3.8–7.2 mmol/L).

During delivery insulin infusion should be suspended while glucose infusion and glucose monitoring should be continued. The neonates of mothers with GDM or with pre-gestational diabetes are at the same risk for complications, particularly those infants born macrosomic (birthweight >4000 g).[62]

A pediatrician experienced in resuscitation of the newborn should be present whether delivery is vaginal or by Cesarean section. As soon as the infant is born, the following actions are essential:

1. Early clamping of the cord, i.e. within 20 seconds from delivery, to avoid erythrocytosis.
2. Evaluate vital signs: determine the Apgar score at 1 and 5 min.
3. Clear oropharynx and nose of mucus. Later empty the stomach: be aware that stimulation of the pharynx with the catheter may lead to reflex bradycardia and apnea.
4. Avoid heat loss; keep the neonate warm and transfer to an incubator pre-warmed to 34°C.
5. Perform a preliminary physical examination to detect major congenital malformations.
6. Monitor heart and respiratory rates, color, motor behavior at least during the first 24 h after birth.
7. Start early feeding, preferably breast milk at 4–6 h after delivery. Aim at full caloric intake (125 kcal/kg and 24 h) at 5 days, divided into six to eight feeds a day.
8. Promote early infant–parents relationship (bonding).

The neonate is usually best cared for in specialized neonatal units. Interference with the infant should be minimal. The neonates should be observed closely after delivery for respiratory distress. Capillary blood glucose should be monitored at 1 h of age and before the first four breast feedings (and for up to 24 h in high risk neonates). Currently, some amperometric blood glucose meters are acceptable for use in neonates, provided that suitable quality control procedures and operator training are in place. A neonatal blood glucose level <36 mg/dL (2.0 mmol/L) needs to be verified by repeat testing (laboratory verification is preferred but should not delay the initiation of treatment). Levels <36 mg/dL (2.0 mmol/L) should be considered abnormal and treated. If the baby is obviously macrosomic, calcium and magnesium levels should be checked on day 2.[11] Breast feeding, as always, should be encouraged in women with GDM.[17]

Postpartum maternal follow-up

Women with GDM have an increased risk to develop diabetes, usually Type 2, after pregnancy. Approximately 10% of GDM women present clinical overt diabetes soon after pregnancy and in the remaining population the incidence rate constantly increases over years from delivery up to 70% at 10 years in specific groups.[63]

Obesity and other factors that promote insulin resistance appear to enhance the risk of Type 2 diabetes after GDM, while markers of islet cell-directed autoimmunity are associated with an increase in the risk of Type 1 diabetes.[64,65]

Another risk factor for developing diabetes after delivery is the need for insulin supplementation to maintain good metabolic control during pregnancy.[66] A study involving 102 women with previous GDM followed for 8 years after pregnancy, showed an increased risk of developing diabetes in those who required bedtime insulin for the presence of persistent fasting hyperglycemia while no difference was seen between those who received only prandial injections in respect to noninsulin-treated controls.[67]

In all women with history of GDM and particularly in those presenting the above-mentioned risk factors the ADA advices a reclassification of the maternal glycemia at 6 weeks after delivery with a 75-g OGTT.[68] If the blood glucose levels are normal, another evaluation should be done after 3 years. In the case of impaired fasting glucose (IFG) or impaired glucose tolerance (IGT), glucose testing is advised every year. These patients should be placed on an intensive MNT, and on an individualized exercise regime due to their very high risk of developing diabetes.[69] Medications that provoke insulin resistance should be avoided if possible. Patients should be educated on symptoms of hyperglycemia and they should be advised to seek medical attention if they should develop such symptoms.[70] They should also be educated on the need for family planning to ensure optimal glycemia control from the start of any subsequent pregnancy. Offspring of women with GDM are at increased risk of obesity, glucose intolerance, and diabetes in late adolescence and young adulthood.[28]

Pre-gestational diabetes

Pre-conceptional care of women with diabetes

Despite progress in diabetes treatment pregnancies in women with either Type 1 or Type 2 diabetes are still associated with poorer outcomes with respect to healthy nondiabetic women.

A survey conducted in the UK covering a period of 12 years from 1990 to 2002 showed that pregnancy in Type 2 diabetic mothers was associated with an increased risk of infant mortality (2-fold for stillbirth up to 6-fold for death within 1 year) and of congenital malformation (11 times) with respect to nondiabetic mothers in the same geographical area.[71]

Another study conducted in the Netherlands in the period 199–2000 showed higher rate of perinatal mortality (2.8%), preterm delivery (32.2%), Cesarean section (44.1%) and congenital malformation (8.8%) in pregnant women with Type 1 diabetes related to the referring general population; they also showed an higher incidence of poor outcomes in unplanned pregnancies.[72]

Elements of an organized program for pre-conceptional care are best based on the various published clinical trials that have been successful in preventing excess spontaneous abortions and major malformations in IDM[3,73,74] when a good metabolic control is achieved. The pre-conceptional care is also provided on the basis of a cost–benefit analysis.

The model for diabetes preconception and early pregnancy health care includes four main elements: (1) education of the patient about the interaction between diabetes, pregnancy, and family planning; (2) education in diabetes self-management skills; (3) physician-directed medical care and laboratory testing; and (4) counselling by a mental health professional, when indicated, to reduce stress and improve adherence to the diabetes treatment plan.[70]

The desired outcome of the preconception phase of care is to lower HbA1c values to a level associated with optimal development during organogenesis. Epidemiological studies indicate that HbA1c test values up to 1% above normal are associated with rates of congenital malformations and spontaneous abortions that are not greater than rates in nondiabetic pregnancies. However, rates of each complication continue to decrease with even lower HbA1c test levels. Thus, the general goal for glycemic management in the preconception period and during the first trimester should be to obtain the lowest HbA1c test level possible without undue risk of hypoglycemia in the mother. In 2003 the ADA stated that the goal for metabolic control in diabetic pregnant should be less than 1% above the upper limit of the normal range.[75]

To obtain these values, there is need for an appropriate meal plan, self-monitoring of blood glucose (SMBG), self-administration of insulin and self-adjustment of insulin doses, treatment of hypoglycemia (patient and family members), incorporation of physical activity, and development of techniques to reduce stress and cope with denial.[70]

A complete anamnesis is imperative before planning for pregnancy. This should include, but not be limited to, questioning for duration and type of diabetes (Type 1 or Type 2), acute complications, including history of infections, ketoacidosis, and hypoglycemia, chronic complications, including retinopathy, nephropathy, hypertension, atherosclerotic vascular disease, and autonomic and peripheral neuropathy, diabetes management, including insulin regimen, prior or current use of oral glucose-lowering agents, SMBG regimens and results, medical nutrition therapy, and physical activity, concomitant medical conditions and medications, thyroid disease in particular for patients with Type 1 diabetes, menstrual/pregnancy history; contraceptive use and support system, including family and work environment.[70] To minimize the occurrence of malformations, standard care for all women with diabetes who have child-bearing potential should include (1) counselling about the risk of malformations associated with unplanned pregnancies and poor metabolic control; (2) use of effective contraception at all times unless the patient is in good metabolic control and actively trying to conceive;[70] (3) integration of the patient into the management of her condition; and (4) identification and treatment of complications of diabetes such as retinopathy, nephropathy, and hypertension.[76]

Diabetic retinopathy, nephropathy, autonomic neuropathy (especially gastroparesis), and coronary artery disease (CAD) can be affected by or can affect the outcome of pregnancy. Thus, physical examination should give particular attention to blood pressure measurement, including testing for orthostatic changes, dilated retinal examination by an ophthalmologist or other eye specialist knowledgeable about diabetic eye disease, and cardiovascular examination for evidence of cardiac or peripheral vascular disease. If found, patients should have screening tests for CAD before attempting pregnancy, to ensure they can tolerate the increased cardiac demands; and a neurological examination, including examination for signs of autonomic neuropathy.

Laboratory evaluation should focus on assessment and detection of diabetic complications that may affect or be affected by pregnancy: serum creatinine and urinary excretion of total protein and/or albumin (albumin-to-creatinine ratio or 24-h excretion rate).

Pregnancy seems not to be correlated with the development of diabetic retinopathy in women who did not have retinopathy before pregnancy.[77] Nevertheless pregnancy is associated with a significant progress towards more severe degrees of retinopathy in those who have pre-proliferative or proliferative retinopathy before pregnancy. All women who present proliferative retinopathy should undergo laser therapy before initiating a pregnancy.[78] Different studies showed a rapid worsening of retinopathy in diabetic mothers when a strict metabolic control is obtained in a short time.[79–81] Intervention in women with severe pre-proliferative or proliferative retinopathy should be tailored to achieve gradual metabolic control in preconception care.

Diabetic nephropathy complicates 5–10% of pregnancies in women with Type 1 diabetes[82] leading to an increased risk of fetal abnormalities, perinatal mortality, and mother morbidity.

Patients with protein excretion >190 mg/24 h have been shown to be at increased risk for hypertensive disorders during pregnancy. Patients with protein excretion >400 mg/24 h also are at risk for intrauterine growth retardation during later pregnancy. No specific treatments are indicated, but patients should be counselled about these risks. Since patients should not take angiotensin-converting enzyme (ACE) inhibitors during pregnancy, these assessments should be carried out after cessation of these drugs.

Women with incipient renal failure (serum creatinine >265.2 μmol/L or creatinine clearance <50 mL/min) should be counselled that pregnancy may induce a permanent worsening of renal function in >40% of patients. In subjects with less severe nephropathy, renal function may worsen transiently during pregnancy, but permanent worsening occurs at a rate no different from the background. Therefore, it should not serve as a contraindication to conception and pregnancy. As mentioned above, the presence of proteinuria in excess of 190 mg/24 h before or during early pregnancy is associated with a tripling of the risk of hypertensive disorders in the second half of pregnancy. ACE inhibitors for treatment of microalbuminuria should be discontinued in women who are attempting to become pregnant.

The presence of autonomic neuropathy, particularly manifested by gastroparesis, urinary retention, hypoglycemic unawareness or orthostatic hypotension may complicate the management of diabetes in pregnancy. These complications should be identified, appropriately evaluated, and treated before conception. Peripheral neuropathy, especially compartment syndromes such as carpal tunnel syndrome, may be exacerbated by pregnancy.

Measurement of serum thyroid stimulating hormone and/or free thyroxin level in women with Type 1 diabetes because of the 5–10% coincidence of hyper- or hypothyroidism and then other tests as indicated by physical examination or history. Successful preconception care programs have used the following pre- and postprandial glycemic goals: (1) *before meals*, values for capillary whole-blood glucose of 70–100 mg/dL (3.9–5.6 mmol/L) or capillary plasma glucose 80–110 mg/dL (4.4–6.1 mmol/L) 2 h; and (2) *after meals*, values for capillary whole-blood glucose of <140 mg/dL (<7.8 mmol/L) at 2 h or capillary plasma glucose <155 mg/dL (<8.6 mmol/L) at 2 h.[75] Implement the treatment plan and monitor HbA1c levels at intervals of 1–2 weeks until stable. Then, counsel the patient about the risk associated with her level. If she does not achieve a low-risk level of <1% above the upper limit of normal, consider modification of the treatment regimen, including addition of postprandial glucose monitoring.[11] Glycemic goals may need to be modified according to the patient's recognition of hypoglycemia and the risk of severe neuroglycopenia. Outpatient management is the appropriate forum for achieving preconception glycemic goals. Once the patient has achieved stable glycemic control (assessed by the HbA1c test) that is as good as she can achieve, then she can be counselled about the risk of malformations and spontaneous abortions. If the risk as well as the status of maternal diabetic complications and any coexisting medical conditions are acceptable, then contraception can be discontinued. If conception does not occur within 1 year, the patient's fertility should be assessed.

Metabolic monitoring during pregnancy

Metabolic and weight targets for diabetic pregnant women are similar to those presented for GDM. Close attention should be paid to the management of insulin doses considering that during pregnancy insulin need progressively increases from the first to the third trimester and that it inversely reduces in the immediate postpartum period. A recent study confirmed also in Type 1 diabetic pregnancy the superiority of 1 h postprandial blood glucose measurements in respect to the pre-prandial monitoring in reducing the risk of maternal and fetal complications.[12] Hypoglycemia occurs more frequently during pregnancy in women with Type 1 diabetes, some evidences correlate maternal hypoglycemia with adverse fetal consequences. Thus although tight glycemic control is desirable during pregnancy efforts should be made to avoid blood glucose below 3.9 mmol/L.[83] Therefore it will be very important to provide educational support for self-management both for the home blood glucose monitoring and for the insulin self-adjustment. Moreover, strict control of blood pressure should be guaranteed. According to the recent classification by the Joint National Committee (JNCV) four levels of blood pressure control are defined.[84] The first stage corresponds to blood pressure of 140–159/90–99 mmHg and indicates the lowest degree of severity. However, due to the fact that diabetic pregnant women have a higher risk of hypertensive disorder some authors suggested starting anti-hypertensive treatment when blood pressure levels are above 135/85 mmHg. The contraindication of treatment with ACE inhibitors during pregnancy has to be reinforced due to the higher risk of fetal malformation. Diuretics and beta blockers should also be avoided during pregnancy. One of the greatest risks for the diabetic mother is the worsening of a pre-existing diabetic retinopathy. In the case of development of proliferative lesions laser treatment can be used during pregnancy. Hospitalization is not an elective choice for pregnant diabetics but it should be considered only in case of severe complications like ketoacidosis, hypoglycemic coma or pre-eclampsia.

Also, for the diabetic pregnant patient Cesarean section should be avoided whenever possible. It is vice versa recommended in the following cases: pre-eclampsia, malformations, abnormal fetal presentation, advanced age of the mother, and previous Cesarean section.

REFERENCES

1. Hawthorne G, Robson S, Ryall EA, et al. Prospective population based survey of outcome of pregnancy in diabetic women: results of the Northern Diabetic Pregnancy Audit, 1994. BMJ 1997; 315: 279–81.

2. Casson IF, Clarke CA, Howard CV, et al. Outcomes of pregnancy in insulin dependent diabetic women: results of a five year population cohort study. BMJ 1997; 315: 275–8.

3. Kitzmiller JL, Buchanan TA, Kjos S, Combs CA, Ratner RE. Pre-conception care of diabetes, congenital malformations, and spontaneous abortions. Diabetes Care 1996; 19: 514–41.

4. Persson B, Hanson U, Lunell NO. Diabetes mellitus and pregnancy. In: Alberti, Zimmet, DeFronzo, eds. International Textbook of Diabetes Mellitus. Chichester: John Wiley; 1997.

5. Metzger BE, Coustan DR. Summary and recommendations of the Fourth International Workshop–Conference on Gestational Diabetes Mellitus. The Organizing Committee. Diabetes Care 1998; 21(suppl. 2): B161–7.

6. Carr SB. Screening for gestational diabetes mellitus. Diabetes Care 1998; 21(suppl 2): B14–8.

7. Orsini Federici M, Mosca A, Testa R, et al., for the Italian Society of Clinical Biochemistry and Clinical Molecular Biology, and the Italian Society of Laboratory Medicine. National survey on the execution of the oral glucose tolerance test (OGTT) in a representative cohort of Italian laboratories. Clin Chem Lab Med 2006; 44: 568–73.

8. HAPO Study Cooperative Research Group. The Hyperglycemia and Adverse Pregnancy Outcome Study. Int J Gynecol Obstet 2002; 78: 69–77.

9. International Diabetes Federation – European Region. Guidelines for diabetes care. A desktop guide to type 2 diabetes mellitus. Walter Wirtz Druck Verlag, Germany, August 1998.

10. Homko CJ, Sivan E, Reece EA. Is self-monitoring of blood glucose necessary in the management of gestational diabetes mellitus? Diabetes Care 1998; 21(suppl 2): B118–22.

11. De Veciana M, Major CA, Morgan MA, et al. Postprandial versus preprandial blood glucose monitoring in women with gestational diabetes mellitus requiring insulin therapy. New Engl J Med 1995; 333: 1237–41.

12. Manderson G, Patterson C, Hadden R, et al. Preprandial versus postprandial blood glucosemonitoring in type 1 diabetic pregnancy: A randomized controlled clinical trial. Am J Obstet Gynecol 2003; 189: 507–12.

13. Gabbe S, Graves R. Management of diabetes mellitus complicating pregnancy. Obstet Gynecol 2003; 102: 857–68.

14. Weisz B, Shrim A, Homko C, et al. One hour versus two hours postprandial glucose measurement in gestational diabetes: a prospective study. J Perinatol 2005; 25: 241–4.

15. Chen R, Yogev Y, Ben-Haroush A, et al. Continuous glucose monitoring for the evaluation and improved control of gestational diabetes mellitus. J Matern Fetal Neonatal Med 2003; 14: 256–60.

16. Buhling KJ, Winkel T, Wolf C, et al. Optimal timing for postprandial glucose measurement in pregnant women with diabetes and a non-diabetic pregnant population evaluated by the Continuous Glucose Monitoring System (CGMS). J Perinat Med 2005; 33: 125–31.

17. American Diabetes Association. Gestational diabetes mellitus. Position Statements. Diabetes Care 2004; 27: S88–S90.

18. Gunton JE, McElduff A. Hemoglobinopathies and HbAlc measurement. Diabetes Care 2000; 23: 1197–8.

19. Madsen H, Ditzel J, Hansen P. Hemoglobin Alc determinations in diabetic pregnancy. Diabetes Care 1981; 4: 541–6.

20. Cefalu WT, Prather KL, Chester DL. Total serum glycosolated proteins in detection and monitoring of gestational diabetes. Diabetes Care 1990; 13: 872–5.

21. Gin H, Vambergue A, Vasseur C, et al. Could blood ketone monitoring be a tool for managing gestational diabetes mellitus? Diabetes Care 2006; 29: 743.

22. Hoffman L, Nolan C, Wilson JD, Oats JJN, Simmons D. Gestational diabetes mellitus – management guidelines The Australasian Diabetes in Pregnancy Society. MJA 1998; 169: 93–7.

23. American Diabetes Association. Gestational diabetes mellitus. Diabetes Care 2001; 24(suppl 1): 77.

24. Franz MJ, Horton ES, Bantle JP, et al. Nutrition principles for the management of diabetes and related complications [Technical review]. Diabetes Care 1994; 17: 490–518.

25. American Diabetes Association. Standards of Medical care in diabetes – 2007. Diabetes Care 2007; 30: S4–S41.

26. American Diabetes Association. Evidence-based nutrition principles and recommendations for the treatment and prevention of diabetes and related complications. Diabetes Care 2003; 26(suppl 1): S51–S61.

27. Luke B, Murtaugh MA. Dietetic treatment. In: Reece EA, Coustan DR eds. Diabetes Mellitus in Pregnancy. New York: Churchill Livingstone; 1998.

28. Lapolla A, Botta RM, Vitacolonna E. Diabete in gravidanza. Diabete 2001; 13: 269–83.

29. Crowther C, Hiller J, Moss J, et al., for the Australian Carbohydrate Intolerance Study in Pregnant Women (ACHOIS) Trial Group. Effect of treatment of gestational diabetes mellitus on pregnancy outcomes. N Engl J Med 2005; 352: 2477–86.

30. Buchanan TA, Kjos Sl, Schafer U, et al. Utility of foetal measurements in the management of gestational diabetes mellitus. Diabetes Care 1998; 21(suppl 2): B99–B106.

31. J Jovanovic L, Ilic S, Pettitt DJ, et al. Metabolic and immunologic effects of insulin lispro ingestational diabetes. Diabetes Care 1999; 22: 1422–7.

32. Persson B, Swahn ML, Hjertberg R, et al. Insulin lispro therapy in pregnancies complicated by type 1 diabetes mellitus. Diabetes Res Clin Pract 2002; 58: 115–21.

33. Owens D, Vora J. Insulin aspart: a review. Expert Opin Drug Metab Toxicol 2006; 2: 793–804.

34. Pettitt DJ, Ospina P, Kolaczynski JW, Jovanovic L. Comparison of an insulin analog, insulin aspart, and regular human insulin with no insulin in gestational diabetes mellitus. Diabetes Care 2003; 26: 183–6.

35. Jovanovic L. Achieving euglycaemia in women with gestational diabetes mellitus: current options for screening, diagnosis and treatment. Drugs 2004; 64: 1401–17.

36. Gottlieb PA, Frias JP, Peters KA, Chillara B, Garg SK. Optimizing insulin therapy in pregnant women with type 1 diabetes mellitus. Treat Endocrinol 2002; 1: 235–40.

37. Price N, Bartlett C, Gillmer M. Use of insulin glargine during pregnancy: a case-control pilot study. Br J Obstet Gynaecol 2007.

38. Graves D, White J, Kirk J. The use of insulin glargine with gestational diabetes mellitus. diabetes care 2006; 29: 471–2.

39. Langer O. Maternal glycaemic criteria for insulin therapy in gestational diabetes mellitus. Diabetes Care 1998; 21(suppl 2): B91–8.

40. Jovanovic L, Peterson CM. The art and science of maintenance of normoglycemia in pregnancies complicated by type 1 diabetes mellitus. Endocr Pract 1996; 2: 130–42.

41. Nachum Z, Ben-Shlomo I, Weiner E, Shalev E. Twice daily versus four times daily insulin dose regimens for diabetes in pregnancy: randomised controlled trial. BMJ 1999; 319: 1223–7.

42. Simmons D, Thompson CF, Conroy C, Scott DJ. Pumps in pregnancies complicated by type 2 diabetes and gestational diabetes in a multiethnic community. Diabetes Care 2001; 24: 2078–82.

43. Carta Q, Meriggi E, Trossarelli GF, et al. Continuous subcutaneous insulin infusion versus intensive conventional insulin therapy in type I and type II diabetic pregnancy. Diabet Metab 1986; 12: 121–9.

44. Kremer C, Duff P. Glyburide for the treatment of gestational diabetes. Am J Obstet Gynecol 2004; 190: 1438–9.

45. Langer O, Yogev Y, Xenakis E, Rosenn B. Insulin and glyburide therapy: Dosage, severity level of gestational diabetes, and pregnancy outcome. Am J Obstet Gynecol 2005; 192; 134–9.

46. Elliot B, Langer O, Schussling F. A model of human placental drug transfer. Am J Obstet Gynecol 1997; 176: 527–30.

47. Cefalo RC. A comparison of glyburide and insulin in women with gestational diabetes mellitus. Obstet Gynecol Survey 2001; 56: 126–7.

48. Kirschbaum TH. Medical complications of pregnancy. In: Yearbook of Obstetrics, Gynecology, and Women's Health. St. Louis, MO: Mosby; 2002, pp. 103–6.

49. Vanky E, Salvesen KA, Heimstad R, et al. Metformin reduces pregnancy complications without affecting androgen levels in pregnant polycystic ovary syndrome women: results of a randomized study. Human Reprod 2004; 19: 1734–40.

50. Brock B, Smidt K, Ovesen P, Schmitz O, Rungby J. Is metformin therapy for polycystic ovary syndrome safe during pregnancy? Basic Clin Pharmacol Toxicol 2005; 96: 410–2.

51. Jovanovic L. Controversies in the diagnosis and treatment of gestational diabetes. Cleve Clin J Med 2000; 67: 481–8.

52. Jovanovic L, Kessler A, Peterson GM. Human maternal and fetal response to graded exercise. J Appl Physiol 1985; 56: 1719–22.

53. Collings C, Curet IB. Fetal heart rate response to maternal exercise. Am J Obstet Gynecol 1985; 151: 498–501.

54. Erkkola R. The physical work capacity of the expectant mother and its effect on pregnancy, labor and newborn. Int J Gynecol Obstet 1976; 14: 153–9.

55. Veille JC, Hohimer RA, Burry K, Speroff L. The effect of exercise on uterine activity in the last eight weeks of pregnancy. Am J Obstet Gynecol 1985; 151: 727–30.

56. Durak EP, Jovanovic-Peterson L, Peterson CM. Comparative evaluation of uterine response to exercise on five aerobic machines. Am J Obstet Gynecol 1990; 162: 754–6.

57. Jovanovic L. American Diabetes Association's Fourth International Workshop–Conference on Gestational Diabetes Mellitus: summary and discussion. Therapeutic interventions. Diabetes Care 1998; 21(suppl. 2): B131–7.

58. Zamorski MA, Biggs WS. Management of suspected foetal macrosomia. Am Fam Physician 2001; 63: 302–5.
59. Coustan DR, for the American College of Obstetricians and Gynecologists Committee on Practice Bulletins – Obstetrics. Gestational Diabetes. ACOG practice bulletin #30. Washington: ACOG; 2001.
60. Coustan DR. Delivery time, mode and management. In: Reece EA, Coustan DR, eds. Diabetes Mellitus in Pregnancy. New York: Churchill Livingstone; 1998.
61. Hod M, Bar J, Peled Y, et al. Antepartum management protocol. Timing and mode of delivery in gestational diabetes. Diabetes Care 1998; 21(suppl. 2): B113–7.
62. Persson B, Hanson U. Neonatal morbidities in gestational diabetes mellitus. Diabetes Care 1998; 21(suppl. 2): B79–B84.
63. Kim C, Newton KM, Knopp RH. Gestational diabetes and the incidence of type 2 diabetes. Diabetes Care 2002; 25: 1862–8.
64. Dalfrà MG, Lapolla A, Masin M, et al. Antepartum and early postpartum predictors of type 2 diabetes development in women with gestational diabetes mellitus. Diabet Metab 2001; 27: 675–80.
65. Dornhorst A, Rossi M. Risk and prevention of type 2 diabetes in women with gestational diabetes. Diabetes Care 1998; 21(suppl. 2): B43–9.
66. Ben-Haroush A, Yogev Y, Hod M. Epidemiology of gestational diabetes mellitus and its association with Type 2 diabetes. Diabet Med 2004; 21: 103–13.
67. Wah N, Cheung T, Helmink D. Gestational diabetes. The significance of persistent fasting hyperglycemia for the subsequent development of diabetes mellitus. J Diabet Comp 2006; 20: 21–5.
68. American Diabetes Association. Report of the expert committee on the diagnosis and classification of diabetes mellitus. Diabetes Care 2003; 26(suppl. 1): S5–20.
69. American Diabetes Association. Report of the Expert Committee on the Diagnosis and Classification of Diabetes Mellitus. Diabetes Care 2002; 25(suppl. 1): S5–20.
70. American Diabetes Association. Preconception care of women with diabetes. Diabetes Care 2002; 25(suppl. 1): S82–4.
71. Dunne F, Brydon P, Smith K, Gee H. Pregnancy in women with Type 2 diabetes: 12 years. outcome data 1990–2002. Diabet Med 2003; 20: 734–8.
72. Evers M, de Valk H, Visser G. Risk of complications of pregnancy in women with type 1 diabetes: nationwide prospective study in the Netherlands. BMJ 2004; 328; 915–20.
73. Rosenn B, Miodovnik M, Combs CA, Khoury J, Siddiqi TA. Glycaemic thresholds for spontaneous abortion and congenital malformations in insulin-dependent diabetes mellitus. Obstet Gynecol 1994; 84: 515–20.
74. Willhoite MB, Bennert HW, Palomaki GE, et al. The impact of preconception counselling on pregnancy outcomes. The experience of the Maine Diabetes in Pregnancy Program. Diabetes Care 1993; 16: 450–5.
75. American Diabetes Association. Preconception care of women with diabetes. Diabetes Care 2003; 26(suppl. 1): S91–3.
76. Elixhauser A, Weschler JM, Kitzmiller JL, et al. Cost–benefit analysis of preconception care for women with established diabetes mellitus. Diabetes Care 1993; 16: 1146–57.
77. Star J, Carpenter MW. The effect of pregnancy on the natural history of diabetic retinopathy and nephropathy. Clin Perinatol 1988; 25: 887–916.
78. Chan WC, Lim LT, Quinn MJ, et al. Management and outcome of sight-threatening diabetic retinopathy in pregnancy. Eye 2004; 18: 826–32.
79. Early worsening of diabetic retinopathy in the Diabetes Control and Complications Trial. Arch Ophthalmol 1998; 116: 874–6.
80. Wang PH, Lau J, Chalmers TC. Meta-analysis of effects of intensive blood glucose control on later complications of type 1 diabetes. Lancet 1993; 341: 1306–9.
81. Jampol LM, Phelps R, Sakol P, et al. Diabetic retinopathy during pregnancy: Role of regulation of hyperglycemia. Ophthalmol Vis Sci 1986; 27: 4.
82. Gordon M, Landon MB, Samuels P, Hissrich S, Gabbe SG. Perinatal outcome and long-term follow-up associated with modern management of diabetic nephropathy. Obstet Gynecol 1996; 87: 401–9.
83. ter Braak E, Evers I, Erkelens D, Visser G. Maternal hypoglycemia during pregnancy in type 1 diabetes: maternal and fetal consequences. Diabetes Metab Res Rev 2002; 18: 96–105.
84. The Fifth Report of the Joint National Committee on Detection and Treatment of High Blood Pressure. Arch Intern Med 1993; 153: 154.

26 Medical nutritional therapy for gestational diabetes mellitus

Emily Albertson and Lois Jovanovic

Introduction

Pregnancy causes a multitude of metabolic changes within a woman's body in order to provide the proper nutrients to the developing fetus. In women with diabetes Type 1, Type 2, and gestational diabetes mellitus (GDM) these metabolic perturbations must be treated distinctly and aggressively to optimize fetal development and health. Pre-gestational diabetes (either Type 1 or Type 2) has the potential to subject the developing fetus to abnormal maternal glucose levels resulting in problems with organogenesis producing congenital abnormalities or spontaneous abortion. Furthermore, gestational diabetes mellitus presents after organogenesis in the second part of pregnancy, therefore the major risk for the fetus is macrosomia. Although the goal for dietary therapy for each of these disorders is the same which is euglycemia, the means to achieve it are very different and somewhat controversial. In the case of gestational diabetes, the mainstay of therapy is medical nutritional therapy whereas in insulin-requiring diabetes, dietary therapy is compensated with pre-meal insulin injections. In this chapter, the metabolic changes in normal pregnancy will be presented followed by the general guidelines for pregnancy. Fetal complications associated with inadequate nutrition or metabolic perturbation will be briefly explored, followed by issues and treatment for gestational diabetes mellitus, with emphasis on specific dietary therapies for GDM.

Metabolic changes in normal pregnancy

During pregnancy, metabolism increases by 15–26% to support both mother and developing fetus.[1] Early pregnancy is characterized by normal glucose tolerance, normal hepatic gluconeogenesis, and normal or improved insulin sensitivity.[1–5] As pregnancy progresses, carbohydrate metabolism becomes altered due to an increase in insulin secretion and decreased insulin sensitivity. Thus, some insulin resistance occurs, by late pregnancy overall insulin action is decreased 50–70% as compared to a nonpregnant women.[5]

Lipid metabolism is also altered in hepatic and adipose tissue. Early pregnancy hormones, estrogen, progesterone, and insulin promote the storage of lipids within maternal tissues. Therefore, in early pregnancy, initially there is a decrease in serum triacylglycerols, fatty acids, cholesterol, lipoproteins, and phospholipids. However, as estrogen and insulin resistance impacts the mother, lipolysis and hypertriglyceremia ensues.[5] For example at week 12, estrogen causes cholesterol, specifically HDL, to be utilized as a major metabolic fuel for the placenta throughout the remaining weeks of pregnancy, thus serum concentrations increase. Furthermore, VLDL is altered in the second and third trimesters due to a change in adipose and hepatic enzyme activity, specifically the decrease of lipoprotein lipase (LPL). Notably, when maternal glucose levels decrease as can be seen during the fasting state, hepatic LPL activity increases allowing the mobilization of lipids and ketones for fetal nutrition.

Human chorionic gonadotropin, prolactin, and glucagon also contribute by stimulating lipolysis in late pregnancy. This serves to preferentially send glucose and protein to the fetus, while the maternal tissues rely more on fatty acid oxidation and ketogenesis to meet their energy requirement. Finally, during the third trimester a change in hepatic gluconeogenesis can be seen. Due to a 10–15 mg/dL decrease in basal rate of glucose and an insulin concentration of two times the concentration seen in a nonpregnant women, the liver must compensate by secreting 16–30% more glucose to meet the energy needs of both the mother and fetus.[3,6,7] Assel et al.[7] found that the maternal hepatic glucose production is dependent upon maternal body weight in a linear fashion. Late pregnancy also is characterized by a rise in the carbohydrate contribution to the overall oxidative metabolism as energy.

In normal pregnancy, metabolic changes occur to shunt nutrients from the mother to the fetus, allowing for optimal development and growth, however as we explore the following sections of this chapter it will become apparent that alteration based on input and dysfunction can alter the body's natural plan and cause both distress to the mother and fetus.

General nutritional guidelines for pregnancy

Normal pregnancy nutritional guidelines focus on several dietary elements. Major topics include: caloric intake, macronutrient proportion, vitamins and minerals, and alcohol consumption. The energy requirements of the fetus must be met to ensure proper development and provide for postpartum lactation without causing excessive maternal weight gain. The energy standard to support a pregnancy has been debated heavily and will be explored in the GDM nutritional therapy section below. The American College of Obstetricians and Gynecologists advocates several basic concepts for a balanced diet for pregnant women. They suggest eating three to four servings of fruits and vegetables, nine servings of whole grains for energy, three servings of dairy for calcium, and three servings of meat to reach daily protein requirements. Vitamin supplementation to achieve daily nutrients, as an adjunct to a healthy diet, is encouraged when recommended by the woman's physician. Certain foods should be avoided in pregnancy due to fetal developmental harm. These include: deli meat, certain preparations of smoked fish, soft cheeses, unpasteurized milk, refrigerated pate, raw meat, and raw eggs, which have been associated with bacterial infections such as *Salmonella*, *Listeria*, and *Escherichia coli*. *Toxoplasma gondii*, the protozoan that causes toxoplasmosis, has also been found as contaminant in unwashed vegetables and raw meat. Fish containing mercury and raw shellfish should be avoided. Caffeine has been associated with miscarriage, premature birth, low birthweight, and withdrawal symptoms in the neonate when consumed in large amounts in pregnancy. However, other studies have implicated caffeine intake in modest levels to be non-detrimental in pregnancy. Until further studies can evaluate the effects of caffeine, it is recommended to be avoided altogether.[8,9] Alcohol should not be used in any amount during pregnancy. *In utero* exposure has been linked to developmental disorders such as fetal alcohol syndrome. Also, alcohol should be avoided postpartum while breast feeding.[10]

Gestational diabetes mellitus

As discussed in the previous section on metabolic changes in pregnancy, the nondiabetic women undergoes drastic and dynamic metabolic changes to provide glucose as the preferential energy source to the developing fetus. Although, the pathophysiological mechanism behind GDM remains unknown, some current theories include a predisposition to future Type 2 diabetes triggered by the changes in metabolism that normally accompany pregnancy, or an increased response by the woman's body to normal metabolic changes of pregnancy. GDM has been defined as 'glucose intolerance of variable severity with onset or first recognized during pregnancy'.[11] It is important to note that GDM does not cause a malfunction in insulin secretion or improper pro-insulin or glucagon activity: insulin resistance remains the prominent characteristic.[12] In the United States, GDM affects 2–14% of the pregnant

population per year depending on the ethnicity of the population studied.[13,14] A women who is most likely to be affected by GDM is one who is obese, >25 years of age, has a family history of diabetes especially in first-degree relatives, has a past medical history for glucose intolerance or metabolism problems and/or miscarriages or other obstetric problems. Additionally, Latino, African, Native American, South or East Asian, and Pacific Islanders are at a higher risk for developing GDM.[15] The Santa Barbara County Health Care Services Program Study[16] found that women who meet several of these criteria, at the greatest risk, should be tested as early as feasible, while those with average risk should be tested at 24–28 weeks gestation. However, GDM can easily appear in low-risk women, therefore universal screening would be ideal.

Screening methods for GDM

The screening methods for GDM are very controversial. The two criteria sets endorsed by the World Health Organization or the US National Diabetes Data Group are each distinct and are primarily based on statistical standard deviations without regarding the level of clinical outcome achieved. An attempt to set international standards and identify those at risk for developing GDM is currently under way in a 5-year, prospective, observational and multi-center study, the Hyperglycemia and Adverse Pregnancy Outcomes Study. It involves 25,000 women in 10 countries and specifically will look at the clinical outcomes with respect to Cesarean delivery, fetal hyperinsulinemia, macrosomia, and neonatal morbidity in correlation to maternal glycemic levels.[17]

Fetal complications of maternal hyperglycemia

Uncontrolled hyperglycemia primarily affects fetal growth on both extremes of the normal growth curve. In those diabetic mothers that have advanced vascular disease, fetal growth deceleration may occur due to placental insufficiency. Fetal growth deceleration is defined as those in lower 5th percentile on a growth curve adjusted for gestational age.[18,19] Macrosomia defined as an absolute birthweight of greater than 4000-g or greater than the 90th percentile (adjusted for gender, ethnicity, and gestational age). Cesarean sections often must be performed when the baby is at term to reduce the risk of birth trauma such as Erb's palsy or Klumpke's paralysis.[20] Cesarean sections also adds risk to the mother's health. As explained by the Pederson hypothesis,[21] the effects of an intrauterine environment of hyperglycemia and hyperinsulinemia include: hypoglycemia, organ developmental problems (especially gastrointestinal), erythrocytosis, iron redistribution, calcium and magnesium deficiencies, respiratory problems (respiratory distress syndrome), cardiac problems (intraventicular hypertrophy and cardiomyopathy or heart failure), hyperbilirubinemia, and neurological sequelae.

A multitude of metabolic problems occur that not only affect the immediate future of the neonate, but as these children mature they have a predisposition of future metabolic problems, such as Type 2 diabetes and metabolic syndrome.[22,23] Subsequently, this pattern of metabolic disease takes a cyclic course affecting future generations.

Does treatment of GDM make a difference in pregnancy outcome?

In June 2005, Crowther and colleagues[24] published the results of a 10-year multi-center randomized clinical trial in Australia and the United Kingdom called the Australian Carbohydrate Intolerance Study in Pregnant Women (ACHOIS) (Table 26.1). The purpose of the ACHOIS was to determine whether medical nutritional therapy, glucose monitoring, and insulin therapy was superior to routine prenatal care with regard to reducing the risk of perinatal complications and postpartum maternal health status. A total 1000 women participated in this trial, 490 in the intervention group, and 510 in the routine care group with eligibility based upon the presence of one or more risk factors for GDM, or a positive 50-g Glucose challenge test (GCT) who did not have an indication of pregestational diabetes, history of GDM, or an active chronic disease. The WHO criteria were used to identify those with GDM, and women with severe glucose impairments were excluded. Therapies provided to the women in the interventional group consisted of dietary counseling with consideration to pre-pregnancy weight, activity level, normal dietary intake, and weight gain. Women were asked to self-monitor their glucose levels four times a day and proceed with insulin therapy dosage adjustments based upon those levels. Women in the routine care group received care from blinded clinicians as to the status of the previously performed oral glucose tolerance test (OGTT). However, if the clinician felt the patient was experiencing glucose intolerance, assessment and treatment could be instituted at his or her discretion.

Otherwise, prenatal care that was specific to the center visited was given. Primary outcomes included one or more perinatal complications defined as death, shoulder dystocia, bone fracture, and nerve palsy. Admission to the neonatal intensive care unit and jaundice that required phototherapy was also assessed. Secondary outcomes included a consideration of the primary outcome, gestational age at delivery, overall birthweight, and birthweight adjusted for gestational age, and the presence of macrosomia or fetal decelerated growth. Maternal outcomes were assessed on the basis of general and mental health including depression, anxiety, gestational age at birth, mode of birth, weight gain during pregnancy, hospital admissions and prenatal visits, and common complications, such as pregnancy induced hypertension.

The ACHOIS study[24] established several significant results both in the neonatal and maternal outcomes. The rate of serious adverse perinatal outcomes was significantly different between the interventional and routine care groups at 1 vs. 4%, respectively ($P < 0.01$). This rate established the number needed to treat at 34 to reduce the incidence of perinatal complication. Newborns in the interventional group were admitted to the neonatal intensive care units more often, at a rate of 71 vs. 61% admission rate in the routine group ($P < 0.01$). No significant difference was seen when considering the length of stay in the NICU or use of phototherapy due to jaundice. Thirty-nine percent of interventional group mothers were induced into labor versus 29% in the routine care group ($P < 0.001$). However, rates and reason for Cesarean sections were similar between the groups.[24]

With regard to the secondary outcomes, the interventional group neonates had significantly lower mean birthweights ($P < 0.01$) and were born earlier presumably due to higher labor induction rates. However, when adjusting for gestational age with respect to birthweight there were significantly fewer neonates born to interventional mothers that qualified in the

---

Table 26.1   Summary of the ACHOIS Study

Maternal and neonate primary, secondary outcomes evaluated	Intervention group, $n = 490$ mothers, 506 neonates	Routine group, $n = 510$ mothers, 524 neonates
Perinatal complications ($P = 0.01$)	1%	4%
NICU admission rate ($P = 0.01$)	71%	61%
Length of stay and phototherapy implementation (NSD)	Median 1 day; Interquartile range: 1–2 days	Median 1 day; Interquarile range: 1–3 days
Labor induction ($P < 0.001$)	39%	29%
Rate of Cesarean section (NSD)	31%	32%
Mean birthweigh t ($P < 0.001$)	3335 g ± 551g	3482g ± 660g
Large for gestational age ($P < 0.001$)	13%	22%
Macrosomia ($P < 0.001$)	10%	21%
Small for gestational age (NSD)	7%	7%
Maternal Edinburgh Postnatal Depression Score >12 ($P = 0.001$)	8%	17%

NSD, No significant difference.
(From Crowther et al.[24])

large for gestational age category. Additionally, macrosomia occurred significantly less often, but the rate of infants in the small for gestational age group did not differ between the interventional and routine care groups. Maternal outcomes regarding maternal perception at 3 months postpartum of health showed an improved quality of life in the interventional mothers specifically with a reduction in the incidence depression, 8 vs. 17% as measured by the Edinburgh Postnatal Depression Scale.[24] (Table 26.1).

The ACHOIS study clearly shows the benefits of using a multi-faceted approach toward managing GDM to the neonate and the mother. Not only does it advocate dietary and insulin therapies, but when one considers the population chosen and the method of randomization, it supports the use of universal screening. Based on the study design, the interventional group would be equivalent to universal screening practices and the routine group would represent those in which GDM screening is not routine. Therefore, by applying the results of the study in the women receiving routine care, only 34 women would need to be treated with interventional therapies to produce one improved neonatal outcome. Given the severity of an adverse neonatal outcome, this finding would support expanding the GDM screening population to include women who would routinely not be screened for GDM.

GDM and nutritional therapy

As demonstrated above, management of GDM is multifaceted. Insulin therapy, exercise, and diet are all vital components toward reducing the incidence of maternal hyperglycemia and ultimately fetal complications. The remainder of this chapter will focus on GDM nutritional therapy. Currently, there is no universally accepted medical nutritional therapy for the treatment of GDM. The American Dietetic Association advocates the standard medical nutritional therapy for a GDM mother to be the standard therapy advocated in nonpregnant adults with the carbohydrate content standard being < 60% carbohydrate per meal. However, when these standards were followed an increase in insulin therapy was seen in more than 50% of the GDM women.[25] Additional studies have supported lower carbohydrate percentages. For example, in a study involving obese GDM women, when the carbohydrate was restricted to 33%, the infants were all within normal birthweight ranges and there was no evidence of maternal ketonemia.

Ketonemia and ketonuria

Following an overnight fast, 10–20% of all pregnant women have ketones in their blood.[26,27] This fasting ketonemia or 'starvation ketonemia' has not been associated to fetal detriment. However, in studies conducted by Rizzo and colleagues, hyperketonemia during pregnancy, which results from maternal diabetes (hyperglycemia) has been implicated to affect the fetus's intellectual and behavioral development as measured by Bayley Scales of Infant Development, and the Stanford–Binet Intelligence Scale, which were administered at ages 2 and 3, 4, and 5 years, respectively. Hence, it was suggested that ketonemia be avoided in all pregnant women.[28]

Buchanan and colleagues contrasted the metabolic response in normal pregnant women without GDM, to those who were obese with GDM. He subjected both groups to an overnight fast and then an extended 18-h total fast. Obese GDM women had a greater decrease in plasma glucose levels and were not more prone to develop ketonemia than the normal pregnant women. This result would support the use of decreasing the frequency of meals in order to achieve lower pre-prandial glucose levels in obese GDM women.[29] In a study of Type 1 diabetic women, Jovanovic and co-workers showed that those infants whose mothers had the lowest beta-hydroxybutyrate levels had the largest infants because mothers' postprandial glucose concentrations where higher due to the increased caloric intake prescribed to avoid the ketonemia.[30]

Caloric restriction

Caloric restriction in pregnant women with GDM is another aspect of medical nutritional therapy that needs to be addressed. When women who are classified as obese or overweight prior to pregnancy, the amount of weight gain in pregnancy differs from those who are at a normal or underweight prior to pregnancy. The National Academy of Science has recommended that for women greater than 150% of ideal body weight, no more than 15 pounds should be gained with pregnancy. Optimal infant birthweight was achieved when less than 3 kg or no weight was gained in these women.[31] Hypo-caloric diets have been explored in women with GDM based upon a 2400 kcal/day diet. Investigators[32] compared a 2400 kcal/day diet to a 1200 kcal/day diet and achieved significant differences in average glucose and fasting insulin levels, but not in fasting or postglucose challenge tests. Those in the 1200 kcal/day group developed ketonemia and ketouria, therefore the study was discontinued due to the controversial association of ketones with fetal developmental harm. Subsequently, in another study conducted by the same investigators, within the first week, when compared with the 2400 kcal/day diet, a 1600 kcal/day diet improved fasting and mean daily glucose values without the development of ketonemia. Further studies have advocated a 1500 kcal/day to 1800 kcal/day diet for obese women with GDM with similar results.[33]

The standards for energy requirements for pregnant women with GDM, as supported by the American College of Obstetrics and Gynecology, determine the amount of energy needed to maintain pregnancy based upon the pre-gravid weight. For GDM women, who are 1.5 times their ideal body weight the caloric intake is 12–15 kcal/kg of the current pregnant weight, while those at less than 0.8 of their ideal body weight are to increase their caloric intake to 35–40 kcal/kg current pregnant weight. For those at 0.8 to 1.2 times their ideal body weight, 30 kcal/kg and those at 1.2–1.5 times ideal body weight, 24 kcal/kg current pregnant weight is the standard.[15] The 'euglycemic diet' advocated the lower range of the spectrum set by the American College of Obstetrics and Gynecology.

Carbohydrate restriction

The Pederson hypothesis attributes fetal macrosomia due to hyperinsulinemia caused by maternal hyperglycemia. Several studies have shown that when maternal glucose levels are well controlled, the incidence of macrosomia, fetopathy, and Cesarean sections decreases.[21,34–36] Currently, there is no set standard for pre- and postprandial levels in GDM women. Optimally, the therapeutic target of glucose levels in a woman with GDM would be the same as those who are pregnant without diabetes. Normoglycemia in the pregnant, nondiabetic, non-obese woman was demonstrated in studies conducted in 2001, by Paretti and colleagues.[35] In this study, the postprandial mean glucose during the third trimester did not exceed 105.2 mg/dL (5.8 ± 0.27 mmol/L). At 28 weeks gestation the l daily mean glucose levels was (71.9 ± 5.7 mg/dL) and at 38 weeks it increased to (78.3 ± 5.4 mg/dL), which would coincide with the normal insulin intolerance increase respectively. Paretti et al.[35] also accessed the clinical outcome of these pregnancies based on fetal growth. They found that 1-h postprandial glucose levels at 28 weeks through the third trimester had a positive correlation to fetal abdominal growth. Furthermore, the results are supportive in attributing the postprandial 1-h glucose levels as a predictor of infant birthweight, fetal macrosomia, fetal hyperinsulinemia and fetal abdominal circumference in nondiabetic pregnancies. Therefore, one may consider the level of insulin resistance as a spectrum, in which those with GDM are affected in the same way as nondiabetic pregnant women but to a greater extent. Hence, the levels of glycemia achieved in nondiabetic pregnant women to decrease incidence of fetal complications and growth would be applicable to those with GDM.

Another study to support the importance of postprandial glucose levels is the Diabetes in Early Pregnancy study, which was conducted with Type 1 diabetic mothers. When postprandial glucose levels increased there was an increased risk of macrosomia. The threshold for the marked increase was seen when postprandial glucose levels reached 120 mg/dL.[36] Thus, a dietary therapy, 'the euglycemic diet' was developed on the basis of this study.

The euglycemic diet takes into account the metabolic changes that occur within the pregnant woman as she goes throughout her day. In the morning a surge of cortisol is seen ('the dawn phenomenon'), which causes the release of glucose from stored sources and hepatic gluconeogenesis, thus the blood glucose is higher to begin with. Therefore, a decreased amount of carbohydrate is needed in the breakfast meal. A small study ($n = 14$), was conducted with GDM women who were greater than 130% of their ideal body weight at 32–36 weeks' gestation. The goal was to achieve a postprandial of 120 mg/dL at 1h. None of the patients were on an insulin regimen and a caloric restriction of 24 kcal/kg/day was established. Patients kept a diary of glucose levels four times a day and food intake. The carbohydrate parameters of the diet were as follows: 12.5% of the total daily carbohydrate at breakfast, 28% at lunch and dinner, with the remainder in three snacks disturbed throughout the day. The postprandial glucoses recorded by the women correlated to the carbohydrate intake.

From this study, the author has adapted this diet to achieve optimal control of glycemic levels in her patients. Most GDM women are very compliant and want to do what is necessary to have a healthy baby. By having patients take an active role in their medical care, they can significantly reduce their risk for fetal macrosomia. In a study conducted by de Veciana et al.[37] when patients monitored their pre- and postprandial glucose levels, the risk of fetal macrosomia decreased from 42 to 12%. Additionally, these patients also had lower hemoglobin A1c levels, therefore supporting that they maintained lower glycemic levels. Hemoglobin A1c is an effective clinical tool for accessing glycemic control and can be performed every 2 weeks to chart management because the turnover rate of the red blood cells during pregnancy is only 90 days as compared with 120 days in the nonpregnant state. Thus a significant improvement in glucose control is manifest by a significantly improved hemoglobin A1c level although the steady state has not been achieved until after 6 weeks.

Patients monitor their pre- and postprandial glucose levels and only proceed with a meal when their pre-prandial glucose levels are 90 mg/dL or less, otherwise insulin is initiated. A pre-prandial glucose of 90 mg/dL and a postprandial of 120 mg/dL may seem controversial or strict, however given the risk of macrosomia and the positive outcomes that have been obtained clinically the authors of this chapter advocate these glycemic goals for medical nutritional therapy.[38]

It is imperative that patients learn which foods have high carbohydrate content, so educational lessons and nutritional food label reading is essential for the success of any therapy that is instituted. A list of high carbohydrate foods is recommended to give patients in order to remind them what needs to be portioned. For example, the 'big 5' are potatoes, rice, pasta, bread/tortillas, and cereal (Figure 26.1). By teaching patients to adhere to a euglycemic diet, not only are they able to control their glucose levels effectively, but also they are able to modify their diet postpartum facilitating weight loss. A simple teaching tool that is used in Santa Barbara County is shown in Figure 26.2. The one-page handout identifies the foods to avoid, foods to eat with caution, and foods that may be eaten which minimally impact on the postprandial glucose concentrations and thus can be eaten liberally. Ideally, a breakfast of less than 33% of the daily carbohydrate intake, lunch at 45%, and a dinner at 55% are suggested to maintain a postprandial glucose level of 120 mg/dL.[39]

Role of fats in GDM therapy

Fat content in the American Diabetic Association's diet consists of less than 25% of the total caloric intake, whereas the euglycemic diet is composed of 40% of the total daily caloric intake. The role of saturated and mono-unsaturated fats in GDM women is different with respect to the uptake of glucose postprandially. In a study comparing these two types of fats, 1-h postprandial glucose levels are approximately equal; however, the duration of the elevated glucose levels differ. In GDM women who consumed mono-unsaturated fat, the glucose levels remained elevated longer and thus insulin dosage had to be adjusted to counteract the maintained

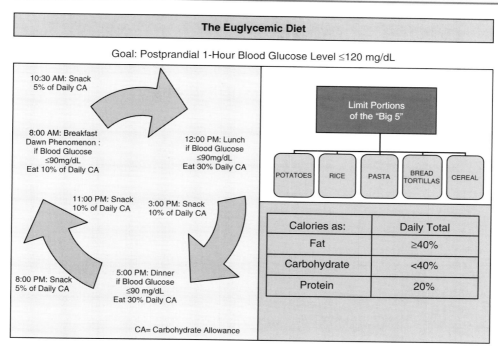

Figure 26.1 The euglycemic diet.

elevated glycemia. Conversely, meals consumed containing saturated fat, had a shorter duration of elevated glucose levels, making them preferential with regard to glycemic control of postprandial glucose levels. Furthermore, lower postprandial durations decrease the risk of macrosomia and the need for increased insulin doses.[40] Advocating saturated fats over mono-unsaturated fats is understandably controversial due to the correlation that has been made with saturated fats and heart disease in nonpregnant individuals. Further studies are needed to answer whether eating a higher proportion of saturated fat during medical dietary therapy for GDM at approximately gestation weeks 24–40 is a significant time period to have adverse long-term effects on the mother versus the benefit of controlling postprandial glucose level duration, which decreases the risk of fetal complication.

Role of protein

Protein content in the ADA diet and euglycemic diet makes up 20% of the total daily caloric intake. Increased satiety has also been correlated with meals that are high in protein content.[41,42] Thus, this aspect could help morbidly obese patients manage their overall caloric intake especially when moderate caloric restriction therapy is being used. Low carbohydrate/ high protein diets in normal pregnant women have been explored notably in the Motherwell studies running from 1938 to 1977. The Motherwell studies suggested a link between increased protein content and low birthweight.[43] Recent studies have expanded the initial Motherwell studies by looking at the offspring of these studies as adults. It has been hypothesized that increased protein intake can stimulate

maternal cortisol production and expose the fetus to high levels of cortisol which may facilitate life long hyper-secretion of cortisol. Herrick and colleagues found a correlation to increased plasma cortisol levels consequently causing hypertension in the adult Motherwell offspring.[44] However, they postulated that the type of protein consumed and the type of carbohydrate paired with it may factor into the physiologic affects seen. Co-factors needed for protein metabolism such as folate and vitamin B6, may be excluded when certain types of carbohydrate are avoided, such as bread and potatoes and green leafy vegetables, as was done in the Motherwell studies. 'In mothers with a limited capacity to synthesize nonessential amino acids, maternal amino acid oxidation could impair fetal growth as a result of reduced availability of nonessential amino acids.'[43] Therefore, the physiologic effect of low birthweight on the fetus would be caused multi-factorially and not just due to high protein consumption. Additional studies will be necessary to determine the role of high protein diets in pregnant women and specifically, in women with GDM.

Conclusion

Gestational diabetes is a period of glucose intolerance that manifests at the beginning of the third trimester. Metabolic changes in the normal pregnant women also have a degree of insulin resistance that shunts glucose preferentially to the fetus. To maintain blood glucose levels within a tight range, the normal pregnant woman must increase her insulin secretion up to 4-fold. When the pancreas is not able to compensate for the increased insulin needs of pregnancy, GDM occurs resulting in hyperglycemia and hyperinsulinemia in both

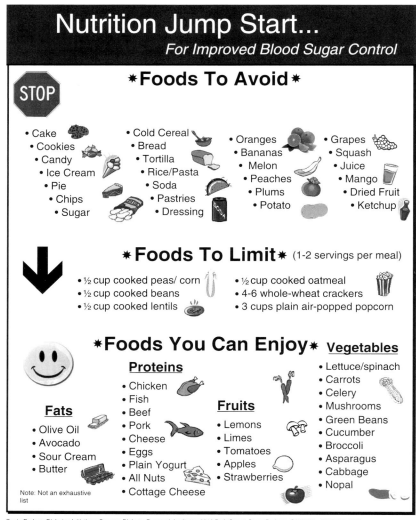

Figure 26.2 The one-page handout used in Santa Barbara county.

mother and fetus. These increased glucose and insulin levels manifest a multitude of fetal and maternal complications, the most prevalent being macrosomia. Other complications include hypoglycemia, erythrocytosis, hypocalcemia and hypomagnesia, hyperbilirubinema, iron redistribution, respiratory distress, and neurological effects. Poor gestational metabolic management can be directly linked to the level of neurological functioning of the child and these children are more prone to develop metabolic syndromes such as Type 2 diabetes. This would affect generations to come as well. The management of gestational diabetes mellitus is based upon the synergistic effects of medical nutritional therapy, exercise, and an insulin regimen when necessary. Therefore, the identification and treatment of GDM is crucial.

Screening tests using at-risk formulations and oral glucose tolerance tests remain a point of controversy. Universal screening would be optimal to identify those with GDM. The research clearly shows the benefit of expanding screening and providing medical nutritional therapy, glucose monitoring, and insulin

therapy to all women who manifest even minor elevations of glycemia. And thereby decrease perinatal complications, such as macrosomia. Maternal postpartum depression rates may also be improved with improved care during pregnancy.

Multiple studies have correlated fetal complications such as macrosomia to 1-h postprandial glucose levels. By restricting carbohydrate concentration in the euglycemic diet and modifying the caloric intake based on pre-gravid weight, success has been achieved in reducing large for gestational age and macrosomic infants. The euglycemic diet targets a pre-prandial glucose of 90 mg/dL or less and a 1-h postprandial of 120 mg/dL. Optimal glucose levels have been heavily debated and there is not currently a universal standard. However, research has shown that normal pregnant women in the third trimester have lower pre-prandial and postprandial glucose concentrations than nonpregnant women. This would support advocating lower standards of ≤90 mg/dL pre-prandially and 120 mg/dL postprandially for women with gestational diabetes.

Hypocaloric diets have been explored and appear safe for the obese gestational diabetic woman. The American College of Obstetrics and Gynecology advocate consideration of the mother's pre-gravid weight when considering the caloric needs per kg per day. The presence of maternal ketonemia and ketouria is controversial with respect to fetal development, and the mechanisms and outcomes associated with ketonemia resulting from uncontrolled glucose levels and starvation may be different with respect to detriment to the fetus.

Fat content also remains controversial although studies have shown that meals with saturated fat as compared to mono-unsaturated fat result in the same-hour postprandial glucose level, but the duration of the level is shorter facilitating lower insulin dosages. High protein/low carbohydrate diets are also controversial and in normal pregnant women have been correlated to lower birthweights and adult offspring increased cortisol levels. However, satiety is also important and protein malnutrition should be avoided in pregnancy. More research is necessary to determine the effect of these macromolecules on normal pregnant individuals and those with GDM.

Overall, medical nutritional therapy is one of the staples of GDM management. Women with GDM are very compliant and most are willing to make dietary changes in their lives for the benefit of their baby. The successful triad of medical nutritional therapy, exercise, and insulin therapy for GDM is essential to achieving, not only healthy babies, but also to assure that generations to will begin life with normal metabolism and thus and future metabolic aberrancy is reduced in the offspring.

REFERENCES

1. Butte NJ, Hopkinson JMM, Mehta N, et al. Adjustments in energy expenditure and substrate utilization during late pregnancy and lactation. Am J Clin Nutr 1999; 69: 299–307.
2. Catalano PM, Tyzbir ED, Roman NM. Longitudinal changes in insulin release and insulin resistance in non-obese pregnant woman. Am J Obstet Gynecol 1991; 165; 1667–72.
3. Catalano PM, Tyzbir ED, Wolfe RR, et al. Longitudinal changes in basal hepatic glucose production and suppression during insulin infusion in normal pregnant women. Am J Obstet Gynecol 1992; 167: 913–9.
4. Catalano PM, Tyzbir ED, Wolfe RR, et al. Carbohydrate metabolism during pregnancy in control subject and women with gestational diabetes. Am J Physiol 1993; 264: E60–7.
5. Butte NJ. Carbohydrate and lipid metabolism in pregnancy: normal compared with Gestational diabetes mellitus [Review]. Am J Clin Nutr 2000; 71(suppl.): 1256S–61S.
6. Kalhan SC, D'Angelo LJ, Savin SM, Adam PAJ. Glucose production in pregnant women at term gestation. Sources of glucose for human fetus. J Clin Invest 1979; 63: 388–94.
7. Assel B, Rossi K, Kalhan D. Glucose metabolism during fasting through human pregnancy. J Clin Invest 1997; 100: 1775–81.
8. Narod SA, De Sanjose S, Victoria C. Coffee during pregnancy: a reproductive hazard? Am J Obstet Gynecol 1991; 164: 1109–14.
9. Leviton A, Cowan L. A review of the literature relating caffeine consumption by women to their risk of reproductive hazards [Review]. Food Chem Toxicol 2002; 40: 1271–310.
10. Abel EL. Prenatal effects of alcohol [Review]. Drug Alcohol Depend 1984; 14: 1–10.
11. Report of the expert committee on the diagnosis and classification of diabetes mellitus. Diabetes Care 2003; 26(suppl. 1): S5–20.
12. Buchanan TM, Metzger BE, Freinkel N. Insulin sensitivity and beta cell responsiveness to glucose during late pregnancy in lean and moderately obese women with normal glucose tolerance or gestational diabetes mellitus. Am J Obstet Gynecol 1990; 162: 1008–14.
13. Coustan DR. Gestational diabetes. In: Harris MI, Cowie CC, Stern MP, et al. eds. Diabetes in America, 2nd edn. Publication 95-1468. Baltimore: National Institutes of Health; 1995, pp. 703–17.
14. Miller E, Hare JW, Clogerty JP, et al. Elevated maternal hemoglobin A_{1c} in early pregnancy and major congenital anomalies in infants of diabetic mothers. N Engl J Med 1981; 304: 1331–5.
15. American College of Obstetrics and Gynecology. Gestational diabetes. Practice bulletin no. 30. Obstet Gynecol 2001; 98: 525–38.
16. Jovanovic L, Bevier W, Peterson CM, for the Santa Barbara County Health Care Services Program. Birth weight change concomitant with screening for and treatment of glucose-intolerance of pregnancy: a potential cost-effective intervention. Am J Perinatol 1997; 14: 221–8.
17. The Hyperglycemia and Adverse Pregnancy Outcome (HAPO) Study. Int J Gynecol Obstet 2002; 78: 69–77.
18. Georgieff MK. Therapy of infants of diabetic mothers. In: Burg FD, Ingelfinger JR, Wald ER, Polin RA, eds. Current Pediatric Therapy, 15th edn. Philedephia: WB Saunders; 1995, pp. 793–803.
19. Creasy RK, Resnik R. Intrauterine growth restriction. In: Creasy RK, Resnick R, eds. Maternal–Fetal Medicine, 4th edn. Philadelphia: WB Saunders; 1999, pp. 569–89.
20. Nold JL, Georgieff MK. Infants of diabetic mothers. Pediatr Clin N Am 2004; 51: 619–37. Schwartz RP. Neonatal hypoglycemia: how low is too low? J Pediatr 1997; 131: 171–3.
21. Pederson J. the Pregnant Diabetic and Her Newborn, 2nd edn. Baltimore: Williams and Wilkins; 1977.
22. Weiss PA, Scholz HS, Haas J, et al. Long term follow-up of infants of mothers with Type I diabetes: evidence for hereditary and non-hereditary transmission of diabetes and precursors. Diabetes Care 2000; 23: 905–11.
23. Boney CM, Verma A, Tucker R, Vohr BR. Metabolic syndrome in childhood: association with birth weight, maternal obesity, and gestational diabetes mellitus. Pediatrics 2005; 115: e290–6.
24. Crowther CA, Hiller JE, Moss JR, et al. Effect of treatment of gestational diabetes mellitus on pregnancy outcomes. N Engl J Med 2005; 352: 2477–86.
25. Kitzmiller JL, Gavin LA, Gin GD, et al. Preconception care of diabetes: glycemic control prevents congenital anomalies. JAMA 1991; 265: 726–31.
26. Knopp RH, Magee M, Raisys V. Hypocaloric diets and ketogenesis in the management of obese gestational diabetic women. J Am Coll Nutr 1991; 10: 649–67.
27. Mills JL, Simpson JL, Driscoll SG, et al. Incidence of spontaneous abortion among normal women and insulin dependent diabetic women whose pregnancies were identified within 21 days of conception. N Engl J Med 1988; 319: 1617.
28. Rizza T, Metzger BE, Urns WJ, et al. Correlations between antepartum maternal metabolism and intelligence of offspring. N Engl J Med 1991; 325: 911–6.
29. Buchanan TA, Metzger BE, Freinkel N. Accelerated starvation in late pregnancy: a comparison between obese women with and without gestational diabetes mellitus. Am J Obtet Gynecol 1990; 162: 1015–20.
30. Jovanovic L, Metztger B, Knopp RH. Beta hydroxybutyrate levels in type 1 diabetic pregnancy compared with normal pregnancy. Diabetes Care 1998; 21: 1–5.
31. King J, Allen L. Nutrition during pregnancy. Washington DC: National Academy Press; 1990.
32. Magee MS, Knopp RH, Benedetti, TJ. Metabolic effects of 1200 kcal diet in obese pregnant women with gestational diabetes. Diabetes 1990; 39; 234–40.
33. Knopp RH, Magee MS, Raisys V. Hypocaloric diets and ketogenesis in the management of obese gestational diabetic women. J Am Coll Nutr 1991; 10: 649–67.
34. Combs CA, Gunderson E, Kitsmiller JL, et al. Relationship of fetal macrosomia to maternal postprandial glucose control during pregnancy. Diabetes Care 1992; 15: 1251–7.
35. Parretti E, Mecacci F, Papini M, et al. Third-trimester maternal glucose levels from diurnal profiles in nondiabetic pregnancies. Diabetes Care 2001; 24: 1319–27.
36. Jovanovic L, Peterson CM, Reed GF, et al. Maternal postprandial glucose levels and infant birth weight: the Diabetes in Early

Pregnancy study. The National institute of Child Health and Human Development – Diabetes in Early Pregnancy Study. Am J Obstet Gynecol 1991; 164: 103–11.

37. de Veciana M, Major CA, Morgan MA, et al. Postprandial versus preprandial blood glucose monitoring in women with gestational diabetes mellitus requiring insulin therapy. N Engl J Med 1995; 333: 1237–41.

38. Jovanovic L, Pettitt, DJ. Contempo updates. Linking evidence and experience: gestational diabetes mellitus. JAMA 2001; 286: 2516–18.

39. Peterson CM, Jovanovic L. Percentage of carbohydrate and glycemia response to breakfast, lunch, and dinner in women with gestational diabetes. Diabetes 1991; 40(suppl. 2): 172–4.

40. Ilic S, Jovanovic L, Pettit DJ. Comparison of the effect of saturated and monounsaturated fat on postprandial plasma glucose and insulin concentration in women with gestatonal diabetes mellitus. Am J Perinatal 2000; 16: 489–95.

41. Hill AJ, Blundell JE. Macronutrients and satiety: the effects of high protein or high carbohydrate meal on subjective motivation to eat and food preferences. Nutr Behav 1986; 3: 133–44.

42. Westerterp-Plantenga MS. The significance of protein in food intake and body weight regulation [Review]. Curr Opin Clin Nutr Metab Care 2003; 6: 635–8.

43. Kerr JF, Campbell-Brown BM, Johnstone FD. A study on the effect of high protein low carbohydrate diet on birthweight on an obstetric population. In: Sutherland HW, Stowers JM, eds. Carbohydrate Metabolism in Pregnancy and the Newborn 1978. Berlin: Springer-Verlag; 1979; pp. 518–34.

44. Herrick K, Phillips DI, Haselden S, et al. Maternal consumption of a high-meat, low-carbohydrate diet in late pregnancy: relation to adult cortisol concentrations in the offspring. J Clin Endocrinol Metab 2003; 88: 3554–60.

27 Insulin therapy in pregnancy

Lois Jovanovic and John L. Kitzmiller

Introduction

Before the advent of insulin, few diabetic women lived to childbearing age. Before 1922, fewer than 100 pregnancies in diabetic women were reported, and most likely these women had Type 1 and not Type 2 diabetes.[1] Even with this assumption, these cases of diabetes and pregnancy were associated with a >90% infant mortality rate and a 30% maternal mortality rate. As late as 1980, physicians were still counseling diabetic women to avoid pregnancy.

This philosophy was justified because of the poor obstetric history in 30–50% of diabetic women. Improved infant mortality rates finally occurred after 1980, when treatment strategies stressed better control of maternal plasma glucose levels, and once self-blood glucose monitoring (SBGM) and glycosylated hemoglobin (A1C) became available. As the pathophysiology of pregnancy complicated by diabetes has been elucidated, and as management programs have achieved and maintained near normoglycemia throughout pregnancy complicated by Type 1 diabetes, perinatal mortality rates have decreased to levels seen in the general population. This review is intended to help the clinician understand the increasing insulin requirements of pregnancy, and to design treatment protocols to achieve and maintain normoglycemia throughout pregnancy.

Glucose toxicity and the role of postprandial hyperglycemia

If the mother has hyperglycemia, the fetus will be exposed to either sustained hyperglycemia or intermittent pulses of hyperglycemia; both situations prematurely stimulate fetal insulin secretion.

Fetal hyperinsulinemia may cause increased fetal body fat (macrosomia) and, therefore, a difficult delivery, or cause inhibition of pulmonary maturation of surfactant and, therefore, respiratory distress of the neonate. The fetus may also have decreased serum potassium levels caused by the elevated insulin and glucose levels, and may therefore have cardiac arrhythmias. Neonatal hypoglycemia may cause permanent neurological damage. There is also an increased prevalence of congenital anomalies and spontaneous abortions in diabetic women who are in poor glycemic control during the period of fetal organogenesis, which is nearly complete by 7 weeks postconception.

Thus, a woman may not even know she is pregnant at this time. It is for this reason that pre-pregnancy counseling and planning is essential in women of childbearing age who have diabetes. Because organogenesis is complete so early on, if a woman presents to her health care team and announces that she has missed her period by only a few days, if the blood glucose levels are immediately normalized then there is still is a chance to prevent cardiac anomalies, although the neural tube defects are already 'set in stone' by the time the first period is missed. These findings emphasize the importance of glycemic control at the earliest stages of conception.[2-4] Ideally, if a diabetic woman plans her pregnancy, then there is time to create algorithms of care that are individualized and a woman can be given choices. When a diabetic woman presents in her first few weeks of pregnancy, there is no time for individualization, but rather rigid protocols must be urgently instituted to provide optimal control within 24–48 h.

After the period of organogenesis, maternal hyperglycemia interferes with normal fetal growth and development during the second and third trimesters.[5] The maternal postprandial glucose level has been shown to be the most important variable to impact on the subsequent risk of neonatal macrosomia.[6-8] The fetus thus is 'overnourished' by the peak postprandial glucose level.[9] This peak response occurs in >90% of woman at 1 h after beginning a meal. Therefore, 1 h after beginning a meal the glucose level needs to be measured and treatment designed to maintain this blood glucose in the normal range. Studies have shown than when the postprandial glucose levels are maintained from the second trimester onward to <120 mg/dL 1 h after beginning a meal, then the risk of macrosomia is minimized.[8]

Diabetogenic forces of normal pregnancy increase insulin requirements[10]

The fetal demise associated with pregnancy complicated by Type 1 diabetes seems to arise from glucose extremes. Elevated maternal plasma glucose levels should always be avoided, because of the association of maternal hyperglycemia with subsequent congenital malformation and spontaneous abortions.[2,5] To achieve normoglycemia, a clear understanding of 'normal' carbohydrate metabolism in pregnancy is paramount.

Thus, the amount of insulin required to treat Type 1 diabetic women throughout pregnancy needs to be sufficient to compensate for (1) increasing caloric needs; (2) increasing adiposity; (3) decreasing exercise; and (4) increasing anti-insulin or diabetogenic hormones of pregnancy. The major diabetogenic hormones of the placenta are human chorionic somatomammotropin (hCS), previously referred to as human placental lactogen (hPL), estrogen and progesterone. Also, serum maternal cortisol levels (both bound and free) are increased. In addition, at the elevated levels seen during gestation, prolactin has a diabetogenic effect.[10] The strongest insulin antagonist of pregnancy is hCS. This placental hormone appears in increasing concentrations beginning at 10 weeks of gestation. By 20 weeks of gestation, plasma hCS levels are increased 300-fold, and by term the turnover rate is 1000 mg/dL. The mechanism of action whereby hCS raises plasma glucose levels is unclear, but probably originates from its growth hormone-like properties. hCS also promotes free fatty acid (FFA) production by stimulating lipolysis, which promotes peripheral resistance to insulin.

Placental progesterone rises 10-fold above nonpregnant levels and is associated with an insulin increase in normal healthy pregnant women by 2- to 4-fold.

Most of the marked rise of serum cortisol during pregnancy can be attributed to the increase of cortisol-binding globulin induced by estrogen. However, free cortisol levels are also increased. This increase potentiates the diurnal fluctuations of cortisol with the highest levels occurring in the early morning hours.

The rising estrogen levels also trigger the rise in pituitary prolactin early in pregnancy. Prolactin's structure is similar to a growth hormone and at concentrations reached by the second trimester (>200 ng/mL) prolactin can affect glucose metabolism. Although there are no studies that have examined prolactin alone as an insulin antagonist, there is indirect evidence that suppressing prolactin in gestational diabetic women with large doses of pyridoxine improves glucose tolerance.

In addition to the increasing anti-insulin hormones of pregnancy, there is also increased degradation of insulin in pregnancy caused by placental enzymes comparable to liver insulinases.

The placenta also has membrane-associated insulin-degrading activity. Concomitant with the hormonally induced insulin resistance and increased insulin degradation, the rate of disposal of insulin slows. The normal pancreas can adapt to these factors by increasing the insulin secretory capacity. If the pancreas fails to respond adequately to these alterations, then gestational diabetes mellitus (GDM) results. In a woman with Type 1 diabetes, her insulin requirement will rise progressively. Failure to increase her insulin doses appropriately will result in increasing hyperglycemia.[10]

Rationale for the use of human insulin during pregnancy

Although controversial, the rate of complications in pregnancies of diabetic women has been tied to the metabolic control of maternal glucose.[1–5] Perhaps the debate remains because some reports claim that neonatal complications occur in spite of excellent metabolic control, although there fail to measure postprandial glucose levels.[11,12] Postprandial glucose control has been suggested as key to neonatal outcome for the pregnant woman with either Type 1 diabetes or GDM.[6–8]

Alternatively, some have suggested that neonatal morbidity is secondary to the variability of maternal serum glucose and the presence of antibodies to insulin.[13] Placental transfer of insulin complexed with immunoglobulin (IgG) has also been associated with fetal macrosomia in mothers with near-normal glycemic control during gestation. Menon et al.[13] reported that antibody-bound insulin transferred to the fetus was proportional to the concentration of antibody-bound insulin measured in the mother.

Also, the amount of antibody-bound insulin transferred to the fetus correlated directly with macrosomia in the infant and was independent of maternal blood glucose levels. In contrast, Jovanovic et al.[14] discovered only improved glucose control, as evidenced by lower postprandial glucose excursions, but not lower insulin antibody levels, correlated with lower fetal weights. They showed that insulin antibodies to exogenous insulin do not influence infant birthweight.

It has been reported that both insulin lispro and insulin aspart, (analogs of human insulin with a peak insulin action achieved within 1 h after injection) significantly improve the postprandial glucose levels in nonpregnant diabetic patients.[15–21] Because normoglycemia is important in the treatment of pregnant diabetic women, the use of insulin analogs would appear beneficial in the care of these women if the safety profile can be documented. This review presents the reports that studied the safety and efficacy of insulin analogs in pregnancy, and offers an opinion as to the utility of insulin analogs for treatment of the diabetes during pregnancy.

Concern about anti-insulin antibody formation during pregnancy

Anti-insulin antibodies that cross the placenta may contribute to hyperinsulinemia *in utero* and thus potentiate the metabolic aberrations in the fetus. Although insulin does not cross the placenta, antibodies to insulin do cross it and may bind fetal insulin; this necessitates the increased production of free insulin to re-establish normoglycemia. Thus, the anti-insulin antibodies may potentiate the effect of maternal hyperglycemia to produce fetal hyperinsulinemia.

Human and highly purified insulins are significantly less immunogenic than mixed beef–pork insulins.[16] Human insulin treatment has been reported to achieve improved pregnancy and infant outcome compared to using highly purified animal insulins.[14] Insulin lispro (which has the amino acid sequence in the beta chain reversed at positions B28 and B29) has been reported to be more efficacious than human regular insulin to normalize the blood glucose levels in GDM women. This insulin rapidly lowered the postprandial glucose levels, thereby decreasing the A1C levels, with fewer hypoglycemic episodes and without increasing the anti-insulin antibody levels.[17] In addition, the safety and efficacy of insulin lispro in the treatment of Type 1 diabetic women throughout pregnancy has recently been reported.[22] Also, insulin aspart has recently been reported to be safe and efficacious in Type 1 diabetic women.[23] However, there are only case reports and a small series of the use of the long-acting insulin analogues[24–27] during pregnancy. They appear to be associated with increased macrosomia, however.[27] The following discussion helps the clinician decide if the newer insulin's benefit outweighs any risks.

Use of rapid-acting insulin analogs in pregnancies complicated by diabetes

Postprandial glucose control in the patient with GDM is important to neonatal outcome.[6–8] The Diabetes in Early Pregnancy (DIEP) Study identified 28.5% of infants from diabetic mothers who were >90th percentile in infant birthweights.[8] The birthweight in this 28.5% correlated positively with fasting blood glucose and A1C. When adjusted for fasting blood glucose and A1C, the nonfasting blood glucose concentration in the third trimester was an even stronger predictor of infant birthweight and fetal macrosomia. Combs et al.[7] confirmed these findings, as they associated macrosomia with higher postprandial glucose concentrations obtained between weeks 29 and 32 of gestation. In addition, they described a higher risk of small-for-gestational-age (SGA) infants in those with lower (<130 mg/dL (7.2 mmol/l)) 1 h postprandial glucose levels. De Veciana et al.[6] described improved fetal outcome and less risk of neonatal hypoglycemia, macrosomia and Cesarean delivery in patients who managed GDM by controlling 1 h postprandial glucose concentrations than in those who managed by only the preprandial glucose concentrations. Therefore, rapid-acting insulin analogs that possess unique properties may make it a valuable therapeutic option in the treatment of GDM and the prevention of neonatal complications. First, the rapid absorption of insulin lispro from the subcutaneous site allows for a faster insulin peak concentration versus regular human insulin.[17,18] This effect more closely mimics the physiologic first-phase insulin release and results in lower postprandial glucose concentrations, and may lead to improved postprandial coverage.[15] In addition, insulin lispro is known to up-regulate insulin receptors.[19,20] In the present authors' study,[17] the postprandial glucose response to the test meal was more frequently within the normal glucose range after a standardized dose of insulin lispro as compared with regular human insulin. Second, the elimination of insulin from the venous space is the same as with regular human insulin, but the faster absorption of insulin lispro allows both the glucose-lowering effect and the patient's exposure to insulin to be less, which may result in a diminished antibody response. Certainly, in clinical trials there has not been any increase in antibody response associated with insulin lispro use.[15,18,19,22] Since placental transfer of insulin occurs when it is complexed with immunoglobulin, the lack of insulin lispro-induced antibody formation could be expected to result in little, if any, placental transfer of insulin lispro to the neonate,

as was demonstrated in the present authors' study. Thus, the overall decrease in circulating insulin as lispro, plus the lower immunogenic response of lispro, leads to less maternal antibody formation and, therefore, less insulin transfer to the fetus with a reduction in risk for physical malformations.[17,21]

Menon et al.[13] attempted to link maternal antibody formation to negative fetal outcomes. Careful review of the paper reveals, instead, better overall control of maternal hyperglycemia with attendant reductions in fetal macrosomia. This may have ultimately diminished the risk of neonatal complications, including macrosomia. Previous investigations have demonstrated that birthweight could be normalized with regular human insulin.[22–24] This aggressive therapeutic intervention may explain the apparent lack of macrosomia in both patient groups. No differences in fetal parameters, as would be expected in the clinical setting where euglycemia is a goal of therapy, reduce risk to the fetus.

Although the present authors were interested in the metabolic effects of insulin lispro in GDM women, the primary concern was safety, specifically the risk of hypoglycemia, hyperglycemia, and antibody production that might cause the insulin to cross the placenta to the fetal side. In the study, 42 GDM women were randomized to receive regular human insulin or insulin lispro prior to consuming a test meal.[17] Throughout the remainder of gestation, subjects received premeal insulin lispro or regular human insulin (with and without basal insulin), and performed blood glucose monitoring before and after each meal. During the test meal, the areas under the glucose curve (AUGC), and those for insulin and C-peptide levels, were significantly lower in the insulin lispro group. The incidence of postprandial hyperglycemia (>120 mg/dL) was significantly lower in the lispro group. Overall metabolic control also improved significantly in the insulin lispro group, which showed the greatest absolute decrease in A1C levels as compared to the regular human group. The reduction from baseline A1C concentrations at 6 weeks was statistically significant for the insulin lispro group but not for the regular human insulin group.[17] To determine the immunologic effects of insulin lispro compared with regular human insulin, three different types of antibodies were studied: (1) lispro-specific antibodies; (2) regularspecific antibodies; and (3) cross-reactive antibodies. Levels of all three antibodies were evaluated at the time of enrollment, 6 weeks after enrollment, at delivery (both in the maternal serum and the umbilical cord blood) and at the postpartum follow-up visit in maternal serum. No statistically significant differences were seen between the insulin lispro and regular human insulin groups.

Now there are several reports of the safety and efficacy of both insulin lispro and insulin aspart in pregnancy to confirm the results of the original report.[17–25] Insulin aspart has also been suited in a similar fashion as insulin lispro. Wyatt et al.[22] have reported that insulin aspart is not immunogenic, improved the area under the curve for the postprandial glucose excursion and facilitates term delivery of a healthy infant. In addition, the patient satisfaction was improved using insulin aspart compared to regular human insulin. Conclusions from these studies are that those women with GDM who are not optimally managed with diet and exercise need insulin therapy. Insulin lispro and insulin aspart cause fewer hypoglycemic events than human regular insulin and it attenuates a greater postprandial response than regular human insulin. Furthermore, the antibody levels are not increased over those seen with regular human insulin, and therefore insulin lispro and insulin aspart may be considered a treatment option in patients with GDM.

Theoretical risks of the use of insulin analogs during pregnancy complicated by pre-gestational diabetes

Diamond and Kormas[28] first questioned the safety of using insulin lispro during pregnancy in 1997. They reported on two patients who used insulin lispro during pregnancies and deliveries. One of these pregnancies was terminated at 20 weeks gestation and the second pregnancy resulted in a seemingly healthy infant after an elective Cesarean delivery, but who subsequently died unexpectedly 3 weeks later. Both infants were discovered to have congenital abnormalities, which led the authors to question whether insulin lispro might have teratogenic effects on the fetus, in which case it should not be used during pregnancy. The report cites concerns about insulin lispro use during pregnancy, yet it does not provide conclusive evidence that insulin lispro was responsible for the malformations of the infants mentioned. In fact, there is sufficient reason to doubt that insulin lispro was to blame, since these isolated case reports were not part of a study and there was no control group. Therefore, the findings should stimulate initiation of clinical trials testing the safety of insulin lispro during pregnancy and not be taken as evidence that it is unsafe. Despite the opinion of Diamond and Kormas[28] that poor glycemic control was not responsible for the abnormalities of the infants in the cases described above, there is insufficient evidence to support this claim. The letter reports that A1C levels were determined every 3 months and that both women had values <7% at each test. However, an A1C of 7% may be associated with an increased risk of fetal malformations. Since organogenesis is complete within the first 7 weeks of pregnancy,[29] and women tend to improve their glycemic control as the pregnancy progresses, an A1C measured at 3 months of pregnancy is a poor reflection of the mother's blood glucose levels at conception and during the critical first organogenic weeks of pregnancy.

The report also indicated that both women maintained a mean blood glucose level of <108 mg/dL. A pregnant woman's target blood glucose should be <90 mg/dL fasting and <120 mg/dL postprandially.[29] If the women measured their fasting blood glucose only, the reported mean is obviously too high. If postprandial measurements were also taken into account, the mean is still too high, although less so. These women would be categorized as being at high risk for bearing infants with malformations. Throughout pregnancy, the second mother was being treated for hypertension and if the malformations were due to a medication it is perhaps unfair to single out insulin lispro. In spite of the medication used, the malformations reported are more indicative of poor glycemic control: situs inversus, one of the abnormalities in the first infant, occurs almost exclusively in children of diabetic mothers.[30,31] During the initial clinical trials testing insulin lispro, pregnant women were excluded.

However, some participants became pregnant unexpectedly during the trials and 19 infants were born by these mothers who were using insulin lispro. Of these births, one child had a right dysplastic kidney but the other 18 were healthy.[32]

Now there is a report that shows that insulin lispro is not teratogenic. Wyatt et al.[22] report has shown that insulin lispro is not associated with increased malformations. This report clearly showed that the 27 malformations that occurred in this data set of 500 exposed pregnancies only occurred in women whose A1C levels were greater than 2 standard deviations above the mean of normal. There were no malformations in the sample of women whose A1C levels were within 2 standard deviations of normal. Thus the null hypothesis has been proven: insulin lispro does not by itself cause malformations. Malformations are only associated with hyperglycemia in the first trimester. Mathiesen et al.[23] have now reported that insulin aspart is safe and efficacious in pregnancy with no increase in malformation rate.

Possible effects of rapid-acting insulin analogs on the mother

There are three situations in life in which rapid normalization of blood glucose levels increase the risk for deterioration of diabetic retinopathy: puberty, pregnancy, and rapid normalization of blood glucose levels. If two of these events occur in the same patient, the risk for retinopathy progression is potentiated.[33,34] All three situations are associated with increased serum concentrations of growth-promoting factors.[33] It is hypothesized that when the blood glucose level is rapidly decreased, there is increased retinal extravasation of serum proteins. If there is a concomitant increase in the concentration of serum growth-promoting factors, a predisposed retina may deteriorate. Pregnancy *per se* is the most frequently reported situation in which rapid normalization of blood glucose is associated with deterioration of retinal status. Normal pregnancy is associated with high concentrations of many growth-promoting factors.[35–40] Hill et al.[37] reported that a potent mitogen and angiogenic factor normally absent from the adult circulation become detectable by 14 weeks of gestation and is maximal at 22–32 weeks of gestational. A placental growth hormone variant had been found to increase throughout pregnancy, along with hCS and prolactin.[38]

Production of maternal insulin-like growth factor (IGF)-I has also been shown to increase significantly above nonpregnant levels.[34] It is well known that diabetes mellitus is associated with perturbations of growth hormone IFG-I in cases of poor metabolic control.[37] Kitzmiller et al.[41] have suggested that treatment with insulin lispro during pregnancies complicated by diabetes may be associated with acceleration of diabetic retinopathy. If treatment with lispro insulin did play a role in the rapid deterioration of retinopathy in the case reports, it most likely was not mediated by IFG-I activity of lispro. Human insulin binds to the IFG-I receptor with an affinity of 0.1–0.2% that of IFG-I. A comparison of insulin lispro and human insulin was made to determine the relative IFG-I receptor binding affinity in human placenta membranes, skeletal muscle, smooth muscle cells, and mammary epithelial cells. Insulin lispro had a slightly higher affinity for the human placenta membranes when compared with human insulin (1.3 times greater than human insulin). No other differences were observed in any other cell lines. Despite the suggested increased affinity, it should be noted that the absolute affinity for the IFG-I receptor is extremely low for both insulin lispro and human insulin. Concentrations >1000 times above the normal physiologic range are needed to reach 50% receptor binding. IFG-I is a much larger protein chain than insulin and there is a 49% homology between human insulin and IFG-I. The reversal of the B28 and B29 amino aids in insulin lispro increases this homology to 51%, because of the analogous position in the IGF molecule. It has been shown that insulin lispro has the same affinity for the IFG-I receptor as does human insulin; also, the dissociation kinetics of insulin lispro on the insulin receptor are identical to those of insulin, indicating that insulin lispro should have no excess mitogenic effect via either the IFG-I or the insulin receptor.[42,43] Patients in the Kitzmiller reports[41] all had elevated levels of IFG-I due to poor control of their diabetes and due to pregnancy *per se*, independent of the possible IFG-I activity of lispro. However, anecdotal cases should never be used to infer a cause–effect relationship. In controlled clinical trials of >2000 patients with insulin lispro, no significant differences in retinopathy were observed, but there were no pregnant women in this trial.[15]

The factors that emerge as the independent risk factors for retinopathy progression include: elevated A1C at baseline, duration of diabetes, significant proteinuria (>300 mg/24 h), pregnancy and rapid normalization of blood glucose (in <14 weeks). In fact, the strongest risk factor for retinopathy progression, independent of baseline retinal status, is baseline elevation of A1C associated with a rapid decline to normal. Of 14 patients who were treated with insulin lispro during pregnancy, described by Kitzmiller et al.,[41] 11 had risk factors, including evidence of baseline retinopathy, which have been associated with progression to proliferative retinopathy during pregnancy. Therefore we can learn the fact that if there is no retinopathy during the first trimester of a pregnancy complicated by diabetes, progression to proliferative retinopathy needing laser therapy is rare, however, many of the cited references above emphasize that baseline elevation of glucose associated with rapid normalization can accelerate retinopathy. Phelps et al.[44] clearly showed that deterioration of retinopathy correlated significantly with the levels of plasma glucose at entry and with the magnitude of improvement in glycemia during the first 6–14 weeks after entry. Although the 13 patients with no retinopathy at baseline did not progress to proliferative retinopathy, one did develop moderate hemorrhages, exudates and intraretinal microaneurysms (IRMA). Of their 20 patients with initial background retinopathy, two progressed to proliferative retinopathy. Laatikainen et al.[45] confirmed that the decrease in A1C levels was most rapid in the

two patients with the worst progression. They concluded that a rapid near normalization of glycemic control during pregnancy could accelerate the progression of retinopathy in poorly controlled diabetic patients. The DIEP Study[34] reported that the 10.3% of diabetic women who progressed, despite no retinopathy at baseline, had an initial A1C elevation of 4 standard deviations (SD) above the mean of a normal population (risk progression 40%, odds ratio (OR) 2.4). Independent of retinal status, the DIEP study also reported that duration of diabetes increased the risk of progression such that after 6 years duration of diabetes the OR was 3.0, by 11–15 years it was 9.7 and >16 years it was 15.0, but hyperglycemia was a stronger risk factor. Additional evidence has been reported by the Diabetes Control and Complications Trial (DCCT).[46] In the conventional care group who became pregnant ($n = 135$), and thus had immediate intensification of glucose control, 47% worsened their retinal status and the OR for progression by the second trimester was 2.6 compared to diabetic women in the conventional group who did not become pregnant. In order to compare the A1C levels reported by the DCCT trial[43] to other published reports, the approximate equivalent baseline A1C levels, using the DCCT normal range, is 7.1, 9.8, and 9.5%, respectively. In addition, the rate of fall of the A1C level in the three case reports was faster than the reported rate of fall associated with deterioration of retinal status.

There is one case report in the literature which clearly shows that the combination of pregnancy and rapid normalization of severe hyperglycemia is sufficient to 'explode' a previously normal retina. Hagay et al.[47] reported a case of a woman with no previously documented hyperglycemia who presented at 8 weeks of gestation with an HbA1C level of 16% and her ophthalmic examination was reported to be 'completely normal'. She was treated with intensive insulin therapy and at 12 weeks her A1C level was 5.9%. By the second trimester she had severe bilateral proliferative diabetic retinopathy needing photocoagulation. In a report by Omori et al.[48] studying Japanese pregnant diabetic women, the prevalence of retinopathy was 34.4% in their Type 2 diabetic population. In addition, the prevalence of proliferative retinopathy was as high in the Type 2 women as in the Type 1 pregnant women, despite the shorter duration of documented diabetes in their Type 2 patients. Need for photocoagulation occurred in 50% of their Type 2 pregnant diabetic women patients with greater than background retinopathy at the beginning of pregnancy.

If insulin lispro did play a role in the progression of retinopathy, it is more likely that the insulin lispro facilitated the rapid normalization of the blood glucose levels. In pregnant diabetic patients, it has been shown that insulin lispro improves glucose control and thus significantly lowers the A1C level compared to patients who are administered human regular insulin.[17,22]

There is danger in normalizing blood glucose quickly, regardless of the type of insulin used, in pregnant women with a long duration of diabetes and elevated A1C levels in the first trimester, in those with proteinuria and perhaps those with Type 1 diabetes. To date there have not been extensive clinical trials on the retinal status of women treated with insulin aspart (or any other insulin analog) in pregnancy. Thus we await clinical trials of the use of all of the insulin analogs in pregnancy to make a decision about the role of analogs in the progression of retinopathy during pregnancy. Busy clinics may have a decreased ability to examine retinae thoroughly. Mild background retinopathy may be missed, even in the best of settings. Any retinopathy increases the risk, especially if the blood glucose level is elevated. Rather than recommending angiography to all women before each pregnancy is planned, in the case of no retinopathy seen on retinal examination, it is prudent to improve the glucose control slowly. These case reports reinforce the need to intensify pre-conceptional care programs to allow the luxury of slowly normalizing the blood glucose and to plan the pregnancy only after the blood glucose levels have been stabilized in the normal range for at least 6 months.[46–48] If a patient presents pregnant, with high A1C levels, regardless of the retinal status, as suggested by these cases, then a retinal specialist needs to be on the team, be vigilant and treat any developing angiopathy while the blood glucose is normalized.

If an insulin analog was available that was not immunogenic and had the rapid action of insulin lispro but had less IFG-I activity than human insulin, then even if there was no proof that the IFG-I activity of the insulin plays a role in the acceleration of diabetic retinopathy when the blood glucose level is normalized quickly, such an insulin would become the treatment of choice. Insulin aspart, an insulin analog that has been shown to produce a peak blood level at 40 min and lowers postprandial glucose levels significantly better than human insulin, has only 69% the IFG-I activity of human insulin.

Long-acting insulin analogs have only recently been used in clinical practice.[49] The first clinically available long-acting insulin analog is insulin glargine. Insulin glargine has a glycine substitution in the alpha chain at the 21 position and two glargines attached to the beta chain terminal at position 30. It is soluble insulin and has been shown to provide peakless, sustained and predictable 24 h action. Of note, insulin glargine has a 6-fold increase in IFG-I activity as compared to human insulin. There are no clinical trials using insulin glargine in pregnancy, nor are there reports of the retinal status in any of the 32 women in the previously published case reports of the use of glargine in pregnancy.[24–27] However, a recent paper[27] describing 118 women treated with glargine during pregnancy showed that the macrosomia rate was increased 4-fold over that reported using human insulins. Of note, insulin glargine has a 6-fold increase in IFG-I activity as compared to human insulin. Another insulin analog that is currently in clinical trials is insulin detemir. Here again there are no trials using this insulin in pregnancy, but the studies show that detemir has the same IFG-I activity as human insulin.[27]

The clinician has to keep in mind that the most important concern is to safely normalize the maternal blood glucose. Before 1985, impure animal insulin was used, with a result that the IgG antibody levels rose the longer the women were treated. After 20 years of diabetes, women had antibody levels >10,000. Purified human insulin has been available for >20 years, so there is a new generation of Type 1 diabetic women who have never been treated with animal insulins, and

thus have negligible antibodies. Before giving these women insulin analogs it must be proved that: (1) they do not cause an immunologic response; (2) they do not cross the placenta; (3) they do not increase the risk of congenital anomalies or spontaneous abortions; and (4) they do not significantly increase the serum IFG-I levels or accelerate diabetic retinopathy.

Definition of normoglycemia based on infant outcome

Previously, glucose control and targets for treatment were based on clinical judgment and concern for hypoglycemia. In fact, most clinicians preferred to maintain hyperglycemia rather than increase the risk of a hypoglycemic reaction. As tools and techniques improved to achieve near-normal glucose levels during pregnancy, the emphasis has changed to strive for the degree of maternal metabolic control that is associated with normal body size and proportions in full-term infants.

Mello et al.[50] published a study in which they investigated the anthropomorphic characteristics of 98 full-term singleton infants born to 98 women with Type 1 diabetes. They reported that those women who had a mean daily blood glucose level <95 mg/dL had normal infants, whereas the women with mean blood glucose levels >95 mg/dL delivered infants with an increased prevalence of being large for gestational age, with a significantly greater ponderal index and thoracic circumference with respect to the control group. Others have confirmed that overall mean glucose levels of <95 mg/dL can avoid alterations in fetal growth.[5]

Jovanovic et al.[51] studied 52 Type 1 diabetic women and found that when the mean blood glucose was maintained between 80 and 84 mg/dL, the outcome of pregnancy was normal. Langer et al.[52] assessed the relationship between optimal levels of glycemic control and perinatal outcome in a prospective study of 334 GDM women and found that when the mean glucose levels were <86 mg/dL, this group had a significantly higher prevalence of small-for-gestational age infants. In contrast, when the mean glucose levels were >105 mg/dL, there was a 20% prevalence of large-for-gestational-age infants.

Hellmuth et al.[53] found that the frequency of hypoglycemia, especially nocturnal hypoglycemia, was seen with a prevalence of 37% in the first trimester of pregnancies treated with intensified insulin therapy. Sacks et al.[53] studied 48 Type 1 and 113 Type 2 diabetic women during pregnancy. They found that the mean glucose levels were higher in the Type 1 patients and at least one daily glucose level was <50 mg/dL during 19% of observational days compared to only 2% of days in the Type 2 group.

Rosenn et al.[54] and Rosenn and Miodovnik[55] published papers on the topic of the increased risk of hypoglycemia during pregnancies complicated by diabetes. They found that at least 40% of mothers reported hypoglycemia during pregnancy. Clinically significant hypoglycemia requiring assistance from another person occurred in 71% of the 84 women studied, with a peak incidence occurring between 10 and 15 weeks of gestation. They did not observe any increase in embryopathy.

Jovanovic et al.[56] then published the first trimester insulin requirements of women studied in the DIEP Study. They showed that there was a drop in insulin requirements during weeks 8–11 of gestation, which was seen in all Type 1 diabetic women whose glucose concentrations were insensitively managed. The majority of decreases in the insulin requirement were seen in the overnight period. It was concluded that the insulin doses needed to be decreased for the overnight insulin requirement to prevent nocturnal hypoglycemia during the late first trimester.

Insulin requirements

Type 1 diabetic women must increase their insulin dosage to compensate for the diabetogenic forces of normal pregnancy. However, the exact pattern of insulin dosage increase is still controversial. Many observers have detected a decline in insulin requirement late in the first trimester of diabetic pregnancies. Jorgen Pedersen, the father of the study of diabetes in pregnancy, was among the first to observe that first trimester hypoglycemia was a symptom of pregnancy and that it was common knowledge among the physicians of the day. Pedersen wrote,

> Those physicians who manage diabetic women should be particularly alert for hypoglycemia in women who have recently become pregnant. About the 10th week of gestation there is an improvement in glucose tolerance manifesting itself as insulin coma, milder insulin reaction or an improvement in the degree of compensation. When a reduction in insulin dosage is called for it amounts to an average of 34%.

Indeed, he even claimed, Once in a while pregnancy may be diagnosed on account of inexplicable hypoglycemic attacks.' In a total of 26 cases of insulin coma collected, all of the cases in his series occurred in months 1–4 of gestation, with the majority occurring at months 2–3. He also noted that by late gestation, regardless of the metabolic control and duration of diabetes, average daily insulin requirements increased 2-fold from earlier in pregnancy.

Early first trimester over-insulinization might explain a later first trimester drop in insulin requirement. One example of this effect may be the significantly greater weight gain seen in the first trimester by diabetic women compared to healthy nondiabetic women. Perhaps the drive to increase caloric intake to prevent hypoglycemia in the first trimester may have been the cause of the first trimester excessive weight gain in the diabetic women compared to the controls. On the other hand, others have not seen the first trimester decrease in insulin requirement.

There are also reports of rising insulin requirement in the first trimester. The present authors have described the insulin requirements during pregnancy of a population of well-controlled Type 1 diabetic women which possibly lends credence to the notion that first trimester over-insulinization may be the cause of the hypoglycemia seen by some workers in the first trimester. In addition, together with the DIEP Study

Group, the present authors have analyzed the insu ment and sub-stratified based on degree of glu in the first trimester.[56] The weekly insulin (as units/kg/day) were examined in the first tri betic women in the DIEP Study with accurate gestationa dating, regular glucose monitoring, daily insulin dose recording and monthly A1C measurements. In pregnancies that resulted in live-born, term, singleton infants, a significant increase in mean weekly dosage was observed in weeks 3–7 ($P < 0.001$), followed by a significant decline in weeks 8–15 ($P < 0.001$). The Friedman nonparametric test localized significant changes to the interval between weeks 7–8 and weeks 11–12. To determine if prior poor glucose control exaggerated these trends, the women were divided based on their A1C values: <2 SD above the mean of a normal population (group 1), 2–4 SD (group 2), and >4 SD (group 3) at baseline. Late first trimester declines in dosage were statistically significant in group 2 ($P = 0.002$) and in groups 2 and 3 together ($P = 0.003$). Similarly, women with body mass index (BMI) >27.0 had a greater initial insulin rise and then fall compared to leaner women. Observations in the DIEP Study cohort disclosed a mid-first trimester decline in insulin requirement in insulin-dependent, diabetic pregnant women. Possible explanations include over-insulinization of previously poorly controlled diabetes and a transient decline in progesterone during the late first trimester luteo-placental shift in progesterone production.

Clinicians should anticipate a reduction in insulin requirement in the 4-week interval between weeks 8 and 12 of gestation. Based on these studies of well-controlled diabetic women, an algorithm for care and an insulin requirement protocol has been created, based on gestational week and the woman's current pregnant body weight. The total daily dose of insulin in the first trimester (weeks 5–12) insulin requirement is 0.7 unit/kg/day; in the second trimester (weeks 12–26) the insulin requirement is 0.8 unit/kg/day; in the third trimester (weeks 26–36) the insulin requirement is 0.9 unit/kg/day; and at term (weeks 36–40) the insulin requirement is 1.0 unit/kg/day (Table 27.1). The insulin needs to be divided throughout the day to provide the basal need (the dose of insulin that keeps a woman normal in the fasting state) and meal-related need. When multiple insulin injections are used to provide the basal need, NPH insulin is preferred because it has a more predictable absorption pattern than lente or Ultralente insulin. Also, the recently developed long-acting insulin analogs (insulin glargine or insulin determir) have not yet been proven to be safe or efficacious in pregnancy. Preferred use of NPH is to give one sixth of the total daily dose of insulin (I) as morning, dinner and bedtime injections (i.e. NPH dose equals 50% of daily dose divided into three equal injections of NPH given every 8 h, or at 8 am, 4 pm, and 12 midnight; Table 27.1).

The other half of the total daily insulin dose should be a rapid-acting insulin (insulin lispro or insulin aspart) given before each meal to control postprandial glycemia (Table 27.1). This dose of rapid-acting insulin can be given using the insulin infusion pump or by multiple doses of subcutaneously injected insulin (Tables 27.1, 27.2, and 27.3). The meal-related insulin dose (one half of the total daily insulin requirement (0.5I)) (Table 27.1). The exact division of this meal-related insulin dose depends on the size of the woman's lunch versus her dinner.

Table 27.1   Insulin dosage regimen for diabetic pregnancy

1. Pregnancy NPH plus rapid-acting insulin schedule   Patient weight in kg =   Date & Time:
"Big I" = total daily units of insulin
Circle One: Gestational weeks = 0–12   13–28   29–34   35–40   OTHER
                              k = 0.7   0.8   0.9   1.0
Calculate desired units of insulin from above line.
        "Big I" = _____ (k units × weight kg)/24 hours
        "Big I" = Basal insulin requirement + Bolus (meal-related) insulin requirement
        Basal = ½ "Big I," Bolus = ½ "Big I"
        Basal: Divide so that ⅙ of "Big I" is NPH given before breakfast, ⅙ of "Big I" is NPH given before dinner, and ⅙ of "Big I" is NPH given before bedtime.
        Bolus: Divide so that ⅙ of "Big I" is rapid-acting insulin given before breakfast, ⅙ of "Big I" is rapid-acting insulin given before lunch, and ⅙ of "Big I" is rapid-acting insulin given before dinner. The rapid-acting insulin is then titrated based on the blood glucose.

        0800 Pre-breakfast: NPH = ⅙"Big I" = _____.
            Check yesterday's pre-dinner BS:
                If yesterday's pre-dinner BS <60, then decrease today's ₐₘ NPH by 2 units.
                If yesterday's pre-dinner BS 61–90, no change in today's ₐₘ NPH.
                If yesterday's pre-dinner BS >91, then increase today's ₐₘ NPH by 2 units.

Do not feed the patient until the blood sugar is below 120 mg/dL.	Rapid-acting insulin = ⅙ "Big I" = _____ to be adjusted according to the following scale: Pre-breakfast BS <60 = _____ = (⅙ "Big I" dose) – 3% of the "Big I." 61–90 = _____ = ⅙ "Big I" dose. 91–120 = _____ = (⅙ "Big I" dose) + 3% of the "Big I." >121 = _____ = (⅙ "Big I" dose) + 6% of the "Big I." If today's BS 1 hour after breakfast is <110, then decrease tomorrow's pre-breakfast rapid insulin by 2 units. If today's BS 1 hour after breakfast is 111–120, no change in tomorrow's pre-breakfast rapid insulin. If today's BS 1 hour after breakfast is >121, then increase tomorrow's pre-breakfast rapid insulin by 2 units.

        1200 Pre-lunch: Rapid-acting insulin is ⅙ "Big I" = _____ to be adjusted according to the following scale:

Do not feed the patient until the blood sugar is below 120 mg/dL.	Pre-lunch BS <60 = _____ = (⅙ "Big I" dose) – 3% of "Big I." 61–90 = _____ = ⅙ "Big I" dose 91–120 = _____ = (⅙ "Big I" dose) + 3% of "Big I." >121 = _____ = (⅙ "Big I" dose) + 6% of "Big I." If today's BS 1 hour after lunch is <110, then decrease tomorrow's pre-breakfast rapid insulin by 2 units. If today's BS 1 hour after lunch is 111–120, no change in tomorrow's pre-breakfast rapid insulin. If today's BS 1 hour after lunch is >121, then increase tomorrow's pre-breakfast rapid insulin by 2 units.

        1700 Pre-dinner: NPH = ⅙"Big I" = _____.
            Rapid-acting insulin is ⅙ "Big I" = _____ to be adjusted according to the following scale:
            If yesterday's pre-bedtime BS <60, then decrease today's dinner NPH by 2 units.
            If yesterday's pre-bedtime BS 61–90, no change in today's dinner NPH.
            If yesterday's pre-bedtime BS >91, then increase today's dinner NPH by 2 units.

Do not feed the patient until the blood sugar is Below 120 mg/dL.	Pre-dinner BS <60 = _____ = (⅙ "Big I" dose) – 3% of "Big I." 61–90 = _____ = ⅙ "Big I" dose 91–120 = _____ = (⅙ "Big I" dose) + 3% of "Big I." >121 = _____ = (⅙ "Big I" dose) + 6% of "Big I." If today's BS 1 hour after dinner is <110, then decrease tomorrow's dinner rapid insulin by 2 units. If today's BS 1 hour after dinner is 111–120, no change in tomorrow's dinner rapid insulin. If today's BS 1 hour after dinner is >121, then increase tomorrow's dinner rapid insulin by 2 units.

        2400 Bedtime NPH: Give ⅙ "Big I" = _____.
            If today's pre-breakfast BS is <60, then decrease today's bedtime NPH by 2 units.
            If today's pre-breakfast BS is 61–90, no change in today's bedtime NPH.
            If today's pre-breakfast BS is >91, then check the 3 ₐₘ BS and, if it is <70 (regardless of today's pre-breakfast BS), decrease today's bedtime NPH by 2 units.
            If today's pre-breakfast BS is >91, and the 3 ₐₘ BS >70, increase today's bedtime NPH by 2 units.
            Also, if the 3 ₐₘ BS is >91, then call the doctor for 3 ₐₘ rapid insulin scale equal to the pre-lunch rapid scale.

Compensatory doses to adjust for high or low glucose levels are calculated as 3% of the total daily insulin requirement. Clinicians should note that hyperglycemia would occur if the patient used only insulin lispro or insulin aspart for the meal-related needs, and if the woman goes a long time between meals. The dose of NPH insulin may not be sufficient to prevent an escape of the blood glucose before the next dose of insulin is given. To prevent this escape of blood glucose when >3 h elapses between injections of the rapid-acting insulin analogs of lispro or aspart, the patient should add 3% of her total daily insulin requirement as regular human insulin to the lispro injection to extend the effectiveness of the rapid-acting component.

Insulin infusion pumps

Insulin infusion pumps have been used for treatment for over two decades.[57] However, the data on the safety and efficacy of

Table 27.2   Basal insulin pump program (using human regular, insulin lispro or insulin aspart)

Period	Basal requirement (B*) (hourly infusion rate)	Rationale
Midnight to 4 am	50% less basal, (B/24 × 0.5)	Maternal cortisol at nadir
4 am to 10 am	50% more basal, (B/24 × 1.5)	Highest level of maternal cortisol
10 am to noon	Basal, (B/24)	

*B = 0.5I (the total daily insulin) or an hourly rate of B/24.
To refine basal settings, have the patient perform self-blood glucose monitoring at the end of each period to determine whether adjustments are needed. For instance, at the 4 am test, the blood glucose level should be 60–90 mg/dL; if blood glucose level is out of this range, dial up or down insulin in increments of 0.10 unit/h. (Consider using 0.1 unit/kg as NPH insulin at bedtime to prevent diabetic ketoacidosis secondary to needle slippage; then decrease the overnight basal from 4 am to 10 am by 0.02 unit/kg/h.)

insulin pumps during pregnancies complicated by diabetes are still in its infancy. Kitzmiller et al.[58] showed that insulin pump therapy did improve glucose control and minimized clinically significant hypoglycemic events to 2.2/week. Coustan et al.[59] then reported a randomized clinical trial of insulin pump therapy versus conventional therapy in pregnancies complicated by diabetes. They showed that there were no differences between the two treatment groups with respect to outpatients mean glucose levels, symptomatic hypoglycemia or HbA1C levels.

They concluded that excellent diabetes control can be achieved with both insulin infusion pumps and with multiple injections of insulin. Carta et al.[60] also performed a randomized trial of continuous subcutaneous insulin infusion versus intensive conventional insulin therapy in Type 1 and Type 2 diabetic pregnant women. They reported that there were not significant differences in mean insulin requirements at the different stages of gestation and that perinatal outcome was satisfactory in both groups, however, in their study, control of fetal growth was better with interfiled convention therapy compared to fetal growth in the pump group. Mancuso et al.[61] studied the efficacy of the insulin pump in the home treatment of pregnant diabetic women. They reported that that using the pump seven Type 1 diabetic women delivered term infants and had no macrosomia or neonatal problems along with normal glucose tolerance tests at two years of life.

Table 27.3   Pre-meal sliding scale dose calculation using rapid-acting insulin*

Pre-meal basal glucose (mg/dL)	Compensatory insulin
<60	Meal-related insulin dose minus 3% I
61–90	Meal-related insulin dose: no adjustment necessary
91–120	Meal-related insulin dose plus 3% I
121	Meal-related insulin dose plus 6% I

*Human regular insulin or insulin lispro or insulin aspart.
†Meal-related insulin is half the total daily insulin dose (I), such that 40% of the dose is at breakfast, 30% is at lunch and 30% is at dinner.

Potter et al.[57] studied continuous insulin infusion in the third trimester of eight pregnancies complicated by diabetes. Compared to historical controls, they concluded that diurnal variations of blood glucose concentrations were dampened. Leveno et al.[62] performed a case controlled trial of insulin pump therapy versus literature intensified conventional therapy, and observed no significant differences between the groups for glucose control, cost and complications. They concluded that insulin pumps were not acceptable to all pregnant diabetic women and that such therapy may not be necessary to improve pregnancy outcome. Caruso et al.[63] treated 12 poorly controlled pregnant diabetic women with insulin infusion pumps and showed that glucose levels could be quickly normalized with a remarkable decrease in variation of glucose excursions. In addition, they showed that amniotic fluid insulin, glucose and C-peptide levels were normal, and none of the infants were macrosomic or had any neonatal problems. They concluded that insulin infusion pump therapy was highly effective compared to intensified conventional treatment. In a nested case-controlled study, Simmons et al.[64] utilized insulin pumps in pregnancies complicated by Type 2 diabetes and GDM in a multiethnic community, and showed in 30 women that none experienced severe hypoglycemia and 79% had improved glycemic control within 1–4 weeks. Mothers using the pump had greater insulin requirements and greater weight gain. Although their infants were more likely to be admitted to the special care unit, they were not heavier nor did they have more hypoglycemic events than control subjects. Jensen et al.[65] reported their series using insulin infusion pump therapy (n = 11) in the pre-conception treatment period in Type 1 diabetic women compared to women treated with conventional therapy (n = 9). Two fetuses born of mothers treated with conventional therapy exhibited early group delay, whereas all 11 fetuses born of mothers treated with pump therapy were normal; there were no malformations in either group. Gabbe et al.[66] published a series of 24 Type 1 diabetic patients and reported no difference in the groups of women treated with pump compared with those treated with intensified insulin therapy for episodes of hypoglycemia, costs, complication, glycemic control or in pregnancy outcome. The advantages seen were all postpartum because those women who were on the pump into their postpartum period sustained better glucose control than those who were on intensified insulin therapy during pregnancy. The conclusion drawn from this review

Table 27.4   Review of the literature on using insulin infusion pump therapy in pregnancies complicated by diabetes

Author and year (reference)	No. on CSII*	Trimester or weeks gestation	Type of DM†	Type of trial/comments
Potter et al. 1980 (57)	8	Third	1	Longitudinal/improved
Kitzmiller et al. 1985 (58)	24	5–10	1	Longitudinal/no difference
Coustan et al. 1986 (59)	22	Second and third	1	Randomized/no difference
Carta et al. 1986 (60)	14	First	1	Case–control/improved
Mancuso et al. 1986 (61)	12	Third	1	Longitudinal/improved
Jensen et al. 1986 (65)	9	Before and all trimesters	1	Case–control
Caruso et al. 1987 (63)	12	Third	1	Longitudinal/improved
Leveno et al. 1988 (62)	11	Second and third	1	Self-selection/no difference
Gabbe et al. 2001 (66)	23	Second, third and postpartum	1	Only postpartum improved
Simmons et al. 2002 (64)	30	Second	GDM and 2‡	Equal

*Continuous subcutaneous insulin infusion.
†Diabetes mellitus.
‡Gestational diabetes mellitus.

of the literature on using insulin pump therapy in pregnant women with diabetes is that pump therapy is not necessary in order to achieve and maintain optimal control (27.4); however, five of the 10 papers suggest that insulin pump therapy has an advantage over intensified multiple injections of insulin. In addition, only 155 patients were reported in these 10 trials and in all but one paper the women had their pump therapy started in the second or third trimester (Table 27.4).

Insulin algorithms for continuous insulin infusion pump therapy in pregnancy

The basal need is usually 50% of the total daily insulin dose (0.5I) and may be delivered using a constant infusion pump (Table 27.2) or by multiple doses of intermediate-acting insulin (Table 27.1). When using a constant infusion pump the basal need is calculated as an hourly rate (Table 27.2) and is delivered such that the calculated rate (0.5I or total dose over 24 h divided by 24) is given between 10 am and midnight. The rate is cut in half (i.e. 0.5I divided by 24 times 0.5) from midnight to 4 am, and increased by another 50% (i.e. 0.5I divided by 24 times 1.5) to counteract the morning rise of cortisol levels that are potentiated during pregnancy. Also, low-dose NPH before bedtime has been used by some clinicians to prevent the possible occurrence of diabetic ketoacidosis if the needle slips out of position during the overnight period. This dose of NPH insulin needs to be sufficient to provide protection from ketosis, or 0.1 unit of NPH times the weight of the women in kilograms. Then the overnight basal insulin needs to be decreased to allow for the NPH dose. The 4 am to 10 am basal insulin should thus be adjusted downward by 0.02 unit/kg/h.

Insulin and glucose treatment during labor

With improvement in antenatal care, intra-partum events play an increasingly crucial role in the outcome of pregnancy.

The artificial beta cell may be used to maintain normoglycemia during labor and delivery, but normoglycemia can be maintained easily by subcutaneous injections. Before active labor, insulin is required, and glucose infusion is not necessary to maintain a blood glucose level of 70–90 mg/dL. With the onset of active labor, insulin requirements decrease to zero and glucose requirements are relatively constant at 2.5 mg/kg/min. From these data, a protocol for supplying the glucose needs of labor has been developed.[67]

The goal is to maintain the maternal plasma glucose between 70 and 90 mg/dL. In cases of the onset of active spontaneous labor, insulin is withheld and an intravenous (i.v.) dextrose infusion is begun at a rate of 2.55 mg/kg/min. If labor is latent, normal saline is usually sufficient to maintain normoglycemia until active labor begins, at which time dextrose is infused at 2.55 mg/kg/min. Blood glucose is then monitored hourly and if it is <60 mg/dL then the infusion rate is doubled for the subsequent hour. If the blood glucose rises to >120 mg/dL, 2–4 units of regular insulin are given i.v. each hour until the blood glucose level is 70–90 mg/dL. In the case of an elective Cesarean section, the bedtime dose of NPH insulin is repeated at 8 am on the day of surgery and every 8 h if the surgery is delayed. A dextrose infusion may be started if the plasma glucose level falls to <60 mg/dL, and 2–4 units of regular insulin given i.v. every hour if the blood glucose rises to >120 mg/dL.[67]

Insulin and glucose requirements postpartum

Maternal insulin requirements usually drop precipitously postpartum, possibly for 48–96 h. Insulin requirements should be recalculated at 0.6 unit/kg based on the postpartum weight and should be started when the 1 h postprandial plasma glucose value is >150 mg/dL or the fasting glucose level is >100 mg/dL. The postpartum caloric requirements are 25 kcal/kg/day, based on the postpartum weight. For women who wish to breast feed, the calculation is 27 kcal/kg/day and insulin requirements are 0.6 unit/kg/day. The insulin requirement during the night drops dramatically during lactation, owing to the glucose siphoning into the breast milk. Thus, the majority of the insulin requirement is needed during the daytime to cover the increased caloric needs of breast feeding. Normoglycemia should especially be prescribed for nursing diabetic women, because hyperglycemia elevates milk glucose levels.[68]

Conclusions

With the advent of tools and techniques to maintain normo-glycemia before, during, and between all pregnancies complicated by diabetes, infants of diabetic mothers now have the same chances of good health as those infants born to the nondiabetic woman. Animal and human studies clearly implicate glucose as the teratogen. These studies, and others, emphasize the need for pre-conception programs and the need for support systems to facilitate the maintenance of normoglycemia throughout pregnancy. The morbidity and subsequent development of the infant of the diabetic mother is associated with hyperglycemia. Therefore, the goal of insulin therapy is to achieve and maintain normo-glycemia before, during and after all pregnancies complicated by diabetes.

REFERENCES

1. Pedersen J. Course of diabetes during pregnancy. Acta Endocr 1952; 9: 342–7.
2. Mills JL, Knopp RH, Simpson JL, et al. Lack of relation of increased malformation rates in infants of diabetic mothers to glycemic control during organogenesis. N Engl J Med 1988; 318: 671–6.
3. Mills JL, Simpson JL, Driscoll SG, et al. Incidence of spontaneous abortion among normal women and insulin-dependent diabetic women whose pregnancies were identified within 21 days of conception. N Engl J Med 1988; 319: 1617–23.
4. Mills JL, Fishl AR, Knopp RH, et al. Malformations in infants of diabetic mothers: problems in study design. Prev Med 1983; 12: 274–86.
5. Jovanovic L, Peterson CM, Saxena BB, et al. Feasibility of maintaining normal glucose profiles in insulin-dependent pregnant diabetic women. Am J Med 1980; 68: 105–12.
6. DeVeciana M, Major CA, Morgan MA, et al. Postprandial versus preprandial blood glucose monitoring in women with gestational diabetes mellitus requiring insulin therapy. N Engl J Med 1995; 333: 1237–41.
7. Combs CA, Gunderson E, Kitzmiller JL, et al. Relationship of fetal macrosomia to maternal postprandial glucose control during pregnancy. Diabetes Care 1992; 15: 1251–7.
8. Jovanovic L, Peterson CM, Reed GF, et al. Maternal postprandial glucose levels and infant birth weight: the Diabetes In Early Pregnancy Study. Am J Obstet Gynecol 1991; 164: 103–11.
9. Jovanovic L. What is so bad about a big baby? [Editorial]. Diabetes Care 2001; 24: 1317–8.
10. Knopp RH. Hormone mediated changes in nutrient metabolism in pregnancy: a physiological basis for normal fetal development. In: Jacobsen MS, Rees JM, Golden NH, Irwin CE, eds. Adolescent Nutritional Disorders: Prevention and Treatment. New York: New York Academy of Sciences; 1997; pp. 251–71.
11. Knight G, Worth RC, Ward JD. Macrosomia despite well-controlled diabetic pregnancy. Lancet 1983; 2: 1431.
12. Visser GHA, van Ballegooie E, Slutter WJ. Macrosomia despite well-controlled diabetic pregnancy. Lancet 1984; 1: 284–5.
13. Menon RK, Cohen RM, Sperling MA, et al. Transplacental passage of insulin in pregnant women with insulin-dependent diabetes mellitus. Its role in fetal macrosomia. N Engl J Med 1990; 323: 309–15.
14. Jovanovic L, Kitzmiller JL, Peterson CM. Randomized trial of human versus animal species insulin in diabetic pregnant women: improved glycemic control, not fewer antibodies to insulin, influences birth weight. Am J Obstet Gynecol 1992; 167: 1325–30.
15. Anderson Jr. JH, Brunelle RL, Koivisto VA, et al. Reduction of postprandial hyperglycemia and frequency of hypoglycemia in IDDM patients on insulin-analog treatment. Diabetes 1997; 46: 265–70.
16. Fineberg SE, Rathbun MJ, Hufferd S, et al. Immunologic aspects of human proinsulin therapy. Diabetes 1988; 37: 276–80.
17. Jovanovic L, Ilic S, Pettitt DJ, et al. The metabolic and immunologic effects of insulin lispro in gestational diabetes. Diabetes Care 1999; 22: 1422–6.
18. Fineberg NS, Fineberg SE, Anderson JH, et al. Immunologic effects of insulin lispro [Lys(B23), Pro (B29)] human insulin in IDDM and NIDDM patients previously treated with insulin. Diabetes 1996; 45: 1750–4.
19. Jehle PM, Fussgaenger RD, Kunze U, et al. The human insulin analog insulin lispro improves insulin binding on circulating monocytes of intensively treated insulin dependent diabetes mellitus patients. J Clin Endocr Metab 1996; 81: 2319–27.
20. Jehle PM, Fussgaenger RD, Seibold A, et al. Pharmacodynamics of insulin lispro in 2 patients with type II diabetes mellitus. Int J Clin Pharmacol Ther 1996; 34: 498–503.
21. Balsells M, Corcoy R, Mauricio D, et al. Insulin antibody response to a short course of human insulin therapy in women with gestational diabetes. Diabetes Care 1997; 20: 1172–5.
22. Wyatt JW, Frias JL, Hoyme HE, et al., IONS Study Group. Congenital anomaly rate in offspring of mothers with diabetes treated with insulin lispro during pregnancy. Diabet Med 2005; 22: 803–7.
23. Mathiesen ER, Kinsley B, Amiel SA, et al., Insulin Aspart Pregnancy Study Group. Maternal glycemic control and hypoglycemia in type 1 diabetic pregnancy: a randomized trial of insulin aspart versus human insulin in 322 pregnant women. Diabetes Care 2007; 30: 771–6.
24. Holstein A, Plaschke A, Egberts EH. Use of insulin glargine during embryogenesis in a pregnant woman with type 1 diabetes. Diabet Med 2003; 20: 779–80.
25. Devlin JT, Hothersall L, Wilkis JL. Use of insulin glargine during pregnancy in a type 1 diabetic woman. Diabetes Care 2002; 25: 1095–6.
26. Dolci M, Mori M, Baccetti F. Use of glargine insulin before and during pregnancy in a woman with type 1 diabetes and Addison's disease. Diabetes Care 2005; 28: 2084–5.
27. Price N, Bartlett C, Gillmer M. Use of insulin glargine during pregnancy: a case–control pilot study. Br J Obstet Gynecol 2007; 114: 453–7. E-pub 25 January 2007.
28. Diamond T, Kormas N. Possible adverse fetal effects of insulin lispro. N Engl J Med 1997; 337: 1009.
29. Mills JL, Baker L, Goldman A. Malformations in infants of diabetic mothers occur before the seventh gestational week: implications for treatment. Diabetes 1979; 23: 292.
30. Jovanovic L. Role of diet and insulin treatment of diabetes in pregnancy. Clin Obstet Gynecol 2000; 43: 46–51.
31. Kucera J. Rate and type of congenital anomalies among offspring of diabetic mothers. J Reprod Med 1971; 7: 61–4.
32. Anderson J, Bastyr E, Wishner K. Response to Diamond and Kormas. N Engl J Med 1997; 337: 1009–12.
33. Jovanovic L. Retinopathy risk: what is responsible? Hormones, hyperglycemia, or humolog? Diabetes Care 199; 22: 846–50.
34. Chew EY, Mills JL, Metzger BE, et al., National Institute of Child Health and Human Development. Metabolic control and progression of retinopathy: The Diabetes in Early Pregnancy Study. Diabetes Care 1995; 18: 631–7.
35. Merimee TJ, Zapf J, Froesch ER. Insulin-like growth factors: studies in diabetics with and without retinopathy. N Engl J Med 1983; 309: 527–31.
36. Larinkari J, Laatikainen L, Ranta T. Metabolic control and serum hormone levels in relationship to retinopathy in diabetic pregnancy. Diabetologia 1982; 22: 327–31.
37. Hill DJ, Clemmons DR, Riley SC, et al. Immunohistochemical localization of insulin like growth factors and IGF binding proteins-1, -2, and -3 in human placenta and fetal membranes. Placenta 1993; 14: 1–12.
38. MacLeod JN, Worsley I, Ray Y, et al. Human growth hormone variant is a biologically active somatogen and lactogen. Endocrinology 1991; 128: 1298–302.
39. Gluckman PD. The endocrine regulation of fetal growth in late gestation: the role of insulin-like growth factors. J Clin Endocr Metab 1995; 80: 1047–50.
40. Holly JMP, Amiel SA, Sandhu RR, et al. The role of growth hormone in diabetes mellitus. J Endocr 1988; 118: 353–64.

41. Kitzmiller J, Main E, Ward B, et al. Insulin lispro and the development of proliferative diabetic retinopathy during pregnancy. Diabetes Care 1999; 22: 874.

42. DiMarchi RD, Chance RE, Long HB, et al. Preparation of an insulin with improved pharmacokinetics relative to human insulin through consideration of structural homology with insulin-like growth factor-1. Horm Res 1994; 41(suppl. 2): 93–6.

43. Llewelyn J, Slieker LJ, Zimmermann JL. Pre-clinical studies on insulin lispro. Drugs Today 1998; 34(suppl. C): 11–21.

44. Phelps RL, Sakol L, Metzger BE, et al. Changes in diabetic retinopathy during pregnancy: correlations with regulation of hyperglycemia. Arch Ophthalmol 1986; 104: 1806–10.

45. Laatikainen L, Teramo K, Hieta-Heikurainen H, et al. A controlled study of the influence of continuous subcutaneous insulin infusion treatment on diabetic retinopathy during pregnancy. Acta Med Scand 1987; 221: 367–76.

46. Lachin J, Clearly P, and the DCCT Research Group. Pregnancy increases the risk of complication in the DCCT. Diabetes 1998; 47(suppl. 1): 1091.

47. Hagay ZJ, Schachter M, Pollack A, Ley R. Development of proliferative retinopathy in a gestational diabetes patient following rapid metabolic control [Case report]. Eur J Obstet Gynecol Reprod Biol 1994; 57: 211–3.

48. Omori Y, Minei S, Tamaki T, et al. Current status of pregnancy in diabetic women. A comparison of pregnancy in IDDM and NIDDM mothers. Diabetes Res Clin Pract 1994; 24: S273–8.

49. Trujillo A. Insulin analogs in pregnancy. Diabetes Spectrum, April, 2007.

50. Mello G, Paretti E, Mecacci F, et al. What degree of maternal metabolic control in women with type 1 diabetes is associated with normal body size and proportions in full-term infants? Diabetes Care 2000; 23: 1494–8.

51. Jovanovic L, Druzin M, Peterson CM. Effect of euglycemia on the outcome of pregnancy in insulin-dependent diabetic women as compared with normal control subjects. Am J Med 1981; 71: 921–7.

52. Langer O, Levy J, Brustman L, Anyaegbunam A, Merkatz R, Divon M. Glycemic control in gestational diabetes mellitus. How tight is tight enough: small for gestational age versus large for gestational age? Am J Obstet Gynecol.1989 Sep; 161(3):646–53.

53. Hellmuth E, Damm P, Molsted-Pedersen L, Bendtson I. Prevalence of nocturnal hypoglycemia in the first trimester of pregnancy in patients with insulin treated diabetes mellitus. Acta Obste Gynecol Scand 2000; 79: 3–5.

54. Rosenn BM, Miodovnik M, Holcberg G, et al. Hypoglycemia: the price of intensified insulin therapy for pregnant women with insulin-dependent diabetes mellitus. Obstet Gynecol 1995; 85: 417–22.

55. Rosenn BM, Miodovnik M. Glycemic control in the diabetic pregnancy: is tighter always better? J Matern Fetal Med 2000; 9: 29–34.

56. Jovanovic L, Mills JI, Knopp RH, et al., and the National Institute of Child Health and Human Development – Diabetes in Early Pregnancy Study Group. Declining insulin requirement in the late first trimester of diabetic pregnancy. Diabetes Care 2001; 24: 1130–6.

57. Potter JM, Beckless JP, Cullen DR. Subcutaneous insulin infusion control of blood glucose concentration in diabetics in third trimester of pregnancy. Br Med J 1980; 26: 1099–101.

58. Kitzmiller JL, Younger MD, Hare JW, et al. Continuous subcutaneous insulin therapy during early pregnancy. Obstet Gynecol 1985; 66: 606–11.

59. Coustan DR, Reece A, Sherwin RS, et al. A randomized clinical trial of the insulin pump versus intensive conventional therapy in diabetic pregnancies. J Am Med Assoc 1986; 255: 631–5.

60. Carta O, Meriggi E, Trossarelli GF, et al. Continuous subcutaneous insulin infusion versus intensive conventional insulin therapy in type 1 and type 2 diabetic pregnancy. Diabetes Metab 1986; 12: 121–9.

61. Mancuso S, Caruso A, Lanzone A, et al. Continuous subcutaneous insulin infusion in pregnant diabetic women. Acta Endocr 1986; 277(suppl.): 112–6.

62. Leveno KJ, Fortunato SJ, Raskin P, et al. Continuous subcutaneous insulin infusion during pregnancy. Diabetes Res Clin Pract 1988; 4: 257–68.

63. Caruso A, Lanzone V, Massidda M, et al. Continuous subcutaneous insulin infusion in pregnant diabetic patients. Prenat Diagn 1987; 7: 41–50.

64. Simmons D, Thompson CF, Conroy C, Scott DJ. Use of insulin pumps in pregnancies complicated by type 2 diabetes and gestational diabetes in a multiethnic community. Diabetes Care 2002; 24: 2078–82.

65. Jensen BM, Kuhl C, Petersen LM, et al. Preconceptional treatment with insulin infusion pumps in insulindependent diabetic women with particular reference to prevention of congenital malformations. Acta Endocr 1986; 277(suppl.): 81–5.

66. Gabbe SG, Holing E, Temple P, Brown ZA. Benefits, risks, costs, and patient satisfaction associated with insulin pump therapy for the pregnancy complicated by type 1 diabetes mellitus. Am J Obstet Gynecol 2000; 182: 1283–91.

67. Jovanovic L, Peterson CM. Insulin and glucose requirements during the first stage of labor in insulin-dependent diabetic women. Am J Med 1983; 75: 607–l2.

68. Jovanovic L. (ed.) Medical Management of Pregnancy Complicated by Diabetes. Alexandria: American Diabetes Assoc. Inc.: 1993; revised 1995 and 2000.

28 Oral anti-diabetic agents in pregnancy: Their time has come

Oded Langer

Introduction

Gestational diabetes mellitus (GDM) continues to be a major public health problem for the mother and unborn fetus with an estimated incidence of 3–10%, depending upon geographic location, affecting at least 105,000–350,000 women annually in the United States. The cornerstone of treatment is diabetic diet and when dietary modifications do not control maternal glycemia, pharmacological therapy is initiated. The administration of short- and long-acting insulin will be required in 20–60% of pregnancies that are complicated by GDM in order to maintain adequate glycemic control. Because of its high efficacy rate (50–80% of patients will achieve good glycemic control) and its purported inability to cross the placenta and adversely affect the fetus, insulin has remained the drug of choice.[1]

Bauman and Yallow,[2] however, have confirmed that older generations of insulin readily cross the placenta as insulin–antibody complexes. The results by Menon et al.[3] correlated insulin antibody passage rates with macrosomia. Therefore, the findings regarding the safety of insulin therapy needs to be addressed. Moreover, the introduction of new insulin analogs (e.g. lispro) requires further investigation to rule out stimulation of antibody production that may assist insulin transfer through the placenta. In addition, insulin administration is inconvenient and expensive which makes this factor of even greater concern in developing countries. Therefore, the continuous search for a safe and effective alternative to insulin therapy has been an ongoing challenge.

The use of oral anti-diabetic agents in nonpregnant Type 2 diabetic women has become the standard of care in the United States (US) to help patients maintain the tight glucose control that lowers their risk for microvascular complications.[4,5] The prevalence of GDM varies in direct proportion to the prevalence of Type 2 diabetes in a given population or ethnic group. In the US, the prevalence rate ranges from 1 to 14%.[6] Among different ethnic groups, both forms have been diagnosed in varying rates. Both Type 2 diabetes and GDM are heterogeneous disorders whose pathophysiology is characterized by peripheral insulin resistance, impaired regulation of hepatic glucose production and declining beta-cell function.

The prime objective for treatment of both pregnant and nonpregnant diabetic patients is to optimize the glycemic profile. Insulin and the oral anti-diabetic agents were designed to reduce the level of glycemia. Although until recently there was paucity of information on the efficacy for the use of oral anti-diabetic agents in pregnancy, and, therefore, its restricted role in the management of GDM in the US, both glyburide and metformin have been widely prescribed in Europe and South Africa without reported adverse side effects to the fetus.[7–17]

Lately, consideration for the use of oral anti-diabetic agents in pregnancy has become 'debatable' in scientific forums in the US. At the 5th International Workshop on GDM and at the North American Study Group, the use of glyburide during pregnancy was endorsed. The historic ban on the use of oral anti-diabetic agents in pregnancy has been based on scant evidence of case reports[18,19] and one study in particular on fetal anomalies in 50 poorly controlled diabetic women prior to pregnancy[20] begging the question: is it the drug or is it the level of glycemia?

The controversy surrounding the management of GDM with oral anti-diabetic agents stems from the lack of data from well-designed studies. The term for emphasizing outcome-based approaches is 'evidence-based medicine'. When doctors continue to question established practices and base decision-making on research evidence rather than on anecdotes and the opinions of 'experts', they can perform at their best. The purpose of this review is to provide the reader with the evidence and the foundation for understanding the use of oral anti-diabetic drugs in pregnancy as an effective alternative to insulin therapy in achieving glycemic control. The concerns of teratogenicity due to possible placental transfer, neonatal and maternal outcome, and basic pharmacological advantages will be addressed.

Oral anti-diabetic agents: Classification and characteristics

In contrast to systematic studies that led to the isolation of insulin, *sulfonylureas* were discovered accidentally. Additional clinical trials led to the discovery of tolbutamide in the 1950s and since that time many agents in this class of drugs have been developed, e.g. chlorpropamide. Second-generation sulfonylureas were subsequently developed that include glyburide and glipizide. In 1997, the first drug in a new class of oral insulin secretagogues called meglitinides (benzoic acid derivatives) was approved for clinical use. The agent repaglinide has gained acceptance as a fast-acting, pre-meal therapy to limit postprandial hyperglycemia.[21]

Biguanides were recognized as early as 1920 but received clinical recognition in the US only in the past decade. Phenformin, the primary drug in this group, was withdrawn from American and European markets because of the side effects of lactic acidosis. Its replacement, metformin, although used extensively in Europe, has only been recognized for use in the US since 1995.[21]

Thiazolidinediones were introduced in 1997. The first agent, troglitazone, was reported to have a high rate of hepatic toxicity, and as a result, was withdrawn from the market in 2000. However, newer agents in this class such as rosiglitazone and pioglitazone are widely used in clinical practice without reported hepatic toxicity. *Alpha-glucosidase inhibitors*, which reduce intestinal absorption of starch and glucose (acarbose), have now been introduced into clinical practice.[21]

The oral anti-diabetic agents act, depending upon the specific group, directly upon the beta cells to increase insulin secretion and/or to decrease hepatic glucose production and to increase peripheral insulin sensitivity. The advantage of using these agents rather than administering exogenous insulin is their ability to have an impact by nutrient availability, extra pancreatic effect and/or to increase insulin availability through the physiological route.

The prevalence of Type 2 diabetes and GDM has increased by 33% in the past decade in the US.[6] This reality may be attributable to the increased rate of obesity in the general population in all ethnic groups and the trend towards advanced maternal age in pregnancy. Because of the relative ease of administration and the low cost involved in overall therapy with oral anti-diabetic agents, they have become the drug of choice in the treatment of Type 2 diabetes. One can assume that their popularity will only increase in the future, especially after confirmation from the large prospective study by the United Kingdom Prospective Diabetes Study (UKPDS) group. The results of the study demonstrated that Type 2 diabetic patients can maintain their desired level of control, thereby lowering their risk for microvascular complications.[22] We, in a randomized study of the use of oral anti-diabetic agents demonstrated that glyburide is an efficacious alternative to insulin in the treatment of diabetes in the pregnant subject.[23]

The reader should consider the following 'drug compass' when contemplating the use of an insulin secretagogue in pregnancy:

1. Will the drug–drug interactions complicate its use with the necessary and commonly administered drugs?
2. Can glycemic control be achieved by using the optimal dose?
3. After nutrient ingestion, can the drug reduce the time lag between the plasma glucose rise and insulin secretion?
4. Can serious postprandial and fasting hypoglycemia be minimized because the drug duration of action is short enough or its dependence on plasma glucose levels sufficient?

5. Are there any side effects that can reduce the long-term beneficial effects?[29]

A major consideration in the efficacy of the drug will be its ability to cross the placenta and, if this is so, what toxicity, if at all, can it cause to the developing fetus. Often, the fear of drug-induced adverse outcome, especially after the thalidomide era in the 1960s, precludes the physician's ability to judge the scientific rationale for using a drug and evaluating it using evidence-based data instead of depending upon dogma. Very few medications have been shown to *not* cross the placental barrier. In fact, a pregnant woman is often exposed to four or five prescription drugs during pregnancy for a variety of complaints. Similar to other epithelial barriers, transfer of drugs across the placenta is affected by several factors: molecular weight, pK_a, lipophilicity, placental blood flow, blood protein binding, elimination half-life, and the specific placental transport system that affects the ability of drugs to enter the fetal compartment.[21,24,25]

Sulfonylureas have been used in the treatment of Type 2 diabetes since 1942 because of their capacity to cause hypoglycemia by stimulating insulin release from pancreatic beta cells. Sulfonylureas bind to specific receptors on beta cells forcing closure of potassium adenosine triphosphate (ATP) channels and opening of calcium channels that cause an increase in cytoplastic calcium that stimulates insulin release. The major effect of these drugs is to enhance insulin secretion.[26–31] Sulfonylureas may also further increase insulin levels by reducing hepatic clearance of the hormone, the main contributor to fasting hyperglycemia. Enhanced insulin secretion diminishes glucose toxicity and improves insulin secretion after meals, thus reducing postprandial hyperglycemia. These drugs can also enhance peripheral tissue sensitivity to insulin.[27–32] The sulfonylureas influence insulin secretion in direct proportion to plasma glucose levels from 60 to 180 mg/dL: they do not stimulate insulin secretion when the plasma glucose is <60 mg/dL.[32,33] The mechanism of action of sulfonyureas is to rapidly facilitate insulin secretion in response to nutritional intake which will result in a minimal to no lag time between the changes in plasma glucose and modification of the insulin secretory rate.[34,35]

Chlorpropamide has been available for >30 years and is a highly effective oral anti-diabetic agent with a very long duration of action. The main side effect for Type 2 nonpregnant patients is a significantly higher rate of severe and protracted hypoglycemia. This complication has not been reported to be a major concern for pregnant patients in previous studies.[7–17] The drug stimulates the antidiuretic hormone secretion, potentiating its effect at the renal tubular level, resulting in water retention and hyponatremia. With the development of second-generation sulfonylurea drugs that do not cross the placenta (glyburide), and with the high rate of hypoglycemia, chlorpropamide should not be recommended for use in pregnancy.[21]

Glyburide (also known as glibenclamide and glybenzcyclamide) is one of the second generation hypoglycemic sulfonylureas; this group also includes glipizide, gliclazide, and glimepiridel. These sulfonylureas are considerably more potent than the earlier agents. When given as a single agent, the peak plasma level of glyburide occurs within 4 h; the absorption of the drug is not affected by food digestion. Metabolism of glyburide occurs in the liver and its metabolites are extracted in bile and urine in equal proportions. Ten hours is the approximate elimination half-life of glyburide. Adverse effects of the drug are infrequent, occurring in <4% of patients receiving second-generation agents.[21] However, in 11–38% of Type 2 nonpregnant patients, the main side effect of glyburide is hypoglycemia, with symptoms being dose related: the older patient is at greater risk of a hypoglycemic episode.

The patient most receptive to glyburide therapy is one who has been hyperglycemic for less than 5 years, is willing to follow a dietary protocol, and is either of normal weight or obese. Characteristic features of both Type 2 diabetes and GDM are beta-cell exhaustion and insulin resistance. Most often, patients of both diabetic types are comparable in obesity, are asymptomatic in the early stages of the disease and have similar prevalence in the same ethnic group. Given the similarity of the phenotypic features of these complications, it is safe to assume that the use of glyburide may be beneficial in the prevention of maternal–fetal GDM complications.

Glimeperide is a new sulfonylurea drug. Both this drug and glyburide displace one another from their respective binding sites. Glimeperide has a 2.5- to 3-fold faster rate of association and an 8- to 9-fold faster rate of dissociation from the beta-cell SUR binding site than glyburide. This results in a more rapid release of insulin and a shorter duration of insulin secretion. Glimeperide significantly increases second-phase insulin secretion, whole-body glucose uptake, and insulin sensitivity.[26,36,37] The increase in insulin sensitivity may be explained by studies demonstrating lower fasting plasma insulin and C-peptide levels in patients using this drug compared to glyburide-treated patients with comparable levels of glycemic control. It should be noted that, to date, glimeperide has not been tested for use in pregnancy.[26,36,37]

Biguanides

Metformin is an oral anti-diabetic drug that is chemically and pharmacologically unrelated to the sulfonylureas. Metformin is a second-generation biguanide that was reintroduced and distributed in the US after biguanide phenformin was withdrawn from the market in the 1970s: both were introduced in 1957. Metformin has been universally shown to be effective in improving the glycemic profile in diabetic patients. Its mechanism of action is thought to include decreased hepatic glucose production and intestinal absorption of glucose, and increased peripheral uptake of glucose and utilization. The two latter mechanisms result in improved insulin sensitivity, i.e. decreased insulin requirements.[38,39] Importantly, metformin does not stimulate insulin secretion and, therefore, does not cause hypoglycemia either in diabetic or control patients. The drug acts by causing the translocation of glucose transporters from the miscrosomal fraction to the plasma membrane of hepatic and muscle cells.[40]

Metformin has no significant effects on the secretion of glucagons, cortisol, growth hormone or somatostatin. The mechanism by which metformin reduces hepatic glucose production is controversial, but the preponderance of data indicates an effect on reducing gluconeogenesis.[40] It has a strong safety and efficacy record, with a frequency of lactic acidosis one-tenth that of the parent drug. The incidence of lactic acidosis with metformin is 0.03 cases/1000 patients annually. The elimination of plasma half-life time is 6 h. Therefore, patients with renal compromise should not receive metformin, since the risk of lactic acidosis increases with the degree of renal impairment and patient age. Metformin should be introduced gradually in 500 or 850 mg increments to a maximum of 2000 mg daily.[38,39]

The peak plasma level when the drug is given as a single agent occurs within 4 h. The extent of absorption is reduced with food intake; however, it should be administered with meals to minimize gastrointestinal intolerance. Metformin is not metabolized and is eliminated unchanged in the urine. It has been effective in reducing plasma triglyceride and cholesterol levels, as well as in promoting weight loss in obese diabetic patients. Hypoglycemia is not an overt side effect of its use. Metformin does not stimulate the fetal pancreas to over-secrete insulin. The efficacy of the drug to reverse known defects responsible for insulin resistance in Type 2 diabetes and its safety with regard to hypoglycemia suggests that it may be an ideal drug for a primary prevention study in GDM.

Thiazolidenediones are a class of drugs which may provide still another pharmacological alternative to insulin therapy, although to date there are no reported data on its use in pregnancy. *Troglitazone*, the first of these agents to be introduced, has been withdrawn from use because it was associated with severe hepatic toxicity, followed by a number of deaths. These oral anti-diabetic agents exert their principal effects by lowering insulin resistance in peripheral tissue. A decrease in systemic and local tissue lipid availability may also contribute to its positive attributes in controlling the effects of diabetes.

Rosiglitazone, another oral agent in this group, is more potent than troglitazone and claims to offer a lower risk of hepatotoxicity. It is absorbed within 2 h but the maximum clinical effect is not observed for 6–12 weeks. It is recommended that liver function be measured before the start of therapy and monitored once initiated. Studies also report considerable weight gain with this drug.[41,42]

Similarities exist between rosiglitazone and glyburide in their pharmacological characteristics, which may suggest that there is a possibility that they do not cross the placenta. If this proves to be the case, rosiglitazone, like metformin, may be an ideal agent for the management of GDM and Type 2 diabetes in pregnancy, as a single therapy or in combination with glyburide.

Alpha-glucosidase inhibitors act by slowing the absorption of carbohydrates from the intestine, thereby reducing the postprandial rise in blood glucose. The postprandial rise is blunted in both normal and diabetic patients. Gastrointestinal side effects require gradual dosage increments over time after initiation of therapy. This group of drugs may be considered a monotherapy in elderly patients but are typically used in combination with other oral anti-diabetic agents and/or insulin. Acarbose, the oral agent in this group currently in use, may be added to most other available therapies.[43,44]

Rationale for the use of oral hypoglycemic agents in the management of gestational diabetes mellitus

The intensified insulin approach in the management of GDM has been shown to result in perinatal outcomes comparable to those in the general population; thus, it has become the method of choice for control of glycemia.[1] A less invasive, efficacious alternative that would achieve similar perinatal outcome while enhancing patient compliance has been a major diabetes research goal for the past 20 years.

The underlying principle for the use of oral anti-diabetic agents in pregnancy has been motivated by three factors, as follows;

First, the similarity between Type 2 diabetes and GDM. In addition to the insulin secretion and resistance abnormalities found in both conditions, there is a loss of the first phase insulin secretion with a striking lag time between the postprandial rise in glucose and the presence of significant insulin at the peripheral sites.[33,34] It results in an early increase in postprandial glucose values. As discussed before, second-generation sulfonylurea agents are rapid in onset and have a short duration of action which makes them ideal agents for treatment in the very early stages of Type 2 diabetes and possibly GDM patients.

Second, GDM and patients with impaired glucose tolerance (IGT) are characterized by a mild hyperglycemia in comparison to Type 2 diabetics. However, this mild hyperglycemia is significantly elevated in comparison to nondiabetic women. As the disease progresses to Type 2 diabetes, there is progressive loss of beta-cell function.[45,46] In the presence of insulin resistance with obesity, pregnancy, and, especially GDM, insulin secretion will initially increase to compensate for the impairment in insulin action. The ensuing decrease in secretion over time will, in turn, result in the progression from normal glucose tolerance to GDM, from there to IGT and to Type 2 diabetes.[46]

Oral anti-diabetic agents have been successfully used to decrease glycemic levels in Type 2 diabetic patients. Since GDM subjects have the mildest form of the glucose tolerance abnormality, it is reasonable to assume that the use of oral anti-diabetic agents in the treatment of GDM should be even more effective than its current use with Type 2 diabetic patients.

Third, The United Kingdom Prospective Diabetes Study (UKPDS) of Type 2 diabetes supported the efficacy of these drugs and in particular the use of glyburide.[22] The study demonstrated that with the use of glyburide, 70% of the patients achieved a desirable level of glucose control with the most favorable effect achieved within the first 5 years of therapy.[22] The study also reported a decrease in microvascular and macrovascular complications. Rather than credit a specific therapy as the factor responsible for reduced risk of complications, the authors concluded that improvement in glycemic control was the crucial factor in treating the disease.

The UKPDS[22] and the Diabetes Control and Complications Trial (DCCT)[47] groups suggest that intensive therapy in patients with Types 1 and 2 diabetes will result in improved glycemic control and a decrease in the complication rate. Thus, intensified therapy can, by itself, provide the primary prevention for diabetic complications. Studies of pregnant diabetic women, including a study of >2000 GDM patients[1] demonstrated that intensified therapy results in improvement in glycemic control and in perinatal outcomes similar to those in the nondiabetic population.

Since GDM is characterized by a milder glycemic profile and occurs 2–10 years earlier than Type 2 diabetes, the use of oral anti-diabetic agents in its treatment should be even more effective. In addition, it is reasonable to expect that the success rate for therapy with GDM patients should be >70%, as achieved with Type 2 diabetics. In evaluating the use of glyburide in comparison to insulin[23] in GDM women, we found that 82% of the glyburide patients and 88% of the insulin patients achieved targeted levels of control. In another randomized study,[14] 80% of subjects treated with oral agents or diet alone maintained targeted blood glucose levels of <150 mg/dL. In contrast, only 38% of the insulin patients were able to achieve this level, probably due to poor compliance. Since these results were reported, multiple studies have reconfirmed that glyburide and insulin have comparable rates in achieving levels of glycemic control and outcome in pregnancy[48–56] (Tables 28.1 and 28.2).

Success in achieving targeted levels of glycemia will vary from study to study because of different doses, administration algorithms, length of therapy, type of patient (severity and ethnicity), and non-comparable groups (compliant versus non-compliant subjects). Finally, to date, there is no evidence that a diabetic medication will be able to maintain targeted levels of glycemic control in all patients.

Table 28.1   Use of oral anti-diabetic agents in pregnancy: glyburide

Reference	Study design	Good glyburide	Contr LGA
Langer et al.[23]	Ramdomized controlled trial	82 and 88%	12 vs. 13%
Lim et al.[50]	Prospective observational	Not significant	Not significant
Conway et al.[51]	Prospective observational	84%	Not applicable
Kremer and Duff[12]	Prospective observational	81%	19%
Chmait et al.[48]	Prospective observational	82%	7%
Gilson et al.[53]	Prospective observational	82%	Not significant
Fines et al.[54]	Retrospective case–control	Not applicable	8 vs. 25%
Velasquez et al.[92]	Case series	82%	16 vs. 29%

Table 28.2   Use of oral anti-diabetic agents in pregnancy: glyburide compared with insulin

Reference	Study design	Glyburide	Regular insulin	Good control	LGA
Pendsey et al.[93]	Randomized controlled trial	23 Repaglinde	23	Improved glycemic control	–
Hellmuth et al.[49]	Prospective	68 Sulfonylurea	42	Poor in all	35–44% ↑PET
Notelovitz et al.[13]	Randomized controlled trial	2 × 52 Tolbutamide Chlorpropamin	52	Oral 80% Insulin 36%	No neonat. hypog.
Yogev et al.[84]	Prospective	25	30	MBG - NS	–
Moore et al.[94]	Randomized controlled trial	31	32	MBG - NS	–
Jacobson et al.[55]	Retrospective	236	316	MBG - NS	–
Kitzmiller et al.[95]	Retrospective	73	Refused insulin	47%	No neota. hypog.
Coetzee and Jacobson et al.[96]	Retrospective	126	–	–	Dec. PMN

The incidence of congenital anomalies in nondiabetic women is 2–3% but increases to 7–9% overall in pregnant diabetic patients. The rate will be even higher in poorly controlled diabetics and as the severity of the disease increases. An unanswered question remains: what is the toxic agent that triggers the development of malformations – is it the glucose or is it the oral anti-diabetic agent? This dilemma has led to several investigations of animal species or tissue cultures as a source for the answers. These types of studies provide the conditions with which to test separately and together the effect of different drug doses in conjunction with varying levels of glucose. However, needless to say, reports from mice studies are not generally applicable to human embryos.

Smithberg and Runner[57] studied different hypoglycemia-inducing treatments, including insulin, tolbutamide, and fasting of prepuberal mice, as well as combination treatments involving nicotinamide plus insulin or tolbutamide. They were all found to be potent teratogens in one or more inbred strains of mice. Teratogenic treatments cause a variable proportion of deaths. The response of different strains of mice to individual treatments relevant to teratogenicity or lethality was highly variable. It is the variability of response elicited from each strain of mouse as a group which may be the most pertinent finding in these experiments. Most noteworthy is the 3% mortality produced by insulin treatment in strain BALB/c as compared to 17% in mouse strain 129. This example demonstrates the variability in study results reported in the literature. It also makes one realize that it was the strain of mouse that was the determining factor in recommending or failing to recommend a particular drug.

However, first-generation sulfonylureas, such as tolbutamide and chlorpropamide, were found to be associated with congenital malformations in the majority of animal studies. Adverse effects appear to be caused by the drugs and not by the hypoglycemia they produce. Chlorpropamide appeared to be embryotoxic in mouse embryos in culture.[56–58] To date, no animal studies have been performed to evaluate second- and third-generation sulfonylureas and their association to fetal malformations.

Denno and Sadler[59] evaluated the effect of biguanides using metformin and phenformin as embryotoxic agents at concentrations equal to serum levels obtained in patients treated with the agent clinically. They found that phenformin is embryotoxic, whereas metformin is not, suggesting that metformin is also the safer drug during pregnancy in patients with non-insulin-dependent diabetes mellitus (NIDDM). However, it should be noted that in the present study, metformin was not without adverse effects since it produced a delay in neural tube closure and also reduced yolk sac protein values at two different concentrations. While delayed closure of the neural tube may not have resulted in gross morphological abnormalities, it was not possible to assess subtler alterations that might result from such a delay using the culture system. Shephard[60] and Schardein[61] reported that metformin did not appear to be a major teratogen because <0.5% of the rat fetuses in mothers administered 500–1000 mg/kg developed anophthalmia and anencephaly. However, evidence of embryo toxicity was evident with higher doses of the drug.

The characteristics of individual drugs will determine their placental transfer capability. These factors will include: molecular weight, pK_a, lipophilicity, placental blood flow, blood protein binding, and elimination half-life.[62–65] Although the cutoff for actual molecular weight passage across the placental barrier has not yet been accurately defined, it is generally agreed that molecular weights ≤1000 Da passively permeate across the placental barrier with sustained maternal blood concentrations.[62–68]

The recirculating single-cotyledon human placental model is widely used to characterize the transport and metabolism of numerous drugs and nutrients. It is a reliable *in vitro* model for human placental transfer since it facilitates the study of intact human placenta independent of fetal metabolism. Experiments can be validated against known substances that freely cross the placenta.[69–73]

In recent studies using the single cotyledon model, it was demonstrated that metformin freely crosses the placenta. In light of this finding and the existence of contradicting data in animal studies regarding the teratogenic effect of metformin, one must be very cautious when prescribing this drug in pregnancy. However, it should also be noted that the majority of drugs used during pregnancy also cross the placenta yet do not cause adverse effects to the fetus.

Unlike other species, the human placental barrier is composed of a single rate-limiting layer of multinucleated cells, the syncytiotrophoblasts. During the formation of the placenta, fetal tissues erode the maternal blood vessels to attain a closer proximity to the maternal circulation. Chorionic villi that contain fetal blood vessels infiltrate the maternal vessels and establish a sinusoid in which the villi are suffused by maternal blood.[62–65] The rate-limiting barrier for penetration across the human placenta is the syncytiotrophoblast layer. Therefore, animal studies addressing placental transfer (e.g. mice) will not necessarily be applicable in humans.[66]

Since animal studies are not conclusive about the safety of the fetus regarding the association between drugs and malformations, additional research approaches are needed to determine drug transfer across the placenta and/or tests of fetal blood for evidence of the drug. Only data that will provide information on the association between metformin or any other drug used clinically in humans will be the final testimony of the existence or absence of teratogenic affect of these agents on the fetus. One can speculate that all oral anti-diabetic drugs will not cross the placenta as is the case with glyburide and will allow us to use a potentially attractive drug because of its multi-systemic response in the treatment of gestational diabetes and in pregnancy in general. However, this wishful thinking is not the reality: some drugs (such as metformin and the glitizone group) cross the placenta. Several animal studies have demonstrated that these drugs cross the placental barrier and cause, in rats, delayed body growth and insulin resistance. One study in an *in vivo* murine model found that rosiglitazone did not impair murine blastocyst development *in vitro* or cause phenotypic harm to the mouse fetus when administered during pregnancy. These findings bring us back to the question previously addressed relevant to metformin: is it enough to declare a drug contra-indicated if the drug crosses the placenta or evidence of no damage to the embryo and fetus should permit us to use newly developed drugs with a potentially high benefit to the embryo, fetus, and mother?!?

We evaluated the ability of first- and second-generation sulfonylureas to cross the placenta.[24,25] Glyburide's molecular weight is 494 units (U); it is one of the largest oral anti-diabetic agents. First, transport and metabolism of glyburide across the human placenta was investigated, with the following results: (1) there was virtually no significant transport of glyburide in either the maternal-to-fetal or fetal-to-maternal directions, with an average transport of 0.26% at 2 h. These levels are 3- to 8-fold higher than the therapeutic peak levels after a 5 mg oral dose in humans. In fact, when cord blood samples were tested using high-performance liquid chromatography (HPLC), glyburide was undetectable in these samples despite maternal plasma levels of 50–150 ng/ml. (2) After increasing the glyburide concentration to 100 times the therapeutic levels, transport was not appreciably altered. Equilibrium dialysis demonstrated that at least 98% of the glyburide was protein bound. (3) Glyburide is neither metabolized nor sequestered by the placenta.

In the second set of studies in 1994[72] and 1997,[73] we demonstrated that second-generation sulfonylureas, especially glyburide, do not significantly cross the diabetic or nondiabetic placenta. Fetal concentrations reached no more than 1–2% of maternal concentrations. Although glipizide crossed the placenta in small amounts, this was significantly higher than glyburide. In contrast, tolbutamide diffused across the placenta most freely. In general, glyburide has not been demonstrated to be teratogenic in animal and human studies. Recently, several laboratory and clinical studies reconfirmed the lack of transfer and adverse affect of glyburide.

Clinical studies

The use of oral anti-diabetic agents was historically contraindicated in the US. This dogma, supported by scant data, was predicated on the assumption that the drugs could cause fetal damage and/or demise. The results of numerous studies during the current decade have systematically revealed the error in the above assumptions. Yet, there persists a group of nay-sayers who are tenacious in their disregard of new research findings thus denying the mother and fetus alternative, more convenient and sometimes even more effective modes of therapy.

Insulin therapy involves daily injections which do not always result in optimal compliance by many women, and women in many developing countries cannot afford insulin therapy. Studies have demonstrated that both diet- and insulin-treated women have comparable psychological profiles in different ethnic groups.[77–79] However, given the choice of insulin injections versus tablets, almost all women will opt for the latter.

Since our original publication in 2000, several investigators reported their clinical experience with glyburide.[48–55] Each demonstrated the effectiveness of glyburide therapy to achieve glycemic control. However, different studies used different criteria to define success rate.

Three issues of concern have been raised: (1) the increased rate of congenital anomalies; (2) the possible induction of fetal macrosomia due to direct stimulation of the fetal pancreas resulting in hyperinsulinemia; and, (3) the increased rate of hypoglycemia due to fetal hyperinsulinemia. The sources for the above concerns were based on clinical observations of case reports or small retrospective studies, the majority published in the 1960s and 1970s. The patient populations were mainly Type 2 diabetics and the drugs used were mainly first-generation sulfonylureas.[18–20] An example of a study used to generate the recommendation that there is an increased risk for neonatal hypoglycemia with the use of these drugs was a case report of three infants whose mothers received chlorpropamide and another mother of an infant given acetohexamide; another case report reported prolonged symptomatic neonatal hypoglycemia.[18,19] The recommendation not to use oral anti-diabetic agents because of an increased rate of anomalies was based on a retrospective study involving 50 Type 2 diabetic patients, all with hyperglycemia prior to conception (glycosylated hemoglobin (HbA1c) levels >8%).[20] The fact that maternal hyperglycemia existed preconception makes it impossible to determine if the increased rate of anomalies found in these study subjects was a result of the medication or of the elevated glucose level.

In contrast, three studies in the past decade have suggested that there is no association between oral anti-diabetic agents and congenital malformations. Towner et al.[81] treated 332 Type 2 diabetic patients with oral anti-diabetic agents or insulin prior to pregnancy. The authors demonstrated, using a stepwise logistic regression, that the mode of therapy did not have an adverse effect, while the level of glycemia and maternal age were significant factors contributing to the rate of anomalies.

We demonstrated similar findings in a retrospective analysis of 850 Type 2 diabetic women exposed to different oral hypoglycemic agents, insulin and diet therapy prior to and during the first trimester of pregnancy.[82] Again, it was the blood glucose and not the mode of therapy that had the net effect on the rate of anomalies. Finally, Koren,[83] at an National Institute Health (NIH) Food and Drug Administration (FDA) conference presented the results of eight studies and concluded that the use of oral anti-diabetic agents have no effect on the rate of fetal anomalies due to a very narrow confidence interval (CI) (odds ratio (OR) 1.0; 95% CI 1.05–1.85).

To date, no randomized study addressing the use of oral anti-diabetic agents during organogenesis has been performed. The results of early small-scale studies suggest that an association exists. However, these studies were not controlled for the level of glycemia. The above large-scale studies, although retrospective, demonstrated that the cause of anomalies is the level of glycemia and not the use of oral anti-diabetic drugs.

It remains unresolved if the treatment of Type 2 diabetes with oral anti-diabetic agents will accelerate the rate of anomalies. On the other hand, is it not an over-reaction to condemn these medications? With existing data, care providers need to objectively present information to patients so that issues are addressed and informed decisions are made. Moreover, there should be diligence in separating data from Type 2 diabetic studies when considering GDM.

In the case of GDM, the issue of anomalies is simpler. GDM patients are diagnosed and enter therapy after the first trimester (after the organogenesis period). There then remains concern about potential fetal hypoglycemia and stimulation for macrosomia if the drug crosses the placenta. However, as previously discussed, glyburide does not cross the placenta and therefore cannot stimulate adverse effects in the fetus. Finally, Langer et al.[23] provided the clinical support for this concern. It was demonstrated that in patients entering therapy after the first trimester, the rate of anomalies was comparable for insulin- and glyburide-treated patients, and similar to the rate reported in the nondiabetic general population.

There are several retrospective and randomized studies in the literature that have evaluated the use of first- and second-generation sulfonylurea drugs and metformin in pregnancy. Notolovitz[14] studied the utility of tolbutamide, chlorpropamine, diet and insulin in a randomized study with a small sample size with relatively low power (each of the four arms of the study contained c. 50 patients). There was no significant difference for perinatal mortality and congenital anomalies. Good glycemic control was defined as a blood glucose level <150 mg/dL. Eighty percent of the subjects using

oral anti-diabetic agents or diet and 36% of the insulin-treated patients achieved the targeted glycemic category (i.e. <150 mg/dL).

Langer et al.[23] performed a randomized study in which 440 GDM women were recruited between 11 and 33 weeks gestation with a singleton pregnancy (Table 28.3). The blood glucose profile was comparable for the glyburide and the insulin-treated groups (114 ± 9 versus 116 ± 22 mg/dL, respectively). Patients were randomly assigned to receive either glyburide (n = 201; initial dose 2.5 mg orally, increasing by 5 mg/week up to a total of 20 mg) or insulin (n = 203; initial dose 0.7 U/kg subcutaneously three times daily, increasing each week as necessary) for glycemic control. Patients were required to measure their glucose values seven times daily. The targets for glycemic control were a mean blood glucose level of 90–105 mg/dL, a fasting blood glucose level of 60–90 mg/dL, a preprandial blood glucose level of 80–95 mg/dL and a postprandial blood glucose level of <120 mg/dL. Both treatments caused significant reductions in blood glucose levels compared with levels measured at home for 1 week prior to initiation of treatment. Mean blood glucose levels in the glyburide group decreased from 114 to 105 mg/dL, whereas those in the insulin group decreased from 116 to 105 mg/dL. Eighty-two percent of the glyburide-treated and 88% of the insulin-treated subjects were able to achieve targeted levels of glycemia. However, eight glyburide-treated women (4%) failed to achieve the desired level of control early in the third trimester and were transferred to insulin therapy. None of the patients developed severe symptoms of hypoglycemia. However, in the insulin-treated group a significantly higher rate of subjects had 1–6% of their self-monitoring blood glucose determinations values <40 mg/dL compared to the glyburide subjects. In another study, using continuous blood glucose monitoring for 3 days, we reconfirmed our original findings; however, the testing time was limited[84] (Figure 28.1). The glyburide and insulin groups had similar rates of pre-eclampsia (6%) and Cesarean sections (23–24%). Neonatal outcomes did not differ significantly between the two groups. The glyburide and insulin

Table 28.3   Selected neonatal outcomes for insulin and glyburide

Outcome	Insulin (%), n = 203	Glyburide (%), n = 201
LGA	12.8	12.4
Macrosomia	4.0	7.0
Ponderal index >2.85	11.8	9.0
Hypocalcemia	1.0	1.0
Hyperbilirub.	3.9	5.5
Polycythemia	2.5	1.5
Intravenous glucose	11.0	14.0
Lung compliance	5.9	7.9
Respiratory support	2.5	1.5
NICU	7.4	5.9

All results were non-significant.
(Modified from Langer et al.[23])

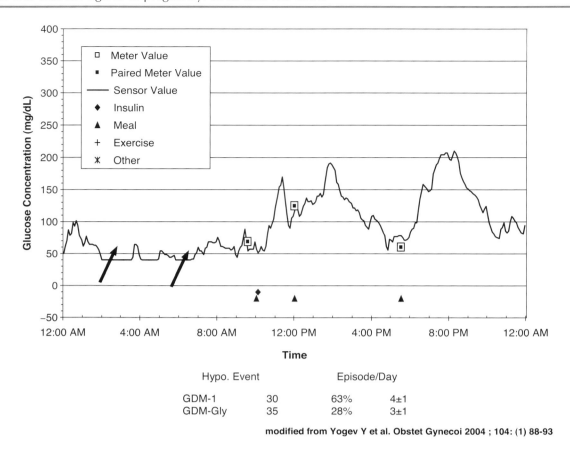

Hypo. Event		Episode/Day	
GDM-1	30	63%	4±1
GDM-Gly	35	28%	3±1

modified from Yogev Y et al. Obstet Gynecoi 2004 ; 104: (1) 88-93

Figure 28.1 CGM asymptomatic hypoglycemic episodes (more than 30 consecutive minutes of reading below 50 mg/dL). (Modified from Yogev et al.[84])

groups had a similar incidence of large-for-gestational-age (LGA) infants (12 vs. 13%) macrosomia (7 vs. 4%) lung complications (8 vs. 6%), hypoglycemia (9 vs. 6%), admission to a neonatal intensive care unit (6 vs. 7%) and fetal anomalies (2 vs. 2%).

This clinical study confirmed basic science studies that glyburide does not cross the placenta in significant amounts. Glyburide was undetectable in cord serum to the level of sensitivity of the test. As a quality control, simultaneous samples of maternal serum were obtained from 12 women at the time of delivery to determine whether sufficient gradient levels for glyburide exist. Maternal levels ranged from 50 to 150ng/ml. To ascertain any potential effect of glyburide on fetal pancreas, insulin umbilical cord levels between the two groups were compared. The mean cord serum insulin concentrations were similar for both groups.

Several clinical trials studied the effect of metformin as a single or combination therapy in pregnancy. The results of the studies indicated a significant mean decline in plasma glucose concentrations.[12,16,17] In one study,[17] the failure of metformin to achieve targeted levels of glycemic control was 53.8% for established diabetics and 28.6% in the GDM patients. Apart from a high incidence of neonatal jaundice requiring phototherapy, the infant morbidity in the metformin group was low. The rate of LGA infants was double the rate found in the authors' general population. However, the LGA

rate was comparable in the metformin- and insulin-treated patients, approaching 20%. Finally, the mothers of the three infants with congenital malformations in the metformin group initiated therapy in the third trimester.

In another study by the same authors, 12 patients treated with metformin and glibenclamide alone, and the combination of diet, metformin and glibenclamide were compared. Patients who failed to achieve glycemic control with the oral anti-diabetic agent therapy were transferred to insulin therapy. The incidences of LGA neonates (>90th percentile) were 15% (metformin), 27% (glibenclamide), 33% (combined therapy group) and 41% (failed oral insulin-treated group). The relative increase in the rate of LGA infants must be explained by the severity of the disease and the higher rate of poorly controlled subjects in the combination- and insulin-treated groups. Neonatal hypoglycemia is defined as <25 mg/dL: the overall rate of neonatal hypoglycemia was 11.5%, with the highest rates for the patients treated with glibenclamide (27%) and combination therapy (glibenclamide and metformin) (18%), and the lowest rate in metformin-treated patients (5%). The high rate of neonatal hypoglycemia corresponds with a rate of LGA infants reported in our study, suggesting that a significant number of their patients were in suboptimal glucose control.

Will glyburide be as effective as insulin at all severity levels of GDM? And, is there a dose limitation above which the efficacy of glyburide will decrease in comparison to insulin? We found that glyburide and insulin are equally efficacious for GDM treatment at all severity levels of diabetes when FPG on a GTT was between 95 and 139 mg/dL. As the level of disease severity increases, the success rate for achieving established levels of glycemic control decreases. The majority of patients (71%) will require, on average, up to 10 mg daily dose of glyburide to achieve established levels of glycemic control. Stratifying patients by GDM severity no significant difference was found in neonatal size, metabolic complications, and the composite outcome between the two treatment modalities.

For adjustment of the potential confounding effects of several factors, we performed logistic regression analysis when the primary outcome was LGA. We found that the mean blood glucose, severity of GDM (categorized by the fasting plasma from the OGTT), previous macrosomia, and weight gain in pregnancy, were the only significant contributors. Again, treatment modality, parity and pre-pregnancy weight (BMI) were found to be non-contributors. Therefore, reaching established levels of glycemic control and not the mode of therapy is the key to improving pregnancy outcome in GDM women.[85]

Several studies have sought to identify the predictors of glyburide therapy failure. Rochon et al.[86] studied 101 GDM women requiring pharmacological therapy while testing 4/daily. Criteria for success was achieving fasting between 60 and 90 mg/dL and 2-h postprandial <120 mg/dL. Seventy-nine percent of the women achieved targeted levels of glycemic control. The authors concluded that 'predicting glyburide failure is difficult, but failure does not appear to be associated with increased adverse pregnancy outcomes.' However, in this study, pregnancy outcome included shoulder dystocia 10%, macrosomia (in the success group) 16%, Cesarean delivery approximately 40%. These outcome rates are higher than expected in well-controlled diabetic women.

Kahn et al.[87] analyzed 95 GDMs receiving glyburide therapy. The overall success rate was 81%. Criteria for failure were 20% of fasting blood glucose determinations at ≥95 mg/dL and 1-h postprandial ≥140 mg/dL. Patients were instructed to take the glyburide 30 min prior to breakfast and dinner when the initial dose was individualized based on patient weight and degree of hyperglycemia. This administration criterion is unconventional and deviates from standard recommendations in the literature. The perinatal outcome was associated with 27% LGA and 12% pre-eclampsia. Their conclusion was that 'glyburide was more likely to fail in women diagnosed in pregnancy of older age, multi-parity, with higher fasting glucose'. Is it possible that with the above perinatal outcomes, the majority of patients were undiagnosed Type 2 diabetic women?

Chmait et al.[48] in 46 patients, evaluated failure of glyburide therapy. Failure was defined when the maximum glyburide dose could not maintain fasting plasma <110 mg/dL and 1-h postprandial <140 mg/dL. Approximately 81% of the patients achieved these goals. Jacobson et al.[55] with 122 women on insulin and 137 treated with glyburide instructed patients to test blood glucose 4/daily: fasting and either 1- or 2-h postprandial (per individual provider preference). Targeted goals were fasting 100 mg/dL, 1-h 155 mg/dL and 2-h 130 mg/dL. Eighty-six percent of glyburide and 63% of insulin patients achieved these goals. However, the reported macrosomia rate was 25%.

Recently, we sought to identify predictors of treatment failure in GDM in 379 glyburide treated women. Failure of glyburide therapy is largely dependent upon the physician's ability to recognize and adequately adjust the glyburide dose. Physician intervention can preclude an avoidable failure. GDM severity, obesity, early gestational age at diagnosis, maternal age, and parity are all known factors that influence the success rate in treatment of the diabetic patient independent of pharmacological agent. All of these were found to be non-contributing variables of the failure rate of glyburide therapy[88] (Figure 28.2).

We found an inverse relation between disease severity and level of glycemia resulting in approximately 40% in the high fasting category achieving targeted levels of glycemic control. This was true for glyburide- and insulin-treated patients at each level of severity. Of note, the success rate in the high severity category is similar to that reported in the nonpregnant Type 2 diabetics.

Obesity, in and of itself, is a precursor of potential adverse outcome in pregnancy. Diet-treated GDM patients, overweight (BMI 26–29) or obese (BMI =30), are associated with adverse pregnancy outcome regardless of the level of glycemic control. In contrast, for those treated with insulin therapy who achieve established glycemic levels in pregnancy, outcome will be comparable to those of normal weight patients.[89] Patients who achieved targeted levels of glycemic control had comparable perinatal outcome for both treatment modalities. Therefore, appropriate utilization of glyburide therapy in obese patients will result in pregnancy outcome comparable with those treated with insulin.[90]

Conclusions

Success in truly achieving level of glycemic control may vary from study to study because of different criteria for success, failure to administer the maximal dose, different doses and administration algorithms, length of therapy, type of patient (severity, ethnicity, and obesity), and comparable groups (compliant vs. non-compliant subjects). Thus, studies reporting

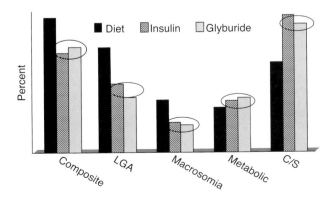

Figure 28.2 Comparison between obese well-controlled GDM by treatment modalities.

similar 'success rates' may result in significantly different perinatal outcomes which in turn may lead to erroneous conclusions on cause and causation.

Different oral anti-diabetic agents act via diverse mechanisms of action. These drug characteristics provide a more physiological approach to the treatment of Type 2 diabetes and GDM. Furthermore, combination therapies will enhance the effect of these drugs on glucose metabolism. Although sulfonylureas are the only oral agents that have been studied in GDM women in randomized controlled trials, other oral anti-diabetic agents may have an even greater therapeutic effect in controlling glycemic levels. Evidence suggests that glyburide is as effective as insulin in maintaining desired glycemic levels and results in comparable outcomes. However, regardless of the mode of therapy, whole-patient care (glucose monitoring, education, diet adherence, etc.) will determine the overall success in managing this disease and maximizing the quality of perinatal outcome.

In our experience, glyburide has become the drug of choice for use in GDM when pharmacological intervention is required, regardless of GDM severity level and obesity. The non-invasive, cost-effective patient-friendly regimen lends itself more readily to potential patient compliance.[91] Although both treatment modalities show comparable perinatal outcome, it appears from our and other investigators' experience that oral therapy is more readily accepted by patients than insulin injections. However, failure to achieve established levels of glycemic control, regardless of the choice of treatment modality and physician failure to provide the appropriate drug algorithm and dose will result in adverse perinatal outcome. In the near future, we will require studies with appropriate sample sizes and power that will evaluate different oral anti-diabetic drugs in comparison to glyburide, combination therapies such as glyburide and acarbose, glyburide and metformin and an oral anti-diabetic agent with insulin to optimize patient/physician choices in the treatment of diabetes in pregnancy.

REFERENCES

1. Langer O, Rodriguez DA, Xenakis EMJ, et al. Intensified vs. conventional management of gestational diabetes. Am J Obstet Gynecol 1994; 170: 1036–47.
2. Bauman WA, Yallow RS. Transplacental passage of insulin complexed to antibody. Proc Natl Acad Sci USA 1981; 78: 4588–90.
3. Menon RK, Cohen RM, Sperling MA, et al. Transplacental passage of insulin in pregnant women with insulin-dependent diabetes mellitus. N Engl J Med 1990; 323: 309–15.
4. Turner RC, Cull CA, Fright V, et al. Glycemic control with diet, sulfonylurea, metformin, or insulin inpatients with type 2 diabetes mellitus: progressive requirement for multiple therapies. J Am Med Assoc 1999; 281: 2005–12.
5. Lebovitz HE. Insulin secretagogues: old and new. Diabetes Rev 1999; 7: 139–53.
6. Coustan DR. Gestational diabetes. In: National Institutes of Diabetes and Digestive and Kidney Diseases. Diabetes in America, 2nd edn. Publication No. 95-1468. Bethesda, Maryland: NIDDK: 1995, pp. 703–17.
7. Douglas CP, Richards R. Use of chlorpropamide in the treatment of diabetes in pregnancy. Diabetes 1967; 16: 60–1.
8. Jackson WPU, Campbell GD, Notelovitz M, Blumson D. Tolbutamide and chlorpropamide during pregnancy in human diabetics. Diabetes 1963; (suppl.): 98–101.
9. Sutherland HW, Bewsher PD, Cormack JD, et al. Effect of moderate dosage of chlorpropamide in pregnancy on fetal outcome. Arch Dis Child 1974; 49: 283–91.
10. Stowers JM, Sutherland HW. The use of sulphonylureas biguinides and insulin in pregnancy. In: Stowers, Sutherland, eds. Carbohydrate Metabolism in Pregnancy and the Newborn. Edinburgh: Churchill Livingstone; 1975, pp. 205–20.
11. Coetzee EJ, Jackson WPU. Oral hypoglycemics in the first trimester and fetal outcome. S Afr Med J 1984; 65: 635–7.
12. Coetzee EJ, Jackson WPU. Pregnancy in established non-insulin-dependent diabetics. S Afr Med J 1980; 61: 795–802.
13. Notelovitz M. Oral hypoglycemic therapy in diabetic pregnancies. Lancet 1974; ii: 902–3.
14. Notelowitz M. Sulfonylurea therapy in the treatment of the pregnant diabetic. S Afr Med J 1971; 45: 226–9.
15. Coetzee EJ, Jackson WPU. The management of non-insulin-dependent diabetes during pregnancy. Diabetes Res Clin Pract 1986; 1: 281–7.
16. Coetzee EJ, Jackson WPU. Diabetes newly diagnosed in pregnancy: a 4-year study at Groote Schuur Hospital. SA Mediese Tydskrif 1979; 467–75.
17. Coetzee EJ, Jackson WPU. Metformin in management of pregnant insulin-independent diabetics. Diabetologia 1979; 16: 241–5.
18. Kemball ML, McIvert C, Milner RDG, et al. Neonatal hypoglycemia in infants of diabetic mothers given sulphonylurea drugs in pregnancy. Arch Dis Child 1970; 45: 696–701.
19. Zucker P, Simon G. Prolonged symptomatic neonatal hypoglycemia associated with maternal chlorpropamide therapy. Pediatrics 1968; 42: 824–5.
20. Piacquadio K, Hollingsworth DR, Murphy H. Effects of in-utero exposure to oral hypoglycemic drugs. Lancet 1991; 338: 866–9.
21. Hardmons J, Limbird X, eds. Goodman and Gillman's The Pharmacologic Basis of Therapeutics, 9th edn. New York: McGraw Hill; 1996, pp. 1712–92.
22. American Diabetes Association. Implications of the United Kingdom Prospective Diabetes Study. Diabetes Care 2000; 23(suppl. 2): S27–31.
23. Langer O, Conway DL, Berkus MD, Xenakis EMJ, Gonzales O. A comparison of glyburide and insulin in women with gestational diabetes mellitus. N Engl J Med 2000; 343(16): 1134–38.
24. Elliot B, Langer O, Schenker S, Jonhson RF. Insignificant transfer of glyburide occurs across the human placenta. Am J Obstet Gynecol 1991; 165: 807–12.
25. Koren G. Glyburide and fetal safety; transplacental pharmacokinetic considerations. Reprod Toxicol 2001; 15: 225–9.
26. Lebovitz HE. Insulin secretagogues: old and new. Diabetes Rev 1999; 7: 139–53.
27. Rossetti L, Giaaccari A, DeFronzo RA. Glucose toxicity. Diabetes Care 1990; 13: 610–30.
28. Simonson DC, Farrannini E, Bevilacqua S, et al. Mechanism of improvement in glucose metabolism after chronic glyburide therapy. Diabetes Care 1984; 33: 838–45.
29. Groop L, Luzi L, Melanger A, et al. Different effects of glyburide and glipizide on insulin secretion and hepatic glucose production in normal and NIDDM subjects. Diabetes 1987; 36: 1320–8.
30. Groop LC, Barzilai N, Ratheiser K, et al. Dose-dependent effects of glyburide on insulin secretion and glucose uptake in humans. Diabetes Care 1991; 14: 724–7.
31. DeFronzo RA, Simonson DC. Oral sulfonylurea agents suppress hepatic glucose production in non-insulin-dependent diabetic individuals. Diabetes Care 1984; 7: 72–80.
32. Kahn SE, McCulloch DK, Porte Jr D. Insulin secretion in normal and diabetic humans. In: Alberti KGMM, Zimmer P, DeFronzo RA, Keen H, eds. International Textbook of Diabetes Mellitus, 2nd edn. Chichester: Wiley; 1997, pp. 337–54.
33. Mitrakou A, Kelley D, Mokan M, et al. Role of reduced suppression of glucose production and early insulin release in impaired glucose tolerance. N Engl J Med 1992; 326: 22–9.
34. Polansky KS, Given BD, Hirsch I, et al. Abnormal patterns of insulin secretion in non-insulin dependent diabetes mellitus. N Engl J Med 1988; 318: 1231–9.
35. Leahy JL. Natural history of beta cell dysfunction in NIDDM. Diabetes Care 1990; 13: 992–1010.
36. Clark HE, Matthews DR. The effect of glimerpiride on pancreatic beta-cell function under hyperglycemic clamp and hyperinsulinaemic, euglycaemic clamp conditions in non-insulin dependent diabetes mellitus. Horm Metab Res 1996; 28: 445–50.
37. van der Wal PS, Draeger KE, van Iperen AM, et al. Beta cell response to oral glimepiride administration during and following a hyperglycaemic clamp in NIDDM patients. Diabet Med 1997; 14: 556–63.

38. Product information. Glucophage. Bristol-Myers Squibb, 1997.
39. Klepser TB, Kelly MW. Metformin hydrochloride: an antihyperglycemic agent. Am J Health-Syst Pharm 1997; 54: 893–903.
40. Stumvoll M, Nurjhan N, Perriello G, et al. Metabolic effects of metformin in non-insulin dependent diabetes mellitus. N Engl J Med 1995; 333: 550–4.
41. Buckingham RE, Al-Barazanji KA, Toseland N, et al. Peroxisome proliferator-activitated receptor-gamma agonist, rosiglitazone, protects against nephropathy and pancreatic islet abnormalities in Zucker fatty rats. Diabetes 1998; 47: 1326–34.
42. Lebovitz HE. Thiazolidinediones. In: Lebovitz HE, ed. Therapy for Diabetes Mellitus and Related Disorders, 3rd edn. Alexandria, VA: American Diabetes Association; 1998, pp. 181–5.
43. Coniff RF, Seaton TB, Shjapiro JA, et al. Reduction of glycosylated hemoglobin and postprandial hyperglycemia by acarbose in patients with NIDDM. Diabetes Care 1995; 18: 817–20.
44. Lebovitz HE. Alpha-glucosidase inhibitors. Endocrinol Metab Clin N Am 1997; 26: 539–51.
45. UK Prospective Diabetes Study Group V. Characteristics of newly presenting type 2 diabetic patients: estimates of insulin sensitivity and islet beta-cell function. Diabet Med 1988; 5: 444–8.
46. UK Prospective Diabetes Study Group 16. Overview of 6 years' therapy of type 2 diabetes: a progressive disease. Diabetes 1995; 44: 1249–58.
47. The Diabetes Control and Complications Trial Research Group. The effect of intensive treatment of diabetes on the development and progression of long-term complications in insulin-dependent diabetes mellitus. N Engl J Med 1993; 329: 977–86.
48. Chmait R, Dinise T, Daneshmand S, et al. Prospective cohort study to establish predictors of glyburide success in gestational diabetes mellitus [Abstract]. Am J Obstet Gynecol 2001; 185.
49. Hellmuth E, Damm P, Molsted-Pedersen L. Oral hypoglycemic agents in 118 diabetic pregnancies. Diabetic Med 2000; 17: 507–11.
50. Lim JM, Tayob Y, O'Brien PM, Shaw RW. A comparison between the pregnancy outcome of women with gestation diabetes treated with glibenclamide and those treated with insulin. Med J Malaysia 1997; 52: 377–81.
51. Conway DL, Gonzales O, Skiver D. Use of glyburide for the treatment of gestational diabetes: the San Antonio experience. J Matern Fetal Neonatal Med 2004; 15: 51–5.
52. Kremer CJ, Duff P. Glyburide for the treatment of gestational diabetes. Am J Obstet Gynecol 2004; 190: 1438–9.
53. Gilson G, Murphy N. Comparison of oral glyburide with insulin for the management of gestational diabetes mellitus in Alaskan native women. Am J Obstet Gynecol 2002; 187: 6:(S), S152.
54. Fines V, Moore T, Castle S. A comparison of glyburide and insulin treatment in gestational diabetes mellitus on infant birth weight and adiposity. Am J Obstet Gynecol 2003; 189: 6(S), S108.
55. Jacobson GF, Ramos G, Ching J, et al. Comparison of glyburide and insulin for the management of gestational diabetes in a large managed care organization. Am J Obstet Gynecol 2005; 193: 118–24.
56. Sivan E, Feldman B, Dolitzki M, et al. Glyburide crosses the placenta in vivo in pregnant rats. Diabetologia 1995; 38: 753–6.
57. Smoak IW. Teratogenic effects of chlorpropamide in mouse embryos in vitro. Teratology 1992; 45: 474.
58. Smoak IW, Sadler TW. Embryopathic effects of short-term exposure to hypoglycemia in the mouse. Am J Obstet Gynecol 1990; 163: 619–24.
59. Denno KM, Sadler TW. Effects of the biguanide class of oral hypoglycemic agents on mouse embryogenesis. Teratology 1994; 49: 260–6.
60. Shepard TH. Catalog of Teratogenic Agents, 8th edn. Baltimore: John Hopkins University Press; 1995, p. 270.
61. Schardein JL. Chemically Induced Birth Defects, 2nd edn. New York: Marcel Dekker; 1993, pp. 417–8.
62. Audus KL. Controlling drug delivery across the placenta. Eur J Pharmacol Sci 1999; 8: 161–5.
63. Dancis J. Placental physiology. In: Kretchmer N, Quilligan EJ, Johnson JD, eds. Prenatal and Perinatal Biology and Medicine, Physiology and Growth, Vol. 1. Chur, Switzerland: Harwood Academic Publishers, 1987, pp. 1–33.
64. Enders AC, Blakenship TN. Comparative placental structure. Adv Drug Del Rev 1999; 38: 3–16.
65. Ala-Kokko TL, Vahakangas K, Pelkonen O. Placental function and principles of drug transfer. Acta Anaesth Scand 1993; 37: 47–9.
66. Sibley CP. Mechanism of ion transfer by the rat placenta: a model for the human placenta? [Review]. Placenta 1994; 15: 675–91.
67. Willis DM, O'Grady JP, Faber JJ, Thornburg KL. Diffusion permeability of cyanocobalamin in human placenta. Am J Physiol 1986; 250: R459–64.
68. Malek A, Blann E, Mattison DR. Human placental transport of oxytocin. J Matern–Fetal Med 1996; 5: 245–55.

69. Brandes JM, Travoloni N, Potter JB, et al. A new recycling technique for human placental cotyledon perfusion: application to studies of the fetomaternal transfer of glucose, insulin, and antipyrine. Am J Obstet Gynecol 1983; 146: 800–6.
70. Schenker S, Johnson R, Hays S, et al. Effects of nicotine and nicotine/ethanol on human placental amino acid transfer. Alcohol 1989; 6: 289–96.
71. Schenker S, Dicke J, Johnson R, et al. Human placental transport of cimetidine. J Clin Invest 1987; 80: 1428–34.
72. Elliot B, Schenker S, Langer O, et al. Comparative placental transport of oral hypoglycemic agents. A model of human placental drug transfer. Am J Obstet Gynecol 1994; 171: 653–60.
73. Elliot B, Langer O, Schussling F. A model of human placental drug transfer. Am J Obstet Gynecol 1997; 176: 527–30.
74. Nanovskaya TN, Nekhayeva IA, Patrikeeva SL, et al. Transfer of metformin across the dually perfused human placental lobule. Am J Obstet Gynecol 2006; 195: 1081–5.
75. Kovo N, Haroutiunian S, Feldman N, et al. Determination of metformin transfer across the human placenta using dually perfused ex-vivo placental cotyledon model [Abstract]. Am J Obstet Gynecol December 2005; 193: S85.
76. Hale TW, Kristensen JH, Hacket LP, et al. Transfer of metformin into human milk. Diabetologia 2002; 45: 1509–14.
77. Sevillano J, Lopez-Perez IC, Herrera E, et al. Englitazone administration to late pregnant rats produces delayed body growth and insulin resistance in their fetuses and neonates. Biochem J 2005; 389: 913–8.
78. Chan LYS, Yeung JH, Lau TK. Placental transfer of rosiglitazone in the first trimester of human pregnancy. Fertil Steril 2005; 83: 955–8.
79. Wareing M, Greenwood SL, Fyfe GK, et al. Glibenclamide inhibits agonist-induced vasoconstriction of placental chorionic plate arteries. Placenta 2006; 27: 660–8.
80. Klinker DR, Lim HJ, Strawn EY, et al. An in vivo murine model of rosiglitazone use in pregnancy. Fertil Steril 2006; 86(suppl. 3): 1074–9.
81. Towner D, Kjos SL, Montoro MM, et al. Congenital malformations in pregnancies complicated by NIDDM. Diabetes Care 1995; 18: 1446–51.
82. Langer O, Conway D, Berkus M, Xenakis EMJ. There is no association between hypoglycemic use and fetal anomalies [Abstract]. Am J Obstet Gynecol 1999; 180: S38.
83. Koren G. Proceedings of the NIH/FDA Toxicology in Pregnancy conference. Toronto, 2000.
84. Yogev Y, Ben-Haroush A, Chen R, et al. Undiagnosed asymptomatic hypoglycemia: Diet, insulin, and glyburide for gestational diabetic pregnancy. Obstet Gynecol 2004; 104: 88–93.
85. Langer O, Yogev Y, Xenakis E, Rosenn B. Insulin and glyburide therapy: Dosage, severity level of gestational diabetes, and pregnancy outcome. Am J Obstet Gynecol 2005; 192: 134–9.
86. Rochon M, Rand L, Roth L, Gaddipati S. Glyburide for the management of gestational diabetes: Risk factors predictive of failure and associated pregnancy outcomes. Am J Obstet Gynecol 2006; 195; 1090–4.
87. Kahn BF, Davies JK, Lynch AM, Reynolds RM, Barbour LA. Predictors of glyburide failure in the treatment of gestational diabetes. Obstet Gynecol 2006; 107: 1303–9.
88. Langer O, Most O, Monga S. Glyburide: Predictors of treatment failure in gestational diabetes [Abstract]. Am J Obstet Gynecol 2006; 195: S136.
89. Langer O, Yogev Y, Xenakis E, Brustman L. Overweight and obese in gestational diabetes: The impact on pregnancy outcome. Am J Obstet Gynecol 2005; 192: 1768–76.
90. Langer O, Monga S, Most O. Obese gestational diabetic women: Comparison of insulin and glyburide therapies [Abstract]. Am J Obstet Gynecol 2006; 195: 136S.
91. Goetzel L, Wilkins I. Glyburide compared to insulin for the treatment of gestational diabetes mellitus: a cost analysis. J Perinatol 2002; 22: 403–6.
92. Velazquez MD, Bolnick J, Cloakey D. The use of glyburide in the management of gestational diabetes. Obstet & Gynecol 2003; (Suppl. 88S): 101–4.
93. Pendsey SP, Sharma RR, Chalkhore SS. Repaglinde: A feasible alternative to insulin in management of gestational diabetes mellitus. Diabetes Res Clin Pract 2002; 56 Suppl. (1); S46 (OR103).
94. Moore L, Clokey D, Briery C, et al. Metformin use in gestational diabetes: efficacy and maternal and neonatal outcomes. Am J Obstet Gynecol 2006; 195(6); S142 (Abs).
95. Kitzmiller J. Limited efficacy of glyburide for glycemic control. Am J Obstet Gynecol 2001; 185: S198.
96. Coetzee EJ, Jackson WPU: Pregnancy in established noninsulin-dependent diabetics. S A Med J 1980; 61: 795–802.

29 Continuous glucose monitoring during pregnancies complicated by diabetes mellitus

Yariv Yogev, Rony Chen and Moshe Hod

Introduction

Gestational diabetes mellitus (GDM), defined as 'carbohydrate intolerance of variable severity with onset or rest recognition during pregnancy'[1] occurs in almost 4% of all pregnancies in the United States, but the actual prevalence may differ with ethnicity and maternal age.[2] Women with high blood glucose levels experience a greater risk of adverse maternal and fetal outcomes, including pre-eclampsia, Cesarean delivery, macrosomia, congenital anomalies and increased risk for future development of Type 2 diabetes.[3] The most common and significant neonatal complication clearly associated with GDM is macrosomia.[4] The greatest danger of macrosomia lies in its association with increased risk of birth injuries and asphyxia. In untreated GDM the risk of macrosomia is as high as 40% of neonates.[5] In addition, neonatal macrosomia is associated with the metabolic syndrome of hyperinsulinemia and deposition of fat in the visceral cavity.[6] The literature has documented that intensified management for GDM reduces the rate of neonatal complications and can normalize birthweight.[7] At the same time, others are concerned that attempts at tight control can increase the risk for severe hypoglycemia that may also compromise the well-being of both mother and fetus.[8] Therefore, the goal of achieving desired levels of glucose became a patient–care provider initiative.

Understanding 'normality': Glycemic profile in normal and diabetic pregnancies

Traditionally, in the management of diabetes complicating pregnancy, various methods of glucose monitoring (urine strips, plasma, capillary and, more recently, continuous glucose monitoring (CGM)) as well as different timing have been proposed, including the measurement of fasting, preprandial, postprandial, and mean 24-h blood glucose concentrations.[1,9,10]

Moreover, several authors have emphasized the association between postprandial glucose determinations and pregnancy outcome.[11,12] Interestingly, these recommendations were not evidently based on the extent of deviation from normal glycemic physiology, but rather on the association between pregnancy outcome and various measures of glucose levels.

Diurnal glycemic profile in nondiabetic pregnancies

Until recently, only a paucity of data existed concerning the normal glycemic profile in nondiabetic pregnancies.[13–15] Moreover, these pioneering studies included small sample sizes in a hospital setting, under strict diet limitations; and in fact, some of the evaluated subjects were diabetic,[13] in addition, collected data included only a single day of evaluation during the third trimester. Moreover, no stratification was performed for maternal obesity. In a more recent study[16] the maternal glycemic profile was evaluated using self-monitoring blood glucose in non-obese nondiabetic women during the third trimester suggesting a gradual increase in daily mean glucose during this time.

In a recent study, Yogev et al.[17] used continuous glucose monitoring in nondiabetic obese and non-obese gravid patients. Fifty-seven gravid women were studied, and eligibility was limited to women with singleton pregnancies, after completion of 20 weeks of pregnancy, with normal GCT (<130 mg/dL) or normal OGTT. Women diagnosed with GDM in prior pregnancies were excluded. During the study period, all women were asked to refrain from lifestyle modification or dietary restriction. Patients were connected for 72 consecutive hours and were unaware of the results of the sensor measurements during the monitoring period. During this period, they also performed fingerstick capillary glucose measurements in the morning after overnight fasting and 2 h after meals (six to eight times per day) using a reflectance monitor and self-coded the data into the monitor.

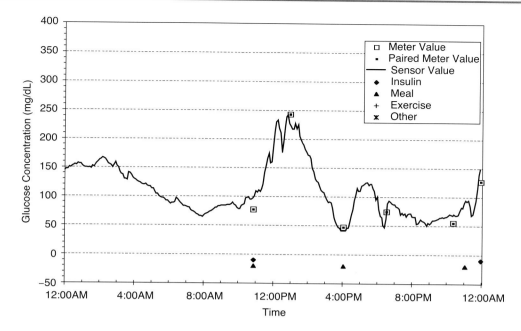

Figure 29.1   Twenty-four-hour glucose monitoring using the continuous glucose monitoring system.

Quality control measures of glucose levels from the meter, sensor, and plasma glucose were performed at the initial time of connection to the continuous glucose monitoring system and again at study completion.

The continuous glucose monitoring system (MiniMed, Sylmar, CA) was used in all cases. The system measures glucose levels in subcutaneous interstitial tissue. It is composed of a disposable subcutaneous glucose-sensing device and an electrode impregnated with glucose oxidase connected by a cable to a lightweight monitor. The system takes a glucose measurement every 10 s, based on the electrochemical detection of glucose by its reaction with glucose oxidase (Figure 29.1), and stores an average value every 5 min, for a total of 288 measurements each day. The time delay between glucose values of venous plasma and subcutaneous concentrations is given with maximal 5 min. The software for the download of the sensor data takes this delay into consideration, avoiding the need for further corrections. It has been demonstrated that the correlation coefficient (r) between the glucose measurements by the sensor and meter was 0.93 ± 0.04, and between the plasma glucose, reflectance meter monitoring, and sensor recording, 0.91 ± 0.02.[18] The patients were instructed to code the time of food intake at the beginning of the meal into the monitor. The patients' level of physical activity was not standardized and all were instructed to go about their normal daily routines.

Approximately 750 glucose determinations were obtained for each subject during this time period. Thus, ambulatory glycemic profile during second half of pregnancy was characterized enabling defining normal glycemia in pregnancy (Table 29.1). When we further analyzed the glycemic profile we found no difference in preprandial values during the day and significantly lower mean blood glucose levels during the night time (23:00 pm to 06:00 am) in comparison to day time (Table 29.1). These findings are lower than previously

reported[13,14] but in agreement with others.[15] Thus, our data may provide the actual unbiased characterization of glycemic profile in the second half of pregnancy which may imply the level of glycemia to be aimed for in the pregnant diabetic in order to mirror normoglycemia.

Postprandial glycemic profile: A hint for improved management?

A review of the literature suggests that the risk of macrosomia rise as maternal glycemia increase.[19–21] Specifically, the risk of macrosomia appears to increase with increasing postprandial glucose levels.[22–24] Thus, the American Diabetes Association (ADA) recommends postprandial glucose monitoring in pregnancies complicated by diabetes.[1]

Table 29.1   Ambulatory glycemic profile and postprandial glucose levels in nondiabetic pregnancies[17]

Parameter	
Mean blood glucose (mg/dL)	83.7 ± 18
Fasting glucose (mg/dL)	75 ± 12
Preprandial glucose (mg/dL)	78 ± 11
Peak postprandial glucose value (mg/dL)	110 ± 16
Peak postprandial time (min)	70 ± 13
Mean blood glucose of 3-h postprandial measurements (mg/dL)	98 ± 12
1-h postprandial glucose value (mg/dL)	105 ± 12
2-h postprandial glucose value (mg/dL)	97 ± 10
3-h postprandial glucose value (mg/dL)	84 ± 14
Mean blood glucose – night-time (mg/dL)	68 ± 10

Additionally, controversy exists regarding the most appropriate postprandial timing that correlates the best to perinatal outcome: 1-h or 2-h postprandial glucose determinations. Same controversy exists with regard to the appropriate threshold (<140 mg/dL in 1-h and <120 mg/dL 2-h postprandial) to define normality.[22,24–26] Ben-Haroush et al.[27] demonstrated that the time interval from meal to peak postprandial glucose levels (approximately 90 min) was similar in all the evaluated types of diabetic pregnancies (Type 1, GDM insulin-treated or diet only) and is not affected by the level of glycemic control. Moreover, no difference was obtained in postprandial glycemic profile between breakfast, lunch or dinner. We recognize that future studies should look for the association between postprandial glucose values at 90 min and pregnancy outcome prior to recommending 90 min as the proper time for postprandial glucose analysis. Now that more rapid-acting insulin analogs are available, it is possible to blunt the peak postprandial glucose response without fear of subsequent hypoglycemia. The timing of the peak response is yet to be agreed upon. Once the timing of the highest blood glucose levels of the day in pregnant diabetic women are known, then treatment strategies to minimize this peak, and thus minimize the risk of macrosomia, can be developed. Yogev et al.[17] demonstrated that in nondiabetic gravid subjects that peak glucose value is achieved at approximately 70 min postprandial at a mean glucose level of 110 mg/dL. Therefore, should the postprandial threshold be modified in GDM patients, or should the targeted postprandial values in the pregnant diabetic remain higher than the postprandial values found in nondiabetic women rationalize further study? The controversy remains, however, as to the exclusive role of maternal glucose in the etiology of macrosomia. In fact, there are still reports that macrosomia can manifest 'despite normoglycemia'.[5,21]

The use of CGM for treatment evaluation

The wide range of glucose values obtained with the use of the CGM provides the opportunity to identify both unrecognized hyperglycemia and hypoglycemic events in comparison to self-monitoring blood glucose.

Undetected hyperglycemia

In pregnancies complicated with Type 1 diabetes, Yogev et al.[18] demonstrated a mean total time (192 ± 28 min/day) of undetected hyperglycemia (glucose levels >140 mg/dL) identified by CGM. The approximate 3-h hyperglycemia recorded throughout the day would not be recognized if self-monitoring blood glucose was used alone. Furthermore, when GDM patients were evaluated[28] the mean total time of hyperglycemia was 132 ± 31 min/day for insulin treated GDM and 94 ± 23 min/day for GDM patients treated with diet only. One possibility that macrosomia has persisted despite intensified care protocols is that we miss times during the day when glucose levels are elevated. These events were discovered to be unscheduled meals not detected by conventional self-blood glucose protocols. Furthermore, these elevations of blood glucose often occurred shortly after patients took fasting and postprandial finger stick glucose determinations that indicated that their glucose levels were in the target ranges. Importantly, no correlation was found between higher levels of HbA1c and hyperglycemic episodes, another finding supporting the weak association between HbA1c and glucose level monitoring in pregnancy.

Undetected hypoglycemia

Despite years of meticulous study, there is still a paucity of information regarding the optimal level of glycemia in diabetic pregnancy which clinicians should target to safely reduce maternal and perinatal morbidity. Strict metabolic control in this patient population has been associated with an increased risk of maternal hypoglycemia. Rosenn et al.[8] reported significant hypoglycemia, defined as hypoglycemia requiring assistance from another person, in 71% of gravid patients with Type 1 diabetes with a peak incidence in the first trimester. In our study, using CGM, in Type 1 gravid patients, hypoglycemic events were recorded in 76% of the patients, most of the episodes were nocturnal, some of them asymptomatic.[18] Interestingly, in all cases, an interval of 1-4 h preceded clinical manifestations. When GDM patients were assessed, hypoglycemic events were recorded in 58% of the patients, all of them insulin-treated.[28] The impact of maternal hypoglycemia on human fetal development and neonatal outcome has not been extensively studied. Although concern about the hazards of hypoglycemia are related primarily to the pregnant mother, the potential effects on the developing fetus need to be considered as well. In order to estimate the prevalence of undiagnosed, asymptomatic hypoglycemic events that occur in diabetic patients and to evaluate whether the rate of asymptomatic hypoglycemic episodes vary under different modalities of treatment for gestational diabetes, Yogev et al.[29] conducted a study using CGM on GDM patients treated with glyburide, insulin or diet only. Asymptomatic hypoglycemic events were found to be common during pharmacological treatment in GDM. However, patients treated with glyburide had significantly fewer asymptomatic hypoglycemic events than insulin-treated patients. Patients treated with diet alone and in nondiabetic women, no hypoglycemic events were identified. Our findings may be explained by treatment modality as the side effect of pharmacological glycemic control during pregnancy rather than by the pathogenesis of the disease.

Algorithms for management using continuous glucose monitoring

Kaufman et al.[30] demonstrated that CGM could serve as a clinical tool for clinical decision-making and glycemic control in children with Type 1 diabetes. In another recent work, Hershkovitz et al.[31] demonstrated the clinical implications of CGM use to assess and manage asymptomatic hypoglycemic events in children with glycogen storage disease. Jovanovic has showed that CGM profiles allowed the physician to identify glucose patterns and to better target diabetic treatment.

The treatment changes would not have been made on the basis of meter data alone.[32]

In a pilot study, Yogev et al.[33] studied eight women with diabetes in pregnancy, of whom six were Type 1 and 2 were GDM. Data derived from the CGM for 72 h were assessed and treatment was adjusted on the basis of the findings. Two to four weeks later, the patients were re-evaluated with CGM. In the second time period, a significant reduction in mean blood glucose, hypoglycemic events and duration of undetected hyperglycemia was demonstrated. Recently, Kerssen et al.[34] reported that since there is a wide variability in the day-to-day glucose levels of pregnant women with Type 1 diabetes, the use of CGM raises a problem for adjustment of therapy. They concluded that fine-tuning of insulin regimens based on 3-day measurements with the CGM method is not advisable.

In order to respond to the subheading query above, several conditions need to be met. A sample size should be large enough to provide data on pregnancy outcome; the study should include at least two groups: one using self-monitoring blood glucose and the second CGM and glucose testing must be performed throughout pregnancy since a 3-day testing cannot predict level of glycemia. These are the limitations of the current research using CMG. However, we need to be mindful that CGM is still an experimental measure and not a routine clinical tool. The frequency needed for CGM monitoring in diabetic pregnancy and its hypothetical advantage over self-monitoring blood glucose in enhancing pregnancy outcome still needs to be demonstrated. A large prospective study on maternal and neonatal outcome is needed to evaluate the clinical implications of this new monitoring technique.

Conclusions

Many physicians have had the experience of managing women with GDM who appeared to have good glycemic control based on their SBGM diaries and HbA1c; nonetheless, these women still delivered a macrosomic infant. It may be that using CGM in GDM women can reveal high postprandial blood glucose levels unrecognized by intermittent blood glucose determinations. CGM shows where and how hyperglycemia that might contribute to neonatal complications is occurring, and provides a useful tool to help educate patients in behavior modifications that can improve compliance with the management regimen.

REFERENCES

1. Metzger BE, Coustan DR. Summary and recommendations of the Fourth International Workshop–Conference on Gestational Diabetes Mellitus. The Organizing Committee. Diabetes Care 1998; 21 (suppl. 2): B161–7.
2. Engelgau M, German R, Herman W, et al. The epidemiology of diabetes and pregnancy in the US, 1988. Diabetes Care 1995; 18: 1029–33.
3. McCance DR, Pettitt DJ, Hanson RL, et al. Birth weight and non-insulin-dependent diabetes: thrifty genotype, thrifty phenotype, or surviving small baby genotype? Br Med J 1994; 398: 942–5.
4. Langer O, Mazze R. The relationship between large-for-gestational-age infants and glycemic control in women with gestational diabetes. Am J Obstet Gynecol 1988; 159: 1478–83.
5. Persson B, Hanson U. Neonatal morbidities in gestational diabetes mellitus. Diabetes Care 1998; 21(suppl. 2): B79–84.
6. Jovanovic L, Crues J, Durak E, Peterson CM. Magnetic resonance imaging in pregnancies complicated by diabetes predicts infant birthweight ratio and neonatal morbidity. Am J Perinatol 1993; 10: 432–7.
7. Jovanovic L, Bevier W, Peterson CM. The Santa Barbara County Health Care Services Program: birth weight change concomitant with screening for and treatment of glucose-intolerance of pregnancy: a potential cost-effective intervention. Am J Perinatol 1997; 14: 221–8.
8. Rosenn BM, Miodovnik M. Glycemic control in the diabetic pregnancy: is tighter always better? J Maternal–Fetal Med 2000; 9: 29–34.
9. Langer O. A spectrum of glucose thresholds may effectively prevent complications in the pregnant diabetic patient. Semin Perinatol 2002; 26: 196–205.
10. Langer O, Berkus M, Brustman L, et al. Rationale for insulin management in gestational diabetes mellitus. Diabetes 1991; 40(suppl. 2): 186–90.
11. Jovanovic-Peterson L, Peterson CM, Reed GF, et al. Maternal postprandial glucose levels and infant birth weight: the Diabetes in Early Pregnancy Study. The National Institute of Child Health and Human Development – Diabetes in Early Pregnancy Study. Am J Obstet Gynecol 1991; 164: 103–11.
12. de Veciana M, Major CA, Morgan MA, et al. Postprandial versus preprandial blood glucose monitoring in women with gestational diabetes mellitus requiring N Engl J Med 1995; 333: 1237–41.
13. Gillmer MD, Beard RW, Brooke FM, et al. Carbohydrate metabolism in pregnancy. Part I. Diurnal plasma glucose profile in normal and diabetic women. Br Med J 1975; 3: 399–402.
14. Cousins L, Rigg L, Hollingsworth D, et al. The 24-hour excursion and diurnal rhythm of glucose, insulin, and C-peptide in normal pregnancy. Am J Obstet Gynecol 1980; 136: 483–8.
15. Phelps RL, Metzger BE, Freinkel N. Carbohydrate metabolism in pregnancy. XVII. Diurnal profiles of plasma glucose, insulin, free fatty acids, triglycerides, cholesterol, and individual amino acids in late normal pregnancy. Am J Obstet Gynecol. 1981; 140: 730–6.
16. Parretti E, Mecacci F, Papini M, et al. Third-trimester maternal glucose levels from diurnal profiles in nondiabetic pregnancies: correlation with sonographic parameters of fetal growth. Diabetes Care 2001; 24: 1319–23.
17. Yogev Y, Ben-Haroush A, Chen R, et al. Diurnal glycemic profile in obese and normal weight non-diabetic pregnant women. Am J Obstet Gynecol 2004; 191: 949–53.
18. Yogev Y, Chen R, Ben-Haroush A, et al. Continuous glucose monitoring for the evaluation of gravid women with type 1 diabetes women. Obstet Gynecol 2003; 101: 633–8.
19. Hod M, Rabinerson D, Peled Y, et al. Gestational diabetes mellitus: is it a clinical entity? Diabetes Rev 1995; 3: 603–13.
20. Ogata ES. Perinatal morbidity in offspring of diabetic mothers. Diabetes Rev 1995; 3: 652–7.
21. Langer O. Is normoglycemia the correct threshold to prevent complications in the pregnant diabetic patient? Diabetes Rev 1995; 4: 2–10.
22. Jovanovic L, Reed GF, Metzger BE, et al. Maternal postprandial glucose levels and infant birth weight: the Diabetes in Early Pregnancy Study. The National Institute of Child Health and Human Development – Diabetes in Early Pregnancy Study. Am J Obstet Gynecol 1991; 164: 103–11.
23. Combs CA, Gunderson E, Kitzmiller JL, et al. Relationship of fetal macrosomia to maternal postprandial glucose control during pregnancy. Diabetes Care 1992; 15: 1251–7.
24. deVeciana M, Major CA, Morgan MA. Postprandial versus pre-prandial blood glucose monitoring in women with gestational diabetes mellitus requiring insulin therapy. N Engl J Med 1995; 333: 1237–41.
25. Langer O, Carver K, Langer M. Postprandial glucose determinations: Are one and two hours the same? Arch Per Med 2002; 8: 7–8.
26. Sivan E, Weisz B, Homko C, et al. One or two hours postprandial glucose measurements: Are they the same? Am J Obstet Gynecol 2001; 185: 604–7.
27. Ben-Haroush A, Yogev Y, Chen R, et al. The postprandial glucose profile in the diabetic pregnancy. Am J Obstet Gynecol 2004; 191: 576–81.

28. Chen R, Yogev Y, Ben-Haroush A, et al. Continuous glucose monitoring for the evaluation and improved control of gestational diabetes mellitus. J Matern Fetal Neonatal Med 2003; 14: 256–60.
29. Yogev Y, Ben-Haroush A, Chen R, et al. Undiagnosed asymptomatic hypoglycemia: diet, insulin, and glyburide for gestational diabetic pregnancy. Obstet Gynecol 2004; 104: 88–93.
30. Kaufman FR, Gibson LC, Halvorson M, et al. A pilot study of the continuous glucose monitoring system: clinical decisions and glycemic control after its use in pediatric type 1 diabetic subjects. Diabetes Care 2001; 24: 2030–4.
31. Hershkovitz E, Rachmel A, Ben-Zaken H, et al, Continuous glucose monitoring in children with glycogen storage disease type-1. J Inherit Metab Dis 2001; 24: 863–9.
32. Jovanovic L. The role of continuous glucose monitoring in gestational diabetes mellitus. Diabetes Tech Therapeut 2000; 2(suppl. 1): S67–71.
33. Yogev Y, Ben-Haroush A, Chen R, et al. Continuous glucose monitoring for treatment adjustment in diabetic pregnancies – a pilot study. Diabet Med 2003; 20: 558–62.
34. Kerssen A, de Valk HW, Visser GH. Day-to-day glucose variability during pregnancy in women with Type 1 diabetes mellitus: Glucose profiles measured with the Continuous Glucose Monitoring System. Br J Obstet Gynaecol 2004; 111: 919–24.

30 Insulin pumps in pregnancy

Ohad Cohen

Introduction

The management of diabetes in pregnancy, as put forward by the 'St. Vincent' declaration, is aimed at achieving near normal pregnancy outcomes.[1] Although a decrease in the rates of major malformations, and spontaneous abortions had occurred vis a vis improvement in glycemic control, the goals have not yet been achieved.[2,3] Only 40–60% of women with pre-existing diabetes achieve optimal glycemic control while pregnant.[4]

One of the major barriers to achieving the St Vincent goals for pregnancy is the failure to timely obtain physiological glycemic targets.[5] Recent studies using continuous glucose sensing technology have shown that physiological glycemic levels are lower than the treatment targets set for the management of diabetes in pregnancy.[6] There is also a discrepancy between the guidelines HbA1c goal of <7% on the one hand and the requirements to maintain blood glucose levels within the normal (nondiabetic) range on the other hand, which entails a HbA1c level of less than 5.5%.[6,7]

Obtaining physiological glucose levels, safely, during pregnancy is difficult as major barriers are:

- Increasing rates of hypoglycemia
- Narrow glycemic range
- Variability in insulin absorption from the nonphysiological subcutaneous insulin delivery depot
- Changing insulin requirements during pregnancy, due to weight gain and increasing insulin resistance
- Pregnancy-related gastrointestinal problems, e.g. hyperemesis gravidarum, reflux disease

This chapter reviews the benefits of using a continuous subcutaneous insulin infusion (CSII) – an insulin pump – for addressing the above obstacles. Given the paucity of studies addressing the use of insulin pump therapy specifically in pregnancy, we also rely on data from nonpregnant Type 1 diabetic patients.

CSII decreases the rates of hypoglycemia

Hypoglycemia is a major problem in pregnant women,[8] secondary to both the intensification of insulin treatment and to the decline of the counter-regulatory response to hypoglycemia during pregnancy. Rates of severe hypoglycemia has

been reported to reach 71% of pregnant women, in whom glycemic goals were set at 100 mg/dL fasting and 140 mg/dL at 90 min post-meal by Rosenn et al.[9] They found an overall incidence of 6.68 episodes per patient per pregnancy of severe hypoglycemia, equivalent to an incidence of 894 episodes per 100 patient-years. The DCCT trial reported fewer cases: 58 cases of severe hypoglycemia per 270 pregnancies.

CSII has been consistent in showing reduction in hypoglycemia while maintaining low HbA1c. Bode et al.[10] demonstrated a significant reduction in major hypoglycemic events during the first year of CSII use when hypoglycemic rates decreased from 138 episodes per 100 patient-years to 22 episodes; a reduction that was sustained for at least 4 years.[10] An approximately 80% drop in hypoglycemic episodes with CSII was similarly described in the UK[11] and Germany.[12] This reduction in hypoglycemia can potentially cause partial recovery of the counter-regulatory response responsible for hypoglycemic awareness,[13] further increasing the safety of intensive insulin therapy. In the only prospective and randomized trial of CSII in pregnancy conducted more than 20 years ago, a trend for less hypoglycemia with pump was noted, although not powered to reach statistical significance.[14]

Increasing awareness of hypoglycemia and prevention of hypoglycemia are, therefore, important indications for the use of CSII in Type 1 diabetic patients, pregnant and nonpregnant alike.

Improvement in glycemic control with CSII

The current goals of glycemic control in pregnancy is defined by the measurements of pre-meal and 1-h post meal capillary glucose levels and HbA1c. Several meta-analyses of randomized controlled trials in nonpregnant Type 1 diabetic patients[15–17] indicate that CSII is advantageous over multiple daily injections of insulin (MDI) to obtain better glycemic control. The average differences between CSII and MDI were reduction in HbA1c of 0.5% and reduction in mean blood glucose concentration of 18 mg/dL. Beyond the improvement in the above glycemic indices, use of CSII also improves glycemic control by decreasing glycemic excursions[18] in nonpregnant diabetics and in pregnancy as well.[19] These glycemic excursions, have recently been implicated as a cause for diabetes related complications and the reduction in glucose excursions is currently gaining importance as a therapeutic goal.[20] Glycemic excursions might also underlie diabetic fetopathy as malformations and macrosomia[7,21] was reported in women with low HbA1c but high excursions.

Though not all agree,[22] it is generally accepted that reducing HbA1c and glycemic excursions are indications for CSII in pregnancy.

CSII decreases variability in insulin absorption

Variability in the action of insulin can cause fluctuations in glucose levels leading to the unpredictability of glucose levels. The cause is multifactorial; among those described[23] are different injections sites, physical activity, insulin preparations, insulin dose, insulin handling and mixing. Continuous subcutaneous insulin infusion offers a precise and a reproducible way of insulin administration resulting in less variability in absorption rates (<3%) in comparison to MDI.[24,25] Contributing factors to the stability of insulin absorption is the single site of a continuous low rate flow of insulin (preferably a short-acting analogue) that prevents inter-regional variation in absorption, prevention of a subcutaneous reservoir formation and thus preventing third-space dynamics. The use of the distended abdominal region during pregnancy is not associated with clinically significant changes in insulin absorption. CSII decreases glycemic variability by stabilizing day-to-day insulin absorption.

CSII and pregnancy-related adjustments in insulin requirements

Insulin requirements during pregnancy change significantly in comparison to the nonpregnant state. These changes are caused by the physiological increase in insulin resistance that accompanies pregnancy and the weight gain. The adjustment of insulin treatment dose is complex because the increase is not linear and there are in-between periods of reduction in the insulin requirements. It is important to follow patients meticulously and to change the insulin doses appropriately. During gestation, the periods of decrease in insulin requirements are around week 12 and during periods when food intake is reduced. Notably, when patients suffer from hyperemesis gravidarum, particularly in the first trimester, and when the pregnancy induces reflux disorders later on in gestation, patients suffer nausea and vomiting and thus decrease their food intake and insulin requirements. These constant changes and the need for sudden dose adjustments is best met by CSII which is currently the most flexible insulin delivery system available.[26]

Disadvantages of CSII

The major disadvantage of CSII is ketoacidosis resulting from disturbance in insulin delivery. Though pump malfunction is rarely the cause for ketoacidosis, occlusions of the infusion sets and/or cannula by a mechanical kink or deposits can cause nondelivery of insulin. In these cases occlusion detectors provide alarms triggered by increasing pressure in the system.

More problematic, are low pressures; the more common cause is dislodgement of the catheter, empty reservoir, air bubbles, and back-flow along the Teflon catheter (tunneling). In these cases the (currently used) alarms are not triggered. When the insulin flow is abruptly stopped a rapid increase in blood glucose is observed, especially when short-acting analogs are used. Furthermore, in 2 h, a significant increase in ketones is observed reaching dangerous levels above 1 mmole/L in 6 h.[27–29] In pregnancy, due to the predisposition towards ketone production, the increase might be earlier, with poor consequences for both the mother and fetus. It is therefore imperative that pregnant diabetic women on CSII be compliant with blood glucose monitoring (at least four times daily), as such monitoring will serve as a timely detection of insulin delivery problems. When appropriate patient selection is fulfilled then an actual decrease in ketoacidosis is observed in pregnant diabetic women on CSII.[30,31]

Additional problems encountered are a wide range of skin reaction from mild irritations ('tape allergy') to subcutaneous abscesses. Proper skin care and adherence to pump-use rules will prevent and treat most of theses reactions. Special hypoallergenic tapes and skin barriers are available to alleviate most problems. Skin reactions are not a significant cause for discontinuation of pump use.

In 2006, the European Association of Perinatal Medicine proposed the following indications and contraindications for the use of CSII in pregnancy:

Indications

- Preconception use of CSII
- Insufficient goal attainment
- Recurrent hypoglycemia
- Instability and significant excursions of glucose levels

Contraindications

- Noncompliance with frequent glucose monitoring
- Non-adherence to follow-up
- Guaranteed supply of disposables and technical support

Insulin pumps: Hardware and disposables

Insulin pumps that are currently available carry the following components:

- Insulin reservoir placed in the housing containing the pump
- Infusion sets
- Teflon cannula to a subcutaneous depot

The insulin pump weighs between 75 and 107 g. It holds the insulin reservoir, the volume of which differs between the models and varies between 2 and 3 mL (200 and 300 U). As the reservoir is changed every 2–3 days, the choice of model is dependent upon the daily insulin dosage. As the daily use of insulin at close to delivery averages 1.2 U/kg it is recommended to choose pumps with 3-mL reservoirs. The different models shown in Figure 30.1 have much in common. Differences can be noted regarding reservoir volume and water compatibility.

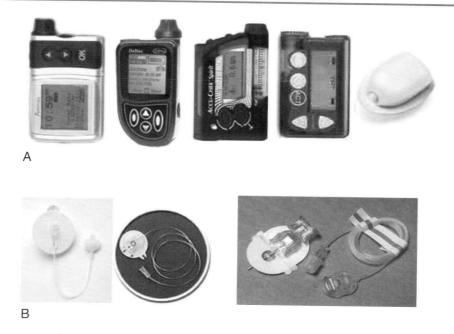

Figure 30.1 (A) Various types of insulin pump. From left to right: Animas IR-1250; Deltec Cozmo; ACCU-CHEK Spirit; Medtronic MiniMed Paradigm 522/722 and OmniPod.(B) Various infusion sets.

Infusion sets have various lengths and the choice will depend on the patient's height and pump positioning preference. Typical lengths of the infusions sets are 23, 24, 31, 42, and 43 inches.

Most cannulas used today are made of Teflon, introduced subcutaneously with a removable metal inserter. Cannulas of older designs used metal needles that were less secured to the skin and, currently, are used on rare occasions when patients have skin reactions to the Teflon tube. The cannulas have two basic designs: a straight in cannula that is inserted perpendicular to the skin, and a slanted design inserted at an angle of 30–45. The length of the cannula varies from 9 to 12 mm for the straight design and 13–17 mm for the slanted design. The typical gauge is 27. Choice of the design depends on the patient's weight and subcutaneous tissue thickness. For pregnancy the 9 mm straight or slanted design is recommended. A approximately 3 mm depth marks the subcutaneous delivery threshold.

The area of choice for insertion is usually the abdominal area where the absorption is rapid and consistent, avoiding areas of tissue scars and proximity (2 cm) to the naval area.

During pregnancy when the abdomen becomes too firm to pinch up subcutaneous tissue, the upper outer thigh or hip may be used instead. The upper arm is also an option, although many people find that dealing with the catheter tubing is quite awkward with an arm placement. The infusion sets should be changed and insertion site rotated every 2–3 days.

Insulin pumps: Bolus calculators and software

Bolus calculators

Strict control of postprandial hyperglycemia in pregnancy requires complex calculation of the meal insulin dose: the bolus dose. Among the multiple factors needed to be considered in determining the bolus dose are (1) target blood glucose, (2) current blood glucose, (3) carbohydrate-to-insulin ratios (CIR), (4) total grams of carbohydrate (CHO) in the meal, and (5) insulin sensitivity factors (ISF).[32]

Some of these factors are modifiable, such as the amount of carbohydrates (CHO) to be consumed and planed exercise; some are non modifiable, such as the insulin sensitivity, which varies with the week of gestation and has diurnal variations. Additional factor to be considered is the insulin-action time (the pharmacodynamics) of the previous injected insulin boluses ('active insulin').

Advanced insulin pumps (e.g. Medtronic Mnimed Paradigm X12 and X22, Animas IR-1250) have integrated bolus calculators that provide bolus decision support to the patients. Using these calculators, the patient provides the modifiable factor – meal CHO and the current capillary blood glucose levels – and the calculator generates a recommended bolus insulin dose based on predefined sensitivity factors, glycemic targets, and considering the active insulin. Use of bolus insulin doses computed by a bolus calculator, has been shown to improve attainment of target postprandial blood glucose but with fewer correction boluses and supplemental carbohydrate.[33]

Insulin pumps: Software

An important component of up-to-date insulin pump therapy is the computer-based information management system. These systems include both the software and the hardware for uploading and downloading data. Incorporation of these systems in the clinical setting enables the integration of the ever-growing data accumulated during the daily use of insulin pumps, and provides a unified platform useful for clinical decision making and as an educational tool. Input includes:

- Health team-generated information – basal rates, carbohydrate to insulin ratios, correction factors
- Information on patient's pattern of insulin use – total daily insulin use, basal/bolus ratios, bolus patterns, pump disconnection periods
- Information on the patient's daily activity – meals, carbohydrate content of meals, exercise
- Glucose measurements either from self-monitoring blood glucose (SMBG) or from continuous glucose monitoring (CGM)

An illustration of such an information management system is shown in Figure 30.2. In this system (e.g. CareLink Medtronic Minimed) the patient can download the data collected on the pump and on the glucose meter either at home or at the clinic. Data is then sent over the Internet to a server that can be accessed by an authorized physician. The integrated data can then be seen and processed by the health-providing team through different screens that enable clinical decision making. As seen in Figure 30.3, the daily detail screen of the CareLink data management system provides, in a single screen, the glucose levels measured by both the glucose meter and by the continuous glucose sensor on the top, the insulin delivered as basal and boluses in the middle, and the estimated carbohydrates ingested at each meal with exercise at bottom of the screen. This comprehensive presentation assists in evaluating and adjusting the needs of therapy (glucose levels, meals, and exercise) with the measures taken: insulin delivery as basal and bolus insulin. Additional computerized support systems are currently under development.

Initiating insulin pump therapy

Timing of initiation of pump therapy

Preconception care to achieve stringent blood glucose has been advocated in order to reduce the rate of malformations.[33] As such, it is recommended that an insulin pump is initiated at the preconception visits mainly to ensure that technical difficulties will be overcome by training prior to conception thus avoiding unnecessary ketosis and hyperglycemia, and to ensure proper patient selection. Nevertheless, initiation during pregnancy, provided proper patients are selected, can be achieved in an outpatient setting.[34]

Initiating basal rate

Management and prescription of insulin delivery by pumps during pregnancy should be performed by experienced health professionals, in a multidisciplinary set-up including a fetal–maternal gynecologist, endocrinologist, diabetes nurse, and a dietitian. Basal insulin is usually based on the following considerations:

- Prevailing basal insulin dose
- Current glycemic control (HbA1c, SMBG)
- Timing in respect of gestational stage (preconception, week of gestation)
- Extent of hypoglycemic events

In establishing the total basal amount, the following points concerning daily insulin have to be considered: total long-term acting insulin (Glargine), total intermediate acting insulin (Determir, NPH), and the relative amount of the intermediate acting insulin in the mixtures used (75% of Humalog75/25, 70% of the Humulin/Novolin/Novalog 70/30, 50% of Humulin/Humalog50/50) (brand names might differ in different countries).

In most cases the total basal insulin will consist of 50–60% of the total mean daily insulin used by the patient. In adjusting the dosage for pump use it is usually recommended to decrease the total dose by 20–25%. This adjustment can vary according to specific circumstances. For example if the HbA1c is higher than the desired a smaller correction (−10%) can be made. On the hand, if the total insulin used is too high, as exemplified by recurrent hypoglycemia, high carbohydrate intake, or when restrictive dietary measures are planned, the reduction of basal insulin dose can be greater.

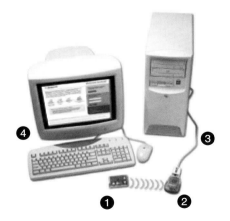

1. Paradigm® 515 or 715 insulin pump
2. Paradigm link® blood glucose monitor
3. Paradigm link interface cable
4. Web-based access to the *medtronic carelink®* *therapy management system for diabetes system*

Figure 30.2   An information management system.

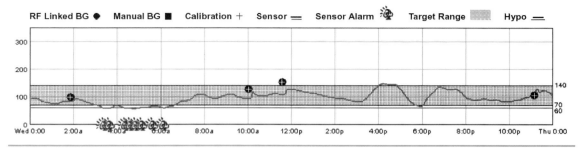

Insulin Delivery

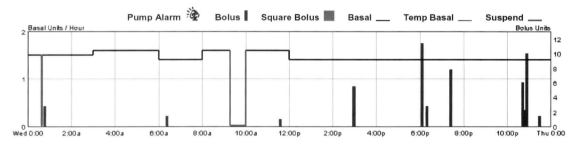

Carbohydrates and Exercise

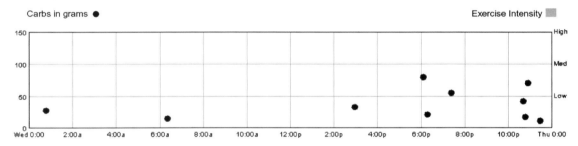

Figure 30.3   Daily details as seen with the CareLink data management system.

Pregnancy is unique in the sense that profound changes in insulin requirement are exhibited during gestation and that these changes are not linear.[35–37] As described in Table 30.1, the first days post-conception are characterized by a slight decline in subcutaneous MDI insulin requirements (median, 0.66 U/kg), following an increase to a first peak of 0.77 U/kg by gestational week 7, declining to 0.69 U/kg at week 15. Thereafter a gradual increase is noted till weeks 36–38 when

the average total dose is 1.0 U/kg ending by a small decrease at 38–40 weeks of gestation. These total insulin dosages are averages and individual 'tailoring' of insulin requirements is needed specifically to accommodate for severe weight gain.

Once the daily insulin requirements are calculated followed by the 20% total dose reduction, 50–60% is then calculated as the basal insulin to be delivered in 24 h. In nonpregnant Type 1 individuals the basal rate is not constant, rather, there is a 3-fold increase in the basal insulin requirements between 6 and 9 a.m. (or earlier depending on the awakening time) requiring changes in basal rate via insulin pumps from 4 to 7.[38] This 'dawn phenomenon' relates to a circadian increase in glucose counter-regulatory hormones mainly GH. A second increase in insulin requirements in noted in the late afternoon ('dusk phenomenon') but the physiological explanation is not as clear. Although no clear evidence for the persistence of the above diurnal variation in basal insulin requirements into pregnancy, in clinical practice, most pregnant women will require at least three infusion rates in a 24-h period,[36] with a low basal rate from midnight to 4 a.m., increasing in the early morning hours and back to the average at around 8–9 a.m.

As an example, a 32-year-old P2G2 Type 1 diabetic patient in her 17th week of gestation is currently using two NPH injections a day, 14 in the morning and 10 at dinner time and

Table 30.1   Variation in insulin requirements from preconception to end of pregnancy

Week	Insulin requirements (U/kg) (median)
Preconception	0.7
4	0.64
7	0.77
15	0.69
16–26	0.8
26–36	0.9
36–38	1.0
38+	0.9

three injections of meal-time Humalog daily. She is refereed for CSII because of poor glycemic control: HbA1c 7.2% (upper normal, 6.5%), mean glucose 152 with night-time hypoglycemia. Her weight is 65 kg. Basal insulin requirements are as follows.

Total daily basal insulin: 14 + 10 = 24 U.
20% basal insulin reduction for CSII: 24 − (24 × 20/100) = 19.2 U
19.2 U in 24 h is equivalent to 19.2/24 = 0.8 U/h

In order to validate the basal insulin calculations they can be compared with the average gestational week insulin requirements:

Average insulin requirements at week 17 = 0.8 U/kg or 0.8 × 65 = 52 U
Decrease by 20% for CSII 52 × 80% = 41.6 U
50% of total insulin requirements as basal is 41.6 × 50% = 20.8 U

The basal insulin dose is close to the average requirements. A suggested basal rate program is given in Table 30.2.

Establishing bolus calculations

Bolus calculations should involve health care professionals experienced in insulin pump therapy and carbohydrate counting and assessment. In general the bolus insulin is composed from the correction bolus, i.e. the amount of insulin needed to decrease a specific level of glucose to the desired glucose level and the meal bolus which is the required amount of insulin to match the glycemic load of the meal.

The correction bolus is determined by an empiric factor formulated by Dr Paul Davidson based on the total daily insulin dose (TDD) and signifies glucose utilization by insulin, i.e. glucose sensitivity (thus some use the term 'sensitivity factor'). If short-acting insulin analogs are used the correction factor is derived by the dividing 1700 by TDD (for human insulin, use 1500). A correction factor approximates the amount of glucose in mg% that will decrease by injecting 1 U of insulin. Thus a correction factor of 50 signifies a 50 mg% reduction per unit of insulin analogue injected. If the patients glucose levels is 150 mg% above the target (i.e. 250 mg%) 3 U of insulin (150/50 = 3) are needed.

The meal bolus is the approximation of the dose of insulin needed per amount of carbohydrate ingested. Much of this

approximation is achieved individually by careful follow-up and adjustments. Here two empirical 'rule of thumbs' apply: the '500 rule'; that is, by dividing 500 by the TDD one can approximate the ratio of ingested carbohydrate (in grams) covered by 1 insulin unit (CIR).

For example, the 32-year-old P2G2 Type 1 diabetic patient in her 17th week of gestation whose TDD is 52 plans to have a lunch consisting of 60 g of carbohydrates, and her current premeal glucose is 145 mg%. In order to approximate her bolus dose one has to calculate the CF and the carbohydrate: insulin ratio (CIR):

Correction factor (CF) is 1700/52 = 32
Carbohydrate:insulin ratio is 500/52 ~ 10
Correction bolus is calculated by subtracting the current glucose levels from the target glucose and then dividing by the CF; 145 − 90 = 55, and 55/32 = 1.7 U
Meal bolus is calculated by dividing the meal carbohydrate content be CIR: 60/10 = 6 U.
Total bolus is therefore the sum of the correction and the meal boluses: 6 + 1.7 = 7.7 U

The advantage in using a bolus calculator built into the insulin pump software is that it enables these calculations to be done simply by inputting the current glucose levels and the amount of carbohydrates in the planned meal. Beyond the advantage of the bolus calculators, simplifying calculations to the patient, one can program different CF and CIR during the day. This is an important feature during pregnancy were the morning insulin needed to cover carbohydrate is noted to be much higher than during the rest of the day. Additionally, as described before, the calculators take into account active insulin from previous boluses, decreasing the amount of active insulin present from the calculated bolus, thus preventing overbolusing when correcting for high blood sugars. A typical program of CIR and CF fed into the bolus calculators is presented in Figure 30.4.

Optimizing insulin therapy during pregnancy

Following the initial set up of the basal rate CF, CIR, and the glucose goals, the patient returns for the fine tuning of the pump. In order to optimize the basal rate one can observe the pattern of the preprandial glucose either from SMBG or from continuous glucose monitoring. The latter is especially useful for determining and fine tuning the overnight basal rate. Additional technique is meal skipping; that is, a meal is postponed and the glucose trend is followed either by SMBG every 30 min or by using continuous sensors. If the glucose trend is upward then an increase in the basal rate is needed, the opposite is needed when a downward trend in noted. Changes are usual done in steps of 0.2 U/h.

For optimizing the bolus dosage there should be track of the food intake either by food diaries or by following the carbohydrate entries downloaded from the pump software. If the diabetic patient's postprandial glucose levels are above target, the adequacy of carbohydrate content estimation of the meal is revised. Further education in carbohydrate counting is called for when the patient cannot estimate adequately the

Table 30.2	Suggested basal rate program
Time of day	**Insulin (U/h)**
0000–0400	0.4
0400–0800	1.4
0800–1800	0.8
1800–2200	1.0
2200–2400	0.8

Bolus wizard settings								
Carbohydrate ratio (grams per unit insulin)			Insulin sensitivity (mg/dl per unit insulin)			Blood glucose target (mg/dl)		
	Time	Setting		Time	Setting		Time	Setting
1	00:00	10	1	00:00	30	1	00:00	80
2	06:00	3	2	06:00	15	2		
3	12:00	6	3	12:00	35	3		
4			4			4		
5			5			5		
6			6			6		
7			7			7		
8			8			8		

Left panel:
- Bolus wizard: ON
- Wizard status: Set
- Carbohydrate units: Grams
- Blood glucose units: mg/dl
- Insulin type: Fast Acting

Figure 30.4   A typical program of carbohydrate:insulin ratio (CIR) and correction factor (CF) fed into the bolus calculators.

carbohydrate content of food. If the carbohydrate content is adequately assessed, than tweaking of the correction factor or carbohydrate insulin ratio is needed. This fine tuning necessitates the estimation of different correction factors at different time periods during the day. For example, the sensitivity factor is usually lower in the morning, so is the carbohydrate:insulin ratio. Throughout the gestation, the total daily insulin dose can be adjusted to match the gestational needs.

Pump use during labor and delivery

Maintaining euglycemia during the peripartum is essential for the prevention of neonatal hypoglycemia. When the pregnant diabetic woman enters active labor the insulin requirements fall drastically while the glucose infusion rate necessary to maintain a blood glucose level of 70–90 mg/dL was found to be constant at 2.55 mg/kg/min.[39] Protocols for maintaining euglycemia during labor are usually based on i.v. infusion of glucose, to maintain glucose consumption, and low rate of insulin (1–4 U/h) with no more subcutaneously administered insulin.

The low rate of insulin required can be administered by the pump using a temporary fixed basal rate. Feldberg et al.,[40] in a small trial, showed a decrease in neonatal hypoglycemia using CSII compared with an intravenous regimen. The choice between i.v. insulin protocol and continuation of CSII depends on the familiarity with insulin pumps and the practice at the maternity ward.

Postpartum there is a rapid decline in insulin resistance, thus patients should be instructed to activate a postpartum basal program following placental expulsion. This basal rate is usually a reduction by 30–50% of their third trimester basal rate. When the mother is nursing the higher level of decrease (50%) will be required. During the period following the delivery, mothers tend to have a more erratic daily schedule, at times neglecting or omitting insulin injections with inevitable decrease in glycemic control. It was therefore a very positive finding that women who opted to continue with CSII postpartum maintained good glycemic control in comparison to those who retuned to insulin injections.[34] Insulin pump therefore is a preferred choice for tight glycemic control during pregnancy and postpartum.

REFERENCES

1. Workshop Report. Diabetes care and research in Europe: The Saint Vincent declaration. Diabet Med 1990; 19: 360.
2. Platt MJ, Stanisstreet M, Casson IF, Howard CV, Walkinshaw S, Pennycook S, McKendrick O. St Vincent's Declaration 10 years on: outcomes of diabetic pregnancies. Diabet Med. 2002; 19: 216–20.
3. Evers IM, de Valk HW, Visser GHA. Risk of complications of pregnancy in women with type 1 diabetes: nationwide prospective study in the Netherlands. BMJ 2004; 328: 915–8.
4. Kauffman RP. The Diabetes in Pregnancy Dilemma: Leading Change with Proven Solutions. J Am Med Assoc 2006; 296: 1530–1.
5. Hadden DR. How to improve prognosis in type 1 diabetic pregnancy. Old problems, new concepts. Diabetes Care.1999; Suppl 2: B104–8.
6. Yogev Y, Ben-Haroush A, Chen R, Rosenn B, Hod M, Langer O Diurnal glycemic profile in obese and normal weight nondiabetic pregnant women.Am J Obstet Gynecol. 2004;191:949–53.
7. Kerssen A, de Valk HW, Visser GHA. Forty-eight-hour first-trimester glucose profiles in women with type 1 diabetes mellitus: a report of three cases of congenital malformation. Prenat Diagn 2006; 26: 123–7.

8. ter Braak EWM, Evers IM, Erkelens DW, Visser GHA. Maternal hypoglycaemia during pregnancy in type 1 diabetes: maternal and fetal consequences. Diabetes Metab Res Rev 2002; 18: 96–105.
9. Rosenn BM, Miodovnik M, Holcberg G, Khoury JC, Siddiqi TA. Hypoglycemia: the price of intensive insulin therapy for pregnant women with insulin-dependent diabetes mellitus. Obstet Gynecol 1995; 85: 417–22.
10. Bode BW, Steed RD, Davidson PC. Reduction in severe hypoglycemia with long-term continuous subcutaneous insulin infusion in type 1 diabetes. Diabetes Care 1996; 19: 324–7.
11. Pickup JC, Kidd J, Burmiston S, Yemane N. Effectiveness of continuous subcutaneous insulin infusion in hypoglycaemia prone type 1 diabetes: implications for NICE guidelines. Pract Diabet Int 2005; 22: 10–4.
12. Linkeschova R, Raoul M, Bott U, Berger M, Spraul M. Less severe hypoglycaemia, better metabolic control, and improved quality of life in Type 1 diabetes mellitus with continuous subcutaneous insulin infusion (CSII) therapy; an observational study of 100 consecutive

patients followed for a mean of 2 years. Diabet Med 2002; 19: 746–51.

13. Fanelli C, Pampanelli S, Lalli C, et al. Long-term intensive therapy of IDDM patients with clinically overt autonomic neuropathy: effects on hypoglycemia awareness and counter-regulation. Diabetes 1997; 46: 1172–81.

14. Coustan DR, Reece E, Sherwin RS, et al. A randomised clinical trial of the insulin pump vs. intensive conventional therapy in diabetic pregnancies. JAMA 1986; 255: 631–6.

15. Pickup JC, Mattock MB, Kerry S. Glycaemic control with continuous subcutaneous insulin infusion compared to intensive insulin injection therapy in type 1 diabetes: meta-analysis of randomised controlled trials. BMJ 2002; 324: 705–8.

16. Weissberg-Benchell J, Antisdel-Lomaglio J, Seshadri R. Insulin pump therapy: a meta-analysis. Diabetes Care 2003; 26: 1079–87.

17. Retnakaran R, Hochman J, DeVries JH, et al. Continuous subcutaneous insulin infusion versus multiple daily injections: the impact of baseline A1c. Diabetes Care 2004; 27: 2590–6.

18. Pickup JC, Kidd J, Burmiston S, Yemane N. Determinants of glycaemic control in type 1 diabetes during intensified therapy with multiple daily insulin injections or continuous subcutaneous insulin infusion: importance of blood glucose variability. Diabetes Metab Res Rev 2006; 22: 232–7.

19. Rudolf MC, Coustan DR, Sherwin RS, et al. Efficacy of the insulin pump in the home treatment of pregnant diabetics. Diabetes 1981; 30: 891–5.

20. Hirsh IB, Brownlee M. Should minimal blood glucose variability become the gold standard of glycemic control? J Diabetes Complications 2005; 19: 178–81.

21. Kerssen A, de Valk HW, Visser GHA. Diurnal glucose profiles during pregnancy in women with type 1 diabetes mellitus; relations with infant birth weight. Thesis, University Utrecht, The Netherlands; 2005.

22. Gottlieb PA, Frias JP, Peters KA, Chillara B, Garg SK. Optimizing insulin therapy in pregnant women with type 1 diabetes mellitus. Treat Endocrinol 2002; 1: 235–40.

23. Gin H, Hanaire-Broutin H. Reproducibility and variability in the action of injected insulin. Diabetes Metab 2005; 31: 7–13.

24. Lauritzen T, Pramming S, Deckert T, Binder C. Pharmacokinetics of continuous subcutaneous insulin infusion. Diabetologia 1983; 24: 326–9.

25. LePore M, Pampanelli S, Fanelli C, et al. Pharmacokinetics and pharmacodynamics of subcutaneous injection of long-acting human insulin analog glargine, NPH insulin, and ultralente human insulin and continuous subcutaneous infusion of insulin lispro. Diabetes 2000; 49: 2142–8.

26. Bode BW, Tamborlane WV, Davidson PC. Insulin pump therapy in the 21st century. Strategies for successful use in adults, adolescents, and children with diabetes. Postgrad Med 2002; 111: 69–71.

27. Guerci B, Meyer L, Sallé A, et al. Comparison of metabolic deterioration between insulin analog and regular insulin after a 5-hour interruption of a continuous subcutaneous insulin infusion in type 1 diabetic patients. J Clin Endocrinol Metab 1999; 84: 2673–8.

28. Pfutzner J, Forst T, Butzer R, et al. Performance of the continuous glucose monitoring system (CGMS) during development of ketosis in patients on insulin pump therapy. Diabet Med 2006; 23: 1124–9.

29. Castillo MJ, Scheen AJ, Lefhbvre PL. The degree/rapidity of the metabolic deterioration following interruption of a continuous subcutaneous insulin infusion is influenced by the prevailing blood glucose level. J Clin Endocrinol Metab 1996; 81: 1975–8.

30. Lapolla A, Dalfra MG, Masin M, et al. Analysis of outcome of pregnancy in type 1 diabetics treated with insulin pump or conventional insulin therapy. Acta Diabetol 2003; 40: 143–9.

31. Nordström L, Spetz E, Wallström K, Walinder O. Metabolic control and pregnancy outcome among women with insulin-dependent diabetes mellitus. Acta Obstet Gynecol Scand 1998; 77: 284–9.

32. Gross TM, Kayne D, King A, Rother C, Juth S. A bolus calculator is an effective means of controlling postprandial glycemia in patients on insulin pump therapy. Diabetes Technol Ther 2003; 5: 365–9.

33. ADA position statement on preconception care of women with diabetes. Diabetes Care 2004; 27: s76–8.

34. Gabbe SG, Holing E, Temple P, Brown ZA. Benefits, risks, costs, and patient satisfaction associated with insulin pump therapy for the pregnancy complicated by type 1 diabetes mellitus. Am J Obstet Gynecol 2000; 182: 1283–91.

35. Jovanovic L, Knopp RH, Brown Z, et al. National Institute of Child Health and Human Development Diabetes in Early Pregnancy Study Group. Declining insulin requirement in the late first trimester of diabetic pregnancy. Diabetes Care 2001; 24: 1130–6.

36. Jovanovic L. Achieving euglycaemia in women with gestational diabetes mellitus. Curr Opt Screen Diagn Treat Drugs 2004; 64: 1401–17.

37. Jovanovic L, Nakai Y. Successful pregnancy in women with type 1 diabetes: from preconception through postpartum care. Endocrinol Metab Clin N Am 2006; 35: 79–97.

38. Clarke WL, Haymond MW, Santiago JV. Overnight basal insulin requirements in fasting insulin-dependent diabetics. Diabetes 1999; 29; 78–80.

39. Jovanovic L, Peterson CM. Insulin and glucose requirements during the first stage of labor in insulin-dependent diabetic women. Am J Med 1983; 75: 607–12.

40. Feldberg D, Dicker N, Samuel D, et al. Intrapartum management of insulin-dependent diabetes mellitus (IDDM) gestants. A comparative study of constant intravenous insulin infusion and continuous subcutaneous insulin infusion pump (CSIIP), Acta Obstet Gynaecol Scand 1988; 67: 333–8.

31 Artificial pancreas and pregnancy: Closing the loop

Eli Kupperman, Howard Zisser and Lois Jovanovic

Insulin requirements during pregnancy

Although women with diabetes need to manage their blood glucose at all times, it is even more important prior to and during pregnancy, as blood glucose extremes can have an enormous effect on the health of the fetus. Preconceptional counseling and care are of extreme importance when a woman with Type 1 diabetes is planning a family. Preconception counseling and glucose control is essential because once pregnancy is diagnosed organogenesis is nearly completed. Poor blood glucose control during organogenesis can lead to both spontaneous abortions and congenital malformations.[1] Frequently, women do not know that they are pregnant prior to the end of organogenesis. Without preconception glucose control, up to 25% of pregnancies may be affected.[2]

When a woman is pregnant, she must avoid both hypoglycemia and hyperglycemia. Severe hypoglycemia has been associated with an increased risk of maternal death.[3] Hyperglycemia on the other hand, while it does not have an immediate affect on the mother, can have drastic affects on the fetus.

Hyperglycemia in the mother leads to hyperinsulinemia in the fetus.[1] Fetal hyperinsulinemia is implicated in fetal complications such as macrosomia (high birthweight), respiratory problems, cardiac myohypertrophy, and birth trauma.[1] According to a study by Jovanovic et al.[4] the best way to prevent macrosomia is to maintain postprandial normoglycemia. The risk of macrosomia is lowest when, during the second and third trimester, mothers are able to keep their glucose levels less than 120 mg/dL 1 h after a meal and less than 90 mg/dL when fasting.

Near the end of the first trimester of pregnancy, maternal insulin needs decrease. This decrease in insulin requirement was first noted by Jorgen Pedersen,[1] who warned other physicians to be aware of hypoglycemic events in women with diabetes, as it might be a sign of pregnancy. While the insulin requirements drop in the end of the first trimester, the woman becomes more insulin resistant and will require increasing amounts of insulin to maintain glucose control throughout the remainder of the pregnancy.[5] The amount of insulin required will almost double by the end of the third trimester.[5]

This increase in insulin resistance is due in large part to the presence of anti-insulin hormones that appear during pregnancy, including prolactin, human chorionic somatomammotropin (hCS), progesterone, and estrogen.[1,6] Thus, additional insulin is required to compensate for this increase in insulin resistance.

One way to achieve this desired control is through the use of standing orders, pre-approved algorithms that determine the amount of insulin to be given to the pregnant woman based on weight, weeks of gestation, and food intake. The following figure is a standing order for calculating the total amount of insulin to be given during a day, broken up between basals and boluses (Table 31.1).[7]

One way to maintain normal glucose levels in women with diabetes during a crucial time such as pregnancy is through the use of an artificial pancreas.

History of the artificial pancreas

If diabetes is caused by nonfunctioning pancreatic beta cells, what could be a better treatment for the disease than mimicking the normal function of those beta cells? This solution is the ultimate goal of many diabetes researchers around the world: the development of an artificial pancreas.

The artificial pancreas, which can either be implanted within the body or placed outside of the body, must have three components. The first component is a device that measures the glucose concentration in the body both with precision and speed. This glucose-sensing unit would record readings continuously in order to make sure the second component of the artificial pancreas, the insulin-delivery component, receives accurate directions. The insulin pump would have to store and deliver precise amounts of insulin based upon the readings of the glucose sensor in a manner that is both safe and timely. A selection of continuous glucose monitors and insulin infusion devices is shown in Figures 31.1 and 31.2. The third, and most complicated piece of the artificial pancreas, is the piece that in essence 'closes the loop'. This component must contain an algorithm or control system that has the ability to take the data gathered by the glucose sensor either directly or wirelessly and determines an appropriate amount of insulin to be delivered by the insulin pump (Figure 31.3).

Table 31.1   Insulin dosage regimen for diabetic pregnancy

Insulin dosage regimen for diabetic pregnancy				
1. Pregnancy NPH plus rapid-acting insulin schedule	Patient weight in kg =			Date & Time:

Big I = total daily units of insulin

Circle One: Gestational weeks =	0–12	13–28	29–34	35–40	OTHER
k =	0.7	0.8	0.9	1.0	

Calculate desired units of insulin from above line.

Big I = _____(k units × weight kg)/24 hours

Big I = Basal insulin requirement + Bolus (meal-related) insulin requirement

Basal = ½ Big I, Bolus = ½ Big I

Basal: Divide so that 1/6 of Big I is NPH given before breakfast, 1/6 of Big I is NPH given before dinner, and 1/6 of Big I is NPH given before bedtime.

Bolus: Divide so that 1/6 of Big I is rapid-acting insulin given before breakfast, 1/6 of Big I is rapid-acting insulin given before lunch, and 1/6 of Big I is rapid-acting insulin given before dinner. The rapid-acting insulin is then titrated based on the blood glucose.

A review article by Shalitin and Phillip[8] gives an excellent history of attempts at and improvements upon the development of an artificial pancreas. The first major attempt at the artificial pancreas was made in the early 1970s with the Biostator™, a glucose-controlled insulin infusion system which relied on glucose-sensing equipment and an algorithm dependent on the rate of change of the glucose readings to determine the amount of insulin to be delivered.[9,10] One major drawback with this system was that the Biostator™ was far from being portable. Both the glucose readings and insulin delivery were performed intravenously. Hence, the system is used only for research purposes such as glucose clamp studies or to study insulin requirements during labor.

Later in the 1970s, the first external portable pumps were introduced.[11] However, these too were excessively large and unreliable. More recently pumps with adjustable basal levels were introduced, closely mimicking normal insulin physiology, as insulin requirements change during different parts of the day. While these newer pumps are portable and more

effective, it is still necessary to regularly maintain the device and to make sure the insulin is being delivered to the body. Possible failures, such as a clogged or dislodged catheter, mean that the patient must still pay close attention to and continually check the effectiveness of the pump.[12] In order to diminish the danger of hyperglycemia resulting from a dislodged catheter, pregnant patients can take NPH insulin at night and turn down their basal. Newer insulin pumps are being tested that are implanted inside of the patient. These pumps are associated with improved glycemia because intraperitoneal delivery of insulin works faster than insulin delivered subcutaneously,[13] though still not as fast as insulin delivered directly into the blood stream.[14]

The glucose sensor remains the main limiting factor in the development of a commercially viable closed-loop system, as presently available sensors fail to demonstrate satisfactory characteristics in terms of reliability and/or accuracy.[15] Many non-invasive methods of obtaining blood glucose concentrations have been tested. One of the first of these methods used the optical sensor that worked on the premise that the absorption of near-infrared light is directly correlated to the concentration of glucose in the body. This device has problems with interference when gathering its data and during the calibration process, thus rendering it an unfeasible option in the development of an artificial pancreas.[16] One glucose sensor

Figure 31.1   A selection of popular continuous glucose monitors.

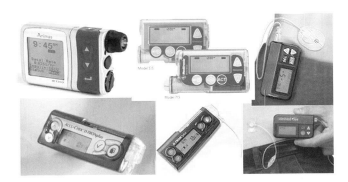

Figure 31.2   A selection of popular insulin infusion devices.

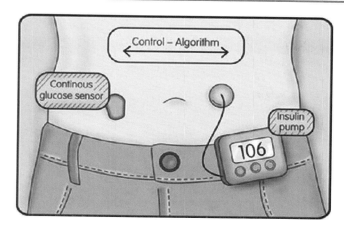

Figure 31.3   A cartoon of a full artificial pancreas.

that performed its job to a satisfactory level is the Gluco Watch™ Biographer. Unfortunately, the GlucoWatch™ Biographer sensor took 2 h and 55 min to calibrate and was associated with skin irritation in up to 20% of the patients. It was impractical for widespread use.[17] Currently, the most practical glucose sensor is the subcutaneous enzymatic continuous glucose monitoring system (CGMS). While implantable glucose sensors are less of a burden on the patient with diabetes, one must be wary of all implantable sensors that test the interstitial fluid. Measurements gathered in this manner may be less accurate than those that come from direct samples of the blood (Table 31.2).[8]

The trickiest part of the artificial pancreas, of course, is getting the insulin pump and the glucose sensor to communicate with one another. This requires a very specific algorithm that takes input from the sensor and then calculates an amount of insulin to be delivered and a speed of delivery. This algorithm must also work continuously, reliably, and without a single failure. The first attempt at this algorithm was made in the 1970s when Albisser et al.[10] used the rate of change of the glucose level to determine the amount of insulin necessary. Since this first attempt, many efforts at achieving a working algorithm have been made. A Japanese group led by Professor Shichiri[18] claims success of their product for a week's worth of time and longer, if the patient calibrates it periodically. The results, however, were never able to be repeated by another group. Medtronic is currently testing closed-loop artificial pancreases using its own algorithm using both an external sensor and an external pump.[19] In addition, a group led by Dr Eric Renard[20] has had a successful 48-h test. Projects are

still ongoing around the world, but a true closed-loop artificial pancreas that consistently shows satisfactory results over long-term trials is still non-existent to date.

Problems with and solutions for the artificial pancreas

Over the many years that researchers have been attempting to create an artificial pancreas, many obstacles have crept in. Early insulin pumps did not have a means of adjusting basal levels throughout the day. Additionally, many glucose sensors were unable to perform their job accurately because of interference or inability to take measurements on a continuous basis. Currently, pumps have adjustable basal rates and glucose sensors, are becoming accurate, but one important component of the artificial pancreas is still far from being perfected. This component is the algorithm that calculates the amount of insulin needed based upon data gathered by the glucose sensor, both the current level of blood glucose and the trends of increase and decrease.

The main reason for the difficulty in finding a precise algorithm is two periods of delay associated with a closed-loop artificial pancreas. The first is the delay in the time it takes to obtain a reading from the subcutaneous glucose-monitoring device. This primary delay creates a difference between the true value of the capillary glucose in current time and the value that the glucose sensor reads in the interstitial fluid. If the sensor takes a measurement every 5 min (common for current continuous glucose monitoring systems), the capillary and interstitial glucose levels could be different by as much as 10 mg/dL. While 10 mg/dL is hardly a reason for much concern, the algorithm that controls the insulin pump may think blood glucose levels are still rising after a meal when in fact they have begun to fall. If the measurement of the sensor is not accurate to the time, the insulin pump could deliver the wrong amount of insulin, and cause either hypoglycemia if too much insulin is delivered or hyperglycemia if the pump does not deliver an adequate amount of the hormone.

One way most continuous glucose sensors abates the affect of this delay is the use of low-pass filters.[14] These low-pass filters allow the control device to read smoother changes in blood glucose level and to estimate rate of change more accurately than if the algorithm simply used the exact readings found by the continuous glucose sensor. This reduction of noise is generally accomplished with one of two types of filters, finite impulse response (FIR) filters or infinite impulse response (IIR) filters.[21] FIR filters work by taking a weighted

Name of sensor	Benefits	Drawbacks
Optical sensor	Non-invasive, simple	Unreliable, inaccurate, prone to interference
GlucoWatch™ Biographer	Accurate, non-invasive	Caused rashes
CGMS	Accurate, reliable	Invasive, can be a burden to user, bulky

Table 31.2   Characteristics of three types of glucose sensor

average of past glucose readings, giving more weight to more recent readings while IIR filters accomplish their task by taking a weighted average of past readings as well as past filter values, thereby utilizing a greater amount of data.[14]

The second delay that causes problems with the development of an algorithm for controlling the artificial pancreas is the delay between the time of insulin infusion and the time when the insulin begins to work. This time delay is about 15 min for initial activity and around an hour for peak effect. The length of these potentially hazardous delays is dependent upon the type of artificial pancreas system. If the patient is using a device with both the glucose sensor and the insulin pump placed externally on the body and taking measurements and infusing insulin subcutaneously, the total delay could be about 100 min.[22–25] For a device with the sensor placed intra-venously and the insulin pump delivering the hormone directly to the intraperitoneal cavity, the total time of the delays is roughly 70 min.[15] It is easy to see that this discordance of glucose sensing and insulin delivery creates a major problem for scientists attempting to devise a working algorithm.

During times of inactivity and fasting, blood glucose levels do not change at a fast rate. Therefore, successful algorithms have already been devised that translate glucose sensor data to insulin infusion amounts for these sedentary times of the day. The problem associated with the artificial pancreas comes into play, however, during meal times and times of physical exercise and illness. For these periods of the day, when blood glucose levels rise and fall at rapid rates, the artificial pancreas would have to react to changes almost instantaneously. For example, if the delay between insulin infusion and maximum utility of that insulin is approximately an hour and the delay between eating and peak blood glucose is also approximately an hour, insulin would need to be delivered around the time when the patient begins to eat. However, because of the delay between when the patient first begins to eat and when glucose levels first show signs of increasing, the pump would deliver insulin late, causing the patient's blood glucose to rise. This pattern means that, in addition to adjusting insulin infusion rates based upon the present blood glucose level and the rate of increase or decrease, the algorithm would need some way to predict when the patient will eat or when the patient will exercise. The most feasible way to do this is through input by the patient prior to eating or exercising. This type of artificial pancreas is known as one with 'closed loop with meal announcement' control or 'semi-closed-loop' control.[15] Therefore, while the artificial pancreas will be self-contained the majority of the time, it should still have the ability to accept input from the patient when needed.

Beta cells in a person without diabetes do not release insulin all at once but rather twice, in 'first' and 'second' phase responses.[26,27] The first phase response is similar to a bolus release of insulin and generally occurs as soon as the meal begins. The second phase response begins shortly after the first phase response and slowly increases until glucose levels are back to normal (Figure 31.4).[14] Two important parameters, the amount of insulin released in the first response and the slope of increase in the second response, are proportional to the increase in the level of blood glucose.[14] Therefore, patients would need to know the approximate amount of carbohydrate

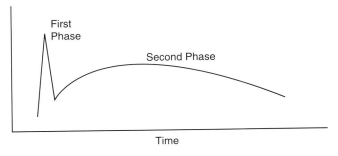

Figure 31.4   Two-phase release of insulin, similar to the release of insulin by beta cells in a person without diabetes.

in their upcoming meal to know how much of an insulin bolus to give. They would still need to, in essence, 'count carbs'. More recent models may use a small pre-prandial bolus to mimic the first phase secretion and then allow the algorithm to control insulin delivery after preset parameters are met.[28]

Multiple models of insulin delivery algorithms have been devised in recent years. The oldest and most widely used algorithm is known as the proportional, integral, and derivate scheme (PID).[14] The formula for a PID controller requires only knowing the difference between the current glucose level and the target glucose level and the time since food intake began along with a few pre-determined constants. The problem with the PID controller, as well as other popular control algorithms including the Biostator™,[9,29,30] and more recent ones such as those by Fischer,[31,32] Kraegen,[33] and Albisser[34] is that while they include a first-phase response that mimics a healthy pancreas well, the second-phase response is constant rather than increasing as is the case in a well-functioning organ.[14]

Should a pregnant woman with diabetes use an artificial pancreas?

The benefits of an artificial pancreas are ever increasing and potentially vast. Current deficiencies with fully functioning models render them imperfect, though improvements are quick to come and it is possible that there could be a fully functioning and accurate model of the entire device within the next few years. Benefits of wearing an artificial pancreas include peace of mind, such as not having to worry about not having enough insulin or having too much insulin, not having to remember to take blood glucose readings multiple times every day, and not having to remember to inject oneself with insulin before every meal and before going to bed. In addition, with an artificial pancreas there would be fewer finger sticks, less counting of calories and carbohydrates, and, if the patient's insulin delivery device and continuous glucose sensor are internal, no devices to clip to one's hip or carry in one's purse.

The risk of diabetic ketoacidosis (DKA) during pregnancy would be lower with a properly functioning artificial pancreas. DKA, a condition in which the blood becomes acidic because of a sharp increase in ketones due to insulin deficiency, is a major reason why in the past diabetic women were urged not to become pregnant. It was feared that the high incidence of DKA in pregnant women with diabetes would carry a significant risk, including death. An external device may add to the risk of DKA. Since there is no long-acting insulin in an insulin infusion device, ketosis develops in a matter of hours, if the infusion set dislodges. To ensure that there is no interruption during the night, it is suggested that when women with Type 1 diabetes are using an external insulin pump, that 0.1 U/kg of NPH be given before bed. Overnight basal

infusion rate should be adjusted appropriately downward to allow for this extra insulin to be on board.

Until a cure for diabetes is found, the next best alternative is the use of an artificial pancreas to replicate the endocrine activity of the pancreas. While current models of closed-loop artificial beta cells are not perfect, trials are ongoing and a fully functional device is just around the corner. The use of these devices will hopefully be widespread and improve the quality of life for many people with diabetes.

REFERENCES

1. Kitzmiller JL, Jovanovic L. Insulin therapy in pregnancy. In: Textbook of Diabetes and Pregnancy. London, New York: Martin Dunitz; 2003, pp. 359–78.
2. Miller E, Hare JW, Cloherty JP, et al. Elevated maternal hemoglobin A1c in early pregnancy and major congenital anomalies in infants of diabetic mothers. New Engl J Med 1981; 304: 1331–4.
3. Hadden DR. Diabetes in pregnancy 1985. Diabetologia 1986; 29: 1–9.
4. Jovanovic L, Peterson CM, Reed GF, et al. Maternal postprandial glucose levels and infant birth weight: the Diabetes in Early Pregnancy Study. Am J Obstet Gynecol 1991; 164: 103–11.
5. Clapp JF. Effects of diet and exercise on insulin resistance during pregnancy. Metab Syndr Relate Disord 2006: 2: 84–90.
6. Knopp RH. Hormone mediated changes in nutrient metabolism in pregnancy: a physiological basis for normal fetal development. In: Jacobsen MS, Rees JM, Golden NH, Irwin CE, eds. Adolescent Nutritional Disorders: Prevention and Treatment. New York: Academy of Sciences; 1997; pp. 251–71.
7. Jovanovic L, Mills JL, Knopp RH, et al., and the National Institute of Child Health and Human Development – Diabetes in Early Pregnancy Study Group. Declining insulin requirements in the late first trimester of diabeteic pregnancy. Diabetes Care 2001; 24: 1130–6.
8. Shalitin S, Phillip M. Closing the loop: combining insulin pumps and glucose sensors in children with type 1 diabetes mellitus. Pediatr Diabet 2006; 7(suppl. 4): 45–9.
9. Clemens AH, Chang PH, Myers RW. The development of Biostator™, a glucose controlled insulin infusion system (GCIIS). Horm Metab Res 1974; 6: 339–42.
10. Albisser AM, Leibel BS, Ewrt TG, et al. An artificial endocrine pancreas. Diabetes 1974; 23: 389–404.
11. Pickup JC, Keen H, Parsons JA, Alberti KGM. Continuous subcutaneous insulin infusion: an approach to achieving normoglycemia. Br Med J 1978; 1: 204–7.
12. Chantelau E, Spraul M, Muhlhauser I, Gause R, Berger M. Long-term safety, efficacy and side-effects of continuous subcutaneous insulin infusion treatment for type 1 diabetes mellitus: a one centre experience. Diabetologia 1989; 32: 421–6.
13. Schade DS, Valentine V. To pump or not to pump. Diabetes Care 1981; 30: 149–55.
14. Steil GM, Penteleon AE, Rebrin K. Closed-loop insulin delivery – the path to physiological glucose control. Adv Drug Deliv Rev 2004; 56: 125–44.
15. Hovorka R. Continuous glucose monitoring and closed-loop systems. Diabet Med 2006; 23: 1–12.
16. Gough DA, Armour JC. Development of the implantable glucose sensor: what are the prospects and why is it taking so long? Diabetes 1995; 44: 1005–9.
17. Potts RO, Tamada JA, Tierney MJ. Glucose monitoring by reverse iontophoresis. Diabetes Metab Res Rev 2002: 18(suppl. 1): s49–s53.
18. Shichiri M, Sakakida M, Nishida K, Shimoda S. Enhanced, simplified glucose sensors: long-term clinical application of wearable artificial endocrine pancreas. Artif Organs 1998; 22: 32–42.
19. Steil GM, Rebrin K, Janowski R, Darwin C, Saad MF. Modeling β-cell insulin secretion – implications for closed-loop glucose homeostasis. Diabetes Technol Ther 2003; 5: 953–64.
20. Renard E, Shah R, Miller M, et al. Sustained safety and accuracy of central IV glucose sensors connected to implanted insulin pumps and short-term closed-loop trials in diabetic patients. Diabetes 2003; 52: A36.
21. Proakis JG, Manolakis DG. Digital Signal Processing: Principles, Algorithms, and Applications. New Jersey: Prentice-Hall; 1996.
22. Plank J, Wutte A, Brunner G, et al. A direct comparison of insulin aspart and insulin lispro in patients with type 1 diabetes. Diabetes Care 2002; 25: 2053–7.
23. Hovorka R, Shojaee-Moradie F, Carroll PV, et al. Partitioning glucose distribution/transport, disposal, and endogenous production during IVGTT. Am J Physiol 2002; 282: E992–1007.
24. Rebrin K, Steil GM, Van Antwerp WP, Mastrototaro JJ. Subcutaneous glucose predicts plasma glucose independent of insulin: implications for continuous monitoring. Am J Physiol 1999; 277: E561–71.
25. Heinemann L. Continuous glucose monitoring by means of the microdialysis technique: underlying fundamental aspects. Diabetes Technol Ther 2003; 5: 545–61.
26. Elahi D. In praise of the hyperglycemic clamp: a method for assessment of B-cell sensitivity and insulin resistance. Diabetes Care 1996; 19: 278–86.
27. King DS, Staten MA, Kohrt WM, et al. Insulin secretory capacity in endurance-trained and untrained young men. Am J Physiol 1990; 259: E155–61.
28. Marchetti G, Massimiliano B, Jovanovic L, Zisser H, Seborg D. An improved PID Switching Control Stratagey for Type 1 Diabetes. Proceedings of the 28th IEEE EMBS Annual International Conference. New York City, USA, 30 Aug to 3 Sept 2006.
29. Calabrese G, Bueti A, Zega G, et al. Improvement of artificial endocrine pancreas (biostator; GCHS) performance combining feedback controlled insulin administration with a pre-programmed insulin infusion. Horm Metab Res 1982; 14: 505–7.
30. Fogt E, Dodd LM, Jenning EM, Clemens AH. Development and evaluation of a glucose analyzer for a glucose controlled insulin infusion system. Clin Chem 1978; 24: 1366–72.
31. Fischer U, Jutzi E, Bombor H, et al. Assessment of an algorithm for the artificial B-cell using the normal insulin-glucose relationship in diabetic dogs and men. Diabetologia 1980; 18: 97–107.
32. Fischer U, Salzsieder E, Freyse EJ, Albrecht G. Experimental validation of a glucose-insulin control model to simulate patterns in glucose turnover. Comput Meth Prog Biomed 1990; 32: 249–58.
33. Kraegen EW, Campbell LV, Chia YO, Meler H, Lazarus L. Control of blood glucose in diabetics using an artificial pancreas. Aust NZ J Med 1977; 7: 280–6.
34. Broekhuyse HM, Nelson JD, Zinman B, Albisser AM. Comparison of algorithms for the closed-loop control of blood glucose using the artificial beta cell. IEEE Trans Biomed Eng 1981; 28: 678–86.

32 Hypoglycemia in diabetic pregnancy

A. Lapolla, M.G. Dalfrà, C. Lencioni and G. Di Cianni

Introduction

Hypoglycemia is a major factor that precludes people with both Type 1 and Type 2 diabetes from achieving near-normal glycemia. The risk of hypoglycemia is due both to the imperfect pharmacokinetic of current therapy, which produces inappropriately high insulin concentrations plus a failure in the protective mechanisms that limit falls in blood glucose concentrations.

Therefore, hypoglycemia is an inevitable price of the good metabolic control and the limiting factor to the best value of the daily glycemic profile, in every condition in which it is required.

The goal of insulin therapy in pregnant women with diabetes is to reduce the risk of maternal–fetal complications to the risk levels found in the nondiabetic population. Therefore, maternal normal glycemia during pregnancy is essential for the health of the fetus and the mother. Strategies to achieve and maintain normal glycemia in pregnancy are onerous but not negotiable and hypoglycemia became nearly inevitable using available strategies. In addition, pregnancy itself may be associated with an impaired counter-regulation system and lack of awareness of hypoglycemia. This could result in an increase of severe hypoglycemic episodes.

The pathophysiology of hypoglycemia, its effects on the mother and on the fetus, and its management in pregnancy, are discussed in detail in this chapter.

Frequency of hypoglycemia

In diabetes

Hypoglycemia is the most frequent acute complication of Type 1 diabetes mellitus therapy. It has been reported that diabetic people live about 10% of their life with glycemic values lower than 60 mg/dL (3.3 mmol/L) and that, on average, once a week they present an episode of symptomatic hypoglycemia. About every 4–5 years a case of these can lead to coma with the need of assistance and admission to hospital.[1] In 2–4% of the cases hypoglycemia causes death for people with Type 1 diabetes mellitus.[2]

Hypoglycemia is a common complication also for people with Type 2 diabetes. The rate of severe hypoglycemia in Type 2

diabetes is 10% of that of Type 1 diabetes. Nevertheless, the prevalence rates rise to 70–80% in clinical trials using insulin to achieve good metabolic control.[3]

More recently, in a cohort of Type 1 and insulin-treated Type 2 diabetic patients surveyed for 4 weeks, a rate of 43 events per patient per year in Type 1 and 16 events per year in Type 2 diabetic subjects was reported. Predictors for hypoglycemia in Type 1 and Type 2 diabetic patients included a history of previous hypoglycemia.[4]

During diabetic pregnancy

In pregnant women with diabetes (Types 1 and 2) good metabolic control before and during pregnancy is essential to reduce maternal–fetal morbidity and mortality. To obtain and maintain an optimal daily glycemic profile and HbA1c levels to near normal values during pregnancy, women with diabetes are at increased risk of severe hypoglycemic episodes.

Rosen and co-workers[5] have reported that in a cohort of 84 pregnant women with Type 1 diabetes, 71% have had significant episodes of hypoglycemia requiring assistance from another person. The peak of incidence occurred from the 10th to 15th week of gestation and blood glucose fluctuations were more frequent in women who have experienced severe hypoglycemia, independently of HbA1c levels.

In another observation performed in 55 Type 1 diabetic women,[6] a prevalence of nocturnal hypoglycemic episodes (blood glucose <3.0 mmol/L) in the first trimester was of 37%; the peak of incidence occurred at 5 a.m. In this study, the best predictive value for the occurrence of nocturnal hypoglycemia,

---

Box 32.1   Causes of hypoglycemia in pregnant diabetic women

- Impairment of glucose counter-regulation
- Increased insulin sensitivity
- Reduced metabolic clearance of insulin
- Intensified insulin therapy
- Low glycemic targets
- Nausea
- Vomiting

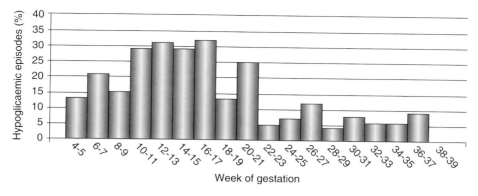

Figure 32.1   Rate of severe hypoglycemia (<35 mg/dL) during pregnancy in Type 1 diabetic women.[6–9]

was a bedtime plasma glucose lower than 6.0 mmol/L (Figure 32.1).

Moreover, Evers et al.[7] compared the frequency of severe hypoglycemic episodes (including hypoglycemic coma) in 278 women registered in the first trimester of pregnancy with that in the four months before pregnancy. Severe hypoglycemia increased from 0.9 ± 2.4 episodes to 2.6 ± 6.3 and coma from 0.3 ± 1.3 to 0.7 ± 3.7 (all $P < 0.05$). Interestingly, the authors focused on the risk indicators predictive for severe hypoglycemia. They showed that severe hypoglycemia was independently related to a positive history of severe hypoglycemic episodes before pregnancy, a longer duration of diabetes, an HbA1c level lower than 6.5%, and finally a higher total daily insulin dose.

Recently, the possibility to use a continuous glucose monitoring system that describes glucose patterns all day during pregnancy, has provided new data on hypoglycemic episodes. In 20 pregnant women affected by Type 1 diabetes studied with continuous glucose monitoring, postprandial hypoglycemic events (glucose ≥ 2.7 mmol/L for over 15 min after the glucose peak time) were recorded in 11.6% of the meals and occurred, without symptoms, 161 ± 46 min after mealtime.[8] The same approach was applied to gestational diabetic pregnant women, making it possible to identify asymptomatic hypoglycemic events in 63% of insulin-treated GDM patients, and in 28% of glyburide-treated GDM. The majority of registered events were nocturnal (83%) in insulin-treated patients, while in glyburide-treated women hypoglycemic values were equally registered during the day as well as in the night.[9]

The results of these clinical studies underline the importance of verifying how the benefits of the good glycemic control during pregnancy can be obtained avoiding the risk of severe hypoglycemia.

Protective response to hypoglycemia

Glucose, in physiological conditions, provides 90% of the necessary energy for brain functioning. Since neurons are not able to synthesize glucose and since their reserves are sufficient only for a few minutes, cerebral functions are totally dependent on circulating glucose. The decrease of glycemic values is associated with a series of redundant neuro-endocrine responses aimed at bringing glycemic levels to the physiological range.[10]

Falling plasma glucose concentrations are sensed in the hypothalamus and other regions of the brain as well as in the hepatic portal vein and the carotid artery. Glucose sensing in visceral sites sends the information to the brain via the cranial nerve (especially vagous nerve) and, as a result of a complex integration within the brain, these signals are responsible for the autonomic response (sympathetic and parasympathetic) organized within the hypothalamus. Through mechanisms that include increased autonomic activity, hypoglycemia causes reduced pancreatic beta-cell insulin secretion and increased alfa-cell glucagon secretion. Hypoglycemia, involving hypothalamo-hypophyseal neuroendocrine mechanisms, also causes an increased secretion of growth hormone and adrenocorticotropin. The exact mechanism involved in this process is not well known. The glucokinase-mediated sensing in pancreatic beta-cells remains the best characterized mechanism of response to glucose falling. Similar mechanisms may be operative at brain neuron levels.[11]

The reduction of glycemia in the physiological area (about 4.4 mmol/L) causes a decline in insulin secretion that favours increased production of glucose from the liver. This represents the initial defense against falling glucose.[12]

Glucagon stimulates hepatic glycogenolysis and it also favors gluconeogenesis but it seems also to determine autonomic inputs. Epinephrine has a similar action to that of glucagon, but it becomes critically important when glucagon secretion is lacking. These two hormones are therefore considered the ones mainly involved in the counter-regulation response; in fact, the development or the accentuation of the hypoglycemic crisis does not take place without these two hormones.

Other hormones, however, such as the growth hormone and cortisol, are involved in counter-regulation, especially in prolonged hypoglycemia. Their effect is carried on by limiting glucose consumption and favoring its production.[10]

Pathophysiology of glucose counter-regulation

In diabetes

The defense mechanisms against hypoglycemia are clearly impaired in Type 1 diabetes. In fact, insulin deficient (Type 1 and advanced Type 2) diabetic patients are not able to decrease insulin levels and the loss of glucagon response to hypoglycemia is the most common defect in these patients. Under these conditions, epinephrine remains critical for counter-regulation. However, many Type 1 diabetic patients, especially after recurrent hypoglycemia and in the presence of long-term diabetes (10–20 years), suffer from reduced responses of epinephrine. Therefore, Type 1 diabetic patients with combined defect of glucagon and epinephrine are at about a 6-fold increased risk for severe iatrogenic hypoglycemia during intensive insulin therapy.[13]

Hypoglycemia in Type 2 diabetes is less frequent than in Type 1 because of insulin resistance and intact counter-regulation, at least in patients with a short duration of diabetes. As the duration of diabetes increases and beta-cell function deteriorates, glucagon responses to hypoglycemia may become abnormal, as in Type 1 diabetes.[14] Therefore, hypoglycemia may occur in Type 2 diabetes, as a consequence of both insulin or sulfonylurea treatment addressed to achieve the goals of intensive treatment.

During diabetic pregnancy

Diabetic pregnancy is characterized *per se* by an impairment of the counter-regulatory response. As observed by experimental studies performed in diabetic dogs, epinephrine and glucagon response to hypoglycemia is impaired during pregnancy.[15] Moreover, these data have also been confirmed in human pregnancy by using the hypoglycemic clamp technique.[16,17] In intensively treated Type 1 diabetic pregnant women a consistent lower epinephrine and glucagon response was found with respect to nondiabetic nonpregnant women. In addition, the glycemic thresholds for epinephrine and growth hormone secretion resulted decreased. This may be the consequence, at least in part, of intensive insulin treatment of the patients. Impaired secretion of both hormones, especially that of glucagon, has also been demonstrated in nondiabetic pregnant women. The exact mechanisms involved in the reduction of glucagon and epinephrine secretion during pregnancy are not completely clear. Nevertheless, as for glucagon, one possibility is that the placental hormones exert a suppressive effect on it. Has to be in this context, it has been reported that the arginin-induced secretion of glucagon is decreased in women using hormonal contraception.[16] These data imply a suppression of these hormones by the high levels of estrogen and progesterone that characterize pregnancy. Moreover, the results of a more recent experimental study suggest that the blunting of glucagon secretion during insulin induced hypoglycemia in pregnancy is related to a generalized impairment of a number of different signals, including parasympathetic and sympathoadrenal stimuli and altered sensing of circulating and/or intraislet insulin.[18] Also, growth hormone response during pregnancy is progressively reduced in both pregnant women with and without diabetes and this can be determined by the progressive increase of placental hormones.[16] Another study using hyperinsulinemic hypoglycemic clamp in Type 1 diabetic pregnant women in the third trimester of pregnancy, showed a significant increase of placental growth hormone during hypoglycemia. These observations indicate that the placenta is an endocrine organ that can play an active role in

acute metabolic processes such as the hormonal counter-regulation of hypoglycemia.[19]

Pathophysiology of hypoglycemia

Type 1 diabetes

Inappropriate hyperinsulinemia, either absolute or relative, is the initiating cause of hypoglycemia in diabetes mellitus. Hyperinsulinemia is the rule in diabetes mellitus, both Type 1 and Type 2, because of the therapeutic delivery of insulin into the peripheral rather than portal circulation and because of the empirical algorithms used to administer insulin. Absolute hyperinsulinemia, due to excessive levels of circulating insulin because of an excess of dosage or irregularity of absorption, causes hypoglycemia more frequently during the hours preceding meals or in the first morning hours. Relative hyperinsulinemia is due to other conditions such as: delayed or inadequate diet (especially as far as the range of carbohydrates is concerned), physical exercise, renal failure, excessive alcohol consumption, delayed gastric emptying. In these conditions usually hypoglycemia occurs after meals.[20]

Nevertheless, as reported by the DCCT, the hyperinsulinemia can explain only a part of the severe hypoglycemic episodes that are observed in people with Type 1 diabetes. In fact, in this study 714 severe hypoglycemic episodes were registered in 216 people (all in intensive treatment) and after multivariate analysis, the conventional factors associated to hyperinsulinemia, explained only 8.5% of the variability.[21]

This suggests that hypoglycemia is the result of a defective balance between excessive insulinemic levels and a deficit of the counter-regulatory system. In fact, many Type 1 diabetic patients show a loss of glucagon response to hypoglycemia and, especially in long-term diabetes, a reduced response of epinephrine. Therefore, Type 1 diabetic patients with a defect in epinephrine response in the setting of defective insulin secretion and glucagon response, are predisposed to severe hypoglycemic episodes.[13]

Moreover, people with Type 1 diabetes in tight metabolic control, require lower values of glycemia to stimulate the counter-regulatory response and to have the alarm symptoms. On the contrary, people with a bad metabolic control already activate the counter-regulatory response at relatively high glycemic levels.[22]

Type 2 diabetes

Type 2 diabetes is characterized by insulin resistance and persistent beta-cell function, which allows insulin secretion to decrease as blood glucose falls, and apparently intact counter-regulation. Consequently, as reported in the literature,[14] the rate of severe hypoglycemia is lower than in Type 1 diabetes. However, the UKPDS study showed that the frequency of hypoglycemia increases over the years with a prolongation of the duration of insulin treatment.[23] Patients with advanced Type 2 diabetes and long duration of insulin treatment have reduced glucagon and sympathoadrenal response to hypoglycemia.[14]

In people with Type 2 diabetes hypoglycemia is often a consequence of the pharmacological treatments with hypoglycemic agents that stimulate pancreatic insulin secretion (sulfonylureas, glinides). Drugs that act on insulin sensitivity (metformin and glitazones) do not cause hypoglycemia.

Diabetic pregnancy

Hypoglycemia during diabetic pregnancy is certainly linked to the intensified insulin treatment useful to reach and maintain the targets of glycemic control recommended in these women. Low blood glucose levels can expose women to the risk of hypoglycemia. Moreover, the impairment of glucose counter-regulation[16–18] and other features such as an increase in insulin sensitivity during the first trimester of gestation,[24] are important in determining an increase in hypoglycemic episodes during pregnancy.

It is well known that the need for insulin increases progressively during pregnancy reaching a maximum, with the largest fluctuations, during the third trimester. In this context, a reduced metabolic clearance of insulin in the third trimester, as reported by Bjorklund et al.[25] can reduce the recovery from hypoglycemia.

Finally, nausea and vomiting, common in the first trimester, can contribute to hypoglycemia by reducing the ingestion of carbohydrate (Box 32.1).

Symptoms

In classical textbooks, hypoglycemia is usually defined as a plasma glucose concentration below 50–55 mg/dL (2.7–3 mmol/L).[26] However, the glycemic thresholds responsible for the activation of the counter-regulatory system is already evident at a plasma glucose concentrations of 65–70 mg/dL (3.6–3.8 mmol/L).[27] Thus a physiological definition of hypoglycemia could be any glycemia below 65 mg/dL. In diabetic people symptoms of hypoglycemia may shift upwards or downwards depending on antecedent glycemic control.

According to the entity of the clinical presentation, hypoglycemia can be classified as symptomatic, light–moderate and severe hypoglycemia both in pregnancy and outside pregnancy.

Symptoms of hypoglycemia, which are the same during pregnancy, are divided into two categories: neurogenic and neuroglycopenic (Figure 32.2). Neurogenic (autonomic) symptoms are triggered by a failing in glucose levels and cause patients to recognize that they are experiencing a hypoglycemic episode. These symptoms are activated by the autonomic nervous system and are mediated by norepinephrine, epinephrine and acetylcholine. Neurogenic symptoms (catecholamine-mediated) include anxiety, palpitations, sweating, shakiness, dry mouth, pallor, pupil dilatation, diaphoresis, hunger, and paresthesia.

The insufficient contribution of glucose to the brain (neuroglycopenia) with an associated cerebral reduction of oxygen, causes neuroglycopenic symptoms. The cognitive function becomes impaired when plasma glucose concentration falls below 50–55 mg/dL (2.7–3 mmol/L).[27] However, this threshold varies depending on the different aspects examined and psychometric tests adopted. These symptoms include abnormal mentation, irritability, difficult speaking, ataxia,

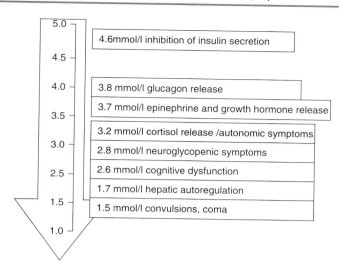

Figure 32.2   Symptoms of hypoglycemia.

paresthesia, headache, stupor, and eventually (if untreated) seizure, coma, and even death. Neuroglycopenic symptoms can also include transient focal neurological deficits (e.g. diplopia, hemiparesis). These symptoms usually represent the alarm signal of a more serious hypoglycemic attack, and they usually precede the alterations of the cortical function.

In this phase the person is completely conscious and can himself/herself interrupt the attack, by rapid intake of carbohydrates.

Severe hypoglycemia appears when glucose levels continue to fall. In these cases the person is incapable of starting treatment for the resolution of the episode and he/she needs rapid and adequate assistance.

Lack of awareness of hypoglycemia

The inability of patients to recognize impending hypoglycemia is a major clinical problem in the management of insulin treated diabetes and it represents an important barrier to tight metabolic control especially in patients that have been encouraged to treat their diabetes intensively. Lack of awareness of hypoglycemia is a common long-term complication of diabetes. Epidemiological surveys in unselected population have reported that around 25% of subjects with Type 1 diabetes experience persistent or intermittent difficulty in recognizing hypoglycemia.[28]

In diabetic people with a long history of diabetes a reduced autonomic activation in response to hypoglycemia cause a lack of neurogenous alarm symptoms (hypoglycemia unawareness). This can lead to severe hypoglycemic crises without the typical alarm signs. Awareness of hypoglycemia is largely the result of sympathetic neural, rather than adrenomedullary, activation.

The exact mechanism of hypoglycemia unawareness is not completely understood. It is thought to be due to an alteration in the relationship between glycemic thresholds of the various components of the physiological response to hypoglycemia, and cognitive functions.[29] Patients who lack awareness demonstrate sympathoadrenal activation at lower glucose concentrations than those who have awareness and, importantly, at a lower level than that for cognitive impairment.

Strong evidence indicates that defective loss of symptoms of hypoglycemia in Type 1 diabetic patients is largely the result of antecedent, frequent hypoglycemia. It seems likely that antecedent hypoglycemic episodes contribute to defective glucagon response and impaired secretion of epinephrine during hypoglycemia. The attenuated epinephrine response to hypoglycemia is a marker of an attenuated autonomic and sympathetic response. It causes the initial loss of the warning symptoms of hypoglycemia and, over time, by a downward vicious spiral including progressively impaired physiological responses and increasing clusters of hypoglycemic episodes, the development of hypoglycemia unawareness.[22]

Diabetic pregnancies are often characterized by hypoglycemia unawareness. The mechanisms operating during pregnancy are not different from those outside pregnancy. In particular the exposure to low blood glucose levels requested to obtain an ideal daily glycemic profile, is the main factor involved in the reduced hypoglycemia awareness of pregnancy.

Maternal hypoglycemia

Fetal consequences

A series of experimental studies in animals have demonstrated a teratogenic effect of maternal hypoglycemia occurring during the embryogenesis. The exposure, in vitro, of mouse embryos to hypoglycemic milieu even for short periods (2 h) in the first stages of embryogenesis, resulted in malformations. This could be explained by the fact that younger embryos are very sensitive to hypoglycemia because they are dependent on uninterrupted glycolisis and do not have developed the ability for aerobic glucose metabolism.[30,31]

Studies regarding a potential teratogenic effect of hypoglycemia in pregnant women are few. Impastato et al.,[32]

more than 40 years ago, reported that six out of 19 normal pregnant women who received insulin coma therapy, for psychiatric disorders, during the early phase of pregnancy, had malformed fetus. The following clinical studies evaluating the potential teratogenic effect of maternal hypoglycemia in diabetic patients, as reported in Table 32.1, showed no increase in the frequency of fetal malformations in women who experienced frequent episodes of hypoglycemia.[33-41]

Anyway, due to the limited data reported in literature, and to the fact that no prospective studies have been performed on this topic, the possibility that severe episodes of hypoglycemia may contribute to congenital malformations cannot be completely excluded (Table 32.1).

Studies aimed to evaluate fetal heart rate (FHR) during hypoglycemia in diabetic pregnant women, are conflicting. While some studies showed fetal tachycardia during maternal hypoglycemic coma,[42] others, showed bradycardia and reduced fetal movements during maternal hypoglycemia.[43] An increased FHR has been demonstrated during hypoglycemic clamp studies, probably as a consequence of maternal increased simpatico-adrenal activity.[44] On the contrary, other studies have reported no changes in FHR and fetal movements, suggesting that the fetus could use alternative substrate during episodes of maternal hypoglycemia.[45] Anyway, with correction of maternal blood glucose levels FHR and fetal activity returned to normal.

Although data regarding congenital malformations and functional cardiac anomalies are not conclusive, it is accepted that low levels of maternal glucose during pregnancy, may cause fetal growth retardation and small for gestational age infants.

Langher has showed that in gestational diabetic pregnant women the frequency of small for gestational age infants was 20% in women with low mean plasma glucose levels (<4.8 mmol/L), significantly higher with respect to normal pregnant women (11%).[46]

In addition, maternal hypoglycemia may also determine impaired fetal beta-cell function. In fact, animal experimental

Table 32.1 Maternal hypoglycaemia and embryogenesis in Type 1 diabetic pregnancies

Study (first author, reference number, and year)	Time of exposure Glycemic levels	Pregnancy outome
Impastato et al.[32] 1964	<10 gw (19 nondiabetic women)	Abortion (2) stillbirth (2), multiple malformations (1), Hirschprung's disease (1)
Molsted-Pedersen et al.[33] 1964	First trimester	Lower frequency of maternal hypoglycemia in malformed infants
Bergman et al.[34] 1986	Whole pregnancy (BG <3.3mmol/L)	No relationship with malformations
Rayburn et al.[35] 1986	Whole pregnancy (altered consciousness requiring assistance by another person)	No relationship with malformations
Mills et al.[36] 1988	5–12 gw BG <2.8 mmol/L or symptoms	No relationship with malformations
Steel et al.[37] 1990	<9 gw Severe hypoglycemia	No relationship with malformations
Kitzmiller et al.[38] 1991	2–8 gw BG <2.7 or symptoms	No relationship with malformations
Kimmerle et al.[39] 1992	Not known Hypoglycemic coma	No relationship with malformations
Rosenn et al.[40] 1995	7–13 gw Severe hypoglycemia	No relationship with malformations
DCCT[41] 1996	First trimester Severe hypoglycemia	No relationship with malformations

BG, blood glucose; gw, gestational week.

studies suggest that a fetus with intrauterine growth restriction caused by chronic placental insufficiency, has impaired insulin secretion, insulin biosynthesis, and insulin content. The fetal beta-cell dysfunction might indicate mechanisms that are developmentally adaptive for fetal survival, but later in life might predispose offspring to adult-onset diabetes.[47]

The degree of glycemic control during pregnancy affects perinatal outcome; nevertheless, data of pregnancy outcome in diabetic women with repeated hypoglycemia are few. Perinatal outcome seems not to be affected by severe episodes of hypoglycemia.[34,39]

Finally, studies in children of mothers who experienced frequent severe hypoglycemic episodes during pregnancy, showed no relation between intellectual performance, psychomotor development, and hypoglycemia. Rizzo et al. studied children of mothers with hypoglycemia during the second and third trimester of pregnancy. They found normal intelligence scores at 2 and 5 years of age.[48]

Maternal risk of hypoglycemia

Severe hypoglycemia can be harmful for the mother because it can be related to the development of coma, seizures and maternal death. Furthermore recurrent hypoglycemic episodes can determine a deterioration of cognitive function.[49]

Treatment

Diabetic people should be educated to identify correctly the alarm symptoms of hypoglycemia and to treat themselves promptly to prevent progression to neuroglycopenia. All hypoglycemic episodes, even in the absence of symptoms, require treatment. The goal of the treatment is to increase the blood glucose to a safe level to avoid clinical consequences.

Relatives, friends, teachers, and co-workers should be taught to recognize symptoms of hypoglycemia and, where there is doubt, they must immediately treat the person who may have hypoglycemia.

Mild-to-moderate hypoglycemia is usually treated with food, oral glucose tablets, or sucrose solutions. It is sufficient to administer 15–20 g of glucose as glucose tablets (3–5 g/10 kg body weight) or soft drinks containing pure glucose to raise blood glucose by 65 mg/dL (3 mmol/L). Fruit juice is absorbed more slowly than glucose and is not as effective in raising the blood glucose levels as tablets or liquid glucose. Likewise, honey is less efficient than glucose because it contains only 40–50% glucose and the same amount of fructose. Sucrose solution as granulated sugar in orange juice or milk does not provide a quick rise in blood glucose levels for rapid symptomatic relief and may require the administration of a larger volume. Moderate hypoglycemia may require a second administration of glucose.

In the case of loss of consciousness, the treatment is 10–25 g (20–50 ml) of 33% glucose solution injected intravenously over 1–3 min. The intravenous infusion of glucose solutions (20–50 mL at 33%) is the advised treatment for the hospitalized patient.

The administration of glucose solutions at 33% must be carefully controlled to avoid phlebitis and pain in case of breaking of the vein.

Glucagon is ideal to use at home and the standard dose is 1 mg given subcutaneously. The maximal blood glucose response occurs after 15 min, with a peak at 20 min to 1 h. When glucagon is used, it is important to remember that post-glucagon nausea and vomiting are common and that careful monitoring of blood glucose levels should be continued until the patient is able to eat normally.

Glucagon does not cross the placenta and its use in pregnancy is not dangerous.[50]

Conclusions

Diabetic pregnancy represents the most important challenge of insulin therapy, requiring a continuous effort to maintain euglycemia and avoid severe hypoglycemic episodes. Frequent exposure to low glucose levels determines an impaired glucose counter-regulation and hypoglycemia unawareness. Hypoglycemia may be dangerous for the mother, but it is unclear whether and to what extent it determines embryopathy. Finally, the worry about hypoglycemic episodes can have a negative impact on the experience of pregnancy for the mother and her partner. Women should avoid hypoglycemic episodes and be able to prevent them. Therefore, women have to be adequately instructed to perform self-glucose monitoring, observance of the diet especially of the inter-meal snacks, and insulin plan. The new therapeutic strategies, including the short-acting insulin analogs, that cover the prandial glucose peaks and reduce the hypoglycemic episodes better than the regular insulin, seem promising in this context.

REFERENCES

1. The DCCT Research Group. Hypoglycemia in the Diabetic Control and Complications Trial. Diabetes 1997; 37: 271–86.
2. Laing SP, Swerdlow AJ, Slater SD, et al. The British Diabetic Association Cohort Study. II. Cause-specific mortality in patients with insulin treated diabetes mellitus. Diabet Med 1999; 16: 466–71.
3. The U.K. Prospective Diabetes Study Group. Intensive blood-glucose control with sulfonylureas or insulin compared with conventional treatment and risk of complication in patients with type 2 diabetes. Lancet 1998; 352: 837–53.
4. Donnelly LA, Morris AD, Frier BM, et al. Frequency and predictors of hypoglycaemia in type 1 and insulin-treated type 2 diabetes: a population based study. Diabet Med 2005; 22: 749–55.
5. Rosenn BM, Miodovnik M, Holcberg G, Khoury JC, Siddiqi TA. Hypoglycemia: the price of intensive insulin therapy for pregnant women with insulin dependent diabetes mellitus. Obstet Gynecol 1995; 85: 417–22.
6. Hellmuth E, Damm P, Molsted-Pedersen L, Bendtson I. Prevalence of nocturnal hypoglycemia in first trimester of pregnancy in patients with insulin treated diabetes mellitus. Acta Obstet Gynecol Scand 2000; 79: 958–62.
7. Evers IM, ter Braak EWMT, de Valk HW, et al. Risk indicators predictive for severe hypoglycemia during the first trimester of type 1 diabetic pregnancy. Diabetes Care 2002; 25: 554–9.

8. Ben-Haroush A, Yogev Y, Chen R, et al. The postprandial glucose profile in the diabetic pregnancy. Am J Obstet Gynecol 2004; 191: 576–81.

9. Yogev Y, ben Haroush A, Chen R, et al. Undiagnosed asymptomatic hypoglycemia: diet, insulin, and glyburide for gestational diabetic pregnancy. Obstet Gynecol 2004; 104: 88–93.

10. Cryer P, Davis S, Shamoon H. Hypoglycaemia in diabetes. Diabetes Care 2003; 26: 1902–12.

11. Cryer PE. The prevention and correction of hypoglycemia. In: Jefferson LS, Cherrington AD, eds. Handbook of Physiology. The Endocrine Pancreas and Regulation of Metabolism. New York: Oxford University Press; 2001, pp. 1057–92.

12. Mitrakou A, Ryan C, Venemen T, et al. Hierarchy of glycemic thresholds for activation of conterregulatory hormone secretion, initiation of symptoms and onset of cerebral dysfunction in normal human. Am J Physiol 1991; 260: E67–74.

13. Fanelli C, Pampanelli S, Lalli C, et al. Long term intensive therapy of IDDM diabetic patients with clinically overt autonomic neuropathy on awareness and counterregulation to hypoglicaemia. Diabetes 1997; 46: 1172–81.

14. Segel SA, Paramore DS, Cryer PE. Hypoglycaemia associated autonomic failure in advanced type 2 diabetes. Diabetes 2002; 51: 724–33.

15. Connolly CC, Aglione LN, Smith MS, Lacy B, Moore MC. Pregnancy impairs the counterregulatory response to insulin-induced hypoglycemia in the dog. Am J Physiol Metab 2004; 287: 480–8.

16. Rosenn BM, Miodovnik M, Khoury JC, Siddiqi TA. Counter-regulatory hormonal responses to hypoglycemia during pregnancy Obstet Gynecol 1996; 87: 568–74.

17. Diamond MP, Reece EA, Caprio S, et al. Impairment of counterregulatory hormone responses to hypoglycemia in pregnant women with insulin-dependent diabetes mellitus. Am J Obstet Gynecol 1992; 166: 70–7.

18. Canniff KM, Smith MS, Lacy DB, Williams PE, Moore MC. Glucagon secretion and autonomic signaling during hypoglycemia in late pregnancy. Am J Physiol Regul Integr Comp Physiol 2006; 223: 4–28.

19. Bjorklund AO, Adauson UK, Calstrom KA, et al. Placental Hormones during induced hypoglycemia in pregnant women with insulin dependent diabetes mellitus: evidence of an active role for placenta in hormonal counter-regulation. Br J Obstet Gynecol 1998; 105: 649–55.

20. Fanelli C, Porcellati F, Pampanelli S, Bolli G. Insulin therapy and hypoglycaemia: the size of the problem. Diabetes Metab Res Rev 2004; 20: S32–42.

21. The Diabetes Control and Complications Trial Research Group. Epidemiology of severe hypoglycaemia in the Diab Control and Complication Trial. Am J Med 1991; 90: 450–9.

22. Cryer PE. Hypoglycaemia-associated autonomic failure in diabetes. Am J Physiol 2001; 281: E115–21.

23. The UKPDS Research Group. Overview of 6 years of therapy of type 2 diabetes: a progressive desease. Diabetes 1995; 44: 1249–58.

24. Di Cianni G, Miccoli R, Volpe L, Lencioni C, Del Prato S. Intermediate metabolism in normal pregnancy and in gestational diabetes. Diab Met Res Rev 2003; 19: 259–70.

25. Bjorklund AO, Adamson UK, Lins PE, Westegren LM. Diminished insulin clearance during late pregnancy in patients with type 1 diabetes mellitus. Clin Sci 1998; 95: 317–23.

26. Foster DW, Rubenstein AH. Hypoglycaemia. In: Wilson JD, Braunwald E, Isselbacher KJ et al. eds. Harrison's Principles of Internal Medicine. New York: McGraw-Hill; 1991, pp. 1759–68.

27. Briscoe VJ, Davis SN. Hypoglycaemia in type 1 and type 2 diabetes: physiology, pathophysiology, and management. Clin Diabetes 2006; 24: 115–21.

28. Pramming S, Thorsteinsson B, Bendstone I, Binder C. Symptomatic hypoglicaemia in 411 type 1 diabetic patients. Diabet Med 1991; 8: 217–22.

29. Heller SR. How should hypoglycaemia unawareness be managed? In: Gill G, Williams G, Pickup J, eds. Difficult Diabetes: Current Management Challenges. Oxford: Blackwell Science; 2001; pp. 168–87.

30. Illsley NP. Glucose transportes in human placenta. Placenta 2000; 21: 14–22.

31. Smoak IW, Sadler TW. Embryopathic effects of short-term exposure to hypoglycemia in mouse embryo in vitro. Am J Obstet Gynecol 1990; 163: 619–24.

32. Impastato DJ, Gabriel AR, Lardaro EH. Electric and insulin shock therapy during pregnancy. Dis Nerv Syst 1964; 23: 542–6.

33. Molsted-Pedersen L, Tygstrup I, Pedersen J. Congenital malformations in newborn infants of diabetic women. Correlation with maternal diabetic vascular complications. Lancet 1964; 23: 1124–6.

34. Bergman M, Seaton TB, Auerhahn CC, et al. The incidence of gestational hypoglycemia in insulin-dependent and non-insulin-dependent diabetic women. NY State J Med 1986; 86: 174–7.

35. Rayburn W, Piehl E, Jacober S, Schork A, Ploughman L. Severe hypoglycaemia during pregnancy: its frequency and predisposing factors in diabetic women. Int J Gynaecol Obstet 1986; 24: 263–8.

36. Mills JL, Knopp RH, Simpson JL, et al. Lack of relation of increased malformation rates in infants of diabetic mothers to glycemic control during organogenesis. N Engl J Med 1988; 318: 671–6.

37. Steel JM, Johnstone FD, Hepburn DA, Smith AF. Can pregnancy care of diabetic women reduce the risk of abnormal babies? BMJ 1990; 301: 1070–4.

38. Kitzmiller JL, Gavin LA, Gin GD, et al. Preconception care of diabetes. Glycemic control prevents congenital anomalies. JAMA 1991; 265: 731–6.

39. Kimmerle R, Heinemann L, Delecki A, Berger M. Severe hypoglycemia incidence and predisponing factors in 85 pregnancies of type 1 diabetic women. Diabetes Care 1992; 15: 1034–7.

40. Rosenn B, Siddiqi TA, Miodovnik M. Normalization of blood glucose in insulin-dependent diabetic pregnancies and the risks of hypoglycemia: a therapeutic dilemma. Obstet Gynecol Surv 1995; 50: 56–61.

41. The Diabetes Control and Complications Trial (DCCT) Group. Pregnancy outcome in the Diabetes Control and Complications Trial. Am J Obstet Gynaecol 1996; 174: 1343–53.

42. Confino E, Ismajovic B, David MP, Gleicher N. Fetal heart rate in maternal hypoglycaemic coma. Int J Gynaecol Obstet 1985; 23: 59–60.

43. Langer O, Cohen WR. Persistent fetal bradycardia during maternal hypoglycaemia. Am J Obstet Gynaecol 1984; 149: 688–90.

44. Bjorlund AO, Adamson UK, Almstrom NH. Effects of hypoglycaemia on fetal heart activity and umbilical artery doppler velocity waveforms in pregnant women with insulin dependent diabetes mellitus. Br J Obstet Gynaecol 1996; 103: 413–20.

45. Lapidot A, Haber S. Effect of acute insulin-induced hypoglycemia on fetal versus adult brain fuel utilization assessed by ^{13}C MRS isotopomer analysis of (U-^{13}C)-glucose metabolism. Dev Neurosci 2000; 22: 444–55.

46. Langer O, Levy J, Brustman L, et al. Glycemic control in gestational diabetes mellitus – how tight is tight enough: small for gestational age versus large for gestational age? Am J Obstet Gynaecol 1989; 161: 646–53.

47. Limesand SW, Rozane PJ, Zerbe GO, Hutton JC, Hav Jr WW. Attenuated insulin release and storage in feal sheep pancreatic islet with intrauterine growth restriction. Endocrinology 2006; 147: 1488–97.

48. Rizzo T, Metzger BE, Burns WJ, Burns K. Correlations between antepartum maternal metabolism and child intelligence. N Engl J Med 1991; 325: 911–6.

49. Deary IJ, Frier BM. Severe hypoglycaemia and cognitive impairment in diabetes. BMJ 1996; 313: 767–8.

50. Rayburn W, Piehl E, Sanfield J, Compton A. Reversing severe hypoglycaemia during pregnancy with glucagon therapy. Am J Perinatol 1987; 4: 259–61.

33 Sonography in diabetic pregnancies

Israel Meizner and Reuven Mashiach

Introduction

Diabetes is the most common medical complication of pregnancy. Patients can be separated into those who were known to have diabetes before pregnancy (overt) and those diagnosed during pregnancy (gestational diabetes mellitus, GDM). GDM is associated with 3–5% of all live births,[1] though the rate may be even higher in selected populations (e.g. Mexican–Americans, Asians, Indians).[2,3] The rate of Type 2 diabetes has increased significantly (approximately 33%) compounded with the presumed parallel risk for obesity.[4] Women with GDM often develop Type 2 diabetes in later life.[5,6] The significant improvement in outcome of diabetic pregnancies since the advent of insulin therapy at the start of the twentieth century is attributable to improved perinatal maternal glycemic control, close antepartum surveillance, and advances in neonatal care. With appropriately treated gestational diabetes, the likelihood of fetal death is no different from that in the general population.[7] Nevertheless, diabetic gravidas are still at high risk of adverse perinatal outcome. The complications include an increase in perinatal mortality, congenital malformations, deviant fetal growth (macrosomia and growth restriction), metabolic complications, birth trauma and the resultant increase in neonatal intensive care unit admission.[8,9] Ultrasonography is important for monitoring diabetic pregnancies and potentially improving both perinatal management and fetal outcome. It is used to assess four major factors:

- Gestational age
- Congenital anomalies
- Growth abnormalities
- Macrosomia
- Intrauterine growth restriction
- Fetal well-being (dynamic assessment)

The evaluation should take the differences between gestational and pregestational diabetes into account and be tailored accordingly.

Gestational age

The evaluation of gestational age is vital to the management of diabetic gravidas because of the increased possibility of growth abnormalities and the importance of delivery at term. The clinical estimation of gestational age has been found to be unsatisfactory in a significantly large number of cases, even when the menstrual history is reliable, and it may therefore be inadequate for critical management decisions.[10] The two most widely used ultrasound measurements for determining gestational age are crown–rump length (CRL) in the first trimester (up to 12 weeks' gestation) and biparietal diameter (BPD) in the second (before 32 weeks' gestation).[11,12] The CRL, assessed with transvaginal sonography, can predict the delivery date to within 5 days.[13] The BPD, assessed by serial ultrasound examinations, is used for confirmation. Femur length is also a valuable predictor of gestational age, especially when it is technically impossible to measure BPD.[14] The first sonographic examination to determine dates should be performed in the first trimester, prior to 12 weeks' gestation whenever possible. These data can assist in the interpretation of gestational-age-correlated biochemical data, such as alpha-fetoprotein and glycosylated hemoglobin levels, as well as in the early detection of fetal malformations. If the findings in the first ultrasound examination differ significantly from clinical dating, the ultrasound examination usually needs to be repeated after at least a 3-week interval. Gestational age can then be determined by the methods of mean projected gestational age or growth-adjusted sonographic age.[15] After 32 weeks' gestation, ultrasound can estimate age only within ±3 weeks. Clinicians should be aware that CRL measurements of fetuses of diabetic gravidas may lag behind those of normal fetuses at the same gestational age.[16] These fetuses also have a higher risk of being malformed.[17–19] Steel et al.[20] reported that early growth delay is probably an artefact of incorrectly estimated ovulation date. These observations can be confirmed only by the study of many diabetic women with conceptually timed pregnancies.

Congenital anomalies

An association between maternal diabetes mellitus and congenital malformations has been suspected since the nineteenth century.[21,22] Despite the considerable advances in the management of the pregnancy complicated by diabetes, the rate of congenital malformations has not changed dramatically. Congenital malformations and their sequelae have replaced intrauterine fetal death and respiratory distress syndrome as the major causes of morbidity and mortality in infants of diabetic mothers.[21] Their estimated frequency is 6–10%, or 3- to 5-fold higher than the rate in the general population.[23] Therefore, perinatal death as a result of congenital malformations account for approximately 40–50% in infants of diabetic mothers.[24,25] Most researchers believe that high rates of severe malformations are the consequence of poorly controlled diabetes, both periconceptionally as well as early in pregnancy,[26,27] though others have failed to totally corroborate these findings.[28–30] The precise mechanism underlying the abnormal development of fetuses of hyperglycemic mothers has not been completely elucidated. The pathogenesis may also involve factors other than hyperglycemia, such as free oxygen radical scavenging enzymes.[31] Diabetes in pregnancy is not associated with a specific fetal phenotype or syndrome, but rather affects multiple organ systems.[32]

The sonographic detection of recognizable congenital anomalies is an important aspect of the management of diabetic pregnancy. Diabetes-associated malformations occur very early in pregnancy, usually before the eighth week of gestation. Therefore, the evaluation should be done in the first trimester of pregnancy and repeated in the second. Cardiovascular anomalies are the most common, especially conotruncal and ventricular septal defects.[33–35] Indeed, maternal diabetes mellitus has been accepted as one of the indications for fetal echocardiography because congenital heart disease occurs four to five times more frequently in the offspring of women with diabetes than in the general population.[36–38] Antenatal identification is important because some defects are ductal-dependent and require immediate therapy after birth.[39] Fetuses of diabetic mothers are at risk for accelerated myocardial growth. The cardiomyopathy is mainly related to poor glycemic control. In adequately controlled glycemia, cardiac growth and ventricular diastolic filling are normal.[40,41] Second in frequency are neural tube defects (NTD). Maternal serum alpha-feto-protein (MSAFP) testing is an important indicator of NTD: second-trimester values in women with pre-gestational diabetes are on average 20% lower than in the general population. In these cases, MSAFP levels are corrected without regard to diabetic control. The sensitivity of ultrasound for the detection of NTDs associated with increased MSAFP values is reporting as high as 94%.[42] Be that as it may, all diabetic pregnancies should be sonographically evaluated for NTDs regardless of MSAFP level. Anencephaly is the most common anomaly affecting the central nervous system, with an incidence of 0.57% in fetuses of diabetic pregnancy, or 3-fold higher than in the normal population (0.19%).[43] Maternal diabetes is also thought to increase the risk of holoprosencephaly, which results from failure of cleavage of the prosencephalon. Interestingly, the lesion most associated with diabetic embryopathy, namely caudal regression syndrome (caudal dysplasia sequence)[44] is actually less common than cardiovascular malformations. However, it is difficult to estimate its incidence because it is often reported together with cases of sirenomelia. The pathogenesis is currently thought to be heterogenous. The primary defect is in the midposterior axis mesoderm. All degrees of severity may occur, depending primarily on the relative length and width of the early caudal deficit.[35]

The most severe form is presumably the consequence of a wedge-shaped early deficit of the caudal blastema.[45] Associated anomalies, in accordance with the severity of the syndrome, may include imperforate anus, absence of external genitalia, renal agenesis, absence of internal genitalia except gonads, a single umbilical artery, absence of bladder, and fusion of the lower limbs. The principal findings of caudal regression syndrome on sonographic radiology are as follows: various types of lower limb anomalies ranging from hip dislocation to frog-leg deformity and equinovarus, hydrocephalus, and Dandy–Walker malformation, complete absence of the spine below L_1, partial or complete absence of the caudal part of the sacrum, intraspinal anomalies in the form of meningomyelocele and sacral lipoma, whereas the pelvis is small owing to the absence of a sacrum, and the iliac bones touch or even fuse.[46] Up to 16% of these cases are associated with diabetes mellitus.[47,48] Although the disorder occurs 200 times more often in infants of diabetic mothers, only 1.3 per 1000 diabetic pregnancies are affected. This anomaly cannot be considered pathognomonic for diabetes since it occurs in other conditions as well. The skeletal, genitourinary, and gastrointestinal systems may also be affected. Defects involving the genitourinary system that show preponderance in infants of diabetic mothers include ureteral duplication, renal agenesis, and hydronephrosis.

Controversy exist as to the optimum time to perform the first ultrasound examination and how many subsequent examinations are needed for identification of fetal malformations.[49] Fetal evaluation cannot be wholly completed during the first anatomical scan. An early scan at 10–14 weeks of gestation permits exclusion of major malformations, and an additional scan at 20–22 weeks is advisable in order to rule previously unrecognized malformations.

Growth abnormalities

Monitoring fetal growth is a challenging and highly inexact process. Today's tools, which involve serial plotting of fetal growth parameters, are superior to earlier clinical estimations, but accuracy is still only about 15%, even with the most sophisticated ultrasound equipment. Particular effort should be directed toward the diagnosis of fetal macrosomia, the most frequent fetal complication (up to 50%) of diabetic pregnancy.[50–54] Macrosomia is a term used rather imprecisely to describe a very large fetus–neonate. There is no universally accepted definition. Macrosomia has been variously defined as a birth weight greater than 4000–4500 g as well as a birth weight greater than 2 standard deviations above the mean for gestational age or above the 90th percentile for population-specific and sex-specific growth curves. It is not only a result of maternal hyperglycemia, an elevated levels of lipids and amino acids, which are also characteristic pregnancies complicated by GDM, can result in fetal overgrowth as well. Fetal organomegaly is also common, affecting the fetal liver, pancreas, heart and adrenal glands.[55] Fetal overgrowth or macrosomia can lead to some of the most common morbidities seen in infants of women with GDM. For example, the incidence of shoulder dystocia, which ranges from 0.2 to 2.8% in the general population[56,57] can be as high as 3–9% in infants of women with GDM.[58] In addition, the growth of these infants tends to be asymmetric, with larger chest/head and shoulder/head ratios than in infants born to women with normal glucose tolerance.[59] Shoulder dystocia may be associated with other birth traumas, such as Erb's palsy, clavicular fracture, fetal distress, low Apgar scores, and birth asphyxia,[60] though 25–75% of brachial plexus injuries are unrelated to antecedent shoulder dystocia.[61] The management of fetal macrosomia has been the subject of much clinical concern and scientific investigation. Over the past 30 years, several investigators have attempted to derive formulas using sonographic measurements of fetal organs to estimate fetal weight. The older formulas used measures of the fetal head, abdomen, and femur, either alone[62] or in combination.[63,64] Some authors demonstrated differences in accuracy and precision among these formulas.[65,66] Although most reported that regardless of the formula used, the accuracy of the fetal weight estimation decreased with increasing birth weight.[67–69] Consequently, alternative sonographic markers for fetal macrosomia have been proposed which take advantage of the presumed correlation between subcutaneous fat deposition and fetal weight. Three-dimensional ultrasound measurements of fetal upper arm volume,[70,71] fetal chest,[72] abdominal[73] and humeral[74] soft tissue thickness, and cheek-to-cheek diameter,[75] as well as of the subcutaneous tissue/femur length ratio,[66,67] have yielded varying screening efficacies for macrosomia. Table 33.1 lists a number of population-based studies that assessed the clinical performance of ultrasound in predicting macrosomia. The data in the last two columns suggest that only 15–81% of babies (median, 67%) predicted to be macrosomic are indeed macrosomic at birth, and that only 50–100% (median, 62%) of all cases

of macrosomia are successfully predicted by sonographic measurements.

Currently, no single sonographic measurement is capable of distinguishing between large-for-gestational-age (LGA) and appropriate-for-gestational-age (AGA) infants of diabetic mothers. The finding of an abdominal circumference above the 90th percentile during the second or third trimester is associated positively with fetal macrosomia, but actual birth weights of the babies predicted to be macrosomic on this basis overlap with those of AGA babies in a substantial proportion of cases.[84]

Other techniques for estimating fetal weight have been reported as well. In one study, magnetic resonance imaging yielded estimates within 3% of the actual birth weight in 11 patients whose babies weighed between 1.6 and 3.3 kg. This compared favorably with the 6.5% error by sonographic examination of the same patients.[85]

The estimation of weight in fetuses of diabetic mothers involves special considerations. Because of this disproportionate contribution of fat to fetal body weight and because fat is less dense than lean body tissue, equations used derived from cross-sectional data may theoretically overestimate fetal weight when applied to the GDM population.[86] Furthermore, the time from examination to delivery may influence the accuracy and precision of the sonographic estimates.[78,79,87]

Clinically, studies have found no significant differences in absolute percent error of birth weight between infants of women with diabetes and those born to women without diabetes.[88] The accuracy of birth weight prediction by ultrasound and by clinical estimates has been analyzed in a number of studies.[89–94] When the sample was limited to babies with an actual birth weight of >4 kg, no significant differences were found between the clinical and ultrasound estimates at or near the onset of labor.

Table 33.1   Sonographic criteria for macrosomia in the general population and in diabetic mothers. Except as indicated, macrosomia was defined as a birth weight ≥4000 g

Sonographic criteria	Number scanned	Inclusion criteria	PPV (%)	Sensitivity (%)
AC, FL[65]	3512	Nondiabetic	15	94
AC, FL[69]	150	37+ weeks	52	54
AC, FL[66]	223	35–42 weeks	67	62
AC, FL, BPD[78]	479	40 4/7 weeks, nondiabetic	67	56
BPD, OFD, ALD, ASD, FL[79]	498	22–50	67	67
Abdominal sub-cutaneous tissue[73]	133	37–42 weeks	59	70
Humeral soft tissue[74]	95	Term, prior macrosomia; diabetic	81	88
	519	≥41 weeks	64	56
	472	≥41 weeks	70	61
AC, FL[80]		Nondiabetic		
AC, FL[81]	406	36+ weeks	51	50
	86	36+ weeks	67	100
AC, FL, BPD, HC[83]*	Nondiabetic			
AC, FL, HC[83]				

PPV, positive predictive value; Sens, sensitivity; AC, abdominal circumference; FL, femur length; BPD, biparietal diameter; HC, head circumference; OFD, occipitofrontal diameter; ALD, abdominal longest diameter; ASD, abdominal shortest diameter; NR, not reported; *Macrosomia defined as birth weight ≥90th percentile for gestational age.

Intrauterine growth restriction (IUGR), broadly defined as a birth weight lower than the 10th percentile for a given gestational age or an infant with evidence of tissue wasting and malnutrition, is not common in diabetic pregnancies. Because IUGR is associated with conditions that predispose the fetus to uteroplacental insufficiency, it is more likely to occur in diabetic pregnancies complicated by severe vasculopathy. The resultant decrease in placental nutrient transfer is thought to be responsible for the IUGR in these infants. Unlike macrosomic fetuses, fetuses with IUGR associated with pancreatic agenesis apparently stop growing at 28–30 weeks' gestation.[95] The relative inaccuracy of clinical means for detecting IUGR may result in misdiagnosis in 50–70% of cases. Serial ultrasonography may be beneficial as it is offered as a routine antenatal procedure.

The use of three-dimensional ultrasonography in the assessment of the diabetic fetus

The growing importance of the three-dimensional method and the extended range of applications in prenatal diagnosis has been underscored by many descriptions published in recent scientific publications. The usefulness of this technology is currently being debated. Some studies suggest that the image information acquired by three-dimensional ultrasound technology is nearly always inferior to the image information obtained by conventional two-dimensional imaging[96] while others support its use.[97,98]

REFERENCES

1. Ventura SJ, Martin JA, Curtin SC, Mathews TJ, Park MS. Births: Final data for 1998. National Vital Statistics Reports, vol. 48; 2000.
2. King H. Epidemiology of glucose intolerance and gestational diabetes in women of childbearing age. Diabetes 1998; 2(suppl. 2): 9–13.
3. Engelgau NM, Herman WH, Smith PI, German RR, Aubert RE. The epidemiology of diabetes and pregnancy in the US. Diabetes Care 1998; 18: 1029–33.
4. Langer O, Yogev Y, Xenakis E, Brustman L. Overweight and obese in gestational diabetes: the impact on pregnancy outcome. Am J Obstet Gynecol 2005; 192: 1768–76.
5. MacNeill S, Dodds L, Hamilton DC, Armson BA, Vandenhof M. Rates and risk factors for recurrence of gestational diabetes. Diabetes Care 2001; 24: 659–62.
6. Conway D, Langer O. Effects of new criteria for type 2 diabetes on the rate of postpartum glucose intolerance in women with gestational diabetes. Am J Obstet Gynecol 1999; 181: 600–14.
7. Metzger BE, Coustan DR. Summary and recommendations of the Fourth International Workshop–Conference on Gestational Diabetes Mellitus. Diabetes Care 1998; 21: B161–75.
8. Suhonen L, Hiilesmaa V, Teramo K. Glycemic control during early pregnancy and fetal malformations in women with type 1 diabetes mellitus. Diabetologia 2000; 43: 79–82.
9. Lauenborg J, Mathiesen E, Ovesen P, et al. Audit on stillbirths in women with pregestational type 1 diabetes. Diabetes Care 2003; 26: 1385–8.
10. Callen PW. Ultrasonography in Obstetrics and Gynecology. Philadelphia: WB Saunders; 2000, pp. 146–70.
11. Robinson HP. Sonar measurements of the fetal crown-rump length as a means of assessing maturity in first trimester pregnancy. Br Med J 1973; 4: 28–31.
12. Campbell S, Newman GB. Growth of the fetal biparietal diameter during pregnancy. J Obstet Gynecol Br Com 1971; 78: 513–6.
13. Robinson HP, Fleming JEE. A critical evaluation of sonar crown–rump length measurements. Br J Obstet Gynecol 1975; 82: 702–6.
14. O'Brien GD, Queenan JT, Campbell S. Assessment of gestational age in the second trimester by real-time ultrasound measurement of the femur length. Am J Obstet Gynecol 1981; 139: 540–4.
15. Kopta MM, Tomich PG, Crane JP. Ultrasound methods of predicting the estimated date of confinement. Obstet Gynecol 1981; 57: 657–60.
16. Pedersen JF, Molsted-Pedersen L. Early growth retardation in diabetic pregnancy. Br Med J 1979; 1: 18–19.
17. Pedersen JF, Molsted-Pedersen L. Early fetal growth delay detected by ultrasound marks increased risk of congenital malformation in diabetic pregnancy. Br Med J 1981; 283: 80–4.
18. Pedersen JF, Molsted-Pedersen L, Mortensen HB. Fetal growth delay and maternal hemoglobin A1c in early diabetic pregnancy. Obstet Gynecol 1984; 64: 351–61.
19. Pedersen JF, Molsted-Pedersen L. The possibility of an early growth delay in White's class A diabetic pregnancy. Diabetes 1985; 34: (suppl. 2): 47–50.
20. Steel JM, Wu PS, Johnstone DF, et al. Does early growth delay occur in diabetic pregnancy? Br J Obstet Gynaecol 1995; 102: 224–7.
21. Mills JL. Malformations in infants of diabetic mothers. Teratology 1982; 25: 385–9.
22. Mills JL, Baker L, Goldman AS. Malformations in infants of diabetic mothers occur before the seventh gestational week: Implications for treatment. Diabetes 1979; 28: 292–6.
23. Hanson U, Persson B. Outcome of pregnancy complicated by Type 1 insulin dependent diabetes in Sweden: Acute pregnancy complications, neonatal mortality, and morbidity. Am J Perinatol 1993; 10: 330–3.
24. Becerra JE, Khoury MJ, Cordero JF, Erickson JD. Diabetes mellitus during pregnancy and the risks for specific birth defects: a population-based controlled study. Pediatrics 1990; 85: 1–9.
25. Landon MB, Gabbe SG. Diabetes and pregnancy. Med Clin North Am 1988; 72: 1493–511.
26. Miller E, Hare JW, Cloherty JP, et al. Elevated maternal hemoglobin A1c in early pregnancy and major congenital anomalies in infants of diabetic mothers. N Engl J Med 1981; 304: 1331–9.
27. Lucas MJ, Leveno KL, Williams ML, Raskin P, Whalley PJ. Early pregnancy glycosylated hemoglobin, severity of diabetes, and fetal malformations. Am J Obstet Gynecol 1989; 161: 426–30.
28. Mills JL, Knopp RH, Simpson JL, et al. National Institute of Child Health and Human Development Diabetes in Early Pregnancy Study: Incidence of spontaneous abortion among normal women and insulin-dependent diabetic women whose pregnancies were identified within 21 days of conception. N Engl J Med 1988; 318: 671–81.
29. Schaefer-Graf UM, Buchanan TA, Xiang A, et al. Patterns of congenital anomalies and relationship to initial maternal fasting glucose levels in pregnancies complicated by type 2 and gestational diabetes. Am J Obstet Gynecol 2000; 182: 313–24.
30. Rose BJ, Graff S, Spencer R. Major congenital anomalies in infants and glycosylated hemoglobin levels in insulin-requiring diabetic mothers. J Perinatol 1988; 8: 309–11.
31. Reece EA, Homko CJ, Wu YK. Multifactorial basis of the syndrome of diabetic embryopathy. Teratology 1997; 54: 171–82.
32. Mills JL. Congenital malformations in diabetes. In: Gabbe SG, Oh W, eds. Infant of the Diabetic Mother. Report of the 93rd Ross Conference on Pediatric Research. Columbus, Ohio: Ross Laboratories; 1987, pp. 12–9.
33. Adams MM, Mulinare J, Dooley K. Risk factors for conotruncal cardiac defects in Atlanta. J Am Coll Cardiol 1989; 14: 432–42.
34. Ferencz C, Rubin JD, McCarter RJ. Maternal diabetes and cardiovascular malformations: Predominance of double outlet right ventricle and truncus arteriosus. Teratology 1990; 41: 319–26.
35. Lowy C, Beard RW, Goldschmidt J. Congenital malformations in babies of diabetic mothers. Diabet Med 1986; 3: 458–62.
36. Rowland TW, Hubbell JP, Nadas AS. Congenital heart disease in infants of diabetic mothers. J Pediatr 1973; 83: 815–20.
37. Ramos-Arroyo MA, Rodriguez-Pinilla E, Cordero JF. Maternal diabetes: The risk for specific birth defects. Eur J Epidemiol 1992; 8: 503–8.

38. Fraser R. Diabetes in pregnancy. Arch Dis Child 1994; 71: 224–38.
39. Ramada SS, Christine HC, Robert PL, Janet SK, Wesley L. Maternal diabetes mellitus: Which views are essential for fetal echocardiography. Obstet Gynecol 1997; 90: 575–9.
40. Kozak-Barany A, Jokinen E, Kero P, et al. Impaired left ventricular diastolic function in newborn infants of mothers with pregestational or gestational diabetes with good glycemic control. Early Hum Dev 2004; 77: 13–22.
41. Jaeggi ET, Fouron JC, Proulx F. Fetal cardiac performancein uncomplicated and well-controlled maternal type I diabetes. Ultrasound Obstet Gynecol 2001; 17: 311–5.
42. Watson WJ, Chescheir NC, Katz VL. The role of ultrasound in evaluation of patients with elevated maternal serum alpha-fetoprotein: A review. Obstet Gynecol 1991; 78: 123–8.
43. Soler NG, Walsh CH, Malins JM. Congenital malformations in infants of diabetic mothers. J Med 1976; 178: 303–7.
44. Lenz W, Maier W. Congenital malformations and maternal diabetes. Lancet 1964; 2: 1124–8.
45. Smith DW, Jones KL. Recognizable Pattern of Human Malformation. Philadelphia: WB Saunders; 1982, pp. 486–7.
46. Meizner I, Bar-Ziv J. In utero diagnosis of skeletal disorders. An atlas of prenatal sonographic and postnatal radiologic correlation. Boca Raton, Florida: CRC Press; 1993, pp. 72–7.
47. Rusnak SL, Driscoll SG. Congenital spinal anomalies in infants of diabetic mothers. Teratology 1965; 25: 385–9.
48. Mills JL. Malformations in infants of diabetic mothers. Teratology 1982; 25: 385–8.
49. American College of Obstetricians and Gynecologists. Practice Bulletin Number 58, December 2004. Washington, DC: ACOG; 2004.
50. Boyd ME, Usher RH, McLean FH. Fetal macrosomia: prediction, risks, proposed management. Obstet Gynecol 1983; 61: 715–22.
51. Lubchenco LO, Hansman C, Dressler M, Boyd E. Intrauterine growth as estimated from liveborn birth-weight data at 24 to 42 weeks of gestation. Pediatrics 1963; 32: 793–800.
52. Spellacy WN, Miller S, Winegar A, Peterson PQ. Macrosomia –maternal characteristics and infant complications. Obstet Gynecol 1985; 66: 185–90.
53. Langer O. Is normoglycemia the correct threshold to prevent complications in the pregnant diabetic patient? Diabetes Rev 1996; 4: 2–10.
54. American College of Obstetricians and Gynecologists. Fetal Macrosomia. ACOG Technical Bulletin no. 159. Washington, DC: ACOG; 1991.
55. Persson B, Hanson U. Neonatal morbidities in gestational diabetes mellitus. Diabetes 1998; 21(suppl. 2): 79–84.
56. Acker DB, Sachs BP, Friedman EA. Risk factors for shoulder dystocia. Obstet Gynecol 1985; 66: 762–7.
57. Langer O, Berkus HD, Huff RW, Sameloff A. Shoulder dystocia: Should the fetus weighing 4000 g be delivered by cesarean section? Am J Obstet Gynecol 1991; 165: 831–7.
58. Elliot JP, Garite TJ, Freedman RK, McQuown DS, Patel JM. Ultrasonic prediction of fetal macrosomia in diabetic patients. Obstet Gynecol Clin North Am 1999; 26: 445–58.
59. Ballard JL, Rosenn B, Khoury JC, Miodovnik M. Diabetic fetal macrosomia: Significance of disproportionate fetal growth. J Pediatr 1993; 122: 445–58.
60. Levine MG, Holroyde S, Woods JR, et al. Birth trauma: Incidence and predisposing factors. Obstet Gynecol 1984; 63: 792–5.
61. Gherman RB, Goodwin TM, Ouzounian JG. Brachial plexus palsy associated with cesarean section: an in utero injury? Am J Obstet Gynecol 1997; 177: 1162–4.
62. Campbell S, Wilkin D. Ultrasonic measurements of fetal abdomen circumference in the estimation of fetal weight. Br J Obstet Gynecol 1975; 82: 689–97.
63. Hadlock FP, Harrist RB, Carpenter RJ, Deter RL, Park SK. Sonographic estimation of fetal weight: The value of femur length in addition to head and abdomen measurements. Radiology 1984; 150: 535–40.
64. Shepard MJ, Richards VA, Berkowitz RL, Warsof RL, Hobbins JC. An evaluation of two equations for predicting fetal weight by ultrasound. Am J Obstet Gynecol 1982; 142: 47–54.
65. Smith GCB, Smith MFS, McNay MB, Fleming JEE. The relation between fetal abdominal circumference and birthweight: findings in 3512 pregnancies. Br J Obstet Gynaecol 1997; 104: 186–90.
66. Shamley KT, Landon MB. Accuracy and modifying factors for ultrasonographic determination of fetal weight at term. Obstet Gyncol 1994; 84: 926–30.
67. Dudley NJ. Selection of appropriate ultrasound methods for the estimation of fetal weight. Br J Radiol 1995; 68: 385–8.
68. Hirata GI, Medearis AL, Horenstein J. Ultrasonographic estimation of fetal weight in the clinically macrosomic fetus. Am J Obstet Gynecol 1990; 162: 238–42.
69. Miller JM, Korndorffer FA, Gabert HA. Fetal weight estimates in late pregnancy with emphasis on macrosomia. J Clin Ultrasound 1986; 14: 437–42.
70. Favre R, Bader A-M, Nisand G. Prospective study on fetal weight estimation using limb circumferences obtained by three-dimensional ultrasound. Ultrasound Obstet Gynecol 1995; 6: 140–4.
71. Liang R-I, Chang F-M, Yao B-L. Predicting birth weight by fetal upper-arm volume with use of three-dimensional ultrasonography. Am J Obstet Gynecol 1997; 177: 632–8.
72. Winn NH, Rauk PN, Petrie RH. Use of the fetal chest in estimating fetal weight. Am J Obstet Gynecol 1992; 167: 448–50.
73. Petrikovsky BM, Oleschuk C, Lesser M. Prediction of fetal macrosomia using sonographically measured abdominal subcutaneous tissue thickness. J Clin Ultrasound 1997; 25: 378–82.
74. Sood AK, Yancey M, Richards D. Prediction of fetal macrosomia using humeral soft tissue thickness. Obstet Gynecol 1995; 85: 937–40.
75. Abramovicz JS, Sherer DM, Woods JR. Ultrasonographic measurements of cheek-to-cheek diameter in fetal growth disturbances. Am J Obstet Gynecol 1993; 169: 405–8.
76. Santolaya-Forgas J, Meyer WJ, Gautier DW. Intrapartum fetal subcutaneous tissue/femur length ratio: An ultrasonographic clue to fetal macrosomia. Am J Obstet Gynecol 1994; 171: 1072–5.
77. Rotmensch S, Celentano C, Liberati M, et al. Screening efficacy of the subcutaneous tissue width/femur length ratio for fetal macrosomia in the non-diabetic pregnancy. Ultrasound Obstet Gynecol 1999; 13: 340–4.
78. O'Reilly-Green CP, Divon MY. Receiver operating characteristics curves of sonographic estimated fetal weight for prediction of macrosomia in prolonged pregnancies. Ultrasound Obstet Gynecol 1997; 9: 403–8.
79. Rossavik IK, Joslin GL. Macrosomatia and ultrasonography: What is the problem? South Med J 1993: 86: 1129–32.
80. Pollack RN, Hauer-Pollack G, Divon MY. Macrosomia in postdates pregnancies: the accuracy of routine ultrasonographic screening. Am J Obstet Gynecol 1992; 167: 7–11.
81. Chervenack JL, Divon MY, Hirsch J. Macrosomia in the postdate pregnancies: is routine ultrasonographic screening indicated? Am J Obstet Gynecol 1989; 161: 753–6.
82. Levine AB, Lockwood CJ, Brown B. Sonographic diagnosis of the large for gestational age fetus at term: does it make a difference? Obstet Gynecol 1992; 79: 55–8.
83. Delpapa EH, Muller-Heubach E. Pregnancy outcome following ultrasound diagnosis of macrosomia. Obstet Gynecol 1991; 78: 340–3.
84. Keller JD, Metzger BE, Doodly SL. Infants of diabetic mothers with accelerated fetal growth by ultrasonography: are they all alike? Am J Obstet Gynecol 1990; 163: 893–7.
85. Baker PN, Johnson IR, Gowland PA. Fetal weight estimation by echo-planar magnetic resonance imaging. Lancet 1994; 343: 644–5.
86. Crane SS, Avallone DA, Thomas AJ. Sonographic estimation of fetal body composition with gestational diabetes mellitus at term. Obstet Gynecol 1996; 88: 849–54.
87. Spinnato JA, Allen RD, Mendenhall HW. Birth weight prediction from remote ultrasonographic examination. Am J Obstet Gynecol 1989; 161: 742–7.
88. Alsulyman OM, Ouzounian JG, Kjos SL. The accuracy of intrapartum ultrasonographic fetal weight estimation in diabetic pregnancies. Am J Obstet Gynecol 1997; 177: 503–6.
89. Raman S, Urquhart R, Yusof M. Clinical versus ultrasound estimation of fetal weight. Aust NZ Obstet Gynaecol 1992; 32: 196–9.
90. Chauhan SP, Cowan BD, Magann EF. Intrapartum detection of a macrosomic fetus: Clinical versus 8 sonographic models. Aust NZ J Obstet Gynaecol 1995; 35: 266–70.
91. Watson WJ, Soisson AP, Harlass FE. Estimated weight of the term fetus. Accuracy of ultrasound vs clinical examination. J Reprod Med 1998; 33: 369–71.
92. Sherman DJ, Arieli S, Tovbin J. A comparison of clinical and ultrasonic estimation of fetal weight. Obstet Gynecol 1998; 91: 212–7.
93. Chauhan SP, Hendrix NW, Magann EF. Limitation of clinical and sonographic estimates of birth weight: experience with 1034 parturients. Obstet Gynecol 1998; 91: 72–7.
94. Johnstone FD, Prescott RJ, Steel JM. Clinical and ultrasound prediction of macrosomia in diabetic pregnancy. Br J Obstet Gynaecol 1996; 103: 747–54.

95. Dourow N, Buyl-Strouvens ML. Agenesis du pancreas. Arch Fr Pediatr 1969; 26: 641–50.

96. Scharf A, Ghazwiny MF, Steinborn A, Baier P, Sohn C. Evaluation of two-dimensional versus three-dimensional ultrasound in obstetrics diagnostics: a prospective study. Fetal Diagn Ther 2001; 16: 333–41.

97. Chan KL, Liu X, Ascah KJ, Beauchesne LM, Burwash IG. Comparison of real-time 3-dimensional echocardiography with conventional 2-dimensional echocardiography in the assessment of structural heart disease. J Am Soc Echocardiogr 2004; 17: 976–80.

98. Cosmi E, Piazze JJ, Ruozi A, et al. Structural tridimensional study of yolk sac in pregnancies complicated by diabetes. J Perinat Med 2005; 33: 132–6.

34 Diabetes in Pregnancy: Is Doppler useful?

Salvatore Alberico, Paolo Bogatti, Gianpaolo Maso and Uri Wiesenfeld

Introduction

The prevalence of diabetes among women is increasing worldwide. Epidemiological studies showed that the incidence of gestational diabetes (GDM) has steadily increased, reaching 6.1% Italy,[1] while pre-gestational diabetes has an incidence of 0.6–1%.

Since 1970 the number of people considered overweight (BMI ≥25) or frankly obese (BMI ≥30) has increased greatly in industrialized countries. This trend has also affected obstetric practice; e.g. in some areas in the USA, pregnant women with BMI ≥30 represent more than 30% of cases.[2] In Italy, at present, about 16% of pregnant women have a BMI ≥25, but this percentage is increasing. Therefore, physicians and the media have began to pay more attention to this problem.

Today, women with diabetic pregnancy assume they have a legitimate right to a pregnancy with a successful outcome. This result is now achievable, whereas in the past there was a high rate of both maternal and fetal complications.

In the management of diabetes in pregnancy it is important to recognize two groups (pre-gestational diabetes and GDM) of women with different genetic and phenotypic aspects, having different risks and therefore requiring different obstetric management. In the first group are women with diabetes associated with polycystic ovarian syndrome (PCOS), which, outside pregnancy, shows several vascular alterations, similar to some forms of diabetes, and which is accentuated by pregnancy. Approximately 5–10% of fertile women have the syndrome,[3] of which 50–80%, either obese or thin, show hyperinsulinemia.[4] Pathogenesis of hyperinsulinemia can be related to peripheral insulin resistance or to decreased hepatic clearance or increased pancreatic sensitivity. Obesity can enhance hyperinsulinemia, which can be further associated with decreased HDL-cholesterol and increased VLDL-cholesterol and triglycerides. Therefore the women show increased cardiovascular risk at a young age, even outside pregnancy.

Another high-risk group is represented by obese women with pre-gestational diabetes or GDM, with an incidence, in our department, of 17.4% in patients with BMI ≥25 and of 33.3% in patients with BMI ≥30.

Insulin resistance determines increased circulating levels of leptin and the inflammatory markers cytokines, interleukins 1–6 and tumor necrosis factor-alfa (TNF-α). The peripheral effects of these substances are an increased intracellular content of fat and decreased insulin sensitivity. The increase of fat induces the proliferation of vasa-vasorum of tunica media of arteries, with macrophage activation and a further increase in cytokine levels. This process can explain the inflammatory condition that provokes vascular damage.[5] Based on this information, Gu et al. examined the death certificates of 14,734 adults (age 25–74 years) with and without diabetes in a national cohort of the US population, showing that in 69% of cases atherosclerosis was associated.[6]

This introduction aimed to stress the importance of vascular changes that occur in a normal pregnancy and therefore the essential role of an absent or atypical vascular modification, which occurs more frequently in GDM or even before pregnancy in women with pre-gestational diabetes. Therefore there is a need for good plasma glucose control to reduce vascular damage that is harmful to the fetus and for good markers of fetal well-being. These markers should be sufficiently robust to preserve the fetus from hypoxic events and be able to quickly determine cerebral lesions, since decreased placental flow can be associated with maternal ketoacidosis.

In the past the main cause of intrauterine deaths was related to maternal ketoacidosis, while today it is associated with fetal macrosomia. This latter condition is related to fetal hyperinsulinemia which has an anabolic effect on nutrients and also affects the production of insulin-like growth factors.[7] Since fetal glucose levels are correlated with maternal levels, maternal hyperglycemia causes fetal hyperglycemia and secondary hyperinsulinemia as a result of beta-cell hyperplasia.

Cordocentesis in diabetic pregnancies demonstrated hyperlactacidemia and acidemia without hypoxemia,[8] the level of acidemia being correlated with the insulin level.[9]

Hyperinsulinemia and hyperglycemia independently increase aerobic and anaerobic glucose metabolism with increased oxygen consumption, lactate production and decreased pH and PO_2. Increased lactate production can be explained by the reduced fetal capacity for oxidative metabolism and low pyruvate dehydrogenase activity. Severe hyperglycemia produces acidemia and hypoxemia where moderate hyperglycemia is associated with acidemia without hypoxemia.[10] However, when mild hypoxemia is present in the fetus, mild hyperglycemia can produce severe acidosis and possibly fetal death.

259

Knowledge of these pathophysiology keypoints is necessary to promote adequate fetal surveillance in the diabetic mother. In this field Doppler flow velocimetry might play an important role, although in different gestational periods, and in different vascular areas, but distinguishing, initially, maternal phenotype and clinical aspects.

The aim of this chapter is to examine the literature concerning the correlation between Doppler flow velocimetry and fetal wellbeing and to identify fetuses at risk for unfavorable outcomes (IUGR, pre-eclampsia, fetal hypoxemia), but we will try mainly to define a flow monitoring 'personalized' by the type of maternal diabetes and by the type of fetal growth (since the combination of the situations described before has also an effect on the fetus). Finally, we will propose a schedule for using this technique, for anticipating the conditions when there is a real risk of fetal damage.

Doppler flow velocimetry of uterine circulation

Maternal blood flow to the intervillous space is supplied by vessels which show deep remodeling in normal pregnancy. Increased vessel diameter and substitution of the muscular layer of the vessel wall by trophoblastic invasion of the distal portion of spiral arteries all lead to a low impedance, high capacity vascular system. These modifications generally occur in two stages: the decidual portion of the vessel is invaded in the first trimester, while the miometrial segment is invaded in the second. As a result the diameter of spiral arteries is increased in pregnancy from 15–20 to 300–500 μm. It is well known that some obstetric pathologies, like pre-eclampsia and intrauterine growth retardation, are associated with failed or insufficient trophoblastic vascular invasion with defective reduction of vascular resistance. An attractive model in pre-eclampsia suggests that reduced placental perfusion is producing some vascular factors which cause the well known multisystem derangements in the mother. The unmodified maternal vessels show typical atherosclerotic lesions with fibrinoid deposition and foam-cell invasion which further reduce placental perfusion. These processes, although pre-eclampsia is clinically evident in late pregnancy, operate months in advance.

Histological studies[11,12] coupled with Doppler studies enabled the recognition that progressive reduction of vascular resistance can be detected by Doppler. The specific manifestation is the increased diastolic component of uterine artery Doppler tracing and concomitant reduction of measured resistance indexes. In failed or incomplete trophoblastic invasion resistance does not decrease and a protodiastolic notch can appear in the sonogram. Unfortunately, heterogeneous and even conflicting results appeared when Doppler flow measurements of the uterine artery in pregnancy were used as a screening test. Gestational age at enrolment, high/low risk pregnant population, definition criteria for a pathological Doppler tracing, Doppler equipment itself, end-point definition and different therapeutic strategies were all responsible for the difficulties encountered in validating Doppler flow measurements in the uterine artery as a screening test.

In diabetic pregnancies a similar effectiveness was found when screening the uterine artery by Doppler as for the complications of defective placentation. Haddad et al.[13] found increased vascular impedance in the uterine artery in 45% of 37 diabetic pregnancies developing pre-eclampsia or growth retardation. Also, Kofinas et al.[14] found good correlation between high impedance in the uterine artery and pre-eclampsia in 31 patients with gestational diabetes and 34 insulin-dependent diabetic patients. No correlation was found with glycemic control, however.

Pietryga et al.[15] found abnormal Doppler results in uterine artery in all the 11 patients with pre-eclampsia out of 146 gestational diabetic women. Vascular impedance was also related to birthweight and placental weight, but not to maternal HbA1c levels. However, abnormal placental vascular impedance was not frequently found in gestational diabetes. This last observation seems very logical since the vast majority of diabetic patients do not show vasculopathy, being gestational diabetics or White's class B/C which show an 8–10% associated pre-eclampsia in comparison with White's class D/F/R which show a 16% risk.[16]

Different findings characterized the cases with pre-gestational diabetes mellitus:[17] 155 pre-gestational diabetic women showed a correlation between increased impedance in the uterine artery and the level of HbA1c, increased impedance being also significantly related to pre-gestational vasculopathy and hence to adverse outcome of pregnancy, being altered placental perfusion detrimental for fetal wellbeing. In contrast to these results other authors found no correlation between uterine artery Doppler and White classification, but this can possibly be explained by the small numbers of women with vasculopathy.[18–21]

Doppler flow velocimetry of umbilical artery

The umbilical cord was the first fetal area to be studied by Doppler and many publications have been concerned with this topic. Umbilical arteries carry 40% of cardiac flow to the placenta and this means that, quantitatively, there is a continuously increasing amount of blood flowing through them, tertiary vascular villi expansion and subsequent reduction in placental vascular resistances being the predisposing factors.

Reduced diastolic velocities can be found in cases of increased placental impedance due to specific placental lesions (reduced number of tertiary villi arteries, increased numbers of obliterated vessels) which can be found in pregnancies complicated by pre-eclampsia and intrauterine growth retardation.[22,23] Reduced placental perfusion reduces oxygen delivery to the fetus, as well as that of glucose and other nutritional elements with compensatory hemodynamic modifications (increased blood flow to the ductus venosus and the so-called 'centralization of the circulation').

In diabetic pregnancies the aim of Doppler studies of umbilical circulation is to determine whether impedance to flow is related to maternal glycemic control and whether there is any correlation with maternal vasculopathy, obstetric complications and fetal compromise.

Olofsson et al.[24] found higher pulsatility in umbilical artery of diabetic pregnancies when compared to nondiabetic. No association was found with the degree of glycemic control and fetal size, but fetal distress in labor was more frequent in cases with increased resistance. Bracero et al.[25] found a significant correlation between maternal glycemia and vascular impedance, the latter being also positively correlated with stillbirths and neonatal morbidity. Bracero et al.[26] also found a 2.6 relative risk for adverse outcome in diabetic pregnancies with increased impedance in umbilical artery. This relative risk was even higher than that of an abnormal biophysical profile and a nonreactive NST.

Landon et al.[27] found no association between umbilical artery resistance and maternal blood glucose or HbA1c levels. Higher indexes were found in women with vascular disease, which was also associated with subsequent discovery of growth retardation. In women without vasculopathy, increased resistance was associated with the development of pre-eclampsia. Similar results were found by Dicker et al.[28]

Reece et al.[29] found higher umbilical pulsatility in diabetic women with vasculopathy and in fetuses with intrauterine growth restriction and neonatal metabolic complications. No correlation was found with glycemic control.

Johnstone et al.[30] found no significant association between downstream resistance in umbilical artery and glycemic control in 128 diabetic pregnancies. Fetal distress occurred both in pregnancies with normal and increased resistance.

Zimmermann et al.[31] evaluated 53 insulin-dependent diabetic mothers using Doppler tracing in umbilical artery. No association was found between vascular resistance and glycemic control or maternal vascular disease.

Pietryga et al.[32] found abnormal umbilical artery blood flow velocity in 5% of 146 gestational diabetic women. Lower impedance was found in macrosomic newborns, while only 2/11 pre-eclamptic patients displayed abnormal umbilical artery Doppler.

Doppler velocimetry of fetal arterial area

The physiopathologic sequence of velocimetric alterations in chronic hypoxemia have been demonstrated: increased placental resistances (telediastolic flow reduced/absent in umbilical artery) are associated with 'brain and heart sparing effects', for preserving an adequate oxygenation of vital organs (heart, brain, adrenal glands) by vascular dilatation accompanied by constriction of fetal somatic vasa (descending thoracic aorta, renal artery, splenic artery, superior mesenteric artery). In extreme conditions of placental insufficiency (inverted telediastolic flow in umbilical artery) there is a 'central decompensation' with loss of adaptation mechanisms in brain (middle cerebral artery) and alteration of Doppler velocimetry in cardiac and venous areas (absent or inverted wave in venous duct).[33]

The abnormal Doppler results in umbilical arteries represent a placental impairment (placental test), but without reflecting the degree of fetal adaptation to this condition, whereas the study of arterial and venous areas seems useful in diabetic pregnancies with vascular involvement (fetal growth restriction and pre-eclampsia).

The modifications of fetal vascular area in pregnancies complicated by growth restriction and/or pre-eclampsia have been demonstrated. Many areas have been studied with Doppler velocimetry, but the majority of the research focused on cerebral area and mainly on middle cerebral artery and on descending thoracic aorta, expression of splanchnic area, with the purpose to show the redistribution of circle that is observed in chronic hypoxemia.

Doppler velocimetry uses commonly qualitative indexes (pulsatility index, showing the resistances afterwards the examined segment, but also depending from blood viscosity, vascular compliance and cardiac contractility) and quantitative indexes (systolic peak velocity and mean velocity).[34]

The objective of qualitative and quantitative evaluations are complementary. Pulsatility index (PI) is commonly used to show the fetal effects of chronic uteroplacental insufficiency: 'brain sparing effect' with reduction of PI due to cerebral vasodilatation and increase of PI in descending thoracic aorta due to peripheral vasoconstriction. Quantitative evaluation (angle depending and therefore prone to methodological errors) has been proposed to find an eventual fetal anemization: in these situations, the correlation between the increased peak of systolic velocity in middle cerebral artery and severe fetal anemia.[35]

In pre-gestational diabetes, Doppler velocimetry of fetal areas is indicated for vascular complications: it seems that temporal sequence leading to fetal hemodynamic modifications depends on the entity of vasculopathy not on diabetes itself.

Different and controversial is the application of fetal velocimetry to gestational diabetes or to insulin depending diabetes without vascular alteration (mainly nephropathy and retinopathy). Salvesen et al.[18,35] used Doppler to examine 48 diabetic pregnancies, well controlled by insulin therapy. Except three pregnancies complicated by pre-eclampsia and/or fetal growth restriction, uteroplacental and fetal flow velocity were normal: no significant differences in velocimetric pattern of uterine, umbilical, middle cerebral arteries and of descending thoracic aorta versus control group. It is interesting to observe that in the majority of diabetic pregnancies with nephropathy, acidemia and hypoxemia were found in cordocentesis although velocimetric patterns were normal. It has been suggested that hypoxemia and acidemia may be the consequence of metabolic alterations of diabetes, leading to hyperlactacidemia in presence of normal fetal growth and in absence of redistribution of circulation.

Other authors studied Doppler velocimetry of middle cerebral artery in pregnancies complicated by insulin-dependent diabetes: pulsatility index was not different from controls and was not correlated to the levels of glycemia, fructosamine or maternal glycosylated hemoglobin.[36]

Other authors evaluated the velocity of systolic peak to predict a polycythemia. Although a physiopathologic background seemed correct (see fetal anemia and increase of systolic peak velocity), no correlation was found between velocimetric pattern and prevalence of hyperbilirubinemia, although the limited number of cases or the lack of cases with severe polycytemia could explain these results.[37]

Reece et al.[38] studied Doppler velocimetry in descending thoracic aorta of insulin-dependent diabetic pregnant women and found no significant association between PI and fetal outcome, concluding that Doppler examination of this area is not useful in clinical practice for recognizing fetuses at risk of imminent damage.

However, other authors considered qualitative and quantitative patterns and showed that higher fetal aortic volume flow occurred in fetuses in diabetic than in nondiabetic pregnancies. The former group developed distress in labor more frequently. It was suggested that there might be an increased placental vascular resistance with a compensatory increase in volume flow, concluding that the pulsatility index can not be considered a characteristic feature of diabetic pregnancy.[39]

An interesting study by Fadda et al.[40] found that multi-area evaluation in diabetic pregnancies (umbilical artery, descending thoracic aorta, middle cerebral artery) may be useful for identifying fetuses at risk for intrapartum fetal distress and neonatal acidosis: the presence of velocimetric alterations in all areas, exposes the fetus, already in a potential subacute hypoxemia/acidemia, to a risk of unfavorable outcome.

Takahashi et al.[41] found the possibility of using Doppler velocimetry to recognize the transient redistribution of circulation induced by maternal ketoacidosis: velocimetric and cardiotocographic alterations disappeared promptly after treatment of maternal hyperglycemia, and pregnancy continued normally.

Doppler velocimetry of fetal cardiac and venous areas

Newborns of diabetic mothers are at risk for hypertrophic miocardiopathy. This condition is characterized by thickening of the interventricular septum,[42] of ventricular walls and by alterations of systolic and diastolic function that can lead to congestive cardiac failure.[43]

Doppler evaluation of fetal heart in diabetic pregnant women has mainly the aim of finding flow abnormalities at the atrioventricular and ventriculoarterial valves, to identify the signs of a potential chronic hypoxemia and to show the consequences of myocardial hypertrophy.

Regarding the first aspect, it has been demonstrated that even in well-controlled diabetes, the means of the middle and maximal velocities measured in fetal atrioventricular valves, are higher compared to normal controls. This aspect is related to an increased cardiac output, in absolute terms or fraction of estimated fetal weight: these conditions seem a compensation mechanism of chronic hypoxemia due to altered oxidative metabolism within placental dismaturity. These hemodynamic modifications may partially explain the mechanism of myocardic hypertrophy.

Studies on insulin-dependent diabetic pregnancies with good glycemic control in the second and third trimesters, found a significant thickening of the interventricular cardiac septum and of the left and right ventricular walls with altered development of cardiac function. In Doppler terms, the alteration of cardiac function determines at the AV level a reduced phase E/A ratio (ratio between early passive atrial filling wave and active atrial filling wave). These findings were observed as independent from maternal glycosylated hemoglobin levels, showing that fetal interventricular septum hypertrophy and deficit of diastolic function are present although diabetes is well controlled.[44] Therefore fetal cardiomegaly may relate to increased insulin sensitivity of fetal myocardium.[45] This hypothesis is strengthened by the evidence of a progressive reduction and affinity of insulin myocardic receptors from fetal to adult age.[46]

The altered E/A ratio shown in atrioventricular valves may be the consequence of altered ventricular compliance due to thickening of cardiac walls and to modification of blood viscosity (pre-load) because of polycythemia. Several studies have shown that these echocardiographic modifications are recognizable from the 12th week and their severity is correlated with the degree of glycemic control.[47]

Intracardiac flow modifications were seen also in aortic and pulmonary tracts: in pregnancies complicated by insulin-dependent diabetes the velocities of systolic peak were significantly higher than in controls. These findings may be the result of increased contractility of myocardium (inotrope effect), as shown by postnatal studies, and of increased volume of intracardiac flow, related to increased cardiac output in fetuses that are large for gestational age.

As expected, hemodynamic cardiac modifications determine velocimetric alterations in venous areas. It has been demonstrated that diastolic function deficit may be responsible for retrograde pulsations in the umbilical vein and significantly reverse flow in the inferior vena cava during atrial contraction. In diabetic pregnancies, pre-load index in the inferior vena cava is increased and significantly associated with umbilical artery pH reduction, to polycytemia at birth, and neonatal morbidity.[48] The velocimetric alteration could be not seen in other fetal areas: this observation confirms the complexity of metabolic and hemodynamic effects in presence of diabetes, which has a different physiopathology from chronic hypoxemia due to uteroplacental insufficiency, characterized by an increase of peripheral resistances (afterload). Significant modifications were found at the venal duct. Doppler qualitative evaluation of PI in this area may have an essential role in timing the delivery in a pregnancy with severe fetal growth restriction: correlation between hypoxemia, acidemia, risk of fetal mortality, and alteration of velocimetric profile of this phase (absent or inverted a wave) has been clearly demonstrated.[33]

The study of the venous duct in diabetic pregnancies showed significant differences in PI in diabetes, with or without interventricular septum hypertrophy. More interesting is the observation of significant differences between the control group (no diabetes) and diabetes without interventricular septum hypertrophy: this finding suggests that other factors, independent of myocardial hypertrophy, may be responsible of diastolic function impairment.[49]

In physiologic pregnancies, the E/A rate at atrioventricular valves tends to decrease with the advancement of pregnancy, as expression of better intracardiac compliance and myocardial contractility, increase of pre-load (volume related to increase of growth of fetal weight) and decrease of afterload (peripheral resistances), reaching at the end of pregnancy a rate of about one. In the first days of neonatal life, this rate is bigger than one.

In newborns of diabetic mothers, the rate can remain smaller than one: the lack of evidence of peripheral alterations (afterload) and of flow volume towards the right sections of heart may suggest an alteration of diastolic function and of ventricular compliance. These hemodynamic aspects may be responsible for the more frequent observation of transient tachypnea, pulmonary edema and cardiovascular disease in the adult (Baker's hypothesis).[50]

Conclusions

- The evaluation of fetal well-being by using Doppler flow must be preceded by a clinical evaluation of maternal conditions, thus recognizing the level of risk related to the type of maternal diabetes and to the capacity to 'normalize' the maternal glycemic profile.
- Doppler velocimetry of uterine and umbilical arteries may be useful for identifying the patients at risk of developing pre-eclampsia and/or fetal growth restriction within diabetic pregnancies.
- There is no evidence that velocimetry of uterine and umbilical arteries is related to maternal glycemic control.
- Physiopathologic events leading to fetal hypoxemia and acidemia are different from those observed in chronic placental insufficiency. Fetuses of diabetic mothers may be markedly hypoxemic without velocimetric modifications of uteroplacental and fetal areas and circle redistribution. In intrauterine growth restriction due to reduced placental function acidemia and hypoxemia are strictly related where

in diabetic pregnancies acidemia can be found without hypoxemia. This simple observation suggests that impaired placental function is unlikely to be the explanation for acidemia in diabetes although decreased villous surface, villous edema and thickening of the basement membrane have all been demonstrated.

- The controversial results found in literature regarding correlation between peripheral fetal and uteroplacental velocimetric patterns and neonatal outcome may be due to potential bias in the study designs (limited number of cases and not severe glycemic levels may justify the absence of flow alterations) and the peculiar pathophysiology of the disease: qualitative more than quantitative indexes may be markers for fetal cardiovascular homeostasis in pregnancies complicated by diabetes mellitus.
- Fetuses of diabetic mothers, regardless of glycemic control, are at risk of developing interventricular septum hypertrophy with deficit of diastolic function: a velocimetric study of the atrio-ventricular and venous area may be useful in addressing the severity of this condition.
- Different methods of fetal surveillance in diabetic pregnancies have been proposed, depending on the type of diabetes (GDM, pre-existing diabetes mellitus), the degree of glycemic control, the type of therapy (diet, insulin): there are no randomized trials addressing which are the best methods and timing of fetal assessment.
- Results from combined tests (cardiotocography, biophysical profile, Doppler velocimetry) might offer the best method of fetal monitoring; their frequency personalized could depending on the type of disease and pattern of fetal growth.

REFERENCES

1. Alberico S, Strazzanti C, De Santo D, et al. Gestational diabetes: universal or selective? J Matern Fetal Neonatal Med 2004; 16: 331–7.
2. Kabiru W, Raynor BD. Obstetric outcomes associated with increase in BMI category during pregnancy. Am J Obstet Gynocol 2004; 191: 928.
3. Franks S. Polycystic Ovary syndrome. N Engl J Med 1995; 333: 853–61.
4. Ciampelli M, Fulghesu AM, Cucinelli F, et al. Heterogeneity in β cell activity, hepatic insulin clearance and peripheral insulin sensitivity in woman. Hum Reprod 1997; 12: 1897–901.
5. Corti R, Hutter R, Badimon JJ, et al. Evolving concepts in the triad of atheroslerosis, inflammation and thrombosis. J Thromb Thrombolysis 2004; 17: 35–44.
6. Gu K, Cowie CC, Harris MI. Mortality in adults with and without diabetes in a national cohort of the U.S. population, 1971–1993. Diabetes Care 1998; 21: 1138–45.
7. Wang HS, et al. The role of insulin-like growth factor I and insulin like growth factor binding protein I in the control of human fetal growth. J Endocrinol 1992; 132: 11–9.
8. Bradley RJ, et al. Fetal acidosis and hyperlacticemia diagnosed by cordocentesis in pregnancies complicated by maternal diabetes mellitus. Diabet Med 1991; 8: 464–8.
9. Salvesen DR, et al. Fetal pancreatic beta cell function in pregnancies complicated by maternal diabetes mellitus. Am J Obstet Gynecol 1993; 168: 1363–9.
10. Robillard JE, et al. Metabolic effect of constant hypertonic glucose infusion in well oxygenated fetuses. Am J Obstet Gynecol 1978; 130: 199–203.
11. Brosens IA, et al. The role of the spiral arteries in the pathogenesis of preclampsia. Obstet Gynecol Ann 1971; 1: 117.
12. Khong TY, et al. Inadequate maternal vascular response to placentation in pregnancies complicated by pre-eclampsia and by small for gestational age infants. Br J Obstet Gynecol 1986; 93: 1049.
13. Haddad B, et al. Predictive value of uterine Doppler waveform during pregnancies complicated by diabetes. Fetal Diagn Ther 1993; 8: 119–25.
14. Kofinas AD, et al. Uteroplacental Doppler flow velocity waveform analysis correlates poorly with glycemic control in diabetic pregnant women. Am J Perinatol 1991; 8: 273–7.
15. Pietryga M, et al. Placental Doppler velocimetry I gestational diabetes mellitus. J Perinat Med 2006; 34: 106–10.
16. Cousins L. Pregnancy complications among diabetic women: review. Obstet Gynecol Surv 1987; 42: 140.
17. Pietryga M, et al. Abnormal uterine Doppler is related to vasculopathy in pregestational diabetes mellitus. Circulation 2005; 112: 2496–500.
18. Salvesen DR, Higueras MT, Mansur CA, et al. Placental and fetal Doppler velocimetry in pregnancies complicated by maternal diabetes mellitus. Am J Obstet Gynecol 1993; 168: 645–52.
19. Johnstone FD, et al. Doppler umbilical artery flow velocity waveforms in diabetic pregnancy. Br J Obstet Gynecol 1992; 99: 135–40.
20. Landon MB, et al. Doppler umbilical artery velocimetry in pregnancy complicated by insulin-dependent diabetes mellitus. Obstet Gynecol 1989; 73: 961–5.
21. Dicker D, et al. Umbilical artery velocimetry in insulin dependent diabetes mellitus pregnancies. J Perinatol Med 1990; 18: 391–5.
22. Fox RY, et al. The correlation of arterial lesions with umbilical artery Doppler velocimetry in the placentas of small for dates pregnancies. Obstet Gynecol 1990; 75: 578.
23. Mc Cowan LM, et al. Umbilical artery flow velocity waveforms and placental vascular bed. Am J Obstet Gynecol 1987; 157: 900.
24. Olofsson P, et al. Fetal blood flow in diabetic pregnancy. J Perinat Med 1987; 15: 545–53.
25. Bracero L, et al. Umbilical artery velocimetry in diabetes and pregnancy. Obstet Gynecol 1986; 68: 654–8.

26. Bracero L, et al. Comparison of umbilical Doppler velocimetry, NST and biophysical profile in pregnancies complicated by diabetes. J Ultrasound Med 1996; 15: 301–8.

27. Landon MB, et al. Doppler umbilical artery velocimetry in pregnancy complicated by insulin-dependent diabetes mellitus. Obstet Gynecol 1989; 73: 961–5.

28. Dicker D, et al. Umbilical artery velocimetry in insulin dependent diabetes mellitus pregnancies. J Perinat Med 1990; 18: 3915.

29. Reece EA, et al. Diabetes mellitus in pregnancy and the assessment of umbilical artery waveforms using pulsed Doppler ultrasonography. J Ultrasound Med 1994; 13: 73–80.

30. Johnstone FD, et al. Doppler umbilical artery flow velocity waveforms in diabetic pregnancy. Br J Obstet Gynecol 1992; 99: 135–40.

31. Zimmermann P, et al. Doppler velocimetry of the umbilical artery in pregnancies complicated by insulin dependent diabetes mellitus. Eur J Obstet Gynecol Reprod Biol 1992; 47: 85–93.

32. Pietryga M, et al. Placental Doppler velocimetry I gestational diabetes mellitus. J Perinat Med 2006; 34: 106–10.

33. Baschat AA. The fetal circulation and essential organs – a new twist to an old tale [Editorial]. Ultrasound Obstet Gynecol 2006; 27: 349–54.

34. Mari G, for the Collaborative Group for Doppler Assessment of the Blood Flow Velocities in Anemic Fetuses. Non invasive diagnosis by Doppler ultrasonograpgy of fetal anemia due to maternal red-cell alloimmunization. N Engl J Med 2000; 342: 9–14.

35. Salvesen DR, Higueras MT, Brudenell JM, et al. Doppler velocimetry and fetal heart rate studies in nephropathic diabetics. Am J Obstet Gynecol 1992; 167: 1297–303.

36. Ishimatsu J, Matsuzaki T, Yakushiji M, et al. Blood flow velocity waveforms of the fetal middle cerebral artery in pregnancies complicated by diabetes mellitus. Kurume Med J 1995; 42: 161–6.

37. Leung WC, Lam H, Lee CP, et al. Doppler study of the umbilical and fetal middle cerebral arteries in women with gestational diabetes mellitus. Ultrasound Obstet Gynecol 2004; 24: 534–7.

38. Reece EA, Hagay Z, Moroder W, et al. Is there a correlation between aortic Doppler velocimetric findings in diabetic pregnant women and fetal outcome? J Ultrasound Med 1996; 15: 437–40.

39. Olofsson P, Lingman G, Marsal K, et al. Fetal blood flow in diabetic pregnancy. J Perinat Med 1987; 15: 545–53.

40. Fadda GM, D'Antona D, Ambrosini G, et al. Placental and fetal pulsatility indices in gestational diabetes mellitus. J Reprod Med 2001; 46: 365–70.

41. Takahashi Y, Kawabata I, Shinohara A, et al. Transient fetal blood flow redistribution induced by maternal diabetic ketoacidosis diagnosed by Doppler ultrasonography. Prenat Diagn 2000; 20: 524–5.

42. Macklon NS, Hop WC, Wladimiroff JW. Fetal cardiac function and septal thickness in diabetic pregnancy: a controlled observational and reproducibility study. Br J Obstet Gynaecol 1998; 105: 661–6.

43. Kozak-Barany A, Jokinen E, Kero P, et al. Impaired left ventricular diastolic function in newborn infants of mothers with pregestational or gestational diabetes with good glycemic control. Early Hum Dev 2004; 77: 13–22.

44. Jaeggi ET, Fouron JC, Proulx F. Fetal cardiac performance in uncomplicated and well-controlled maternal type I diabetes. Ultrasound Obstet Gynecol 2001; 17: 311–5.

45. Rizzo G, Arduini D, Romanini C. Accelerated cardiac growth and abnormal cardiac flow in fetuses of type I diabetic mothers. Obstet Gynecol 1992; 80: 369–76.

46. Thorsson AV, Hintz RL. Insulin receptors in the newborn: Increase in receptor affinity and number. N Engl J Med 1977; 297; 908–12.

47. Rizzo G, Arduini D, Capponi A, et al. Cardiac and venous blood flow in fetuses of insulin-dependent diabetic mothers: evidence of abnormal hemodynamics in early gestation. Am J Obstet Gynecol 1995; 173: 1775–81.

48. Rizzo G, Arduini D, Romanini C. Cardiac function in fetuses of type I diabetic mothers. Am J Obstet Gynecol 1991; 164: 837–43.

49. Zielinsky P, Marcantonio S, Nicoloso LH, et al. Ductus venosus flow and myocardial hypertrophy in fetuses of diabetic mothers. Arq Bras Cardiol 2004; 83: 51–6.

50. Seppanen MP, Ojanpera OS, Kaapa PO, et al. Delayed postnatal adaptation of pulmonary hemodynamics in infants of diabetic mothers. J Pediatr. 1997; 131: 545–8.

35 Fetal lung maturity

Antonio Cutuli, Graziano Clerici and Gian Carlo Di Renzo

Introduction

The immaturity of lung tissue and function leads to an acute progressive breathing failure, the so-called respiratory distress syndrome (RDS). The diabetic pregnancy, and particularly poorly controlled maternal diabetes, represents one of the most important risk condition for RDS.

Though the perinatal mortality rate in pregnancies complicated by diabetes has declined, conditions such as congenital malformation, prematurity, hypoglycemia and respiratory distress are still common problems of the newborns (Table 35.1).[1–5]

Despite the considerable improvement in neonatal care, the morbidity for respiratory complications such as RDS in the infants born to diabetic mothers is considerable, as is the financial burden of the resulting care.[5,6]

According to recent figures, 10–20% of all RDS cases result from elective interference with normal pregnancy. In high-risk pregnancy the planning of the optimal timing of the therapy, of the delivery and the adequate fetal surveillance is even more critical[7] to improve the offspring outcome.[8] The improved outcome of diabetic pregnancies depends in a large measure on accurate timing of delivery which is determined by metabolic control, fetal well-being and documentation of fetal lung maturity.

Until recently, RDS was the most common and most serious disease in infants of diabetic mothers. In the 1970s, improved management of diabetic pregnancies resulted in a decline in its incidence from 31 to 3%.[7,9]

The observation of Kulovich indicates that the nondiabetic fetus achieves pulmonary maturity at a mean gestational age of 34–35 weeks. By 37 weeks, more than 99% of normal newborns have mature lung profiles as assessed by phospholipid assays.

In a diabetic pregnancy, however, it is unwise to assume that the risk of respiratory distress has passed until after 38.5 gestational weeks have been completed.[7,9]

Clinical studies investigating the effect of maternal diabetes on fetal lung maturation have produced no univocal data. In a series of 805 infants of diabetic mothers delivered over a 10-year period, Robert et al.[9] found the corrected risk for RDS was nearly six times that of mothers without diabetes mellitus. With the introduction of protocols that have emphasized glucose control and antepartum surveillance, RDS has become a less common complication in infants of diabetic mothers.

Several studies agree that, in well-controlled diabetic women delivered at term, the risk of RDS is no higher than that observed in the general population.[10,11]

In conclusion, the risk of hyaline membrane disease at any given gestational age before week 38 is five to six times higher in infants of diabetic mothers than in infants of nondiabetic mothers.

Pathophysiology of fetal lung maturation in diabetic pregnancies

Neonatal pulmonary function of the infants of diabetic mothers is suboptimal compared with infants of nondiabetic women matched for gestational age.[10,11]

The mechanism by which maternal diabetes affects pulmonary development remains unknown. An extensive review of the literature confirms that hyperglycemia and hyperinsulinemia are involved in delayed pulmonary maturation influencing pulmonary surfactant biosynthesis.[12]

Table 35.1 Perinatal morbidity in diabetic pregnancy

Morbidity	Gestational diabetes	Type I diabetes	Type II diabetes
Hyperbilirubinemia	29%	55%	44%
Hypoglycemia	9%	29%	24%
Respiratory distress	3%	8%	4%
Transient tachypnea	2%	3%	4%
Hypocalcemia	1%	4%	1%
Cardiomyopathy	1%	2%	1%
Polycythemia	1%	3%	3%

(From California Department of Health Service, 1991.)

This may be due to inadequate production of alveolar surfactant or abnormal lung maturation and function.

In vitro studies have documented that insulin can interfere with substrate availability for surfactant biosynthesis. Smith et al.[13] demonstrated that when insulin was added to fetal lung cell cultures with cortisol present, steroid-enhanced lecithin synthesis was abolished. Engle et al.[14] found that higher levels of insulin resulted in diminished glucose and choline uptake by fetal rat type II alveolar cells.

Carlson et al.[15] have shown that insulin blocks cortisol action at the level of the fibroblasts by reducing the production of fibroblast–pneumocyte factor.

Other authors[16] reported abnormal timing of phospholipid production in diabetic pregnancy, as indicated by a delay in the appearance of phosphatidylglycerol in the amniotic fluid only in gestational diabetes (White's class A patients). Smith[17] postulated that insulin interferes with normal timing of glucocorticoid-induced pulmonary maturation in the fetus.

Some investigators have disagreed with these findings, reporting that fetal lung maturation occurred later in pregnancies with poor glycemic control regardless of class of diabetes.[18–22] Bourbon et al.[23] proposed that elevated maternal plasma level of myoinositol in diabetic women may inhibit or delay the fetal production of phosphatidylglycerol.

It is suspected that neonatal respiratory problems in these infants have a histologic basis in addition to biochemical origin. Pinter et al.[24] demonstrated decreased fluid clearance and lack of thining of the lung's connective tissue compared with controls in the fetal lung of diabetic rat. Bhavnani et al.[25] reported higher lung glycogen levels and reduced pulmonary compliance in offspring of diabetic rabbits compared with controls.

Glucose balance has an effect on the incidence of the hyaline membrane disease (Figure 35.1). Several studies have attempted to explain the mechanism of hyaline membrane disease. Hawdon and Aynsely-Green,[26] in an investigation of type II pneumocytes in rats and rabbits, showed that insulin inhibits the cortisol-dependent production of phosphatidyl-choline, apparently as a consequence of the inhibited production of one of the prerequisites of phosphatidylcholine, fibroblast–pneumocyte factor. In rats, high glucose levels block the transformation of choline to phosphatidylcholine, and butyrate blocks the translation of mRNA into surfactant proteins.

Evaluation of fetal lung maturity

Fetal lung maturity assessment has become a very important tool in the management of high-risk pregnancies, especially the diabetic ones.

In the past, elective preterm delivery to avoid unexpected intrauterine death was common. This practice often resulted in high incidence of neonatal morbidity and mortality. With improvement of glycemic control and better techniques of antepartum surveillance, most patients with diabetes now deliver at term.[25]

In view of the risk of lung immaturity in fetuses of diabetic mothers, the assessment of fetal lung maturity is essential.[27] A number of diagnostic methods with high degree of accuracy and predictability have been developed and are now available.

Unless excellent gestational dating has been established in a well controlled patient who has reached 39 weeks' gestation,

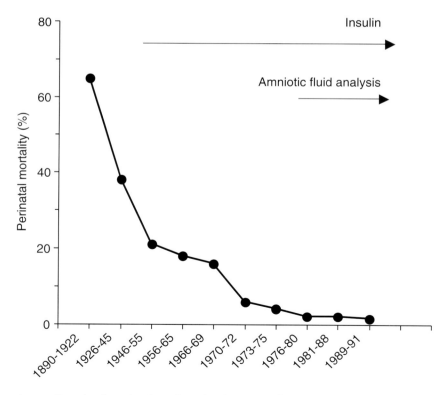

Figure 35.1   Perinatal mortality after introduction of insulin therapy and amniotic fluid analysis. (Modified from Moore.[32])

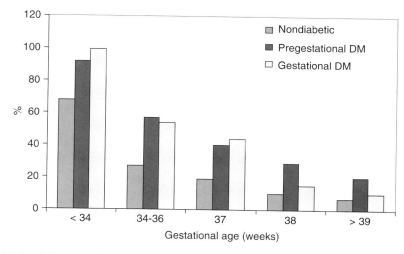

Figure 35.2   Pulmonary immaturity rates. DM: diabetes mellitus. (Modified from Langer.[30])

an amniocentesis should be performed before elective delivery to assess fetal pulmonary maturity.

Several controversies exist surrounding fetal lung maturity in diabetes pregnancies. Berkowitz et al.[28] concluded that biochemical maturation of the fetal lung in diabetic pregnancies strongly correlated with gestational age and did not appear to be significantly delayed when compared to nondiabetic ones.

Moore[29] found that the degree of delay in lung maturity testing appeared to be greater among those patients with pre-existing diabetes compared with those with gestational diabetes mellitus. In contrast, Langer[30] found no difference in pre-existing diabetes and gestational diabetes in pulmonary immaturity rates (Figure 35.2).

A prospective study on determination of fetal lung maturity in diabetic mothers demonstrates that irrespective of fetal lung maturity testing, RDS is extremely rare in this large cohort of term infants born to gestational and pre-gestational diabetic women. In this study up to 15–25% of term diabetic pregnancies will have 'immature' fetal lung maturity testing utilizing various measurements of surfactant, but rarely do these infants exhibit RDS.[31]

In normal pregnancies, any test of gestational age or general fetal maturation state correlates well with the degree of fetal lung maturity because maturational events are normally linked closely with gestational age (Table 35.2). A test of lung maturation in the abnormal pregnancy, such as diabetic one, is not a test of gestational age. Tests of fetal lung maturation depend on amniotic fluid composition reflecting the status of the fetal lung.

Phospholipids

The lecithin–sphingomyelin ratio (L/S ratio) was introduced by Gluck and colleagues in the 1971.[33] The test depends on the flow of fetal lung fluid into amniotic fluid changing in this phospholipid composition. The result is expressed as the ratio of a lecithin (phosphatidylcholine) to sphingomyelin.

Sphingomyelin is a general membrane lipid and is not related to lung maturational events. The sphingomyelin content in amniotic fluid tends to fall from about 32 weeks' gestational age to term, whereas the more satured lecithin concentration (a large part from the fetal lung) increases.

The L/S ratio for normal pregnancies is less than 0.5 at 20 weeks, gradually increases to 1.0 at 32 weeks and around 35 weeks achieves a value of 2.0 correlating it with fetal lung maturity, empirically RDS is unlikely if it is more than 2.0 (Figures 35.3 and 35.4).

The evaluation of the L/S ratio by chromatography is standardized and the determination methods show a sensitivity of 83–97% and a specificity of 98%.[36–38] This approach, nevertheless, is problematic due to the difficulty of performing it as a routine activity: it requires expertise and special laboratory tools.

Table 35.2   Accuracy of tests to assess fetal lung maturity

Parameter	Measurement made
Sensitivity	Ability of test to correctly identify all fetus at risk for RDS
Specificity	Ability of test to correctly identify all fetuses not at risk for RDS
False-positive rate	Percentage of fetuses identified as being at risk for RDS but do not develop RDS
False-negative rate	Percentage of fetuses identified as not being at risk for RDS but develop RDS

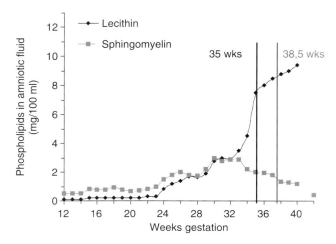

Figure 35.3 Changes in the concentrations of lecithin and sphingomyelin in the amniotic fluid. The vertical lines indicate achieved pulmonary maturity in nondiabetic (black) and diabetic (gray) pregnancy.

Many factors can affect the L/S ratio. Lecithin is found in many body fluids including blood, vaginal secretions, and gastrointestinal fluid.

The value of the L/S ratio has been questioned in diabetic pregnancies where there is an increase of false negatives which could reach a quarter of cases, varying from 3 to 30%. Most series, however, report a low incidence of RDS with a mature L/S ratio.[9]

Some authors show that the L/S ratio may not be a reliable indicator of pulmonary maturity in diabetic pregnancies,[10] Gindes et al.[39] affirm that a ratio above 2.0 does not guarantee for lung maturation. Diabetes may affect the secretion of the fetal lung fluid, resulting in a higher removal of phospholipids from alveolar lining and in an increase false-negative rate.[40]

Other authors reported no difference between diabetic patients and controls.[41,42] When maternal diabetes is well controlled during pregnancy, the L/S ratio can be reliably used to establish the risk of neonatal RDS.[43,44]

Surfactant of mature lungs contains phosphatidylglycerol (PG), which is absent early in gestation and only appears at about 35 weeks' gestational age.[35] Phosphatidylglycerol is virtually present only in lung tissue and surfactant. Thus, amniotic fluid contaminated with blood or meconium can be analysed for this substance.[45] When PG is present, RDS does not occur except possibly in case of intrapartum acidemia and hypoxemia or other fetal disease. With trace amounts of PG in amniotic fluid, an incidence of RDS <1% has been reported.[46] Many authors confirmed that the addition of detection of PG decreases the rate of false positives significantly and improves the specificity of the L/S ratio.[46]

The appearance of the acidic phospholipid phosphatidylglycerol may be delayed by fetal hyperinsulinemia and it is associated with an increased incidence of RDS. Although the appearance of PG has been reported to be delayed in pregnancies of diabetic women, it remains a reliable predictor of pulmonary maturity.[47] However, the absence of PG in diabetic pregnancy does not imply the diagnosis of pulmonary immaturity, since PG fails to appear in 10% of amniotic fluid samples by 40 weeks' gestation[48] and the presence of PG is reported in only half of samples studied for both diabetic and nondiabetic patients with mature L/S ratios and gestation of 34 weeks or beyond.

Prior to lung maturation, phosphatidylinositol (PI) increases in amniotic fluid from about 26 weeks to 35 weeks. PG appears in amniotic fluid as the percentage of phosphatodylinositol decreases.[35]

The 'lung profile' is a test that combines the L/S ratio with measurements of the percentage of disaturated (acetone precipitable) lecithin (phosphatidylcholine), phosphatidylinositol and phospsphatidylglycerol in the amniotic fluid.[16] The information provided by this profile enhances the accuracy of diagnosing fetal lung maturity and provides further details on lung development. In a small group of cases, the specificity

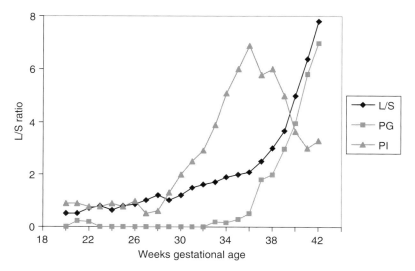

Figure 35.4 L/S ratio, phosphatidylglycerol (PG) and phosphatidylinositol (PI) in amniotic fluid from normal pregnancies. (From Gluck et al.[34] and Hallman et al.[35])

was increased from 69 to 93% by substituting the lung profile for the L/S ratio.[36]

The introduction of immunological (Amniostat-FLM) evaluation of phosphatidylglycerol provides rapid results with minimal equipment needs.[49–51] However, this method has a false-positive rate >50%. Literature data confirm the utility of this approach as a screening test for its rapidity and simplicity of execution, particularly in cases of contamination and/or in diabetic patients. The results of phosphatidylglycerol assay by thin-layer chromatography and Amniostat-FLM were reported to be concordant in 90–95% of the cases.[52]

Proteins

The predominant protein involved in surfactant metabolism is a 35-kDa protein, called surfactant associated protein 35 (SAP-35). This protein originates from type II alveolar cells. An increase in amniotic fluid occurs near term and a significant correlation with pulmonary maturity has been reported.[53,54] The measurement of this protein is simply available using an ELISA method and a specific monoclonal antibody. For Hallman et al.[54] the test predicted an RDS with an accuracy similar to that of L/S ratio. In high-risk pregnancies such as diabetes or hypertension, the levels of SAP-35 have less correlation with fetal pulmonary maturity and are probably not highly reliable in these situations.[54]

Lipids

In amniotic fluid at term cholesterol palmitate is present. Its role is not known but it could serve as a transport mode for palmitic acid which is used in the synthesis of saturated phosphatidycholine. A simple method for determining this substance in amniotic fluid has been reported, using thin-layer chromatography and densitometry.[55] In a small group of patients, levels of cholesterol palmitate were correlated with fetal lung maturity. However, a similar correlation was not demonstrated in diabetic pregnancies.[56]

Fluorescence polarization

There are at present two systems used to measure fluorescence polarization: the FELMA microviscometer and the TDX system. The fluorescence polarization of amniotic fluid is in large part determined by binding of the probe to phospholipid structures and to the predominant protein, albumin.[57] Fluorescence polarization of amniotic fluid is inversely related to the L/S ratio.[58,59] The specificity of this method to predict RDS ranges from 50 to 70%.[60,61] The technique is not reliable when amniotic fluid is contaminated by blood or meconium. The fluorescence polarization values are not significantly affected by high-risk pregnancy except for maternal diabetes, which has variable effects on values, and is an unreliable indicator of fetal maturity.[62]

In a multicenter study of the TDX system, a sensitivity of 96% and a specificity of 88% were obtained with a cutoff value for maturity set at 50 mg/g (surfactant/albumin value). In this evaluation the corresponding sensitivity and specificity for L/S ratio was 96 and 83%, respectively.[63] In insulin-dependent diabetic patients, a TDX–FLM value of at least 70 mg/g is not associated with RDS requiring intubation.[64,65] Parvin et al. showed that the incorporation of gestational age into the evaluation of fetal lung monitoring allows for individualized, gestational age-specific risk assessment and provides gestational age-specific cutoffs with increased specificity. In fact, the odds of RDS decrease by 31% for each increasing week of gestational age and decrease by 67% for each 10 mg/g increase in the TDX–FLM II ratio. Gestational age specific TDX–FLM II cutoffs are provided with sensitivities between 84 and 100%.[66]

Other tests

Another method used to assay fetal lung maturation is the evaluation of lamellar-body (LB) concentrations contained in surfactant where LB are secreted by type II pneumocytes; thus LB count is easy to quantify and requires no special instrumentation (Coulter counter).[67] Cutoff values of ≥30,000–35,000/ml have a sensitivity of almost 100% and a specificity of 96%. More recent studies suggest that LB count more than 50,000/µl predicts pulmonary maturity. The negative predictive value of this cutoff is 93% and positive predictive value is 48%; the sensitivity for prediction of RDS is 85% and specificity 70%.[68] According to Ghidini et al.[69] the LB count >37,000 is an optimal diagnostic threshold for the diagnosis of lung maturity in nondiabetic pregnant women.

In a recent study[70] considering high-risk pregnancies, such as diabetic mothers, they found that LB count is a screening test for predicting neonatal lung maturity as good as maturity assay by fluorescence polarization and it is more reliable than the foam stability index test.

Nevertheless, there are no large data on the ability of this method to assess fetal lung maturity in diabetic pregnancies. The use of LB count in pregnancies complicated by diabetes mellitus was evaluated by DeRoche et al.[71] These authors found that a LB count of 37,000/µl has a sensitivity of 80% and a specificity of 100% in the prediction of fetal lung maturity by standardized methods of phospholipid analysis. Such a count (≥37,000/µl) correlated with the lecitin/sphingomyelin ratio and phosphatidyglycerol values in pregnancies of diabetic patients.

Stable microbubble test on amniotic fluid is recognized as a rapid, simple and reliable procedure that can identify infants who are likely to develop RDS.[72] In this test, a rating of microbubble ≥20/mm² indicates that idiopathic RDS will not occur after delivery. Complete absence of stable microbubble suggests high risk of RDS. Bubbles formed by agitation with Pasteur pipette were examined in hanging drops under a microscope using 10× power.[72,73] There are no studies dealing with the application of a stable microbubble test on diabetic pregnancy.

In the amniotic fluid there are some specific protein such as apoprotein A (SP-A), which combined with dipalmitoylphosphatidylcholine and phosphatidylglycerol forms an active complex. SP-A increases in amniotic fluid in parallel with phospholipids. Several immunological tests have been proposed to measure it, and a specific enzyme-linked immunoassay has been developed.[74] No data are available regarding its use in diabetic pregnancy.

Table 35.3   Comparison of fetal lung indices between diabetic pregnancies and matched controls at different gestational age

Test	28–34 weeks			35–38 weeks		
	Diabetic pregnancies (n = 18)	Controls (n = 18)	P	Diabetic pregnancies (n = 27)	Controls (n = 27)	P
Shake test	2.1:1 ± 1.4	2.6:1 ± 1.1	NS	3.7:1 ± 0.9	3.0 ± 1.2	NS
Planimetric L/S	3.0 ± 1.9	2.8 ± 0.9	NS	3.8 ± 1.2	4.6 ± 1.9	NS
Stoichiometric L/S	5.8 ± 1.7	3.8 ± 1.7	NS	9.8 ± 7.2	8.4 ± 6.6	NS
Phosphatidylglycerol*	33%	26%	NS	70%	79%	NS
Lamellar bodies count (×10³/μl)	37.2 ± 38.4	34.2 ± 10.6	NS	45.3 ± 32.7	50.0 ± 32.4	NS

Values are mean ± SD.
*Percent of phosphatidylglycerol present on chromatography.
(From Piper.[79])

For testing fetal lung maturity, the foam stability index and the so-called 'shake' test have been introduced, based on the formation of a stable layer of foam in a test tube containing a mixture of amniotic fluid and ethanol. The presence of blood or meconium interferes with these tests. These are simple tests but they are not widely employed overall in high-risk pregnancies.[75]

Summary

Caution must therefore be used in planning the delivery of patients with a mature >L/S ratio and absent PG. The L/S ratio can be used to assess fetal lung maturity when glucose levels have been well controlled in a diabetic pregnancy. But when control has been erratic or is difficult to assess, positive phosphatidylglycerol or higher L/S ratio (>2.5) should be used to predict fetal lung maturity.[76]

A study[77] has compared fetal lung maturity as determined by amniotic fluid test in diabetic pregnancies under euglycemic control, with matched controls. The authors found no statistical difference when comparing fetal lung maturity indices between diabetic pregnancies and controls (Table 35.3).

Furthermore, comparing Type I and Type II diabetes with respective controls, the only significant difference detected was for a higher proportion of PG presence in the type II group compared to controls (Table 35.4).

Ghidini et al.[78] affirm that an L/S ratio of ≥3.0 represented the optimal trade-off between sensitivity (68%) and false-positive rate (6%) in the prediction of presence of PG. Similarly, a significant relationship exists between LB count values and presence of PG. A LB count of ≥50,000 represents the optimal trade-off between sensitivity (92%) and false positive rate (0) in the prediction of presence of PG. Then, in diabetic pregnant patients, the presence of PG in the amniotic fluid more closely corresponds to an L/S ratio of ≥3.0 or to a lamellar body count of ≥50,000.

According to Piper[79] amniotic fluid analysis is not necessary at or beyond 38 weeks of gestation well-dated diabetic pregnancies with good glycemic control. This limits the potential need for amniotic fluid assessment in order to planning elective delivery in cases in which lung maturation is anticipated to be delayed nor in cases with late or inadequate prenatal care resulting in unconfirmed dates. However, this

Table 35.4   Comparison of fetal lung indices in Type 1 and Type 2 gestational diabetes

Test	Type 1 diabetes (IDDM)			Type 2 diabetes (GDM)		
	IDDM (n = 19)	Controls (n = 19)	P	GDM (n = 26)	Controls (n = 26)	P
Shake test	2.6:1 ± 1.4	2.0:1 ± 1.1	NS	4.0:1 ± 0.6	3.0 ± 1.2	NS
Planimetric L/S	3.1 ± 1.0	3.3 ± 1.1	NS	3.5 ± 1.4	4.3 ± 2.5	NS
Stechiometric L/S	7.6 ± 4.7	6.0 ± 4.4	NS	5.9 ± 3.4	8.8 ± 7.5	NS
Phosphatidylglycerol*	47%	42%	NS	53%	46%	0.01
Lamellar bodies count (×10³/μl)	32.0 ± 20.7	34.0 ± 24.0	NS	39.4 ± 30.7	37.1 ± 27.1	NS

Values are mean ± SD.
*Percent of phosphatidylglycerol presence on chromatography.
(From Piazze et al.[77])

author confirms the ability of PG to more accurately detect lung maturity and immaturity in diabetic pregnancies.

Ventolini et al. proposed a fetal lung maturity algorithm recommended when an elective delivery is planned before 39 weeks' gestation.[75,80] The first test to be used is the LB count, results being available within 10–15 min. A count of 50,000 or more indicates maturity. A count below 15,000 indicates immaturity. When the LB count falls between 15,000 and 50,000 it is classified as transitional. In these circumstances, a TDX–FLM II test should be performed on the same sample. This test requires longer processing time. A value of 55 mg/g is considered mature and a value of <40 mg/g is considered immature. When the TDX–FLM II result falls between 40 and 55 mg/g, it is considered borderline, and the amniotic fluid should be further tested for the presence of PG and L/S ratio. The presence of PG or a L/S ratio of ≥2.5 indicates that the fetal lungs are mature. Confirmation of fetal lung maturity should be obtained before delivery and planned Cesarean section. Moore[32] has suggested that six points be ascertained in order to fulfil this requirement (Box 35.1).

Induction of fetal lung maturity

When fetal lungs are immature, the infant will most likely develop respiratory distress syndrome, and about 25% of untreated infants die within 28 days of birth, and another 25% will develop chronic lung disease (bronchopulmonary dysplasia).

Box 35.1 Confirmation of fetal maturity before induction of labor or planned cesarean section in diabetic pregnancy

1. Phosphatidylglycerol >3% in amniotic fluid collected from vaginal pool or by amniocentesis
2. Completion of 38.5 weeks' gestation
3. Normal last menstrual period
4. First pelvic examination before 12 weeks confirms dates
5. Sonogram before 24 weeks confirms dates
6. Documentation of more than 18 weeks of unamplified (fetoscope) fetal heart tones

Since 1972, when Liggins and Howie reported decreased RDS in newborns from mother who received a prenatal administration of corticosteroids,[81] several randomized trials have utilized steroids (and/or other drugs) to induce and/or improve pulmonary maturity. Many reports have confirmed the original findings that antenatal administration of glucocorticoids to the mother is associated with a statistically significant reduction in the incidence of RDS.[82] Almost all have demonstrated the efficacy of corticosteroids treatment for reducing perinatal morbidity and mortality, as confirmed by a recent meta-analysis on the role of corticosteroids to prevent RDS.[83] During the last decade, the strategy for the prevention of RDS has been directed towards the acceleration of fetal lung maturity by administering various hormones to the mother.

Box 35.2 Guidelines produced in 1994 and revised in 2000: National Institutes of Health[92,93]

Antenatal Corticosteroids

Clinical Recommendations
- All pregnant women between 24 and 34 weeks gestation who are at risk of preterm delivery within 7 days should be considered candidates for antenatal treatment with a single course of corticosteroids.
- Treatment consists of two doses of 12 mg of betamethasone given intramuscularly 24 hours apart or four doses of 6 mg of dexamethasone given intramuscularly 12 hours apart, as recommended by the consensus panel in 1994. There is no proof of efficacy for any other regimen.
- Because of insufficient scientific data from randomized clinical trials regarding efficacy and safety, repeat courses of corticosteroids should not be used routinely. In general, it should be reserved for patients enrolled in randomized controlled trials. Several randomized trials are in progress.

What additional information should be obtained?
- The following research is recommended:
  - Well-designed randomized clinical trials which are of sufficient power to evaluate efficacy and safety are needed.
  - In light of the possible risks, the design of randomized clinical trials should minimize the exposure of mothers and fetuses while protecting the integrity of the research design.
- These trials should assess:
  - clinically important neonatal morbidities, such as respiratory distress syndrome, chronic lung disease, and brain injury
  - clinically important maternal morbidities, such as infection and adrenal suppression
  - the effects of repeat courses of corticosteroids on patterns of fetal and postnatal growth
  - the potential effects of incremental courses on benefits and risks, since the benefits of repeat courses of antenatal corticosteroids are likely to decrease with advancing gestational age
  - the efficacy and safety of rescue therapy
  - the interaction of repeat courses of antenatal corticosteroids with postnatal corticosteroid therapy
  - long-term growth and neuropsychological outcome up to at least school age, using state-of-the-art techniques.
- In addition: animal studies should evaluate the pathophysiologic and metabolic mechanisms of potential benefits and risks, including the effects of repeat corticosteroids on central nervous system myelination and brain development.

Box 35.3   Guidelines from the RCOG[94] on the antenatal use of glucocorticosteroids

Guidelines of Royal College of Obstetricians and Gynecologists

Antenatal corticosteroids to prevent Respiratory Distress Syndrome
Effectiveness
- Antenatal corticosteroids are associated with a significant reduction in rates of RDS, neonatal death and intraventricular hemorrhage. *Evidence level Ia*
- The cost and duration of neonatal intensive care is reduced following corticosteroid therapy. *Evidence level III*
- The optimal treatment–delivery interval for administration of antenatal corticosteroids is after 24 h but fewer than 7 days after the start treatment. *Evidence level Ia*
- The use of antenatal corticosteroids in multiple pregnancies is recommended, but a significant reduction in rates of RDS has not been demonstrated.
- If a tocolitic is used, ritodrine no longer seems to be the best choice. Atosiban or nifedipine appear to be preferable, as they have fewer adverse effects and seem to have comparable effectiveness. *Evidence level Ia*

Safety
- Women may be advised that the use of a single course of antenatal corticosteroids does not appear to be associated with any significant maternal or fetal adverse effects. *Evidence level Ib*
- The use of antenatal corticosteroids in pregnancies complicated by maternal diabetes mellitus is recommended, but a significant reduction in rates of RDS has not been demonstated.

Strict glycaemic control prior to conception and during pregnancy has been shown to reduce the incidence of neonatal RDS to that of matched control. Women with either insuline-dependent diabetes or gestational diabetes were not entered into randomized controlled trials of antenatal corticosteroids therapy, so there is no evidence that antenatal corticosteroid therapy is either safe or effective in these circumstances. In view of the adverse effect of maternal hyperglycemia on fetal lung maturity it is possible that any benefit corticosteroids could be offset by corticosteroid-induced hyperglycemia.

Indications for antenatal corticosteroid therapy. Evidence level Ia
Every effort should be made to initiate antenatal corticosteroid therapy in women between 24 and 34 weeks of gestation with any of the following:
- Threatened preterm labor
- Antepartum hemorrhage
- Preterm rupture of the membranes
- Any condition requiring elective preterm delivery

Between 35 and 36 weeks obstetricians might want to consider antenatal steroid use in any of the above conditions although the numbers needed to treat will increase significantly.

Contraindications
- Corticosteroid therapy is contraindicated if a woman suffers from systemic infection including tuberculosis. Caution is advised if suspected chroioamnionitis is diagnosed.

Dose and route of administration
- Betamethasone is the steroid of choice to enhance lung maturation. Recommended theraphy involves two doses of betamethasone 12 mg, given intramuscularly 24 h apart. *Evidence level III*

A large observational study suggested that antenatal exposure to betamethasone, but not dexamethasone, is associated with a decrease risk of cystic periventricular leucomalacia among premature infants born at 24–31 weeks of gestation.

Repeated doses
- The use of repeated courses of antenatal corticosteroids has not been shown to have any significant benefit. *Evidence level III*

Effectiveness of thyrotrophin-releasing hormone
- The use of thyrotropin-releasing hormone is not recommended in combination with antenatal corticosteroids. *Evidence level Ia*

Classification of evidence levels
The evidence used in this guideline was graded using the scheme below and the recommendations formulated in a similar fashion with a standardised grading scheme.
- Ia   Evidence obtained from meta-analysis of randomized controlled trials.
- Ib   Evidence obtained from at least one randomized controlled trial.
- IIa   Evidence obtained from at least one well-designed controlled study without randomization.
- IIb   Evidence obtained from at least one other type of well-designed quasi-experimental study.
- III   Evidence obtained from well-designed non-experimental descriptive studies, such as comparative studies, correlation studies and case studies.
- IV   Evidence obtained from expert committee reports or opinions and/or clinical experience of respected authorities.

Grades of recommendations
- Requires at least one randomized controlled trial as part of a body of literature of overall good quality and consistency addressing the specific recommendation. (Evidence levels Ia, Ib).
- Requires the availability of well controlled clinical studies but no randomized clinical trials on the topic of recommendations. (Evidence levels IIa, IIb, III).
- Requires evidence obtained from expert committee reports or opinions and/or clinical experiences of respected authorities. Indicates and absence of directly applicable clinical studies of good quality. (Evidence level IV).

Good Practice Point
- Recommended best practice based on the clinical experience of the guideline development group.

Gojnic et al.[84] tried to reduce or even eliminate the risks of fetal macrosomia by accelerating fetal maturation and delivery before the 36th week (34th to 36th week). Acceleration of fetal maturation was achieved by endogenous release of thyrotropin-releasing hormone stimulated by periodic fluctuations in fetal oxygenation resulting from oxytocin-induced uterine contractions. This approach needs further evaluation. At present, glucocorticoids remain the most widely used and the safest agents.

A recent Cochrane review[85] of antenatal corticosteroids for accelerating fetal lung maturation included 21 studies (comprising a total of 3885 women and 4269 infants) and demonstrated that treatment with antenatal glucocorticosteroids (AGC) does not increase the risk of chorioamnionitis or puerperal sepsis or of death to the mother. Treatment with antenatal corticosteroids is associated with an overall reduction in neonatal death, RDS, cerebroventricular hemorrhage, necrotizing enterocolitis, respiratory support, intensive care admissions, and systemic infections in the first 48 h of life.[85,86] A complete course of AGC has been found to be independently associated with a decreased risk for severe IVH also in preterm very low birthweight infants from multiple pregnancies.[87] For every 11 fetuses treated with AGC there will be one fewer case of RDS and a similar reduced need for postnatal surfactant treatment. There will be also one fewer death in the neonatal period for every 23 treated fetuses and a similar reduction in IVH. Since it is unlikely that further prospective controlled trials on AGC will ever be performed, the results of the meta-analysis by Crowley[88] represent the definitive evidence-based proof of the effects of AGC. In a well performed study, betamethasone was found to reduce periventricular leukomalacia PVL, whereas dexamethasone tended to increase the risk (1.5, 0.8–2.9).[89] Furthermore, only betamethasone was associated with reduced mortality (0.52; 0.39–0.70) whereas dexamethasone was not (0.89; 0.60–1.32).[89] The optimal dosage to administer has been fixed as two doses of 12 mg of betamethasone given i.m. 24 h apart or four doses of 6 mg of dexamethasone i.m. given every 12 h. For infants born at 29–34 weeks' gestation, treatment with AGC clearly reduces the incidence of RDS and of overall mortality. While AGC do not clearly decrease the incidence of RDS in infants born at 24–28 weeks' gestation, they reduce its severity. More importantly, AGC clearly reduce mortality and the incidence of IVH in this group. All fetuses between 24 and 34 weeks' gestation should be considered candidates for this treatment, unless immediate delivery is imminent or AGC may have an adverse effect on the mother.[90] The only absolute contraindications

> **Box 35.4 Key Guidelines from European Association of Perinatal Medicine on antenatal use of corticosteroids[90]**
>
> - Administration of one single-course of ACG is the most important treatment to prevent RDS and brain injury and increase survival that can be provided by the obstetrician to patients at risk of preterm delivery at 24–34 weeks of gestation
> - Based on observational clinical and animal studies, betamethasone is preferable to dexamethasone
> - There is no direct evidence that tocolytic treatment *per se* might affect the risk of perinatal brain injury or adverse neurological outcome

to the use of AGC are chorioamnionitis, peptic ulcer and tuberculosis. In infants born beyond 34 weeks' gestation the risk of neonatal mortality, RDS, and IVH is low. The use of AGC in mothers expected to deliver at more than 34 weeks is not recommended, unless there is evidence of pulmonary immaturity using amniotic fluid FLM tests.[91]

We report the Guidelines produced by the National Institute of Health in the United States in 1994 and revised in 2000[93] on the effect of corticosteroids for fetal lung maturation on perinatal outcomes (Box 35.2), and those of The Royal College of Obstetricians and Gynaecologists on the same issue, published in 1996 and revised in 2004 (Box 35.3).[94] Finally, we report the summary of current recommendations on the use of AGC from the European Association of Perinatal Medicine[90] (Box 35.4).

Conclusions

If a pregnant woman has diabetes under poor control, the infant is at risk for RDS because of delayed lung maturation, which includes a delay in the appearance of surfactant and, probably, delayed lung structural maturation as a result of both high insulin and glucose effects on fetal lung parenchima. However, concerns about reliability of the lung maturity tests in diabetic pregnancies has decreased as management of the pregnant diabetic has focused on good control of blood glucose levels.[95]

Strict blood glucose control should be maintained during pregnancy, and the timing of delivery should be taken only when a combination of tests for the prediction of fetal lung maturity and eventually induction of this has been performed.

REFERENCES

1. Diabetes care and research in Europe: the Saint Vincent declaration. Diabetic Med 1990; 7: 360.
2. Greene MF, Hare JW, Krache M, et al. Prematurity among insulin-requiring diabetic gravid women. Am J Obstet Gynecol 1989; 161: 106–11.
3. Hanson U, Persson B. Outcome of pregnancies complicated by type 1 insulin-dependent diabetes in Sweden: acute pregnancy complications, neonatal mortality and morbidity. Am J Perinatol 1993; 10: 330–3.
4. Landon MB, Gabbe SG, Piana R, Mennuti MT, Main EK. Neonatal morbidity in pregnancy complicated by diabetes mellitus: predictive value of maternal glycemic profiles. Am J Obstet Gynecol 1987; 156: 1089–95.
5. Reece EA, Homko CJ. Infant of the diabetic mother. Semin Perinatol 1994; 18: 459–69.
6. Livingstone EG, Herbert WNP, Hage ML. Use of the TDx-FLM assay in the evaluating fetal lung maturity in an insulin-dependent diabetic population. Obstet Gynecol 1995; 86: 826–9.
7. Di Renzo GC, Anceschi MM, Guidetti R, Cosmi EV. Requirements of perinatal prevention and treatment of respiratory distress syndrome. Eur Respir J 1989; 2(suppl. 3): 68s–72s.

8. Frantz III ID, Epstein MF. Fetal lung development in pregnancies complicated by diabetes. In: Merkatz IR, Adam PAJ, eds. The diabetic pregnancy: a perinatal perspective. New York: Grune and Stratton; 1979.
9. Robert MF, Neff RK. Association between maternal diabetes and the respiratory distress syndrome in the newborn. New Engl J Med 1976; 294: 357–60.
10. Kjos SL, Walther FJ, Montoro M. Prevalence and etiology if respiratory distress in infants of diabetic mothers: predictive value of fetal lung maturation tests. Am J Obstet Gynecol 1990; 163: 898–903.
11. Piper JM, Langer O. Does maternal diabetes delay fetal lung maturit? Am J Obstet Gynecol 1993; 168: 783.
12. Bourbon JR, Farrell PM. Fetal lung development in the diabetic pregnancy. Pediatric Res 1985; 19: 253–67.
13. Smith BT, Giroud CJP. Insulin antagonism of cortisol action on lecithin synthesis by cultured fetal lung cells. J Pedatr 1975; 87: 953–5.
14. Engle M, Langan SM. The effects of insulin and hyperglycemia on surfactant phospholipid biosynthesis in organotypic cultures on type II pneumocytes. Biochem Biophys Acta 1983; 753: 6–13.
15. Carlson KS, Smith BT. Insulin acts on the fibroblast to inhibit glucocorticoid stimulation of lung maturity. J Appl Physiol 1984; 57: 1577–9.
16. Kulovich MV, Gluck CKL. The lung profile: II. Complicated pregnancy. Am J Obstet Gynecol 1979; 136: 64.
17. Smith BT. Pulmonary surfactant during fetal development and the neonatal adaptation: hormonal control. In: Robertson B, Van Golde LMG, Batemburg JJ, eds. Pulmonary surfactant. Amsterdam: Elsevier; 1984, pp. 357–81.
18. Ferroni KM, Gross TL, Sokol RJ. What affects fetal pulmonary maturation during diabetic pregnancy? Am J Obstet Gynecol 1984; 150: 270.
19. Tyden O, Berne C, Erikkson UJ. Fetal maturation in strictly controlled diabetic pregnancy. Diabetes Res 1984; 1: 1314.
20. Landon MB, Gabbe SC, Piana R. Neonatal morbidity in pregnancy complicated by diabetes mellitus: predictive value of maternal glycemic profiles. Am J Obstet Gynecol 1987; 156: 1089–93.
21. Cunningam MD, Desai NS, Thomson SA. Amniotic fluid phosphatidyl-glycerol in diabetic pregnancy. Am J Obstet Gynecol 1978; 131: 712.
22. Ylinen K. High maternal levels of hemoglobin A1c associated with delayed fetal lung maturation in insulin-dependent diabetic pregnancies. Acta Obstet Gynecol Scand 1987; 66: 263–6.
23. Bourbon JR, Doucet E, Rieutort M. Role of myo-inositol in impairment of fetal lung phosphatidylglycerol biosynthesis in the diabetic pregnancy: physiological consequences of phosphatidylglycerol deficient surfactant in the newborn rat. Exp Lung Res 1986; 11: 195.
24. Pinter E, Peyman JA, Snow K. Effects of maternal diabetes on fetal rat lung ion transport: contribution of alveolar and bronchiolar epithelial cells to Na+,K+ ATPase expression. J Clin Invest 1991; 87: 821–30.
25. Bhavnani BR, Enhorning G, Ekelund L. Maternal diabetes and its effect on biochemical and functional development of rabbit fetal lung. Biochem Cell Biol 1988; 66: 396–404.
26. Hawdon JM, Aynsley-Green A. Neonatal complications, including hypoglycemia. In: Dornhorst A, Hadden DR, eds. Diabetes and Pregnancy: An International Approach to Diagnosis and Management. New York: John Wiley; 1996, pp. 303–18.
27. Cosmi EV, Di Renzo GC. Diagnosis of fetal lung maturity. In Cosmi EV, Scarpelli EM, eds. Pulmonary Surfactant System. Amsterdam: Elsevier; 1983, pp. 77–98.
28. Berkowitz K, Reyes C, Saadat P. Comparison of biochemical indices in gestational diabetes and non diabetic pregnancies, J Reprod Med 1997; 42: 793–800.
29. Moore TR. A comparison of amniotic fluid fetal pulmonary phospholipids in normal and diabetic pregnancy. Am J Obstet Gynecol 2002; 186: 641–50.
30. Langer O. The controversy surrounding fetal lung maturity in diabetes in pregnancy: a re-evaluation. J Matern Fetal Neonat Med 2002; 12: 428–32.
31. Kjos SL, Berkowitz KM, Kung B. Prospective delivery of reliably dated term infants of diabetic mothers without determination of fetal lung maturity: comparison to historical control. J Matern Fetal Neonatal Med 2002; 12: 433–37.
32. Moore TR. Diabetes in pregnancy. In: Creasy RK, Resnik R, eds. Maternal Fetal Medicine, 4th edn. Phildelphia: Saunders; 1999, pp. 964–95.
33. Gluck L, Kulovich MV, Boerer Jr RC. Diagnosis of the respiratory distress syndrome by amniocentesis. Am J Obstet Gynecol 1971; 109: 440.
34. Gluck L, Kulovich MV, Borer RC. The interpretation and significance of the leithin/sphingomyelin ratio in amniotic fluid. Am J Obstet Gynecol 1974; 120: 142.

35. Hallman M, Kulovich M, Kirkpatrick E. Phosphatidylinositol and phosphatidylglycerol in amniotic fluid: indices of lung maturity. Am J Obstet Gynecol 1976; 125: 613.
36. Harvey D, Parkinson C, Campbell S. Risk of respiratory distress syndrome. Lancet 1975; 1: 42
37. Kulovich MV, Hallman MB, Gluck L. The lung profile. I. Normal pregnancy. Am J Obstet Gynecol 1975; 135: 57.
38. Di Renzo GC, Cutuli A, De Graaf O, et al. Problematiche diagnostiche nella valutazione della maturità fetale. In AOGOI, 7° Corso di aggiornamento in Medicina Perinatale, Bormio 1997, 75–7.
39. Gindes L, Chen R, Perri T, et al. Perinatal morbidity in offspring of diabetic mothers. Isr J Obstet Gynecol 2002; 12: 165–71.
40. Tsai MY, Marshall JG. Phosphatidylglycerol in 261 samples of amniotic fluid from normal and diabetic pregnancies, as measured by one-dimensional thin layer chromatography. Clin Chem 1979; 25: 682–5.
41. Gluck L, Kulovich MV. Lecithin/sphingomyelin ratios in amniotic fluid in normal and abnormal pregnancy. Am J Obstet Gynecol 1973; 115: 539: 46.
42. Sigh EJ, Mejia A, Zuspan FP. Studies of human amniotic fluid phospholipids in normal, diabetic and drug abuse pregnancy. Am J Obstet Gynecol 1974; 119: 623–9.
43. Tabsh KMA, Brinkman CR, Bashore RA. Lecithin/sphingomyelin ratio in pregnancies complicated by insulin-dependent diabetes mellitus. Obstet Gynecol 1982; 59: 353–8.
44. Farrell PM, Engle MJ, Curet LB. Satured phospholipids in amniotic fluid of normal and diabetic pregnancies. Obstet Gynecol 1984; 64: 77–85.
45. Dubin SB. The laboratory assessment of fetal lung maturity. Am J Clin Pathol 1992; 97: 836.
46. Plauche WC, Faro S. Letellier R. Phosphatidylglycerol and fetal lung maturity. Am J Obstet Gynecol 1982; 144: 167.
47. Curet LB, Olbson RV, Schneider JM, Zachman RD. Effects of diabetes mellitus on amniotic fluid lecithin/sphingomyelin ratio and respiratory distress syndrome. Am J Obstet Gynecol 1979; 135: 10–3.
48. Golde SH, Mosley GH. A blind comparison study of the lung phospholipid profile, fluorescence microviscosimetry and the lecithin-sphingomyelin ratio. Am J Obstet Gynecol 1980; 126: 222.
49. Garite TJ, Yabusaki KK, Moberg LJ. A new rapid slide agglutination test for amniotic fluid phosphatidylglycerol. Am J Obstet Gynecol 1983; 147: 681–6.
50. Lockitch G, Wittmann BK, Mura SM, Hawkley LC. Evaluation of Amniostat-FLM assay for assessment of fetal lung maturity. Clin Chem 1984; 159: 65–8.
51. Benoit J, Merrill S, Rundell C. An intial clinical trial with both vaginal pool amniocentesis samples. Am J Obstet Gynecol 1993; 169: 573–6.
52. Saad SA, Fadel HF, Fahmy K, et al. The reliability and clinical use of a rapid phosphatidylglycerol assay in normal and diabetic pregnancies. Am J Obstet Gynecol 1987; 157: 1516–20.
53. McMahon MJ, Mimouni F, Miodovnik M. Surfactant associated protein (SAP-35) in amniotic fluid from diabetic and non dibetic pregnancies. Obstet Gynecol 1987; 70: 94–8.
54. Hallman M, Arjomaa P, Mizumoto M, Akino T. Surfactant proteins in the diagnosis of fetal lung maturity. Am J Obstet Gynecol 1988; 158: 531–5.
55. Ludimir J, Alvarez JG, Mennuti MT. Cholesterol palmitate as a predictor of fetal lung maturity. Am J Obstet Gynecol 1987; 157: 84–8.
56. Ludimir J, Alvarez JG, Landon MB. Amniotic fluid cholesterol palmitate in pregnancies complicated by diabetes mellitus. 1988; 72: 360–2.
57. Tait JF, Franklin RW, Simpson JB, Ashwood ER. Improved fluorescence polarization assay for use in evaluating fetal lung maturity. I. Development of the assay procedure. Clin Chem 1986; 32: 248–54.
58. Russell JC. A calibrated fluorescence polarization assay for assessment of fetal lung maturity. Clin Chem 1987; 33: 1177–84.
59. Blumenfeld TA, Stark RI, James LS, George JD. Determination of fetal lung maturity by fluorescence polarization of amniotic fluid. Am J Obstet Gynecol 1978; 130: 782–7.
60. Golde SH, Vogt JF, Gabbe SG, Cabal LA. Evaluation of the FELMA in icroviscometer in predicting fetal lung maturity. Obstet Gynecol 1979; 54: 639–42.
61. Ashwood ER, Tait JF, Foerder CA. Improved fluorescence polarization assay for use in evaluating fetal lung maturity. III. Clin Chem 1986; 32: 260.
62. Barkau G, Hashiach S, Lanzer D. Detrmination of fetal lung maturity from amniotic fluid microviscosity in high risk pregnancy. Obstet Gynecol 1982; 59: 615–23.
63. Russell JC, Cooper CM, Ketchun CH. Multicenter evaluation of TDx test for assessing fetal lung maturity. Clin Chem 1980; 35: 1005.
64. Livingston EG, Herbert WN, Hage ML, for the Diabetes and Fetal Maturity Study Group. Use of the TDx-FLM assay in evaluating fetal

lung maturity in an insulin-dependent diabetic population. Obstet Gynecol 1995; 86: 826–9.

65. Tanasijevic MJ, Winkelman JW, Wybenga DR. Prediction of fetal lung maturity in infants of diabetic mothers using FLM S/A and disaturated phosphatidylcholine tests. Am J Clin Pathol 1996; 105: 17–22.

66. Parvin CA, Kaplan LA, Chapman JF, McManamon TG, Gronowski AM. Predicting respiratory distress syndrome using gestational age and fetal lung maturity by fluorescent polarization. Am J Obstet Gynecol 2005; 192: 199–207.

67. Ahwood ER, Palmer SE, Taylor JS. Lamellar body counts for rapid feal lung maturity testing. Obstet Gynecol 1993; 81: 619.

68. Khazardoost S, Yahayazadeh H, Borna S, et al. Amniotic fluid lamellar body count and its sensitivity and specificity in evaluating of fetal lung maturity. J Obstet Gynecol 2005; 25: 257–9.

69. Ghidini A, Poggi Sh, Spong Cy, et al. Role of lamellar body count for the prediction of neonatal respiratory distress syndrome in non-diabetic pregnant women. Arch Gynecol Obstet 2005; 27: 325–8.

70. Abd El Aal DE, Elkhirshy AA, Atwa S, El-Kabsh MY. Lamellar body count as a predictor of neonatal lung maturity in high-risk pregnancies. Int J Gynaecol Obstet 2005; 89: 19–25.

71. DeRoche ME, Ingardia CJ, Guerette PJ, et al. The use of lamellar body counts to predict fetal lung maturità in pregnacies complicated by diabetes mellitus. Am J Obstet Gynecol 2002; 187: 908–12.

72. Pattle RE, Kratzing CC, Parkinson CE, et al. Maturity of fetal lungs tested by production of stable microbubbles in amniotic fluid. Br J Obstet Gynaecol 1979; 86: 615–22.

73. Kumazawa K, Hiramatsu Y, Masuyama H, et al. Prediction markers for respiratory distress syndrome: evaluation of the stable microbubble test, surfactant protein-A and hepatocyte growth factor levels in amniotic fluid. Acta ??ed Okayama 2003; 57: 25–32.

74. Kuroki Y, Takahashi H, Fukuda Y. Two-site "simultaneous" immuno-assay with monoclonal antibodies for the determination of surfactant apoproteins in human amniotic fluid. Pediatr Res 1985; 19: 1017.

75. Ventolini G, Neiger R, Hood D, Belcastro C. Update on assessment of fetal lung maturity. J Obstet Gynaecol 2005; 25: 535–8.

76. Bartelsmeyer JA. Fetal lung maturity. In: Winn HN, Hobbins JCH, eds. Clinical Maternal–Fetal Medicine. London: Parthenon; 2000.

77. Piazze JJ, Anceschi MM, Maranghi L, et al. Fetal lung maturity in pregnancies complicated by insulin-dependent and gestational diabetes: matched cohort study. Eur J Obstet Gynecol 1999; 83: 145–50.

78. Ghidini A, Spong CY, Goodwin K, Pezzullo JC. Optimal thresholds of the lecithin/sphingomyelin ratio and lamellar body count for the prediction of the presence of phosphatidyl glycerol in diabetic women. J Matern Fetal Neonat Med 2002; 12: 95–8.

79. Piper JM. Lung maturation in diabetes in pregnancy: if and when to test. Semin Perinatol 2002; 26: 206–9.

80. Ventolini G, Neiger R, Hood DL, Belcastro MR. Changes in the threshold of fetal lung maturity testing and neonatal outcome of infants delivered electively before 39 weeks gestation: implications and cost-effectiveness. J Perinatol 2006; 26: 264–7.

81. Liggins GC, Howie RN. A controlled trial of antepartum glucocorticoid treatment for prevention of the respiratory distess syndrome in premature infants. Pediatrics 1972; 50: 515–25.

82. Anceschi M, Maranghi L, Cosmi E. Prevention of fetal and neonatal lung immaturity. In: Kurjak A, Chervenak F, eds. Textbook of Perinatal Medicine. Oxford: Information Health Care; 2006, pp. 1433–45.

83. Crowley P. Prophylactic corticosteroids for preterm birth (Cochrane Review). In: The Cochrane Library. Oxford. Update Software 2003; 3.

84. Gojnic M, Pervulov M, Petkovic S, Mostic T, Jeremic K. J Mater Fetal Neonatal Med 2004; 16: 11–4.

85. Roberts D, Dalziel S. Antenatal corticosteroids for accelerating fetal lung maturation for women at risk of preterm birth. Cochrane Database Syst Rev 2006; 19: CD004454.

86. Neilson JP. Cochrane Update: Antenatal corticosteroids for accelerating fetal lung maturation for women at risk of preterm birth. Obstet Gynecol 2007; 109: 189–90.

87. Blickstein I, Reichman B, Lusky A, Shinwell ES. Israel Neonatal Network. Plurality-dependent risk of severe intraventricular hemorrhage among very low birth weight infants and antepartum corticosteroid treatment. Am J Obstet Gynecol 2006; 194: 1329–33.

88. Crowley P. Prophylactic corticosteroids for preterm birth (Cochrane review). Wiley, Chichester: The Cochrane Library, 2004.

89. Baud O, Foix-L'Helias L, Kaminski M, et al. Antenatal glucocorticoid treatment and cystic periventricular leukomalacia in very premature infants. N Engl J Med 1999; 341: 1190–6.

90. Di Renzo GC, Roura LC. European Association of Perinatal Medicine Study Group on Preterm Birth. Guidelines for the management of spontaneous preterm labor. J Perinat Med 2006; 34: 359–66.

91. DI Renzo GC, Al Saleh E, Mattei A, Koutras I, Clerici G. Use of tocolytics: what is the benefit of gaining 48 hours for the fetus? BJOG 2006; 113(suppl. 3): 72–7.

92. NIH Consensus Conference. Corticosteroids for fetal maturation on perinatal outcome. J Am Med Assoc 1995; 275: 413–7.

93. Antenatal corticosteroids revisited: repeat courses. NIH Consensus Statement 17; 2000, p. 1.

94. Royal College of Obstetricians and Gynecologists. Antenatal corticosteroids to prevent respiratory distress syndrome. Guideline No. 7. Revised February 2004. Link: http: //www.rcog.org.uk/index.asp?PageID=511

95. Wunder D, Durig P. Diabetes mellitus and pregnancy: screening and therapy. Schweiz Rundsch Med Prax 2003; 92: 591–6.

Monitoring in labor

Roberto Luzietti and Karl G. Rosén

Introduction

Alteration of fetal carbohydrate metabolism may contribute to intrauterine asphyxia. There is considerable evidence linking hyperinsulinemia and fetal hypoxemia. Hyperinsulinemia induced in fetal lambs by an infusion of exogenous insulin produces an increase in oxygen consumption and a decrease in arterial oxygen content. The fetus of the diabetic mother is also at increased risk of asphyxia because of other factors such as increased fetal metabolic rate and oxygen requirement, ketoacidosis and the increased incidence of certain pathological conditions in the diabetic pregnancy, e.g. pre-eclampsia and vasculopathy, which can result in a reduction in placental blood flow and fetal oxygenation.

All these factors make intrapartum fetal surveillance in pregnancies complicated by maternal diabetes of fundamental importance. In this chapter the basis and current development of intrapartum fetal monitoring, with particular reference to ST waveform analysis of the fetal electrocardiogram (ECG), will be reviewed. The twentieth century saw dramatic developments in medical care as technological advances were applied to both diagnosis and treatment. However, some areas of obstetrics have been slow to benefit from these advances, and none more so than the care of the fetus in labor. Fetal surveillance during labor constitutes a challenge in information management. To give birth is a natural process for women. For the child it may constitute a threat for intact survival and ominous changes may appear within minutes, putting labor-ward management in the forefront of medical high-risk management. The nurse/midwife/obstetrician manages this complex situation by visual analysis of a host of information, both clinical and that directly recorded, from the fetus in particular. The current situation is far from satisfactory and a new strategy has to be developed and implemented to take obstetric management further into this century.

What information is required?

The capacity of fetuses to handle hypoxemia may differ greatly, depending not only on the condition prior to labor but also due to events during labor which may affect the ability to mobilize these defense systems. Therefore, it may be difficult to rely only on the actual level of oxygenation. Instead, it may be more rewarding to try to interpret the reactions taking place in a high-priority organ like the heart or the brain.

Much would be gained if there were continuous information available providing direct measure on the ability of the fetus to respond to the stress of labor. The fetal ability to adapt to hypoxemia, hypoxia, and asphyxia involves multiple defense mechanisms. These consist primarily of behavioral changes, i.e. reduced active sleep with fewer fetal movements and enhanced extraction of available oxygen. Cardiovascular compensation that increases blood flow to the most important organs, i.e. the brain, the heart, and the adrenals, is of importance during hypoxia, as is the metabolic defense of anaerobic metabolism. It is only when these compensatory mechanisms are insufficient that asphyxia will develop and along with it the possibility of central nervous system damage and handicap (for review see Greene and Rosén[1]).

Available techniques

To achieve a change, we need to analyze what were the shortcomings when electronic fetal monitoring (EFM) was introduced some 30 years ago. With EFM obstetricians hoped to prevent the delivery of dead or impaired babies who had suffered from birth asphyxia. It is now realized that cardiotocography (CTG) does not provide all the information required to do this.[2,3] Misinterpretation of the CTG not only causes an increase in unnecessary intervention but is also implicated in a large proportion of patients with birth asphyxia and avoidable perinatal morbidity.[4] Misinterpretation could be corrected with improved understanding and enhanced identification of specific events in fetal heart rate (FHR) patterns. The automatic assessment of FHR variability and reactivity antenatally provides a good example of the latter. Physiologically, there are a multitude of factors influencing FHR in the term fetus and it should not be anticipated that there are FHR features that are specific enough to discriminate between different levels of hypoxia. However, at the same time, EFM provides relevant information of fetal reactiveness, i.e. a fetus showing a completely normal CTG should have matters under control. At the same time, a CTG pattern with complete lack of FHR variability and reactivity (Figure 36.1) should serve as the best indicator of a fetus that has lost its ability to respond and is in a preterminal situation.

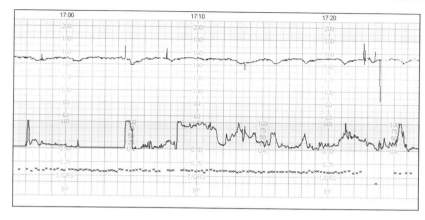

Figure 36.1   Para 1, normal pregnancy, spontaneous onset at 39 weeks gestation, oligohydramnios plus decreased fetal movements noted by the mother. Emergency Cesarean section for fetal distress at 17:43. Female 2900 g, Apgar score 1-3-5, cord artery data not obtained, cord vein data – pH 7.29, pCO_2 6.5 kPa, BDecf (base deficit in the extra cellular fluid) 2.5 mmol/l. Initial ventilation by mask followed by intubation, meconium in upper airways. Adequate breathing at 25 minutes of age. Marked hypoglycemia (0.5 mmol/l) initially. No sign of meconium aspiration or RDS (respiratory distress syndrome). Increased neuromuscular tone but normal electroencephalogram. No suctioning reflex initially. Normal behavior after 4 days. Discharged home after 15 days.

Fetal blood sampling

Fetal blood sampling (FBS) can be used along with CTG monitoring to assess the fetal acid–base status during labor and can reduce operative intervention,[5] but it requires additional expertise, is time consuming, and gives only intermittent information; therefore, it is not widely used.[3]

Considering the need to improve understanding of the process of intrapartum hypoxia, very little new information has emerged with regard to the analysis of scalp pH since the early work by Rosén et al.[6] At the same time as EFM and FBS have been shown to improve outcome, the use of FBS has also been questioned by analyzing outcome measures in a large clinical service where the rate of FBS decreased from 1.76 to 0.03% without any change in the Cesarean section rate or an increase in indicators of perinatal asphyxia.[7] Thus, the attitude towards the clinical usefulness of FBS and scalp pH is, after 30 years, still unclear.

To what extent should a scalp pH add to our ability to identify fetuses at risk of intrapartum hypoxia? The limitation of a scalp pH is that it will always reflect the status of the peripheral blood where an acidosis is inherent due to the accumulation of CO_2. Respiratory acidemia is generated in the blood, whereas metabolic acidemia is generated in the tissues. This means that a scalp sample *per se* will not always reflect the state of the tissues. If the aim is to identify those fetuses suffering from metabolic acidosis, a scalp blood pH may be a poor predictor. Furthermore, the effectiveness of FBS in clinical practice is another problem. In the Plymouth trial, despite the use of a strict protocol, 39% of cases had FBS performed unnecessarily and 33% of cases did not have it performed when it was indicated.[5] The decision to perform FBS depends on the interpretation of the CTG: if the level of CTG interpretation is suboptimal, the value of monitoring by FBS is limited.[8]

Pulse oximetry

Pulse oximetry is focused on recording the actual level of fetal hypoxemia and relates the level of oxygenation of organ function as indicated by FHR.[9] A US multicenter randomized trial of 1010 women in labor with a non-reassuring FHR tracing showed a reduction in emergency Cesarean sections from 10 to 5%. However, unexpectedly, the study also showed an increase in the Cesarean section rate for failure to progressin the test group, 19 vs. 9%, and the overall Cesarean section rates were not different between the test and control groups.

The current literature holds somewhat diverging views on the information available from fetal pulse oximetry during labor. The issue still to be resolved is the ability of CTG + pulse oximetry to provide diagnostic capacity on fetal metabolic acidosis.[10,11] Thus, the situation may arise where the two parameters in combination may not be specific enough to enable the obstetrician to grade the impact of hypoxemia on fetal organ function.

A different approach to assess fetal condition during labor is that based on evaluation of high-priority organ function. ST analysis of the ECG during exercise testing is well proven in assessing myocardial function in the adult.[10]

Fetal ECG

Similar to the adult stress test, ST waveform analysis of the fetal ECG, affected by the stress of labor, should provide key information about the ability of the high-priority organ, i.e. the fetal heart, to respond. This assumption seems to hold true and ST analysis has emerged not as an alternative to CTG but as a support tool, allowing more accurate interpretation of intrapartum events along the lines depicted in Figure 36.2. Furthermore, the fetal ECG is readily obtainable during labor from the same scalp electrode used to obtain the FHR and no alterations are required in the patient handling routines.

Figure 36.3 indicates those parts of the ECG that provide specific information on the fetal response to hypoxia. The waveform marked P corresponds to the contraction of the atrium; the next sequence is the contraction of the ventricles, illustrated by the waveforms Q, R and S.

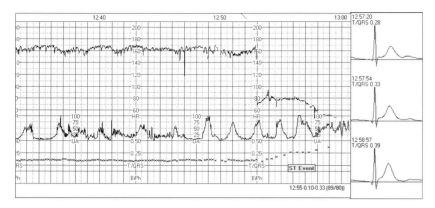

Figure 36.2 STAN recording during the second stage of labor. Uneventful pregnancy at term. At 12:53 the midwife, who was a trained STAN user, noted as abrupt shift in the fetal heart rate (FHR) recording. She immediately informed the clinician about the situation of an emerging acute asphyxia. The clinician, who had not been trained, choose to verify that the FHR was recorded by applying an external sensor. The baby was delivered 14 min after the end of the recording, with Apgar scores of 3 at 1 min and of 5 at 5 min, and developed signs of neonatal encephalopathy with seizures. Acute placental abruption with an immediate stop in cord vein blood flow was the cause of this acutely emerging intrapartum asphyxia.

Physiology

The ST segment and the T wave relate to the repolarization of myocardial cells in preparation for the next contraction, a process that is energy consuming. An *increase* in T-wave height, quantified by the ratio between T and QRS amplitudes (the T/QRS ratio) (Figure 36.2), occurs when the energy balance within the myocardial cells threatens to become negative.[1,8,12] A negative energy balance means a situation where the amount of oxygen supplied to the cells no longer covers the energy required for metabolic activity. During hypoxia this balance becomes negative and the cells produce energy by the beta-adrenoceptor-mediated anaerobic breakdown of glycogen reserves.[6] The ability of these cells to produce energy in this manner, and thereby maintain myocardial function, is a vital compensatory defense mechanism.[13] This process not only produces lactic acid but also potassium ions (K^+), which affects myocardial cell membrane potential and causes a rise in the ST waveform (Figure 36.3).[12] Thus, the rise in T-wave amplitude and the increase in the T/QRS ratio reflect the rate of myocardial glycogenolysis and the utilization of a key fetal defense to hypoxia.

Hypoxemia is just one way in which this myocardial energy balance changes, so producing ST waveform changes. Another

mechanism by which these ST changes may occur is the general surge of stress hormones (adrenaline) occurring in response to the squeezing and squashing of labor. This will stimulate the heart to increase its pumping activity, and at the same time induce glycogenolysis and high T waves. This general arousal is part of normal labor and in these cases the healthy fetus will display a reactive CTG, ensuring normality.[14]

Biphasic ST events

ST depression with negative T waves has been observed during hypoxia experiments in experimentally growth-retarded guinea pigs.[7] Clinically, these changes have emerged as a specific sign of myocardial hypoxic stress, reflecting a myocardium either unable or with insufficient time to mobilize its defense to hypoxemia. The result is a decrease in myocardial activity and a risk of cardiovascular failure.

The physiology behind biphasic ST events is related to the mechanical performance of the myocardium, and the relationship between the inner (endocardium) and outer (epicardium) layers of the walls of the ventricles in particular. As we know it, biphasic ST illustrates an imbalance between these two layers, the reason being that the perfusion pressure of the endocardium is always lower when the mechanical strain is greater. This means that unless the myocardium is generally activated (beta-receptor activation and enhanced Frank–Starling relationship, i.e. the ability of the myocardium to respond to volume load), any decrease in performance will cause biphasic ST. Thus, not only may hypoxia *per se* cause biphasic ST as a sign of maladaptation, but so will all factors substantially altering the balance and performance characteristics within the myocardial wall. Basically, biphasic ST is the pattern to be expected whenever the myocardium is exposed to factors that may decrease its ability to respond.

Probably the most clinically important aspect of biphasic ST is that once it has been identified, then a situation of potentially reduced myocardial performance has also been identified and 'classical' signs of fetal reactions to an emerging

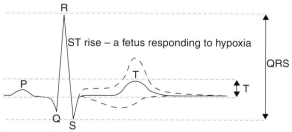

Figure 36.3 The ECG, with a schematic presentation of hypoxia-related changes; the T/QRS ratio measurement is also indicated.

hypoxia should not be expected. From what is stated above, it should be noted that a fetus displaying biphasic ST events is not usually in a situation of immediate hypoxia and metabolic acidosis. However, with further progress of labor, especially during the second stage, these fetuses will suffer.

Recently, Westgate et al.[15] reported on ST-waveform changes during repeated umbilical cord occlusions in near-term fetal sheep. As expected, they found an increase in the T/QRS ratio with cord occlusions that became more marked when the level of hypoxia was increased by reducing the time between occlusions from 5 to 2.5 min. Fetuses no longer capable of maintaining their cardiovascular response reacted with negative ST changes in between occlusions. The authors concluded that an increase in the T/QRS ratio indicated hypoxic stress, and that the appearance of biphasic and negative waveforms between contractions may be a useful marker for the development of severe fetal decompensation.

Clinical research

The concept of ST analysis has been developed through a continuous validation process, starting with experimental research followed by bioengineering developments and the generation of a dedicated medical device.

Plymouth randomized controlled trial

This was the first randomized controlled trial (RCT) where 2400 high-risk term deliveries were studied, comparing CTG monitoring plus ST-waveform analysis (CTG + ST) with standard CTG monitoring.[14] Strict clinical guidelines were developed and initially tested in the Plymouth RCT of CTG + ST versus CTG, which showed a safe reduction in operative deliveries for fetal distress (ODFD) by 46%, with fewer babies born with signs of intrapartum hypoxia. The trial also showed the need to improve data presentation, as three cases in the CTG + ST arm had clinical signs of asphyxia in spite of ST events which were missed. To improve the detection of ST events, a new STAN recorder was developed utilizing modern software to improve signal quality and allow for automatic identification of significant ST events. This work required extensive signal processing and not until fast-processing capacity became available (at reasonable costs) in the 1990s was the next step taken: the introduction of the event log.

This approach was tested in a European multicenter prospective trial of 320 high-risk pregnancies. The cases were managed according to the routine CTG with blinded ST information (data stored on a PC connected to a STAN prototype unit). There were six cases of marked hypoxia, all of which showed ST-waveform changes of a magnitude to signify immediate delivery.[16]

This ST log function in combination with the CTG + ST clinical guidelines was recently shown to accurately identify all 15 babies with marked oxygen deficiency among a group of 574 Swedish and Norwegian babies. Although conventional CTG monitoring was used to assess the condition of the babies these cases were still missed and, as a consequence, three of them are likely to suffer permanent brain damage.[9] These results have recently been verified in a second large randomized trial.

Swedish multicenter RCT

The aim of this large trial was to test the hypothesis that intrapartum monitoring of term fetuses with CTG + ST results in a reduced rate of both ODFD and of newborns with metabolic acidosis, as compared with CTG alone.[10,17]

The primary outcome of this RCT was published recently.[17] It showed a significant reduction in ODFD from 8.0 to 5.9%, at the same time as the risk of being born with cord artery metabolic acidosis, defined as cord artery pH < 7.05 and BDecf (base deficit in extracellular fluid) >12 mmol/L, was reduced from 1.44 to 0.57%.

The Swedish RCT was designed with a power to assess potential improvements in neonatal outcome. The trial design also allowed testing of the effects of growing, with the new STAN technology in the three busy labor ward units with cases managed by >300 midwives and physicians. The current analysis summarizes the findings associated with the 351 babies that were admitted to the Special Care Baby Unit (SCBU).

Results

Table 36.1 gives neonatal outcome according to intention to treat. The case of intrapartum death after retraining in the CTG + ST arm had second-stage CTG and ST changes that were not recognized; the scalp electrode was disconnected due to ventouse extraction for failure to progress and a severely asphyxiated baby was delivered after 23 min. The other case had 10 min of a T/QRS ratio rise before a normal delivery, the Apgar score was normal and the baby was observed for 3 h in the SCBU due to cord metabolic acidosis. All patients except for the one in the CTG + ST arm had intrapartum events detected as abnormal by the STAN clinical guidelines: this patient had had the STAN recorder disconnected 3.5 h before delivery.

Fetal scalp pH (i.e. FBS) has hitherto been regarded as the method of reference for detection of intrapartum hypoxia; 495 cases from both arms had fetal scalp pH samples. Of a total of 46 cases with metabolic acidosis at delivery, only six had FBS data. The ST waveform could be assessed in five of these six babies, showing abnormalities lasting from 25 to 276 (median 119) min before delivery. In only one case was an abnormal FBS obtained (pH 7.13), at which point ST events had been recorded for 80 min. In the other five cases, the scalp pH was normal (>7.20) and not repeated as labor progressed.

A 1600 cases interim analysis revealed six cases where ST events had been ignored and the fetus exposed to hypoxia. This observation showed that ST analysis improved the sensitivity of detecting adverse events in labor and it was decided to continue with the trial, with the addition of regular staff meetings to discuss cases.

According to the protocol, a secondary analysis was made, with the exclusion of neonates with severe malformations and inadequately monitored cases (those monitored for <20 min and cases where the monitoring was interrupted >20 min before delivery). Table 36.2 shows the outcomes among adequately monitored neonates during the second phase of the trial.

Thus, irrespective of what outcome measure was applied, the Swedish RCT documented marked improvements in neonatal outcome after retraining with enhanced experience of ST analysis. The improvements in the diagnosis of intrapartum

Table 36.1   Distribution of cases with adverse/complicated neonatal outcome, related to the method of intrapartum fetal surveillance and their occurrence in relationship to retraining

	CTG		CTG + ST	
	Before (*n* = 1250)	After retraining (*n* = 1197)	Before (*n* = 1333)	After retraining (*n* = 1186)
Perinatal death	1 (asphyxia)	0	1 (sepsis)	1 (asphyxia)
Outcome of SCBU visit				
Neuromuscular symptoms				
Seizures	1	2	0	0
Increased neuromuscular tone	1	3	0	0
Irritability only	1	0	3	0
Met acid + other symptoms	3	7	4	1
Total	7	12	8	2

OR 0.17, 95% CI 0.03–0.78, *P* = 0.01.
met acid, metabolic acidosis.

hypoxia during the second phase of the trial also enabled a 44% reduction in ODFD, from 8.7 to 5.0% (*P* = 0.001).

The data from these two large RCTs, including 6826 cases, have shown that, with the support of fetal ECG ST-waveform analysis, the number of babies born with cord metabolic acidosis could be reduced from 1.43 to 0.57% [odds ratio (OR) 0.39, 95% confidence interval (CI) 0.21–0.72, *P* = 0.0017] whilst at the same time ODFD were reduced from 8.4 to 5.6% (OR 0.65, 95% CI 0.53–0.78, *P* < 0.001).

EU project

The expectation of society is that the application of the results of health technology assessment will improve the quality of care and ensure that available resources are used effectively. The objective of the EU project is to develop and validate a model whereby the user aspects are put to the fore to stimulate postgraduate training and an appropriate management structure.

Today, there are no specific requirements regarding the implementation of a medical device knowledge transfer process. Action according to regulatory requirements is only required when things go wrong, obviously too late in a situation such as labor, when oxygen deficiency may institute a threat to life and intact survival. The prime objective of the

EU-supported FECG project is to develop a model whereby 10 academic centers across Europe, as a joint effort, are made active partners of this knowledge-transfer process. These centers of excellence then become their regions' hubs of experience.

Methodology

The aim of the STAN concept is to provide a more thorough understanding of fetal reactions to the stress and strain of labor. The EU-supported FECG (fetal ECG) project includes the development and testing of educational material, such as a trainer/simulator that allows midwives and doctors to gain experience from displaying real cases virtually from a database. This enables exposure to rare but important cases, not otherwise easily experienced. Multimedia-based teaching, together with conventional written material, is also used. In parallel to the educational efforts, STAN S21 fetal heart recorders are used clinically.

Results and discussion

Table 36.3 gives the initial data from the 10 obstetric units participating in the project. One neonate developed increased neuromuscular tone during the first 24 h, with signs of metabolic acidosis at 1 h of age (no cord data available). The STAN recording showed an abnormal CTG + baseline rise in the

Table 36.2   Neonatal outcome among adequately recorded cases during the second phase of the Swedish RCT

	CTG		CTG + ST		
	n	%	*n*	%	OR, 95% CI, *P*
Total	1049		1054		
Apgar score 1 min <4	23	2.19	8	0.76	0.34, 0.14–0.80, 0.011
Apgar score 5 min >7	13	1.24	8	0.76	0.61, 0.23–1.58, 0.37
Apgar score 5 min <4	5	0.48	0	0.00	*P* = 0.031
Admissions to SCBU	78	7.44	54	5.12	0.67, 0.46–0.98, 0.036
Cord artery metabolic acidosis	14	1.54	4	0.44	0.28, 0.08–0.92, 0.032

Table 36.3   The FECG project: outcome of intrapartum fetal monitoring to April 2001 (corresponding data from the Swedish RCT are also given)

	EU project, incidence (%), *n* = 2181	Swedish RCT incidence (%)	
		CTG + ST, *n* = 2228	CTG, *n* = 2164
ODFD, STAN indication	7.2		
ODFD, CTG indication	9.1		
ODFD, fetal scalp pH	1.3		
ODFD, total	17.6	5.9	8.0
Cord artery metabolic acidosis (pH < 7.05 and BDecf >12 mmol/L)	0.66 (1921 cases with cord data available)	0.57	1.44
Neuromuscular symptoms, metabolic acidosis plus neonatal care	0.23	0.13	0.74

T/QRS ratio that was missed for 60 min. The material includes another 13 cases with cord artery metabolic acidosis (pH < 7.05 and BDecf >12 mmol/L), corresponding to 0.66%. Four of those required special neonatal care but no neuromuscular abnormalities were noted. All but one of these five cases with signs of complicated neonatal outcome had ST events lasting ≥20 min. Only two of the 13 cases with cord metabolic acidosis did not show ST events, nor were the CTG abnormal. These data are comparable to those noted in the Swedish RCT. Thus, standard CTG recording would cause a metabolic acidosis incidence of 1.4%. The results achieved in the FECG project clearly indicate that the 0.6% incidence may be achieved even from the first day of STAN usage.

Conclusions

The primary aim of intrapartum fetal monitoring is to reduce the risk of babies being affected by oxygen deficiency during labor. The appropriate clinical use of combined CTG + ST of fetal ECG allow this to be achieved by improving the detection and prevention of intrapartum hypoxia, with consequent improvements in perinatal outcomes.

Appendix: Case report

Para 0, complicated pregnancy with maternal diabetes and pre-eclampsia. Induction after 35 + 6 weeks gestation. The recording starts during the first stage of labor.

Already, at the onset of recording, a biphasic ST event is noted. The FHR is normal and there was no need for intervention according to STAN clinical guidelines. However, the biphasic pattern was repeating itself at 15:00, indicating that the fetal myocardium is operating under stress. A reason would be the early gestational age or cardiac malformation/dystrostophy and the lessened ability of the fetal heart to manage the strain of labor.

The recording continued and another ST event, consisting of a baseline rise in the T/QRS ratio, was noted at 17:17. At this point CTG abnormalities were noted and intervention was required according to CTG + ST guidelines. This pattern is often the initial sign of impending hypoxia and indicates of the inability of the placenta to meet the demands of the fetus. The fetus is not acidotic but the resources are inadequate to meet the further stress of active pushing in particular.

At 17:38, late decelerations commenced and another ST rise was indicated at 18:25. When the physician was informed by the midwife at 18:25, it was decided to continue with further augmentation of labor.

The last 30 min of the recording illustrate the occurrence of progressive hypoxia with a continuing rise in the T/QRS ratio. At 19:21, the head was delivered but shoulder dystocia occurred: the baby was delivered at 19:26. Apgar score 0–0–0; birthweight 4650 g; cord artery data, pH 6.90, PCO_2 11.6 kPa, BDecf 14.1 mmol/L. The baby responded to resuscitation with heart activity at 12 min of age but died within the first 24 h, no autopsy was performed.

Comments

This case illustrates the main problems of an uncontrolled diabetic pregnancy with a large-for-date fetus developing intrapartum hypoxia and shoulder dystocia. Furthermore, data are now available to continuously assess the condition of a fetus at risk to allow for a safe delivery, provided that STAN clinical guidelines are followed.

REFERENCES

1. Greene KR, Rosén KG. Intrapartum asphyxia. In: Levene MI, Bennett MJ, Punt J, eds. Fetal and Neonatal Neurology and Neurosurgery. Edinburgh: Churchill Livingstone; 1995, pp. 265–72.
2. Larsen JF. Why has conventional intrapartum cardiotocography not given the expected results? J Perinat Med 1996; 24: 15–23.
3. Nelson KB, Dambrosia JM, Ting TY, Grether JK. Uncertain value of electronic fetal monitoring in predicting cerebral palsy. N Engl J Med 1996; 334: 613–8.
4. Greene KR. Intelligent fetal heart rate computer systems in intrapartum surveillance. Curr Opin Obstet Gynaecol 1996; 8: 123–7.

5. Murphy KW, Johnson P, Moorcraft J, et al. Birth asphyxia and the intrapartum cardiotocograph. Br J Obstet Gynaecol 1990; 97: 470–9.
6. Rosén KG, Dagbjartsson A, Henriksson BA, et al. The relationship between circulating catecholamines and ST waveform in the fetal lamb electrocardiogram during hypoxia. Am J Obstet Gynaecol 1984; 149: 190–5.
7. Rosén KG, Isaksson O. Alterations in fetal heart rate and ECG correlated to glycogen, creatine phosphate and ATP levels during graded hypoxia. Biol Neonate 1976; 30: 17–24.
8. Rosén KG, Kjellmer I. Changes in the fetal heart rate and ECG during hypoxia. Acta Physiol Scand 1975; 93: 59–66.
9. Rosén KG, Luzietti R. Intrapartum fetal monitoring – its basis and current developments. Prenat Neonat Med 2000; 5: 155–68.
10. Sokolow M, McIlroy MB. In: Clinical Cardiology. Los Altos, CA: Lange Medical Publications; 1981, pp. 97–112.
11. Sundström A-K, for the Swedish STAN study group. Randomised controlled trial of CTG versus CTG+ST analysis of the fetal ECG. J Obstet Gynaecol 2001; 21: 18–9.
12. Hökegård KH, Eriksson BO, Kjellmer I, et al. Myocardial metabolism in relation to electrocardiographic changes and cardiac function during graded hypoxia in the fetal lamb. Acta Physiol Scand 1981; 113: 1–7.
13. Dawes GS, Mott JC, Shelley HJ. The importance of cardiac glycogen for the maintenance of life in fetal lambs and newborn animals during anoxia. J Physiol 1959; 146: 516–38.
14. Westgate J, Harris M, Curnow JSH, Greene KR. Plymouth randomised trial of cardiotocogram only versus ST waveform plus cardiotocogram for intrapartum monitoring: 2,400 cases. Am J Obstet Gynecol 1993; 169: 1151–60.
15. Westgate JA, Bennet L, Brabyn C, et al. ST waveform changes during repeated umbilical cord occlusions in near-term fetal sheep. Am J Obstet Gynecol 2001; 184: 743–51.
16. Luzietti R, Erkkola R, Hasbargen U, et al. European community multi-center trial 'Fetal ECG analysis during labor': ST plus CTG analysis. J Perinat Med 1999; 27: 431–40.
17. Amer-Wåhlin I, Hellsten C, Norén H, et al. Intrapartum fetal monitoring: cardiotocography versus cardiotocography plus ST Analysis of the Fetal ECG. A Swedish randomized controlled trial. Lancet 2001; 358: 534–8.

37 Timing and mode of delivery

Oded Langer

Introduction

In the United States a full term baby dies in 1 out of 500 deliveries, and a mother dies in 1 in 10,000. If this were 1940, more than 15,000 mothers would have died in childbirth and 120,000 newborns! In the past it was risky for the mother and her unborn fetus but safe for the obstetrician. Today, it is safe for the mother and child but in light of malpractice, risky for the physician. Herein lies the paradox.

There is an additional paradox. Today, the yardstick for the advancement of a profession is the model of evidence-based medicine, i.e. the idea that nothing should be introduced into practice unless it has withstood peer review from a rigorous randomized clinical trial. Yet, in a ranking of medical specialties according to their use of evidence drawn from randomized clinical trials, obstetrics came in last. Even when such trials are conducted, the results are invariably ignored by practitioners.

This state of affairs is the result of several factors. Neonatal complications, especially shoulder dystocia and stillbirth on the one hand and the potential for maternal trauma associated with these complications on the other hand has over-ridden evidence-based data in the reality of the delivery room. Often in obstetrics, a well-seasoned obstetrician will apply a strategy that appears worthwhile and not wait for the results of a clinical trial; obstetricians and their fellow professionals establish guidelines of care based on their acumen and beliefs. They simply try the technique to see if it improves outcome. As a rule of thumb, the fear from obstetrical complications, i.e. shoulder dystocia and its potential for an accompanying malpractice suit over-rides the fear from complications associated with a Cesarean delivery. In addition, the new fashion that supports Cesarean delivery by request has further diminished the use of evidence-based data for managing the timing and mode of delivery for the pregnant diabetic.

In this chapter, the existing data will be evaluated and recommendations made for the treatment approach that optimizes pregnancy outcome for the diabetic mother. Waiting for the results of clinical trials that may never materialize is a fruitless endeavor. This approach has made child delivery safer and has evolved despite the increasing age of the mother, obesity, and the risk factors associated with diabetic pregnancies.[1] The decision about the optimum time to deliver the baby in the pregnancy complicated by diabetes has to consider the balance between the perceived risks of late intrauterine death and shoulder dystocia and the consequences of unnecessary prematurity and Cesarean section delivery.

It is essential to stress the issue of fetal demise in pregnancy. Fetal death, excluding congenital anomalies, has been found to be associated with the level of glycemic control in the pregnant diabetic woman. The level of glycemia is one of the factors that will mandate timing of delivery in these patients. A brief review of the literature reveals that approximately 80% of the studies in obstetrics are observational[2] while about 11% are randomized studies. Since studies evaluating perinatal mortality due to diabetes in pregnancy are under the constraints of strict ethical standards that prevent randomized trials, it is necessary that the basic characteristics of both the study and control populations be comparable, e.g. incidence of prolapse of cord, medical complications, parity, ethnicity, and prenatal care. Only then does the disease in question, diabetes, become the main cause for the difference in rates between the groups in perinatal outcome.

Fetal demise in the pregnant diabetic is often defined as 'unexplained fetal death'. The demise is the result of the metabolic acidosis developed in the fetal compartment in the presence of an abnormal glucose level rather than the traditional explanation of fetal hypoxia. The second and up to the middle of the third trimesters account for minimal rates of fetal demise; the majority of fetal deaths occur late in the third trimester. This mortality pattern is associated with fetal development and increase in insulin sensitivity during pregnancy. Although insulin can be detected as early as the latter part of the first trimester, the affinity to insulin action becomes significant at or about the 28th week of gestation resulting in fetal hyperinsulinemia that leads to fetal acidemia and hyperlacticemia without evidence of fetal hypoxia. Supporting this concept, Pettitt et al.[3] found that of 236/1000 fetal deaths, the majority occurred in large-for-gestational age (LGA) infants of gestational diabetes mellitus (GDM) mothers. Needless to say, fetal hypoxemia can occur in all types of diabetes, especially pregnancies associated with hypertensive disorder and microvascular complications (Types 1 and 2). Maternal insulinemia alone can be a cause for vasoconstriction and fetal hypoxia.[2,3]

The association between level of glycemia and fetal demise during the antepartum period was demonstrated by O'Sullivan et al.[4] They found that GDM compared to nondiabetic pregnancies had a 4-fold higher perinatal mortality. Pettitt et al.[3] found similar mortality rates for GDM and pre-existing diabetic subjects (59/1000 vs. 43–125/1000, respectively). Karlsson and Kjellmer[5] evaluated relationships between the degree of glycemic control and perinatal mortality and

Table 37.1　Diabetes and stillbirths in the United States, 1995–1997

	Fetal death rate			
Birthweight (g)	Nondiabetic (n = 10,733,983)	Diabetic (n = 271,691)	RR	95% CI
4000–4249	0.6	2.9	3.6	2.7–5.1
4250–4499	0.7	3.7	3.7	2.7–5.1
4500–4749	0.9	7.1	6.4	4.4–9.3
4750–4999	2.0	8.6	3.1	1.9–5.1
5000–5249	3.7	15.9	3.4	1.9–6.1
5250–5499	5.2	21.6	3.6	1.5–8.6
>5500	18.3	38.9	1.8	1.7–1.9

(From Mondestin.[7])

found a 3.8% perinatal mortality rate for the blood group <100 mg/dL, 16% in the group of 100–150 mg/dL, and 24% in the group with >150 mg/dL. Finally, keeping a mean blood glucose threshold of <100 mg/dL during the prenatal period will result in the lowest rate of fetal demise and provides the opportunity to avoid unnecessary early deliveries. In a recent study,[6] Schmidt reported a 3.4 higher relative risk for GDM patients. In addition, Mundestin et al.[7] demonstrated a 3- to 6-fold increase in perinatal mortality when the majority of patients were GDM. The data were driven from all deliveries in the USA including 230,000 GDM and 3,000,000 nondiabetic (Table 37.1).

In the past, there was a false belief that infants of diabetic mothers matured earlier. The reasoning behind this view was a classic example of the wrong conclusion being drawn from a study that described two major changes in management. On the one hand, they delivered all babies at 36 weeks; but this was part of a regimen that paid much closer attention to the control of the mother's diabetes during pregnancy. The perinatal outcomes from their study showed that in comparison to other units in Great Britain, there was a greater than 50% reduction in the fetal death rate from 29.4 to 11.3%. The overall perinatal mortality in comparison with the other units decreased from 40.1 to 25.5% and in their own unit from 37%. The key outcome parameter that was not given due importance was the rise in neonatal death from 10.7 to 14.2%.[8,9]

In 1979, Roversi et al.[10] in Italy challenged this nearly 30-year-old regimen demonstrating that it was meticulous attention to blood glucose control that was the key factor in reducing perinatal mortality and, in particular, late intrauterine fetal death. Using the maximum dose of insulin that could be tolerated by the mother, they carried 94% of the pregnancies to 38 weeks or more, 19% not being delivered until after 40 weeks. The only late fetal death occurred at 37 weeks in a woman with diabetic nephropathy. At the same time, Drury et al.[11] at the National Maternity Hospital in Dublin, reported their experience of the first 141 diabetic pregnancies managed using a regimen of tight control and not delivering the baby before full term irrespective of the severity of the diabetes unless obstetric complications necessitated intervention. This was done without the use of either cardiographic surveillance or ultrasonic assessment of fetal well-being. Spontaneous

labor ensued in 57% of cases, the Cesarean section rate was 20% and perinatal mortality was 31/1000. A subsequent analysis of this management policy and outcome by Rasmussen et al.[12] showed that the only deaths in normally formed infants occurred with evidence of poor metabolic control, clinical macrosomia or polyhydramnios.

Furthermore, the report from Murphy et al.[13] demonstrated that the additional benefit in allowing the pregnancies of women with diabetes to go to full term was that there was a 4-fold increase in the rate of spontaneous vaginal delivery. This came without a significant increase in the emergency Cesarean section rate and a modest fall in elective Cesarean section rate (Figures 37.1 and 37.2). A later update from the Dublin group[14] showed that between 1981 and 1994 their conservative policy maintained a high vaginal delivery rate of 93% (90.5% of these being normal deliveries), with a Cesarean section rate of 7% compared with the nondiabetic population rate of 3.4%. The perinatal mortality rate had fallen to 13.5/1000. In Australia[15] in 1999, fetal demise not associated with congenital anomalies accounted for 15% of the total. The cause of death in most diabetic pregnancies is not known (except for those associated with diabetic ketoacidosis); it is possible that they are in fact unrelated to maternal diabetes per se. Consequently, it is not realistic to expect that all deaths can be prevented with the currently available tools for fetal surveillance.

Further reassurance for taking the pregnancy to term comes from a study by Sheiner et al.[16] In a multiple logistic regression analysis of 72,875 singleton deliveries, no association was found between intrapartum fetal death and maternal diabetes. The significant factors were maternal age >35 years, polyhydramnios, congenital malformations, pathologic presentation, abruptio placentae, and cord prolapse.

Lung maturation and iatrogenic prematurity

As mentioned above, the fear of stillbirths in the past, and even in current practice in several maternity units in the United States and Europe, encouraged the policy of planned

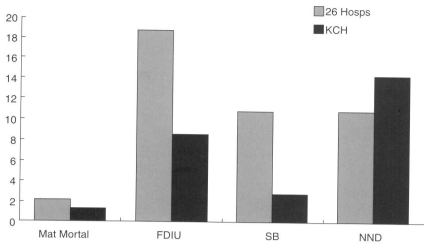

Figure 37.1   Comparison of the outcome of diabetic pregnancies managed at King's College Hospital, London and at 26 other UK hospitals.[1]

delivery of these patients at approximately 34–37 weeks' gestation. Indeed, this policy significantly decreased the stillbirth rate but, in contrast, resulted in iatrogenic prematurity with the accompanying neonatal complications, especially respiratory distress syndrome (RDS) (formerly known as hyaline membranous disease). The policy decreased stillbirths but created a higher rate of neonatal morbidity and mortality. All this led to the development of fetal maturity lung testing, which is addressed at length elsewhere in the book. However, in the past two to three decades, lung maturity testing has enabled us to significantly decrease iatrogenic prematurity and to comprehend the impact of the level of glycemic control and the delay in lung maturation.

We now have the technology to synchronize planned deliveries and lung maturity in a relatively safe mode. In addition, the modern approach to fetal surveillance testing and the recognition of the importance of glucose control presented an opportunity to avoid planned deliveries due to fear

of fetal demise. On the other hand, perhaps there is now an opportunity to consider planned delivery for the oversized fetus (macrosomia) in order to prevent shoulder dystocia and its accompanying complications.[17–19]

In our institution, we currently use the following approach for lung maturity testing. In patients who achieved the targeted level of glycemic control with imminent or no fetal compromise by specific abnormal patterns of surveillance testing or severe maternal complications that require immediate delivery/termination of pregnancy, delivery will occur without lung testing. In cases where the targeted level of glycemia was not met and the indication does not pose an immediate risk to mother and fetus, e.g. previous Cesarean section or growth restriction but normal fetal surveillance testing results, only in the presence of positive lung maturity testing does delivery occur. If test results are negative, patients should be under strict surveillance and lung maturity testing repeated within a week.

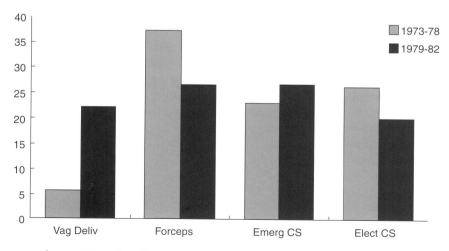

Figure 37.2   The effect of change of management on mode of delivery.

Glycemic control should always be considered in the decision process to perform/not to perform lung maturity testing. In cases of poor glycemic control, regardless of gestational age, amniocentesis for lung maturity testing should be performed. On the other hand, in the presence of good glycemic control and reassuring dates for patients after 37 weeks gestation, delivery can be performed without prior testing. This approach will decrease the number of unnecessary invasive procedures performed to confirm/refute lung maturity.

Fetal overgrowth in the diabetic pregnancy

The other major factor that influences the decision on the timing of delivery is the likelihood of shoulder dystocia and particularly permanent brachial plexus nerve palsy. Shoulder dystocia has been aptly described as 'the infrequent, unanticipated, unpredictable nightmare of the obstetrician'.[20] The major dilemma for the obstetrician is the poor predictive power of methods of fetal weight assessment and particularly shoulder width in the fetus. Coupled with this is the dynamic interaction between the maternal pelvic girdle, the power of the uterine contractions, maternal expulsive efforts and the fetal diameters that will ultimately determine whether the shoulders pass easily through the outlet of the maternal pelvis. Fetal weight alone is a poor predictor. Approximately 40–50% of shoulder dystocia will occur within the infant group weighing <4000 g.[21] However, it should be noted that pregnancies with infants weighing <4000 g are the majority, while the total number of infants weighing >4000 g is about 8–10%. Furthermore, although macrosomia is one of the classic markers of diabetes in pregnancy, a larger number of macrosomic babies will be identified in the general population while the prevalence of diabetes is 3–5%. Thus, policies for timing and method of delivery should consider the total population that may be affected.[20,21]

The overgrown fetus of a diabetic mother is at an increased risk for serious adverse outcome due to shoulder dystocia during vaginal delivery. Traditionally, authors have emphasized Erb's palsy as the single most significant complication when shoulder dystocia occurs. However, the prevalence of Erb's palsy is relatively low. Shoulder dystocia without Erb's palsy remains a serious complication involving bone fractures, asphyxia and even fetal death. Cesarean delivery greatly reduces the likelihood of such outcomes and may, therefore, be used as the primary prevention approach. However, it should be noted that Cesarean delivery itself is not free of fetal and/or maternal complications, which may include increased maternal blood loss, traumatic organ injury (ureters), infection, as well as other long-term complications. Therefore, in light of the fact that Cesarean section rates are increasing universally, the benefit–risk ratio should be assessed for any given complication before surgery.

In diabetic patients, the majority of shoulder dystocia cases occur among macrosomic infants born vaginally. In a cohort study of nearly 75,000 nondiabetic women, the rate of macrosomic infants was 7.6% compared to 20.6% in the 1500 diabetic women.[20] Nondiabetic women had an overall shoulder dystocia rate of 0.5%, compared to 3.2% in diabetic women. The shoulder dystocia rate was 0.3% when birthweight was <4000 g and 4.9% when it was >4000 g in diabetic patients. Macrosomic infants of diabetic mothers had a more than 3-fold higher risk of shoulder dystocia than macrosomic infants of nondiabetic pregnancies (14.7 vs. 4.4%). However, within each 250 gram birthweight category over 4000 g, diabetics had significantly more shoulder dystocia than nondiabetics.

Anthropometric differences explain the discrepancy in the risk for shoulder dystocia between diabetic and nondiabetic women. In nondiabetic women, macrosomia is constitutional in origin thus resulting in a proportionally larger infant. In contrast, for the diabetic macrosomic infant, its overgrowth is due to continuous fetal hyperinsulinemia resulting in disproportional growth and organomegaly in the majority of organs with the exception of the brain. It has been found that there is a significant difference in several anthropomorphic measures such as abdominal and shoulder circumference, as well as an increase in fetal fat mass distribution. Organ overgrowth is used as the marker to identify the fetus compromised by diabetic macrosomia.[20,22,23] As compared to a macrosomic fetus of a nondiabetic woman, the macrosomic fetus in a diabetic pregnancy is proportionately large, with much of the excess weight distributed in the trunk and shoulders. This increased chest–head and shoulder–head size discrepancy results in a higher risk for shoulder dystocia.[24,25]

Just as the shoulder dystocia rate goes up with increasing birthweight so too does the risk of injury when shoulder dystocia occurs. Ecker et al.[26] found a relative risk for brachial plexus injury of 9.6 for infants weighing >4000 g vs. <4000 g; the relative risk increased to 17.9 and 45.2 at birthweight thresholds >4500 and 5000 g, respectively. Increasing birthweight, maternal diabetes, and vaginal delivery were all independently associated with an increased risk for brachial plexus injury.

Using ultrasonography to detect fetal overgrowth

The accurate prediction of fetal weight in intrauterine life is an attractive approach to identify the fetus at risk. Unfortunately, it has been demonstrated that the error in weight estimation is relatively high (10–20%); thus, mothers are being subjected to often unnecessary interventions. Nevertheless, ultrasonographic estimation of fetal weight is commonly employed in clinical practice. In a survey of practitioners, approximately 75% of maternal–fetal specialists and almost 66% of general obstetricians utilized ultrasound to estimate fetal size prior to the delivery of the diabetic woman.[27]

Recently, it was demonstrated that 31 different sonographic estimations of fetal weight formulae had comparably poor accuracy for prediction of macrosomia. The 1986 formula devised by Ott had the lowest total score. Using Ott's formula, an estimated fetal weight (EFW) of >4000 g had a sensitivity of 45% to predict macrosomia and a positive predictive value

(PPV) of 81%. In order to achieve 90% sensitivity using this formula, it would have required a diagnosis of macrosomia with an EFW >3535 g, but this would have comprised 46% of the population with a 42% false-positive rate.[28]

When EFW was predicted by ultrasound to be >4000 g, 75–85% of infants were macrosomic at birth.[29,30] In the author's experience, ultrasonic EFW by the Shepard formula correctly predicted the presence or absence of macrosomia in 87% of diabetic pregnancies.[31] Maternal obesity, a common co-morbidity in a diabetic population, does not appear to diminish the accuracy of fetal weight estimation by ultrasound.[32] In general, overestimation of fetal weight would seem to make the practice less beneficial.

Using a combination of approaches to detect fetal macrosomia in a population of both diabetic and nondiabetic women, Chauhan et al.[33] compared the performance of various methods, including a standard formula for calculating fetal weight, clinical estimation and measures of fetal subcutaneous tissue by ultrasound. Using receiver operating characteristic curves to assess these diagnostic modalities, they found traditional fetal weight estimation by ultrasound to perform the best, and shoulder soft tissue width to perform the worst. Therefore, although formulae for fetal weight estimation used in daily clinical practice lack the level of accuracy in predicting fetal overgrowth that we would like to achieve, they appear to be the best tools available, and they do not require special expertise or equipment to obtain them.

Cohen et al.[34] proposed the abdominal diameter (AD) minus the biparietal diameter (BPD) as a predictor of whether a fetus will be compromised by shoulder dystocia at delivery. The authors used severe shoulder dystocia as their end point, retrospectively examining the AD – values obtained from infants of diabetic mothers with EFW of 3800–4200 g within 2 weeks of delivery. Infants with shoulder dystocia had significantly larger AD – BPD measurements despite finding no difference in birthweight between the shoulder dystocia and normal delivery groups. No infant with an antenatal AD – BPD value <2.6 cm suffered shoulder dystocia. However, the PPV for this cut-off was only 30%. Prospective studies using comparable models may provide improved predictors of shoulder dystocia.[35]

Benefits of Cesarean delivery in preventing shoulder dystocia and fetal injury

Avoidance of vaginal delivery for the large fetus of a diabetic mother eliminates the possibility of shoulder dystocia and should, therefore, eliminate the risk of nerve and bone injury, as well as the more serious outcomes of birth asphyxia and intrapartum death resulting from shoulder dystocia. Although it is recognized that brachial plexus injury can occur in the setting of Cesarean delivery,[36,37] the risks associated with vaginal birth are much greater.[38] Indeed, a population-based study of births in Washington State, USA, revealed no reported cases of brachial or Erb's palsy in over 13,000 consecutive Cesarean deliveries.[39] Therefore, it is reasonable to conclude

that performance of a Cesarean section will prevent Erb's–Duchenne palsy in the vast majority of cases. It is for this reason that Cesarean delivery has been proposed as the preferred route of delivery for the large fetus.

Among diabetic women, 84% of shoulder dystocia cases occur in infants with birthweights >4000 g. Among nondiabetic women, only 60% of deliveries complicated by shoulder dystocia involve a macrosomic fetus.[20] Thus, avoidance of vaginal delivery of macrosomic fetuses of diabetic mothers would eliminate most cases of shoulder dystocia, while the same practice in nondiabetic mothers would eliminate just over half of the cases. The practicality of this plan in the clinical setting is hampered by two factors: firstly, accurate antenatal identification of macrosomia is difficult to accomplish; and, secondly, most cases of shoulder dystocia do not result in permanent damage to the infant. We are currently unable to select those cases in which the fetus is excessively large much less detect which overgrown fetus is at risk for handicap or death due to shoulder dystocia. This fact has diminished the enthusiasm of some authors for Cesarean delivery for suspected macrosomia.[40]

Rouse et al.,[40] using a decision analysis methodology abstracting information available in the literature, calculated the probability of shoulder dystocia according to birthweight in both diabetic and nondiabetic pregnancies. It is noteworthy that for birthweights ≥4500 g, the probability is 52% in diabetic pregnancies compared with 14% in nondiabetic pregnancies. The mean probability that a neonatal brachial plexus injury will persist was 6.7% (range 0–19%).[41] Rouse et al.[40] calculated that to prevent one case of permanent brachial plexus injury in babies weighing ≥4500 g would necessitate performing 153 Cesarean deliveries in diabetic mothers and 419 in nondiabetics. If a cutoff of 4000 g is used, then 169 Cesarean sections would be required in diabetics and 654 in nondiabetics.

Rouse and Owen[41] updated their initial analysis by factoring in information from recent population-based studies on the frequency of brachial plexus injury, both transient and persistent. These calculations suggest that an even greater number of Cesarean sections would need to be performed in order to prevent permanent palsies. However, Erb's palsy should not be the only consideration in evaluation of morbidity prevention by Cesarean section. Although Erb's palsy is a severe complication, bone fractures, asphyxia, respiratory complications requiring neonatal intensive care admission, and neonatal and fetal demise should be considered when calculating the cost of Cesarean sections performed to prevent shoulder dystocia and adverse outcomes. In fact, when the composite outcome approach is used, 81% of shoulder dystocia cases of the infants of diabetic mothers will be identified compared to 34% for infants of nondiabetic mothers.[20]

Applying the same types of calculations to an actual obstetric population, Mullin et al.[42] examined the results of their policy of offering Cesarean deliveries to all diabetic women with EFW >4250 g (by sonographic or clinical means). Of 72 women meeting this fetal weight threshold during a 3-year period, 61% elected for Cesarean delivery. Seventeen of the remaining women delivered vaginally (39% Cesarean section rate in women who labored), and four of these deliveries were complicated by shoulder dystocia (24%). Based on previously reported rates of brachial plexus injuries, the investigators then calculated the number of Cesarean sections needed to prevent one case of permanent Erb's palsy. In diabetic women, approximately 100–400 Cesarean sections would result in avoidance of one case of permanent palsy. This number is somewhat more favorable toward a policy of prophylactic Cesarean section than that estimated by Rouse et al.[40] and Rouse and Owen.[41] This highlights the fact that cost–benefit ratios of prophylactic Cesarean sections for suspected macrosomia in diabetic women may be most meaningful when calculated for, and applied to, an individual population taking into account overall morbidity rather than a single outcome parameter. Moreover, different diabetic programs report different rates of macrosomia (poor glycemic control) which affects the rate of shoulder dystocia. Probably, achievement of adequate glycemic control will be a major factor in decreasing the rate of this complication in diabetic mothers.

Theoretical models provide a foundation for clinical studies. However, paucity of information exists on the actual clinical impact of a policy of prophylactic Cesarean sections in reducing the frequency of shoulder dystocia events. If there is no significant decrease in shoulder dystocia rate, there cannot be an accompanying decrease in brachial plexus injury and other adverse outcomes. In one of the few published reports, Conway and Langer[31] in a prospective study addressed this issue. Diabetic women underwent Cesarean delivery when EFW by ultrasound was >4250 g, a threshold chosen to reduce unnecessary intervention due to sonographic error. Labor inductions of LGA fetuses with birthweights <4250 g were also performed. Although only 11% of the diabetic population underwent Cesarean section or inductions for macrosomia, the shoulder dystocia rate among diabetic women dropped significantly on implementing this procedure compared to the previous 3-year period [1.5 vs. 2.8%; odds ratio (OR) 0.5, range 0.3–1.0]. Among macrosomic infants, the shoulder dystocia rate dropped from 19 to 7% (OR 0.3, range 0.1–1.0). The Cesarean delivery rate among diabetics rose from 21.7 to 25.1%. Conway and Langer's[31] study demonstrated the possibility of reducing the rate of shoulder dystocia in diabetic women using prophylactic Cesarean delivery for the macrosomic fetus.

Ultrasonic estimation of fetal weight needs to take into account whether or not the mother has diabetes. Otherwise, there is a significant underestimation of fetal weight of >10% using conventional weight prediction tables.[43] Diabetic pregnancies, because of the larger fetal weight, are five times more likely to be complicated by shoulder dystocia than nondiabetic pregnancies (5 vs. 1.1% for birthweights ≥4000 g). Brachial plexus injuries are four times more likely in diabetic pregnancies. However, due to the paucity of long-term follow-up, the prevalence of the permanency of the injury is not yet well established.[41,44]

The concern that delaying delivery until full-term results in a greater morbidity rate led Kjos et al.[45] to conduct a randomized controlled trial (RCT) of 200 pregnancies complicated by GDM. Patients were assigned either to elective delivery at 38 weeks or to expectant management, which included twice weekly cardiotocography and amniotic fluid volume evaluation. The Cochrane review[46] of this trial found that the risk of having a Cesarean section was similar for both groups [relative risk (RR) 0.81, 95% confidence interval (CI) 0.52–1.26]. The risk of macrosomia was reduced in the elective delivery group (RR 0.56, 95% CI 0.32–0.98) and there were three cases of mild shoulder dystocia in the expectant management group. They concluded that due to the limited number of studies, there is little evidence to support either elective delivery at 38 weeks or expectant management.

Cesarean section rates for women with diabetes are significantly greater than for their nondiabetic counterparts in most series. Remsberg et al.[47] conducted a detailed analysis of 42,071 singleton births in South Carolina, USA. Diabetic mothers comprised 3.6% of the series, 80% of which had GDM. Of the pre-existing diabetic patients, 51.3% underwent a Cesarean section, as did 34.4% of those with GDM. For nondiabetic women, 22.9% of births were by Cesarean section. Regression analysis showed an association between diabetes and Cesarean section that was not mediated by infant size alone. The strongest reported associations were with disproportion, previous Cesarean delivery, failed induction and malpresentation. These results and those from other studies[14,48] suggest that the practice patterns of the clinicians and not macrosomia itself are the major factors in the high Cesarean section rates.

One of the major contributors to the Cesarean section rate is the presence of a previous Cesarean section scar. Two studies have examined the outcome of vaginal birth after Cesarean (VBAC) in women with diabetes. In Coleman et al.[49] study, VBAC was offered if the sonographically EFW was <4000 g. Overall, the successful VBAC rate was lower in women with diabetes (64.1 vs. 73.2%; OR 1.90, range 1.20–2.99). This was not due to the higher induction rate in women with diabetes (OR 2.16, range 1.37–3.40). Women with diabetes who delivered vaginally were more likely to have an operative vaginal delivery, forceps (OR 2.71, range 1.15–6.45); vacuum (OR 2.59, range 0.89–7.73). Most importantly, there were no significant differences between the two groups in the incidence of shoulder dystocia, pre-eclampsia, pelvic lacerations or prolonged hospitalization, and the only two ruptured uteri occurred in the control group.

In another study, Blackwell et al.[50] compared diabetic women with/without a previous Cesarean section delivery. In the previous Cesarean section group, the rate of repeat Cesarean section was doubled (56.3 vs. 26.3%) with a successful VBAC rate of 43.7%. From these two studies it can be concluded that for women with diabetes who have had a previous Cesarean delivery, it is reasonable and safe to offer both a VBAC and induction of labor.

Returning to the debate about mode of delivery and EFW, the use of elective Cesarean section to prevent shoulder dystocia remains controversial. As discussed above, the dilemma is that current methods of determining the EFW have inherent inaccuracies. Furthermore, 50% of brachial plexus injuries occur in the absence of shoulder dystocia and can occur with a Cesarean delivery, which suggests that ante- and intrapartum factors are at least as important etiologically as shoulder dystocia.[51]

Cesarean section, although associated with maternal morbidity (e.g. infection, bleeding) is often a physician-driven decision rather than a complication of the disease. The Cesarean section rate has evolved as part of the criteria to evaluate disease in general and GDM in particular. Today Cesarean section rates are continuously rising with more repeat Cesarean sections, Cesarean section by demand and elective Cesarean section for breech delivery. It will not be surprising if, in the near future, the rate of Cesarean section begins to reach 40–50% for all deliveries. Indeed, many centers have already outstripped these numbers for both diabetic and nondiabetic patients. Therefore, Cesarean section rate should not be used as an endpoint in GDM because the procedure is not directly related to the morbidity of the disease. It is directly related to physician decision making and performance and as such has become a self-fulfilling prophecy in the treatment of GDM, i.e. knowing one has a GDM patient gives the physician license to opt for a Cesarean delivery.

This has been demonstrated by Naylor et al. that the Cesarean section rate is not related to the rate of large infants in GDM. One of the problems inherent in studying the natural history of a treatable entity is that knowledge of the diagnosis may change the clinician's behavior. In the Toronto study the authors looked at the Cesarean delivery rate. Approximately 34% of patients with diagnosed GDM delivered by Cesarean section, compared with 20% of women with normal results on screening tests and OGTTs. However, this 70% increase in the Cesarean delivery rate was not caused by macrosomia. In fact, the macrosomia rate among pregnancies with diagnosed gestational diabetes mellitus was about 10%, similar to that in the control group.

On the other hand, physicians are not automatically influenced by the GDM diagnosis. They instead weigh the presenting conditions of the disease. In one of our own studies, evaluating the intensified approach to the management of gestational diabetes involving 1145 intensified treated GDM and 1316 conventional treated GDMs compared to 4922 nondiabetic controls, the Cesarean section rate in the intensified treated patients was similar to the rate of the general population. In another study we prospectively performed elective Cesarean section for fetal weight >4250 g as a prophylactic measure to decrease the rate of shoulder dystocia. The study revealed that the Cesarean section rate in the GDM population increased from 21 to 25% but the shoulder dystocia decreased from 2.6 to 1.1% (a decrease of 70%).[53]

It is not possible to offer advice to the clinician with any degree of certainty on what should be the threshold for performing an elective Cesarean delivery in women with diabetes with the currently available evidence. Certainly, a past history of shoulder dystocia should influence the decision on the mode of delivery unless the EFW is significantly less than the previous birthweight. Unless obstetric complications dictate otherwise, the uncomplicated (normal estimated birthweight, amniotic fluid volume, and metabolic control) diabetic pregnancy, both pre-gestational and gestational, can be left to go into spontaneous delivery at full term. Induction of labor and planned VBAC carry no greater risks than for the nondiabetic pregnancy. Elective Cesarean section for the pregnant diabetic patient should be actively considered if the EFW is ≥4250 g,[20,31] although some authors recommend an EFW of 4000 g.

Summary

The timing of delivery of the diabetic patient is a balancing act between potential intrauterine death, shoulder dystocia, and the consequences of premature delivery. Achieving targeted levels of glycemic control will reduce rates of fetal demise. Stillbirths are not limited to late third trimester; therefore, the care provider needs to be vigilant to the level of glycemic control and fetal surveillance testing. For diabetic women in poor glycemic control, regardless of gestational age, lung maturity testing should be performed. For diabetic women in good glycemic control and reassuring dates after completing 37 weeks gestation, delivery can be performed without prior lung testing. In diabetic pregnancies, the majority of shoulder cases occur in fetuses >4000 gm (84%); 58% in nondiabetic pregnancies. Achieving glycemic control will decrease the macrosomia and the subsequent shoulder dystocia rates. For nondiabetic women, trial of vaginal delivery with EFW >4000 g may be considered; liberal policy towards Cesarean section is a consideration in the presence of labor abnormalities. For diabetic patients, elective Cesarean section delivery is strongly recommended when EFW 4000–4250 g; the decision may be individualized in this weight range.

REFERENCES

1. Gawande A. The Score. Annals of Medicine. The New Yorker: October 9, 2006; 58–67.
2. Gerstein HC, Haynes RB. Evidence-based Diabetes Care. London: BC Decker; 2001, pp. 1–48.
3. Pettitt DJ, Knowler WC, Baird HR, et al. Gestational diabetes: infant and maternal complications of pregnancy in relation to third-trimester glucose tolerance in the Pima Indians. Diabetes Care 1980; 3: 458–64.
4. O'Sullivan JB, Charles D, Mahan CM, et al. Gestational diabetes and perinatal mortality rate. Am J Obstet Gynecol 1973; 1: 901–4.
5. Karlsson K, Kjellmer I. The outcome of diabetic pregnancies in relation to the mother's blood sugar level. Am J Obstet Gynecol 1972; 112: 213–20.
6. Schmidt MI, Duncan BB, Reichelt AJ, et al. Gestational diabetes mellitus diagnosed with a 2-h 75-g oral glucose tolerance test and adverse pregnancy outcomes. Diabetes Care 2001; 24: 1151–3.
7. Mondestin M, Ananth C, Smulian J, et al. Birth weight and fetal death in the United States: The effect of maternal diabetes during pregnancy. Am J Obstet Gynecol 2002; 187: 922–6.
8. Peel J, Oakley WG. Transactions of the 12th British Congress of Obstetrics and Gynaecology 1949; 161.
9. Peel J. A historical review of diabetes and pregnancy. J Obstet Gynecol Br Commun 1972; 79; 385–95.
10. Roversi GD, Gargulio M, Nicolini U, et al. A new approach to the treatment of diabetic pregnant women. Am J Obstet Gynecol 1979; 135: 567–76.
11. Drury MI, Stronge JM, Foley ME, MacDonald DW. Pregnancy in the diabetic patient: timing and mode of delivery. Obstet Gynecol 1983; 62: 279–82.
12. Rasmussen MJ, Firth R, Foley M, Stronge JM. The timing of delivery in diabetic pregnancy: a 10-year review. Aust NZ J Obstet Gynecol 1992; 32: 313–7.

13. Murphy J, Peters J, Morris P, et al. Conservative management of pregnancy in diabetic women. Br Med J 1984; 288: 1203–5.
14. McAuliffe FM, Foley M, Firth R, et al. Outcome of diabetic pregnancy with spontaneous labour after 38 weeks. Irish J Med Sci 1999; 168: 160–3.
15. Nassar N, Sullivan EA. Australia's mothers and babies 1999. AIHW Cat No. PER 19, Perinatal Statistics Series no. 11. Sydney: AIHW National Perinatal Statistics Unit; 2001.
16. Sheiner E, Hallak M, Shomam-Vardi I, et al. Determining risks for intrapartum fetal death. J Reprod Med 2000; 45: 419–24.
17. Langer O, Conway, D. Level of glycemia and perinatal outcome in pregestational diabetes. J Matern–Fetal Med 2000; 9: 35–41
18. Langer O. A spectrum of glucose thresholds may effectively prevent complications in the pregnant diabetic patient. Semin Perinatol 2002; 26: 196–205.
19. Piper JM. Lung maturation in diabetes in pregnancy: if and when to test. Semin Per 2002; 26: 206–9.
20. Langer O, Berkus MD, Huff RW, Samueloff A. Shoulder dystocia: should the fetus weighing ≥4,000g be delivered by cesarean section? Am J Obstet Gynecol 1991; 165: 831–7.
21. Keller JD, Lopez-Zeno JA, Dooley SL, Socol ML. Shoulder dystocia and birth trauma in gestational diabetes: a five-year experience. Am J Obstet Gynecol 1991; 165: 928–30.
22. Langer O. Macrosomia in the fetus of the diabetic mother. In: Divon M, ed. Abnormal Fetal Growth. New York: Elsevier Science Publishers; 1991, pp. 99–110.
23. Susa JB, McCormick KL, Widness JA, et al. Chronic hyperinsulinemia in the fetal rhesus monkey: effects on fetal growth and composition. Diabetes 1979; 28: 1058–63.
24. McFarland MB, Trylovich CG, Langer O. Anthropometric differences in macrosomic infants of diabetic and nondiabetic mothers. J Matern–Fetal Med 1998; 7: 292–5.
25. Modanlou HD, Komatsu G, Dorchester W, et al. Large-for-gestational-age neonates: anthropometric reasons for shoulder dystocia. Obstet Gynecol 1982; 60: 417–23.
26. Ecker JL, Greenberg JA, Norwitz ER, et al. Birth weight as a predictor of brachial plexus injury. Obstet Gynecol 1997; 89: 643–7.
27. Landon MB. Prenatal diagnosis of macrosomia in pregnancy complicated by diabetes mellitus. J Matern–Fetal Med 2000; 9: 52–4.
28. Combs CA, Rosenn B, Miodovnik Siddiqi TA. Sonographic EFW and macrosomia: is there an optimum formula to predict diabetic fetal macrosomia? J Matern–Fetal Med 2000; 9: 55–61.
29. Tamura RK, Sabbagha RE, Dooley SL, et al. Real-time ultrasound estimations of weight in fetuses of diabetic gravid women. Am J Obstet Gynecol 1985; 153: 57–60.
30. Benson CB, Doubilet PM, Saltzman DH. Sonographic determination of fetal weights in diabetic pregnancies. Am J Obstet Gynecol 1987; 156: 441–4.
31. Conway DL, Langer O. Elective delivery of infants with macrosomia in diabetic women: reduced shoulder dystocia versus increased cesarean deliveries. Am J Obstet Gynecol 1998; 178: 922–5.
32. Field NT, Piper JM, Langer O. The effect of maternal obesity on the accuracy of fetal weight estimation. Obstet Gynecol 1995; 86: 102–7.
33. Chauhan SP, West DJ, Scardo JA, et al. Antepartum detection of macrosomic fetus: clinical versus sonographic, including soft-tissue measurements. Obstet Gynecol 2000; 95: 639–42.

34. Cohen B, Penning S, Major C, et al. Sonographic prediction of shoulder dystocia in infants of diabetic mothers. Obstet Gynecol 1996; 88: 10–3.
35. Jaffe R. Identification of fetal growth abnormalities in diabetes mellitus. Semin Perinatal 2002; 26: 190–5.
36. Morrison JC, Sanders JR, Magann EF, et al. The diagnosis and management of dystocia of the shoulder. Surg Gynecol Obstet 1992; 175: 515–22.
37. Bar J, Dvir A, Hod M, et al. Brachial plexus injury and obstetrical risk factors. Int J Gynecol Obstet 2001; 73: 21–5.
38. Gregory KD, Henry OA, Ramicone E, et al. Maternal and infant complications in high and normal weight infants by method of delivery. Obstet Gynecol 1998; 92: 507–13.
39. Mocanu EV, Greene RA, Byrne BM, et al. Obstetric and neonatal outcome of babies weighing more than 4.5 kg: an analysis by parity. Eur J Obstet Gynecol Reprod Biol 2000; 92: 229–33.
40. Rouse DJ, Owen J, Goldenberg RL, et al. The effectiveness and costs of elective cesarean delivery for fetal macrosomia diagnosed by ultrasound. J Am Med Assoc 1996; 276: 1480–6.
41. Rouse DJ, Owen J. Prophylactic cesarean delivery for fetal macrosomia by means of ultrasonography – a Faustian bargain? Am J Obstet Gynecol 1999; 181: 332–8.
42. Mullin P, Gherman R, Melkumian A, et al. The relationship of shoulder dystocia to estimated fetal weight. Presented at the 68th Annual Meeting of the Pacific Coast Obstetrical and Gynecological Society, Ashland, OR, 2001.
43. Wong SF, Chan FY, Cincotta RB, et al. Sonographic estimation of fetal weight in macrosomic fetuses: diabetic versus non-diabetic pregnancies. Aust NZ J Obstet Gynaecol 2001; 41: 429–32.
44. American College of Obstetricians and Gynecologists: Task Force on Cesarean Delivery Rates: Evaluation of cesarean delivery. Washington, DC: American College of Obstetricians and Gynecologists; 2000.
45. Kjos SL, Henry OA, Montoro M, et al. Insulin requiring diabetes in pregnancy: a randomised trial of active inductioiin of labor and expectant management. Am J Obstet Gynecol 1993; 169: 611–5.
46. Boulvain M, Stan C, Irion O. Elective delivery in diabetic pregnant women. Cochrane Database of Systematic Reviews [computer file]. (2): CD 001997, 2000.
47. Remsberg KE, McKeown RE, McFarland KF, Irwin LS. Diabetes in pregnancy and cesarean delivery. Diabetes Care 1999; 22: 1561–7.
48. Blackwell SC, Hassan SS, Wolfe HW, et al. Why are cesarean delivery rates so high in diabetic pregnancies? J Perinat Med 2000; 28: 316–20.
49. Coleman TL, Randall H, Graves W, Lindsay M. Vaginal birth after cesarean among women with gestational diabetes. Am J Obstet Gynecol 2001; 184: 1104–7.
50. Blackwell SC, Hassan SS, Wolfe HM, et al. Vaginal birth after cesarean in the diabetic gravida. J Reprod Med 2000; 45: 987–90.
51. Gherman EM, Forouzan I, Morgan MA. A retrospective analysis of Erb's palsy cases and their relationship to birth weight and trauma at delivery. Am J Obstet Gynecol 1998; 178: 423–7.
52. Langer O, ed. The Diabetes in Pregnancy Dilemma: Leading Changes with Simple Solutions. New York: University Press of America, Inc.; 2006.
53. Langer O, Rodriguez DA, Xenakis EMJ, et al. Intensfied vs. conventional management of gestational diabetes. Am J Obstet Gynecol 1994; 170: 1036–47.

38 Prevention of fetal macrosomia

Giorgio Mello, Elena Parretti and Moshe Hod

Introduction

The developing fetus depends for its growth on the passage of nutrients from the mother via the placenta. Alterations or imbalance of glucose, amino acids, and lipids present in the mother's blood will be reflected in fetal development as well as in later life.

The main growth substance, glucose, which the fetus cannot synthesize for itself, is received from the maternal circulation by means of facilitated diffusion through the placenta.[1] This diffusion is regulated principally through maternal plasma glucose levels. The maternal metabolic condition is therefore the first determinant of fetal growth.

In normal pregnancies insulin sensitivity to nutrients decreases in all women with advancing gestation. The result of the decreases in insulin sensitivity is greater nutrient availability and higher ambient insulin concentrations for the developing fetoplacental unit.

Maternal metabolic disorders of glucohomeostasis, ranging from slightly impaired glucose tolerance to overt diabetes, since they provide an excess of substrates, are able to provoke an increased stimulation of the fetal beta cells with consequent hyperinsulinemia, which is in turn responsible for fetal hypersomatism by selectively accelerating fuel utilization and storage in insulin-sensitive fetal tissues leading to a higher incidence of fetal macrosomia.[2]

Types of macrosomia

The term macrosomia is often used to describe a birthweight >4000 g or ≥90th percentile for gestational age,[3–5] a weight exceeding 4000 g is found in approximately 5.5–10% of all infants,[6] although the incidence is much higher in newborns from diabetic women (10–33%).[4–7]

However, there are two types of macrosomia: the first type is constitutional, or symmetric, macrosomia. This accounts for 70% of cases, and is the result of genetic factors and does not therefore imply an abnormal supply of nutrients in utero.[8,9] The fetus is big but normal and the only potential problem is to avoid trauma during delivery. In contrast, the second type of macrosomia is asymmetric and accounts for 30% of cases. This form is the typical picture related to maternal diabetes and is characterized by organomegaly and should be considered a pathological entity.[8,9] This type of macrosomia is associated with an abnormal thoracic and abdominal circumference, which are relatively larger than the head circumference.[10] These infants also differ in terms of their body proportions when compared with neonates of mothers with normal glucose metabolism.[11] As a result, disproportion between the head and shoulder girdle of the fetus, causing difficulty in delivery of the shoulders, predisposes to birth trauma (shoulder dystocia, clavicular fracture, and brachial palsy) and, as a consequence, an increased rate of Cesarean sections. In addition, it has been postulated that asymmetric macrosomia could have long-term consequences for the offspring, including obesity, coronary heart disease, hypertension, and Type 2 diabetes.[12–14]

Definitions of macrosomia

For these reasons the classical definition of macrosomia based on weight and gestational age is not perhaps appropriate to identify features of disproportionate growth in the fetuses of mothers with abnormal glucose metabolism.[15] In this respect the use of weight-to-length ratios such as the ponderal index[15] and the birth symmetric index[16] gives a more accurate description of fetal overgrowth. In addition, recent advances in ultrasound techniques have made possible the precise measurement of fetal insulin-sensitive tissue growth and thereby an accurate analysis of fetal body composition in terms of lean body mass and fat body mass.[16–18] The human body is classically divided into lean and fat body mass components.

Genetic factors may have a stronger relationship with lean body mass. Catalano has shown that lean body mass can comprise 86% of mean birthweight and account for 83% of the variance in birthweight.[19] The in utero environment may correlate better with fetal fat body mass, and comprise only 14% of birthweight but account for 46% of the variance in birthweight.[19] Fat accretion occurs essentially from week 27 of gestation until term.

Measurement of fetal body composition

These findings suggest the potential usefulness of estimates of fetal body composition, with particular reference to fat mass,

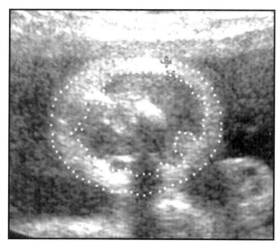 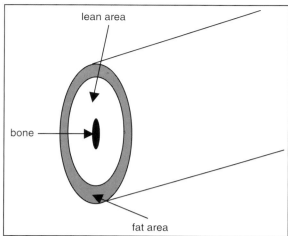

Figure 38.1 Mid-thigh lean and fat areas.

for the determination and evaluation of growth abnormalities. The use of an index of fat mass as a predictor of morbidity has been widely used in neonates.[20]

It is possible to make ultrasound measurements of both lean and fat body mass. Head circumference, femur length, mid-upper arm and mid-thigh central areas (Figure 38.1), can be measured for lean body mass, and anterior abdominal wall thickness (Figure 38.2), subscapular thickness, mid-upper arm and mid-thigh subcutaneous areas (Figure 38.1) can be measured for fat body mass.[21]

Measurements using this technique, comparing fat and lean body mass measurements during gestation, have shown significant correlations with both birthweight and estimates of neonatal lean and fat mass.[20,21] Both accuracy and reproducibility of lean and fat mass measurements have been demonstrated in various studies, suggesting that the technique is reliable.

In the clinical context, these measurements can reveal the effects of different maternal metabolic conditions on fetal growth and provide indications for intervention or therapy.

The distinction between symmetric and asymmetric overgrowth is important because efforts should be directed to the asymmetric overgrown fetus and to methods of primary prevention of this abnormality by appropriate management approaches for the mother and the fetus.[8]

Preventing fetal macrosomia

The issue of 'preventing fetal macrosomia' requires closer scrutiny; it would seem that, for some obstetricians, identification of the oversized fetus is viewed simply in terms of reducing the birth risk of shoulder dystocia and the rate of Cesarean section. This clinical approach stems partly from the perceived lack of accurate diagnostic tools to identify all diabetic pregnant women at risk of macrosomia, as well as lack of effective measures to control intrauterine fetal growth. However it is important to stress that the perspective should be rather that of 'preventing not only intrapartum but also postpartum complications associated with fetal macrosomia by appropriate management of the macrosomic fetus.' Identification of the overgrown fetus allows treatment of the overgrown fetus. In addition, the risk of delivering the infant early to stop the accelerated *in utero* growth with potential complications related to prematurity, such as hyperbilirubinemia, hypocalcemia and respiratory distress,[22] could also be reduced since the estimation of fetal body composition method allows the distinction between symmetric but normal growth and pathological overgrowth.

The problem of sonographic estimation of fetal weight, which is less accurate the heavier the fetus is, reaching a mean error of ±20% for fetuses close to 4000 g, thus increases diagnostic uncertainty precisely where accuracy is most needed, can be overcome by adopting estimation of fetal body composition as outlined above.

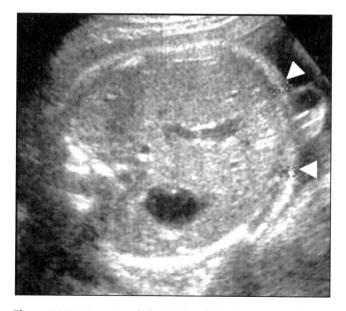

Figure 38.2 Anterior abdominal wall thickness (arrowhead).

Treatment strategies

In the prevention of asymmetric fetal overgrowth in mothers with abnormal glucose metabolism, treatment strategies must be targeted to prevent overnutrition of the fetus.[23] The goal of management in pregnancy complicated by altered glucose tolerance must be to maintain the blood glucose level as near to normal as possible in order to achieve normalization of fetal growth. Indeed, glycemia is the single maternal metabolic parameter routinely assessed in diabetic pregnancies, and the criteria for metabolic control and therapeutic strategies of diabetes in pregnancy are based on maternal glucose levels,[24] since normoglycemia in pregnancy is associated with normal levels of other nutrients such as aminoacids and lipids.[25] However perhaps 'glucose is merely an easily assessed covariate among other more dominant fetal growth determinants.'[26]

Maternal plasma amino acid levels are important for fetal growth, because they provide essential substrate. For example, a study has shown that mothers who had higher protein turnover at 18 weeks' gestation had infants with increased lean body mass, as illustrated by birth length. After adjustment for significant covariables such as the duration of gestation and the baby's sex, 26% of the variation in length at birth was accounted for by maternal protein synthesis at 18 weeks' gestation.[27] In addition, diabetes in pregnancy has been shown to have a profound impact on maternal circulating lipids in pregnancy, promoting their transfer to the fetus by increasing the maternal–fetal concentration gradient, especially of FFA and triglycerides. This may contribute to an increase in body fat mass in newborns of diabetic mothers.[28]

In many studies of glucose levels in diabetic pregnancy, however, the rate of macrosomia was still high despite apparent rectification of glycemia. As a consequence, recently, the time period for most effective daily blood glucose monitoring with respect to the impact on perinatal outcome has come under closer investigation in order to ascertain which period gives the most useful correlation: fasting; preprandial; 1 h postprandial; 2 h postprandial; bedtime; mean daily glucose value; HbA1c have all been examined although so far none of these has been shown to be unequivocally superior to the others.

Value of normoglycemia

Importantly, the value of normoglycemia in nondiabetic pregnancy has now been determined. A study has provided the true definition of normoglycemia during the third trimester in normal nondiabetic pregnancies.[29] Overall daily mean glucose levels showed a slight but progressive increase from 28 (71.9 ± 5.7) to 38 (78.3 ± 5.4) weeks and mean postprandial glucose levels never exceeded 105.2 mg/dL; in addition, 1 h postprandial glucose values were found to positively correlate with fetal abdominal growth as early as 28 weeks' gestation, and this correlation was maintained through the third trimester. These glucose values have been confirmed in another study which characterized the daily glucose profile in nondiabetic pregnancies using continuous glucose monitoring.[30] Although demonstrating the safety and the accuracy of using this method, this study, however, made no correlation between glycemic profiles and fetal growth.[30] The correlation

between 1 h postprandial maternal blood glucose concentration in the third trimester and fetal growth now demonstrated in normal pregnancy matches the situation of diabetic pregnancies, where maternal 1 h glucose values are considered a strong predictor of both infant birthweight and fetal macrosomia.[31–33] Also, in diabetic pregnancies, fetal hyperinsulinism and birthweight have been found to correlate best with 1 h postprandial glucose values, as the postprandial glucose peak breaches the placental barrier;[34] in this context, the results from normoglycemic pregnancies seem to suggest that fetal abdominal circumference, that is a parameter of growth of insulin-sensitive tissues, is influenced by postprandial glucose peaks even in glucose tolerant women, and this observation would confirm that glycemia in pregnancy can be regarded as a 'continuum', ranging from normal glucose metabolism to overt diabetes, and that the consequences of hyperglycemia in terms of clinical outcome can be understood as an exaggeration of a mechanism that actually occurs also in normoglycemic pregnancies.[29] In the study of normal pregnancies by Parretti et al. mean postprandial glucose levels never exceed 105.2 mg/dL, a value well below the currently accepted thresholds for good metabolic control in diabetic pregnancies, thus suggesting that blunting the peak postprandial response to such an extent can result in a decreased rate of macrosomia and lead to the absolute normalization of fetal growth. Nonetheless, the American Diabetes Association guidelines for pregnant diabetic women suggest that glucose levels can be as high as 140 mg/dL at the 1-h and 120 mg/dL at the 2-h postprandial time point, recommending action only when the glucose is in hyperglycemic ranges.[35] According to Jovanovic,[36] maintaining such high thresholds for action in the treatment of diabetic pregnant women may have contributed to sustained increased prevalence of macrosomia in infants of diabetic mothers despite 'good glucose control', and in this respect this 'macrosomia despite normoglycemia' would be better described as 'macrosomia because of undetected and therefore undertreated hyperglycemia.'[37,38]

Period of pregnancy

However, another important point needs to be taken into consideration: the period of pregnancy at which normalization of glycemic control is established in order to achieve normalization of fetal growth. In a study of 262 women with gestational diabetes mellitus (GDM) treated with different therapeutic regimes, the introduction of insulin therapy before 32 weeks of gestation achieved a progressive slowing down of fetal abdominal wall thickness and mid-thigh subcutaneous area (Figure 38.3) from 27 to 32 weeks to reach a perfectly comparable rate of growth with that of the normal, nondiabetic control group by 32 weeks and which continued until the end of pregnancy.[39] In contrast, for women who began insulin therapy after 32 weeks of gestation and for those who followed only diet therapy, the initial difference apparent between these two groups and both the pre-32 weeks insulin and normal women at entry widened until the end of pregnancy. In parallel, the difference in glycemic patterns evident at entry (Figure 38.4A) before onset of therapy was modified in the pre-32 weeks women to become perfectly comparable with the

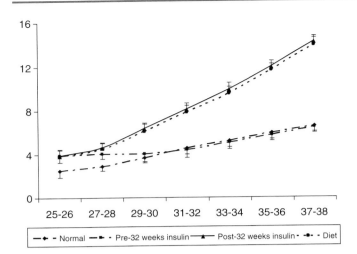

Figure 38.3   Fat body mass: mid-thigh subcutaneous area. Repeated measures of ANOVA *P* <0.002. Normal vs. pre-32 weeks insulin vs. post-32 weeks insulin, diet.

normal group by 32 weeks (Figure 38.4B) while the post-32 weeks insulin therapy women reached a normalization of glycemic values which matched that of the normal control group only at 38 weeks of gestation (Figure 38.4C).[39]

In this study normalization of fetal growth was achieved through a tight glycemic control which matched the patterns of nondiabetic pregnancies before 32 weeks of gestation. It is worth pointing out that although the control was tight, it did not produce under-nourished fetuses resulting in under-weight neonates. The incidence of small for gestational age (SGA) infants in the diabetic groups was not different from that of the control group. The risk of producing under-nourished fetuses with too tight a glycemic control has often been the fear following an influential study of Langer et al.[40] Langer's study, however, focussed on the mean daily glucose level and did not explicitly consider the relevance of excursions. If we look more carefully at Langer's results,[40] we may actually see an interesting observation: 'The mothers with SGA infants were found to have the most stable level of

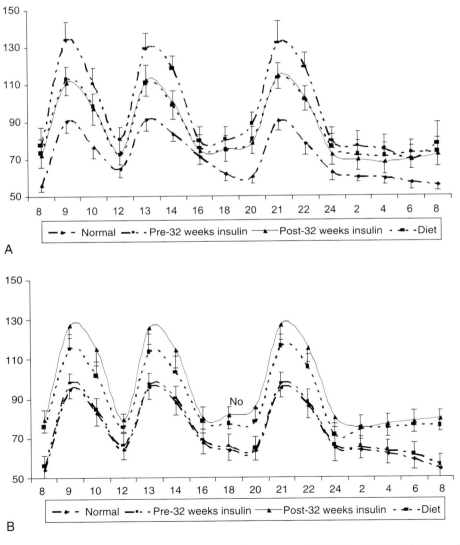

Figure 38.4   (A) 24-h maternal glycemic profiles at entry. Repeated measures of ANOVA, *P* <0.0034. Normal vs. post-32 weeks insulin, diet vs. pre-32 weeks insulin. (B) 24-h maternal glycemic profiles at 32 weeks of gestation. Repeated measures of ANOVA, *P* <0.0076. Normal, pre-32 weeks insulin vs. post-32 weeks insulin vs. diet.

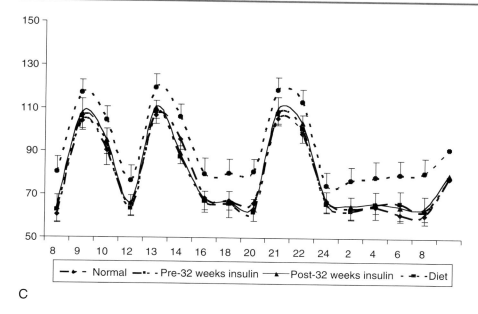

Figure 38.4   cont'd, (C) 24-h maternal glycemic profiles at 38 weeks of gestation. Repeated measures of ANOVA, $P < 0.0092$. Normal, pre-32 weeks insulin, post-32 weeks insulin vs. diet.

glycemic control, the lowest mean blood glucose, with a narrow variability indicated by a 27 mg range.' That is, the SGA mothers did not demonstrate the excursions which are to be seen in the patterns of nondiabetic pregnancy glycemia, and which indeed are necessary in order to eat nutritiously, as Lois Jovanovic has observed: 'To eat nutritiously, patients require a 40 mg/dL blood glucose excursion after each meal.'[23] What is necessary to normalize diabetic fetal growth is the normalization of the glycemic pattern, including normal postprandial excursions. If the preprandial values are relatively low, the necessary postprandial peak will not reach a level to alter fetal growth.

Summary

From the point of view of prevention of fetal macrosomia, our aims should be to provide for the fetus of a mother with altered glucose tolerance a development environment which resembles that of a mother with normal glucose tolerance.

Now that we have been able to establish what the normal intrauterine state is with respect to glucose levels, what we should be aiming for is normalization of the patterns of glycemic level. While we should be cautious of creating undernourished fetuses, we must certainly be cautious of creating over-nourished fetuses.

In our attempts to normalize body composition, we should aim to mimic growth and body composition of the normal fetus which may be best achieved through a maternal metabolic state characterized by a daily glucose circadian rhythm with a 1 h postprandial peak of about 30–40 mg/dL, nonetheless never exceeding a mean of 105 mg/dL, with relative nocturnal hypoglycemia.[29]

It should be remembered that the overgrown fetus of a diabetic mother is not only at immediate risk of birth injury but also, in the long term, has a higher risk of developing obesity, cardiovascular disease, and Type 2 diabetes. With extra care in the intrauterine environment today, we can break the vicious circle of maternal disease–fetal disease and assure a better chance of health for the offspring of women with diabetes.

REFERENCES

1. Aerts L, Pijnenborg R, Verhaeghe J, Holemans K, Van Assche FA. Fetal growth and development. In: Dornhorst A, Hadden DR, eds. Diabetes and Pregnancy: An International Approach to Diagnosis and Management. Chichester: John Wiley; 1996, pp. 77–97.
2. Kalkhoff RK. Impact of maternal fuels and nutritional status on fetal growth. Diabetes 1991; 40:(suppl. 2): 61–5.
3. Langer O, Michael D, Berkus MD, et al. Shoulder dystocia: should the fetus weighing > 4000 grams be delivered by cesarean section? Am J Obstet Gynecol 1991; 165: 831–7.
4. Keller DJ, Lopez-Zeno JA, Dooley SL, et al. Shoulder dystocia and birth trauma in gestational diabetes: a five-year experience. Am J Obstet Gynecol 1991; 165: 928–30.
5. Combs AC, Navkaran BS, Khoury J. Elective induction versus spontaneous labor after sonographic diagnosis of fetal macrosomia. Obstet Gynecol 1993; 81: 492–6.
6. William's Obstetrics, 19th edn. New York: Appleton & Lange; 1993, pp. 493–520.
7. Kaufmann RC, McBride P, Amankwah KS, Huffman DG. The effect of minor degrees of glucose intolerance on the incidence of neonatal macrosomia. Obstet Gynecol 1992; 80: 97–101.
8. Langer O. Fetal macrosomia: etiologic factors. Clin Obstet Gynecol 2000; 43: 283–97.
9. Aschkenazi S, Chen R, Perri T, et al. Size matters: management of the macrosomic infants. Isr J Obstet Gynecol 2001; 12: 159–64.
10. Schwartz R. Hyperinsulinemia and macrosomia. N Engl J Med 1990; 323: 340–2.
11. Mello G, Parretti E, Mecacci F, et al. Anthropometric characteristics of full-term infants: effects of varying degrees of 'normal' glucose metabolism. J Perinat Med 1997; 25: 197–204.

12. Van Assche FA, Holemens K, Aerts L. Fetal growth and consequences for later life. J Perinat Med 1998; 26: 337–46.
13. Godfrey KM, Barker DJ. Fetal nutrition and adult diseases. Am J Clin Nutr 2000; 71(suppl. 5): 1344S–52S.
14. Van Assche EA. Symmetric and asymmetric fetal macrosomia in relation to long-term consequences. Am J Obstet Gynecol 1997; 177: 563.
15. Lepercq J, Lahlou N, Timsit J, et al. Macrosomia revisited: ponderal index and leptin delineate subtypes of fetal overgrowth. Am J Obstet Gynecol 1999; 181: 621–5.
16. Landon MB, Sonek J, Foy P, Hamilton L, Gabbe GG. Sonographic measurement of fetal humeral soft tissue thickness in pregnancy complicated by GDM. Diabetes 1991; 40(suppl. 2): 66–70.
17. Bernstein IM, Catalano PM. Ultrasonographic estimation of fetal body composition for children of diabetic mothers. Invest Radiol 1991; 26: 722–6.
18. Winn HN, Holcomb NL. Fetal nonmuscular soft tissue: a prenatal assessment. J Ultrasound Med 1993; 4: 107–99.
19. Catalano PM, Tyazbir ED, Allen SR, McBean JH, McAuliffe TL. Evaluation of fetal growth by estimation of body composition. Obstet Gynecol 1992; 79: 46–50.
20. Bernstein IM, Goran MI, Amini SB. Differential growth of fetal tissues during the second half of pregnancy. Am J Obstet Gynecol 1997; 176: 28–32.
21. Parretti E, Carignani L, Cioni R, et al. Sonographic evaluation of fetal growth and body composition in women with different degrees of normal glucose metabolism. Diabetes Care 2003; 26: 2741–8.
22. Jovanovic L, Pettitt DJ. Gestational diabetes mellitus. JAMA 2001; 286: 20.
23. Jovanovic L. Optimization of insulin therapy in patients with gestational diabetes. Endocr Pract 2000; 6: 98–100.
24. Buchanan TA, Kitzmiller JL. Metabolic interactions of diabetes and pregnancy. Annu Rev Med 1994; 45: 245–60.
25. Reece EA, Coustan DR, Sherwin RSL. Does intensive glycemic control in diabetic pregnancies result in normalization of other metabolic fuels? Am J Obstet Gynecol 1991; 165: 126–30.
26. Sacks DA, Liu AI, Wolde-Tsadik G, et al. What proportion of birth weight is attributable to maternal glucose among infants of diabetic women? Am J Obstet Gynecol 2006; 194: 501–7.
27. Duggleby SL, Jackson AA. Relationship of maternal protein turnover and lean body mass during pregnancy and birth length. Clin Sci 2001; 101: 65–72.
28. Herrera E. Lipid metabolism in the fetus and the newborn. Diabetes Metab Res Rev 2000; 16: 202–6.
29. Parretti E, Mecacci F, Papini M, et al. Third-trimester maternal glucose levels from diurnal profiles in nondiabetic pregnancies: correlation with sonographic parameters of fetal growth. Diabetes Care 2001; 24: 1319–23.
30. Yogev Y, Ben-Haroush A, Chen R, et al. Diurnal glycemic profile in obese and normal weight nondiabetic pregnant women. Am J Obstet Gynecol 2004; 191: 949–53.
31. Jovanovic L, Peterson CM, Reed GF, and the National Institute of Child Health and Human Development – Diabetes In Early Pregnancy Study. Maternal postprandial glucose levels and infant birth weight: the Diabetes in Early Pregnancy Study. Am J Obstet Gynecol 1991; 164: 103–11.
32. DeVeciana M, Major CA, Morgan MA. Postprandial versus preprandial blood glucose monitoring in women with gestational diabetes mellitus requiring insulin therapy. N Engl J Med 1995; 333: 1237–41.
33. Combs CA, Gunderson E, Kitzmiller JL. Relationship of fetal macrosomia to maternal postprandial glucose control during pregnancy. Diabetes Care 1992; 15: 1251–7.
34. Weiss PAM, Haeusler M, Kainer F, et al. Toward universal criteria for gestational diabetes: relationships between seventy-five and one hundred gram glucose loads and between capillary and venous glucose concentrations. Am J Obstet Gynecol 1998; 178: 830–5.
35. American Diabetes Association: Clinical Practice Recommendations 2006. Diabetes Care 2006; 29(suppl. 1).
36. Jovanovic L. Response to Fraser [Letter]. Diabetes Care 2002; 25: 1104–5.
37. Jovanovic L. What is so bad about a big baby? Diabetes Care 2001; 24: 1317–8.
38. Mello G, Parretti E, Cioni R. Responce to Fraser [Letter]. Diabetes Care 2002; 25: 1105–6.
39. Parretti E, Mello G, Tondi F, et al. Normalization of fetal fat mass in gestational diabetic women. 5th international Workshop–Conference on Gestational Diabetes, 11–13 November, 2005; American Diabetes Association, Abstract 37: 110.
40. Langer O, Levy J, Brustman L, et al. Glycemic control in gestational diabetes mellitus – How tight is tight enough: small for gestational age versus large for gestational age? Am J Obstet Gynecol 1989; 161: 646–53.

39 Timing and delivery of the macrosomic infant: Induction versus conservative management

David A. Sacks

Introduction

The title of this chapter is admittedly ambiguous. First, there is no universally accepted definition of the term 'fetal macrosomia'. Second, given recent changes in attitude toward elective Cesarean delivery, an appropriate subtitle might be 'Deciding when and by what route the suspected macrosomic infant of a diabetic mother should be delivered.' Third, given the number of clinical factors that go into deciding the timing and route of delivery of any infant of a diabetic mother (IDM), finding a study that controls for all of these independent variables is extremely difficult. This chapter will present an overview of current opinions and rationales for elective near-term versus term delivery of the IDM suspected to be large, and present some of the data supporting these opinions.

Existing guidelines

Published guidelines reflect a lack of consensus regarding timing and route of delivery for infants of diabetic women. The American Diabetes Association's Clinical Practice Recommendation for gestational diabetes advises delivery during the 38th week of pregnancy in an effort to prevent further *in utero* growth having achieved maturity.[1] In contrast, the American College of Obstetricians and Gynecologists (ACOG) states that there is no good evidence to support routine delivery prior to 40 weeks gestation in women who have gestational diabetes.[2] The same organization suggests that in the absence of diabetic nephropathy, retinopathy, poor glycemic control or prior stillbirth, infants of pre-gestational diabetic women be delivered at term.[3] Similarly, the Australasian Diabetes in Pregnancy Society (ADIPS) recommends delivery at term for pre-gestational diabetic women who are in good metabolic control and who do not have such complications as pre-eclampsia, intrauterine growth retardation, and hydramnios.[4] Both the ACOG and ADIPS suggest consideration of Cesarean delivery when the estimated fetal weight exceeds 4250 g[4] to 4500 g.[3,4]

Rationale for delivery prior to spontaneous onset of labor

As for any pregnant woman, intercurrent complications of pregnancy such as pre-eclampsia, non-reassuring antepartum testing or premature rupture of membranes at term are indications for delivery regardless of whether or not the mother has diabetes. However, two potential complications of pregnancy which may occur with greater frequency in pregnancies complicated by diabetes are fetal demise and excessive fetal growth. These will be examined individually.

Fetal demise

For several years it has been assumed that intrauterine fetal death occurred more frequently among IDMs than among infants of nondiabetic mothers (INDMs). A population-based study of 271,691 diabetic pregnancies among 10,733,983 deliveries confirmed that while the rates of fetal death for IDMs and INDMs progressively declined from 29 weeks on, the rate of fetal demise among the former consistently exceeded that among the latter from 32 weeks on. The nadir in fetal demise for IDMs was achieved at 38 weeks while that of the NIDMs occurred at 40 weeks (Figure 39.1).[5] At first sight these data would appear to support delivery of IDMs at 38 weeks. However, because of the influence of confounding variables, this inference may not be justified. One such variable is the type of diabetes. While some[6,7] have found no differences in perinatal mortality between Type 1 and Type 2 diabetic pregnancies, others[8] reported a higher rate among the latter. Ethnicity and its concomitant, socioeconomic status, are two other potential confounders, with some reporting variation in perinatal mortality among diabetic women of the same

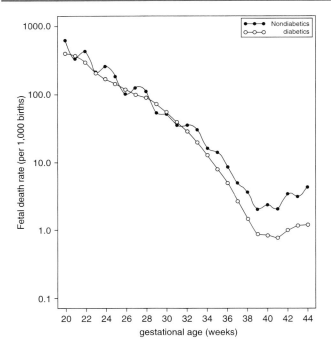

Figure 39.1   Gestational age-specific rates of fetal death (per 1000 births) among infants born to diabetic and nondiabetic patients: United States 1995–1997. (From: Mondestin et al.,[5] with permission from Elsevier.)

diagnostic type but different ethnicities.[6,8] Maternal obesity has been found to have a positive relationship with fetal demise. In one study of 24,505 unselected births a pre-pregnancy body mass index of 30 or greater was found to be independently associated with fetal demise. Because only three of the 112 fetal deaths occurred in diabetic women, it was not possible to determine if this relationship persisted among the latter subgroup.[9]

A baby of a woman who has diabetes is at greater risk of having major birth defects than is that of a woman who does not have diabetes. Historically, anomalous fetuses constituted a major proportion of fetal deaths. With the advent of diagnostic ultrasound, many such anomalies are being identified, and a proportion of anomalous fetuses are aborted prior to achieving a gestational age at which survival is possible.[7] This might serve to decrease the proportion of IDM stillbirths in which anomalies are found. There is substantial variability in the incidence of anomalies among IDM stillbirths in the few recent studies reporting these data (Table 39.1). Because most of these anomalies are compatible with survival till birth, the inference that a given anomaly was contributory to fetal demise may not be valid.

To conclude that delivery prior to 38 weeks will prevent fetal demise, one must review the proportion of unexplained fetal deaths among non-anomalous IDMs occurring at or beyond 38 weeks. Of those studies reporting these data, one[8] found 6/10 (60%) occurring within this time frame, while another[10] found 1/12 (8%) occurred in the 38th week. A third study[7] reported 13/64 (20%) non-anomalous fetal deaths between 37 and 40 weeks.

Two major confounders in the analysis of factors contributing to fetal demise are the level of maternal glycemia, particularly during third trimester, and the utilization of antepartum fetal testing. Only one study[10] included both these factors in their analyses. Mothers of nine of the 12 deaths in non-anomalous fetuses had suboptimal glycemic control during third trimester, the latter defined as a hemoglobin A1c greater than 7.5%. All six normal non-stress tests performed within a week of fetal demise occurred in the three women in good glycemic control carrying non-anomalous fetuses. The deaths in these three occurred at 34, 36, and 38 weeks, respectively.[10]

Excessive fetal growth

Two terms are generally used to define excessive fetal growth. Macrosomia is defined by a birthweight exceeding a certain

Table 39.1   Intrauterine fetal demise (IUFD) among infants of diabetic mothers and controls

	Diabetes		IUFD in diabetic pregnancies			IUFD in nondiabetic pregnancies			
Reference	DM types	Number of DMs	Total (rate)	Anom (%)	GA @ IUFD (weeks)	Number of NDMs	Total (rate)	Anom (%)	P
8	1,2	594	10 (16.8)	1 (10)	32–42	82,025	NR	NR	NR
10	1	1361	25 (18.4)	7 (28)	25–38	NR	NR	NR	NR
11	1	459	14 (30.5)	4 (29)	NR	NR	NR	NR	NR
12	GD,1,2	83	4 (48.2)	NR	NR	NR	NR	NR	NR
13	GD,1,2	733	21 (28.6)	NR	NR	NR	NR	NR	NR
14	2	182	2 (12.2)	0 (0)	NR	NR	NR (6.1)	NR	0.47
15	1	213	4 (18.5)	0 (0)	NR	NR	NR (5.2)	NR	NR
16	1.2	2356	63 (26.8)	NR	NR	620,841	3539 (5.7)	NR	4.7(3.7–6.1)*
17	1	323	4 (12.4)	1 (25)	24–36	NR	NR	NR	NR

IUFD rate is the rate of stillbirths per 1000 neonates born.
Anom (%) refers to the percent of fetal demise in which a fetal anomaly was reported.
P-values and rate ratio indicate a comparison between fetal demises in diabetic and nondiabetic pregnancies.
*Rate ratio. DM = diabetes, IUFD = intrauterine fetal demise, NDM = nondiabetic mothers, Anom = anomalous fetuses,
NR = not reported, GA = gestational age (weeks), GD = gestational diabetes.

number of grams, e.g. 4000 or 4500. While easy to remember, this definition fails to consider the influence of gestational age. The latter is taken into consideration by the term 'large for gestational age' (LGA), which is usually defined as a birthweight exceeding the 90th percentile for a given gestational age within a given population [18 Multiple studies have established that at any gestational age, the birthweight of an IDM exceeds that of an INDM.[5,11,12,14,15] It is also clear that however excessive fetal growth is defined, it occurs with greater frequency among IDMs. Why this is so has been the subject of several investigations.

A number of factors have been associated with excessive fetal growth. Besides maternal glucose intolerance, a positive association with birthweight has been reported for maternal age, ethnicity, parity, pre-pregnancy weight, pregnancy weight gain, male gender, and gestational age at birth, while a negative association has been found with maternal hypertensive disorders and smoking.[19,20] In one multivariate analysis of all of these factors only maternal third trimester glucose values and pre-pregancy body mass index were found to be independently associated with birthweight percentile among infants of insulin-requiring Type 2 and gestational diabetic women.[21]

In the United States, adult obesity has progressively increased over the last two decades.[22] Maternal obesity is associated with both diabetes and fetal overgrowth. An analysis of over 53,000 pregnancies found a 20% increase in maternal weight at first prenatal visit from 1980 to 1999. In that study, whether defined by an absolute weight (e.g. 106, 114, and 136 kg) or a body mass index (BMI) greater than 29 kg/m^2 the incidence of maternal obesity also increased over that time period. While the risk of gestational diabetes and large for gestational age neonates did not vary over time for the obese mothers, the risk of these two adverse outcomes which was attributable to maternal obesity did.[22]

Two other studies reported a progressive increase in gestational diabetes,[23] pre-gestational and gestational diabetes[24] and birthweight over 4000 g in parallel with progression in maternal BMI from the overweight to obese[24] and obese to morbidly obese[23] categories.

Whether either maternal obesity or glucose intolerance has a more dominant effect in determining whether a neonate of a diabetic mother will experience excessive growth has received some scrutiny. In one multivariate analysis, gestational diabetes was found to be unassociated with LGA neonates, whereas a maternal pre-pregnancy BMI of 26.1 was.[25] In another study of nondiabetic gravidas, 37% of whom had a 50-g, 1-h postglucose challenge test result which equaled or exceeded 7.2 mmol/L, multiple logistic regression analysis found a significant association between birthweight ≥4000 g and maternal obesity, but not glucose challenge test result.[26] In contrast, a smaller study found that maternal height and a fasting glucose ≥5.5 mmol/L but not maternal obesity were associated with neonatal macrosomia.[27] That other maternal anthropometric or metabolic factors may be associated with LGA neonates was suggested in two other studies. In one, obese women with normal glucose tolerance had a significantly greater incidence of LGA neonates than did normal weight women who had either impaired glucose tolerance or

gestational diabetes (27.6 vs. 13.3%; $P < 0.05$).[28] In another, well-controlled (mean capillary glucose 5.0–5.6 mmol/L) diet-treated but not insulin-treated overweight and obese gestationally diabetic women had an increased frequency of LGA neonates in univariate analysis. In multivariate analysis, both maternal obesity and mean maternal glucose levels were found to be independently associated with the incidence of LGA neonates.[29] Thus maternal body habitus and treatment modality in addition to weight, height, and glycemic control may need consideration in determining the probability of having a large birthweight neonate.

Infants of women who have glucose intolerance are distinguished from those of women with normal glucose tolerance not only by increased weight at a given gestational age but also by differences in fetal and neonatal body composition. Although lean body mass does not differ between the two, fat constitutes a greater proportion of fetal and neonatal weight for the former than the latter. This difference in body fat is apparent on ultrasound from second trimester to term,[30,31] increases progressively with advancing gestational age[31] and is found in appropriate[32] as well as large for gestational age IDMs.[31] LGA neonates of IDMs have larger skinfold thicknesses than LGA (but similar weight) INDMs.[33] The differences in proportion of weight that is fat as well as in fat distribution may explain why in one study the authors found that for every 250 g increment in birthweight above 3750 g the cumulative incidence of shoulder dystocia was significantly greater for infants of diabetic women[34] (Figure 39.2). These findings have led to the suggestion that fetuses of women who have diabetes who are estimated to be above a designated estimated weight threshold should have Cesarean deliveries prior to the onset of labor.[35] Arresting fetal growth in IDMs has also been used as a rationale to justify induction of labor prior to term.[1]

Method and route of delivery

Cesarean delivery

Given contemporary obstetrics practice, it is not possible to discuss early and/or elective delivery without inclusion of a discussion of the role of Cesarean delivery. In recent years the overall rate of Cesarean deliveries has dramatically increased. Rates from 1 to 37% of all deliveries have been reported from different parts of the globe,[35] with some hospitals reporting rates in excess of 50%.[36] That the increase in Cesarean deliveries may not be of maternal or fetal benefit is suggested by a continent-wide study in which 49% of Cesareans were elective, yet an increase in procedure-related, risk-adjusted maternal morbidity and prematurity-adjusted neonatal intensive care unit admissions was associated with an increase in Cesarean delivery rate.[36]

As with excessive fetal growth, maternal overweight and obesity appear to have independent relationships with Cesarean delivery rates. In one study, over a 20-year period the proportion of Cesarean deliveries attributable to maternal obesity increased in parallel with increasing maternal weight.[22] In another, adjusting for confounders such as fetal macrosomia and maternal diabetes, the Cesarean delivery rate

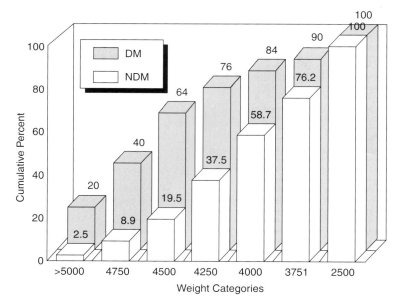

Figure 39.2 Percent cumulative incidence of shoulder dystocia at or above stated birthweight for diabetic (DM) and nondiabetic (NDM) pregnant women. For each birthweight threshold ≥3751 g cumulative incidence of shoulder dystocia was significantly higher in diabetic subjects. (From Langer et al.,[34] with permission from Elsevier.)

was higher for overweight and obese women than for women with average BMIs.[24] In a third, both elective and non-elective Cesarean rates were found to be higher among obese compared with non-obese nondiabetic women, regardless of their 50-g 1-h glucose screening test results.[26]

Overall, the likelihood of having a Cesarean delivery is greater for a woman who has diabetes than is the background risk. The overall risk of Cesarean delivery appears to be less in series analyzing data of women who have only gestational diabetes than in those which include or exclusively consider data of pre-gestationally diabetic women (Table 39.2). A variety of factors either separately or collectively may serve as indications for Cesarean delivery. These include one or more prior Cesarean deliveries, arrest of labor, placental abruption, placenta previa, fetal malpresentation, estimated large fetal

weight, and patient demand. Unfortunately, few studies list the primary indication for Cesarean delivery. Those that do list prior Cesarean delivery[37–39] pre-eclampsia,[37–39] dystocia,[37–40] estimated macrosomia,[40] fetal distress,[37,39,40] placenta previa,[37] failed induction,[37] and malpresentation.[39] None mention diabetes as a primary indication. Thus estimating to what extent, if any, maternal diabetes is considered in deciding whether or not a patient is delivered by Cesarean is no simple task. That maternal diabetes is independently associated with Cesarean delivery has been established in multivariate analyses which controlled for maternal demographics and obstetric complications.[41–45] This association does not establish that diabetes *per se* entered into the decision for route of delivery. However, one other study approached this question from a somewhat different angle. This study compared treated

Table 39.2   Cesarean deliveries among diabetic women

Reference	Diabetes type(s)	Number DM	Mean birthweight (g)	Number (%) LGA	Number (%) CS	Number (%) 1° CS*	Number (%) CS* before labor onset	Number (%) CS* for failed induction
14	2	182	3246	57 (32)	95 (53)	NA	41 (43)	21 (22)
17	1	323	3459	170 (53)	138 (43)	75 (54)	NA	33 (24)
28	GDM, IGT	250	3281	50 (20)	84 (34)	NA	NA	NA
37	GDM	1092	3300	NA	216 (20)	NA	126 (58)	5 (2)
41	GDM,1, 2	4643	3466	NA	1051 (23)	1051 (100)[a]	427 (9)[b]	NA
42	GDM	2755	3460	NA	686 (25)	NA	NA	NA
40	GDM, 1, 2,	148	3570	NA	46 (31)	46 (100)[a]	0	32 (70)
43	GDM, 1, 2,	624	3266	209 (23)	263 (42)	NA	NA	NA

*Percent of total CS. [a]None of the patients had had a prior CS. [b]32% of these 427 were done for suspected macrosomia.
LGA = large for gestational age. CS = Cesarean delivery. 1° CS = primary Cesarean delivery. NA = not available, GDM = gestational diabetes IGT = impaired glucose tolerance.

women who had gestational diabetes with untreated women who had a lesser degree of glucose intolerance. Despite the fact that the second group's babies had an increased rate of macrosomia than the first, there was no significant difference in the frequency of Cesarean delivery between the two groups. This finding suggests the possibility that the obstetrician's threshold to deliver by Cesarean may be lowered merely by the knowledge that the patient has diabetes.[46]

Shoulder dystocia is perhaps the most feared complication of vaginal delivery of the infant of a diabetic mother. The relationship of gestational age at delivery, glucose intolerance, and the prevalence of shoulder dystocia has been explored in a few publications. In one observational study no significant difference in either birthweight or the incidence of shoulder dystocia was found between gestational diabetics who were delivered at a mean of 37 weeks and pre-gestational diabetic women who were delivered at a mean of 36 weeks.[43] In a prospective randomized trial of early delivery of insulin-treated diabetic women, those delivered at a mean of 38 weeks did weigh less than those delivered at a mean of 39 weeks. While the incidence of shoulder dystocia was not statistically significantly different between groups, the three shoulder dystocias in the study occurred in the latter group.[47] A third time series did find a progressive diminution in birthweight and shoulder dystocia over the four time epochs examined. However, over time there was a reduction not only in weeks gestation at delivery but also in targeted glucose values and in estimated fetal weight as an indication for Cesarean delivery, making difficult ascertainment of the independent contribution of early delivery to the reduction in shoulder dystocia.[48]

Shoulder dystocia and fetal macrosomia are dominant risk factors for brachial plexus palsy.[49] Infants born after shoulder dystocia are at greater risk of brachial plexus injury if they have greater birthweight than if they do not. A greater proportion of macrosomic babies are born to diabetic women than to nondiabetic women. For babies born after shoulder dystocia who weigh ≥4000 g, the absolute risk of brachial plexus injury is from 12 to 35%.[50] Of the latter, from 5 to 7% will not spontaneously resolve.[50,51] Surgical restoration of shoulder and elbow function is possible in about 75% of those not resolving spontaneously.[51]

Because of the risks of shoulder dystocia especially among macrosomic infants of diabetic women, the strategy of attempting to identify macrosomic fetuses of these women and performing prophylactic Cesarean deliveries for them prior to the onset of labor has been explored. This strategy is premised on the assumption of the availability of a tool which will predict macrosomia with a reasonable degree of accuracy. Of the three tools utilized for this purpose (clinical, maternal, and sonographic) estimating fetal weight by sonography has been a major focus. Because the accuracy of prediction of a given outcome (positive predictive value) depends on the prevalence of that outcome in the population under study, and because, however defined, macrosomic fetuses are more prevalent in a population of diabetic women than in the nondiabetic population, the accuracy of sonographic prediction of fetal macrosomia is greater among diabetic than nondiabetic women.[50,52] However, even among diabetic women, the range of positive predictive values of sonographically estimated fetal

weight is wide (from 44 to 81% in one review[52]). Furthermore, the already high Cesarean rate among diabetic women (Table 39.2) likely diminishes the benefit of prophylactic Cesarean deliveries in that among those who have Cesareans during labor are women whose macrosomic fetuses are destined to develop shoulder dystocia.[50] Considering the prevalence of fetal macrosomia, shoulder dystocia, and brachial plexus injury among diabetic women, a calculated estimate of the number of Cesarean deliveries needed to prevent one permanent brachial plexus injury was 489 for estimated fetal weights above 4000 g and 443 using a 4500-g threshold.[50]

The clinical utility of incorporating fetal weight estimates in deciding route of delivery was evaluated in one prospective clinical trial. At 37 to 38 weeks gestation fetuses sonographically estimated to weigh ≥4250 g within 7 days of estimated delivery date were delivered by Cesarean prior to onset of labor. Those who were large for gestational age but whose estimated weight was less than 4250 g had their labors induced. Historical controls were used for comparison. The incidence of shoulder dystocia among the group managed by protocol, 1.5%, was significantly less than the 2.8% in the control group. However, of the 53 fetuses estimated to weigh ≥4250 g, 25 (47%) weighed less than 4000 g. The overall Cesarean rate rose significantly from 22% among the controls to 25% during the study period.[53] Two reviews concluded that insufficient data exists to support prophylactic Cesarean delivery above any designated weight threshold.[50,52]

Induction of labor

In discussing the relative merits of labor induction for diabetic women, two fundamental issues must be addressed. First, a comparison should be made of the risks and benefits of awaiting spontaneous onset of labor versus those of delivery prior to the onset of labor. Second, among the latter, the risks and benefits of induction versus Cesarean delivery should be compared. Only one randomized controlled trial examining the relative merits of induction at 38 weeks versus awaiting spontaneous onset of labor has been published.[47] Of the 200 subjects, 187 were insulin-requiring gestationally diabetic women and the remainder pre-gestationally diabetic women without vasculopathy. All were in good metabolic control, had estimated fetal weights less than 3800 g and were at least 38 weeks at entry into the study. Mean birthweight of the induced group was less than that of the expectantly managed group (3446 vs. 3672 g; $P < 0.01$ when adjusted for gestational age and maternal age and weight). The three mild shoulder dystocias all occurred in the expectantly managed group. Of interest is that the rate of Cesarean deliveries between groups was not significantly different. Of those who had Cesarean deliveries, 24% in the induction group and 39% in the expectantly managed group had either failed induction or an arrest disorder as the primary indication for surgery ($P = NS$).[47] Two other observational studies reported similar findings. One consisted of insulin-requiring gestationally diabetic women managed with two different protocols during two different time periods. The study group had their labors induced at 38 weeks. Patients in the historical control group had their labors induced at 40 weeks only if they had a non-reassuring antepartum test, a favorable cervix, or an estimated fetal weight ≥4000 g. While there was a significant difference in weeks gestation at delivery between the study and control groups (38 vs. 39 weeks, respectively, $P < 0.001$) there were no significant differences in birthweight, shoulder dystocia, or rate of Cesarean deliveries.[54] In another retrospective study, gestationally diabetic women who required medication to control their glycemia were compared with those who did not. Women in the former group had their labors induced at 37 weeks; those in the latter group had their labors induced at or beyond 38 weeks for indications similar to the first study. As in that study, women in the induction group delivered earlier than those in control group (38 vs. 39 weeks; $P < 0.001$) but there were no differences between groups in birthweight, shoulder dystocia, or Cesarean deliveries.[55]

An important question is whether diabetic women undergoing labor induction are more likely to ultimately deliver by Cesarean than are nondiabetic women undergoing labor induction. A retrospective comparison of two groups of women undergoing induction found that despite the greater parity and earlier gestational age of the diabetic compared with the nondiabetic group, there were no significant between-group differences in birthweights and in the frequencies of Cesarean deliveries.[56] Because of their earlier gestational age and greater parity one might anticipate a lower Cesarean rate in the diabetic group. However, another study found that among 3392 diabetic women those undergoing labor induction had a significantly lower primary Cesarean rate than those whose labor was not induced. However, the overall Cesarean rate was greater for women who did, as opposed to those who did not have diabetes.[57] From these two data sets one may infer that diabetic women undergoing labor induction may have higher rates of Cesarean deliveries, but that within a group of diabetic women the risks of Cesarean delivery may be unaffected or decreased for those whose labor is induced.

A final question pertains to the comparative risks of Cesarean delivery following induction of labor versus those for women having Cesarean deliveries prior to the onset of labor. While no analysis of this question limited to diabetic women is available, a study of nulliparous women who had no medical problems found that those undergoing Cesarean delivery following labor induction had both unadjusted and adjusted increased risks of intraperative trauma and composite morbidity than those whose Cesareans were performed prior to the onset of labor.[58]

Concluding comments

Delivery at 38 weeks gestation may prevent some intrauterine fetal deaths, particularly among women in poor glycemic control. However, most fetal deaths in pregnancies in diabetic women occur prior to 38 weeks. Maternal obesity and glycemic control appear to be associated with excessive fetal growth. While the former is not subject to modification after onset of pregnancy, the latter usually is. Whether estimates of fetal weight should be incorporated in determining method and route of delivery remains controversial. The reduction in shoulder dystocia using this approach is balanced by an increased rate of Cesarean deliveries. While labor induction for the woman who has diabetes has not been demonstrated to increase the rate of Cesarean deliveries, performing Cesareans prior to the onset of labor is associated with less morbidity than is performing the operation after labor has been initiated.

Clearly much remains to be learned about the timing and method of delivery of women who have diabetes. Hopefully, well-controlled prospective randomized studies will assist in guiding the peripartum care of women burdened with this increasingly prevalent problem.

REFERENCES

1. American Diabetes Association. Gestational diabetes mellitus. Diabetes Care 2004; 27(suppl. 1): S88–S90.
2. American College of Obstetricians and Gynecologists. Gestational Diabetes. ACOG Practice Bulletin No. 30. Washington, DC: ACOG; 2001.
3. American College of Obstetricians and Gynecologists. Pregestational Diabetes Mellitus. ACOG Practice Bulletin No. 60. Washington, DC: ACOG; 2005.
4. McElduff A, Cheung NW, McIntyre HD, et al. The Australasian Diabetes in Pregnancy Society consensus guidelines for the management of type 1 and type 2 diabetes in relation to pregnancy. Med J Aust 2005; 183: 373–7.
5. Modestin MAJ, Ananth CV, Smulian JC, et al. Birth weight and fetal death in the United States: The effect of maternal diabetes during pregnancy. Am J Obstet Gynecol 2002; 187: 922–6.
6. Verheijen ECJ, Critchley JA, Whiteclaw DC, et al. Outcomes of pregnancies in women with pre-existing type 1 or type 2 diabetes, in an ethnically mixed population. Br J Obstet Gynaecol 2005; 112: 1500–3.
7. Macintosh MCM, Flemming KM, Doyle P, et al. Perinatal mortality and congenital anomalies in babies of women with type 1 or type 2 diabetes in England, Wales, and Northern Ireland: population based study. BMJ, doi; 10.1136/bmj.38856.692986.AE (published 16 June 2006).
8. Cundy T, Bamble G, Townsend K, et al. Perinatal mortality in type 2 diabetes mellitus. Diabet Med 2000; 17: 33–9.

9. Kristensen J, Vertergaard M, Wisborg K, et al. Pre-pregnancy weight and the risk of stillbirth and neonatal death. Br J Obstet Gynaecol 2005; 112: 403–8.
10. Lauenborg J, Mathiesen E, Ovesen P, et al. Audit on stillbirths in women with pregestational type 1 diabetes. Diabetes Care 2003; 26: 1385–9.
11. Platt MJ, Stanissreet M, Casson IF, et al. St Vincent's Declaration 10 years on: outcomes of diabetic pregnancies. Diabet Med 2002; 19: 216–20.
12. Sobande AA, Al-Bar H, Archiboug EI. Diabetes and perinatal loss. Saudi Med J 2000; 21: 161–3.
13. Huddle KM. Audit of the outcome of pregnancy in diabetic women in Soweto, South Africa, 1992–2002. S Afr Med J 2005; 95: 789–94.
14. Dunne F, Brydon P, Smith K, et al. Pregnancy in women with type 2 diabetes: 12 years outcome data 1990–2002. Diabet Med 2003; 20: 734–8.
15. Penney GC, Mair G, Pearson DWM. Outcomes of pregnancies in women with type 1 diabetes in Scotland: a national population-based study. Br J Obstet Gynaecol 2003; 110: 315–8.
16. Confidential Enquiry into Maternal and Child Health (CEMACH). Pregnancy in women with type 1 and type 2 diabetes in 2002–2003, England, Wales and Northern Ireland. London: CEMACH; 2005.
17. Evers IM, V de Valk H, Visser GHA. Risk of complications of pregnancy in women with type 1 diabetes: nationwide prospective study

in the Netherlands. BMJ. doi: 1136/bmj.583160.EE (published 5 April 2004).

18. American College of Obstetricians and Gynecologists. Fetal Macrosomia. ACOG Practice Bulletin No. 22. Washington, DC: ACOG; 2000.

19. Okun N, Verma A, Mitchell BF, et al. Relative importance of maternal constitutional factors and glucose intolerance of pregnancy in the development of newborn macrosomia. J Matern Fetal Med 1997; 6: 285–90.

20. Stotland NE, Caughey AB, Breed EM, et al. Risk factors and obstetric complications associated with macrosomia. Int J Gynecol Obstet 2004; 87: 220–6.

21. Sacks DA, Liu AI, Wolde-Tsadik G, et al. What proportion of birth weight is attributable to maternal glucose among infants of diabetic women? Am J Obstet Gynecol 2006; 194: 501–7.

22. Lu GC, Rouse DJ, Dullard M, et al. The effect of the increasing prevalence of maternal obesity on perinatal morbidity. Am J Obstet Gynecol 2001; 185: 845–9.

23. Weiss JL, Malone FD, Emig D, et al. Obesity, obstetric complications and cesarean delivery rate – a population-based screening study. Am J Obstet Gynecol 2004; 190: 1091–7.

24. Rode L, Nilas L, Wejdemann K, et al. Obesity-related complications in Danish single cephalic term pregnancies. Obstet Gynecol 2005; 105: 537–42.

25. Ricart W, López J, Mozas J, et al. Body mass index has a greater impact on pregnancy outcomes than gestational hyperglycaemia. Diabetologia 2005; 48: 1736–42

26. Yogev Y, Langer O, Xenakis EMJ, et al. The association between glucose challenge test, obesity and pregnancy outcome in 6390 non-diabetic women. J Matern–Fetal Neonat Med 2005; 17: 29–34.

27. van Hoorn J, Dekker G, Jeffries S. Gestational diabetes versus obesity as risk factors for pregnancy-induced hypertension disorders and fetal macrosomia. Aust NZ J Obstet Gynaecol 2002; 42: 29–34.

28. Bo S, Menato G, Signorile A, et al. Obesity or diabetes: what is worse for the mother and for the baby? Diabetes Metab 2003; 29: 175–8.

29. Langer O, Yogev Y, Xenakis EMJ, et al. Overweight and obese in gestational diabetes: the impact on pregnancy outcome. Am J Obstet Gynecol 2005; 192: 1768–76.

30. Parretti E, Carignani L, Cioni R, et al. Sonographic evaluation of fetal growth and body composition in women with different degrees of normal glucose metabolism. Diabetes Care 2003; 26: 2741–8.

31. Wong SF, Chan FY, Oats JJN, et al. Fetal growth spurt and pregestational diabetic pregnancy. Diabetes Care 2002; 25: 1681–4.

32. Catalano PM, Thomas A, Huston-Presley L, Amini SB. Increased fetal adiposity: a very sensitive marker of abnormal in utero development. Am J Obstet Gynecol 2003; 189: 1698–704.

33. Vohr BR, McGarvey ST, Coll CG. Effects of maternal gestational diabetes and adiposity on neonatal adiposity and blood pressure. Diabetes Care 1995; 18: 467–75.

34. Langer O, Berkus MD, Huff RW, et al. Shoulder dystocia: should the fetus weighing ≥4000 grams be delivered by cesarean section? Am J Obstet Gynecol 1991; 165: 831–7.

35. World Health Organization. Health Service Coverage. In: World Health Organization, World Health Statistics 2006. Geneva: World Health Organization; 2006. pp. 34–41.

36. Villar J, Valladares E, Wojdyla D, et al. Cesarean delivery rates and pregnancy outcomes: The 2005 WHO global survey on maternal and perinatal health in Latin America. Lancet 2006; 367: 1819–29.

37. Moses RG, Knights SJ, Lucas EM, et al. Gestational diabetes: is a higher cesarean section rate inevitable? Diabetes Care 2000; 23: 15–7.

38. Gunton JE, McElduff A, Sulway M, et al. Outcome of pregnancies complicated by pre-gestational diabetes mellitus. Aust NZ J Obstet Gynaecol 2000; 40: 38–43.

39. Wylie BR, Kong J, Kozak SE, et al. Normal perinatal mortality in type 1 diabetes mellitus in a series of 300 consecutive pregnancy outcomes. Am J Perinatol 2002; 19: 169–76.

40. Blackwell SC, Hassan SS, Wolfe HW, et al. Why are cesarean delivery rates so high in diabetic pregnancies? J Perinat Med 2000; 28: 316–20.

41. Kjos SL, Berkowitz K, Xiang A. Independent predictors of cesarean delivery in women with diabetes. J Matern–Fetal Neonat Med 2004; 15: 61–7.

42. Xiong X, Saunders LD, Wang FL, et al. Gestational diabetes mellitus: prevalence, risk factors, maternal and infant outcomes. Int J Gynecol Obstet 2001; 75: 221–8.

43. Ray JG, Vermeulen MJ, Shapiro JL, et al. Maternal and neonatal outcomes in pregestational and gestational diabetes mellitus, and the influence of maternal obesity and weight gain: the DEPOSIT study. QJ Med 2001; 94: 147–56.

44. Ehrenberg HM, Durnwald CP, Catalano P, et al. The influence of obesity and diabetes on the risk of cesarean delivery. Am J Obstet Gynecol 2004; 191: 969–74.

45. Patel RR, Peters TJ, Murphy DJ, et al. Prenatal risk factors for caesarean section. Analysis of the ALSPAC cohort of 12,944 women in England. Int J Epidemiol 2005; 34: 355–67.

46. Naylor CD, Sermer M, Chen E, et al. Cesarean delivery in relation to birth weight and gestational glucose tolerance. JAMA 1996; 275: 1165–70.

47. Kjos SL, Henry OA, Montoro M, et al. Insulin-requiring diabetes in pregnancy: a randomized trial of active induction of labor and expectant management. Am J Obstet Gynecol 1993; 169: 611–5.

48. Peled Y, Perri T, Chen R, et al. Gestational diabetes mellitus – implications of different treatment protocols. J Pediatr Endocrinol Metab 2004; 847–52.

49. Mollberg M, Hagberg H, Bager B, et al. High birthweight and shoulder dystocia: the strongest risk factors for obstetrical brachial plexus palsy in a Swedish population-based study. Acta Obstet Gynecol Scand 2003; 84: 654–9.

50. Rouse DJ, Owen J. Prophylactic cesarean delivery for fetal macrosomia diagnosed by means of ultrasonography – a Faustian bargain? Am J Obstet Gynecol 1999; 181: 332–8.

51. Conway DL. Choosing route of delivery for the macrosomic infant of a diabetic mother: Cesarean section versus vaginal delivery. J Matern–Fetal Neonat Med 2002; 12: 442–8.

52. Chauhan SP, Grobman WA, Gherman RA, et al. Suspicion and treatment of the macrosomic fetus: A review. Am J Obstet Gynecol 2005; 193: 332–46.

53. Conway DL, Langer O. Elective delivery of infants with macrosomia in diabetic women: Reduced shoulder dystocia versus increased cesarean deliveries. Am J Obstet Gynecol 1998; 178: 922–5.

54. Luria S, Inslev V, Hagay ZJ. Induction of labor at 38 to 39 weeks of gestation reduces the incidence of shoulder dystocia in gestational diabetic patients class A2. Am J Perinatol 1996; 13: 293–6.

55. Rayburn W, Sokkary N, Clokey DE, et al. Consequences of routine delivery at 38 weeks for A-2 gestational diabetes. J Matern–Fetal Neonat Med 2005; 18: 333–7.

56. Yogev Y, Ben-Haroush A, Chen R, et al. Active induction management of labor for diabetic pregnancies at term; mode of delivery and fetal outcome – a single center experience. Eur J Obstet Gynecol Reprod Biol 2004; 114: 166–70.

57. Levy AL, Gonzalez JL, Rappaport VJ, et al. Effect of labor induction on cesarean section rates in diabetic pregnancies. J Reprod Med 2002; 47: 931–2.

58. Allen VM, O'Connell CM, Baskett TF. Maternal morbidity associated with cesarean delivery without labor compared with induction of labor at term. Obstet Gynecol 2006; 108: 286–94.

40 Management of the macrosomic fetus

Gerard H.A. Visser, Inge M. Evers and Giorgio Mello

Introduction

Fetal macrosomia is a frequent complication in pregnancies of women with diabetes. Its incidence depends, among other things, on the definition of macrosomia. On the one hand, birthweight centiles (>90th or >97.7th centile) are used and, on the other, weight (i.e. >4000 g or >4500 g) are used. The use of centiles is preferable from an epidemiological point of view, since such a definition is independent of gestational age. However, weight is more directly related to complications during labor. National studies show an incidence of a birthweight >90th centile in pre-gestational diabetic pregnancies of 20% (Sweden 1982–1985), 33.5% (Sweden 1991–1996), 45% (the Netherlands, 1999–2000) and 51% (UK, 2002–2003).[1–4] These data suggest that there might have been an increase of macrosomia during the past decade: regional and/or multicenter studies show an incidence of 19–43%.[4–10] A birthweight of >4000 g occurs in c. 20–25% of infants of women with insulin-dependent diabetes[3,4,12–14] and a weight >4500 g in 7–10%.[3,13,15]

Macrosomia is related to glucose control [glycosylated hemoglobin (HbA1c) levels] during pregnancy, but the percentage of variance in weight explained by HbA1c values is limited (i.e. <10%).[3] Macrosomia in diabetic pregnancy is related to unexplained death *in utero*, prolonged labor, shoulder dystocia and, as a consequence, fetal asphyxia, clavicle fracture, and/or Erb's palsy. Macrosomic newborns are at increased risk of hypoglycemia, hyperbilirubinemia, and hypertrophic cardiomyopathy.[2,3,16–18] Prevention of macrosomia is therefore of great importance. This should be achieved by reducing weight (centiles); however, since this seems as yet impossible – at least at a nationwide level – a timed early delivery may be an option.

Obstetric management

Management of the macrosomic fetus depends on several factors, such as actual fetal weight (and/or centile) at which perinatal risks increase and the reliability of fetal weight estimation. Moreover, as to the timing of delivery, gestational age (and fetal maturity) and the cervix score are of importance.

Stillbirth

Stillbirth is more frequent in macrosomic fetuses and data from the Swedish Medical Birth Register from 1991 to 1996 show an incidence of 2.4% in large-for-date infants as compared to 1.2% for appropriate-for-date infants of insulin-dependent diabetic women.[2] Prevention of stillbirth in the macrosomic fetus is, apart from improving maternal glucose control and intensified fetal monitoring, only possible through a relatively early delivery. There is a debate on the gestational age at which stillbirth may occur in diabetic pregnancies. Apparently, an older English survey showed that 'all' stillbirths in diabetic pregnancies occurred before 36 weeks,[19,20] whereas more recent data show a clustering *c.* 38 weeks (Table 40.1). However, these data do not take into account the number of infants delivered at the different gestational ages. A large UK nationwide cohort of 2400 pregnancies of women with Type 1 or Type 2 diabetes showed a stillbirth rate of 19/739 (2.6%) in normally formed infants delivered between 32 and 36 weeks and of 13/1420 (0.9%) in infants delivered between 37 and 41 weeks.[4] A timed delivery at or after 38 weeks will, therefore, not prevent most cases.

Shoulder dystocia

Shoulder dystocia is infrequent in fetuses weighing <3500 g (<0.2%). Its incidence is gradually increasing with increasing weight and is *c.* 2–3% with a fetal weight of 4000–4500 g. In infants weighing >4500 g, shoulder dystocia may occur in 10–20% of cases.[13,21] There is strong evidence that maternal diabetes is an independent risk factor for shoulder dystocia in infants weighing >4250 g.[13,24] Langer et al.[13] even found a 3-fold increase in the weight categories of infants weighing >4500 g (Table 40.2). This higher incidence is likely to be due to a higher shoulder-to-head and chest-to-head ratio in these infants,[22] i.e. with the same weight, the head of an infant of a woman with diabetes is born easier than that of a nondiabetic mother, but the shoulders are larger and get stuck more easily. Large babies of nondiabetic women are more likely to be born by Cesarean section, since the bigger head is likely to result in a failure to progress during the first or second stage of labour.

In a recent Dutch nationwide study on pregnancy outcome in Type 1 diabetes, shoulder dystocia was found in 25 of

Table 40.1 Stillbirth in diabetic pregnancy. Number of cases and age of occurrence (gestational age >30 weeks only)

Author (reference)	n	Gestational age (weeks)								
		33	34	35	36	37	38	39	40	41
Lowy et al.[19]	22 (all <36 weeks)									
Garner et al.[33]	3						2	1		
Landon et al. [34]	1					1				
Lagrew et al.[35]	3	1					2			
McAuliffe et al. (from 17)	2								1	1
Evers et al.[8]	2				1		1			
Evers et al.[36]	2				1		1			
Total	13	1			2	1	6	1	1	1

179 vaginally delivered infants (14%; Table 40.3). Its incidence was already 14% in infants weighing 3500–4000 g and 38% in infants with a higher birthweight. There was one case of Erb's palsy and this occurred in one of the nine infants weighing >4500 g. Others found Erb's palsy in 12 of 157 vaginally delivered infants weighing ≥4500 g (7.5%).[21] In the recent Uk nationwide study on Type 1 and Type 2 diabetes shoulder dystocia occurred in 22% of infants with a birthweight of 4000–4250 g, in 25% of infants weighing 4250–4500 g and in 43% in heavier infants.[4] The incidence of Erb's palsy in the general obstetrical population is c. 1–2 per 1000 infants.[23]

By doing a Cesarean section in all diabetic women with an estimated fetal weight >4250 g, c. 80% of shoulder dystocia would be prevented. In contrast, in nondiabetic women such a policy would only prevent 40% of dystocia, with a sharp rise in the incidence of Cesarean sections.[12] This difference between diabetics and nondiabetics is due to the higher prevalence of shoulder dystocia in heavy infants of diabetic mothers and to the different weight distribution of the overall population.

A policy of elective Cesarean sections in case of fetal macrosomia is only effective if fetal weight can be assessed accurately. Unfortunately that is not the case and deviations of up to 15–20% of actual weight have been described with the various ultrasound methodologies used. This also holds true for diabetic cases.[23] In other words, with an estimated fetal weight of 4250 g, 25–30% of infants will weigh <4000 g [95% confidence internal (CI) c. 3500–5000 g]. On the other hand, in order not to miss one infant weighing 4250 g, a Cesarean section should be performed in all cases with an estimated fetal weight of ≥3500 g, since the 95% CI at this weight estimation is 2800–4300 g. This would imply that at least 50% of diabetic women would need a Cesarean section to prevent the vaginal birth of infants weighing >4250 g.[24,25]

This 'inaccuracy' further discourages elective Cesarean sections in nondiabetic fetal macrosomia. However, given the high incidence of shoulder dystocia in diabetics with a fetal weight >4250 g (±25%), a Cesarean section is recommended in these cases.[13,26] Ultrasound estimation of fetal weight is likely to be more accurate if longitudinal measurements and trends are taken into account, rather than an individual measurement. Moreover, ultrasound fetal weight estimation is more accurate when performed at 34–37 weeks of gestation than at term, with an error in birthweight prediction of less than 15% in 91% of cases.[27] In a longitudinal study we found that all infants with an estimated weight on ultrasound >90th centile before 30 weeks, were severely macrosomic at birth (>97.7th centile).[28]

Table 40.2 The incidence of shoulder dystocia in relation to birthweight in a large general population (n = 74,390) and in a diabetic population (n = 1589) in Texas in between 1970 and 1985

Birthweight (g)	Nondiabetic (%)	Diabetic (g)
2500–3750	0.2	0.5
3750–4000	1.0	1.2
4000–4250	2.6	3.0
4250–4500	5.0	6.9
4500–4750	7.5	21.8
>4750	13.0	37.0

(Adapted from Langer et al.[13])

Lung maturation

When considering an elective early delivery because of fetal macrosomia – either induction of labor or a Cesarean section – due account of sufficient fetal maturation has to be taken. Elective Cesarean sections before 39 weeks are known to be associated with conditions like 'wet-lung' or respiratory distress syndrome (in the nondiabetic population too).[29,30] Assessment of fetal lung maturation should therefore be made if a Cesarean section before that time is considered. It is not known if the same holds for a planned induction of labor, since labor itself might stimulate fetal lung maturation. However, it is the present authors' policy to perform lung maturity testing if labor is induced before 38 weeks of gestation. It is uncertain if antenatal corticosteroids,

Table 40.3   The occurrence of shoulder dystocia, clavicle fracture and Erb's palsy according to birthweight in a Dutch nationwide study on Type 1 diabetes and pregnancy between 1999 and 2000

Birthweight (g)	Number	Vaginal delivery	Shoulder dystocia	Clavicle fracture	Erb's palsy
<3000	69	32	–	–	–
3000–3500	79	52	2	–	–
3500–4000	96	56	8	1	–
4000–4500	58	30	9	1	–
≥4500	22	9	6	2	1
Total	324	179 (56%)	25 (14%)	4	1

(From Evers.[36])

given to enhance fetal lung maturation, are effective after 36 weeks of gestation.[31]

Timing of delivery

There is no convincing data as to the optimal timing of delivery of the macrosomic fetus of the woman with diabetes. Gestational age, estimated fetal weight and the degree of glucose control all play a role. In one randomized controlled trial in 200 low-risk women with insulin dependent (pre)gestational diabetes, a lower incidence of Cesarean sections, large-for-gestional age infants and shoulder dystocia was found in case of induction of labor at 38 weeks as compared to expectant management.[32]

The present authors start delivering infants with an estimated fetal weight >97.7th centile from 36 weeks onwards, after determination of fetal lung maturation. Labor may be induced in the case of a favorable cervix. Poor glucose control and excessive fetal weight may result in an even earlier intervention; good glucose control may lead to a later intervention. If longitudinal ultrasound measurements of fetal weight indicate an estimated weight >4250 g, then a Cesarean section is considered. Others consider a Cesarean section if estimated

weight >4000 g (M. Hod, personel communication). It is obvious that also factors, such as obstetrical history and maternal height have to be taken into account.

Conclusions

- The problem of fetal macrosomia in maternal Type 1 and Type 2 diabetes is increasing rather than decreasing.
- Intrauterine death occurs more often of large-for-gestational-age fetuses than of appropriate-for-gestational-age fetuses. There is some evidence that the highest incidence of stillbirth occurs c. 37–39 weeks of gestation.
- Complicated vaginal delivery of infants with shoulder dystocia occurs more often in diabetic women than in nondiabetic women when the infant weighs >4000 or 4250 g.
- In Type 1 diabetes an elective Cesarean section is recommended in cases where the estimated fetal weight is >4250 g, despite limitations in fetal weight estimation.
- In cases where an elective delivery is considered before 38 weeks of gestation, then fetal lung maturity testing is recommended.

REFERENCES

1. Hanson U, Persson B. Outcome of pregnancies complicated by type-1 insulin dependent diabetes in Sweden: acute pregnancy complications, neonatal mortality and morbidity. Am J Perinatol 1993; 4: 330–3.
2. Djerf P, Hanson U. Perinatal complications in large-for-gestational age (LGA) infants compared to non LGA-infants of type-1-diabetic mothers. Abstracts Diabetic Pregnancy Study Group of the EASD, 32nd meeting, Galilee, Israel, 2000, p. 38.
3. Evers IM, De Valk HW, Visser GHA. Macrosomia despite good glycemic control in type-1 diabetic pregnancy; results of a nationwide prospective study. Diabetologia 2002; 45: 1484–9.
4. Macintosh MC, Fleming KM, Bailey JA, et al. Perinatal mortality and congenital anomalies in babies of women with type 1 or type 2 diabetes in England,Wales and Nothern Ireland; population based study. BMJ 2006; 333: 177.
5. Nordström L, Spetz E, Wallström K, Wålinder O. Metabolic control and pregnancy outcome among women with insulin-dependent diabetes mellitus. A twelve-year follow-up in the country of Jåmtland, Sweden. Acta Obstet Gynecol Scand 1998; 77: 284–9.
6. GDF study group – France. Multicenter survey of diabetic pregnancy in France. Gestation and Diabetes in France Study Group. Diabetes Care 1991; 14: 994–1000.
7. Vääräsmäki MS, Hartikainen A, Anttila M, et al. Factors predicting peri- and neonatal outcome in diabetic pregnancy. Early Hum Dev 2000; 59: 61–70.
8. Evers IM, Bos AME, Aalders AL, et al. Pregnancy in women with type 1 diabetes mellitus; still maternal and perinatal complications in spite of good blood sugar control. Ned T Geneesk 2000; 144: 804–9.
9. Leads from the MMWR. Diabetes in Pregnancy Project – Maine, 1986–1987. J Am Med Assoc 1987; 258: 3495–6.
10. Casson IF, Clarke CA, Howard CV, et al. Outcomes of pregnancy in insulin dependent diabetic women: results of a five year population cohort study. Br Med J 1997; 315: 275–8.
11. Hawthorne G, Robson S, Ryall EA, et al. Prospective population based survey of outcome of pregnancy in diabetic women: results of the Northern Diabetic Pregnancy Audit. Br Med J 1994; 315: 279–81.

12. Jervell J, Bjerkedal T, Moe N. Outcome of pregnancies in diabetic mothers in Norway 1967–1976. Diabetologia 1980; 18: 131–4.
13. Langer O, Berkus MD, Huff RW, Samueloff A. Shoulder dystocia: should the fetus weighing ≥4000 grams be delivered by cesarean section? Am J Obstet Gynecol 1991; 165: 831–7.
14. Gabbe SG. Management of diabetes mellitus in pregnancy. Am J Obstet Gynecol 1985; 153: 824–8.
15. DCCT group. Pregnancy outcomes in the Diabetes Control and Complications Trial. The DCCT Research Group. Am J Obstet Gynecol 1996; 174: 1343–53.
16. Berk MA, Mimouni F, Miodovnik M, et al. Macrosomia in infants of insulin-dependent diabetic mothers. Pediatrics 1989; 86: 1029–34.
17. Small M, Cameron A, Lunan CB, MacCuish AC. Macrosomia in pregnancy complicated by insulin-dependent diabetes mellitus. Diabetes Care 1987; 10: 594–9.
18. Gutgesell HP, Speer ME, Rosenberg HS. Characterization of the cardiomyopathy in infants of diabetic mothers. Circulation 1980; 61: 441–50.
19. Lowy C, Beard RW, Goldschmidt J. Congenital malformations in babies of diabetic mothers. Diabet Med 1986; 3: 458–62.
20. Lowy C. Type 1 diabetes and pregnancy. Lancet 1995; 346: 966–7.
21. Lipscomb KR, Gregory K, Shaw K. The outcome of macrosomic infants weighing at least 4500 grams: Los Angeles + University of Southern California experience. Obstet Gynecol 1995; 85: 558–64.
22. Modanloü HD, Komatsu G, Dorchester W, et al. Large-for-gestational age neonates: anthropometric reasons for shoulder dystocia. Obstet Gynecol 1982; 60: 417–23.
23. Foran AM, Donnelly V, Eligott MMc, et al. Erb's palsy, prevalence, prediction and management [Abstract]. J Matern Fetal Neonat Med 2002; 11(suppl. 1): 46.
24. McLaren RA, Puckett JL, Chauhan SP. Estimations of birth weight in pregnant women requiring insulin: a comparison of seven sonographic models. Obstet Gynecol 1995; 85: 565–9.
25. Watson W, Seeds J. Sonographic diagnosis of macrosomia. In: Divon MR, ed. Abnormal Fetal Growth. New York: Elsevier; 1991, pp. 237–42.
26. Carrera JM, Mallafré J. Macrosomia: obstetric management. In: Kurjak A, ed. Textbook of Perinatal Medicine. London: Parthenon Publishing Group; 1998, pp. 1294–5.
27. Best G, Pressman EK. Ultrasonographic prediction of birth weight in diabetic pregnancies. Obstet Gynecol 2002; 99: 740–4.
28. Kerssen A, de Valk HW, Visser GHA. Diurnal glucose profiles during pregnancy in women with type 1 diabetes mellitus; relations with infant birth weight. Diabet Care 2006.
29. Graziosi GC, Bakker CM, Brouwers HAA, Bruinse HW. Elective cesarean section is preferred after the completion of a minimum of 38 weeks of pregnancy. Ned T Geneesk 1998; 142: 2300–3.
30. Donaldsson S, Thorkelsson T, Bergsteinsson H, et al. The effect of gestational age at the time of delivery on the incidence of respiratory dysfunction in neonates born by elective caesarean section without labour. J Matern Fetal Neonat Med 2002; 11(suppl. 1): 20.
31. Roberts D, Dalziel S. Antenatal corticosteroids for accelerating fetal lung maturation for women at risk of preterm birth. Cochrane Database Syst Rev 2006 Jul 19; 3: CD004454.
32. Kjos SL, Henry OA, Montoro M, et al. Insulin-requiring diabetes in pregnancy: a randomized trial of active induction of labor and expectant management Am J Obstet Gynecol 1993; 169: 611–5.
33. Garner PR, D'Alton ME, Dudley DK, et al. Preeclampsia in diabetic pregnancies. Am J Obstet Gynecol 1990; 163: 505–8.
34. Landon MB, Langer O, Gabbe SG, et al. Fetal surveillance in pregnancies complicated by insulin dependent diabetes mellitus. Am J Obstet Gynecol 1992; 167: 617–21.
35. Lagrew DC, Pircon RA, Towers MD, et al. Antepartum fetal surveillance in patients with diabetes: when to start? Am J Obstet Gynecol 1993; 168: 1802–6.
36. Evers IM. Pregnancy outcome in women with type-1 diabetes mellitus: a nationwide study in the Netherlands. PhD thesis, University of Utrecht, 2002.

41 Hypertensive disorders and diabetic pregnancy

Jacob Bar and Moshe Hod

Metabolic syndrome: When hypertension and diabetes meet

The striking increase in the prevalence of obesity, diabetes mellitus (DM), hypertension, and cardiovascular disease in the last two decades[1] has led to the concept of the metabolic syndrome.[2] Also termed syndrome X,[3] insulin resistance syndrome,[4] and the deadly quartet,[5] metabolic syndrome is characterized by a constellation of well-documented risk factors for cardiovascular disease, namely, glucose intolerance, insulin resistance, central obesity, dyslipidemia, and hypertension, that co-occur in individuals at a higher rate than expected by chance. Extensive research has still not completely elucidated the precise cause of the syndrome, although some strong positions have been taken. Nevertheless, it is widely recognized that a combination of genetic predisposition and environmental factors, particularly those associated with socioeconomic status is involved. The environmental factors include both postnatal life habits and nutrition, and – no less important – intrauterine conditions. Indeed, there is plentiful evidence linking low birth weight due to intrauterine growth restriction (IUGR) with an increased risk of vascular disease in later adult life.[6]

Intrauterine factors in metabolic syndrome: The fetal origin of adult disease

Barker[6] pioneered the idea that the epidemic of coronary heart disease in Western countries in the twentieth century, which paradoxically coincided with improved standards of living and nutrition, originated in fetal life. He postulated that the low birthweight and impaired fetal growth which were characteristic of deprived regions in the 1900s may have predisposed the survivors to heart disease in later life. Support was provided by studies conducted in Hertfordshire, England, showing a higher rate of cardiovascular mortality in men who had been small at birth and at 1 year of age.[6] Thereafter, at least seven retrospective cohort studies reported an association of low birthweight with high risk of later ischemic heart disease[7–12] and stroke,[13,14] or impaired glucose tolerance and

DM.[15,16] It was also found to be associated with high blood pressure (BP) in childhood[17,18] and adult life.[19] The evidence was strongest for blood pressure and glucose tolerance,[20] which could be measured earlier in life and for which more data, and sometime also prospective data, were available.[19,21] The evidence was weaker, though still convincing for heart disease, for which data were sparse and often confined to men. The findings in the few studies on stroke, particularly the hemorrhagic type, were consistent.[14]

In another study, Barker et al.[22] observed that the effects of impaired fetal growth are modified by subsequent growth. As such, individuals who were small at birth but became overweight in adulthood were at the highest risk of heart disease and Type 2 DM (a physiological resistance to insulin action). This finding led to the second part of the hypothesis, the thrifty phenotype (Figure 41.1). The authors proposed that the process of adaptation to undernutrition in fetal life leads to permanent metabolic and endocrine changes. These are beneficial if the undernutrition persists after birth, but may predispose the individual to obesity and impaired glucose tolerance if it does not. The most unfavorable growth pattern is smallness and thinness at birth, continued slow growth in early childhood, followed by an acceleration of growth so that height and weight approach the population means, with a continued rise in body mass index above the mean. The growth pattern differs by sex[6,23] and ponderal index.[6] However, as birthweight and ponderal index, as well as body mass index, are only crude measures of the manner in which fetal nutrition affects body composition and the balance of lean body mass to fat, the true impact of fetal growth on later disease remains unclear. Be that as it may, there is no doubt that low birthweight and high body mass index interact and that their effects on BP and impaired glucose tolerance are multiplicative.[6]

The thrifty phenotype paradigm has stimulated a wealth of animal and human research on fetal growth restriction and its sequelae. The hypothesis predicts that a population undergoing a transition from poor to better nutrition will be characterized by more heart disease and impaired glucose tolerance. This is epitomized by the rapidly rising incidence of Type 2 DM, ischemic heart disease, and obesity in increasingly urbanized India.[24–26] Indian infants are exceptionally small, with a mean birthweight of 2700 g, and their mothers tend to be

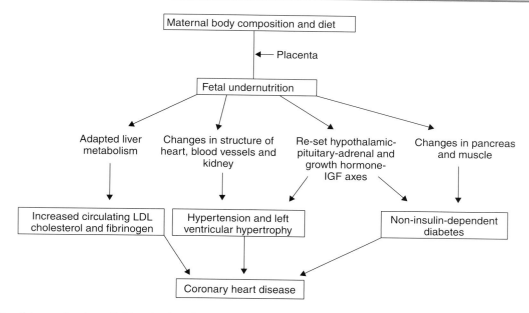

Figure 41.1   Possible mechanisms linking fetal undernutrition and coronary artery disease. IGF, insulin growth factor.

short and underweight. The infants also have low muscle mass, small viscera, and a relative excess of fat – a body composition particularly likely to lead to insulin resistance.[27] In a cohort study in Indian children, Yajnik et al.[28] showed that lower weight at birth and higher body mass index in childhood were associated with impaired glucose tolerance. Although improving the growth and nutrition of the mother before pregnancy would seem to be the ideal strategy to improve fetal growth, animal studies have shown that more than one generation of improved maternal nutrition may be necessary for an optimal outcome.[29,30] Thus, in India, where women begin childbearing already in their teens, before they are fully grown, postponing marriage might be a good first step.[31] There is only limited evidence that nutritional supplements in pregnancy improve fetal growth in undernourished mothers.[32] Furthermore, the effect of supplements varies according to the stage of pregnancy: giving them early in pregnancy may even worsen fetal growth.[6]

Stene et al.,[33] in a large population-based cohort study, noted a relatively weak but significant and nearly linear association between birthweight and risk of Type 1 DM. The ratio of children with a birthweight of 4500 g or more to children with a birthweight of less than 2000 g was 2.21. This finding raised the possibility that perinatal factors influence the risk of Type 1 DM. The underlying mechanisms of this association are unknown, but they probably differ from those responsible for the association between low birthweight and later onset of Type 2 DM.

There may also be factors other than nutrition that play a role in the casual pathway leading to high BP, cardiovascular disease, or Type 2 DM.

The fetal origin hypothesis of adult disease assumes that a poor nutrient supply during a critical period of *in utero* life may 'program' a permanent structural or functional change in the fetus, altering the distribution of cell types, gene expression, or both. Some researchers have accused the authors who

formulated the hypothesis of incorrect statistical interpretations because of chance, artifacts, or confounding factors in later life, but these have been resolved.[34] Nevertheless, it should be emphasized that support for the hypotheses comes mainly from studies in rodents[35] which cannot rule out environmental causes, particularly those associated with socioeconomic status,[36,37] genetic predisposition to low birthweight or hypertension and hypertension-related diseases, and postnatal factors.[38,39] Unfortunately, testing these parameters in humans is neither ethical nor practical.

In an attempt to separate genetic from extrauterine environmental influences, some researchers have studied multiple pregnancies. For example, the Tasmanian Infant Health Survey of a cohort of monozygotic, dizygotic, and singleton pregnancies reported a stronger association between birthweight and BP in children from multiple pregnancies.[40] The association also held true within the monozygotic pairs, suggesting that a genetic predisposition may need to be combined with specific mechanisms within the fetoplacental unit.[40] A study of 492 pairs of female twins showing an inverse relationship of birthweight and adult BP[41] proved further corroboration for the assumption that restricted intrauterine growth is due to placental dysfunction rather than inadequate maternal nutrition or genetic factors.

Two other studies stress the importance of primary prevention of high BP and cardiovascular disease and the controversy still surrounding Barker's fetal origin hypothesis. In the first, school children with a history of low birthweight were found to have impaired endothelial function and a trend towards carotid stiffness, which may represent early expressions of vascular compromise.[42] However, another group of investigators showed no difference in flow-mediated endothelial-dependent vasodilatation (early stage in the development of atherosclerosis) between adolescents who had a low birthweight and controls.[43]

An additional factor that may underlie the proposed contribution of the intrauterine environment to adult disease is the reduced nephron mass documented in infants in disadvantaged populations with intrauterine growth restriction and exposure to maternal diabetes and vitamin A deficiency. A lower nephron mass may impair nephrogenesis, thereby increasing the susceptibility of the infant to later kidney damage from diseases such as hypertension and diabetes, which also commonly affect disadvantaged people.[44]

Mechanisms underlying metabolic syndrome

Metabolic syndrome is characterized by a cluster of clinically recognizable physiological abnormalities: glucose intolerance, high BP, and unfavorable lipid profile – all alterations induced by the compensatory hyperinsulinemia. It also involves biochemical abnormalities.[45] Up-regulation of the inflammatory cascade has recently been recognized as an additional risk factor for the impaired cardiovascular component of the syndrome.[46]

Insulin resistance now appears to be the epidemiological link between high BP and obesity. Insulin resistance induces hypertension via mechanisms at the cellular, circulatory, and neurological levels, as well as via possible polygenic factors. Acquired or transient insulin resistance is associated with certain physical conditions, such as pregnancy, obesity, oral contraceptive use, and severe distress. Type 2 DM is a state of increased insulin secretion caused by the physiological resistance of insulin action and a lower-than-normal beta-cell reserve. Diabetes in pregnancy or gestational DM (GDM) may precede the clinical expression of Type 2 DM in the nonpregnant state, even by several years. Pre-eclampsia and other hypertensive disorders, which are known to have a higher incidence in GDM, can be linked to increased insulin resistance.[47]

Insulin resistance and hypertension in the nonpregnant state

To understand the association between insulin resistance and hypertensive disorders in pregnancy, we first need to elucidate the role of insulin resistance in hypertensive disorders in the nonpregnant state. The pathogenesis of essential hypertension is multifactorial, involving complex interactions between endocrine, metabolic, and genetic factors.

The obesity component

The worldwide obesity epidemic has been a major driving force in the recognition of metabolic syndrome.[45] Several of the definitions proposed for metabolic syndrome include increased waist circumference.[48–50] This factor is known to be associated with a relative predominance of visceral over subcutaneous adipose tissue,[51,52] which results in a higher rate of

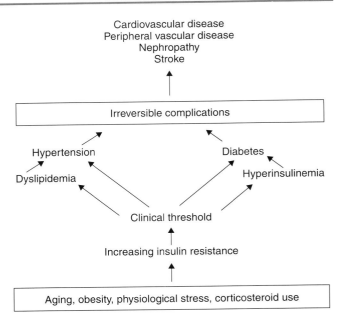

Figure 41.2 Factors influencing the generation of insulin resistance and its clinical correlates in the nonpregnant state.

flux of adipose-tissue-derived free fatty acids to the liver through the splanchnic circulation, thereby effecting glucose production, lipid synthesis, and prothrombotic protein secretion – all features of metabolic syndrome.[53] Obesity, aging, and diabetes can amplify genetic tendencies toward the clinical expression of the disorder (Figure 41.2). Familial clustering of DM and hypertension has been reported by several investigators, who also observed a close association of insulin resistance with obesity-related hypertension.[54,55]

The dyslipidemia component

Several other metabolic disturbances, such as elevated levels of triglycerides, decreased levels of high-density lipoproteins (HDL), high cholesterol level, glucose intolerance, and hyperuricemia, have also been related to hyperinsulinemia.[56] The metabolic consequences of these disturbances include changes in the lipid profile resulting in atherosclerosis, increased deposition of body fat, and proliferation of vascular smooth muscle cells, which place the hypertensive, hyperinsulinemic individual at increased risk of cardiac complications and stroke.[57] Studies of the evolution of the clinical and biological disturbances in women with a polycystic ovary (PCO) support the view that insulin resistance, dyslipidemia, and hypertension are all manifestations of a single syndrome. Often obese, these women have hyperinsulinemia which disrupts sex hormone production,[58] resulting in androgenization and clinical manifestations of hirsutism and infertility. During pregnancy, they have more glucose intolerance[59] and pregnancy-induced hypertension (PIH).[60] Later in life, women with PCO acquire a male-pattern risk profile for coronary artery disease, including dyslipidemia and hypertension.[61]

The inflammatory component

The association of the metabolic syndrome with inflammation is well documented.[62] The increase in proinflammatory cytokines, including interleukin 6, resistin, tumor necrosis factor-alfa (TNF-α), and C-reactive protein,[63] reflects an overproduction by monocyte-derived macrophages and possibly other cells within the expanded adipose tissue mass.[64–66]

Mechanisms of action

Physiologic studies suggest that insulin resistance occurs primarily in the peripheral muscles and is mediated through the nonoxidative intracellular pathways of glucose disposal.[67–69] Insulin modulates BP through several pathways, including stimulation of sympathetic neural activity, direct vasculopathic actions, changes in cellular ion flux, and promotion of sodium retention.

Effect on the sympathetic nervous system

Insulin stimulates the release of plasma norepinephrine,[70] increases heart rate and systolic pressure, and stimulates vascular tone. In younger subjects and in subjects with acute hyperinsulinemia,[71] these effects appear to over-ride insulin's direct vasodilatory effect on the vascular beds. The observation that insulin administration sometimes leads to hypotensive episodes in diabetic patients with autonomic neuropathy is proof of insulin's vasodilatory ability. The complexity of the situation is apparent from the finding that insulin therapy normalizes angiotensin responsiveness[72] and increases pressor responses.[73] Therefore, the possible attenuating effect of insulin on vasoconstrictor responses may be blunted in the presence of a pathological resistance to insulin action at the cellular level.[74]

Effect on vascular smooth muscle and epithelium

Hyperinsulinemia triggers hypertrophy of the vascular smooth muscle cells, leading to vasoconstriction and stiffening of the blood vessels and the development of left ventricular hypertrophy.[75] The additional hyperinsulinemia-induced lipid changes also promote atherosclerosis, with further stiffening and narrowing of the arteries. Evidence regarding the role of insulin resistance and hyperinsulinemia in the pathogenesis of endothelial dysfunction is less clear. McCarthy[76] presumed that the dysregulation of the transmembranous electrolyte pumps, which causes increased basal vascular tone, is a result of relative lack of insulin rather than hyperinsulinemia at the smooth muscle level.

Effect on the transmembranous electrolyte pump

In acute hyperinsulinemic states, transmembranous calcium (Ca) influx is usually lowered and vascular tone is decreased. However, the effect of chronic hyperinsulinemia on Ca^{2+}-adenosinetriphosphatase, Na^+K^+-adenosinetriphosphate, and the Na^+–H^+ countertransport mechanism may actually culminate in a rise in intercellular Ca^{2+} levels and increased vascular tone.[77,78] Studies have shown that erythrocyte sodium–lithium countertransport is elevated in hypertensive patients with insulin resistance and hyperinsulinemia.

At the cellular level, levels of cytosolic calcium increase, along with smooth muscle proliferation.[79]

Genetic components in insulin resistance

Type 2 DM has a strong genetic component. The genetic contribution varies from population group to population group, suggesting that more than one gene is involved and that more than one gene defect may cause similar phenotypic clinical syndromes.[80,81] Research in this area has concentrated on the steps in the insulin-signaling cascade between receptor and transport protein, but a lack of information about a specific postreceptor signaling currently hampers these efforts.

Clinical consequences of insulin resistance

Insulin resistance impairs glucose tolerance while promoting dyslipidemia, obesity, hypertension, and atherosclerosis. Its effects on salt handling by the kidneys predisposes the individual to renal dysfunction. Obesity, glucose intolerance, hyperinsulinemia, hypertension, and dyslipidemia represent cumulative risk factors that generate an escalating cycle of vascular compromise and collapse. Patients with three or more of these risk factors have an increased incidence of stroke, nephropathy, ischemic heart disease, and peripheral vascular disease.[82] Long-term diabetic complications are the most common cause of blindness, renal failure, and limb amputation in the United States today. Meticulous glycemic control has been shown to decrease the incidence of eye disease among diabetic patients. Antihypertensive therapy, specifically with angiotensin converting enzyme inhibitors (ACE-I), is effective in reducing the rate of progression of diabetic kidney disease. To prevent the peripheral vascular remodeling that results in stroke, limb loss, and heart disease, the underlying pathophysiologic mechanism needs to be reversed. This has become possible with the introduction of metformin[83] and troglitazone,[84] which are prototypes of the new classes of insulin-sensitivity-enhancing agents. These drugs are an important addition to the weight loss, exercise, and diet modification programs used to date, lifestyle habits which are effective but rarely adhered to for more than a few years.

Insulin resistance and Type 1 DM

The recent acceptance of the role of insulin resistance in Type 1 DM was supported by the concurrent rise in the incidence of the disease with a steady increase over the last 20–30 years in overweight and sedentary habits in children and adolescents in many populations. Medical evidence of the link between Type 1 DM and insulin resistance/metabolic syndrome continues to grow. The insulin resistance associated with the rising prevalence of weight gain may reflect a more aggressive form of autoimmune disease mediated by the same immuno-inflammatory factors that mediate beta-cell destruction, namely TNF-α and interleukin-6.[85] Moreover, the onset of diabetic nephropathy might contribute to insulin resistance/metabolic syndrome via mechanisms of low-grade inflammation and increased oxidative stress.[86,87] These concepts are included in the 'accelerator hypothesis' on the role of insulin resistance and overweight in Type 1 DM.[88]

Insulin resistance and hypertension in pregnancy

In normal pregnancy, insulin resistance results in a metabolic advantage for the fetus. The mother enters a state of accelerated starvation in which she increases her reliance on lipolysis and protein catabolism as a source of energy. Thus, glucose is reserved for the fetus, which uses it as its primary fuel.[89] A steady supply of glucose is essential for the growing fetomaternal unit; normally, pregnant women are able to increase their insulin secretion to three times that of nonpregnant women.[90] In GDM, however, there is no increase in maternal insulin secretion in reaction to the increasing insulin resistance.[91] Some investigators believe this effect is due to a metabolically limited beta-cell reserve.[92,93] In most women with GDM, insulin sensitivity is restored after pregnancy. However, some may later develop Type 2 DM. The reported cumulative incidence rate of Type 2 DM after GDM is approximately 50% after 5 years.[94,95] It is even higher in women with excessive weight gain or with repeated pregnancies, who continue to experience insulin resistance.[96] Thus, the strong association between insulin resistance, hypertension, obesity and dyslipidemia, as part of the metabolic syndrome or sharing a common pathway in intrauterine life, may explain the higher incidence of hypertensive complications in diabetic pregnancy. Researchers reported that metabolic syndrome may also involve other metabolic abnormalities besides hyperglycemia, hyperinsulinemia, and dyslipidemia, namely, increased concentrations of plasminogen activator inhibitor (PAI)-1,[97] leptin,[98] and TNF-α.[99] Although these markers are surrogate measures of insulin sensitivity, they have been associated with a risk of hypertension in pregnancy. In fact, the normal physiological response to pregnancy has several components, such as insulin resistance, hyperlipidemia, increase in coagulation factors, and upregulation of the inflammatory cascade, that may contribute to a transient and earlier than expected excursion into metabolic syndrome[47] (Figure 41.3).

Gestational diabetes and hypertensive disorders

The study of both GDM and PIH has suffered from the lack of international consensus about classification, definitions, and nomenclature, leading to difficulties in comparing studies that used different diagnostic criteria. Nevertheless, epidemiological and physiological evidence suggests that GDM and PIH are etiologically distinct entities and that GDM is strongly associated with insulin resistance and glucose intolerance, whereas pre-eclampsia is probably not.

Epidemiological studies

Diabetic pregnancy is associated with a higher rate of hypertensive complications than normal pregnancy,[100,101] and a slightly increased risk of pre-eclampsia (15–20% vs. 5–7%).[102–104] The latter holds true even when the diagnosis of GDM is based on the 2-h 75-g oral glucose tolerance test (OGTT).[105] Mean arterial pressure is further increased in the presence of early diagnosis of GDM and the need for insulin therapy.[106] The increased risk of hypertensive disorders in GDM is probably a result of the

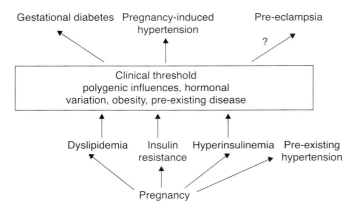

Figure 41.3 Risk factors for vascular disease and metabolic syndrome in pregnancy.

combination of insulin resistance and a genetic predisposition (Figure 41.4). A genetic predisposition to PIH was described in southwestern Navajo Indians, who like other Native Americans, are also at increased risk of hypertension, obesity, and DM.[107] Pre-eclampsia was also reported to be associated with increased fasting plasma insulin levels in African–American women.[108] However, these findings have not been confirmed in more heterogenous populations.[109]

Physiological studies

Patients with the severest form of glucose intolerance are more likely to exhibit pre-eclampsia[110] than patients with milder forms.[109] Controlled studies of the association between insulin resistance and pre-eclampsia have been performed in several populations. Martinez et al.[111] found that among women with normal glucose tolerance in the third trimester, those who subsequently developed severe pre-eclampsia had similar fasting and postprandial glucose levels to normotensive controls, but their fasting plasma insulin levels were 2-fold higher and their post-load insulin concentrations, 4-fold higher. Moreover, Joffe et al.[112] reported that the level of plasma glucose at 1 h after a 50-g oral glucose challenge was

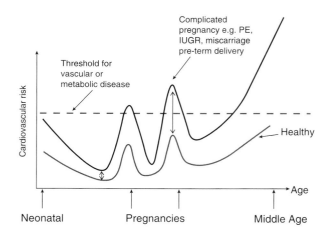

Figure 41.4 Factors influencing the generation of insulin resistance and its clinical correlates during pregnancy. (Sattar et al.[47])

an important predictor of pre-eclampsia, even if it was within the normal range. This suggests that there is a continuum of insulin resistance also in women with normal glucose tolerance that may predispose them to hypertensive disease. This assumption was supported by a similar study in China wherein higher serum insulin concentrations were detected in women with pre-eclampsia.[113] Besides insulin resistance, women with GDM and women with pre-eclampsia have similar hemodynamic profiles, namely, significant left ventricular hypertrophy and reduced diastolic function.[114] The mechanism by which insulin resistance may link these physiological findings is still unknown. One possibility is an interference of insulin resistance with the function of an endogenous solium pump inhibitor or digitalis-like factor. Graves et al.[115] demonstrated that levels of serum digoxin-like immunoreactive factor are higher in women with preexisting diabetes and pre-eclampsia than in normotensive diabetic women.

In hypertensive diabetic patients, some of the physiological changes that occur during pregnancy may persist after pregnancy. In one study, women with a pre-eclamptic pregnancy showed greater plasma insulin responses and steady-state plasma glucose levels 2 months after delivery than women with uncomplicated pregnancy.[116] A longer-term study reported persistent mild hyperinsulinemia in women 17 years after a pre-eclamptic pregnancy, despite their current normoglycemic state.[117] Other investigators, however, failed to detect these changes at 3–6 months after delivery.[118]

Pregestational diabetes and hypertensive complications

In most cases, pregestational diabetes refers to Type 1 DM. The incidence of Type 1 DM in pregnancy ranges from 0.2 to 0.5%.[119,120] Affected women contribute a heterogenous group in terms of duration of diabetes, White's classification, presence of hypertension, and end-organ damage, especially to the eye (retinopathy) and kidney (nephropathy). Pregnancy in women with Type 1 DM is associated with increased risks of pre-eclampsia, IUGR, neonatal morbidity, and perinatal mortality.[110–127] The diagnosis of pre-eclampsia is difficult in women with preexisting hypertension and proteinuria,[120] and women with chronic hypertension are at increased risk of

superimposed pre-eclampsia independent of the presence of diabetes.[128] The rate of hypertensive disorders (PIH and pre-eclampsia) in the various studies ranged from 9 to 66%. The lowest rate occurred in women with milder forms of DM (class B), and the highest in women with diabetic nephropathy. Table 41.1 summarizes the reported rates of pre-eclampsia in women with Type 1 DM.[119,121,129–132] Four of the six studies noted that rates of pre-eclampsia increased with an increasing severity of diabetes, with a mean of 16% (range 9–24%). Rates were higher in patients with diabetic nephropathy (mean 52%, range 35–66%) (Table 41.2). The risk factors identified for pre-eclampsia in women with Type 1 DM were as follows: duration of diabetes, preexisting hypertension, microalbuminuria prior to pregnancy, glycemic control prior to 20 weeks, nulliparity, minimal proteinuria (190–499 mg/dL) before 20 weeks, and nephropathy.[109,122,123,133–135] Siddiqi et al.[122] listed nulliparity, duration of diabetes, and poor glycemic control, and Caritis et al.,[133] nulliparity and mean arterial pressure. Combs et al.[123] added glycohemoglobin (HbAlc) level >9% at 12–16 weeks of gestation and proteinuria >190 mg/dL. Accordingly, Hanson and Persson[119] noted a pre-eclampsia rate of 31% when HbA1c levels were >10.1%, and a rate of 10.2% when HbA1c levels were <10.1%. These findings indicate that PIH/pre-eclampsia might be preventable by aggressive control of maternal BP before and during pregnancy, and prevention of microalbuminuria or reduction of proteinuria level in women with diabetic nephropathy. Recently, researchers found that suboptimal control of hypertension in early pregnancy was associated with a significant risk of preterm delivery.[136]

ACE-I seems to be the ideal agent for the treatment of hypertension.[135,137] According to one long-term follow-up study, the survival of patients with diabetic nephropathy has increased from 5 to 7 years to a median of 21.7 years, most likely because of improvements in aggressive antihypertensive treatment and glycemic control.[138] The same group of investigators showed that pregnancy itself has no adverse impact on kidney function and survival in patients with preserved renal function and diabetic nephropathy.[139] Therefore, in women with Type 1 DM and preexisting hypertension and proteinuria, stringent glycemic control should be started at least 6 months before conception in order to achieve a good pregnancy

Table 41.1   Rate of pre-eclampsia in women with Type 1 diabetes (excluding those with nephropathy)

Authors	Number of women	White's class	Pre-eclampsia* Number	%
Hanson and Persson[119]	463	B–R	53	11.5
Garner[120]	107	B, C	13	12.2
Green et al.[121]	361	B–R	86	23.8*
Miodovnik et al.[129]	136	B–R	12	9.0
Kovilam et al.[130]	238	B–D	36	15
Sibai et al.[131]	462	B–D	92	20
Total	1767		292	16.4

*Includes women with pregnancy-induced hypertension.

Table 41.2   Rate of pre-eclampsia in women with diabetic nephropathy

Authors	Number of women	Pre-eclampsia* Number	Pre-eclampsia* %
Hanson and Persson[119]	31	18	58
Greene et al.[121]	59	39	66
Gordon et al.[124]	45	24	53
Reece et al.[125]	31	11	35
Miodovnik et al.[129]	46	30	65
Kovilam et al.[130]	73*	32	44
Sibai et al.[131]	58	21	36
Bar et al.[135]	24	11	46
Total	367	186	52

*Includes women with retinopathy and nephropathy.

outcome and long-term effect.[135] However, contrary to findings in earlier studies of a nonteratogenic effect of ACE-I in early pregnancy,[140,141] in 2006, Cooper et al.[142] reported an increased risk of major congenital malformations in infants who were exposed to ACE-I in the first trimester compared to infants who were not (OR = 2.71, 95% CI 1.72–4.27). Nevertheless, ACE-I are still useful for patients with diabetic nephropathy for a planned pregnancy. Since conception can take months, preventing the administration of ACE-I during this period may enhance long-term renal function and pregnancy outcome. Patients should be advised to use sensitive pregnancy kits for the earliest possible detection of pregnancy, when the ACE-I must be immediately stopped. The preconception medication should be accompanied by strict glycemic control.[135] Some authors suggested the use of low-dose aspirin to prevent pre-eclampsia, since alterations in the metabolism of prostacyclin and thromboxane A2 have been reported in DM.[120,143] However, Caritis et al.,[143] in a study of 462 women with Type 1 DM, found no significant differences in the rate of pre-eclampsia between the aspirin and placebo groups, although there was a nonsignificant trend toward a lower rate of pre-eclampsia in the aspirin group (19 vs. 32%, respectively). Larger studies in patients with diabetic nephropathy are needed to clarify this issue.

Microalbuminuria, diabetes, and hypertension in pregnancy

The role of microalbuminuria in DM has been established over the last 20 years. At the early stage of DM, when glucose metabolism is not controlled, the increase in glomerular plasma flow and intraglomerular pressure is probably responsible for the increased protein excretion.[144] Some authors believe these hemodynamic alterations are major determinants of both the initiation and progression of diabetic nephropathy.[145] Several studies have reported that patients with Type 1[146] or Type 2 DM[147] who have above-normal urinary albumin excretion rates are more likely to acquire diabetic nephropathy, eventually progressing to renal failure.[148] Microalbuminuria is also associated with an excess of known and potential cardiovascular risk factors, and it is a marker of established cardiovascular disease in both hypertensive[149] and nonhypertensive[150] individuals. Its role in diabetic and hypertensive pregnancy is less clear,[151] but becoming increasingly recognized. One study found that the presence of microalbuminuria in the early third trimester was predictive of pre-eclampsia in pregnant women at risk.[152] Furthermore, a significantly higher rate of women whose pregnancy was complicated by pre-eclampsia, had microalbuminuria 5 years later (40%) than women with uncomplicated pregnancy.[153] Microalbuminuria was also noted in 30% of 72 women who had not conceived since a previous GDM pregnancy 5–8 years previously – a significantly higher rate than in women who did not have a history of GDM.[154] Ekbom[134] in a study of 68 women with Type 1 DM, found that pre-eclampsia developed in 60% of those who had microalbuminuria before pregnancy. When the data were fitted to a logistic regression model, a significant association was revealed between microalbuminuria and duration of diabetes and pre-eclampsia. As in patients with hypertension, the progression to diabetic nephropathy in patients with Type 1 DM and microalbuminuria can be slowed by blockage of the renin–angiotensin system. Angiotensin II receptor antagonists were also recently shown to be renoprotective in patients with Type 2 DM and microalbuminuria.[155] This finding and other preliminary results[135,137] further suggest that pregnancy outcome may be improved with pre-pregnancy ACE-I treatment (discontinued at conception) in diabetic patients with overt proteinuria or microalbuminuria.

REFERENCES

1. Zimmet P, Alberti KG, Shaw J. Global and social implications of the diabetic epidemic. Nature 2001; 414: 782–7.
2. Kylin E. Studien. Hypertonie–Hyperglykamie–Hyperurikamiesyndrome. Zentralblatt for innere Medizine 1923; 44.
3. Reaven GM. Banting lecture 1988. Role of insulin resistance in human disease. Diabetes 1988; 37: 1595–607.
4. DeFronzo RA, Ferrannini E. Insulin resistance. A multifaceted syndrome responsible for NIDDM, obesity, hypertension, dyslipidemia, and atherosclerotic cardiovascular diseases. Diabetes Care 1991; 14: 173–94.
5. Kaplan NM. The deadly quartet. Upper-body obesity, glucose intolerance, hypertriglyceridemia, and hypertension. Arch Intern Med 1989; 149: 1514–20.
6. Barker DJP. Mothers, Babies and Health in Later Life. London: Churchill Livingstone; 1998.
7. Leon DA, Lithell HO, Vagero D, et al. Reduced fetal growth rate and increased risk of death from ischaemic heart disease: cohort study of 15,000 Swedish men and women born 1915–29. Br Med J 1998; 317: 241–5.
8. Rich-Edwards JW, Stampfer MJ, Manson JE, et al. Birth weight and risk of cardiovascular disease in a cohort of women followed up since 1976. Br Med J 1997; 315: 396–400.
9. Stein CE, Fall CHD, Kumaran K, et al. Fetal growth and coronary heart disease in south India. Lancet 1996; 348: 1269–73.
10. Eriksson JB, Forsen T, Tuomilehto J, et al. Catch-up growth in childhood and death from coronary heart disease: longitudinal study. Br Med J 1999; 318: 427–31.
11. Forsen T, Eriksson JG, Tuomilehto J, et al. Growth in utero and during childhood among women who develop coronary heart disease: longitudinal study. Br Med J 1999; 319: 1403–7.

12. Frankel S, Elwood P, Sweetnam P, et al. Birth weight, adult risk factors and incident coronary heart disease: the Caerphilly study. Public Health 1996; 110: 139–43.
13. Eriksson JG, Forsèn T, Tuomilehto J, et al. Early growth and coronary heart disease in later life: longitudinal study. Br Med J 2001; 322: 949–53.
14. Martyn CN, Barker DJP, Osmond C. Mothers' pelvic size, fetal growth, and death from stroke and coronary heart disease in men in the UK. Lancet 1996; 348: 1264–8.
15. Barker DJP, Hales CN, Fall CHD, et al. Type 2 (non-insulin-dependent) diabetes mellitus, hypertension and hyperlipidaemia (syndrome X): relation to reduced fetal growth. Diabetologia 1993; 36: 62–7.
16. Bavdekar A, Chittaranjan S, Fall CHD, et al. Insulin resistance syndrome in 8-year-old Indian children. Small at birth, big at 8 years, or both? Diabetes 1999; 48: 2422–9.
17. Law CM, de Swiet M, Osmond C, et al. Initiation of hypertension in utero and amplification throughout life. Br Med J 1993; 306: 21–7.
18. Moore WM, Miller AG, Boulton TJ, et al. Placental weight, birth measurements, and blood pressure at age 8 years. Arch Dis Child 1996; 74: 538–41.
19. Barker DJ, Osmond C, Golding J, et al. Growth in utero, blood pressure in childhood and adult life, and mortality from cardiovascular disease. Br Med J 1989; 298: 564–7.
20. Hales CN. Non-insulin-dependent diabetes mellitus. Br Med Bull 1997; 53: 109–22.
21. Whincup P, Cook D, Papacosta O, et al. Birth weight and blood pressure: cross-sectional and longitudinal relations in childhood. Br Med J 1995; 311: 773–6.
22. Barker DJP, Martyn CN, Osmond C, et al. Abnormal liver growth in utero and death from coronary heart disease. Br Med J 1995; 310: 703–4.
23. Taylor SJ, Whincup PH, Cook DG, et al. Size at birth and blood pressure: cross-sectional study in 8–11 year old children. Br Med J 1997; 311: 475–80.
24. Gupta R, Gupta VP, Ahluwalia NS. Educational status, coronary heart disease, and coronary risk factor prevalence in a rural population of India. Br Med J 1994; 309: 1332–6.
25. McKeigue PM, Shah B, Marmot MG. Relation of central obesity and insulin resistance with high diabetes prevalence and cardiovascular risk in South Asians. Lancet 1991; 337: 382–6.
26. Pais P, Pogue J, Gerstein H, et al. Risk factors for acute myocardial infarction in Indians: a case–control study. Lancet 1995; 346: 778–9.
27. Hales CN, Barker DJP, Clark PMS, et al. Fetal and infant growth and impaired glucose tolerance at age 64. Br Med J 1991; 303: 1019–22.
28. Yajnik CS, Fall CHD, Vaidya U, et al. Fetal growth and glucose and insulin metabolism in four-year-old Indian children. Diabet Med 1995; 12: 330–6.
29. McLeod KJ, Goldrick RB, Whyte HM. The effect of maternal malnutrition on the progeny in the rat: studies on growth, body composition and organ cellularity in first and second generation progeny. Aust J Exp Biol Med Sci 1972; 50: 435–46.
30. Lemonnier D, Suquet J, Aubert R, et al. Long term effect of mouse neonate food intake on adult body composition, insulin and glucose serum levels. Horm Metab Res 1973; 5: 223–4.
31. Wallace JM, Aitken RP, Milne JS, et al. Nutritionally mediated placental growth restriction in the growing adolescent: consequences for the fetus. Biol Reprod 2004; 71: 1055–62. E-Pub 16 June 2005.
32. Moore SE, Halsall I, Howarth, et al. Glucose, insulin and lipid metabolism in rural Gambians exposed to early malnutrition. Diabet Med 2001; 18: 646–53.
33. Stene LC, Magnus P, Lie RT, et al. Birth weight and childhood onset type 1 diabetes: population based cohort study. Br Med J 2001; 322: 889–92.
34. Leon D. Twins and fetal programming of blood pressure [Editorial]. Br Med J 1999; 319: 1313–4.
35. Langley-Evans SC, Gardner DS, Welham SJ. Intrauterine programming of cardiovascular disease by maternal nutritional status. Nutrition 1998; 11: 39–47.
36. Kramer MS. Determinants of low birth weight: methodological assessment and meta-analysis. Bull WHO 1987; 65: 663–737.
37. Gliksman MD, Kawachi I, Hunter D, et al. Childhood socioeconomic status and risk of cardiovascular disease in middle aged US women: a prospective study. J Epidemiol Community Health 1995; 19: 10–15.
38. Susser M, Levin B. Ordeals for the fetal programming hypothesis. Br Med J 1999; 318: 883–6.
39. Lucas A, Fewtrell MS, Cole TJ. Fetal origins of adult disease – the hypothesis revisited. Br Med J 1999; 319: 245–9.
40. Dwyer T, Blizzard L, Morley R, et al. Within pair association between birth weight and blood pressure at age 8 in twins from a cohort study. Br Med J 1999; 219: 1325–9.
41. Poulter NR, Chang CL, MacGregor AJ, et al. Association between birth weight and adult blood pressure in twins: historical cohort study. Br Med J 1999; 319: 1330–3.
42. Martin H, Hu I, Gennser G, et al. Impaired endothelial function and increased carotid stiffness in 9-year-old children with low birth weight. Circulation 2000; 102: 2739–44.
43. Singhal A, Kattenhorn M, Cole TJ, et al. Preterm birth, vascular function, and risk factors for atherosclerosis. Lancet 2001; 358: 1159–60.
44. Nelson RB. Intrauterine determinants of diabetic kidney disease in disadvantaged populations. Kidney Int 2003; 63(suppl. 83): S13–6.
45. Eckel RH, Grundy SM, Zimmet PZ. The metabolic syndrome. Lancet 2005; 365: 1415–28.
46. Haffner SM. Do interventions to reduce coronary heart disease reduce the incidence of type 2 diabetes? A possible role for inflammatory factors. Circulation 2001; 103: 346–7.
47. Sattar N, Greer IA. Pregnancy complications and maternal cardiovascular risk: opportunities for intervention and screening? Br Med J 2002; 325: 157–60.
48. Alberti KG, Zimmert PZ. Definition, diagnosis and classification of diabetes mellitus and its complications. Part 1: Diagnosis and classification of diabetes mellitus provisional report of a WHO consultation. Diabet Med 1998; 15: 539–53.
49. Executive Summary of the Third Report of the National Cholesterol Education Program (NCEP) Expert Panel on Detection, Evaluation, and Treatment of High Blood Cholesterol in Adults (Adult Treatment Panel III). JAMA 2001; 285: 2486–97.
50. Balkau B, Charles MA. Comment on the provisional report from the WHO consultation. European Group for the Study of Insulin Resistance (EGIR). Diabet Med 1999; 16: 442–3.
51. Bajaj M, Banerji MA. Type 2 diabetes in South Asians: a pathophysiologic focus on the Asian-Indian epidemic. Curr Diab Rep 2004; 4: 213–8.
52. Tanaka S, Horimai C, Katsukawa F. Ethnic differences in abdominal visceral fat accumulation between Japanese, African-Americans, and Caucasians: a meta-analysis. Acta Diabetol 2003; 40(suppl. 1): 302–4.
53. Aubert H, Frere C, Aillaud MF, et al. Weak and non-independent association between plasma TAFI antigen levels and the insulin resistance syndrome. J Thromb Haemost 2003; 1: 791–7.
54. Modan M, Halkin H, Almog S, et al. Hyperinsulinemia: A link between hypertension, obesity and glucose intolerance. J Clin Invest 1985; 75: 809–17.
55. O'Hare JA. The enigma of insulin resistance and hypertension. Am J Med 1988; 84: 505–11.
56. Schmidt MI, Watson RL, Duncan BB, et al. Clustering of dyslipidemia, hyperuricemia, diabetes and hypertension and its association with fasting insulin and central and overall obesity in a general population. Atherosclerosis Risk in Communities Study Investigators. Metabolism 1996; 45: 699–706.
57. Harano Y, Suzuki M, Shinozaki K, et al. Clinical impact of insulin resistance syndrome in cardiovascular diseases and its therapeutic approach. Hypertens Res 1996; 19(suppl. 1): 81–5.
58. Crave J, Fimbal S, Lejeune H, et al. Effects of diet and metformin administration on sex hormone binding globulin, androgens, and insulin in hirsute and obese women. J Clin Endocrinol Metab 1995; 80: 2057–62.
59. Lanzone A, Caruso A, Disimone N, et al. Polycystic ovarian disease: A risk factor for gestational diabetes? J Reprod Med 1995; 40: 312–6.
60. Urman B, Sarac E, Dogan L, et al. Pregnancy in infertile PCOD patients: Complications and outcome. J Reprod Med 1997; 42: 501–5.
61. Talbott E, Guzick D, Cleria A, et al. Coronary heart disease in women with polycystic ovarian syndrome. Arteroscler Thrombovasc Bio 1995; 15: 821–6.
62. Sutherland J, McKinnley B, Eckel RH. The metabolic syndrome and inflammation. Metabolic Syndr Rel Disord 2004; 2: 82–104.
63. Fernandez-Real JM, Ricart W. Insulin resistance and chronic cardiovascular inflammatory syndrome. Endocr Rev 2003; 24: 278–301.
64. Trayhurn P, Wood IS. Adipokinesis: inflammation and the pleiotropic role of white adipose tissue. Br J Nutr 2004; 92: 347–55.
65. Weisberg SP, McCann D, Desai M, et al. Obesity is associated with macrophage accumulation in adipose tissue. J Clin Invest 2003; 112: 1796–808.

66. Xu H, Barnes GT, Yang Q, et al. Chronic inflammation in fat plays a crucial role in the development of obesity-related insulin resistance. J Clin Invest 2003; 112: 1821–30.
67. Capaldo B, Lembo G, Napoli, et al. Skeletal muscle is a primary site of insulin resistance in essential hypertension. Metabolism 1991; 40: 1320–2.
68. Levy J, Zemel MB, Sowers JR. Role of cellular calcium metabolism in abnormal glucose metabolism and diabetic hypertension. Am J Med 1989; 87(suppl. 6A): 7–16.
69. Resnick LM. Cellular ions in hypertension, insulin resistance, obesity and diabetes: A unifying theme. J Am Soc Nephrol 1992; 3: S78–85.
70. O'Hare JA, Minaker K, Young JB, et al. Insulin increases plasma norepinephrine (NE) and lowers plasma potassium equally in lean and obese men. Clin Res 1985; 33: 441A.
71. Rowe JW, Young JB, Minaker K, et al. Effect of insulin and glucose infusions on sympathetic nervous system activity in normal man. Diabetes 1981; 30: 219–25.
72. Christlieg AR. Renin, angiotensin and norepinephrine in alloxan diabetes. Diabetes 1974; 23: 962–70.
73. Weidmann P, Beretta-Piccoli C, et al. Pressor factors and responsiveness in hypertension accompanying diabetes mellitus. Hypertension 1985; 7(suppl. II): 33–42.
74. Zemel MB. Insulin resistance vs. hyperinsulinemia in hypertension: Insulin regulation of Ca2+ transport and Ca(2+)- regulation of insulin sensitivity. J Nutr 1995; 125(suppl. 6): 1738–43.
75. Weidmann P, Bohlen L, de Courten M. Insulin resistance and hyperinsulinemia in hypertension. J Hypertens 1995; 13(suppl. 2): 65–72.
76. McCarthy MF. Insulin resistance – not hyperinsulinemia – is pathogenic in essential hypertension. Med Hypotheses 1994; 42: 226–36.
77. Byyny RL, Lo Verde M, Lloyd S, et al. Cytosolic calcium and insulin resistance in elderly patients with essential hypertension. Am J Hypertens 1992; 5: 459–64.
78. Weidmann P, de Courten M, Boehlen L. Insulin resistance, hyperinsulinemia and hypertension. J Hypertens 1993; 11(suppl. 5): 27–38.
79. Canessa M. Erythrocyte sodium–lithium countertransport: Another link between essential hypertension and diabetes. Curr Opin Nephrol Hypertens 1994; 3: 511–7.
80. Olefsky JM. Pathogenesis of non-insulin dependent diabetes (type II). In: DeGRoot LJ, Besser GM, Cahill JC, eds. Endocrinology, 2nd edn. Philadelphia: WB Saunders; 1989. pp. 1369–98.
81. Rotter JL, Vadheim CM, Rimoin DL. Genetics of diabetes mellitus. In: Rifkin H, Porte D JR, eds. Diabetes Mellitus: Theory and Practice. New York: Elsevier; 1990, pp. 378–413.
82. Gilbert RE, Jerums G, Cooper ME. Diabetes and hypertension: Prognostic and therapeutic considerations. Blood Press 1995; 4: 329–38.
83. DeFronzo RA, Goodman AM. Efficacy of metformin in patients with non-insulin dependent diabetes mellitus. N Engl J Med 1995; 333: 541–9.
84. Nolan JJ, Ludvik MD, Beerdsen RN, et al. Improvement in glucose tolerance and insulin resistance in obese subjects treated with troglitazone. N Engl J Med 1995; 331: 1188–93.
85. Banerji MA. Impaired beta-cell and alpha-cell function in African-American children with type 2 diabetes mellitus – "Flatbush diabetes". J Pediatr Endocrinol Metab 2002; 15: 493–501.
86. Thorn LM, Forsblom C, Fagerudd J, et al. Metabolic syndrome in type 1 diabetes: association with diabetic nephropathy and glycemic control (the FinnDiane study). Diabetes Care 2005; 28: 2019–24.
87. Svensson M, Eriksson JW. Insulin resistance in diabetic nephropathy – cause or consequence? Diabetes Metab Res Rev 2006; 22: 401–10.
88. Wilkin TJ. The accelerator hypothesis: weight gain as the missing link between Type I and Type II diabetes. Diabetologia 2001; 44: 914–22.
89. Kalkhoff RK, Kissebah AH, Kim HJ. Carbohydrate and lipid metabolism during normal pregnancy: Relationship to gestational hormones. In: Merkatz IR, Adam PAJ, eds. The Diabetic Pregnancy: A Perinatal Perspective. New York: Grune & Stratton; 1979.
90. Bergmann RN, Phillips LS, Cobelli C. Physiologic evaluation of factors controlling glucose tolerance in man. Measurement of insulin sensitivity and beta-cell sensitivity from the response to intravenous glucose. J Clin Invest 1981; 68: 1456–67.
91. Buchanon TA, Metzger BE, Freinkel N, et al. Insulin sensitivity and beta-cell responsiveness to glucose during late pregnancy in lean and moderately obese women with normal glucose tolerance or mild gestational diabetes. Am J Obstet Gynecol 1990; 162: 1008–14.
92. Freinkel N, Metzger BE, Phelps RL, et al. Gestational diabetes mellitus: Heterogeneity of maternal age, weight, insulin secretion, HLA, antigens, and islet cell antibodies and the impact of maternal metabolism on pancreatic beta-cell function and somatic growth in the offspring. Diabetes 1985; 34(suppl. 2): 1–7.
93. Yen SCC, Tsai CC, Vela P. Gestational diabetogenesis: Quantitative analysis of glucose–insulin interrelationship between normal pregnancy and pregnancy with gestational diabetes. Am J Obstet Gynecol 1971; 111: 792–800.
94. Metzger BE, Cho NH, Roston SM, et al. Prepregnancy weight and antepartum insulin secretion predict glucose tolerance five years after gestational diabetes mellitus. Diabetes Care 1995; 16: 1598–605.
95. O'Sullivan JB. The Boston gestational diabetes studies: Review and perspectives. In: Sutherland HW, Stowers JM, Pearson DWM, eds. Carbohydrate Metabolism in Pregnancy and the Newborn. London: Springer-Verlag; 1989, pp. 287–94.
96. Peters RK, Kjos SL, Xiang A, et al. Long-term diabetogenic effect of a single pregnancy in women with prior gestational diabetes mellitus. Lancet 1996; 347: 227–30.
97. Abbasi F, McLaughlin T, Lamendola C, et al. Comparison of plasminogen activator inhibitor-1 concentration in insulin-resistant versus insulin-sensitive healthy women. Arterioscler Thromb Vasc Biol 1999; 19: 2818–21.
98. Segal KR, Landt M, Klein S. Relationship between insulin sensitivity and plasma leptin concentration in lean and obese men. Diabetes 1996; 45: 988–91.
99. Fernandez-Real JM, Broch M, Ricart W, et al. Plasma levels of the soluble fraction of tumor necrosis factor receptor 2 and insulin resistance. Diabetes 1998; 47: 1757–62.
100. Greco P, Loverro G, Selvaggi L. Does gestational diabetes represent an obstetric risk factor? Gynecol Obstet Invest 1994; 37: 242–5.
101. Rudge MV, Calderon IM, Ramos MD, et al. Hypertension disorders in pregnant women with diabetes mellitus. Am J Perinatol 1997; 44: 11–5.
102. Sacks DA, Greenspoon JS, Abu-Fadil S, et al. Toward universal criteria for gestational diabetes: the 75-gram glucose tolerance test in pregnancy. Am J Obstet Gynecol 1995; 172: 607–14.
103. Sermer M, Naylor CD, Gare DJ, et al. Impact of increasing carbohydrate intolerance on maternal–fetal outcomes in 3637 women without gestational diabetes. Am J Obstet Gynecol 1995; 173: 146–56.
104. Pennison EH, Egerman RS. Perinatal outcomes in gestational diabetes: A comparison of criteria for diagnosis. Am J Obstet Gynecol 2001; 184: 1118–21.
105. Schmidt MI, Duncan BB, Reichelt AJ, et al. Gestational diabetes mellitus diagnosed with a 2-h 75-g oral glucose tolerance test and adverse pregnancy outcomes. Diabetes Care 2001; 24: 1151–5.
106. Schaffir JA, Lockwood CJ, Lapinski R, et al. Incidence of pregnancy-induced hypertension among gestational diabetics. Am J Perinatol 1995; 12: 252–4.
107. Levy MT, Jacoaber SJ, Sowers JR. Hypertensive disorders of pregnancy in southwestern Navajo Indians. Arch Intern Med 1994; 154: 2181–3.
108. Sowers JR, Saleh AA, Sokol RJ. Hyperinsulinemia and insulin resistance are associated with pre-eclampsia in African–American women. Am J Hypertens 1995; 8: 1–4.
109. Cioffi FJ, Amorosa LF, Vintzileos AM, et al. Relationship of insulin resistance and hyperinsulinemia to blood pressure during pregnancy. J Matern Fetal Med 1997; 6: 174–9.
110. Solomon CG, Graves SW, Greene MF, et al. Glucose intolerance as a predictor of hypertension of pregnancy. Hypertension 1994; 23(6, pt 1): 717–21.
111. Martinez AE, Gonzales OM, Quninones GA, et al. Hyperinsulinemia in glucose-tolerant women with pre-eclampsia: A controlled study. Am J Hypertens 1996; 9: 610–4.
112. Joffe GM, Esterlitz JR, Levine RJ, et al. The relationship between abnormal glucose tolerance and hypertensive disorders of pregnancy in healthy nulliparous women. Am J Obstet Gynecol 1998; 179: 1032–7.
113. Gu H, Rong L, Sai JY. Insulin resistance and pregnancy-induced hypertension. Chung Hua Fu Chan Ko Tsa Chih 1994; 29: 711–3.
114. Oren S, Golzman B, Reitblatt T, et al. Gestational diabetes mellitus and hypertension in pregnancy: Hemodynamics and diurnal arterial pressure profile. J Hum Hypertens 1996; 10: 505–9.
115. Graves SW, Lincoln K, Cook SL, et al. Digitalis-like factor and digoxin-like immunoreactive factor in diabetic women with pre-eclampsia, transient hypertension of pregnancy and normotensive pregnancy. Am J Hypertens 1995; 8: 5–11.

116. Fuh MM, Yin CS, Pei D, et al. Resistance to insulin-mediated glu-cose uptake and hyperinsulinemia in women who had pre-eclampsia in pregnancy. Am J Hypertens 1995; 8: 768–71.

117. Laivuori II, Tikkanen MJ, Ylikorkala O. Hyperinsulinemia 17 years after pre-eclamptic first pregnancy. J Clin Endocrinol Metab 1996; 81: 2908–11.

118. Jacober SJ, Morris DA, Sower JR. Postpartum blood pressure and insulin sensitivity in African–American women with recent pre-eclampsia. Am J Hypertens 1994; 7(10, pt 1): 933–6.

119. Hanson U, Persson B. Epidemiology of pregnancy-induced hyperten-sion and preeclampsia in type 1 (insulin-dependent) diabetic preg-nancies in Sweden. Acta Obstet Gynecol Scand 1998; 77: 620–4.

120. Garner PR. Type 1 diabetes mellitus and pregnancy. Lancet 1995; 346: 152–61.

121. Greene MF, Hare JW, Krache M, et al. Prematurity among insulin-requiring diabetic gravid women. Am J Obstet Gynecol 1989; 161: 106–11.

122. Siddiqi T, Rosenn B, Mimouni F, et al. Hypertension during preg-nancy in insulin-dependent diabetic women. Obstet Gynecol 1991; 77: 514–9.

123. Combs CA, Rosenn B, Kitmiller JL, et al. Early-pregnancy protein-uria in diabetes related to preeclampsia. Obstet Gynecol 1993; 82: 802–7.

124. Gordon M, Landon MB, Samuels P, et al. Perinatal outcome and long-term follow-up associated with modern management of dia-betic nephropathy. Obstet Gynecol 1996; 87: 401–9.

125. Reece EA, Coustan DR, Hayslett JP, et al. Diabetic nephropathy: pregnancy performance and fetomaternal outcome. Am J Obstet Gynecol 1988; 59: 56–66.

126. Hanson U, Persson B. Outcome of pregnancies complicated by type 1 insulin-dependent diabetes in Sweden: acute pregnancy complications, neonatal mortality and morbidity. Am J Perinatol 1993; 10: 330–3.

127. Diamond MP, Shah DM, Hester RA, et al. Complication of insulin-dependent diabetic pregnancies by preeclampsia and/or chronic hypertension: analysis of outcome. Am J Perinatol 1985; 2: 263–7.

128. Sibai BM, Lindheimer ML, Hauth J, et al. Risk factors for preeclampsia, abruptio placentae, and adverse neonatal outcomes among women with chronic hypertension. N Engl J Med 1998; 339: 667–71.

129. Miodovnik M, Rosenn BM, Khoury JC, et al. Does pregnancy increase the risk for development and progression of diabetic nephropathy? Am J Obstet Gynecol 1996; 174: 1180–91.

130. Kovilam O, Rosenn B, Miodovnik M, et al. Is proliferative retinopa-thy a risk factor for adverse pregnancy outcome in women with Type 1 diabetes? J Soc Gynecol Invest 1997; 4:(suppl.) 152A.

131. Sibai BM, Caritis S, Hauth J, et al. Risks of preeclampsia and adverse neonatal outcomes among women with pregestational dia-betes mellitus. Am J Obstet Gynecol 2000; 182: 364–9.

132. Garner PR, D'Alton ME, Dudley DK, et al. Preeclampsia in diabetic pregnancies. Am J Obstet Gynecol 1990; 163: 505–8.

133. Caritis S, Sibai B, Hauth J, et al. Predictors of preeclampsia in women at high risk. National Institution of Child Health and Human Development Network of Maternal-Fetal Medicine Units. Am J Obstet Gynecol 1998; 179: 949–51.

134. Ekbom P. Pre-pregnancy microalbuminuria predicts preeclampsia in insulin-dependent diabetic patients mellitus. Copenhagen Preeclampsia in Diabetic Pregnancy Study Group. Lancet 1999; 353: 377.

135. Bar J, Chen R, Schoenfeld A, et al. Pregnancy outcome in patients with insulin dependent diabetes mellitus and diabetic nephropathy

136. Carr DB, Koontz GL, Gardella C, et al. Diabetic nephropathy in pregnancy: Suboptimal hypertensive control associated with preterm delivery. Am J Hypertens 2006; 19: 513–9.

137. Hod M, van Dijk DJ, Karp M, et al. Diabetic nephropathy and preg-nancy: the effect of ACE inhibitors prior to pregnancy on fetomater-nal outcome – preliminary report. Nephrol Dialysis Transplant 1995; 10: 2328–33.

138. Astrup AS, Tarnow L, Rossing P, et al. Improved prognosis in type 1 diabetic patients with nephropathy: a prospective follow-up study. Kidney Int 2005; 68: 1250–7.

139. Rossing K, Jacobsen P, Hommel E, et al. Pregnancy and progression of diabetic nephropathy. Diabetologia 2002; 45: 36–41.

140. Bar J, Hod M, Merlob P. Angiotensin-converting enzyme inhibitors use in the first trimester of pregnancy. Int J Risk Safety Med 1997; 9: 1–4.

141. Feldkamp M, Jones KL, Ornoy A, et al. ACE inhibitors use in the first trimester of pregnancy. MMWR 1997; 46: 240–2.

142. Cooper WO, Hernandez-Diaz S, Arbogast PG, et al. Major congen-ital malformations after first-trimester exposure to ACE inhibitors. N Engl J Med 2006; 354: 2443–51.

143. Caritis S, Sibai B, Hauth J, et al. Low-dose aspirin to prevent preeclampsia in women at high risk. N Engl J Med 1998; 339: 667–71.

144. Viberti CC, Mackintosh D, Keen H. Determinants of the penetration of proteins through the glomerular barrier in insulin-dependent dia-betes mellitus. Diabetes 1983; 32(suppl. 2): S92–5.

145. Hostetter TH, Rennke HG, Brenner BM. The case for intrarenal hypertension in the initiation and progression of diabetic and other glomerulopathies. Am J Med 1982; 72: 375–80.

146. Viberti GC. Prognostic significance of microalbuminuria in insulin dependent diabetes mellitus. Kidney Int 1992; 41: 836–9.

147. Schmitz A, Vaeth M. Microalbuminuria: a major risk factor in non-insulin-dependent diabetes. A 10 year follow-up study of 503 patients. Diabetic Med 1988; 5: 126–34.

148. Viberti GC, Hill BD, Jarrett RJ, et al. Microalbuminuria is a predic-tor of clinical nephropathy in insulin dependent diabetes mellitus. Lancet 1982; 2: 1430–2.

149. Parving HH, Jensen H, Mogensen CE, et al. Increased urinary albu-min excretion rate in benign essential hypertension. Lancet 1974; 1: 1190–2.

150. Yudkin JS, Forrest RD, Jackson CA. Microalbuminuria as a predic-tor of vascular disease in non-diabetic subjects. Islington Diabetic Survey. Lancet 1988; 2: 530–3.

151. Bar J, Hod M, Erman A, et al. Microalbuminuria: Prognostic and therapeutic implications in diabetic and hypertensive pregnancy. Diabet Med 1995; 12: 649–56.

152. Bar J, Hod M, Erman A, et al. Microalbuminuria as an early predic-tor of hypertensive complications in pregnant women at high risk. Am J Kidney Dis 1996; 28: 220–5.

153. Bar J, Kaplan B, Wittenberg C, et al. Microalbuminuria after preg-nancy complicated by pre-eclampsia. Nephrol Dial Transplant 1999; 14: 1129–32.

154. Friedman S, Rabinerson D, Bar J, et al. Microalbuminuria following gestational diabetes. Acta Obstet Gynecol Scand 1995; 74: 176–81.

155. Parving HH, Lehnert H, Brochner-Mortensen J, et al. The effect of Irbesartan on the development of diabetic nephropathy in patients with Type 2 diabetes. N Engl J Med 2001; 345: 870–8.

treated with ACE inhibitors before pregnancy. J Pediatr Endocrinol Metab 1999; 12: 659–65.

42 Diabetic retinopathy

Nir Melamed, Tamar Perri, Nino Loia and Moshe Hod

Introduction

Diabetic retinopathy is the most common chronic complication of diabetes mellitus,[1] and is the most common cause of blindness in middle-aged subjects in the United States and the United Kingdom.[2–5] The mutual effects of pregnancy and retinopathy, though long a subject of research and debate, remain unclear, and data on methods of diagnosis and management in pregnancy remain scarce.[6–10] The purpose of this chapter is to review the current literature on the effects of pregnancy on diabetic retinopathy, and to provide guidelines for the management of pregnancies complicated by diabetic retinopathy.

Diabetic retinopathy in nonpregnant patients

Epidemiology

The prevalence of diabetic retinopathy is almost 100% in patients with Type 1 diabetes and over 60% in patients with Type 2 diabetes in whom the disease has been present for more than 20 years.[11–13] In the population-based Wisconsin Epidemiologic Study of Diabetic Retinopathy, the prevalence of proliferative diabetic retinopathy was 1.2 and 67% in persons with Type 1 diabetes for less than 10 years and more than 35 years, respectively.

It is estimated that 20–30% of diabetic women in the reproductive age group has some evidence of retinopathy.[1] Risk factors for diabetic retinopathy include longer duration of the disease, onset of disease before 30 years of age, poor glycemic control manifested by higher levels of glycosylated hemoglobin, hypertension, hypertriglyceridemia, anemia, and evidence of diabetic nephropathy.[4,11,14–21]

Classification of diabetic retinopathy

Diabetic retinopathy is a progressive disorder, and is generally categorized as either *nonproliferative* (NPDR, or background) or *proliferative* (PDR), although more detailed grading systems exist,[22,23] as presented in Table 42.1. Grading is performed according to the semi-quantitative assessment of the morphological lesions on fundus photographs. The grading system considers mainly the type and number of retinopathy lesions, while the diagnostic value of the regional distribution of the lesions is largely unknown.[24]

Pathogenesis and natural history

Diabetic retinopathy is the result of several pathological processes that include loss of capillary pericytes, damage to capillary wall resulting in increased permeability and weakness of capillary wall, microvascular occlusion leading to retinal ischemia, and proliferation of new blood vessels. [25–28] It is currently believed that chronic hyperglycemia is the primary cause of diabetic retinopathy.[29–31] Although the exact mechanisms by which hyperglycemia initiates these pathological processes remain unclear, putative mechanisms include impaired autoregulation of retinal blood flow,[32] increased production of sorbitol by the enzyme aldose reductase,[33] accumulation of advanced glycation end-products,[34] oxidative stress,[35–37] increased platelets aggregation and hypercoagulability,[38] and alteration in cell signaling pathways such as diacylglycerol-induced protein kinase C activity.[39–41]

Nonproliferative diabetic retinopathy

Microaneurysms, hypercellular outpouchings from the capillary wall, are the earliest signs of diabetic retinopathy. They appear as small red dots (Figure 42.1), and can be identified in 2 and 98% of the patients with Type 1 diabetes in whom disease has been present for 2 and 15 years, respectively.[42] Possible mechanisms for the formation of microaneurysms include weakness of capillary wall and increased intraluminal pressure.[25,26] Rupture of microaneurysms results in retinal hemorrhages which may appear as either small dots or larger flame-shaped hemorrhages. As a result of the increased capillary permeability, lipids and proteins leak into the outer retina, appearing as well defined yellow-white deposits, known as hard exudates (Figure 42.2). Extravasation of fluids may lead to retinal thickening and edema. Although, in general, nonproliferative retinopathy does not impair vision, hard exudates or retinal edema involving the macular area may lead to severe loss of central vision.[43] Thus, diabetic macular edema (DME) is the most common cause of vision loss in nonproliferative diabetic retinopathy.[44]

318

Table 42.1 Diabetic Retinopathy Severity Scale

Classification	Description
Normal	No evidence of retinopathy
Nonproliferative	
Minimal	Microaneurysms only
Mild	Microaneurysms plus hard exudates, soft exudates (cotton wool spots), mild retinal hemorrhages, venous loops
Moderate	Microaneurysms plus mild intraretinal microvascular abnormalities (IRMA), moderate retinal hemorrhages, venous beading
Severe	Microaneurysms plus moderate to severe intraretinal microvascular abnormalities (IRMA), severe retinal hemorrhages, venous beading
Proliferative	
Proliferative	New vessels in the retina or on the optic disc
High-risk proliferative	Proliferative plus preretinal hemorrhage, fibrous tissue or other high risk characteristics
Advanced diabetic eye disease	Proliferative plus vitreous hemorrhage, retinal detachment or rubeosis iridis

Adapted from the Early Treatment Diabetic Retinopathy Study (ETDRS).[22]

Pre-proliferative diabetic retinopathy

As the disease progresses, retinal capillaries become occluded, leading to retinal ischemia. This stage, known as pre-proliferative retinopathy, is characterized by the appearance of white–grayish cotton-wool spots (soft exudates), reflecting the accumulation of axoplasmic debris due to ischemia-induced interruption of axoplasmic transport, and by the presence of microvascular abnormalities such as venous beading and loops.[22]

Proliferative diabetic retinopathy

The hallmark of proliferative retinopathy is retinal and pre-retinal neovascularization which occurs in response to the increased retinal ischemia (Figure 42.3).[45] Presumably, the nutrient-starved retina sends out a chemical message to stimulate the growth of new blood vessels (neovascularization).

These vessels often grow on the surface of the retina, at the optic nerve, or on the iris, and are characterized by increased fragility. They may penetrate the outlining membrane of the retina and become adherent, with their accompanying fibrovascular tissue, to the posterior vitreous. Visual loss in patients with proliferative retinopathy may be caused by either vitreous hemorrhage (VH), tractional retinal detachment following vitreous contraction, or neovascular glaucoma.[44,46,47] Several growth factors have been shown to be involved in the process of neovascularization, including vascular endothelial growth factor (VEGF),[48–57] insulin-like growth factor I (IGF-I),[58–65] growth hormone (GH),[66–72] pigment-epithelium-derived factor (PEDF),[73–79] placental growth factor (PGF),[80] basic fibroblast growth factor (bFGF),[81] hepatocyte growth factor (HGF),[82–84] and, recently, also erythropoietin (EPO).[85–87]

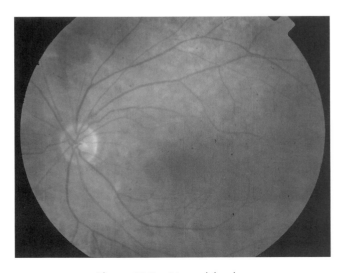

Figure 42.1 Normal fundus.

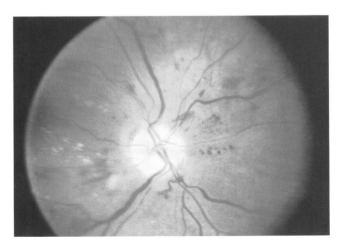

Figure 42.2 Nonproliferative diabetic retinopathy.

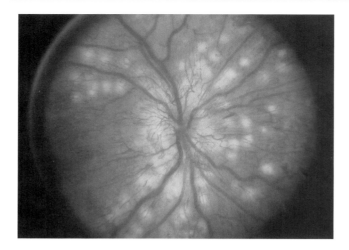

Figure 42.3   Proliferative retinopathy, after photocoagulation treatment.

The Diabetic Retinopathy Study Research Group[88] has identified four risk factors for severe visual loss in diabetic retinopathy, as shown in Box 42.1. Untreated, affected patients have a 30 and 50% risk of visual acuity deterioration to less than 5/200 within 3 and 5 years, respectively.

Treatment of diabetic retinopathy

Several preventative and therapeutic interventions have been shown to be effective in reducing the morbidity associated with diabetic retinopathy. Nevertheless, because of the limitations of these interventions, efforts are being made to improve the understanding of the mechanisms responsible for diabetic retinopathy. This may lead to the development of new therapies, several of which are currently under clinical trials.

Glycemic control

Preventing diabetic retinopathy from developing is the most effective approach to preserve vision. The results of the Diabetes Control and Complications Trial (DCCT)[30,89] have provided clear evidence that intensive glycemic control is associated with a remarkable reduction in the development and progression of diabetic retinopathy in patients with Type 1 diabetes. Subsequent studies supported this finding[90] and demonstrated similar beneficial effects in patients with Type 2 diabetes.[91–93]

Unexpectedly, it was found that some of the patients with pre-existing retinopathy had a transient worsening of their retinopathy after the institution of intensive glycemic control.[30,94–97] This deterioration manifested as an increase in soft exudates and blot hemorrhages, but progression to proliferative retinopathy was uncommon. Although the reason for this transient worsening in not clear, possible mechanisms include reduced plasma volume, or increased levels of growth factors such IGF-I and VEGF.[98–100] Among patients with mild to moderate nonproliferative retinopathy, the long-term benefits of intensive glycemic control exceed the risk of this transient worsening. However, in patients with severe nonproliferative or proliferative retinopathy, photocoagulation may be indicated before intensive glycemic control is initiated.[94]

Multifactorial risk reduction

Control of hypertension, a risk factor for diabetic retinopathy, appears to delay the progression of retinopathy in patients with Type 2 diabetes.[16,21,101] High serum lipid levels are associated with increased risk of hard exudates, macular edema, and proliferative retinopathy.[102,103] Normalization of lipid levels may reduce this risk.

Antiplatelet agents

The increased platelet aggregation observed in diabetic patients and the evidence of microthromboses in retinal capillaries[38] suggested that treatment with antiplatelet agents may be beneficial in diabetic retinopathy. However, in the Early Treatment of Diabetic Retinopathy Study (ETDRS), treatment with daily aspirin had no effect on the development or progression of diabetic retinopathy.[104,105]

Laser photocoagulation

Argon-laser photocoagulation, which was introduced in the 1950s, is the primary treatment for advanced retinopathy. In the Diabetic Retinopathy Study (DRS), panretinal photocoagulation in patients with proliferative retinopathy was associated with 50% reduction in severe vision loss.[88,106,107] In the ETDRS, the use of panretinal photocoagulation at earlier stages of retinopathy (mild to moderate nonproliferative retinopathy) was not found to be beneficial, and was associated with significant loss of visual acuity and peripheral vision.[108] However, focal photocoagulation in areas of vascular abnormality was found to be effective in reducing the risk of moderate visual loss in cases of macular edema.[108] Although the mechanism responsible for the beneficial effect

---

Box 42.1   High-risk characteristics for severe visual loss from proliferative retinopathy*

1. New vessels on or within one disc diameter of the optic disc and at least one-fourth of the disc area in extent, with or without pre-retinal or vitreous hemorrhage.
2. Any new vessels on or within one disc diameter of the optic disk, with pre-retinal or vitreous hemorrhage.
3. New vessels anywhere in the retina more than one disc diameter from the optic disk and at least one-half of the disc area in extent (including the total area of all new vessels in the ocular fundus), with pre-retinal or vitreous hemorrhage.
4. Extensive pre-retinal or vitreous hemorrhage that hides probable new vessels meeting the above criteria.

*The Diabetic Retinopathy Study Research Group. Arch Ophthalmol 1979.

of panretinal photocoagulation is unclear, it was suggested that the destruction of hypoxic regions in the peripheral retina reduces the stimulus for neovascularization.[29] Because of the possible side effects associated with panretinal photocoagulation (loss of peripheral vision and impaired night vision), this treatment is usually recommended only in cases of high-risk proliferative retinopathy.[108] However, patients with Type 2 diabetes can benefit from laser photocoagulation at earlier stages of the disease (severe nonproliferative or early-proliferative retinopathy).[108,109]

Vitrectomy

Vitrectomy, which includes removal of the vitreous gel and may be accompanied by removal of fibrous tissue and repair of retinal detachment, is associated with dramatic improvement of vision in cases of severe vitreous hemorrhage (VH),[110–112] as well as in cases of very severe neovascularization with no evidence of VH.[113–117]

Experimental therapies

Better understanding of the mechanisms and factors involved in the pathogenesis of diabetic retinopathy (as described earlier) has led to exploration of new drugs directed against these factors, some of which are currently under clinical trials. Examples include aldose reductase inhibitors,[33,118–120] protein kinase C inhibitors, antioxidants, inhibition of nonenzymatic glycation of proteins (aminoguanidine),[121] VEGF inhibitors,[122,123] intraocular gene therapy with the PEDF gene,[124,125] and somatostatin analogues (reduce GH and IGF-I levels).[126]

Inhibition of VEGF has been shown to prevent neovascularization in animal models.[122,127,128] In a phase 2 clinical trial, Pegaptanib, a VEGF inhibitor approved by the Food and Drug Administration (FDA) for the treatment of exudative age-related macular degeneration, was associated with improved visual acuity, decreased retinal thickness, and decreased need for photocoagulation.[123]

Diabetic retinopathy in pregnancy

Impact of pregnancy on the development and progression of diabetic retinopathy

Understanding the effect of pregnancy on diabetic retinopathy is essential for determining the optimal management of pregnancies complicated by diabetic retinopathy. However, whether pregnancy influences the development or progression of diabetic retinopathy is still unanswered. Several studies have reported that pregnancy is associated with progression of retinopathy in 17 to 70% of the cases,[129–139] whereas other studies have failed to support these findings.[140–144]

Studies supporting a deteriorating effect of pregnancy on diabetic retinopathy

Moloney et al.[131] prospectively followed 53 pregnant women with Type 1 diabetes every 6 weeks during pregnancy and until 6 months postpartum. Of the 20 women who had no evidence of retinopathy, eight (40%) developed retinopathy during pregnancy. Progression of pre-existing retinopathy during pregnancy was common, with a moderate increase in the number of microaneurysms, and the appearance of retinal hemorrhages and soft exudates in 56 and 28% of the cases, respectively. The risk for the development and progression of retinopathy was related to the duration of diabetes.

Dibble et al.[130] followed 55 pregnant diabetics who were managed by strict glycemic control. Progression of retinopathy was related the duration of diabetes and the severity of retinopathy before pregnancy. Thus, progression of retinopathy occurred in 16% (3 of 19) of the women with minimal or mild nonproliferative retinopathy, compared with 86% (6 of 7) of the women with untreated pre-existing proliferative retinopathy. Similarly, in a prospective cohort study of 145 pregnant women with Type 1 diabetes,[135] Serup found that none of the women with White classes B or C (no evidence of retinopathy) developed persistent retinopathy as a consequence of pregnancy, while deterioration was noticed in 50% of the women with pre-existing retinopathy. Additional support to the role of the severity of retinopathy as a risk factor for progression during pregnancy comes from a retrospective study of 23 pregnant diabetic women.[132] While none of the women with either no evidence of retinopathy (n = 10) or nonproliferative retinopathy (n = 8) experienced progression of retinopathy during pregnancy, four of the five women with proliferative retinopathy required photocoagulation during pregnancy due to progression of retinopathy.

In a prospective study of 234 intensively treated pregnant diabetics,[129] Jervell et al. reported that the development or progression retinopathy occurred in 68 women (29%). Nevertheless, progression was rarely associated with loss of visual acuity.

In order to quantify the effect of pregnancy on diabetic retinopathy, Soubrane et al. followed 22 pregnant diabetics using serial fluorescein angiography examinations.[133] The mean number of microaneurysms increased from 42.7 before pregnancy to 56.7 at the 28th week and to 79.7 at the 35th week. This number decreased to 62.7 and 60.3 at 6 and 15 months postpartum, respectively. Similarly, Hellstedt et al.[139] followed the number of microaneurysms in 21 diabetic women with mild retinopathy. Microaneurysms were assessed during pregnancy and at 3 and 6 months postpartum using red-free photographs. The number of microaneurysms increased progressively during pregnancy and peaked at 3 months postpartum. This increase was related to degree of improvement in glycemic control.

Phelps et al.[134] prospectively studied 35 pregnant women with Type 1 diabetes under tight glycemic control. Progression of nonproliferative retinopathy, noticed in 55% of the women, correlated with the levels of plasma glucose at entry, and with the magnitude of improvement in glycemic control.

Klein et al.[136] assessed the effect of pregnancy on diabetic retinopathy using a control group of nonpregnant Type 1 diabetic women. In addition to poor glycemic control, pregnancy *per se* was a significant and independent risk factor for progression of retinopathy.

Rosenn et al.[137] reported a progression rate of 33% in a prospective study of 154 pregnant women with Type 1 diabetes. They have found that hypertension, either chronic or pregnancy-induced, was a significant and independent risk factor for progression of retinopathy. Level of glycemic control and improved glycemic control in early pregnancy were also associated with progression of retinopathy.

In the Diabetes in Early Pregnancy Study (DIEPS),[138] the risk of progression was strongly correlated with the severity of retinopathy before pregnancy. Thus, progression of more than two steps was noted in 10.3, 21.1, 18.8, and 54.8% of the women with no retinopathy, minimal (microaneurysms only), mild, and moderate-to-severe retinopathy at baseline, respectively. Progression to proliferative retinopathy was observed in 6.3 and 29% of the women with mild and moderate-to-severe retinopathy, respectively. Other factors associated with progression of retinopathy included elevated baseline glycosylated hemoglobin and the magnitude of improvement of glycemic control in early pregnancy.

In another prospective study,[8] 65 diabetic women were followed during pregnancy and 12 months postpartum. While the overall progression rate was 77.5%, only 26% of the women with no retinopathy at baseline had evidence of retinopathy during pregnancy. Duration of diabetes, poor glycemic control, anemia, and elevated systolic blood pressure were also risk factors for progression of retinopathy.

Lovestam-Adrian et al.[142] retrospectively compared a group of 65 pregnant women with Type 1 diabetes with a matched group of nonpregnant women. They have found pre-eclampsia to be a potent independent risk factor for progression of retinopathy.

Studies not supporting a significant effect of pregnancy on progression of retinopathy

There are several studies that failed to demonstrate a significant effect of pregnancy on the natural history of diabetic retinopathy. In another group of studies, although retinopathy progressed during pregnancy, complete or partial regression was observed after delivery.

Stephens et al.[140] found the rate of development of retinopathy during pregnancy to be as low as 2%. Horvat et al.,[141] in a prospective study extending over 12 years, followed 172 diabetic women during pregnancy. Of the 40 women with nonproliferative retinopathy, only four (10%) progressed to proliferative retinopathy. They have found retinopathy to fluctuate during pregnancies, with simultaneous progression and regression of retinopathy in different parts of the same eye. Their conclusion was that pregnancy is not associated with an increased risk for progression of retinopathy and visual loss.

In a retrospective study,[142] the progression of retinopathy in 65 pregnant women with Type 1 diabetes was compared to a matched control group of 56 nonpregnant Type 1 diabetic women. The rate of sight-threatening deterioration of retinopathy was similar for the two groups (13%, 11%, respectively).

Temple et al. prospectively studied 179 pregnancies of Type 1 diabetic women.[144] The overall rate of progression of retinopathy during pregnancy was only 5%, and the rate of progression to proliferative retinopathy necessitating laser therapy was 2.2%.

In the Diabetes Control and Complications Trial (DCCT),[143] although pregnancy was associated with a greater risk for worsening of retinopathy, this worsening was transient, and the long-term risk for progression of retinopathy does not appear to be increased by pregnancy.

Some of the studies cited earlier have reported partial or complete regression of the pregnancy-related worsening of retinopathy. Moloney et al.[131] reported that by 6 months postpartum, the nonproliferative changes had regressed to control levels, and neovascularization showed some regression. Similarly, Serup et al.[135] reported that postpartum regression was common and that proliferative changes that developed during pregnancy disappeared spontaneously after delivery in most of the cases. For this reason, the authors recommended that treatment with photocoagulation during pregnancy and in the early postpartum period should be restricted. In the study of Rosenn et al.,[137] postpartum regression was observed in 13 of the 51 women (25%) in whom progression of retinopathy occurred during pregnancy.

Suggested mechanism

Several mechanisms have been suggested by which pregnancy may lead to progression of retinopathy. Pregnancy is associated with a dramatic change in the hormonal milieu. Human placental lactogen (hPL) is produced in enormous amounts by the placenta, reaching a production rate of about 1 g/day at term. Due to its growth hormone-like activity, hPL may play an important role in the effect of pregnancy on diabetic retinopathy, as mentioned earlier.[66,67,69] The vascular changes induced by the elevated levels of estrogen and progesterone during pregnancy may also contribute to progression of retinopathy.

Pregnancy is also associated with marked physiological changes. The pregnancy-induced increase in cardiac output may lead to increased retinal blood flow, which could damage diabetic vessels. Chen et al.studied the changes in retinal blood flow (RBF) during pregnancy in diabetic and nondiabetic women using laser Doppler velocimetry.[145] Among the diabetic women, only those whose retinopathy progressed had a significant increase in RBF during pregnancy. However, as these patients also had worse glycemic control (higher glycosylated hemoglobin levels prior to and throughout pregnancy), it is not clear if the deterioration can be attributed to the increase in retinal blood flow alone.

As mentioned earlier, hypertension is a risk factor for the progression of diabetic retinopathy.[11,14,16,20,21,137] Hypertensive disorders are common in diabetic pregnancies, complicating up to 40% of pregnancies in Type 1 diabetic women.[146] Thus, hypertension may contribute to the progression of retinopathy during pregnancy.

Another possible mechanism is the improved glycemic control achieved by most of the diabetic women before or at the onset of pregnancy. As discussed earlier, rapid normalization of blood glucose is associated with progression of retinopathy both in nonpregnant[94–97] and pregnant[134,137–139] patients.

Summary

In summary, it appears that pregnancy is associated with progression of diabetic retinopathy, and that the risk for progression is related the factors presented in Table 42.2. One major

Table 42.2   Risk factors for progression of retinopathy during pregnancy

Risk factor	References
Non-modifiable	
Duration of diabetes	8, 130, 131
Severity of retinopathy before conception	130, 135, 138
Poor glycemic control before conception	8, 134, 137, 138
Modifiable	
Chronic or pregnancy induced hypertension	8, 137, 142
Rapid normalization of blood glucose values	134, 137, 138, 139
Anemia	8

drawback of many of thee studies presented above is the lack of a matched control group of nonpregnant diabetic women. The progression of retinopathy during pregnancy may be the result of the normal hormonal and physiological changes during pregnancy, as well as the improved glycemic control and high rate of hypertensive disorders observed in diabetic pregnancies. Nevertheless, these changes may regress postpartum, especially in cases of nonproliferative retinopathy, and may not affect the long-term progression of retinopathy.[143]

Diabetic retinopathy and perinatal outcome

Several investigators have addressed the issue of a possible relationship between diabetic retinopathy and perinatal outcome. Moloney et al.[131] noted that maternal retinal hemorrhages or neovascularization were associated with increased infant morbidity. McElvy et al.[147] performed a prospective study of 205 pregnant women with Type 1 diabetes. Development or progression of retinopathy during pregnancy was significantly associated with reduced fetal growth, manifested by lower mean birthweight and a higher rate of small for gestational age (SGA) and low birthweight (LBW) infants. There was no correlation between progression of retinopathy and gestational age at delivery, preterm delivery, respiratory distress syndrome, neonatal hypoglycemia, or neonatal death.

Klein et al.[148] reported adverse perinatal outcome in 33 of 179 diabetic pregnancies. Severity of retinopathy was the only variable that significantly predicted adverse perinatal outcome.

Lauszus et al.[149] reviewed the records of 26 diabetic pregnancies with pre-existing proliferative retinopathy. Proliferative retinopathy was associated with increased preterm delivery rate (27%) and serious neonatal morbidity.

Management of diabetic retinopathy during pregnancy

As discussed earlier, diabetic retinopathy can worsen during pregnancy. Thus, patients with diabetic retinopathy should undergo preconception counseling and follow-up during pregnancy by a multidisciplinary team that includes a perinatologist, endocrinologist, and ophthalmologist that are experienced in the management of diabetic retinopathy.

Preconception counseling

Patients with diabetes who are planning to become pregnant should be given a thorough explanation on the risk of development or progression of diabetic retinopathy during pregnancy, and the importance of glycemic control throughout pregnancy. Patients with high-risk characteristics (longstanding diabetes, severe retinopathy, coexisting hypertension, poor glycemic control) should be identified and followed appropriately.

A comprehensive eye examination prior to conception should be performed by an ophthalmologist experienced in the care of diabetic retinopathy. This examination carries great importance since it determines the risk for progression of retinopathy, the frequency of follow-up visits during pregnancy, as well as the need for laser photocoagulation prior to conception.

Glycemic control should be achieved prior to conception in order to reduce the risk of progression of retinopathy, as well as to avoid the adverse maternal and fetal outcome associated with poorly controlled diabetes during pregnancy. One goal is to achieve a glycosylated hemoglobin level of less than 6 standard deviations above normal prior to conception.[138] In the presence of proliferative or severe nonproliferative retinopathy, normalization of blood glucose levels should be achieved gradually over a period of weeks to months in order to avoid progression of retinopathy that may result form rapid normalization. However, in patients presenting after conception, blood glucose should be normalized as soon as possible, since the benefits of good glycemic control in early pregnancy far outweigh the risk of transient progression of retinopathy. Other risk factors, such as uncontrolled chronic hypertension, should be followed and treated adequately prior to conception.

One question that needs to be answered is the role of laser photocoagulation prior to conception. As discussed earlier, the ETDRS have found that in Type 1 diabetes, panretinal photocoagulation is beneficial mainly in cases of high-risk proliferative retinopathy and clinically significant macular edema. However, it is recommended that in cases of impending pregnancy, during which rapid progression of retinopathy may occur, photocoagulation should be instituted at earlier stages, as in cases of severe nonproliferative or early proliferative retinopathy.[108,109] In one study of women with proliferative retinopathy, treatment with laser photocoagulation before conception was associated with significant progression of retinopathy in 26% of the women, compared with 58% when treatment was initiated in early pregnancy.[150]

Antenatal follow-up

The frequency of eye examinations during pregnancy depends on the severity of retinopathy prior to conception, evidence of progression of retinopathy, glycemic control, duration of diabetes, and the presence of other risk factors such as hypertension. Thus, patients with no or minimal retinopathy should be evaluated in the first and third trimesters. Patients with mild to moderate retinopathy should undergo evaluation each trimester. In cases of severe nonproliferative or proliferative retinopathy, when there is evidence of progression of retinopathy, and in patients with poor glycemic control or hypertension, follow up may be needed every 2 to 4 weeks. [136,138,143,151,152]

Fluorescein angiography is a sensitive tool to assess the extent of capillary nonperfusion and early neovascularization, and may aid in guiding treatment of macular edema, although ophthalmoscopic examination is satisfactory in most of the cases for the diagnosis of proliferative retinopathy. In addition, although detrimental effects of fluorescein dye on the fetus have not been documented,[153] fluorescein does cross the placenta into the fetal circulation. Thus, fluorescein angiography during pregnancy is generally not indicated.

Laser photocoagulation during pregnancy

The use of laser photocoagulation during pregnancy is controversial. In general, the indications for treatment and the response to laser photocoagulation are the same as for non-pregnant women.[154,155] As described above, several studies reported that postpartum regression of the pregnancy-induced progression of retinopathy is common,[131,135] and the authors recommended that treatment with photocoagulation during pregnancy and in the early postpartum period should be restricted. In contrast, others believe that because the progression of retinopathy during pregnancy can be at times rapid and aggressive, treatment with laser photocoagulation should be applied during pregnancy and after delivery when indicated.[130,156,157] Thus, the decision whether to treat should be made on an individual basis, taking into account the severity of retinopathy, evidence of progression, lack of glycemic control, the presence of additional risk factors, and, on the other hand, the risks and side effects associated with laser photocoagulation.

According to the ETDRS,[158] in patients with diabetic macular edema, focal photocoagulation should be performed during pregnancy, because spontaneous regression rarely occurs after delivery. If the edema does not respond well to photocoagulation, hospitalization is required, with diuretic treatment and occasionally steroids.[159]

Insulin analogues during pregnancy and diabetic retinopathy

In addition to its metabolic effects that are mediated by the insulin receptor, insulin also has a mitogenic effect, currently thought to be mediated by the IGF-I receptor. The possible role of IGF-I in the pathogeneses of diabetic retinopathy (discussed earlier) and the change in the relative affinity of the insulin analogues toward the IGF-I receptor have raised concerns regarding the effect of these analogues on diabetic retinopathy. Insulin lispro has a 1.5-fold higher affinity toward the IGF-I receptor compared with human insulin, and the initial suggestion that insulin lispro may worsen retinopathy was made by Kitzmiller et al.[160] In this study, of the ten patients who were treated with insulin lispro and had no evidence of retinopathy prior to conception, three developed bilateral proliferative changes, and two developed vitreous hemorrhage during pregnancy. However, these patients had poor glycemic control at baseline and experienced significant improvement

in glycemic control during pregnancy, two major risk factors that may be responsible for the progression of retinopathy in these cases. Subsequent studies did not support an effect of insulin lispro on retinopathy.[161–164] Insulin aspart is similar to insulin lispro in many aspects, although its affinity to the IGF-I receptor is the same as human insulin.[165] There is only little data on insulin aspart in pregnancy, and currently it remains a category C medication for pregnancy.[161] The results of multicentric study now in progress on the efficacy and safety of insulin aspart in Type 1 pregnant diabetic patients will provide important information on the safety of insulin aspart during pregnancy.[166] Insulin glargine has a higher affinity to IGF-I receptor and a greater mitogenic activity compared with human insulin (6.5-fold and 8-fold, respectively),[165] which raised concerns on its effects diabetic retinopathy. Two randomized trials demonstrated an increased risk of progression of retinopathy[167] and a higher incidence of new onset macular edema.[168] However, there was lack of consistency between the methods of assessment, and a subsequent prospective randomized studies did not support this observations. A large 5-year randomized multicenter study is in progress.[161] For the moment, the use of insulin glargine during pregnancy is not recommended. The affinity of insulin detemir to IGF-I receptor is 5-fold lower than human insulin, and its mitogenic activity is reduced by 10-fold.[165] There are no data on the use of insulin detemir in pregnancy.

Delivery

Earlier studies recommended early delivery, as soon as lung maturation was achieved, in pregnancies complicated by retinopathy and other vascular diseases. However, more recent research has shown that a well-controlled diabetic pregnancy can be allowed to continue to term in order to avoid iatrogenic prematurity, the risk of amniocentesis, failed induction of labor due to unfavorable cervix, and unnecessary Cesarean section.[169]

The Valsalva maneuver during labor might induce vitreous hemorrhage from active neovascularization.[170,171] The role of elective Cesarean section in these cases is controversial. The mode of delivery should be discussed in advance between patient and obstetrician. A summary of recommendations for management is presented in Figure 42.4.

Summary

Diabetic retinopathy is the most common chronic complication of diabetes mellitus, and it is estimated that 20–30% of diabetic women in the reproductive age group has some evidence of retinopathy.

The purpose of this chapter was to review the current literature on the effects of pregnancy on diabetic retinopathy, and to provide guidelines for the management of pregnancies complicated by diabetic retinopathy.

It appears that pregnancy is associated with progression of diabetic retinopathy, especially in women with the risk factors presented in Table 42.2, although these changes may regress postpartum, especially in cases of nonproliferative retinopathy, and may not affect the long-term progression of retinopathy. In addition, the presence of diabetic retinopathy is associated with adverse pregnancy outcome, including fetal growth restriction, and preterm delivery.

Patients with diabetic retinopathy should undergo preconception counseling and follow-up during pregnancy by a multidisciplinary team as summarized in Figure 42.4. It is now clear that White's advice in 1971 to terminate pregnancies in diabetic patients with progressive proliferative retinopathy is no longer valid,[172] and that with careful professional care, a favorable pregnancy outcome can usually be expected with minimal or no deterioration in ophthalmologic status. Ongoing trials may provide better answers regarding the use of laser photocoagulation and the safety of insulin analogues during pregnancy.

Preconception Counseling

- **Patient education** - explanation on the risk of development or progression of diabetic retinopathy during pregnancy, and the importance of glycemic control during pregnancy.

- **Risk stratification** –identification of patients with high-risk characteristics

- **Comprehensive eye examination**

- **Improve of glycemic control** – should be achieved gradually, especially in patients with advanced retinopathy.

- **Control of co-existing hypertension**

- **Laser photocoagulation** should be considered in patients with severe non-proliferative or proliferative retinopathy

Antenatal Care

- **Multidisciplinary team** - perinatologist, endocrinologist and ophthalmologist that are experienced in the management of diabetic retinopathy.

- Frequency of eye **examinations**:

No – minimal retinopathy	1st, 3rd trimesters
Mild – moderate retinopathy	1st, 2nd, 3rd trimesters
Severe NPDR, PDR Evidence of progression Poor glycemic control Other risk factors	Every 2-4 weeks

- **Fluorescein angiography** is usually avoided during pregnancy

- **Laser photocoagulation** – Because postpartum regression is common, laser photocoagulation should be considered in cases severe non-proliferative or proliferative retinopathy on an individual basis considering the severity of retinopathy, evidence of progression, lack of glycemic control, and the presence of additional risk factors.

- **Macular edema** should be treated with focal laser photocoagulation, diuretics, or steroids.

Delivery

- There is no need for labor induction in women with good glycemic control.

- In cases of high-risk proliferative retinopathy, **elective cesarean section** or **shortening of the second stage** should be considered due to the risk of vitreous hemorrhage.

Figure 42.4   Recommendations for the management of pregnancies complicated by diabetic retinopathy.

REFERENCES

1. Reece EA, Homko CJ, Hagay Z. Diabetic retinopathy in pregnancy. Obstet Gynecol Clin North Am 1996; 23: 161–71.
2. Kahn HA, Hiller R. Blindness caused by diabetic retinopathy. Am J Ophthalmol 1974; 78: 58–67.
3. Foulds WS, McCuish A, Barrie T, et al. Diabetic retinopathy in the West of Scotland: its detection and prevalence, and the cost-effectiveness of a proposed screening programme. Health Bull (Edinb.) 1983; 41: 318–26.
4. Kahn HA, Bradley RF. Prevalence of diabetic retinopathy. Age, sex, and duration of diabetes. Br J Ophthalmol 1975; 59: 345–9.
5. Klein R, Klein B. Vision disorders in diabetes. Diabetes in America. (DHHS publication number 85-1468). United States Government Printing Office, 1985.
6. Cassar J, Kohner EM, Hamilton AM, Gordon H, Joplin GF. Diabetic retinopathy and pregnancy. Diabetologia 1978; 15: 105–11.
7. Elman KD, Welch RA, Frank RN, Goyert GL, Sokol RJ. Diabetic retinopathy in pregnancy: a review. Obstet Gynecol 1990; 75: 119–27.
8. Axer-Siegel R, Hod M, Fink-Cohen S, et al. Diabetic retinopathy during pregnancy. Ophthalmology 1996; 103: 1815–9.
9. Hare JW, White P. Pregnancy in diabetes complicated by vascular disease. Diabetes 1977; 26: 953–5.
10. Carstensen LL, Frost-Larsen K, Fugleberg S, Nerup J. Does pregnancy influence the prognosis of uncomplicated insulin-dependent diabetes mellitus? Diabetes Care 1982; 5: 1–5.
11. Klein R, Klein BE, Moss SE, Davis MD, DeMets DL. The Wisconsin epidemiologic study of diabetic retinopathy. II. Prevalence and risk of diabetic retinopathy when age at diagnosis is less than 30 years. Arch Ophthalmol 1984; 102: 520–6.
12. Aiello LP, Gardner TW, King GL, et al. Diabetic retinopathy. Diabetes Care 1998; 21: 143–56.
13. Fong DS, Aiello L, Gardner TW, et al. Diabetic retinopathy. Diabetes Care 2003; 26(suppl. 1): S99–102.
14. Klein R, Klein BE, Moss SE, Cruickshanks KJ. The Wisconsin Epidemiologic Study of Diabetic Retinopathy: XVII. The 14-year incidence and progression of diabetic retinopathy and associated risk factors in type 1 diabetes. Ophthalmology 1998; 105: 1801–15.
15. Nguyen HT, Luzio SD, Dolben J, et al. Dominant risk factors for retinopathy at clinical diagnosis in patients with type II diabetes mellitus. J Diabetes Complications 1996; 10: 211–9.
16. Okudaira M, Yokoyama H, Otani T, Uchigata Y, Iwamoto Y. Slightly elevated blood pressure as well as poor metabolic control are risk factors for the progression of retinopathy in early-onset Japanese Type 2 diabetes. J Diabetes Complications 2000; 14: 281–7.
17. Klein R, Klein BE, Moss SE. The Wisconsin epidemiological study of diabetic retinopathy: a review. Diabetes Metab Rev 1989; 5: 559–70.
18. Klein R, Moss SE, Klein BE, Davis MD, DeMets DL. The Wisconsin epidemiologic study of diabetic retinopathy. XI. The incidence of macular edema. Ophthalmology 1989; 96: 1501–10.
19. Henricsson M, Berntorp K, Berntorp E, Fernlund P, Sundkvist G. Progression of retinopathy after improved metabolic control in type 2 diabetic patients. Relation to IGF-1 and hemostatic variables. Diabetes Care 1999; 22: 1944–9.
20. Rand LI, Krolewski AS, Aiello LM, et al. Multiple factors in the prediction of risk of proliferative diabetic retinopathy. N Engl J Med 1985; 313: 1433–8.
21. Knowler WC, Bennett PH, Ballintine EJ. Increased incidence of retinopathy in diabetics with elevated blood pressure. A six-year follow-up study in Pima Indians. N Engl J Med 1980; 302: 645–50.
22. Grading diabetic retinopathy from stereoscopic color fundus photographs – an extension of the modified Airlie House classification. ETDRS report number 10. Early Treatment Diabetic Retinopathy Study Research Group. Ophthalmology 1991; 98: 786–806.
23. Wilkinson CP, Ferris 3rd FL, Klein RE, et al. Proposed international clinical diabetic retinopathy and diabetic macular edema disease severity scales. Ophthalmology 2003; 110: 1677–82.
24. Bek T, Helgesen A. The regional distribution of diabetic retinopathy lesions may reflect risk factors for progression of the disease. Acta Ophthalmol Scand 2001; 79: 501–5.
25. Engerman RL. Pathogenesis of diabetic retinopathy. Diabetes 1989; 38: 1203–6.
26. Frank RN. On the pathogenesis of diabetic retinopathy. A 1990 update. Ophthalmology 1991; 98: 586–93.
27. Palmberg P, Smith M, Waltman S, et al. The natural history of retinopathy in insulin-dependent juvenile-onset diabetes. Ophthalmology 1981; 88: 613–8.
28. Mizutani M, Kern TS, Lorenzi M. Accelerated death of retinal microvascular cells in human and experimental diabetic retinopathy. J Clin Invest 1996; 97: 2883–90.
29. Frank RN. Diabetic retinopathy. N Engl J Med 2004; 350: 48–58.
30. The effect of intensive treatment of diabetes on the development and progression of long-term complications in insulin-dependent diabetes mellitus. The Diabetes Control and Complications Trial Research Group. N Engl J Med 1993; 329: 977–86.
31. Sheetz MJ, King GL. Molecular understanding of hyperglycemia's adverse effects for diabetic complications. JAMA 2002; 288: 2579–88.
32. Kohner EM, Patel V, Rassam SM. Role of blood flow and impaired autoregulation in the pathogenesis of diabetic retinopathy. Diabetes 1995; 44: 603–7.
33. A randomized trial of sorbinil, an aldose reductase inhibitor, in diabetic retinopathy. Sorbinil Retinopathy Trial Research Group. Arch Ophthalmol 1990; 108: 1234–44.
34. Brownlee M, Cerami A. The biochemistry of the complications of diabetes mellitus. Annu Rev Biochem 1981; 50: 385–432.
35. Kunisaki M, Bursell SE, Clermont AC, et al. Vitamin E prevents diabetes-induced abnormal retinal blood flow via the diacylglycerol–protein kinase C pathway. Am J Physiol 1995; 269: E239–46.
36. Bursell SE, Clermont AC, Aiello LP, et al. High-dose vitamin E supplementation normalizes retinal blood flow and creatinine clearance in patients with type 1 diabetes. Diabetes Care 1999; 22: 1245–51.
37. Kowluru RA, Tang J, Kern TS. Abnormalities of retinal metabolism in diabetes and experimental galactosemia. VII. Effect of long-term administration of antioxidants on the development of retinopathy. Diabetes 2001; 50: 1938–42.
38. Boeri D, Maiello M, Lorenzi M. Increased prevalence of microthromboses in retinal capillaries of diabetic individuals. Diabetes 2001; 50: 1432–9.
39. Xia P, Inoguchi T, Kern TS, et al. Characterization of the mechanism for the chronic activation of diacylglycerol–protein kinase C pathway in diabetes and hypergalactosemia. Diabetes 1994; 43: 1122–9.
40. Derubertis FR, Craven PA. Activation of protein kinase C in glomerular cells in diabetes. Mechanisms and potential links to the pathogenesis of diabetic glomerulopathy. Diabetes 1994; 43: 1–8.
41. Ishii H, Jirousek MR, Koya D, et al. Amelioration of vascular dysfunctions in diabetic rats by an oral PKC beta inhibitor. Science 1996; 272: 728–31.
42. Klein R. The epidemiology of diabetic retinopathy: findings from the Wisconsin Epidemiologic Study of Diabetic Retinopathy. Int Ophthalmol Clin 1987; 27: 230–8.
43. Klein R, Klein BE, Moss SE, Cruickshanks KJ. The Wisconsin Epidemiologic Study of Diabetic Retinopathy. XV. The long-term incidence of macular edema. Ophthalmology 1995; 102: 7–16.
44. Fong DS, Ferris 3rd FL, Davis MD, Chew EY. Causes of severe visual loss in the early treatment diabetic retinopathy study: ETDRS report no. 24. Early Treatment Diabetic Retinopathy Study Research Group. Am J Ophthalmol 1999; 127: 137–41.
45. Garner A. Histopathology of diabetic retinopathy in man. Eye 1993;7(pt 2): 250–3.
46. Davis MD. Vitreous contraction in proliferative diabetic retinopathy. Arch Ophthalmol 1965; 74: 741–51.
47. Tolentino FI, Lee PF, Schepens CL. Biomicroscopic study of vitreous cavity in diabetic retinopathy. Arch Ophthalmol 1966; 75: 238–46.
48. Sydorova M, Lee MS. Vascular endothelial growth factor levels in vitreous and serum of patients with either proliferative diabetic retinopathy or proliferative vitreoretinopathy. Ophthalmic Res 2005; 37: 188–90.
49. Caldwell RB, Bartoli M, Behzadian MA, et al. Vascular endothelial growth factor and diabetic retinopathy: role of oxidative stress. Curr Drug Targets 2005; 6: 511–24.
50. Rakoczy PE, Brankov M, Fonceca A, et al. Enhanced recombinant adeno-associated virus-mediated vascular endothelial growth factor expression in the adult mouse retina: a potential model for diabetic retinopathy. Diabetes 2003; 52: 857–63.
51. Hogeboom van Buggenum IM, Polak BC, Reichert-Thoen JW, et al. Angiotensin converting enzyme inhibiting therapy is associated with

lower vitreous vascular endothelial growth factor concentrations in patients with proliferative diabetic retinopathy. Diabetologia 2002; 45: 203–9.

52. Simo R, Lecube A, Segura RM, Garcia Arumi J, Hernandez C. Free insulin growth factor-I and vascular endothelial growth factor in the vitreous fluid of patients with proliferative diabetic retinopathy. Am J Ophthalmol 2002; 134: 376–82.

53. Hernandez C, Burgos R, Canton A, et al. Vitreous levels of vascular cell adhesion molecule and vascular endothelial growth factor in patients with proliferative diabetic retinopathy: a case-control study. Diabetes Care 2001; 24: 516–21.

54. Funatsu H, Yamashita H, Shimizu E, Kojima R, Hori S. Relationship between vascular endothelial growth factor and interleukin-6 in diabetic retinopathy. Retina 2001; 21: 469–77.

55. Hammes HP, Lin J, Bretzel RG, Brownlee M, Breier G. Upregulation of the vascular endothelial growth factor/vascular endothelial growth factor receptor system in experimental background diabetic retinopathy of the rat. Diabetes 1998; 47: 401–6.

56. Burgos R, Simo R, Audi L, et al. Vitreous levels of vascular endothelial growth factor are not influenced by its serum concentrations in diabetic retinopathy. Diabetologia 1997; 40: 1107–9.

57. Clermont AC, Aiello LP, Mori F, Aiello LM, Bursell SE. Vascular endothelial growth factor and severity of nonproliferative diabetic retinopathy mediate retinal hemodynamics in vivo: a potential role for vascular endothelial growth factor in the progression of nonproliferative diabetic retinopathy. Am J Ophthalmol 1997; 124: 433–46.

58. Loukovaara S, Immonen IJ, Koistinen R, et al. The insulin-like growth factor system and Type 1 diabetic retinopathy during pregnancy. J Diabetes Complications 2005; 19: 297–304.

59. Poulaki V, Joussen AM, Mitsiades N, et al. Insulin-like growth factor-I plays a pathogenetic role in diabetic retinopathy. Am J Pathol 2004; 165: 457–69.

60. Simo R, Hernandez C, Segura RM, et al. Free insulin-like growth factor 1 in the vitreous fluid of diabetic patients with proliferative diabetic retinopathy: a case-control study. Clin Sci (Lond) 2003; 104: 223–30.

61. Inokuchi N, Ikeda T, Imamura Y, et al. Vitreous levels of insulin-like growth factor-I in patients with proliferative diabetic retinopathy. Curr Eye Res 2001; 23: 368–71.

62. Janssen JA, Jacobs ML, Derkx FH, et al. Free and total insulin-like growth factor I (IGF-I), IGF-binding protein-1 (IGFBP-1), and IGFBP-3 and their relationships to the presence of diabetic retinopathy and glomerular hyperfiltration in insulin-dependent diabetes mellitus. J Clin Endocrinol Metab 1997; 82: 2809–15.

63. Wang Q, Dills DG, Klein R, Klein BE, Moss SE. Does insulin-like growth factor I predict incidence and progression of diabetic retinopathy? Diabetes 1995; 44: 161–4.

64. Arner P, Sjoberg S, Gjotterberg M, Skottner A. Circulating insulin-like growth factor I in type 1 (insulin-dependent) diabetic patients with retinopathy. Diabetologia 1989; 32: 753–8.

65. Chantelau E. Evidence that upregulation of serum IGF-1 concentration can trigger acceleration of diabetic retinopathy. Br J Ophthalmol 1998; 82: 725–30.

66. Powell ED, Frantz AG, Rabkin MT, Field RA. Growth hormone in relation to diabetic retinopathy. N Engl J Med 1966; 275: 922–5.

67. Goebel FD, Ehrenreich H. Growth hormone and diabetic retinopathy. Lancet 1985; 2: 666.

68. Hattori N, Moridera K, Ishihara T, et al. Is growth hormone associated with diabetic retinopathy? J Diabetes Complications 1993; 7: 12–4.

69. Alzaid AA, Dinneen SF, Melton 3rd LJ, Rizza RA. The role of growth hormone in the development of diabetic retinopathy. Diabetes Care 1994; 17: 531–4.

70. McGowan LM, Kiser WR. Regarding the role of growth hormone in the development of diabetic retinopathy. Diabetes Care 1995; 18: 422–3.

71. Growth Hormone Antagonist for Proliferative Diabetic Retinopathy Study Group. The effect of a growth hormone receptor antagonist drug on proliferative diabetic retinopathy. Ophthalmology 2001; 108: 2266–72.

72. Chantelau E. Effect of a growth hormone receptor antagonist on proliferative diabetic retinopathy. Ophthalmology 2002; 109: 2187; author reply 2187–8.

73. Ogata N, Tombran-Tink J, Nishikawa M, et al. Pigment epithelium-derived factor in the vitreous is low in diabetic retinopathy and high in rhegmatogenous retinal detachment. Am J Ophthalmol 2001; 132: 378–82.

74. Ogata N, Nishikawa M, Nishimura T, Mitsuma Y, Matsumura M. Unbalanced vitreous levels of pigment epithelium-derived factor

and vascular endothelial growth factor in diabetic retinopathy. Am J Ophthalmol 2002; 134: 348–53.

75. Boehm BO, Lang G, Feldmann B, et al. Proliferative diabetic retinopathy is associated with a low level of the natural ocular anti-angiogenic agent pigment epithelium-derived factor (PEDF) in aqueous humor. a pilot study. Horm Metab Res 2003; 35: 382–6.

76. Boehm BO, Lang G, Volpert O, et al. Low content of the natural ocular anti-angiogenic agent pigment epithelium-derived factor (PEDF) in aqueous humor predicts progression of diabetic retinopathy. Diabetologia 2003; 46: 394–400.

77. Zhang SX, Wang JJ, Gao G, Parke K, Ma JX. Pigment epithelium-derived factor downregulates vascular endothelial growth factor (VEGF) expression and inhibits VEGF–VEGF receptor 2 binding in diabetic retinopathy. J Mol Endocrinol 2006; 37: 1–12.

78. Yamagishi S, Matsui T, Nakamura K, Inoue H. Pigment epithelium-derived factor is a pericyte mitogen secreted by microvascular endothelial cells: possible participation of angiotensin II-elicited PEDF downregulation in diabetic retinopathy. Int J Tissue React 2005; 27: 197–202.

79. Matsuoka M, Ogata N, Minamino K, Matsumura M. Expression of pigment epithelium-derived factor and vascular endothelial growth factor in fibrovascular membranes from patients with proliferative diabetic retinopathy. Jpn J Ophthalmol 2006; 50: 116–20.

80. Khaliq A, Foreman D, Ahmed A, et al. Increased expression of placenta growth factor in proliferative diabetic retinopathy. Lab Invest 1998; 78: 109–16.

81. Frank RN, Amin RH, Eliott D, Puklin JE, Abrams GW. Basic fibroblast growth factor and vascular endothelial growth factor are present in epiretinal and choroidal neovascular membranes. Am J Ophthalmol 1996; 122: 393–403.

82. Katsura Y, Okano T, Noritake M, et al. Hepatocyte growth factor in vitreous fluid of patients with proliferative diabetic retinopathy and other retinal disorders. Diabetes Care 1998; 21: 1759–63.

83. Hernandez C, Carrasco E, Garcia-Arumi J, Maria Segura R, Simo R. Intravitreous levels of hepatocyte growth factor/scatter factor and vascular cell adhesion molecule-1 in the vitreous fluid of diabetic patients with proliferative retinopathy. Diabetes Metab 2004; 30: 341–6.

84. Simo R, Lecube A, Garcia-Arumi J, Carrasco E, Hernandez C. Hepatocyte growth factor in the vitreous fluid of patients with proliferative diabetic retinopathy: its relationship with vascular endothelial growth factor and retinopathy activity. Diabetes Care 2004; 27: 287–8.

85. Demiroglu H. The balance between anemia, erythropoietin treatment, and elevated erythrocyte aggregation in patients with diabetic retinopathy and nephropathy: a hematologic point of view. Am J Ophthalmol 2003; 136: 776; author reply 776–7.

86. Katsura Y, Okano T, Matsuno K, et al. Erythropoietin is highly elevated in vitreous fluid of patients with proliferative diabetic retinopathy. Diabetes Care 2005; 28: 2252–4.

87. Watanabe D, Suzuma K, Matsui S, et al. Erythropoietin as a retinal angiogenic factor in proliferative diabetic retinopathy. N Engl J Med 2005; 353: 782–92.

88. The Diabetic Retinopathy Study Research Group. Four risk factors for severe visual loss in diabetic retinopathy. The third report from the Diabetic Retinopathy Study. Arch Ophthalmol 1979; 97: 654–5.

89. The Diabetes Control and Complications Trial/Epidemiology of Diabetes Interventions and Complications Research Group. Retinopathy and nephropathy in patients with type 1 diabetes four years after a trial of intensive therapy. N Engl J Med 2000; 342: 381–9.

90. Reichard P, Nilsson BY, Rosenqvist U. The effect of long-term intensified insulin treatment on the development of microvascular complications of diabetes mellitus. N Engl J Med 1993; 329: 304–9.

91. Klein R, Klein BE, Moss SE. Relation of glycemic control to diabetic microvascular complications in diabetes mellitus. Ann Intern Med 1996; 124: 90–6.

92. Ohkubo Y, Kishikawa H, Araki E, et al. Intensive insulin therapy prevents the progression of diabetic microvascular complications in Japanese patients with non-insulin-dependent diabetes mellitus: a randomized prospective 6-year study. Diabetes Res Clin Pract 1995; 28: 103–17.

93. UK Prospective Diabetes Study (UKPDS) Group. Intensive blood-glucose control with sulphonylureas or insulin compared with conventional treatment and risk of complications in patients with type 2 diabetes (UKPDS 33). Lancet 1998; 352: 837–53.

94. Early worsening of diabetic retinopathy in the Diabetes Control and Complications Trial. Arch Ophthalmol 1998; 116: 874–86.

95. Dahl-Jorgensen K, Brinchmann-Hansen O, Hanssen KF, Sandvik L, Aagenaes O. Rapid tightening of blood glucose control leads to transient deterioration of retinopathy in insulin dependent diabetes mellitus: the Oslo study. Br Med J (Clin Res Ed) 1985; 290: 811–5.

96. Lauritzen T, Frost-Larsen K, Larsen HW, Deckert T. Effect of 1 year of near-normal blood glucose levels on retinopathy in insulin-dependent diabetics. Lancet 1983; 1: 200–4.

97. The Kroc Collaborative Study Group. Diabetic retinopathy after two years of intensified insulin treatment. Follow-up of the Kroc Collaborative Study. JAMA 1988; 260: 37–41.

98. Chantelau E, Kohner EM. Why some cases of retinopathy worsen when diabetic control improves. BMJ 1997; 315: 1105–6.

99. Lu M, Amano S, Miyamoto K, et al. Insulin-induced vascular endothelial growth factor expression in retina. Invest Ophthalmol Vis Sci 1999; 40: 3281–6.

100. Carnesecchi S, Carpentier JL, Foti M, Szanto I. Insulin-induced vascular endothelial growth factor expression is mediated by the NADPH oxidase NOX3. Exp Cell Res 2006; 312: 3413–24.

101. UK Prospective Diabetes Study Group. Tight blood pressure control and risk of macrovascular and microvascular complications in type 2 diabetes: UKPDS 38. BMJ 1998; 317: 703–13.

102. Klein BE, Moss SE, Klein R, Surawicz TS. The Wisconsin Epidemiologic Study of Diabetic Retinopathy. XIII. Relationship of serum cholesterol to retinopathy and hard exudate. Ophthalmology 1991; 98: 1261–5.

103. Ferris 3rd FL, Chew EY, Hoogwerf BJ. Early Treatment Diabetic Retinopathy Study Research Group. Serum lipids and diabetic retinopathy. Diabetes Care 1996; 19: 1291–3.

104. Early Treatment Diabetic Retinopathy Study Research Group. Effects of aspirin treatment on diabetic retinopathy. ETDRS report number 8. Ophthalmology 1991; 98: 757–65.

105. Chew EY, Klein ML, Murphy RP, Remaley NA, Ferris 3rd FL. Effects of aspirin on vitreous/preretinal hemorrhage in patients with diabetes mellitus. Early Treatment Diabetic Retinopathy Study report no. 20. Arch Ophthalmol 1995; 113: 52–5.

106. The Diabetic Retinopathy Study Research Group. Preliminary report on effects of photocoagulation therapy. Am J Ophthalmol 1976; 81: 383–96.

107. The Diabetic Retinopathy Study Research Group. Photocoagulation treatment of proliferative diabetic retinopathy. Clinical application of Diabetic Retinopathy Study (DRS) findings, DRS Report Number 8. Ophthalmology 1981; 88: 583–600.

108. Early Treatment Diabetic Retinopathy Study Research Group. Early photocoagulation for diabetic retinopathy. ETDRS report number 9. Ophthalmology 1991; 98: 766–85.

109. Ferris F. Early photocoagulation in patients with either type I or type II diabetes. Trans Am Ophthalmol Soc 1996; 94: 505–37.

110. Machemer R, Norton EW. A new concept for vitreous surgery. 3. Indications and results. Am J Ophthalmol 1972; 74: 1034–56.

111. Machemer R. A new concept for vitreous surgery. 2. Surgical technique and complications. Am J Ophthalmol 1972; 74: 1022–33.

112. Machemer R, Parel JM, Buettner H. A new concept for vitreous surgery. I. Instrumentation. Am J Ophthalmol 1972; 73: 1–7.

113. Two-year course of visual acuity in severe proliferative diabetic retinopathy with conventional management. Diabetic Retinopathy Vitrectomy Study (DRVS) report #1. Ophthalmology 1985; 92: 492–502.

114. The Diabetic Retinopathy Vitrectomy Study Research Group. Early vitrectomy for severe vitreous hemorrhage in diabetic retinopathy. Two-year results of a randomized trial. Diabetic Retinopathy Vitrectomy Study report 2. Arch Ophthalmol 1985; 103: 1644–52.

115. The Diabetic Retinopathy Vitrectomy Study Research Group. Early vitrectomy for severe proliferative diabetic retinopathy in eyes with useful vision. Results of a randomized trial–Diabetic Retinopathy Vitrectomy Study Report 3. Ophthalmology 1988; 95: 1307–20.

116. The Diabetic Retinopathy Vitrectomy Study Research Group. Early vitrectomy for severe proliferative diabetic retinopathy in eyes with useful vision. Clinical application of results of a randomized trial–Diabetic Retinopathy Vitrectomy Study Report 4. Ophthalmology 1988; 95: 1321–34.

117. Early vitrectomy for severe vitreous hemorrhage in diabetic retinopathy. Four-year results of a randomized trial: Diabetic Retinopathy Vitrectomy Study Report 5. Arch Ophthalmol 1990; 108: 958–64.

118. Kador PF, Akagi Y, Takahashi Y, et al. Prevention of retinal vessel changes associated with diabetic retinopathy in galactose-fed dogs by aldose reductase inhibitors. Arch Ophthalmol 1990; 108: 1301–9.

119. Robinson Jr. WG, Laver NM, Jacot JL, et al. Diabetic-like retinopathy ameliorated with the aldose reductase inhibitor WAY-121,509. Invest Ophthalmol Vis Sci 1996; 37: 1149–56.

120. Sorbinil Retinopathy Trial Research Group. The sorbinil retinopathy trial: neuropathy results. Neurology 1993; 43: 1141–9.

121. Brownlee M, Vlassara H, Kooney A, Ulrich P, Cerami A. Aminoguanidine prevents diabetes-induced arterial wall protein cross-linking. Science 1986; 232: 1629–32.

122. Aiello LP, Pierce EA, Foley ED, et al. Suppression of retinal neovascularization in vivo by inhibition of vascular endothelial growth factor (VEGF) using soluble VEGF-receptor chimeric proteins. Proc Natl Acad Sci U S A 1995; 92: 10457–61.

123. Cunningham Jr. ET, Adamis AP, Altaweel M, et al. A phase II randomized double-masked trial of pegaptanib, an anti-vascular endothelial growth factor aptamer, for diabetic macular edema. Ophthalmology 2005; 112: 1747–57.

124. Mori K, Duh E, Gehlbach P, et al. Pigment epithelium-derived factor inhibits retinal and choroidal neovascularization. J Cell Physiol 2001; 188: 253–63.

125. Rasmussen H, Chu KW, Campochiaro P, et al. Clinical protocol. An open-label, phase I, single administration, dose-escalation study of ADGVPEDF.11D (ADPEDF) in neovascular age-related macular degeneration (AMD). Hum Gene Ther 2001; 12: 2029–32.

126. Grant MB, Mames RN, Fitzgerald C, et al. The efficacy of octreotide in the therapy of severe nonproliferative and early proliferative diabetic retinopathy: a randomized controlled study. Diabetes Care 2000; 23: 504–9.

127. Adamis AP, Shima DT, Tolentino MJ, et al. Inhibition of vascular endothelial growth factor prevents retinal ischemia-associated iris neovascularization in a nonhuman primate. Arch Ophthalmol 1996; 114: 66–71.

128. Robinson GS, Pierce EA, Rook SL, et al. Oligodeoxynucleotides inhibit retinal neovascularization in a murine model of proliferative retinopathy. Proc Natl Acad Sci USA 1996; 93: 4851–6.

129. Jervell J, Moe N, Skjaeraasen J, Blystad W, Egge K. Diabetes mellitus and pregnancy – management and results at Rikshospitalet, Oslo, 1970-1977. Diabetologia 1979; 16: 151–5.

130. Dibble CM, Kochenour NK, Worley RJ, Tyler FH, Swartz M. Effect of pregnancy on diabetic retinopathy. Obstet Gynecol 1982; 59: 699–704.

131. Moloney JB, Drury MI. The effect of pregnancy on the natural course of diabetic retinopathy. Am J Ophthalmol 1982; 93: 745–56.

132. Price JH, Hadden DR, Archer DB, Harley JM. Diabetic retinopathy in pregnancy. Br J Obstet Gynaecol 1984; 91: 11–7.

133. Soubrane G, Canivet J, Coscas G. Influence of pregnancy on the evolution of background retinopathy. Preliminary results of a prospective fluorescein angiography study. Int Ophthalmol 1985; 8: 249–55.

134. Phelps RL, Sakol P, Metzger BE, Jampol LM, Freinkel N. Changes in diabetic retinopathy during pregnancy. Correlations with regulation of hyperglycemia. Arch Ophthalmol 1986; 104: 1806–10.

135. Serup L. Influence of pregnancy on diabetic retinopathy. Acta Endocrinol Suppl. (Copenh.) 1986; 277: 122–4.

136. Klein BE, Moss SE, Klein R. Effect of pregnancy on progression of diabetic retinopathy. Diabetes Care 1990; 13: 34–40.

137. Rosenn B, Miodovnik M, Kranias G, et al. Progression of diabetic retinopathy in pregnancy: association with hypertension in pregnancy. Am J Obstet Gynecol 1992; 166: 1214–8.

138. Chew EY, Mills JL, Metzger BE, et al. Metabolic control and progression of retinopathy. The Diabetes in Early Pregnancy Study. National Institute of Child Health and Human Development Diabetes in Early Pregnancy Study. Diabetes Care 1995; 18: 631–7.

139. Hellstedt T, Kaaja R, Teramo K, Immonen I. The effect of pregnancy on mild diabetic retinopathy. Graefes Arch Clin Exp Ophthalmol 1997; 235: 437–41.

140. Stephens JW, Page OC, Hare RL. Diabetes and pregnancy. A report of experiences in 119 pregnancies over a period of ten years. Diabetes 1963; 12: 213–9.

141. Horvat M, Maclean H, Goldberg L, Crock GW. Diabetic retinopathy in pregnancy: a 12-year prospective survey. Br J Ophthalmol 1980; 64: 398–403.

142. Lovestam-Adrian M, Agardh CD, Aberg A, Agardh E. Pre-eclampsia is a potent risk factor for deterioration of retinopathy during pregnancy in Type 1 diabetic patients. Diabet Med 1997; 14: 1059–65.

143. The Diabetes Control and Complications Trial Research Group. Effect of pregnancy on microvascular complications in the diabetes control and complications trial. Diabetes Care 2000; 23: 1084–91.

144. Temple RC, Aldridge VA, Sampson MJ, et al. Impact of pregnancy on the progression of diabetic retinopathy in Type 1 diabetes. Diabet Med 2001; 18: 573–7.

145. Chen HC, Newsom RS, Patel V, et al. Retinal blood flow changes during pregnancy in women with diabetes. Invest Ophthalmol Vis Sci 1994; 35: 3199–208.

146. Cundy T, Slee F, Gamble G, Neale L. Hypertensive disorders of pregnancy in women with Type 1 and Type 2 diabetes. Diabet Med 2002; 19: 482–9.

147. McElvy SS, Demarini S, Miodovnik M, et al. Fetal weight and progression of diabetic retinopathy. Obstet Gynecol 2001; 97: 587–92.

148. Klein BE, Klein R, Meuer SM, Moss SE, Dalton DD. Does the severity of diabetic retinopathy predict pregnancy outcome? J Diabet Complications 1988; 2: 179–84.

149. Lauszus FF, Gron PL, Klebe JG. Pregnancies complicated by diabetic proliferative retinopathy. Acta Obstet Gynecol Scand 1998; 77: 814–8.

150. Sunness JS. The pregnant woman's eye. Surv Ophthalmol 1988; 32: 219–38.

151. Diabetic Retinopathy: Preferred Practice Pattern. American Academy of Ophthalmology. 2003: 1–36.

152. Puza SW, Malee MP. Utilization of routine ophthalmologic examinations in pregnant diabetic patients. J Matern Fetal Med 1996; 5: 7–10.

153. Halperin LS, Olk RJ, Soubrane G, Coscas G. Safety of fluorescein angiography during pregnancy. Am J Ophthalmol 1990; 109: 563–6.

154. Hercules BL, Wozencroft M, Gayed II, Jeacock J. Peripheral retinal ablation in the treatment of proliferative diabetic retinopathy during pregnancy. Br J Ophthalmol 1980; 64: 87–93.

155. Frank RN. Diabetic retinopathy: current concepts of evaluation and treatment. Clin Endocrinol Metab 1986; 15: 933–69.

156. Conway M, Baldwin J, Kohner EM, Schulenburg WE, Cassar J. Postpartum progression of diabetic retinopathy. Diabetes Care 1991; 14: 1110–1.

157. Chan WC, Lim LT, Quinn MJ, et al. Management and outcome of sight-threatening diabetic retinopathy in pregnancy. Eye 2004; 18: 826–32.

158. Early Treatment Diabetic Retinopathy Study Research Group. Treatment techniques and clinical guidelines for photocoagulation of diabetic macular edema. Early Treatment Diabetic Retinopathy Study Report Number 2. Ophthalmology 1987; 94: 761–74.

159. Cassar J, Hamilton AM, Kohner EM. Diabetic retinopathy in pregnancy. Int Ophthalmol Clin 1978; 18: 179–88.

160. Kitzmiller JL, Main E, Ward B, Theiss T, Peterson DL. Insulin lispro and the development of proliferative diabetic retinopathy during pregnancy. Diabetes Care 1999; 22: 874–6.

161. Zib I, Raskin P. Novel insulin analogues and its mitogenic potential. Diabetes Obes Metab 2006; 8: 611–20.

162. Persson B, Swahn ML, Hjertberg R, et al. Insulin lispro therapy in pregnancies complicated by type 1 diabetes mellitus. Diabetes Res Clin Pract 2002; 58: 115–21.

163. Buchbinder A, Miodovnik M, McElvy S, et al. Is insulin lispro associated with the development or progression of diabetic retinopathy during pregnancy? Am J Obstet Gynecol 2000; 183: 1162–5.

164. Bhattacharyya A, Vice PA. Insulin lispro, pregnancy, and retinopathy. Diabetes Care 1999; 22: 2101–4.

165. Kurtzhals P, Schaffer L, Sorensen A, et al. Correlations of receptor binding and metabolic and mitogenic potencies of insulin analogs designed for clinical use. Diabetes 2000; 49: 999–1005.

166. Lapolla A, Dalfra MG, Fedele D. Insulin therapy in pregnancy complicated by diabetes: are insulin analogs a new tool? Diabetes Metab Res Rev 2005; 21: 241–52.

167. Rosenstock J, Schwartz SL, Clark Jr. CM, et al. Basal insulin therapy in type 2 diabetes: 28-week comparison of insulin glargine (HOE 901) and NPH insulin. Diabetes Care 2001; 24: 631–6.

168. Yki-Jarvinen H, Dressler A, Ziemen M. Less nocturnal hypoglycemia and better post-dinner glucose control with bedtime insulin glargine compared with bedtime NPH insulin during insulin combination therapy in type 2 diabetes. HOE 901/3002 Study Group. Diabetes Care 2000; 23: 1130–6.

169. Jovanovic R, Jovanovic L. Obstetric management when normoglycemia is maintained in diabetic pregnant women with vascular compromise. Am J Obstet Gynecol 1984; 149: 617–23.

170. Kassoff A, Catalano RA, Mehu M. Vitreous hemorrhage and the Valsalva maneuver in proliferative diabetic retinopathy. Retina 1988; 8: 174–6.

171. Jones WL. Valsalva maneuver induced vitreous hemorrhage. J Am Optom Assoc 1995; 66: 301–4.

172. White P. Pregnancy and diabetes. In: Marble A, White P, Bradley RF, eds. Joslins Diabetes Mellitus. Philadelphia: Lea & Febiger; 1971, pp. 581–98.

43 Diabetic vascular complications in pregnancy: Nephropathy

Elisabeth R. Mathiesen and Peter Damm

Introduction

Twenty years ago the general medical opinion was against pregnancy in women with diabetic nephropathy and diabetic nephropathy was a contraindication to pregnancy in many centers. With new technology, the widespread use of antihypertensive treatment and increasing experience, maternal and perinatal mortality and morbidity rates in pregnancies complicated by diabetic nephropathy have declined substantially during the last decade. Successful pregnancy outcome with fetal survival rates of up to 95% are now achievable in diabetic women with diabetic nephropathy and a living fetus in first trimester.[1–3] But even with the best care maternal and perinatal complications in women with diabetic nephropathy are consistently more frequent than in diabetic women with normal urinary albumin excretion at conception. Furthermore the question regarding the possible short-term and long-term effects on maternal morbidity and mortality must be borne in mind.

Pathophysiology and treatment of diabetic nephropathy

Diabetic nephropathy is a progressive disease that affects approximately 30% of patients with diabetes and it is the most common cause of end stage renal disease in USA. The first clinical sign is increased excretion of albumin in the urine, so called microalbuminuria in the range 30–300 mg/24 h, corresponding to a spot urine albumine to creatinine ratio of 30 mg/μg. Untreated microalbuminuria progresses to overt diabetic nephropathy characterised by persistent proteinuria, hypertension and a relentless decline in glomerular filtration rate.[4] Histological changes in the glomeruli with increased basal membrane thickness and glomerulosclerosis are characteristics, but universal leakage of albumin over the endothelium in the whole body is also present. Progression to end stage renal disease occurs with a median duration of 7 years after onset of diabetic nephropathy, if let untreated. The introduction of inhibition of the renin–angiotensin system in combination with other antihypertensive has improved the poor prognosis considerably. Progression of manifest diabetic nephropathy can be slowed down by strict antihypertensive treatment with angiotensin converting enzyme (ACE) inhibitors or angiotensin II receptor blockers as first line drugs. It is often necessary to combine the treatment with diuretics, beta-blockers and/or calcium antagonists in order to control the blood pressure and the albumin excretion sufficiently. Strict antihypertensive treament in patients with diabetic nephropathy results in preservation of kidney function documented by a reduction in the decline in glomerular filtration rate to less than one-third of the decline in untreated patients.[4] Inhibition of the rennin angiotensin system with i.e. ACE inhibitors already at the stage of microalbuminuria prior to development of hypertension is also demonstrated effectfull in delaying the progression of the disease and might even reduce the albumin excretion to normal values.[5–7] The aim for the treatment includes blood pressure <130/80 mmHg and albumin excretion as near to normal as possible. In addition to antihypertensive treatment many women with microalbuminuria or diabetic nephropathy are treated with low dose aspirin and statins to reduce the risk of macrovascular complications such as stroke and acute myocardial infarction.

Effects of pregnancy on diabetic nephropathy

Few studies have examined the long-term effect of pregnancy on renal function in women with diabetic nephropathy after strict antihypertensive treatment has been widely used and improved the survivial. The most recent is a case–control study including 26 pregnant women with diabetic nephropathy and normal serum creatinine followed for up to 13 years and the decline in kidney function was compared to women with diabetic nephropathy who did not became pregnant in the study period.[8] The women were offered strict antihypertensive treatment as routine treatment.during the whole study period. They found that in women with serum creatinine within the normal range, pregnancy did not accelerate the decline in kidney function or impair the long-term survival of the mother.[8] However, in women with a reduced creatinine clearance reports suggest that there is an increased risk of deterioration of kidney function during pregnancy.[9,10] The long-term survival of a mother with diabetic nephropathy has improved considerably in recent years, but the chance for the mother of being alive with normal vision and free of renal replacement therapy when the child grows up, is still reported to be reduced.[8]

Effect of diabetic nephropathy on pregnancy outcome

The presence of diabetic nephropathy significantly affects the outcome of pregnancy, primarily due to three reasons: (1) the increased risk of maternal hypertensive complications; (2) the increased risk of preterm delivery due to deteriorating maternal blood pressure and pre-eclampsia; and (3) the increased risk of intrauterine fetal growth restriction and fetal distress caused by placental dysfunction. Severe malformations have been described with a slightly higher prevalence in women with diabetic nephropathy compared to diabetic women with normal kidney function. However, this is most likely due to the poorer metabolic control early in pregnancy often found in these women.

The risk of perinatal mortality in pregnancies complicated by diabetic nephropathy is now close to that of women with Type 1 diabetes without diabetic nephropathy.[1-3] The rate of pre-eclampsia in women with diabetic nephropathy is high 53–64%[1,2,3,11] especially when reduced kidney function,[12] hypertension at onset of pregnancy or severe nephrotic proteinuria is present.[2,3] Moreover, also women with Type 1 diabetes and microalbuminuria have increased risk of developing pre-eclampsia compared to women with Type 1 diabetes and normal urinary albumin excretion.[12] Pre-eclampsia often leads to preterm delivery[11] and preterm delivery before week 34 has been reported in up to 45% of the cases.[11,13] Severe handicap of the children born to mothers with diabetic nephropathy has been described. In a follow-up of 35 children born between 1982 and 1992, the majority were normally developed but seven (20%) had psychomotor retardation when examined at a mean age of 4.5 years.[13] The risk of neuro-developmental problems was highest in children born preterm weighing less than 2000 g. The pathogenesis of pre-eclampsia and preterm delivery in women with diabetic nephropathy is sparsely investigated, but universal endothelial damage seems to be of importance.[14]

Treatment of women with diabetic nephropathy during pregnancy

Strict metabolic control during pregnancy is of utmost importance but may be difficult because women with Type 1 diabetes and diabetic nephropathy often have an increased risk of severe hypoglycaemia. Close surveillance of blood pressure and urinary albumin excretion is central while 24 h ambulatory blood pressure recording has not been shown to be of benefit in the care of these women.[15] Early onset and strict antihypertensive treatment as in the nonpregnant state might improve the outcome. In patients with microalbuminuria introduction of early onset antihypertensive treatment with methyldopa in normotensive pregnant women with Type 1 diabetes and microalbuminuria resulted in a significant reduction in preterm delivery before gestational week 34.[16] Furthermore, early onset and strict antihypertensive treatment in women with diabetic nephropathy most likely also reduce the severity of pre-eclampsia end preterm delivery. Our center recommends initiating antihypertensive treatment in pregnant women with diabetes and elevated urinary albumin excretion at one of the following clinical indications: blood pressure exceeding 135/85; a doubling of urinary albumin excretion; or urinary albumin excretion exceeding 300 mg/24 h.[16] ACE inhibitors or angiotensin receptor blockers used before pregnancy should be changed to other antihypertensive treatment, e.g. methyldopa unless urinary albumin excretion is within the normal range or very low in the microalbuminuric range, where the women can be observed without antihypertensive treatment. It is often necessary to use a combination of different antihypertensive drugs in order to control blood pressure and albumin excretion. Methyldopa, beta blockers (labetalol), calcium antagonists (nifedipine and diltiazem) are often used.[16,17] Like Kimmerle et al.[13] we have the clinical experience that women with diabetic nephropathy receiving early onset intensive antihypertensive treatment have a better pregnancy outcome compared to women initiating antihypertensive treatment late in pregnancy. In late pregnancy close obstetrical surveillance is important to diagnose complications, prevent stillbirths and plan the time of delivery. In other high risk groups for developing pre-eclampsia treatment with low dose aspirin might have some preventive effect. Theoretically low dose aspirin treatment therefore could of benefit in women with diabetic nephropathy. Thus we use low dose aspirin treatment in these women although this is not documented by randomized controlled trials.

Counseling women with diabetic nephropathy

Careful counseling of the woman and her partner of the risk for herself and the newborn is important before the couple can take a well-considered decision regarding pregnancy. An updated diabetes status including hemoglobin A1c, risk of hypoglycemia, degree of retinopathy, serum creatinine, blood pressure, and proteinuria is necessary to estimate the risk for complications during pregnancy. The number of antihypertensive drugs to control the blood pressure sufficiently prior to pregnancy is also of importance, since there has to be room for further intensification of antihypertensive treatment in late pregnancy, if necessary.

Pre-pregnancy treatment with ACE inhibitors combined with strict metabolic control for at least 6 month resulting in low levels of albumin excretion has been found to be associated with a high rate of successful pregnancy outcome.[3] In this study

ACE inhibition was discontinued immediately after the positive pregnancy test and only four out of 24 women delivered preterm. Severe handicap or late infant death was seen in two cases.[3] However, treatment with ACE inhibitors in early pregnancy has recently been shown to be associated with increased risk of congenital malformations.[18] Furthermore ACE inhibition during the last part of pregnancy is associated with abnormal fetal renal development and neonatal renal failure.[19] Treatment with ACE inhibitors or angiotensin II blockers should therefore in general be stopped prior to conception.[18,19] It is often wise to change to other types of antihypertensive treatment that is regarded safe in pregnancy i.e. methyldopa, beta blockers such as labetalol or calcium antagonists. Although the use of diuretics throughout pregnancy is controversial[20] we have good clinical experience with continuation of an ongoing diuretic treatment in stable doses during pregnancy in these women.[16] Statin treatment is associated with malformations and should be discontinued prior to pregnancy.[21] Low-dose aspirin treatment might prevent pre-eclampsia and can be continued or initiated after organogenesis.

Besides the kidney function, focus on retinopathy is very important in these women since severe diabetic retinopathy is prevalent in this group of patients. Laser treatment for diabetic retinopathy should be performed to stabilize the retinopathy prior to pregnancy, when requested.

Box 43.1   Facts regarding pregnancy in diabetic nephropathy

- A take-home baby rate of 95% in women with diabetic nephropathy
- Pregnancy does not deteriorate kidney function in women with diabetic nephropathy and normal serum creatinine
- Hypertensive complications in pregnancy and preterm delivery is prevalent
- ACE inhibition prior to pregnancy and early antihypertensive treatment in pregnancy seems to reduce the risk of pregnancy complications
- ACE inhibition, angiotensin II blockers or statins should not be used during pregnancy
- Careful counseling of women with diabetic nephropathy prior to pregnancy is important

Hope for the future

Strict metabolic control combined with ACE inhibition prior to pregnancy and with early onset intensive antihypertensive treatment during pregnancy, possibly in combination with low dose aspirin, might improve the pregnancy outcome in women with diabetic nephropathy further (Box 43.1).

REFERENCES

1. Reece EA, Leguizaman G, Homko C. Stringent control in diabetic nephropathy associated with optimization of pregnancy outcomes. J Matern–Fetal Med 1998; 7: 213–6.
2. Dunne FP, Chowdhury TA, Hartland A, et al. Pregnancy outcome in women with insulin-dependent diabetes mellitus complicated by nephropathy. Q J Med 1999; 92: 451–4.
3. Bar J, Chen R, Schoenfeld A, et al. Pregnancy outcome in patients with insulin dependent diabetes mellitus and diabetic nephropathy treated with ACE inhibitors before pregnancy. J Pedriatr Endocrinol metab 1999; 12: 659–65.
4. Parving H-H, Smidt UM, Hommel E, et al. Effective antihypertensive treatment postpones renal insufficiency in diabetic nephropathy. Am Kidney Dis 1993; 22; 188–95.
5. Mathiesen ER, Rønn B, Storm B, Foght H, Deckert T. The natural course of microalbuminuria in insulin dependent diabetes – A 10 year prospective study. Diabet Med 1995; 12: 482–7.
6. Mathiesen ER, Hommel E, Giese J, Parving H-H. Efficacy of captopril in postponing nephropathy in normotensive insulin dependent diabetic patients with microalbuminuria. BMJ 1991; 303: 81–7.
7. Mathiesen ER, Hommel E, Hansen HP, Parving H-H. Preservation of normal GFR with long term captopril treatment in normotensive IDDM patients with microalbuminuria. BMJ 1999; 319: 24–5.
8. Rossing K, Jacobsen P, Hommel E, et al. Pregnancy and progression of diabetic nephropathy. Diabetologia 2002; 45: 36–41.
9. Biesenbach G, Stroger H, Zazgornik J. Influence of pregnancy on progression of diabetic nephropathy and subsequent requirement of renal replacement treatment in femal type 1 diabetic patients with impaired renal function. Nephrol Dial Trans 1992; 7: 105.
10. Purdy LP, Hantsch CE, Molitch ME, et al. Effect of pregnancy on renal function in patients with moderate-to-severe diabetic renal insufficiency. Diabetes Care 1996t; 19: 1067–74.
11. Ekbom P, Damm P, Feldt-Rasmussen B, et al. Pregnancy outcome in Type 1 diabetic women with microalbuminuria. Diabetes Care 2001; 24: 1739–44.
12. Khoury JC, Miodovnik M, LeMasters G, Sibai B. Pregnancy poutcome and progression of diabetic nephropathy. What's next? J Matern–Fetal Neonat Med 2002; 11: 238–44.
13. Kimmerle R, Zass RP, Cupisti S, et al. Pregnancies in women with diabetic nephropathy: Long-term outcome for mother and child. Diabetologia 1995; 38: 227–35.
14. Clausen P, Ekbom P, Damm P, et al. Signs of maternal vascular dysfunction precede preeclampsia in type 1 diabetic women.
15. Ekbom P, Damm P, Nørgård K, et al. Urinary albumin excretion and 24-hour blood pressure as predictors of preeclampsia in type 1 diabetes. Diabetologia 2000; 43: 927–31.
16. Nielsen LR, Muller C, Damm P, Mathiesen ER. Reduced prevalence of preterm delivery in women with diabetes type 1 and microalbuminuria – possible effect of early antihypertensive treatment during pregnancy. Diabet Med 2006; 23: 426–31.
17. Khandelwal M, Kumanova M, Gaughan JP, Reece EA. Role of diltiazem in pregnant women with chronic renal disease. Matern–Fetal Neonatal Med 2002; 6: 408–12.
18. Cooper WO, Hernandez-Diaz S, Arbogast PG, et al. Major congenital malformations after first trimester exposure to ACE-inhibitors. N Engl J Med 2006; 354: 2443–51.
19. Tabacova S, Little R, Tsong Y, Vega A, Kimmel CA. Adverse pregnancy outcomes associated with maternal enalapril antihypertensive treatment. Pharmacoepidem Drug Saf 2003; 12: 633–46.
20. Sibai BM. Chronic hypertension in pregnancy. Obest Gynecol 2002; 100: 369–77.
21. Edison RJ, Muenke M. Mechanistic and epidemiologic considerations in the evaluation of adverse birth outcomes following gestational exposure to statins. Am J Med Genet A 2005; 131: 287–98.

44 Diabetic ketoacidosis in pregnancy

Yariv Yogev, Avi Ben-Haroush and Moshe Hod

Introduction

Diabetic ketoacidosis (DKA) is a serious metabolic complication of diabetes with high mortality if undetected. Its occurrence in pregnancy compromises both the fetus and the mother profoundly. Although predictably more common in patients with Type 1 diabetes, it has been recognized in those with Type 2 diabetes as well as gestational diabetes.

DKA is characterized by accelerated gluconeogenesis and ketogenesis. It occurs most often in the presence of predisposing factors such as insulin deficiency (absolute or relative), excess counter-regulatory hormones, fasting and dehydration; infection is a common catalyst.

The principles of management include rehydration, insulin therapy, electrolyte replacement, and identification and treatment of the underlying cause. DKA in pregnancy is an acute metabolic situation, jeopardizing both maternal and fetal well-being. DKA affects 1–3% of pregnancies complicated with diabetes, and is rare in women with previously undiagnosed diabetes.

DKA in pregnancy warrants assessment of fetal well-being during management of the mother. The pathophysiology, effect on the fetus, and management of DKA in pregnancy are discussed in detail in this chapter.

Prevalence, precipitating factors and prognosis

DKA during pregnancy occurs more often in women with insulin-dependent diabetes mellitus (IDDM) than in women with Type 2 or gestational diabetes mellitus (GDM).[1] As the majority of studies on DKA during pregnancy have been done on samples of <30 patients, the actual prevalence has to be extrapolated from that data. According to the National Diabetes Data Group, the incidence of DKA in nonpregnant diabetics indicates an annual incidence of 3–8 episodes/1000 diabetic patients.[2] However, pregnant diabetic women are at greater risk of DKA than nonpregnant diabetic women.[3] DKA usually appears in the second and third trimesters, when there is an increase in insulin resistance,[4] and it is more frequent in undiagnosed new-onset diabetic gravida. The rate of maternal mortality secondary to diabetes has fallen remarkably from 50 to 60% in the pre-insulin era to <1% today.[4] The maternal mortality rate secondary to DKA is not well established, owing to the relatively low prevalence of DKA, but most likely ranges from 5 to 15%.[4,5] Gabbe et al.[4] reported seven maternal deaths among 24 cases of metabolic complications during pregnancy, four of which were related to DKA. Fetal mortality has also decreased markedly since the introduction of the routine use of insulin, although it is still excessively high, ranging from 30 to 90%.[6,7] Montoro et al.[8] reported a fetal death rate of 35% in 20 pregnant women with Type 1 diabetes and DKA on admission; however, once therapy was begun, none of the remaining 13 women sustained fetal loss. Kilvert et al.[9] reported only one fetal loss in seven cases of DKA occurring after the first trimester. In a study of 26 pregnant women with brittle diabetes (i.e. recurrent DKA episodes and frequent hospitalizations) and 27 pregnant women with stable disease, Kent et al.[10] noted 15 (54%) live births, 10 (48%) spontaneous abortions and one (5%) stillbirth in the first group, compared to 25 (95%) live births and no stillbirths in the second group. Confidential inquiries into maternal deaths in the UK for the period between 1979 and 1990 revealed 10 diabetes related deaths, of which three were due to diabetic ketoacidosis.[11]

Increased insulin requirements and accelerated ketosis imposed by pregnancy predisposes the pregnant diabetic patient to an increased risk of DKA. Several factors predispose pregnant diabetic women to ketoacidosis: accelerated starvation, dehydration secondary to emesis, lowered buffering capacity (respiratory alkalosis of pregnancy), increased insulin resistance and stress. Box 44.1 summarizes the precipitating factors for the development of DKA in diabetic pregnancies.

Rodgers and Rodgers[12] reviewed these clinical variables and found that emesis and the use of beta-sympathomimetic drugs were etiologic in 57% of cases, and patient non-compliance and physician management errors were etiologic in 24% of cases and contributory in 16% of cases. Thirty percent of the patients with emesis on admission had a pre-pregnancy history of diabetic gastroenteropathy, thus identifying this group as being at particularly high risk for DKA. This finding emphasizes the importance of patient education and early initiation of treatment in pregnant diabetic patients with emesis. Using tocolytic agents such as beta-adrenergic drugs and steroids for fetal lung maturation should be approached cautiously.

Smoking has been demonstrated to have ketogenic effect (increased production of 3-hydroxybutyric acid) in diabetic women that has not been reproducible in healthy pregnant controls.[13]

Pathogenesis

DKA can result from either a relative or an absolute lack of insulin in the presence of glucose counter-regulatory hormones,

resulting in an overproduction of glucose and ketones in the liver, with release of free fatty acids from adipose tissue (Figure 44.1).

Pregnancy by itself is a state of insulin resistance. Insulin sensitivity has been demonstrated to fall by as much as 56% through 36 weeks of gestation.[14] The production of insulin antagonistic hormones like human placental lactogen, prolactin, and cortisol, all contribute to this. The insulin requirement, for this reason, progressively rises during pregnancy explaining the higher incidence of diabetic ketoacidosis in the second and third trimesters. In addition the physiological rise in progesterone with pregnancy decreases gastrointestinal motility that contributes to an increase in the absorption of carbohydrates thereby promoting hyperglycemia.

Glucagon seems to be the primary insulin antagonist in the development of DKA; Gerich et al.[15] demonstrated that in patients with Type 1 diabetes acute withdrawal of insulin and suppression of glucagon secretion by somatostatin prevented the development of ketoacidosis, whereas in the control group ketoacidosis occurred. These findings indicate that it is not only the lack of insulin that leads to fulminant diabetic ketoacidosis but that glucagon, by means of its gluconeogenic, ketogenic and lipolytic actions, is a prerequisite for its development. Support for this has been provided by studies in pancreatomized humans with low insulin levels, in whom glucose levels rise only slightly in direct correlation with blood glucose and glucagon levels.[16]

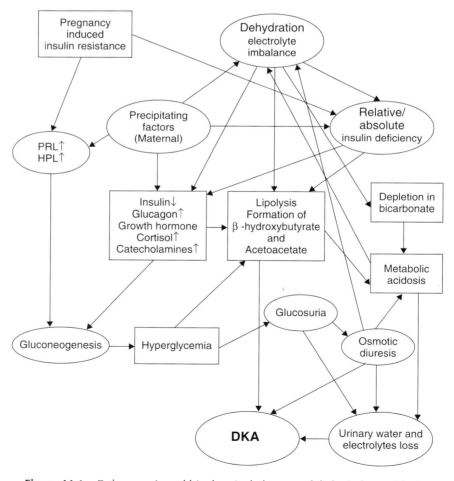

Figure 44.1   Pathogenesis and biochemical changes of diabetic ketoacidosis.

Other glucose counter-regulatory hormones include catecholamines, growth hormone and cortisol. In advancing gestation, human placental lactogen and prolactin also play a role, and have been incriminated in the pathogenesis of DKA. Owing the relative lack of insulin, increased levels of catecholamines and cortisol (due to stress and dehydration) result in significantly increased lipolysis in the adipose tissue and delivery of free fatty acids to the liver. Beta-oxidation of these fatty acids leads to the formation (up to 300%) of ketone bodies, namely β-hydroxybutyrate and acetoacetate, concomitant with a decrease in ketone used by muscle. As ketone bodies are acidic, ion concentrations in body fluids increases and so the pH decreases.

Acidosis is further exacerbated by the decrease in bicarbonate levels owing to bicarbonate neutralization of the ketone bodies prior to their excretion in urine.[5] As a result, a compensatory respiratory alkalosis is added to the baseline relative respiratory alkalosis and metabolic acidemia (renal excretion of bicarbonate) of pregnancy. Thus, the already diminished buffering capacity of pregnancy is compounded by the reduction in ketone use and severe impairment in bicarbonate regeneration. Acidosis, if untreated, leads to pronounced dehydration, oliguria and electrolyte imbalance. Hyperglycemia due to the accumulation of carbohydrates leads to an increase in serum osmolarity, profound osmotic diuresis (when glucose levels exceed those of the renal threshold), a decrease in cardiac output with a drop in blood pressure, and loss of sodium and potassium. Dehydration and severe hyperosmolarity may be further aggravated by the loss of water and electrolytes through acidosis-related vomiting. In advanced DKA, all body compartments become dehydrated, with significant depletion in water, sodium, potassium, chloride, magnesium, phosphate, and bicarbonate. Although the total body sodium deficit is high, the serum sodium level can be low, normal or high. The apparent hyponatremia ('pseudohyponatremia') is secondary to the hyperglycemic and hypertriglyceridemic state; this may be corrected by increasing measured sodium by 1.6 mEq/L for each 100 mg/dL of glucose above normal.[18] The drop in pH is compensated, in part, by the intracellular shift of hydrogen ions from the extracellular space in balance with the potassium flux from the intracellular space. Therefore, although the true serum potassium level is low, the measured serum potassium level will be at the upper end of the normal range. Shock secondary to the depleted intravascular volume may ensue, with decreased tissue perfusion and increased lactic acid production.

Diagnosis

A high index of suspicion and prompt diagnosis is the key to improved outcome of both the fetus and the mother. The clinical presentation of diabetic ketoacidosis in pregnancy is similar to that of nonpregnant diabetics. The classic presentation of DKA in pregnancy consists of vomiting, thirst, polyuria, weakness, altered sensorium, and air hunger. Malaise, headache, weight loss, nausea, and abdominal pain occur less frequently. Importantly, symptoms can vary in severity. On examination, patients will have a characteristic fruity acetone breath odor with rapid and deep respiration (to release more carbon dioxide and prevent further pH deterioration). The diagnosis is confirmed by laboratory documentation of hyperglycemia, acidosis, and ketonuria. Importantly, DKA in this patient population may be followed by euglycemia or mild hyperglycemia.[8,19] In a 10-year study of 11 cases of DKA in pregnancy, Cullen et al.[20] noted symptoms of nausea, vomiting and decreased caloric intake in 10 patients (90%), and plasma glucose levels <200 mg/dL in four patients (36%). Ketonemia and pre-renal azotemia with elevations in blood urea nitrogen and creatinine levels are also common findings. Arterial blood gas analysis revealed acidosis, with the pH usually <7.30, along with an anion gap of 12 mEq/L or greater; serum bicarbonate is often =15 mEq/L. As described earlier, sodium and potassium levels can vary significantly.

Fetal effects of diabetic ketoacidosis

The greatest hazard facing the pregnant diabetic patient with DKA is fetal loss. The exact fetal loss rate is difficult to assess because of the small reported series in the literature. Historically, the reported fetal mortality ranged between 30 and 90%[7] but remarkable progress has been made both in fetal assessment techniques and in the treatment of DKA, and mortality rates in more recent reviews are 10%.[20] Needless to say, fetal loss is primarily related to the severity of the maternal illness and the degree of metabolic decompensation. Most fetal losses occur prior to diagnosis and therefore to the onset of efficient treatment. As ketone bodies freely cross the placenta, maternal acidosis is assumed to cause fetal acidosis; however, the exact mechanism by which maternal DKA affects the fetus remains unclear. Suggestions include a decrease in uterine blood flow and fetal hypoxemia, maternal hyperketonemia inducing fetal hypoxemia, and fetal hyperglycemia causing an increased fetal oxidative mechanism and a decreased fetal myocardial contractility. Indeed, fetal potassium deficit has been found to lead to fetal cardiac arrest.[7] Fetal hypoxia may also be attributed to a DKA-associated phosphate deficit which leads to depletion of red cell 2,3-diphosphoglycerate and consequent impairment of oxygen delivery. The risk of fetal distress, and even death, during the maternal DKA state makes it mandatory to continuously monitor the fetal heart and to assess the biophysical score, and to evaluate the fetal acid–base balance by cordocentesis if necessary. In the few case reports of fetal monitoring during maternal DKA, a nonreassuring pattern with tachycardia, reduced variability and late decelerations was reported.[21,22] LoBue and Goodlin[23] found that the administration of just sodium bicarbonate for 2 h led to the resolution of the late deceleration and decreased variability of uterine contractions. Hughes[22] reported the resolution of a similar fetal heart rate pattern 40 min after intravenous administration of insulin with no mention of maternal rehydration. Other researchers reported that a combination of massive intravenous hydration, insulin therapy and intensive care of the mother lead to resolution of fetal acidosis and on improvement in fetal heart rate monitoring.

The long-term effects of DKA episodes during pregnancy on the fetus remain unclear, but a relationship between plasma ketone levels in the pregnant diabetic women and a lower intelligence quotient in the child has been suggested.[24]

Treatment

Prompt and vigorous treatment in an obstetric intensive care unit is generally needed to decrease the high maternal and fetal mortalities accompanying DKA. All treatment protocols are based on correcting volume depletion, supplying insulin, correcting acidosis and electrolyte imbalance, and, most importantly, identifying and correcting any possible precipitating factor. Continuous fetal heart rate monitoring and biophysical assessment are essential to assess fetal well-being during the third trimester. Induction of labor or an emergency Cesarean section should be done only after maternal stabilization. In the event of preterm labor, magnesium sulfate is the tocolytic drug of choice, as beta-mimetic drugs only exacerbate the metabolic disorder. Major consideration should be given to the use of steroids for lung maturation, as they also worsen the metabolic consequences. A search for a source of infection or other severe illness must be undertaken concomitant with onset of treatment.

Several protocols have recently been suggested for the treatment of DKA. It should be borne in mind, however, that these protocols are only general guidelines and the therapeutic regimen must be tailored to the individual patient on the basis of her prominent clinical features. Only the therapeutic rationale and the physiological basis are outlined in this chapter.

An estimated 4–10 L of deficit occurs in DKA,[25] therefore fluid administration is considered the first priority of treatment in order to improve renal perfusion and thereby increase glucosuria. The initial therapy should be based on isotonic saline for effective restoration of the intravascular volume. In cases of hypernatremia, other isotonic solutions may be used. Importantly, it has been postulated that using hypotonic saline as initial treatment may cause a rapid drop in plasma osmolarity that can lead to fatal cerebral edema, which is a rare event among adults. Thus, when serum glucose falls to <250 mg/dL, the intravenous fluids can be changed to 5% dextrose solution.

There are many dosing regimens for insulin replacement in DKA, and each has its advantages and disadvantages. In recent years, the constant low-dose regimen rather than the high-dose bolus therapy has become popular,[3,26] owing both to its simplicity and to the lower rates of complications of hypoglycemia and hypokalemia. However, bolus or continuous infusion therapy also works well, and the clinician should choose the method with which they have the most experience.[3]

Acidemia in DKA takes longer to correct than the hyperglycemic state. Therefore, insulin therapy should be continued even when normal glucose levels have been achieved. When blood glucose reaches 150–200 mg/dL, a 5% dextrose solution should be used along with insulin.[27] Plasma electrolytes should be frequently evaluated, and once adequate renal function is established, potassium should be replaced, bearing in mind that the often normal or elevated serum potassium level may not reflect the true total deficit of 5–15 mEq/kg of body weight. Potassium is usually administered for 1–3 h, when the level begins to normalize due to the intracellular shift. It is noteworthy that the serum potassium level can fall rapidly as a result of vigorous potassium loss in urine and correction of academia.[28]

If phosphorus is low, replacement of 10–20 mEq/L of potassium phosphate for each 10–20 mEq/L of potassium chloride should be used.

The use of bicarbonate is the most controversial area in the treatment of DKA.[3,23,24] Routine bicarbonate therapy may be unnecessary, as the retained ketone bodies are metabolized and regenerated to bicarbonate. Overzealous replacement should be avoided in order to prevent rapid and complete maternal acidemia that may actually increase fetal P_{CO_2} levels and reduce oxygen delivery to maternal tissues.[7] Bicarbonate therapy should probably be used only in patients with severe acidosis (pH <7.1 or 7.0). There is currently no evidence to support a beneficial effect of bicarbonate in patients with a pH >6.9, though some authors recommend it only for such cases.[27]

Importantly, alkali therapy is associated with many side effects, e.g. hypokalemia, sodium overload, reduction in oxygen delivery capacity and a decrease in cerebrospinal fluid pH.

Prevention

Preconception counseling, intensive metabolic control, prenatal care in a combined obstetric and diabetic clinic, and education are important in preventing this catastrophic complication in diabetic pregnancies. Education of patients specifically aimed at improving their understanding of the risks of pregnancy and the requirements for successful outcome must be emphasized during each visit. Similarly, obstetric and midwifery staff require a high index of suspicion to identify patients early in the course of their illness since the development of diabetic ketoacidosis in pregnancy can be rapid and can also occur at lower blood glucose levels compared to nonpregnant women. The use of reagent strips to detect ketones in urine (ketonuria) when blood glucose levels are high, or if symptoms of intercurrent illness appear, may be one way of early identification of this complication. However, the presence of minor ketonuria in normal pregnancy, especially in the presence of significant emesis, should be borne in mind during evaluation of such patients. The use of reagent strips to detect ketones in blood may help in the differentiation of these two conditions, although this needs validation for its use in routine clinical practice. Certainly, if there are any signs of decompensation, early hospitalization is essential.

Conclusions

DKA is an extreme condition in the spectrum of decompensated diabetes mellitus. Its pathogenesis is related to an absolute or relative deficiency in insulin levels and elevations in insulin counter-regulatory hormones that lead to altered metabolism of carbohydrate, protein, and fat, and varying degrees of osmotic diuresis and dehydration, ketosis, and acidosis. Clinical presentation is characterized by insulin deficiency and ketoacidosis, and insulin therapy is the cornerstone of therapy. The therapeutic regimen is tailored to the prominent clinical features of the individual patient. In gravid patients, rapid correction of the metabolic abnormalities and, consequently, of hyperosmolarity by administration of

hypotonic fluids and insulin should be avoided to decrease the risk for precipitating cerebral edema. Intensive care unit admission is indicated in the management of DKA, in the presence of cardiovascular instability, an inability to protect the airway, obtundation, the presence of blood pressure instability, or if there is not adequate capacity to provide the frequent and necessary monitoring that must accompany its use. Prompt diagnosis and early treatment, along with continuous monitoring of fetal well-being, is well correlated with favorable outcomes of both mother and infant.

REFERENCES

1. Cousins L. Pregnancy complications among diabetic women. Review, 1965–1985. Obstet Gynecol Surv 1987; 42: 140–9.
2. Fishbein HA. DKA, hyperosmolar coma, lactic acidosis and hypoglycemia. In: Harris MI, Hammon RF, eds. Diabetes in America. Washington, DC: US Dept. of Health and Human Sciences; 1985, XII.I–XII.19.
3. Hollingsworth DR. Medical and obstetrics complications of diabetic pregnancies: IDDM, NIDDM, and GDM. In: Brown C-L, Mitchell, eds. Pregnancy, Diabetes and Birth: A Management Guide, 2nd edn. Baltimore: Williams & Wilkins; 1992.
4. Gabbe SG, Mestman HJ, Hibbard LT. Maternal mortality in diabetes mellitus: an 18 year survey. Obstet Gynecol 1976; 48: 549–54.
5. Goto Y, Sato S, Masuda M. Causes of death in 3151 diabetic autopsy cases. Tohoku J Exp Med 1974; 112: 3390–343.
6. Drury MI, Greene AT, Stronge JM. Pregnancy complicated by clinical diabetes mellitus: a study of 600 pregnancies. Obstet Gynecol 1977; 49: 519–24.
7. Kitzmiller JL. Diabetic ketoacidosis and pregnancy. Contemp Obstet Gynecol 1982; 20: 141–5.
8. Montoro MN, Myers VP, Mestman JH, et al. Outcome of pregnancy in diabetic ketoacidosis. Am J Perinatol 1993; 10: 17–21.
9. Kilvert JA, Nicholson HO, Wright AD. Ketoacidosis in diabetic pregnancy. Diabet Med 1993; 10: 278–81.
10. Kent LA, Gill GV, Williams G. Mortality and outcome of patients with brittle diabetes and recurrent ketoacidosis. Lancet 1994; 17: 778–81.
11. Department of Health. Confidential enquiries into maternal deaths: 1979–1981, 1982–1984, 1985–1987, and 1988–1990. London: Department of Health, UK.
12. Rodgers BD, Rodgers DE. Clinical variables associated with diabetic ketoacidosis during pregnancy. J Reprod Med 1991; 36: 797–800.
13. Nylund L, Lunell NO, Persson B, et al. Smoking exerts a ketogenic influence in diabetic pregnancy. Gynecol Obstet Invest 1988; 25: 35–7.
14. Catalano PM, Tyzbir ED, Roman NM. Longitudinal changes in insulin release and insulin resistance in nonobese pregnant women. Am J Obstet Gynecol 1991; 165: 1667–72.
15. Gerich JE, Lorenzi M, Bier DM, et al. Prevention of human diabetic ketoacidosis by somatostatin. Evidence for an essential role of glucagon. N Engl J Med 1975; 8: 985–9.
16. Machoff CD, Pohl SL, Kaiser DL, et al. Determinants of glucose and ketoacid concentration in acutely hyperglycemic diabetic patients. Am J Med 1984; 77: 275–85.
17. Riley Jr LJ, Cooper M, Narins RG. Alkali therapy of diabetic ketoacidosis: biochemical, physiologic, and clinical perspectives. Diabetes Metab Rev 1989; 5: 627–36.
18. Katz MA. Hyperglycemia-induced hyponatremia – calculation of expected serum sodium depression. N Engl J Med 1973; 18: 843–4.
19. Clark JD, McConnell A, Hartog M. Normoglycaemic ketoacidosis in a woman with gestational diabetes. Diabet Med 1991; 8: 388–9.
20. Cullen MT, Reece EA, Homko CJ, Sivan E. The changing presentations of diabetic ketoacidosis during pregnancy. Am J Perinatol 1996; 13: 449–51.
21. Hagay ZJ, Weissman A, Lurie S, Insler V. Reversal of fetal distress following intensive treatment of maternal diabetic ketoacidosis. Am J Perinatol 1994; 11: 430–2.
22. Hughes AB. Fetal heart rate changes during diabetic ketosis. Acta Obstet Gynecol Scand 1987; 66: 71–3.
23. LoBue C, Goodlin RC. Treatment of fetal distress during diabetic keto-acidosis. J Reprod Med 1978; 20: 101–4.
24. Stehbens JA, Baker GL, Kitchell M. Outcome at ages 1, 3, and 5 years of children born to diabetic women. Am J Obstet Gynecol 1977; 15: 408–13.
25. Raskin P, Unger RH. Hyperglucagonemia and its suppression. Importance in the metabolic control of diabetes. N Engl J Med 1978; 31: 433–6.
26. Foster DW, McGarry JD. The metabolic derangement and treatment of diabetic ketoacidosis. N Engl J Med 1983; 21: 159–69.
27. Walker M, Marshall SM, Alberti KG. Clinical aspects of diabetic ketoacidosis. Diabetes Metab Rev 1989; 5: 651–63.
28. Owen OE, Licht JH, Sapir DG. Renal function and effects of partial rehydration during diabetic ketoacidosis. Diabetes 1981; 30: 510–8.

45 Gestational diabetes in multiple pregnancies

Yenon Hazan and Isaac Blickstein

Introduction

Two main reasons – infertility treatment and advanced maternal age – account for the increased incidence of multiple births. In most developed countries, the incidence is two to four times greater then the rate in developing countries and is presently as high as 2–4%.[1] Effective infertility treatment has the most striking effect and according to the East Flanders Prospective Twin Survey, the ratio of induced to spontaneous twins increased from nearly 1:50 in the early 1970s in to the rate of 1:2 in the late 1990s. Moreover, in centers with busy infertility clinics, induced conceptions presently comprise the majority of multiple pregnancies.[1–4] These iatrogenic multiple pregnancies are more frequent among older women with reduced fecundity; however, advanced age is by itself a significant risk for twin pregnancies.[5]

Multiple pregnancies are characterized by greater elevation of hormones with insulin–antagonist activity and therefore may increase the pro-diabetic potential. In addition, the advanced age of the mothers and the greater weight gain in multiple pregnancies are all risk factors for developing gestational diabetes mellitus (GDM). Thus, the combined effect of older maternal age, increased body mass index, and the effect of multiple pregnancy-related increased placental size (the so-called hyperplacentosis) is expected to increase the incidence of GDM during these gestations. Indeed, a recent retrospective large cohort of Canadian births, covering the peak of the epidemic of iatrogenic multiples, found that multiple pregnancies were associated with increase risk of gestational diabetes.[6] However, there is otherwise little information about the potential association between GDM and the epidemic of iatrogenic multiple pregnancies.

This chapter discusses the available data related to GDM and multiple pregnancies and intends to propose possible lines of further research.

Data that may support higher GDM rate in multiples

GDM is one of the most frequent pregnancy complications and is related to co-morbidities such as premature delivery, fetal macrosomia, birth trauma, unexplained antepartum fetal demise, pregnancy-induced hypertension, and placental abruption. Specifically, a retrospective population-based study of twins conceived by *in vitro* fertilization (IVF) found that patients who developed severe pre-eclampsia were more likely to have GDM.[7]

Hyperplacentosis presumably increases hormonal levels in multiple pregnancies and these hormones, in turn, are presumably involved in the increased susceptibility to GDM whereby changes in carbohydrate metabolism during multiple pregnancy promote a pro-diabetic state. Spellacy et al.[8] compared levels of the pro-diabetic hormone human placental lactogen (hPL) in singleton and twin pregnancies. They established serum hPL levels by radioimmunoassay in 75 singleton and 37 twin pregnancies. The results showed a significantly increased hPL level at 30 weeks (7.0 vs. 6.0 mcg/mL) as well as at 36 weeks (9.2 vs. 7.4 μg/mL) in twins vs. the singletons, respectively. The study supported the theory that twin pregnancies are associated with increased level of the principal diabetogenic hormone. Another support to this view comes from the evaluation of carbohydrate metabolism by Spellacy and co-workers who compared between 24 twin and 24 singleton (controls) pregnancies.[9] Cases and controls were similar in age, parity, weight, and gestational age. A 25-g glucose tolerance test was carried out in the second half of gestation and measurements of blood glucose, hPL and plasma insulin levels were established. The hPL levels were significantly higher whereas the fasting, the 5 and 15 min insulin levels were significantly lower in women with twins. The effect of hPL in twin as compared with singleton pregnancies may also be indirectly appreciated by its augmentation of erythropoietin effect as measured by the age distribution shift of erythrocytes in women with twin gestation.[10]

Casele and co-workers conducted a 40-h metabolic study in nondiabetic gestations and compared the response to normal meal eating and the vulnerability to starvation ketosis in 10 twin and 10 singletons, matched for age and pre-pregnancy weight.[11] Glucose, β-hydroxybutyrate, and insulin levels in response to meal eating from 8 a.m. to 12:00 noon on day 1 were similar in twin and singleton pregnancies. On day 2, however, when breakfast was delayed, a progressive but not significantly different decrement in glucose was observed in both twin and singleton pregnancies. On the other hand, a significantly greater progressive rise in β-hydroxybutyrate in twins compared to singletons was observed. These observations may point to the vulnerability of twin gestations to the accelerated starvation of late normal pregnancy.

If hyperplacentosis were the link between multiple gestation and GDM, one may expect that the frequency of GDM will correlate with the number of fetuses. Marconi et al. evaluated glucose disposal rates in a small series of one triplet, five twin, and 11 singleton pregnancies.[12] Maternal fasting glucose concentration and the total fetal and placental weight significantly correlated with increased maternal glucose disposal rate but glucose concentration and total pregnancy weight were interdependent variables.

It could be hypothesize that the difference between multiples and singletons may be the result of a plurality-dependent larger metabolic demand of the multiple gestation. The association between GDM and plurality was examined by Sivan et al.[13] who evaluated the effect of multifetal pregnancy reduction (MFPR) on the incidence of GDM. The authors studied 188 consecutive triplet pregnancies born during the period 1994–1998, of which 103 continued as triplets whereas 85 pregnancies underwent MFPR to twins. The frequency of GDM was significantly higher in the triplet group than in the (reduced) twin group (22.3% vs. 5.8%), leading to the conclusion that plurality influences the frequency of GDM. However, one may consider an alternative explanation whereby the increased frequency of GDM in triplets might be attributed to familial history of diabetes (44% vs. 25%) and BMI at the end of pregnancy (30.3 ± 5 vs. 27.6 ± 3.95). Interestingly, these authors repeated the methodology of Skupski and associates[14] who compared the risk for preeclampsia in triplet and in (reduced from triplets) twin gestations. As with GDM, the triplet group had a higher rate of severe preeclampsia (26.3%) compared with the twin group (7.9%); however, the authors did not find a difference in other maternal complications of pregnancy. In these two studies, both cases and controls started as triplets and MFPR was performed during the early second trimester.[13,14] This methodological construct excludes an early effect of the trophoblastic mass and may indirectly point to a later effect, whereby fetal number, placental mass, or factors unrelated to the success of implantation are more important to the development of preeclampsia and GDM than is successful implantation alone. Geva et al.[15] evaluated the pregnancy outcome of selective second trimester MFPR ($n = 38$) to first trimester MFPR ($n = 70$), (19.7 ± 3.3 and 11.7 ± 0.7 weeks, respectively). The rate of GDM was lower, but not significantly different, among second trimester MFPR (0 vs. 6%).

Using the 1995 to 1997 Multiple Birth File of the United States, Wen et al.[16] compared the maternal morbidity and obstetric complications of 152,238 twins, 5491 triplets and 432 quadruplets or more pregnancies. After an adjustment for important confounding factors, the risk of pregnancy-associated hypertension and eclampsia, anemia, diabetes mellitus, abruptio placenta, premature rupture of membrane, and Cesarean delivery was increased in women with triplet pregnancies and higher-order multiple pregnancies than in women with twin pregnancies. A dose–response relationship was observed for GDM (as well as for pregnancy-associated

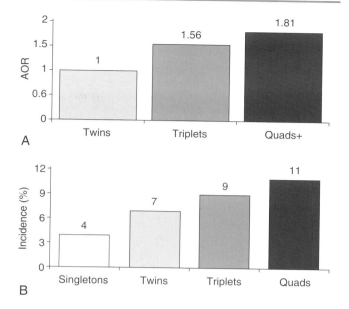

Figure 45.1   Risk of GDM by plurality. (A) Data adapted from Wen et al.[16]; AOR = adjusted odds ratio. (B) Data adapted from Newman and Luke.[17]

hypertension and placental abruption). Newman and Luke[17] complied data from numerous reports on the frequency of GDM in multiple pregnancies. Admittedly, this compilation of data is derived from diverse populations and different time periods. As such, it may not represent the definite frequency of GDM according to plurality, but it unquestionably shows a clear trend. However, Figure 45.1(A and B) suggests that both analyses clearly show similar plurality-dependent trends in the incidence of GDM.

The relationship between zygosity and GDM was not adequately studied mainly because accurate zygosity determinations are simple not available. In his study, Hoskins used the Weinberg rule to estimate zygosity.[18] A higher proportion of unlike-sex (3.5%) than like-sex twin pregnancies (1.6%) were complicated by GDM, resulting in an estimated risk for dizygotic relative to monozygotic pregnancies of 8.6 (95% CI = 3.5–21.0). The higher risk of GDM among mothers of dizygotic twins was attributed to the presence of two placentas which may support the development of greater insulin antagonism than the single placenta in the mother of monozygotic twins.

Conflicting data suggesting the same GDM rate in multiples

In almost three decades research failed to prove a clear-cut higher rate of GDM in multiple pregnancies. Naicker et al.[19] compared 26 women carrying twins with 26 women carrying singletons matched for age, parity, and gestational age. Each woman had an oral glucose tolerance test. Venues blood glucose levels and insulin response were not significantly different between the two groups. The same researcher subsequently reported on 21 twins and 21 matched for age, weight, parity, and gestational age singletons.[20] All 42 subjects had a 100-g glucose tolerance test. The only difference was lower plasma insulin level at 60 min in the twin group, but again, no significant differences in venous plasma glucose response and insulin levels were found between singletons and twins pregnancies. It is unknown, however, if cases in the two studies[19,20] were not the same.

Similar results were reported from the same group using a third trimester intravenous glucose tolerance test (of 0.5 g/kg body weight).[21] The comparison between 20 twin and 20 matched for age, weight, parity, and gestational age singleton pregnancies. Neither significant differences in mean venous insulin levels nor differences in glucose response were found between the groups.

One of the largest surveys was performed by Spellacy and his colleagues who assessed the risk of GDM in a cohort of 101,506 pregnancies, including 1253 twins.[22] The twin gestations were compared with a 5% random sample of singleton pregnancies ($n = 5119$). The data showed that twin pregnancies had no increased risk for GDM.

Henderson et al.[23] used a 50-g 1-h oral glucose challenge test to screen 9185 pregnancies, including 138 (1.5%) twin gestations. GDM was diagnosed when abnormal screens (>129 mg/dL) were followed by two or more abnormal values on the 3-h, 100-g glucose tolerance test (National Diabetes Data Group criteria). The incidence of GDM was similar for singleton and twin gestations: 5.8 and 5.4%, respectively.

Another source of information comes from the longitudinal study of Sameshima et al.[24] who followed eight triplet pregnancies with repeated 75-g glucose tolerance tests performed at all three trimesters as well as postpartum. Glucose values improved during the third trimester compared to the second trimester and postpartum, suggesting that a fetoplacental glucose drain may counterbalance maternal insulin resistance. Another approach was used by Blickstein and Weissman[25] who evaluated 56 twin pregnancies representing the tenth deciles of the mean twin birth weight distribution to investigate whether 'macrosomic' twins face the same increased perinatal risk, as do macrosomic singletons. In both study and control groups, GDM was infrequent and could not explain the increased birth weight among twins.

The lack of an association between multiples and GDM was also evaluated by Anwar et al.[26] and Syeda Zaib-un-Nisa et al.[27] in twins who conceived through IVF. When compared to spontaneous twins, the former had a similar incidence of GDM.

The potential relationship of GDM and antecedent conditions was evaluated by Mikola et al.[28] in 99 pregnancies of woman with polycystic ovarian syndrome (PCOS) compared to an unselected control population. Patient with PCOS often need infertility treatments and a high incidence of multiples is expected. Indeed, this study shows that twin and GDM rates were both increased (9.9 vs. 1.1% and 20 vs. 8.9%, in the PCOS group and in controls, respectively). At the same time, the BMI, a potential confounder for GDM, was also greater in PCOS patients than in controls (25.6 vs. 23). These results may suggest that the higher rate of GDM in patients with PCOS, often related to insulin resistance and hyperinsulinemia, may be attributed to the antecedent PCOS and not to the multiple pregnancies.

GDM in multiple pregnancy

The question whether twin pregnancies with GDM should by controlled in special manner was evaluated by Schwartz et al.[29] who compared the frequency, maternal age, weight, 1-h screen, glucose tolerance test results, post-treatment blood glucose values, insulin requirements and insulin dose in twin and singleton pregnancies associated with GDM and carbohydrate intolerance. These authors found that insulin requirements were not different, but there is an increased incoherence of GDM among twins (7.7 vs. 4.1%). This observation suggests a mild disturbance of carbohydrate tolerance in twins, which may be effectively managed by similar strategies used to control blood glucose in singletons. Ihara et al.[30] compared the effect of twin gestation on carbohydrate metabolism using a 75-g oral glucose tolerance test in 63 twin and 3791 singleton gestations during the third trimester. Plasma glucose concentrations were measured before (i.e. fasting) and at 30 min, 1 h and 2 h after a 75 g glucose oral load and the insulin concentration was measured before (i.e. fasting) and at 30 min after glucose ingestion. Women with twin gestation showed significantly lower plasma glucose concentrations during fasting and at 30 min after the glucose load, but no significant difference in serum glucose levels were found in the other parameters. This study could not find any significant difference in plasma glucose levels as used to define a pathologic OGTT between

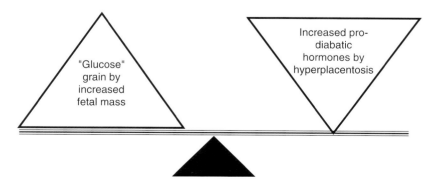

Figure 45.2   The occurrence of GDM might be the net effect between increased levels of pro-diabetic placental hormones counterbalanced by the increase in 'glucose' drain produced by the plurality-dependent increase in total fetal mass.

Box 45.1   Clinical data related to GDM and multiple pregnancies

Data supporting higher GDM rate in multiples
- Hyperplacentosis and higher hPL levels
- Exaggerated response to fasting and food
- Higher age
- Higher BMI and weight gain in multiple gestations
- Plurality-dependent frequency of GDM

Conflicting data concerning GDM and multiple pregnancies
- Similar prevalence of GDM in twin and singleton pregnancies
- No difference in glucose challenge and tolerance tests between twins and singleton pregnancies
- Management of twin and singleton gestations complicated by GDM is similar
- Similar insulin requirements in twin and singleton pregnancies complicated by GDM
- Higher rate of PCOS in multiple pregnancies

twin and singleton pregnancies except for fasting values. This observation suggests a lower tolerance to fasting in twin pregnancies but same glucose tolerance and insulin levels compare to singletons.

The data concerning the effect of GDM on perinatal outcome in multiple pregnancies is scant. Tchobroutsky et al.[31] reported on a high frequency of fetal malformations in type I diabetic women with twin pregnancies; however, the small number of cases precludes a final conclusion. Keller et al.[32] compared 13 twin pregnancies complicated with GDM to matched-by- gestational age twin pregnancies. There was a trend of greater likelihood of respiratory distress syndrome, hyperbilirubinemia and prolonged neonatal intensive care nursery admission in the diabetic group. More recently, Zaw and Stone[33] reported on twins born to a mother with pre-gestational diabetes and complicated with rare fetal anomaly related to diabetic pregnancy: caudal regression syndrome. In this unusual case – which may have long-term neurological, urologic, and orthopedic complications – is only one of a set of monozygotic twins. This report casts some doubt on the pathogenesis of this malformation and suggests an as yet unidentified factor other than hyperglycemia as a potential cause of this complication.

Epilogue

At this stage of our knowledge, the data related to a potential association between GDM and multiple pregnancies are conflicting. However, it may well be that these inconsistent data are a result of two mechanisms affecting the net result in opposite ways (Figure 45.2). On one hand, the increased placental mass is expected to increase pro-diabetic hormonal levels, and on the other, the increased total fetal mass works as a 'glucose' drain and offset this effect. Regrettably, the data presented in this chapter are not appropriate to draw any conclusions and do not support a clear-cut association between GDM and multiple pregnancies despite the inherent logical expectations (Box 45.1). In fact, there are several reservations concerning the available data.

First, some of the available studies are old and do not include multiples resulting from the current epidemic of iatrogenic conceptions. The remarkable difference between mothers, particularly in terms of age, before and after the 1990s[1,2] cast serious doubts if the prevalence cited in older studies is still valid today. Second, most, if not all information are hospital-based and not population-based data. Accordingly, prospective studies on maternal adaptation to carbohydrate metabolism during a multiple pregnancy are flawed by a small sample size and lack of sufficient statistical power. Moreover, time-lead bias, which overlooks changes in management over time have not been considered. For example, it would be interesting to know how the rate of PCOS in mothers of multiple pregnancies influences insulin resistant and GDM rates and how recommendations for excess weight gain during early stages of a multiple pregnancy[17] would influence carbohydrate metabolism.

As a final point, there is striking deficiency of studies related to high-order multiples, especially triplet pregnancies. Obviously, high-order multiples are of negligible importance in the Third World but this is not true any more in most developed countries.[1,2] This chapter clearly suggests that further study is needed to answer these and many other uncertainties related GDM and a multiple pregnancy.

REFERENCES

1. Blickstein I, Keith LG. The spectrum of iatrogenic multiple pregnancy. In: Blickstein I, Keith LG, eds. Iatrogenic multiple pregnancies: Clinical implications. New York: Parthenon Publishing; 2001, pp. 1–7.
2. Blickstein I, Keith LG. The epidemic of multiple pregnancies. Postgrad Obstet Gynecol 2001; 21: 1–7.
3. Loos R, Derom C, Vlietinck R, Derom R. The East Flanders Prospective Twin Survey (Belgium): a population-based register. Twin Res 1998; 1: 167–75.
4. Ventura SJ, Martin JA, Curtin SC, et al. Births: final data for 1998. Nat Vital Stat Rep 2000; 28: 1–100.
5. Beemsterboer SN, Homburg R, Gorter NA, et al. The paradox of declining fertility but increasing twinning rates with advancing maternal age. Hum Reprod 2006; 21: 1531–2.
6. Walker MC, Murphy KE, Pan S, Yang Q, Wen SW. Adverse maternal outcomes in multifetal pregnancies. Br J Obstet Gynaecol 2004; 111: 1294–6.

7. Erez O, Vardi IS, Hallak M, et al. Preeclampsia in twin gestations: association with IVF treatments, parity and maternal age. J Matern Fetal Neonatal Med 2006; 19: 141–6.

8. Spellacy WN, Buhi WC, Birk SA. Human placental lactogen levels in multiple pregnancies. Obstet Gynecol 1978; 52: 210–2.

9. Spellacy WN, Buhi WC, Birk SA. Carbohydrate metabolism in women with a twin pregnancy. Obstet Gynecol 1980; 55: 688–9.

10. Lurie S, Blickstein I. Age distribution of erythrocyte population in women with twin pregnancy. Gynecol Obstet Invest 1993; 36: 163–5.

11. Casele HL, Dooley SL, Metzger BE. Metabolic response to meal eating and extended overnight fast in twin gestation. Am J Obstet Gynecol 1996; 175: 917–21.

12. Marconi AM, Davoli E, Cetin I, et al. Impact of conceptus mass on glucose disposal rate in pregnant women. Am J Physiol 1993; 264: 514–8.

13. Sivan E, Maman E, Homko CJ, et al. Impact of fetal reduction on the incidence of gestational diabetes. Obstet Gynecol 2002; 99: 91–4.

14. Skupski DW, Nelson S, Kowalik A, et al. Multiple gestations from in vitro fertilization: successful implantation alone is not associated with subsequent preeclampsia. Am J Obstet Gynecol 1996; 175: 1029–32.

15. Geva E, Fait G, Yovel I, et al. Second-trimester multiple pregnancy reduction facilitates prenatal diagnosis before the procedure. Fertil Steril 2000; 73: 505–8.

16. Wen SW, Demissie K, Yang Q, et al. Maternal morbidity and obstetric complications in triplet pregnancies and quadruplet and higher-order multiple pregnancies. Am J Obstet Gyncol 2004; 191: 254–8.

17. Newman RB, Luke B, Multifetal pregnancy. Philadelphia: Lippincott, Williams & Wilkins; 2000.

18. Hoskins RE. Zygosity as a risk factor for complications and outcomes of twin pregnancy. 1995; 44: 11–23.

19. Naicker RS, Subrayen KT, Jialal I, et al. Carbohydrate metabolism in twin pregnancy. S Afr Med J 1983; 63: 538–40.

20. Moodley SP, Jialal I, Moodley J, et al. Carbohydrate metabolism in African women with twin pregnancy. Diabetes Care 1984; 7: 72–4.

21. Naidoo L, Jailal I, Moodley J, Desai R. Intravenous glucose tolerance tests in women with twin pregnancy. Obstet Gynecol 1985; 66: 500–2.

22. Spellacy WN, Handler A, Ferre CD. A case–control study of 1253 twin pregnancies from a 1982–1987 perinatal data base. Obstet Gynecol 1990; 75: 168–71.

23. Henderson CE, Scarpelli S, LaRosa D, Divon MY. Assessing the risk of gestational diabetes in twin gestation. Natl Med Assoc 1995; 87: 757–8.

24. Sameshima H, Higo T, Ikenoue T. Longitudinal changes in plasma glucose values of the 75 g glucose tolerance test in triplet pregnancies. Am J Perinatol 2004; 21: 49–55.

25. Blickstein I, Weissman A. 'Macrosomic' twinning: a study of growth-promoted twins. Obstet Gynecol 1990; 76: 822–4.

26. Nassar AH, Usta IM, Rechdan JB, et al. pregnancy outcome in spontaneous twins versus twines who were conceived through in vitro fertilization. Am J Obstet Gynecol 2003; 189: 513–8.

27. Zaib-un-Nisa S, Ghazal-Aswad S, Badrinath P. Outcome of twin pregnancies after assisted reproductive techniques – a comparative study. Eur J Obstet Gynecol Reprod Biol 2003; 109: 51–4.

28. Mikola M, Hiilesmaa V, Halttunen M, el al. Obstetric outcome in women with polycystic ovarian syndrome. Hum Reprod 2001; 16: 226–9.

29. Schwartz DB, Daoud Y, Zazula P, et al. Gestational diabetes mellitus: metabolic and blood glucose parameters in singleton versus twin pregnancies. Am J Obstet Gynecol 1999; 181: 912–4.

30. Ihara M, Mitao M, Yamasaki H, et al. Analysis of glucose tolerance in twin gestations using oral glucose load. Horm Metab Res 2002; 34: 338–40.

31. Tchobroutsky C, Vray M, Papoz L. Fetal malformations in twin pregnancies of type I diabetic women. Lancet 1991; 337: 1358.

32. Keller JD, Utter GO, Dooley SL, et al. Northwestern University Twin Study X: Outcome of twin gestations complicated by gestational diabetes mellitus. Acta Genet Med Gemellol 1991; 40: 153–7.

33. Zaw W, Stone DG. Caudal Regression Syndrome in twin pregnancy with type II diabetes. J Perinatol 2002; 22: 171–4.

46 Thyroid diseases in pregnancy

Jorge H. Mestman

Introduction

It is estimated that 5–20% of women of childbearing age suffer from autoimmune thyroid diseases. Women with diabetes Type 1 are three to five times more likely to be affected as non-diabetic women. In this chapter, we present a brief description of thyroid physiopathology in pregnancy, different aspects of their clinical manifestations, its repercussions on maternal, fetal and neonatal wellbeing and potential long-term effect on the offspring. It is imperative that a team approach be used in the management of these conditions, based on the one that has successfully improved the care of diabetic women. Preconception education and proper diagnosis and management of thyroid dysfunction early in pregnancy are of paramount importance in order to prevent complications during gestation and in the offspring.

In early pregnancy, the maternal thyroid gland needs to increase thyroxine production by approximately 50% as compared to the preconception state. The adaptation is accomplished by three main factors: (1) an increase in thyroxine-binding globulin (TBG) in the first few weeks after conception; (2) the stimulatory effect of hCG on the TSH thyroid receptor with a peak effect between 8 and 14 weeks gestation; and (3) the supply of iodine available to the thyroid gland.[1] The suggested total daily iodine ingestion for pregnant women is 229 µg a day and for lactating women 289 µg daily; prenatal vitamins should contain at least 150 µg of iodine.[2]

The normal thyroid gland is able to compensate for the increase in thyroid hormones demands by increasing their secretion and maintaining the serum levels of free hormones within normal limits throughout gestation. However, in those situations in which there is a subtle pathologic abnormality of the thyroid gland, such as in chronic autoimmune thyroiditis or in hypothyroid women on thyroid hormone therapy, the normal increase in the production of thyroid hormones is not met. As a consequence, the women are at risk of becoming hypothyroid.

Active secretion of thyroid hormones by the fetal thyroid gland commences at about 18 weeks gestation, although iodine uptake occurs between 10 and 14 weeks.[3] Transfer of thyroxine from the mother to the embryo occurs from early pregnancy. Maternal thyroxine has been demonstrated in coelomic fluid at 6 weeks gestation.[4] This maternal transfer continues until delivery, but only in significant amounts in the presence of fetal hypothyroidism.[5] Later in pregnancy the placenta plays in important role on transferring thyroxine due to the presence of the enzyme type 3 iodothyronine deiodinase (MID-III). Thyroid hormone receptor gene expression has been shown in human fetal brain by 8 weeks gestation, supporting the important role of maternal thyroid hormone during the first trimester of human pregnancy in fetal brain development.[6] Mild maternal thyroid deficiency in the first trimester could result in long-term neuropsychological damage to the offspring.[7]

The levels of maternal thyroid hormone concentrations, both total thyroxine (TT_4) and total triiodothyronine (TT_3) increase from early pregnancy, with a slight increase in free hormones in the first trimester with a corresponding lowering of serum TSH. Early in gestation, TSH values below the normal reference range may be seen in up to 15% of uncomplicated pregnancies, returning to normal levels by 18–20 weeks, but in a few situations may remain low until later in pregnancy.[1]

Human chorionic gonadotropin is a weak thyroid stimulator, acting on the thyroid TSH receptor. It is estimated that a 10,000 IU/L increment in circulating hCG corresponds to a mean T_4 increment in serum of 0.1 ng/dL, and in turn to a lowering of TSH of 0.1 mU/L, as seen in the first trimester of gestation. In situations in which there is a high production of hCG, or changes in its biological potency, such as in cases of multiple pregnancies, hydatidiform mole, and hyperemesis gravidarum (HG), serum T_4 concentrations rise to levels seen in thyrotoxicosis with a suppression in serum TSH values.

Thyroid function tests

Measurement of serum TSH is the most practical, simple, and economic screening test for thyroid dysfunction. Serum TSH concentrations are dependent on gestational age; it is lower in the first trimester as compared to the second and third trimester of pregnancy. There is significant clinical data at the present time to support a serum TSH value of 2.5 mIU/L as the upper limit of normal in first trimester of pregnancy, the lower limit of normal is 0.1 mIU/L.[1] There is a fairly good inverse correlation between TSH and hCG concentrations. As mentioned above, low or suppressed TSH values are present in about 15% of pregnant women in the first trimester of gestation. In the presence of an abnormal serum TSH value, the determination of FT_4 or its equivalent free thyroxine index (FT_4I), is necessary for the proper assessment of thyroid function. A word of caution regarding the determination of free thyroxine levels in different trimesters of pregnancy. There is a significant inconsistency among the different commercial assay of serum FT_4 because of methodology used and also because of variation in dietary iodine intake among the different populations studied. Currently none of the manufacturers of the automated free T4 assays has provided trimester specific reference ranges, therefore the determination of total T4 adjusted by a factor of 1.5 for pregnant patients has been suggested as a better estimation of serum free thyroxine concentration.[8] A better alternative is to estimate the free T4, by the free T4 index (FT_4I), calculated using the total T4 value and an indirect determination of serum TBG concentration..

The determination of TSH receptor antibodies (TRAb) is indicated in very special circumstances during pregnancy (Box 46.1). These antibodies are immunoglobulins, usually of the IgG subclass, having different functional activity: thyroid stimulating antibodies (TSI) in most patients with Graves' disease or blocking antibodies, in some patients with Hashimoto's thyroiditis, particularly in those without goiter. They do cross the placental barrier and when present in high titers may affect fetal thyroid function.[9] The chances for the offspring to be affected by these maternal antibodies are very low (up to 2% of mothers with autoimmune thyroid disease). However, if mothers with high titers are not properly identified, the consequences for the infant could be irreversible neurologic and metabolic sequelae. A value of TSRAb five times greater than normal is considered predictive of neonatal or fetal thyroid dysfunction.

Thyroid peroxidase antibodies (TPO) or antimicrosomal antibodies (AMA), markers of chronic autoimmune thyroiditis are present in 5–20% of women of childbearing age.

Goiter is commonly seen in pregnancy in areas of iodine deficiency. However, in the United States and other areas of the world with sufficient iodine intake, the thyroid gland does not clinically increase in size during pregnancy. Therefore, the detection of a goiter in pregnancy is an abnormal finding that needs

---

Box 46.1   Indications for maternal determination of TSI* or TRAb in Graves' disease (TSI)**

- Fetal or neonatal hyperthyroidism in previous pregnancies
- Active disease, on treatment with antithyroid drugs
- Euthyroid, postablation, in the presence of:
  - Fetal tachycardia
  - Intrauterine growth restriction
  - Incidental fetal goiter on ultrasound
- Incidental fetal goiter on ultrasound
- Infant born with congenital hypothyroidism

TSI*: Thyroid stimulating Immunoglobulin; TRAb**, TSH receptor antibodies**.

Box 46.2   Indications for thyroid testing in pregnancy

- Symptoms of thyroid dysfunction
- Family history of autoimmune thyroid disease
- Women on thyroid therapy
- Presence of goiter
- Previous history of:
  - High-dose neck radiation
  - Hyperthyroidism
  - Postpartum thyroid dysfunction
  - Hypothyroidish
  - Chronic Thyroiditis
  - Infertility
  - Miscarriages
  - Per-term delivery
- Previous birth of an infant with thyroid disease
- Type 1 diabetes mellitus
- Autoimmune diseases

---

careful evaluation. The most common cause of diffuse goiter is chronic autoimmune thyroiditis or Hashimoto's thyroiditis.

The indications for requesting TFTs are represented in Box 46.2. Whether routine thyroid screening in pregnant women is necessary remains a controversial issue; in a recent publication of a group of 40 pregnant women diagnosed with hypothyroidism early in pregnancy, 30 % of them were not considered to be in a high risk group for thyroid disease based on clinical history.[10]

Pre-pregnancy counseling

The physician may be faced with different clinical situations when counseling a woman with thyroid disease contemplating pregnancy.

Hyperthyroidism on antithyroid drug treatment

If the woman decides to continue antithyroid drug therapy, PTU is the drug of choice in view of rare cases of methimazole embriopathy (see section on hyperthyroidism). She should be made aware of the importance of frequent testing during gestation to achieve target serum thyroxine levels and the potential side effects on the fetus. Alternative therapies, ^{131}I ablation or thyroidectomy should be discussed. If the patient opts for ablation therapy, there is no long-term effect of ^{131}I therapy on the offspring. However, it is customary to wait 6 months after the therapeutic dose is administered before pregnancy is contemplated. Regardless of the form of therapy chosen, it is important for the patient to be euthyroid at the time of conception.

Previous ablation treatment for Graves' disease

Women treated with ablation therapy and on thyroid replacement therapy will need to increase levothyroxine doses soon after conception to avoid hypothyroidism.[11] In spite of remaining euthyroid on replacement hormonal therapy, in a subgroup of patients, high maternal titers for TSI or TSHRAb may be present, with the fetus being at risk of developing hyperthyroidism despite the mother being euthyroid (Box 46.1). Close follow-up during pregnancy and communication between the obstetrician and endocrinologist is essential.

Previous treatment with ^{131}I for thyroid carcinoma

With very few exceptions, pregnancy does not affect the natural history of women previously treated for thyroid cancer. Spontaneous miscarriages have been reported to be as high as 40% in the first year after radiation treatment as compared with 18% in women who have received no radiation.[12]

Hypothyroidism

Most hypothyroid women on thyroid hormone therapy will require higher doses soon after conception.[11] The increase in requirements is observed in the first 4–8 weeks of gestation. The physician should advise them to obtain thyroid function tests soon after conception. Some physicians suggest to empirically increase the dose of levothyroxine by 25–50 µg day as soon as pregnancy is suspected. Following delivery, the dose should be reduced to pre-pregnancy levels.

Euthyroid chronic thyroiditis

Patients with Hashimoto's thyroiditis are at greater risk of developing hypothyroidism very early in pregnancy because of the increase demand in thyroid hormones; if not properly managed they are at risk of developing the same complications as poorly treated hypothyroid mothers, mainly spontaneous abortions, preterm delivery, and pregnancy-induced hypertension (PIH). One recent study showed a significant decrease of miscarriages and preterm delivery in euthyroid chronic thyroiditis women treated with levo-thyroxine in the first 10 weeks of gestation as compared to euthyroid chronic thyroiditis mothers receiving no treatment and a control population.[13] In the untreated women a significant number of them developed subclinical hypothyroidism. Therefore it appears reasonable to treat euthyroid and subclinical hypothyroidism mothers with levo-thyroxine before or very early in pregnancy to prevent the above complications.

Maternal–placental–fetal interactions

Studies in the last two decades have shown an important role of maternal thyroid hormones in embryogenesis.[14] Maternal thyroxine crosses the placenta in the first half of pregnancy at the time when the fetal thyroid gland is not functional. Maternal TSH does not cross the placenta. TRH does cross the placental barrier, but its physiologic significance is unknown. Methimazole (MM) and propylthiouracil (PTU), cross the placenta, and if given in inappropriate doses may produce fetal goiter and hypothyroidism.[15]

Hyperthyroidism

Hyperthyroidism due to Graves' disease affects pregnancy in about 0.2% of patients[16] (Box 46.3). Gestational

Box 46.3   Etiologies of hyperthyroidism in pregnancy

- Graves' disease
- Nodular thyroid disease
- Subacute thyroiditis
- Iatrogenic
- Gestational thyrotoxicosis:
  - Hyperemesis gravidarum
  - Molar disease
- Rare:
  - Iodine induced
  - TSH-producing pituitary tumor

hyperthyroidism is define as a transient nonimmune hyperthyroidism due in the majority of cases to high levels of hCG or and increased in its biological activity. Single toxic adenoma and multinodular toxic goiter are found in less than 10% of cases. Subacute thyroiditis is rarely seen during gestation.

Transient hyperthyroidism of hyperemesis gravidarum

One of the most clinically recognized forms of gestational thyrotoxicosis is transient hyperthyroidism of hyperemesis gravidarum (THHG). It is characterized by severe nausea and vomiting, with onset between 4 and 8 weeks' gestation, requiring in many cases frequent visits to the emergency room and sometimes repeated hospitalizations for intravenous hydration. Weight loss of at least 5 kg, ketonuria, abnormal liver function tests, and hypokalemia are common findings, depending on the severity of vomiting and dehydration. Free thyroxine levels are elevated, sometimes up to four to six times the normal values, whereas FT_3 is elevated in up to 40% of affected women, values not as high as serum FT_4. The T_3/T_4 ratio is less than 20, as compared with Graves' hyperthyroidism, where the ratio is over 20. Serum TSH concentrations are very low or suppressed.[17] TPO antibodies are negative. In spite of the significant biochemical hyperthyroidism, signs and symptoms of hypermetabolism are mild or absent. Significant in the medical history is the lack of hyperthyroid symptoms before conception, since patients with Graves' disease diagnosed for the first time during gestation give the history of hypermetabolic symptoms antedating several months before pregnancy. Spontaneous normalization of hyperthyroxinemia parallels the improvement in vomiting and weight gain, with most of the cases resolving spontaneously between 14 and 20 weeks' gestation, suppressed serum TSH may lag for a few more weeks after normalization of free thyroid hormone levels. Antithyroid drugs are not effective in ameliorating the symptoms. Correction of vomiting, hydration and electrolytes imbalance is recommended until vomiting subsides and thyroid tests returned to normal.

Hyperthyroidism due to Graves' disease

In the vast majority of patients in whom the diagnosis is made for the first time during pregnancy, hyperthyroid symptoms antedate conception. The clinical diagnosis of thyrotoxicosis may present difficulties during gestation, since many symptoms and signs are commonly seen in normal pregnancy, such as mild palpitations, heart rate between 90 and 100 beats/min, mild heat intolerance, shortness of breath on exercise, and warm skin. Clinical clues for hyperthyroidism are presence of goiter, ophthalmopathy, proximal muscle weakness, tachycardia with a pulse rate over 100 beats/min, and weight loss or inability to gain weight in spite of a good appetite. When hyperthyroidism is properly managed throughout pregnancy, the outcome for mother and fetus is good; however, maternal and neonatal complications for untreated or poorly controlled mothers are significantly increased.[18]

Almost every patient with Graves' disease will have an elevated FT_4 concentration. A suppressed TSH value in the presence of a high FT_4 or FT_4 index confirms the diagnosis of hyperthyroidism. In some unusual situations, the serum FT_4 may be at the upper limit of normal or be slightly elevated, in which case the determination of FT_3 or the FT_3 index will confirm the diagnosis of hyperthyroidism. Thyroid peroxidase antibodies (anti-TPO) or thyroid antimicrosomal antibodies, are positive in the vast majority of patients.

Significant maternal and perinatal morbidity and mortality were reported in early studies.[19] In the last 20 years, however, there has been a significant decrease in the incidence of maternal and fetal complications directly related to improve control of maternal hyperthyroidism.[16,18,20] The most common maternal complication is PIH. In women with uncontrolled hyperthyroidism, the risk of severe preeclampsia was five times greater than in those patients with controlled disease.[18] Other complications include preterm delivery, placental abruption, and miscarriage. Congestive heart failure may occur in women untreated or treated for a short period of time in the presence of PIH or operative delivery.

Fetal and neonatal complications are also related to maternal control of hyperthyroidism. Intrauterine growth restriction (IUGR), prematurity, stillbirth, and neonatal morbidity are the most common complications. Uncontrolled hyperthyroidism during the entire gestation is associated with a 9-fold greater incidence of low-birth-weight infants as compared with the control population[18] (Figure 46.1). It was almost 2.5 times greater in those whose hyperthyroidism was treated

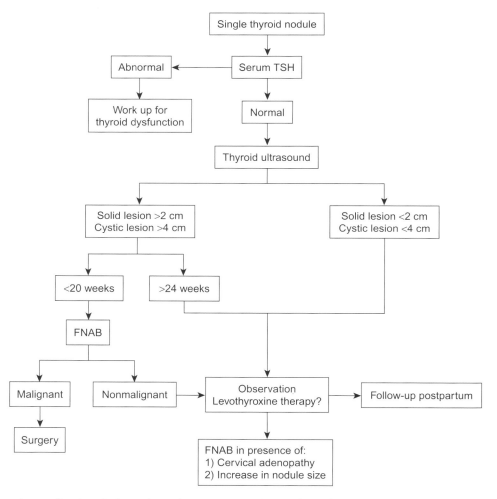

Figure 46.1   Perinatal complications in hyperthyroid women according to thyroid status at time of delivery. RR, relative risks. (Adapted from Millar, et al.[17])

during pregnancy and became euthyroid at some time during gestation. In those mothers achieving a euthyroid state before or early in pregnancy, the incidence of low-birth-weight infants was no different from that in the control population.

The goal of treatment is normalization of thyroid tests as soon as possible and to maintain euthyroidism with the minimum amount of antithyroid medication. Patients should be monitored at regular intervals and the dose of their medications adjusted to keep the FT_4 or preferable the FT_4I in the upper one third of the range of normal.[20] For this purpose, thyroid tests should be performed every 2 weeks at the beginning of treatment and every 2–4 weeks when euthyroidism is achieved. Patients with small goiters, short duration of symptoms, and on minimal amounts of antithyroid medication will be able to discontinue antithyroid drugs by 34 weeks' gestation or beyond and remain euthyroid.

In the USA, the two antithyroid drugs available are PTU and methimazole (Tapazole). Both drugs are effective in controlling symptoms. Aplasia cutis, an unusual scalp lesion, occurred in a small group of patients taking methimazole. A few reports have described a specific embryopathy in infants from mothers treated during the first trimester of pregnancy with methimazole but not with PTU.[21] This has been called 'methimazole embryopathy' and includes cloanal atresia and/or esophageal atresia, minor dimorphic features and development delay. Although these complications were not reported in relatively large series of pregnant women treated with PTU it appears prudent to avoid Tapazole in the first trimester of pregnancy if PTU is available.

The starting dose of PTU is 100–450 mg/day, in three daily doses; methimazole dose is 10–40 mg/day divided in two daily doses.[16] Those mothers with large goiters and longer duration of the disease may need larger doses at initiation of therapy. In patients with minimum symptoms, an initial dose of 10 mg of Tapazole daily or PTU 50 mg two or three times a day may be initiated, with normalization to chemical euthyroidism in 3–7 weeks.[22] Resistance to drug therapy is unusual, most likely due to poor patient compliance.[23] Once clinical improvement occurs, mainly weight gain and reduction in tachycardia, the dose of antithyroid medication may be reduced by half of the initial dose. The daily dose is adjusted every few weeks according to the clinical response and the results of thyroid tests. Serum TSH remains suppressed despite the normalization of thyroid hormone levels. Normalization of serum TSH is an indicator to reduce the dose of medication. If there is an exacerbation of symptoms or worsening of the thyroid tests, the amount of antithyroid medication is doubled. The main concern of maternal drug therapy is the potential side effect on the fetus; mainly, goiter and hypothyroidism. In most studies this has been prevented by using doses no greater than 200 mg PTU or 20 mg methimazole in the last few weeks of gestation. However, small elevations in serum TSH in the neonate have been reported even with low doses of antithyroid medication.[24]

Side effects of antithyroid drugs occur in 3–5% of treated patients. The most common complications of both drugs are pruritus and skin rash. They usually resolve by switching to the other antithyroid medication. In general, the rash occurs 2–6 weeks after initiation of therapy. Much rarer complications are migratory polyarthritis, a lupus-like syndrome, and

cholestatic jaundice. Agranulocytosis, a serious but unusual complication, has been reported in 1 in 300 patients receiving the drug. It is manifested by fever, malaise, gingivitis, and sore throat. Agranulocytosis occurs in the first 12 weeks of therapy and appears to be related to the dose of medication.[25] Routine blood counts are not recommended.

β-Adrenergic blocking agents (labetalol 100 mg twice a day or atenolol 25–50 mg/day) are very effective in controlling hyperdynamic symptoms and are indicated for the first few weeks in symptomatic patients.[16]

Thyroidectomy in pregnancy is effective in managing the disease; indications for surgical treatment are few: allergy to both antithyroid drugs,[26] very large goiters, patient preference, and the exceptional case of resistance to drug therapy.

[131]I therapy is contraindicated in pregnancy since, when given after 10 weeks' gestation, it produces fetal hypothyroidism.[27] A pregnancy test is essential in any woman of childbearing age before a therapeutic dose of ^{131}I is administered.

Assessment of fetal well-being with the use of ultrasonography, nonstress test, and/or biophysical profile is indicated for cases in poor metabolic control, in the presence of fetal tachycardia and/or intrauterine growth restriction, in pregnancies complicated by PIH or any other obstetrical or medical complications. Excessive amounts of antithyroid drugs have induced fetal hypothyroidism and goiter. Ultrasonography for monitoring the size of the fetal thyroid gland as an indicator of therapeutic targets may be useful in women considered high risk (presence of TSH receptor antibody, on ATD therapy); fetal goiter was detected in 11 out of 41 women with active or past history of Graves' disease, 4 fetuses were hyperthyroid and seven were hypothyroid; all of them benefit from adjusting maternal drug therapy. The authors of the study concluded that ultrasonography of the fetal thyroid gland by an experienced ultrasonographer is an excellent diagnostic tool, in conjunction with close teamwork, to ensure normal fetal thyroid function and proper development.[28]

Breast feeding is permitted if the daily dose of PTU or methimazole is less than 200 mg/day or 20 mg/daily, respectively. It is prudent to give the total amount in divided doses after each feeding.[29]

Neonatal hyperthyroidism

Neonatal hyperthyroidism is infrequent, with an incidence of less than 1% of infants born to mothers with Graves' disease, therefore affecting 1 in 50,000 neonates. The disease is caused by the placental transfer of stimulating thyroid antibodies (TSIs) from mother to fetus. High serum maternal TSI titers (a 3- to 5-fold increase over baseline), in the third trimester of pregnancy are predictors of neonatal hyperthyroidism.[30] If the mother is treated with antithyroid medications, the fetus benefits from maternal therapy, remaining euthyroid during pregnancy. However, the protective effect of the antithyroid drug is lost after delivery, and neonatal hyperthyroidism may develop within a few days after birth. If neonatal hyperthyroidism is not recognized and treated properly, neonatal mortality may be as high as 30%. Since the half-life of the antibodies is only a few weeks, complete resolution of neonatal hyperthyroidism is the rule.[28]

Sporadic cases of neonatal hyperthyroidism without evidence of the presence of circulating TSI in mother or infant have recently been published.[31] Activation of mutations in the TSH receptor molecule are the cause of this entity.

Fetal hyperthyroidism

In mothers with a history of Graves' disease previously treated with ablation therapy, either surgery or ^{131}I, concentrations of TSI may remain elevated, in spite of maternal euthyroidism. The concentration of these IgG immunoglobulins in the fetus reaches levels similar to the mother by 26–30 weeks gestation. Therefore, the symptoms of fetal hyperthyroidism are not evident until 22–24 weeks of gestation. Fetal hyperthyroidism is characterized by fetal tachycardia, IUGR, oligohydramnios, and a goiter may be identified on ultrasonography.[28,32] The diagnosis may be confirmed by measuring thyroid hormone levels in cord blood obtained by cordocentesis.[33] Treatment consisted of antithyroid medication given to the mother, PTU 100–400 mg/day or methimazole 10–20 mg/day. The dose is guided by the improvement and resolution of fetal tachycardia and normalization of fetal growth, both of which are indicators of good therapeutic response. Fetal ulreasonography in experts hands could be a valuable diagnostic tool.

Neonatal central hypothyroidism

Infants of untreated hyperthyroid mothers may be born with transient central hypothyroidism (pituitary or hypothalamic origin).[34] High levels of thyroxine crossing the placenta barrier, feedback to the fetus pituitary with suppression of fetal pituitary TSH. The diagnosis is made in the presence of low FT_4 and normal or low TSH in cord blood. This is another complication easily avoidable with proper management of maternal hyperthyroidism.

Hypothyroidism

The incidence of maternal hypothyroidism is between 0.19 and 2.5%.[35] Subclinical hypothyroidism (normal FT_4 and elevated TSH) is more often encountered than clinical hypothyroidism (low FT_4 and elevated TSH). Mild elevations in serum TSH are frequently detected in hypothyroid women on thyroid replacement therapy soon after conception because of the increased demand for thyroid hormones in the first weeks of gestation.[11]

The two most common etiologies of primary hypothyroidism are autoimmune thyroiditis (Hashimoto's or chronic thyroiditis) and post-thyroid ablation therapy, surgical or ^{131}I induced.

As in the case of hyperthyroidism, the most common complication in hypothyroid pregnant women are PIH, prematurity and low birth weight. No significant complications were seen in those women achieving euthyroidism before 24 weeks' gestation.[36–38]

The impact of maternal hypothyroidism on the intellectual development of the offspring has been the subject of several studies.[7,39] In the study by Haddow et al.[7] children born of mothers with mild elevations of serum TSH, measured between 16 and 18 weeks' gestation, were studied at age 7–9. They reported a four-point decrease in IQ score on the Wechsler Intelligence Scale for Children for the whole group; a seven-point was reported in children whose mothers were not teated and in 19% of them the IQ score was less than 85.

Levothyroxine, or L-thyroxine, is the drug of choice for the treatment of hypothyroidism. In view of the complications mentioned above, it is important to normalize thyroid tests. An initial daily dose of 100–150 µg of levothyroxine is well tolerated by the majority of young hypothyroid patients. In those with severe hypothyroidism, there is a delay in the normalization of serum TSH, but normal serum FT_4 or FT_4I values are achieved in the first 2 weeks of therapy. The maintenance dose required for most patients is between 100 and 250 µg of levothyroxine per day. Higher doses may be required for patients after total thyroidectomy for thyroid carcinoma, since the goal in these cases is low values or suppression of serum TSH.

Patients on thyroid therapy before conception should have their TSH checked on their first visit and the amount of levothyroxine adjusted accordingly. The serum TSH should be repeated every 4–6 weeks during the first 20 weeks, at 24–28 weeks and at 32–34 weeks gestation. Increase in thyroid requirements is seen in about 20–30% of patients in the second half of pregnancy. Immediately after delivery, they should return to pre-pregnancy dosage. Iron and calcium tablets taken at the same time with levothyroxine interfere in its absorption. Therefore it is recommended to be taken 2 h apart, preferably with an empty stomach.

Single nodule of the thyroid gland

Nodular thyroid disease is clinically detectable in 10% of pregnant women. In most cases, it is discovered during the first routine clinical examination or detected by the patient herself. The chances for a single or solitary thyroid nodule to be malignant are between 5 and 10%, depending on risk factors such as previous radiation therapy to the upper body, rapid growth of a painless nodule, patient age, and family history of thyroid cancer. Papillary carcinoma accounts for almost 75–80% of malignant tumors, and follicular neoplasm for 15–20%; a few percent are represented by medullary thyroid carcinoma. There is a paucity of information in the literature regarding the management and timing of the work-up in the presence of thyroid nodularity.[40,41] It is generally agreed that elective surgery should be avoided in the first trimester and after 24 weeks' gestation because of the potential risks of spontaneous abortion and premature delivery, respectively.

A hard, painless nodule, measuring more than 2 cm in diameter, is suspicious of malignancy. High-resolution realtime ultrasound is very helpful in defining the size of the lesion, characterizing the dominant one, and identifying microcalcifications suspicious for either papillary or medullary thyroid carcinoma. Fine-needle aspiration biopsy is routinely used for diagnostic purposes.

In a retrospective study, a conservative approach to the management of a single thyroid nodule was recommended.[42] In the study, 61 women were pregnant at the time of the diagnosis of a differentiated thyroid carcinoma. The diagnosis was papillary cancer in 87% of them and follicular cancer in 13%. Fourteen women were operated on during pregnancy, whereas the other 47 women underwent surgical treatment 1–84 months after delivery. The outcome was compared with a group of 598 nonpregnant women matched for age. The median follow-up was 22.4 years as compared with 19.5 years in the nonpregnant group. Treatment and outcome were similar in both groups, those operated on during pregnancy and those in whom thyroidectomy was performed postpartum. The authors concluded that both diagnostic studies and initial therapy might be delayed until after delivery in most patients.

In the presence of a single thyroid nodule detected on physical examination, the following approach is recommended in our institution (Figure 46.2).

The above protocol has been used in our institution for many years. In view of a recent publication discussed previously,[42] it is imperative for the physician to discuss the different therapeutic options with the patient and her family. The anxiety of the patient and her family, and their wishes should be considered in making the final decision. The long-term prognosis of most thyroid cancers is exceptionally good, but patients should be followed for many years.

Chronic autoimmune thyroiditis (Hashimoto's thyroiditis)

Chronic autoimmune thyroid disease is more common in women with other autoimmune diseases, particularly Type 1 diabetes. The prevalence of positive TPO antibodies in women of childbearing age is between 3- and 5-fold higher in Type 1 diabetes.[43]

The clinical picture is characterized by the presence of a goiter, moderate in size, bilateral in most cases, with one lobe

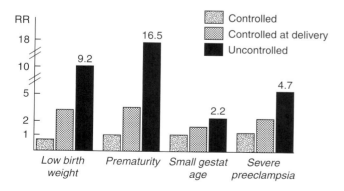

Figure 46.2 Evaluation of single thyroid nodules in pregnancy. (Adapted from Mestman JH. Thyroid and parathyroid diseases in pregnancy. In: Obstetrics: Normal and Problem Pregnancies, 5th ed. Gabbe SG, Niebyl JR, Simpson JL, eds. Elsevier Publishing, Philadelphia, PA 2007 (in print).

larger than the other, firm, rubbery consistency, and moving freely on swallowing. It is painless, although rapid growth of the gland may elicit some tenderness on palpation. Absence of goiter (atrophic thyroiditis) may be present in 30% of patients

The importance of diagnosing chronic thyroiditis in women of childbearing age relates to the potential maternal and fetal complications. Women with chronic thyroiditis are at higher risk for spontaneous abortion, development of hypothyroidism for the first time in pregnancy, premature delivery and postpartum thyroiditis.[44]

Negro et al.[13] recently studied a group of euthyroid women with chronic thyroiditis early in pregnancy. Of 984 pregnant women, 11.7% were TPO antibody positive. Fifty-seven of these women were treated with levothyroxine throughout gestation (0.5 µg/kg daily for a TSH less than 1.0 mIU/L, 0.75 µg/kg for TSH between 1.0 and 2.0 mIU/L and 1 µg/kg for TSH higher than 2 mIU/L or TPO titer exceeding 1500 kIU/L). Seventy-nine percent of patients started the treatment by the 12th week of gestation. Fifty-eight women received no treatment. The mean serum TSH in both groups by 10 weeks gestation was 1.6 ± 0.5 in the treated group and 1.7 ± 0.5 in the untreated one. The TSH value was significantly different than a group of pregnant women with negative antibodies (1.1 ± 0.4) When compared to the untreated women, the incidence of miscarriage and premature delivery (less than 37 weeks gestation) was significantly decrease in the treated mothers. This is the first study showing a beneficial therapeutic effect of levothyroxine therapy in euthyroid women with chronic thyroiditis.

In a very small subset of women with chronic thyroiditis, particularly those without a goiter (atrophic form), antibodies to the TSH receptor with blocking capabilities are present (TRBAb). These antibodies cross the placenta, and at high titers may block the action of TSH in the fetal thyroid, causing transient congenital hypothyroidism, which occurred in 1 of 180,000 live births. The neonatal disease resolves spontaneously over 3–6 months as the maternal antibody is degraded.[45]

Universal screening vs. case-finding cases

Universal vs. case-finding case screening for thyroid disease in pregnancy is controversial.[46] Those women at risk (Box 46.2) should be screened before or early in pregnancy, with the determination of serum TSH and TPOAb. If the serum TSH is elevated a free thyroxine tests should be added. In a recent publication, 40 women out of 1560 consecutive pregnant women (2.6%) had an elevated serum TSH, and 70% of them were in the high-risk group, while 30% of them had no risk factors based on medical history. This study along with a previous one[7] appears to support universal thyroid screening early in pregnancy.

Postpartum thyroid dysfunction

Thyroid dysfunction, hyper- and hypothyroidism, affects 5–10% of women in the 12 months following delivery, or following spontaneous or medically induced abortions.[48] Most of the cases are due to intrinsic thyroid disease, with a few due to hypothalamic or pituitary lesions Patients with autoimmune thyroid disease, chronic thyroiditis, and Graves' disease are most frequently affected.

The clinical diagnosis is not always obvious and the clinician should be concerned about nonspecific symptoms such as tiredness, fatigue, depression, palpitations, and irritability in women following the birth of their child or a miscarriage or abortion. Fatigue is the most common complaint. In some cases, the clinical symptoms resemble the syndrome of postpartum depression. Indeed, thyroid antibodies have been found more frequently in euthyroid women with postpartum depression, but this is still a controversial issue.

Postpartum thyroiditis rarely develop in women with negative antibodies.[47] In about one-third of the cases, mild symptoms of hyperthyroidism develop between 2 and 4 months postpartum. A goiter is felt in the majority of cases, firm and nontender to palpation. Thyroid tests are in the hyperthyroid range and thyroid antibodies, anti-TPO antibody titers, are elevated. Spontaneously, without specific therapy, hyperthyroidism resolves, followed in a few weeks by hypothyroidism, with spontaneous recovery and return to a euthyroid state by 7–12 months following delivery. Antibody titers have a tendency to increase during this process, and a change in the size of the goiter is usually noted. In a few patients, permanent hypothyroidism may develop. About 50% of patients, however, will develop permanent hypothyroidism within 5 years of the diagnosis of PPT.[49,50]

In one-third of patients, the course of PPT is different, characterized by an initial episode of hypothyroidism between 3 and 7 months postpartum without the initial hyperthyroid phase. In the other one third of patients, the initial episode of hyperthyroidism is followed by a return to normal thyroid function.

Postpartum thyroid dysfunction may also occur in patients with a known history of Graves' disease.[51] It is common for women with Graves' disease to have an exacerbation of their symptoms in the first 2 months postpartum. The symptoms of hyperthyroidism are more severe than those in patients with PPT. They may present with ophthalmopathy and hypermetabolic findings. Therapy with antithyroid medications is needed in these cases. On the other hand, patients with Graves' disease may have a bout of hyperthyroidism secondary to a concomitant episode of PPT. The differential diagnosis in this situation is important, since the treatment is different. If not contraindicated (breast-feeding mothers), a 4- or 24-h thyroid radioactive iodine uptake (RAIU) is helpful. It will be very low in patients with PPT, whereas it is high normal or elevated in patients with recurrent hyperthyroidism due to Graves' disease. When it is due to recurrent Graves' disease, treatment with antithyroid medications is indicated, or the physician may advise ablation therapy with [131]I.

It is recommended that a diagnosis of PPT be considered for any thyroid abnormality occurring within 1 year after delivery or miscarriages.

Since most cases of postpartum thyroid dysfunction recover spontaneously, treatment is indicated for symptomatic patients. In the presence of hyperthyroid symptoms, β-adrenergic-blocking drugs (propranolol 20–40 mg every 6 h or atenolol 25–50 mg every 24 h) are effective in controlling the symptoms. Antithyroid medications are not effective, because the hyperthyroxinemia is secondary to the release of thyroid hormones due to the acute injury to the thyroid gland (destructive hyperthyroidism). For hypothyroid symptoms, small amounts of levothyroxine 0.050 mg/day will control symptoms, allowing for a spontaneous recovery of thyroid function after discontinuation of the drug. PPT may recur in future pregnancies, with a recurrence rate between 30 and 70%.[48]

In view of the potential pregnancy complications seen in women with chronic thyroiditis, it is advisable for them to continue with Thyroxine therapy during their childbearing age, even if thyroid tests returned to normal after discontinuation of L-thyroxine therapy.

Acknowledgment

The author wishes to thank Elsa C. Ahumada for her secretarial assistance.

REFERENCES

1. Glinoer D. The regulation of thyroid function during normal pregnancy: importance of the ioding nutrition status. Best Pract Res Clin Endocrinol Metab 2004; 18: 133–52.
2. Glinoer D. Iodine nutrition requirements during pregnancy. Thyroid 2006; 16: 947–8.
3. Thorpe-Beeston JG, Nicolaides KH, Felton CV, et al. Maturation of the secretion of thyroid hormone and thyroid stimulating hormone in the fetus. N Engl J Med 1991; 324: 532.
4. Contempre B, Jauniaux E, Calvo R, et al. Detection of thyroid hormones in human embryonic cavities during the first trimester of pregnancy. J Clin Endocrinol Metab 1993; 77: 1719.
5. Vulsma T, Gons MH, DeVijlder JJM. Maternal fetal transfer of thyroxine in congenital hypothyroidism due to a total organification defect or thyroid agenesis. N Engl J Med 1989, 321: 13.
6. Iskaros J, Pickard M, Evans I, et al. Thyroid hormone receptor gene expression in first trimester human fetus brain. J Clin Endocrinol Metab 2000; 85: 2620.
7. Haddow JE, Palomaki GE, Allan WC, et al. Maternal thyroid deficiency during pregnancy and subsequent neuropsychological development of the child. N Engl J Med 1999; 341: 549.
8. Spencer C, Lee R, Kazarosyan M, et al. Thyroid reference ranges in pregnancy: Studies on an iodine sufficient cohort [Abstract]. Thyroid 2005; 15(suppl. 1): S16.
9. McKenzie JM, Zakarija M. Fetal and neonatal hyperthyroidism and hypothyroidism due to maternal TSH receptor antibodies. Thyroid 1992; 2: 155.
10. Vaidya B, Anthony S, Bilous M, et al. Detection of thyroid dysfunction in early pregnancy: universal screening or targeted high-risk case finding? J Clin Endocrinol Metab 2007; 92: 203–7.
11. Alexander EK, Marqusee E, Lawrence J, et al. Timing and magnitude of increases in levothyroxine requirements during pregnancy in women with hypothyroidism. N Engl J Med 2004; 351: 241–9.
12. Schlumberger M, Vathaire F, Ceccarelli C, et al. Exposure to radioactive iodine 131 for scintigraphy or therapy does not preclude pregnancy in thyroid cancer patients. J Nucl Med 1996; 37: 606.
13. Negro R, Formoso G, Mangieri T, et al. Levothyroxine treatment in euthyroid pregnant women with autoimmune thyroid disease: effects of obstetrical complications. J Clin Endocrinol Metab 2006; 91: 2587–9.

14. Morreale de Escobar G, Obregon MJ, Escobar del Rey F. Maternal thyroid hormones early in pregnancy and fetal brain development. Best Pract Res Clin Endocrinol Metab 2004; 18: 225–48.

15. Perelman AH, Johnson RL, Clemons RD, et al. Intrauterine diagnosis and treatment of fetal goitrous hypothyroidism. J Clin Endocinrol Metab 1990; 71: 618.

16. Mestman JH. Hyperthyroidism in pregnancy. Best Pract Res Clin Endocrinol Metab 2004; 18: 267–88.

17. Goodwin TM, Montoro MN, Mestman JH. Transient hyperthyroidism and hyperemesis gravidarum: clinical aspects. Am J Obstet Gynecol 1992; 167: 648.

18. Millar LK, Wing DA, Leung AS, et al. Low birth weight and preeclampsia in pregnancies complicated by hyperthyroidism. Obstet Gynecol 1994; 84: 946.

19. Bell GO, Hall J. Hyperthyroidism in pregnancy. Med Clin North Am 1960; 44: 363.

20. Momotani N, Noh J, Oyangi H, et al. Antithyroid drug therapy for Graves' disease during pregnancy: optimal regimen for fetal thyroid status. N Engl J Med 1986; 315: 24.

21. Johnsson E, Larsson G, Ljunggren M. Severe malformations in infants born to hyperthyroid mothers on methimazole. Lancet 1997; 350: 1520.

22. Wing DA, Miller LK, Koonings PP. A comparision of propylthiouracil versus methimazole in the treatment of hyperthyroidism in pregnancy. Am J Obstet Gynecol 1994; 170: 90.

23. Cooper DS. Propylthiouracil levels in hyperthyroid patients unresponsive to large doses. Ann Intern Med 1985; 192: 328.

24. Momotani N, Noh JY, Ishikawa N, et al. Effects of propylthiouracil and methimazole on fetal thyroid status in mothers with Graves' hyperthyroidism. J Clin Endocrinol Metab 1997; 82: 3633.

25. Cooper DS, Golminz D, Levin AA, et al. Agranulocytosis associated with antithyroid drugs: effects of patient's age and drug dose. Ann Intern Med 1983; 98: 26.

26. Bruner J, Landon MB, Gabbe SG. Diabetes mellitus and Graves' disease in pregnancy complicated by maternal allergies to antithyroid medication. Obstet Gynecol 1988; 72: 443.

27. Stoffer SS, Hamburger JI. Inadvertent 131I therapy for hyperthyroidism in the first trimester of pregnancy. J Nucl Med 1976; 17: 146.

28. Polak M, Le Gac I, Vuillard E, et al. Fetal and neonatal thyroid function in relation to maternal Graves' disease. Best Pract Res Clin Endocrinol Metab 2004; 18: 289–302.

29. Azizi F, Khoshniat M, Bahrainian M, Hedayati M. Thyroid function and intellectual development of infants nursed by mothers taking methimazole. J Clin Endocrinol Metab 2000; 85: 3233–8.

30. Peleg D, Cada S, Peleg A, Ben-Ami M. The relationship between maternal serum thyroid stimulating immunoglobulin and fetal and neonatal thyrotoxicosis. Obstet Gynecol 2002; 99: 1040–3.

31. Kopp P, Van Sande J, Parma J, et al. Brief report: congenital hyperthyroidism caused by a mutation in the thyrotropin receptor gene. N Engl J Med 1995; 322: 150.

32. Zimmerman D. Fetal and neonatal hyperthyroidism. Thyroid 1999; 9: 727.

33. Nachum Z, Rakover Y, Weiner E, Shalev E. Graves' disease in pregnancy: prospective evaluation of a selective invasive treatment protocol. Obstet Gynecol 2003; 189: 159–65.

34. Kempers MJE, van Tijn DA, van Trotsenburg ASP, et al. Central congenital hypothyroidism due to gestational hyperthyroidism: detection where prevention failed. J Clin Endocrinol Metab 2003; 88: 5851–7.

35. Mandel SJ. Hypothyroidism and chronic autoimmune thyroiditis in the pregnant state: maternal aspect. Best Pract Res Clin Endocrinol Metab 2004; 18: 213–24.

36. Davis LE, Leveno KJI, Cunningham FG. Hypothyroidism complicating pregnancy. Obstet Gynecol 1988; 72: 108.

37. Leung AS, Millar LK, Koonings PP, et al. Perinatal outcome in hypothyroid pregnancies. Obstet Gynecol 1993; 81: 349.

38. Abalovich M, Gutierrez S, Alcaraz G, et al. Overt and subclinical hypothyroidism complicating pregnancy. Thyroid 2002; 12: 63–8.

39. Poop VJ, Brouwers EP, Vader HI, et al. Maternal hypothyroxinemia during early pregnancy and subsequent child development: a 3 year follow up study. Clin Endocrinol (Oxf) 2003; 59; 282–8.

40. Doherty CM, Shindo ML, Rice DH, et al. Management of thyroid nodules during pregnancy. Laryngoscope 1995; 105: 251.

41. Rosen IB, Korman M, Walfish CM. Thyroid nodular disease in pregnancy: current diagnosis and management. Clin Obstet Gynecol 1997; 40: 81–9.

42. Moosa M, Mazzaferri EL. Outcome of differentiated thyroid cancer diagnosed in pregnant women. J Clin Endocrinol Metab 1997; 82: 2862.

43. Stagnaro-Green A. Postpartum thyroiditis. Best Pract Res Clin Endocrinol Metab 2004; 18: 303–16.

44. Abramson J, Stagnaro-Green A. Thyroid antibodies and fetal loss: an evolving story. Thyroid 2001; 11: 57–63.

45. Brown RS, Bellisario RL, Botero D, et al. Incidence of transient congenital hypothyroidism due to maternal thyrotropin receptor-blocking antibodies in over one million babies. J Clin Endocrinol Metab 1996; 81: 1147–51.

46. Casey BM. Subclinical hypothyroidism and pregnancy. Obstet Gynecol Sur 2006; 61: 415.

47. Nicholson WK, Robinson KA, Smallridge RC, Ladenson PW, Powe NR. Prevalence of postpartum thyroid dysfunction: a quantitative review. Thyroid 2006; 16: 573–82.

48. Alvarez-Marfany M, Roman SH, Drexler AJ, et al. Long term prospective study of postpartum thyroid dysfunction in women with insulin dependent diabetes mellitus. J Clin Endocrinol Metab 1994; 79: 10.

49. Kuipens JL, Pop VJ, Vader HL, et al. Prediction of postpartum thyroid dysfunction: can it be improved? Eur J Endocrinol 1998; 139: 36.

50. Premawardhana LDKE, Parkes AB, Ammari F, et al. Postpartum thyroiditis and long term thyroid status prognostic influence of thyroid peroxidase antibodies and ultrasound echogenicity. J Clin Endocrinol Metab 2000; 85: 71.

51. Momotani N, Noh J, Ishikawa N, et al. Relationship between silent thyroiditis and recurrent Graves' disease in the postpartum period. J Clin Endocrinol Metab 1994; 79: 285.

47 Short-term implications: The neonate

Paul Merlob and Moshe Hod

Introduction

An estimated 0.1–0.5% of all pregnancies are complicated by maternal pre-gestational diabetes mellitus (Types 1 and 2) and another 1–5% by gestational diabetes (carbohydrate intolerance first recognized during pregnancy).[1,2] The 1988 National Maternal and Infant Health Survey[3] reported a 4% rate of live-birth diabetic pregnancies: 88% gestational diabetes, 8% pre-gestational Type 2 (noninsulin-dependent) and 4% pre-gestational Type 1 (insulin-dependent).

One of the major goals of the Saint Vincent Declaration for Diabetes Care and Research in Europe[4] was to achieve a pregnancy outcome in diabetic women close to that in non-diabetic women. Thanks to advances in obstetric and neonatologic care, the perinatal mortality and neonatal morbidity associated with diabetic pregnancy have been significantly reduced. However, maternal diabetes still poses numerous metabolic, hematologic and anatomic risks to fetus and newborn (Table 47.1).[1,2,5] Their short-term implications during the first days after birth are discussed in detail in this chapter from a neonatological point of view. Macrosomia and congenital malformations are discussed in separate chapters.

It should be emphasized that the reported prevalence of short-term neonatal complications of maternal diabetes (pregestational or gestational) varies among different studies, mostly because of the lack of control of confounding variables, such as gestational age, maternal age, parity and body mass index (BMI).[6] Comparative evaluations are further impeded by differences in ethnic origin and socioeconomic status of the study samples, differences in diagnostic criteria, and the type and intensity of interventions during pregnancy.[6]

Neonatal hypoglycemia

Definition

The definition of neonatal hypoglycemia has changed over the last 20 years and still remains elusive. There is no accepted threshold for plasma glucose concentration below which neurologic impairment or injury is inevitable. The cutoff of 44 mg% (2.6 mmol/L) is now currently used as the working definition.[7–9] This 'operational threshold'[9] is not a diagnosis of a disease, but an indication for action.

Prevalence

The reported prevalence of neonatal hypoglycemia in diabetic pregnancy varies because of variations in the definition of the disorder; this is in addition to differences in methods of glucose examination, maternal control of diabetes during pregnancy and labor, and neonatal treatment, particularly feeding. It is not surprising in the light of these great variations that the previous figures for neonatal hypoglycemia in infants of diabetic mothers (IDM) have only historical significance. During the last 10 years, in well-controlled diabetic mothers and using the 'operational definition' of neonatal hypoglycemia,

Table 47.1 Effects of maternal diabetes on fetus and neonate

Period of exposure	Effects
1st trimester (embryo) embryogenesis	1. Spontaneous abortions 2. Early growth delay 3. Congenital malformations
2nd and 3rd trimester (fetus)	1. Macrosomia 2. Organomegaly 3. CNS development delay 4. Chronic hypoxemia 5. Stillbirth
Delivery	1. Preterm birth 2. Birth injury
Neonate	**Metabolic** 1. Hypoglycemia 2. Hypocalcemia 3. Hypomagnesemia 4. Other metabolic disorders **Hematologic** 5. Polycythemia 6. Hyperbilirubinemia 7. Other hematologic anatomic disorders; 8. Macrosomia 9. Respiratory distress syndrome 10. Vascular thrombosis 11. Transient disorders 12. Congenital malformations

the prevalence of early neonatal hypoglycemia was still high, particularly in those mothers who were long-standing diabetics. In 2000, Agrawal et al.[10] reported 47% prevalence, but they used a threshold of only 2 mmol/L (c. 34 mg%). Cordero et al[1] noted a 47% prevalence in macrosomic IDM (Type 1) but only 20% in non-macrosomic infants. In infants of gestational diabetes mothers (IGDM), the rate is c. 25%,[10] although some estimates are as high as 40%.[11] In the present authors' population, neonatal hypoglycemia was found in 26.3% of infants whose diabetic mothers maintained strict glycemic control throughout pregnancy and delivery.

Risk factors

The degree of neonatal hypoglycemia in IDM is affected by several maternal and neonatal factors. Early postnatal blood glucose concentrations have been negatively correlated with maternal blood glucose concentrations at delivery and to cord plasma glucose levels. Hypoglycemia did not occur when the maternal blood glucose at delivery was less than 7.1 mmol/L (c. 120 mg%).[6] Maternal glycemic control during labor and delivery is also important: early postnatal hyperglycemia has been described in infants whose nondiabetic mothers received i.v. glucose during labor.[6] Neonatal risk factors include perinatal distress, small for gestational age, polycythemia, and individual susceptibility.

Etiology

The most accepted explanation for the development of neonatal hypoglycemia in IDM is the Pedersen hypothesis or the maternal hyperglycemia–fetal hyperinsulinemia theory.[5] This hypothesis claims that even in women under close observation, the episodic diurnal hyperglycemia characteristic of diabetes is the major factor predisposing the fetus to hyperglycemia because of the direct relationship between the maternal and fetal blood glucose concentrations. The fetal hyperglycemia stimulates the release of insulin by fetal islet cells, giving rise to persistent fetal hyperinsulinemia. After birth, the hyperinsulinemia and inadequate or absence of glucose intake lead to neonatal hypoglycemia. Fetal hyperinsulinemia is also associated with suppression of plasma free-fatty-acid levels and hepatic glucose output.

The Pedersen hypothesis has been extended by Freinkel[12] who has examined the role of other nutrients that provide a substrate mixture for the fetus. Freinkel[12] introduced the concept of 'pregnancy as a tissue culture experience', proposing that the placenta and the fetus develop in an 'incubation medium' that is totally derived from maternal fuels. All these fuels (glucose, amino acids, lipids) transverse the placenta in a concentration-dependent fashion and thus delimit the 'incubation medium' in the fetal circulation. Since all these constituents are regulated by maternal insulin, disturbances in its supply or action will influence the whole nutrient composition to which the fetus is exposed and may lead to fetal hyperinsulinemia.

Other hormones may also play a role. Defective counterregulation by catecholamines and/or glucagon (i.e. failure of their release in response to hypoglycemia) results in both increased glucose clearance and diminished glucose production. These, together with the hyperinsulinemia, decrease hepatic production of glucose, increase peripheral glucose uptake, and impair lipolysis, resulting in hypoglycemia in the neonate.

Clinical manifestations

The clinical manifestations of neonatal hypoglycemia in IDM and IGDM are not specific, and there is no pathognomonic sign. Symptoms may be neurologic (tremor, jitteriness, high-pitched cry, eye-rolling, convulsions), respiratory signs (cyanosis, tachypnea, apnea), cardiac-related (tachycardia, cardiomegaly, cardiac failure), digestive (refusal to feed), or metabolic (hypothermia, sweating), alone or in combination. However, many infants, even those with very low plasma glucose levels, are asymptomatic, probably because of the initial brain glycogen stores, although the exact biochemistry is still unclear. The characteristics of neonatal hypoglycemia in IDM are: very early onset (first hour after birth); generally asymptomatic, non-recurrent and good response to i.v. glucose.[9] However, some cases have been reported even after the first 24 h.[13]

There is no well-defined method for predicting which newborns will have severe hypoglycemia, so all IDM and IGDM must be screened after birth. Blood glucose concentrations should be determined by laboratory measures (stick or glucometer is not reliable for newborns) at 1, 2 and 4 h after birth and then again before feeding until stabilization.

Complications

Early diagnosis and prompt and adequate therapy are essential to prevent the late consequences of severe neonatal hypoglycemia in IDM. Studies in both animals and humans clearly show that severe, prolonged neonatal hypoglycemia leads to acute neurologic injury, often with permanent sequelae. The neuropathological findings in hypoglycemic brain damage include acute degeneration of neurons and glia cells throughout the cerebral cortex and especially the occipital lobes.[14] The damage involves layers 2 and 3 (in contrast to ischemia, which usually affects pyramidal cells in laminae layers 3 and 5–6).[15] On computed tomography (CT) and magnetic resonance imaging (MRI), extensive cerebral loss can be seen, most marked in the occipital regions (in contrast to hypoxic–ischemic injuries, in which parasagittal 'watershed' areas are more evident in the frontal and parieto-occipital regions). Long-term follow-up data are still lacking on IDM in general and asymptomatic hypoglycemic infants in particular. No specific late central nervous system complications have been directly attributed to neonatal hypoglycemia in IDM.

Treatment

The key to the management and treatment of neonatal hypoglycemia is prevention. Feeding should begin as soon as possible after birth. Breast feeding is preferred; for infants with poor sucking, gavage feeding should be provided. If after the initial oral feeding, glucose levels remain <44 mg%, or if the infant is mildly symptomatic, i.v. infusion of glucose 10% (6–8 mg/kg/min) should be started. More severe symptomatic neonatal hypoglycemia is treated with infusion of 2 mL/kg/glucose 10% as a bolus administered slowly over a period of 2–4 min, followed by continuous i.v. infusion of glucose 10% (6–8 mg/kg/min). If hypoglycemia persists, higher rates of glucose administration (8–12 mg/kg/min) may be necessary. Once the plasma glucose level stabilizes above 44 mg%, the infusion may be slowly decreased while oral feeding is increased. A prompt response to therapy is good evidence that the hypoglycemia was indeed the cause of the symptoms.

In a few newborns, when the first-line treatment (early feeding and i.v. glucose) is not sufficient, hormonal treatment with either glucocorticoids, hydrocortisone or glucagon may be started.[9]

Neonatal hypocalcemia

Definition and prevalence

Hypocalcemia is defined as a serum level of calcium below 8 mg% in the full-term infant and below 7 mg% in the preterm infant, or an ionized calcium level below 0.75–1.1 mmol/L (c. 3–4 mg%). Hypocalcemia occurs frequently in IDM and IGDM, even accounting for perinatal distress, such as asphyxia and/or premature delivery.[16] However, the reported rate of 50% for IDM and 10–20% for IGDM in the first 3 days of life were published before tight glucose control in diabetic pregnancy became the accepted policy. Studies have since shown that the frequency and severity of neonatal hypocalcemia is directly related to the severity of the maternal diabetes,[17] and that the rate can be reduced with strict glycemic control.[18]

Risk factors

Acidosis requiring bicarbonate correction, pregnancy-induced hypertension and oral glucose administration are all potential risk factors for hypocalcemia in IDM.

Etiology

Several explanations for alterations in calcium homeostasis in IDM have been suggested.

Prolonged functional hypoparathyroidism

Prolonged functional hypoparathyroidism was proposed as the main explanation for hypocalcemia in IDM. As a result, there is a failure of an appropriate rise in parathyroid hormone (PTH) concentrations in response to hypocalcemia. PTH concentrations are significantly lower in IDM than in infants of nondiabetic mothers during the first 4 days of life, and therefore the PTH response to hypocalcemia occurs later, in the third or fourth day of life.

Hypomagnesemia

Hypomagnesemia may be another explanation for hypocalcemia. It has been suggested that the glucosuria-induced loss in maternal urinary magnesium and the resulting magnesium deficiency in both mother and fetus, inhibits PTH secretion and leads to hypocalcemia.[17] Pregnant diabetic women had significantly lower serum magnesium concentrations throughout

pregnancy than nondiabetic women. Also, lower whole blood ionized magnesium concentrations in hypocalcemic infants of gestational diabetic mothers was demonstrated.[19]

Physicochemical reaction to hyperphosphatemia

Another mechanism that may be at least partially responsible for hypocalcemia is the physicochemical reaction to hyperphosphatemia during the initial 48 h after birth. The intense postnatal erythrocyte breakdown increases the serum level of phosphate, which in turn, decreases the calcium ion concentration by their combination and bone deposition, a process made possible by the inadequate postnatal parathyroid gland response.[20]

High levels of calcitonin

Persistently high levels of calcitonin after birth, possible alterations in vitamin D metabolism and anomalies related to PTH-related protein may also contribute to the complex mechanism of hypocalcemia in IDM.

Clinical manifestations

Clinically, hypocalcemia usually presents between 24 and 72 h after birth. The minimum calcium level is reached at about the end of the first day (22–26 h). In general, hypocalcemia is asymptomatic and self-limited. Symptomatic IDM have a high frequency of neuromuscular signs, such as tremor, jitteriness, hyperirritability, hypertonicity, hoarse cry, clonus, and also convulsions.

Treatment

Treatment consists of the administration of calcium gluconate 10% per os (0.5–1 g/kg/day) divided into four to six doses. Infants who received glucose infusion for correction of hypoglycemia may be treated with a slow infusion of calcium gluconate 10% (500 mg/kg/day). For more severe symptoms, $MgSO_4$ i.m. is used. However, in a randomized, controlled trial, Mehta et al.[21] demonstrated that the administration of $MgSO_4$ i.m. to infants of well-controlled diabetic mothers with a cord magnesium level of <1.8 mg/dL does not reduce the incidence of neonatal hypocalcemia. If promptly and correctly treated, IDM with hypocalcemia have a good prognosis, even those with convulsions.

Neonatal hypomagnesemia

Definition and prevalence

Neonatal hypomagnesemia is defined as a serum magnesium level of less than 1.5 mg/dL (0.62 mmol/L). The frequency and severity of neonatal hypomagnesemia is correlated with the maternal status. A prevalence of up to 37.5% was reported before tight control of maternal diabetes was instituted,[22] and recent figures are much lower.

Etiology

Tsang et al.[22] observed that decreased serum magnesium in IDM is associated with decreased maternal serum magnesium (due to an increase in renal loss secondary to diabetic glycosuria), in addition to decreased neonatal ionized and total calcium, increased serum phosphate, and decreased parathyroid function. In the diabetic pregnancy, the amniotic fluid magnesium concentrations (which reflect mainly the fetal urine) are significantly lower than in nondiabetic pregnancy,[23] which demonstrates a state of fetal magnesium deficiency. The fetal hypomagnesemia, in turn, suppresses parathyroid activity, thereby also inducing hypocalcemia.

Clinical manifestations

The clinical manifestations of neonatal hypomagnesemia in IDM (onset first 3 days of life) are similar to those of hypocalcemia and consist mostly of neuromuscular hyperexcitability (tremor, jitteriness, hyperactivity, hypertonicity, and seizures). However, decreased serum magnesium alone or with decreased ionized or total calcium did not correlate with neuromuscular irritability in these infants. The lack of correlation of these clinical signs with serum levels of magnesium suggests that jitteriness may not be related to hypomagnesemia in IDM. The long-term potential deleterious effects of hypomagnesemia are also unknown.

Treatment

The treatment of hypomagnesemia consists of the administration of $MgSO_4$ i.m. at a dose of 0.2 mL/kg for 2 to 3 days, with close monitoring of serum magnesium levels. Maintenance therapy consists of $MgSO_4$ 25% per os at a dose of 0.25 mL/kg/day, diluted to c. 10% concentration, with monitoring of stools (possible diarrhea).

Other metabolic disorders

In addition to disorders of fuel metabolism (glucose, free-fatty acids, and amino acids), alterations in trace elements and vitamins status also occur in diabetic pregnancy. They are linked to alterations in fetal growth and congenital malformations.

Hyperzincuria

Hyperzincuria is present in Type 1 diabetes. A linear relationship between the magnitude of urinary zinc excretion and the severity of diabetes has been established. However, hyperzincuria is not associated with lower plasma zinc levels. Increased zinc absorption, decreased intestinal zinc excretion, or increased tissue catabolism may account for this finding. Studies in diabetic animals have demonstrated reductions in total fetal body zinc concentrations, particularly in the liver, which persisted despite maternal zinc supplementation during pregnancy.[24] The zinc deficiency resulted in a pattern of malformations similar to that seen in human diabetic pregnancy.

Chromium deficiency

Chromium deficiency is associated with Type 1 diabetes, and increased chromium losses have been noted in diabetic

pregnancy. Treatment with chromium supplementation improves glucose tolerance, insulin levels, and serum lipid profiles. Chromium deficiency has been implicated in diabetic teratogenicity (via mediation of glycemic control) as well as cardiovascular disease.[24]

Thiamin deficiency

Since thiamin plays a role in glucose metabolism, blood thiamin status was examined in gestational diabetic pregnancies and the neonates.[25] Thiamin hypovitaminemia was found in 19% of the 72 pregnancies despite vitamin supplementation and treatment for gestational diabetes. All neonates born to mothers with hypovitaminemia were also thiamin deficient. However, all neonatal blood had significantly higher thiamin concentration than gravidas. Cord blood from neonates born to mothers treated with insulin had significantly higher thiamin concentration than other neonates in the study. Perhaps increased thiamin supplementation during pregnancy seems warranted to avoid metabolic stress in mother and fetus due to thiamin hypovitaminemia.[25]

Neonatal polycythemia and hyperviscosity

Definition and prevalence

Neonatal polycythemia is generally defined as a venous hematocrit above 65%. When time of sampling is taken into account, neonatal polycythemia is diagnosed when venous hematocrit is >70% at age 2 h, >68% at 6 h, and >65% at 12–18 h.[26] A venous hematocrit of =65% has been reported in 20% of IDM[26] and 5% of IGDM[1] during the first days of life. In a prospective study, Mimouni et al.[27] reported a prevalence of 29.4% in IDM after excluding possible confounding factors (site of blood sampling, time of sampling, time of cord clamping, gestational age, mode of delivery and asphyxia at birth).

Etiology

Several explanations for the development of neonatal polycythemia in IDM and IGDM have been suggested.

Intrauterine hypoxemia

The main contributory factor is apparently the intrauterine hypoxemia associated with diabetic pregnancy, which causes an increase in erythropoietin production and, thereby, secondary high erythropoiesis. In a study of fetal blood samples obtained by cordocentesis, Salvessen et al.[28] noted significantly higher levels of fetal plasma erythropoietin in IDM than normal controls. There was a significant association between fetal erythropoietin and erythroblast count, and between erythroblasts and hemoglobin levels. Widness et al.[29] reported a direct relationship between antepartum maternal glucose control and fetal erythropoietin levels. These authors also found that IDM have increased concentrations of plasma erythropoietin, which were correlated with glucose and insulin levels in the amniotic fluid and cord blood.

Placento-fetal blood distribution

Another explanation involves a change in placento-fetal blood distribution. As a result of intrapartum hypoxia, there is a shift in blood flow between the placental and fetal compartments, so that only 25% of the blood volume remains in the placenta (instead of the usual 35%), with the remainder going to the fetus. This mechanism has not yet been studied in depth, but it is apparently associated with changes in blood-vessel resistance.

Decrease in fetal erythrocyte deformability

Blood viscosity in IDM may be affected by a decrease in fetal erythrocyte deformability due to the different metabolic and hormonal conditions in these babies. This hypothesis has not yet been confirmed.

Clinical manifestations

Clinically, neonatal polycythemia may present as erythrocyanosis, cardiorespiratory and neurological signs, alone or in combination. In symptomatic infants, neurological signs (jitteriness, irritability, hypertonicity, seizures) and cardiorespiratory signs (tachypnea, cyanosis, respiratory distress, tachycardia, cardiomegaly) are predominant. However, many infants are asymptomatic. The main pathophysiologic problem in neonatal polycythemia is hyperviscosity which, in IDM, leads to decreased blood perfusion, sludging of erythrocytes, and increased platelet aggregation – all factors associated with the formation of intravascular thrombi. As a result, vascular thromboses occur in various places in the body: brain, retina, heart, lungs, kidneys (renal vein thrombosis), adrenal glands, mesenteric (necrotizing enterocolitis) and peripheral vessels.

Treatment

Treatment of neonatal polycythemia (symptomatic or venous hematocrit >70%) consists of partial dilutional exchange transfusion with albumin 5% or saline. It should be administered as early as possible (preferably 2–4 h after birth) and with an adequate quantity of albumin or saline to quickly reduce the hematocrit and blood viscosity. There is an urgent need for a double-blind, randomized, controlled study to establish the still-controversial indications for dilutional exchange transfusion in asymptomatic polycythemia and to determine if early diagnosis and treatment prevent serious sequelae later in life.

Neonatal hyperbilirubinemia

Definition and prevalence

Neonatal hyperbilirubinemia is defined as a total serum bilirubin level greater than 12 mg/dL (205 mmol/L). Indirect neonatal hyperbilirubinemia develops in 20–25% of IDM. The risk is much higher in IDM and IGDM than in infants of nondiabetic mothers.

Etiology

The pathogenesis of neonatal hyperbilirubinemia remains uncertain, although a number of determinant and contributory factors have been suggested. Determinant factors are:

- Increased hemoglobin catabolism and, as a result, increased bilirubin production. It was demonstrated that in IDM, carbon monoxide production is increased as a result of increased hemoglobin breakdown and bilirubin production.[30]
- The increased rate of erythrocyte breakdown in IDM is probably linked to an altered erythrocyte membrane composition resulting from changes in maternal fuel availability. As a result, red cell membranes of IDM may be more susceptible to oxidation or physical damage than those of normal infants.
- The increased erythropoietin concentration as a result of *in utero* hypoxemia stimulates the production of erythrocytes.

Contributory factors are:

- Polycythemia, a frequent occurrence in IDM, contributes to neonatal hyperbilirubinemia because it makes more red blood cells available for breakdown.
- Bruising, hematomas or birth trauma secondary to fetal macrosomia will result in resorption of more blood, and thereby, hyperbilirubinemia.
- If enteral feeding is delayed, decreased intestinal motility and increased entero-hepatic circulation of bilirubin may also be contributory factors.

Clinical manifestations

Neonatal hyperbilirubinemia is manifested clinically as cutaneous jaundice and, rarely, splenomegaly. It is essential to prevent levels of indirect hyperbilirubinemia that can lead to brain damage. Therefore, all IDM and IGDM need to undergo careful screening of bilirubin levels.

Treatment

Early feeding, correction of metabolic conditions (hypoglycemia, hypoxia, polycythemia) that may exacerbate the hyperbilirubinemia, and timely initiation of phototherapy are adequate treatment measures. In the great majority of cases, they may prevent the need for exchange transfusion.

Other hematologic disorders

In addition to the well-known hematologic disorders (polycythemia, hyperbilirubinemia) of IDM, other problems have been observed in individual blood components.

- In a study of 79 IDM, Green and Mimouni[31] observed a significantly higher nucleated red blood cell count than in normal controls. In the absence of hemolysis or blood loss, this finding could be a result of chronic intrauterine hypoxia.
- Relative leukocytosis, a shift to the left and decreased neutrophil chemotaxis have been described. Reduced cord

blood neutrophil motility and phagocytic bactericidal activity in term neonates born to gestational diabetic mothers were also described.[32] These anomalies were not influenced by maternal insulin therapy.[32]

- Salvessen et al.[33] obtained umbilical venous blood within 24 h of elective delivery from 40 women with diabetic pregnancy at 36–40 weeks' gestation. Mean platelet count was significantly lower in the IDM than the corresponding reference values. However, values a little lower than 150,000/mm^3 were observed in only four IDM (10%).

- In IDM, clot formation is facilitated by characteristic abnormalities in the hemostatic mechanism, such as increased platelet aggregation and high fast antiplasmin levels. The reason for these alterations are not clear.

- IDM, who are large for gestational age and have hypoglycemia at birth have a >90% prevalence of abnormal iron indexes which include decreased serum ferritin and iron concentrations, and increased total iron-binding capacity and free erythrocyte protoporphyrin concentrations.[34] These abnormalities are associated with elevations in cord blood erythropoietin and hemoglobin concentrations and may reflect a redistribution of iron from plasma and storage pools into an expanded pool. They are also related to a chronic state of intrauterine hypoxia, most likely a result of fetal hyperglycemia and hyperinsulinism. IDM with abnormal iron indexes at birth require close developmental follow-up because they are at increased developmental risk.[34]

Respiratory distress syndrome

Definition

Respiratory distress syndrome describes a characteristic constellation of clinical (tachypnea, grunting, costal retractions, nasal flares, and cyanosis), laboratory (metabolic acidosis and hypoxemia) and radiological findings (air bronchogram and reticulo-granular pattern on chest X-ray). It is caused by deficient surfactant production which determines decreased lung compliance with resultant hypoxia. Other causes of respiratory distress in IDM are transient tachypnea of the newborn, meconium aspiration syndrome, polycythemia, and hypertrophic cardiomyopathy.

Prevalence

Diabetes *per se* predisposes IDM to respiratory distress syndrome. Roberts et al.[35] found a 5.6-fold higher risk of respiratory distress syndrome in IDMs than in infants of nondiabetic mothers when confounding variables were excluded. The overall risk of respiratory distress syndrome has dropped significantly from 31% to 3% with the introduction of strict glucose control during pregnancy and delivery at term or near-term. Nevertheless, it remains a potentially severe complication in preterm infants of the diabetic mothers.

Etiology

The increased risk of respiratory distress syndrome in infants born to mothers with uncontrolled or poorly controlled diabetes is due in great part to fetal hyperinsulinemia. Fetal hyperinsulinemia can block the normal enzyme-inducing action of cortisol on the type II fetal pneumocyte production of surfactant, apparently as a consequence of the inhibited production of one of the prerequisites of phosphatidylcholine, fibroblast–pneumocyte factor. Insulin may impair fetal surfactant synthesis by shunting glycerol-β-phosphate toward pyruvate and acetyl-CoA, which decreases its availability for phospholipid biosynthesis. Insulin also seems to interfere with the conversion of phosphatidic acid to phosphatidylglycerol (PG), which has a stabilizing effect on surfactant. When PG is found in amniotic fluid, respiratory distress syndrome is generally absent. Even in gestational diabetic pregnancies, PG appears later in the amniotic fluid than in normal pregnancies.

Fetal hyperglycemia without hyperinsulinemia may also affect surfactant synthesis. Studies in fetal rat lung explants demonstrated that high glucose concentrations inhibited the incorporation of choline into phosphatidylcholine and that butyrate blocks the transcription of messenger ribonucleic acid (mRNA) for surfactant proteins.[36]

Identification and treatment

The standard methods used to assess antenatal lung maturity may not be applicable to diabetic pregnancy. The lecithin/sphingomyelin (L/S) ratio in the amniotic fluid may not accurately predict lung maturity in diabetic pregnancies because respiratory distress syndrome may develop in these offspring despite an L/S ratio greater than 2:0. Kulovitch and Gluck[37] found a significant delay in the appearance of PG that was unrelated to maturation of lecithin. As PG signals final maturation of lung surfactant, once it appears, IDM and IGDM can be delivered safely without risk of respiratory distress syndrome. Therefore, in the event of elective delivery before 38–39 weeks, fetal lung maturity must be documented by amniocentesis, by either the presence of PG (1% risk of respiratory distress syndrome), or a L/S ratio of 2:0 or greater (3% risk of respiratory distress syndrome).[38] These tests are unnecessary beyond 38–39 weeks' gestation in women with good glycemic control, when the risk of respiratory distress syndrome approaches that of the normal population.[39] To minimize respiratory complications in IDM, obstetricians should aim to deliver each infant as close to term as possible (provided that fetal well-being is assured and there are no other antenatal complications), to allow delivery to occur after spontaneous onset of labor (to avoid transient tachypnea), and to prescribe antenatal steroid treatment for mothers who may deliver before term.

Ventricular septal hypertrophy

Definition

Ventricular septal hypertrophy is defined as a septal thickness of more than 2 SD above the normal mean. Septal size during diastole increases in a linear and statistically significant fashion from the 20th week of gestation to term.[40] In IDM, however, cardiac hypertrophy develops late in gestation (at 34–40 weeks), even in the presence of good glycemic control.[41]

Prevalence

Veille et al.,[40] in a study of 64 pregnant women with diabetes, recorded a 75% rate of septal hypertrophy. However, this high prevalence may apply only to patients with less than optimal glucose control. In the present authors' diabetic population with strict glycemic control, ventricular septal hypertrophy was noted in only 7.5% of IDM. Ventricular septal hypertrophy is more prevalent in macrosomic than normal-sized infants (8.3 vs. 1.8%). Mehta et al.[42] found that IGDM had significantly lower left ventricular dimensions during systole and diastole than healthy infants. They also exhibited altered diastolic filling patterns despite the absence of left ventricular or septal hypertrophy, indicating poor myocardial relaxation or decreased passive compliance of the ventricular myocardium. All these IGDM were asymptomatic; however, if exposed to significant stress, they could be at risk of higher morbidity.

Etiology

Cardiac hypertrophic changes can occur in IDM as a result of the fetal hyperinsulinemic state acting on insulin or insulin-like growth factor (IGF)-II receptors, which are present in high density in the heart, particularly in the intraventricular septum.[43] The fetal insulin stimulation leads to an increase in myocardial nuclei, cell number and fibers, and thereby, septal hypertrophy, with decreased left ventricular function and left ventricular outflow obstruction.[1] Echocardiography suggests a left ventricular obstruction to blood outflow caused by the opposition of the thickened interventricular septum to the atrioventricular valves during systole. On non-invasive Doppler ultrasonography, there is a strong negative correlation between septal thickness and cardiac output.

Clinical manifestations

Most infants with ventricular septal hypertrophy are asymptomatic. The septal thickness is detected only by echocardiography and electrocardiography, because cardiomegaly and septal hypertrophy *per se* do not necessarily translate into poor myocardial function. A small number of infants may have left outflow obstruction severe enough to cause left ventricular failure. In these cases, there may be cardiac insufficiency and signs of respiratory distress, such as tachypnea, tachycardia, increase in oxygen consumption, and defective feeding.

Treatment

Ventricular septal hypertrophy usually resolves spontaneously after 3–6 months without sequelae (no permanent effects on the myocardium). Infants with obstructive heart failure should be treated with propranolol (not digoxin!) and supportive care; those who survive the initial period with medical management will also show spontaneous improvement in the hypertrophy.

Ovarian cyst

Prevalence and type

Ovarian cysts are common in the general neonatal population. Using three-dimensional ultrasound, Cohen et al.[44] noted an 84% rate of ovarian cysts in consecutive infants aged one day to 24 months. The prevalence is even higher in IDM. Antenatal sonographic detection of ovarian cysts and polyhydramnios should raise a suspicion of maternal diabetes.[45]

There are different histological types of neonatal ovarian cysts, but the most frequent are follicular cysts.

Etiology

The exact etiology of ovarian cysts is unknown, but it probably involves an endocrinological disturbance (imbalance) of the ovarian anterior pituitary axis, with excessive stimulation of the fetal ovary by placental and maternal hormones. Elevated circulating estradiol levels in neonatal ovarian cysts was recently demonstrated by Arisaka et al.[46] The high rate of ovarian cysts in IDM is presumably due to hypersecretion of the placental human chorionic gonadotropin (HCG) or increased permeability of placenta to HCG.

Clinical manifestations

Clinically, ovarian cysts appear as a smooth, non-tender and freely movable mass in the lower abdomen, usually unilaterally. They measure a few millimeters to more than 20 cm in diameter. Polyhydramnios is observed in 5–12% of cases and is presumed to result from the mass compressing the small intestine.

Complications

In the absence of complications, ovarian cysts usually involute or regress spontaneously. There are three types of complications: primary, secondary, and maternal. Primary complications are torsion, hemorrhage or rupture. Torsion has been noted in 42% of patients, often with asymptomatic cysts detected antenatally. Large cysts may cause secondary complications such as incarceration into an inguinal hernia, bowel or urinary tract obstruction, or thorax compression. Maternal complications are polyhydramnios and vaginal dystocia with cyst rupture.

Treatment

In IDM, treatment of ovarian cysts depends largely on cyst size, sonographic characteristics, and potential risk of complications. Single ovarian cysts of less than 4 cm diameter can be followed expectantly by serial ultrasound scans as they usually regress spontaneously. Ovarian cysts with a diameter of more than 5 cm should be treated. Management options include cystectomy, laparoscopic needle aspiration or laparoscopy. Very large cysts may require intrauterine aspiration to reduce the risk of secondary pulmonary hypoplasia. When surgery is performed, it is important to preserve as much gonadal tissue as possible and, if practical, merely to remove the cyst.

Small left colon

Definition

Neonatal small left colon is a functional transient disease which produces the typical signs and symptoms of low intestinal obstruction. It was first described by Davis et al.[47] in 1974, in 20 full-term infants with symptoms and signs of low colonic obstruction and a barium enema picture of a uniformly narrowed colon from anus to splenic flexure (caliber <1 cm) with abrupt transition at the splenic flexure to a dilated right colon. The small colon had smooth margins without the usual tortuosities, and was smaller than normal. Eight of these newborns (40%) were IDM. Further investigation of 12 asymptomatic IDM yielded 6 (50%) with the same colon configuration.

Etiology

The etiology of neonatal small left colon is unknown, but it may involve neurohumoral imbalances between the autonomic nervous system and glucagon. Fetal and neonatal hypoglycemia is associated with significant hyperglucagonemia with a resultant inhibition of left colon activity.[48] Presumably, the immature intramural ganglion cells are unable to respond to sympathetic stimulation (secondary to hypoglycemia), thereby compounding the ileus.[49] Other suggested causes of in utero neonatal small left colon are hypermagnesemia (after maternal $MgSO_4$ treatment), immaturity of the myenteric plexus in the left bowel wall, and maternal ingestion of psychotropic drugs.

Clinical manifestations

Clinically, neonatal small left colon occurs in the first 24–48 h after birth with abdominal distension and delayed passage of meconium. The diagnosis is based on radiographic findings observed after water-soluble contrast enema, as described by Davis et al.[47] The infant can retain the contrast medium for 24–48 h. Neonatal small left colon is considered to have a benign course. The prognosis is good in absence of complications. The colon returns to normal size after 5–7 days, either spontaneously or after repeated daily saline enemas. Neonatal small left colon should be distinguished from Hirschprung's disease (congenital megacolon), which has a different prognosis and requires different treatment.

Complications

Complications are usually seen in severe cases (hypoglycemic cardiomyopathy, cyanosis, and persistent fetal circulation shortly after birth), and include cecal or ileal perforations and intussusception.

Treatment

Treatment is conservative, except when complications are present. Water-soluble contrast enema examination, done for diagnosis in newborns who develop clinical signs and symptoms of colon obstruction, is also therapeutic.[47] Repeated daily saline enemas have a permanent curative effect.

Strict glycemic control and short-term neonatal complications

It was hypothesized that the early detection (preconceptional) of maternal diabetes, with subsequent normoglycemia before conception and strict metabolic control during pregnancy could prevent the occurrence of most short-term neonatal complications, including congenital malformations.[50,51] Fuhrman et al.[50] in a prospective controlled study tried to verify this hypothesis and showed a statistically significant reduction in the prevalence of congenital malformations in the strict metabolic control group. Another 12 similar prospective studies in the world literature have explored the incidence of preconception normoglycemia and postconception strict glycemic control on the prevalence of major congenital malformations and some of them on short-term neonatal complications.[51] A significant reduction in neonatal morbidity, particularly severe disorders, such as respiratory distress syndrome and major malformations, has been reported; nevertheless, rates remain twice those seen in the general population. Also, the short-term neonatal complications cannot be completely prevented. In 160 diabetic women treated and followed at the Diabetes and Pregnancy Center, Perinatal Division, Rabin Medical Center, during the period 1998–2000, the present authors' group were able to reduce, but not completely exclude, short-term neonatal complications (Table 47.2). However, it is important to emphasize that almost all neonatal complications of maternal diabetes can

Table 47.2 Neonatal short-term implications of 160 mothers with very strict control of pre-gestational diabetes

Implication	Definition	Prevalence (%)
Macrosomia	>4000 g	13.7
Hypoglycemia	<44 mg%	26.3
Hypocalcemia	<8 mg% in full-term <7 mg% in preterm	7.5
Polycythemia	>70% (at 2–4 h) >68% (at 6 h) >65% (at >12 h)	7.5
Hyperbilirubinemia	>12 mg%	19.4
Thrombocytopenia	<150,000	5.0
Respiratory distress syndrome	Clinical findings + blood gases + chest X-ray	3.7
Ventricular septal hypertrophy	Echocardiography Septal thickness >2 SD	7.5

be efficiently reduced or, at least, can be detected very early and treated promptly, thus avoiding later consequences. Some other ways and therapeutic measures are necessary in the future in order to fulfill the goal of the Saint Vincent Declaration: to achieve a pregnancy outcome in the diabetic woman close to that of the nondiabetic woman.

With regard to the effectiveness of treatment of gestational diabetes on perinatal outcomes, two recent studies[52,53] concluded that untreated gestational diabetes carries significant risk for perinatal morbidity in all severity levels of the disease. The rate of perinatal complications was significantly higher in the untreated gestational diabetes (2- to 4-fold increase) with no difference between nondiabetic mothers and treated subjects.[52,53]

Breastfeeding and maternal diabetes

Fifteen observational studies have been written about the role of breastfeeding in IDM and IGDM.[54] There is no contraindication to breastfeeding in these infants, and diabetic women should have the same opportunity to breastfeed as women without diabetes. Higher rates of pregnancy and neonatal complications among diabetic women can pose significant challenges to breastfeeding. Thus, women with diabetes should be strongly encouraged to breastfeed because of maternal and childhood benefits specific to diabetes that are above and beyond other known benefits of breastfeeding.[54]

The milk composition of diabetic mothers is not significantly different from that of the nondiabetic population in total nitrogen, lactose, fat and calories, given the wide variations normally found in control subjects.[55] The only differences reported were a slightly elevated sodium level (140 vs. 100 mcg/g) and a significantly higher glucose concentration.[55] A lower fat content and higher concentrations of polyunsaturated fatty acid have also been found.

Although maternal hypoglycemia does not cause a reduction in breast milk lactose level, it does lead to increased secretion of epinephrine, which inhibits milk production and the ejection reflex. In addition, elevated acetone levels can be expressed in breast milk, placing stress on the newborn liver.[55] As a result, the diabetic mother should be well instructed in order to achieve the right adjustment of diabetes to lactation, and to understand the issues of diet and insulin. These problems are not related to breastfeeding *per se* but to the overall management of diabetes.

Establishing very early breastfeeding is paramount, since colostrum, like breast milk, provides a generous concentration of glucose. The most important factor in success is the time lapsed from birth to the first feeding. Furthermore, the duration of lactation is inversely related to the delay in first feeding. Therefore, good hospital management is critical to successful lactation in diabetic mothers. Intensive-care hospitalization should be kept to a minimum (to avoid mother–infant separation) and a breast pump and other assistance should be provided by the staff, in order to maximize the chances of successful long-term breastfeeding.

REFERENCES

1. Cordero L, Treuer SH, Landon M, Gabbe SG, Management of infants of diabetic mothers. Arch Pediatr Adolesc Med 1998; 152: 249–54.
2. Hod M, Merlob P, Friedman S, et al. Prevalence of congenital anomalies and neonatal complications in the offspring of diabetic mothers in Israel. Isr J Med Sci 1991; 27: 498–502.
3. Engelgau MM, Herman WH, Smith PJ, et al. The epidemiology of diabetes and pregnancy in the U.S. Diabetes Care 1995; 18: 1029–33.
4. Diabetes Care and Research in Europe, The Saint Vincent Declaration, Diabetic Med 1990; 7: 360.
5. Merlob P, Reisner SH. Fetal effects from maternal diabetes, In: Buyse ML, ed. Birth Defects Encyclopedia, 1st edn. Cambridge: Blackwell Scientific; 1990, pp.700–2.
6. Persson B, Hanson U. Neonatal morbidities in gestational diabetes mellitus. Diabetes Care 1998; 21: B79–84.
7. Koh THHG, Aynsley-Green A, Tarbit M, Eyre JA. Neural dysfunction during hypoglycemia. Arch Dis Child 1998; 63: 1353–8.
8. Lucas A, Morley R, Cole T. Adverse neurodevelopmental outcome of moderate neonatal hypoglycemia. BMJ 1988; 297: 1304–8.
9. Cornblath M, Ichord R. Hypoglycemia in the neonate. Semin Perinatol 2000; 24: 136–49.
10. Agrawal RK, Lui K, Gupta JM. Neonatal hypoglycemia in infants of diabetic mothers. J Paediatr Child Health 2000; 36: 354–6.
11. Hagay Z, Reece EA. Diabetes mellitus in pregnancy. In: Reece EA, Hobbins JC, eds. Medicine of the Fetus and Mother, 2nd edn. Philadelphia: Lippincott-Raven; 1999, pp. 1055–91.
12. Freinkel N. Banting Lectures 1980: Of pregnancy and progeny. Diabetes 1980; 29: 1023–35.
13. Schwartz R, Teramo KA Effects of diabetic pregnancy on the fetus and newborn. Semin Perinatol 2000; 24: 120–35.
14. Anderson JM, Milner RDG, Strich SJ. Effects of neonatal hyperglycemia on the nervous system: a pathological study. J Neurol Neurosurg Psychiatry 1967; 30: 295–310.
15. Banker BQ. The neuropathological effects of anoxia and hypoglycemia in the newborn. Dev Med Child Neurol 1967; 9: 544–50.
16. Tsang RC, Kleinman LI, Sutherland JM, Light IJ. Hypocalcemia in infants of diabetic mothers. J Pediatr 1972; 80: 384–95.
17. Reece EA, Homko CJ. Infant of diabetic mother. Semin Perinatol 1994; 18: 459–69.
18. Demarini S, Mimouni F, Tsang RC, et al. Impact of metabolic control of diabetes during pregnancy on neonatal hypocalcemia: a randomized study. Obstet Gynecol 1994; 83: 918–22.
19. Banerjee S, Mimouni FB, Mehta R, et al. Lower whole blood ionized magnesium concentrations in hypocalcemic infants of gestational diabetic mothers. Magnes Res 2003; 16: 127–30.
20. Merlob P, Amir J. Pathogenesis of hypocalcemia in neonatal polycythemia. Med Hypothesis 1989; 30: 49–50.
21. Mehta KC, Kalkwarf HJ, Mimouni F, et al. Randomized trial of magnesium administration to prevent hypocalcemia in infants of diabetic mothers. J Perinatol 1998; 18: 352–6.
22. Tsang RC, Strub R, Brown DR, et al. Hypomagnesemia in infants of diabetic mothers: perinatal studies. J Pediatr 1976; 89: 115–9.
23. Mimouni F, Miodovnik M, Tsang RC, et al. Decreased amniotic fluid magnesium concentration in diabetic pregnancy. Obstet Gynecol 1987; 69: 12–4.
24. Meyer BA, Palmer SM. Pregestational diabetes. Semin Perinatol 1990; 14: 12–23.
25. Baker H, Hockstein S, DeAngelis S, Holland BK. Thiamin status of gravidas treated for gestational diabetes mellitus compared to their neonates at parturition. Int J Vitam Nutr Res 2000; 70: 317–20.
26. Shohat M, Reisner SH, Mimouni F, Merlob P. Neonatal polycythemia: II. Definition related to time of sampling. Pediatrics 1984; 73: 11–3.
27. Mimouni F, Miodovnik M, Siddigi TA, et al. Neonatal polycythemia in infants of insulin-dependent diabetic mothers. Obstet Gynecol 1986; 68: 370–2.

28. Salvessen DR, Brudenell JM, Snijders RJM, et al. Fetal plasma erythropoietin in pregnancies complicated by maternal diabetes mellitus. Am J Obstet Gynecol 1993; 168: 88–94.

29. Widness JA, Teramo KA, Clemons GK, et al. Direct relationship of antepartum glucose control and fetal erythropoietin in human type I (insulin-dependent) diabetic pregnancy. Diabetologia 1990; 33: 378–93.

30. Stevenson DK, Bartoletti AL, Ostrander CR, Johnson JD. Pulmonary excretion of carbon monoxide in the human infant as an index of bilirubin production, II. Infants of diabetic mothers. J Pediatr 1979; 94: 956–8.

31. Green DW, Mimouni F. Nucleated erythrocytes in healthy infants and in infants of diabetic mothers. J Pediatr 1990; 116: 129–31.

32. Mehta R, Petrova A. Neutrophil function in neonates born to gestational diabetic mothers. J Perinat 2005; 25: 178–81.

33. Salvessen DR, Brudenell MJ, Nicolaides KH. Fetal polycythemia and thrombocytopenia in pregnancies complicated by maternal diabetes mellitus. Am J Obstet Gynecol 1992; 166: 1287–92.

34. Amarnath UM, Ophoven JJ, Mills MM, et al. The relationship between decreased iron stress, serum iron and neonatal hypoglycemia in large-for-date newborn infants. Acta Paediatr Scand 1989; 78: 538–43.

35. Robert MF, Neff RK, Hubbell JP, et al. Association between maternal diabetes and the respiratory distress syndrome in the newborn. N Engl J Med 1976; 294: 357–60.

36. Gewold IH. High glucose causes delayed fetal lung maturation in vitro. Exp Lung Res 1993; 19: 619–30.

37. Kulovitch MV, Gluck L. The lung profile, II. Complicated pregnancy. Am J Obstet Gynecol 1979; 135: 64–70.

38. Hallman M, Teramo K, Kankaanpää, et al. Prevention of respiratory distress syndrome: current view of fetal lung maturity studies. Ann Clin Res 1980; 12: 36–44.

39. Ojomo EO, Coustan DR. Absence of evidence of pulmonary maturity at amniocentesis in term infants of diabetic mothers. Am J Obstet Gynecol 1990; 163: 954–7.

40. Veille JC, Sivakoff M, Hanson R, Fanaroff AA. Interventricular septal thickness in fetuses of diabetic mothers. Obstet Gynecol 1992; 79: 51–4.

41. Weber HS. Cardiac growth in fetuses of diabetic mothers with good metabolic control. J Pediatr 1991; 118: 103–7.

42. Mehta S, Nuamah I, Kalhan S. Altered diastolic function in asymptomatic infants of mothers with gestational diabetes. Diabetes 1991; 40: 56–60.

43. Breitwesser JA, Meyer RA, Sperling MA, et al. Cardiac septal hypertrophy in hyperinsulinemic infants. J Pediatr 1980; 96: 530–9.

44. Cohen JL, Shapiro MA, Mandel FS, Shapiro ML. Normal ovaries in neonates and infants: a sonographic study of 77 patients 1 day to 24 months old. Am J Roentgenol 1993; 160: 583–6.

45. Nguyen KT, Reid RL, Sauerbrei E. Antenatal sonographic detection of a fetal theca lutein cyst: a clue to maternal diabetes mellitus. J Ultrasound Med 1986; 5: 665–7.

46. Arisaka O, Kanazawa S, Ohyama M, et al. Elevated circulating estradiol level in neonatal ovarian cyst. Arch Pediatr Adolesc Med 1999; 153: 1202–3.

47. Davis WS, Allen RP, Favara BE, Slovis TL. The neonatal small left colon syndrome. Am J Roentgenol 1974; 120: 322–9.

48. Philippart AI, Reed JO, Georgeson KE. Neonatal small left colon syndrome. J Pediatr Surg 1975; 10: 733–40.

49. Stewart DR, Nixon W, Johnson DG, Condon VR. Neonatal small left colon syndrome. Ann Surg 1977; 186: 741–5.

50. Fuhrmann K, Reiher H, Semmler K, et al. Prevention of congenital malformations in infants of insulin-dependent diabetic mothers. Diabetes Care 1983; 6: 219–23.

51. Hod M, Merlob P. A meta-analysis of perinatal complications of maternal diabetes, Can they be prevented? Early Preg: Biol Med 1996; 2: 15–7.

52. Langer O, Yogev Y, Most O, Xenakis EMJ. Gestational diabetes: the consequences of not treating. Am J Obstet Gynecol 2005; 192: 989–97.

53. Crowther CA, Hiller JE, Moss JR, et al. Effect of treatment of gestational diabetes mellitus on pregnancy outcomes. N Engl J Med 2005; 352: 2477–86.

54. Taylor JS, Kacmar JE, Nothnagle M, Lawrence RA. A systematic review of the literature associating breastfeeding with type 2 diabetes and gestational diabetes. J Am Coll Nutr 2005; 24: 320–6.

55. Lawrence RA. Breast-Feeding: A Guide for the Medical Profession, 5th edn. New York: Mosby Publishers Inc.; 1999.

48 Long-term implications: Child and adult

Dana Dabelea and David J. Pettitt

Introduction

Exposure to the diabetic intrauterine milieu during gestation has been long recognized to have important consequences for the fetus and the newborn. However, it was only recently that long-term effects of such exposure on the child, adolescent and young adult offspring of the diabetic mother have been acknowledged. It is becoming increasingly clear that the effects of the diabetic intrauterine environment extend beyond those apparent at birth.

The long-term changes that may result from development in a diabetic intrauterine environment can be divided into three categories:

1. *Anthropometric.* Growth rates for both weight and height are excessive during the latter stages of gestation and also during childhood and early adulthood, resulting in development of *macrosomia, overweight, and obesity.*
2. *Metabolic and vascular.* Glucose homeostasis is deregulated and glucose tolerance is more likely to be abnormal than that observed in offspring of nondiabetic women, resulting in development of *impaired glucose tolerance and diabetes mellitus.* More recently, *sub-clinical cardiovascular abnormalities* have also been described.
3. *Neurological and psychological.* Offspring of high-risk pregnancies often have neurological deficits, which are usually relatively minor, but which may be significant; psychological and intellectual development may also be affected.

Obesity

Pima Indian study

The offspring of women with diabetes during pregnancy are not only more likely to be large newborns, but are more obese during childhood and adolescence as well. The data from the longitudinal follow-up of offspring of diabetic Pima Indian women demonstrate this clearly.[1–6] Figure 48.1 shows data on Pima Indians who were examined at birth and then followed repeatedly during childhood.[4] The offspring of diabetic women are larger for gestational age at birth, and, at every age before age 20 years, they are heavier for height than are the offspring of prediabetic women, i.e. women who developed

diabetes only after the child was born, or of nondiabetic women. Relative weight in these latter two groups is similar. Figure 48.2 shows the prevalence of severe obesity,[7] defined as a weight ≥140% of the standard weight for height. After the age of 20 years, the differences between the offspring of diabetic women and the other two groups are much less, reflecting the high rates of obesity that are present in this population regardless of the intrauterine environment,[8] although, it is important to keep in mind that, at older ages, the obese offspring of the diabetic women are likely to have been obese much longer than the obese offspring of the nondiabetic and prediabetic women. As duration of obesity is a risk factor for diabetes in this population,[9] this will inevitably increase the risk for developing diabetes in the offspring of diabetic women.

From the data presented in Figure 48.1, it is not clear whether the diabetic intrauterine environment leads to childhood obesity directly or simply results in a large birth weight that in turn leads to the childhood obesity. However, from Figure 48.3 it can be seen that, in the subset of the population that had a normal birthweight, the large size at birth was not a prerequisite for childhood obesity.[6] Even these normal birthweight offspring of the diabetic women were heavier by age 5–9 years than the offspring of nondiabetic and prediabetic women.

The comparison between offspring of diabetic and prediabetic women is an attempt to control for any potential association between a genetic predisposition to obesity and a genetic predisposition to diabetes. However, the ideal way to approach

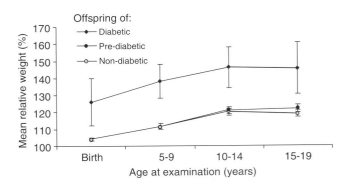

Figure 48.1 Mean relative weight for height in offspring by age and mothers diabetes. (Reprinted with permission from Pettitt et al.[4])

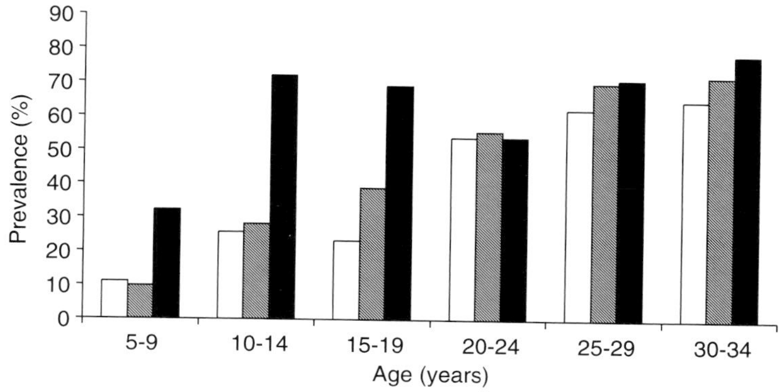

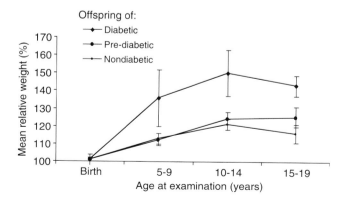

Figure 48.2 Prevalence of severe obesity (weight ≥140% of standard weight for height) in offspring by age and mothers diabetes. Open bars = offspring of nondiabetic mothers; hatched bars = offspring of pre-diabetic mothers; solid bars = offspring of diabetic mothers. (Reprinted with permission from Dabelea et al.[7])

this question is to examine sibling pairs in which one sibling is born before and one born after the onset of their mother's diabetes. Figure 48.4 shows the results of such an analysis.[1] The mean body mass index in the 62 siblings born after the onset of the mother's diabetes, i.e. the offspring of the diabetic woman was significantly higher than among the 121 siblings who were born before the onset of the mother's diabetes and who were therefore not exposed to diabetes *in utero*.

There is some suggestion that relative hyperinsulinemia may be a precursor to childhood obesity. At age 5–9 years, Pima offspring of women with diabetes or impaired glucose tolerance during pregnancy have higher fasting insulin concentrations than the offspring of women with better glucose tolerance during pregnancy.[2] Although this difference is no longer apparent at older ages, a follow-up of children and adolescents found that the fasting insulin concentration at age 5–9 years was significantly correlated with the rate of weight gain during follow-up.[10]

The Diabetes in Pregnancy Center at Northwestern University in Chicago

This is the other longitudinal study that has reported excessive growth in the offspring of women with diabetes during pregnancy.[11,12] In this study, amniotic fluid insulin was

collected at 32–38 weeks of gestation. At the age of 6 years there was a significant association between the amniotic fluid insulin and childhood obesity, as estimated by the symmetry index. The insulin concentrations in 6-year-old children who had a symmetry index of less than 1.0 (86.1 pmol/L) or between 1.0 and 1.2 (69.9 pmol/L) were only half what was measured in the more obese children who had a symmetry index greater than 1.2 (140.5 pmol/L, $P < 0.05$ for each comparison).

Children who were born during this study were examined at birth, at age six months and annually to age 8 years.[12] The symmetry index, which was normal at 1 year of age, deviated increasingly from the norm during follow-up so that by age eight the mean symmetry index was almost 1.3, i.e. the children were, on average, 30% heavier than expected for their height.

This study has added unique insight into the cause of the excessive growth and provided confirming evidence that the diabetic intrauterine environment plays an important role. Amniotic fluid insulin is of fetal origin and is directly correlated with the amount of fetal insulin that is being produced. Fetal insulin, in turn, is correlated with the amount of the circulating glucose, which is of maternal origin and is directly correlated with mother's diabetes control. Thus, this study demonstrates a direct correlation between an objective measure of the diabetic intrauterine environment and the degree of obesity in children and adolescents.[13]

Although the two studies detailed above are of very different design and the patient populations are quite different, the effect on the offspring is similar. Figure 48.5 shows the age-specific symmetry index in offspring from both studies.[2,13,14] From birth to age eight years, the offspring of diabetic women from the Diabetes in Pregnancy Center in Chicago, while less obese than the Pima offspring of diabetic women, have a steady increase in their mean symmetry index that parallels that seen in the Pimas. After the age of 5 years, the symmetry index in the Chicago group exceeds that in the Pima children whose mothers did not have diabetes during pregnancy.

Figure 48.3 Mean relative weight for height in offspring by age and mothers diabetes in normal birthweight offspring (birthweight = 90–109% of the median weight for gestational age). (Reprinted with permission from Pettitt et al.[6])

Other studies

Freinkel, in his 1980 American Diabetes Association Banting lecture,[15] summarized the evidence available at that time,

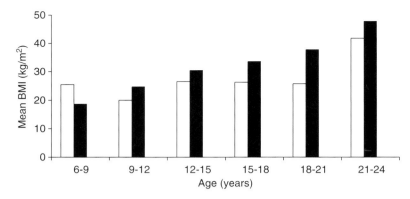

Figure 48.4 Mean BMI by age in siblings exposed and not exposed to diabetic intrauterine environment. (Reprinted with permission from Dabelea et al.[1])

before the data from the longitudinal studies described above were available. In this classic paper, he postulated that we should expect permanent changes in habitus or anthropometric modifications in the offspring of diabetic women.

Most studies have not systematically had a longitudinal follow-up from birth of the offspring of diabetic women, but many provide evidence that these offspring are prone to obesity. In 1959, Hagbard et al.[16] reported the stature of 239 children with an average age of 5 years who were born after the onset of their mothers' diabetes and 68 with an average age of 16 years who were born before the onset of the diabetes. Since the two groups of children were of quite different ages, each was compared with age-appropriate normal data. Those born after the mothers got diabetes were significantly shorter and significantly heavier than normal for their age while those born before showed no deviation from normal.

Cummins and Norrish[17] reported the heights and weights for 50 four- to 13-year-old offspring of diabetic women. The children tended to be tall and heavy, with 68% being above the 50th percentile for height and 70% being above the 50th percentile for weight. In addition, there was an excess of children with excessive weight for height; 32% were above the 90th percentile for weight while only 20% were over the 90th percentile for height.

Vohr et al.[18] examined 7-year-old offspring of diabetic and control women and found that the offspring of diabetic women were significantly more likely to be have a weight for height index above 1.2. Most of these heavy children had been

large for gestational age at birth, probably indicating poor diabetes control during pregnancy.

Gerlini et al.[19] looked at heights and weights of infants of diabetic mothers at birth, during the first year of life and annually up to age 4 years. They found that by age 4 years, the children of mothers with poor metabolic control during pregnancy were significantly heavier and had a significantly higher weight for height ratio than the offspring of women who had been well controlled. The difference was smallest at six months and increased progressively during the 4 years of observation. Interestingly, the differences were larger in the female offspring.

Many previous studies of obesity in the offspring have not specified the type of diabetes, have used mixed samples, or have limited the data to offspring of women with either gestational or Type 2 diabetes. Recently, Weiss et al.[20] have studied the offspring of women with Type 1 diabetes and reported that they have a significantly higher body mass index and symmetry index than the offspring of control women. These measures of obesity were significantly correlated with fasting and post-load blood glucose.

Using total body electrical conductivity estimates of body composition, Catalano et al.[21] showed that newborn infants of women with mild glucose intolerance (i.e. gestational diabetes, GDM) have 20% higher body fat than do infants of women with normal glucose tolerance, regardless of birthweight. Fasting glucose level at the time of maternal oral glucose tolerance test was the strongest single correlate of neonatal adiposity. Taken together, these findings may be regarded as evidence of early effects of exposure to diabetes *in utero* on obesity risk, effects that seem to be amplified during further development.

Some studies have failed to show clear associations between maternal GDM and offspring obesity,[22,23] perhaps because they studied populations with lower diabetes risk. Therefore, most information relating exposure to diabetes *in utero* and childhood outcomes is based on special populations: the Pima Indian study and a specialized pregnancy clinic population in Chicago without an internal comparison group. There is a need to evaluate the effects of exposure to diabetes *in utero* on childhood growth and body size among ethnically diverse youth. This issue is critical to resolve, as programming of offspring adiposity by maternal glucose–insulin metabolism could lead to a

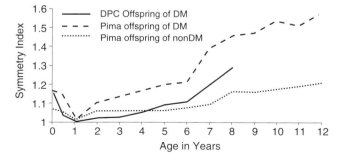

Figure 48.5 Symmetry index by age in offspring of diabetic mothers from the Diabetes in Pregnancy Center (Silverman ODM), offspring of diabetic Pima Indians (Pima ODM) and offspring of nondiabetic Pima Indians (Pima ONDM). (Reprinted with permission from Pettitt et al.[14])

'vicious cycle of increasing childhood obesity and later gestational diabetes over each subsequent generation.[3]

Impaired glucose tolerance and diabetes mellitus

The Pima Indian study

Among the Pima Indians of Arizona, the population with the highest reported prevalence and incidence of Type 2 diabetes in the world, individuals at particular risk include those whose parents developed diabetes at an early age[24] and those whose mothers had diabetes during pregnancy.[25] For more than 30 years, Pima Indian women have had oral glucose tolerance tests during pregnancy as well as on a routine basis approximately every 2 years. Consequently, extensive maternal diabetes information based on glucose data rather than on assessment of family history of diabetes is available for offspring of women who had diabetes before or during pregnancy (diabetic mothers) as well as of those who developed diabetes only after pregnancy (prediabetic mothers) or remained nondiabetic.

Figure 48.6 shows the prevalence of Type 2 diabetes by age group in offspring of diabetic, pre-diabetic, and nondiabetic mothers.[7] By age 5–9 and 10–14 years, diabetes was almost exclusively present among the offspring of diabetic women. In all age groups there was significantly more diabetes in the offspring of diabetic women than in those of prediabetic and nondiabetic women, and there was only a small difference in diabetes prevalence between offspring of prediabetic and nondiabetic women. The small difference may be due to differences in the genes inherited from the mothers, while the large difference in prevalence between the offspring of diabetic and prediabetic mothers, which have presumably inherited the same genes from their mothers, is the consequence of exposure to the diabetic intrauterine environment.[3] These differences persisted after adjusting for presence of diabetes in the father, age at onset of diabetes in either parent, and obesity in the offspring.

A significant correlation between the 2-h post-load plasma glucose in 15–24 year old Pima women and their mother's 2-h glucose during pregnancy has also been described,[2] suggesting that the diabetic intrauterine environment has effects on offspring's plasma glucose that are in addition to genetic or other familial effects.

The congenital effects acquired during development *in utero* may be confounded by genetic factors. Women who develop diabetes at an early age might carry more susceptibility genes than those who develop the disease later in life and, therefore, they might transmit greater genetic susceptibility to their offspring. Thus, the greater frequency of diabetes in the offspring of diabetic pregnancies might be due to greater genetic susceptibility in such offspring. To determine the role of exposure to the diabetic intrauterine environment that is in addition to genetic transmission of susceptibility, the prevalence of Type 2 diabetes was compared in Pima Indian siblings born before and after their mother developed diabetes.[1] Selection of nuclear families was based on having at least one sibling born before and at least one after the mother was diagnosed with Type 2 diabetes. Nineteen families with 58 siblings and 28 sib-pairs discordant both for diabetes and for diabetes exposure were informative for the analysis. In 21 of the 28 sib-pairs, the diabetic sibling was born after mother's diabetes and in only seven of the 28 pairs, the diabetic sibling was born before (odds ratio 3.0, $P < 0.01$, Figure 48.7). In contrast, among 84 siblings and 39 sib-pairs from 24 families of diabetic fathers, the risk for Type 2 diabetes was similar in the sib-pairs born before and after father's diagnosis of diabetes (Figure 48.7). It is evident that, within the same family, siblings born after mother's diagnosis of diabetes have a much greater risk of developing diabetes at an early age than siblings born before the diagnosis of diabetes in the mother. Since siblings born before and after carry a similar risk of inheriting the same susceptibility genes, the different risk reflects the effect of intrauterine exposure to hyperglycemia. Since these differences were not seen in the families of diabetic fathers, it is unlikely that these findings are due to cohort or birth order effects.

In Pima Indian children aged 5–19 years, the prevalence of Type 2 diabetes has increased 2- to 3-fold over the last 30 years.[26] The percent of children who have been exposed to diabetes *in utero* has also increased significantly over the same

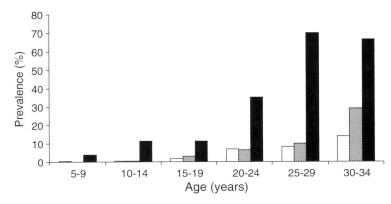

Figure 48.6 Prevalence of Type 2 diabetes, by mother's diabetes during and following pregnancy in Pima Indians aged 5–34 years. Open bars = offspring of nondiabetic mothers; hatched bars = offspring of pre-diabetic mothers; solid bars = offspring of diabetic mothers. (Reprinted with permission from Dabelea et al.7)

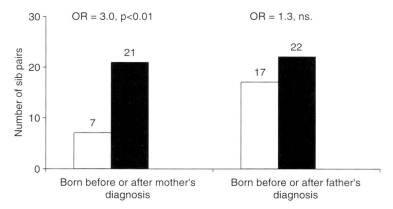

Figure 48.7   Pima Indian sib pairs discordant for diabetes and exposure to diabetes *in utero* diabetes. (Reprinted with permission from Dabelea et al.[69])

time period and this is associated with a doubling of the amount of diabetes in children that may be attributed to this exposure (from 18.1% in 1967–1976 to 35.4% in 1987–1996). The 'epidemic' of Type 2 diabetes in Pima Indian children was almost entirely accounted for, statistically, by the increase in exposure to diabetes during pregnancy and the increase in obesity. Exposure to intrauterine maternal hyperglycemia was the strongest single risk factor for Type 2 diabetes in Pima Indian youth (odds ratio 10.4, $P < 0.0001$).

These data strongly suggest that maternal hyperglycemia, extreme enough to be recognized as diabetes, is a clear risk factor glucose intolerance and Type 2 diabetes in the offspring. However, since maternal fuel supply across a population is a continuum, the relationship between maternal glycemia and offspring risk for Type 2 diabetes may be present across the entire distribution of maternal glucose concentrations. A recent study in Pima Indian pregnant women, who were not diabetic and had glucose levels in the normal range, found a direct linear association between maternal fasting glucose during the third trimester of pregnancy and risk of Type 2 diabetes in their offspring, as well as confirming the direct linear association between maternal glucose and offspring birthweight in nondiabetic pregnancies.[27]

The Diabetes in Pregnancy Center at Northwestern University in Chicago

This follow-up study enrolled offspring of women with pregestational diabetes (both insulin-dependent and noninsulin-dependent) and gestational diabetes from 1977 to 1983. Plasma glucose and insulin were measured both fasting and after a glucose load yearly from 1.5 years of age in offspring of diabetic mothers and one time at ages 10–16 years in control subjects.[28] On their most recent evaluation (age 12.3 years) offspring of diabetic mothers had a significantly higher prevalence of impaired glucose tolerance (IGT) than the age- and sex-matched control group (19.3 vs. 2.5%, Figure 48.8), and two female offspring had developed Type 2 diabetes, at ages 7 and 11 years. Interestingly, in this cohort, the predisposition to IGT was associated with maternal hyperglycemia, regardless of whether it was caused by gestational diabetes or pre-existing insulin-dependent or noninsulin-dependent diabetes.

Moreover, excessive insulin secretion *in utero*, assessed by the amniotic fluid concentration measured at 32–38 weeks' gestation was a strong predictor of impaired glucose tolerance in childhood.

Other Studies

Most,[29–34] although not all,[35–37] family studies have shown a greater transmission of Type 2 diabetes to offspring from mothers than from fathers with Type 2 diabetes. Both genetic and environmental effects have been advanced to explain this excess maternal transmission.

A higher frequency of maternal than of paternal transmission of diabetes has been demonstrated in GK rats.[38] In these rats the diabetic syndrome is produced by strepotozotocin injection or glucose infusion. They do not have any genetic predisposition for diabetes, nor can their diabetes be classified as Type 1 or 2. These studies have demonstrated that hyperglycemia in the mother during pregnancy leads to impairment of glucose tolerance, and decreased insulin action and secretion in adult offspring.[39–41]

The mechanisms by which exposure to diabetes *in utero* increases the risk of impaired glucose tolerance and Type 2 diabetes are still uncertain. Several studies performed in newborns of diabetic mothers have shown an enhanced insulin

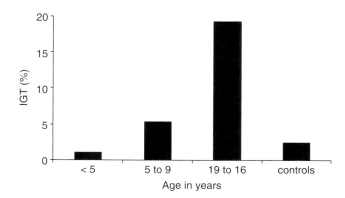

Figure 48.8   Prevalence of IGT in offspring of diabetic mothers in 3-age groups and in control subjects aged 10–16 years. (Reprinted with permission from Silverman et al.[28])

secretion to a glycemic stimulus in these neonates[42] and, accordingly, Van Assche and Gepts[43] and Heding et al.[44] described hyperplasia of the beta cells in newborns of diabetic mothers. Whether this is a transient phenomenon, as suggested by Isles et al.,[45] or leads to impaired glucose tolerance later in life when insulin resistance becomes important, is still uncertain. Impaired insulin secretion[46] has also been proposed as a possible mechanism. Among 104 normal glucose tolerant Pima Indian adults, insulin secretion rates were lower in individuals whose mothers had developed diabetes before the age of 35 years compared with those whose parents remained nondiabetic until the age of 49 years. The acute insulin response was approximately 40% lower in individuals whose mothers had diabetes during pregnancy than in those whose mothers developed diabetes at an early age but after the birth of the subject.[47] These results suggest that exposure to the diabetic intrauterine environment is associated with impaired insulin secretion. Based on the observation made in rats and supported by the Pima Indian findings, it may be hypothesized that exposure to hyperglycemia during critical periods of fetal development 'programs' the developing pancreas in a way that leads to a subsequent impairment in insulin secretion.

Is the situation different if the mother has Type 1 diabetes? There is a two to five fold higher risk for Type 1 diabetes in offspring of fathers than in offspring of mothers with Type 1 diabetes.[48] There are several possible explanations for this finding:[49] genetic transmission with differential susceptibility (imprinting) depending on which parent supplies the predisposing genes; true maternal protection against Type 1 diabetes in offspring; or increased perinatal mortality of babies who have inherited the susceptibility genes for Type 1 diabetes from their mothers. In the cohort of adolescent offspring of diabetic mothers followed by Silverman and colleagues,[28] however, the predisposition to impaired glucose tolerance was only associated with maternal hyperglycemia, and not with the type of diabetes in the mother. Moreover, the prevalence of impaired glucose tolerance was similarly increased in infants (ages 1–4 years) and children (ages 5–9 years) of mothers with pre-gestational Type 1 diabetes and in those of mothers with gestational diabetes.[50]

The metabolic effects of the diabetic intrauterine environment on the fetus might be similar regardless of whether the mother has Type 1 or Type 2 diabetes. Recent data suggest that effects of maternally transmitted diabetes genes may be modified by congenital influences in both Type 1 and Type 2 diabetes, though perhaps in a different direction. A report from the Framingham Offspring Study[51] showed that paternal and maternal Type 2 diabetes conferred equivalent risks for offspring Type 2 diabetes. Offspring of diabetic mothers with an age of onset <50 years, however, had higher risk for both Type 2 diabetes and impaired glucose tolerance than offspring of diabetic fathers. Based on comparable effect sizes among maternal and paternal Type 2 diabetes, the authors concluded that fathers may transmit unique genetic factors of similar strength to maternal environmental effects. An association between paternal, but not maternal, Type 2 diabetes, low birthweight, and Type 2 diabetes was reported in Pima Indian offspring.[52] Using family-based association methods in parent–offspring trios with Type 2 diabetes, Huxtable et al.[53] reported a relationship between the insulin gene and Type 2 diabetes that was mediated exclusively through paternally transmitted class III variable number tandem repeat (VNTR) alleles.

Cardiovascular abnormalities

Animal studies have shown that exposure to diabetes *in utero* can induce cardiovascular dysfunction in adult offspring.[54] Few human studies have examined cardiovascular risk factors in offspring of diabetic pregnancies. By 10–14 years, offspring of diabetic pregnancies enrolled in the Diabetes in Pregnancy follow-up study in Chicago had significantly higher systolic and mean arterial blood pressure than offspring of nondiabetic pregnancies.[12] Manderson et al. reported higher concentrations of markers of endothelial dysfunction (ICAM-1, VCAM-1, E-selectin), as well as cholesterol-to-HDL ratio among offspring of mothers with Type 1 diabetes than among offspring of nondiabetic pregnancies, independent of current body mass index.[55] Recently, the Pima Indian investigators have shown that, independent of adiposity, 7- to 11-year-old offspring exposed to maternal diabetes during pregnancy have significantly higher systolic blood pressure than offspring of mothers who did not develop Type 2 diabetes until after the index pregnancy.[56] These data suggest that *in utero* exposure to diabetes confers risks for the development of cardiovascular disease later in life that are independent of adiposity and may be in addition to genetic predisposition to diabetes and cardio-vascular disease.

Neurological and psychological development

Reports of long-term neurological deficits in the offspring of diabetic mothers include impaired visual motor function, Erb's palsy, seizure disorders, cerebral palsy, mental retardation, speech disturbances, reading difficulties, behavior disturbances and deafness.[57–63] Mechanisms potentially involved in the occurrence of such problems are: (1) birth trauma, especially trauma to the head and neck because of large infant size and shoulder dystocia;[64] (2) prolonged, severe neonatal hypoglycemia, which may damage the central nervous system with potentially permanent deficits;[65] (3) neonatal hyperbilirubinemia, which leads to kernicterus;[57] and (4) abnormal fuel metabolism during gestation, which may cause long-term aberrations in neurological and psychological development.

Major neurological dysfunction has been related to uncontrolled severe diabetes in pregnancy.[58] However, even in the newborn offspring of women with well-controlled diabetes, Rizzo et al.[62] found a significant inverse correlation between maternal blood glucose concentrations during pregnancy and newborn behavior. A correlation between acetonuria during pregnancy and diminished intelligence quotients (IQ) in the offspring of diabetic mothers has been reported in at least two studies.[58,66] In one of these, birthweight was also predictive of IQ, with smaller infants at birth having lower IQ scores at age 5 years.[58] Rizzo et al.,[61] found no correlation between maternal acetonuria and the child's IQ, however, he reported an inverse correlation between maternal second trimester β-hydroxybutyrate concentrations and the offspring's mental development index scores at age 2 years. The mothers of these children had well-controlled diabetes during pregnancy and only infrequent acetonuria.

The offspring of the 1977 to 1983 gravida enrolled in the Northwestern University Diabetes in Pregnancy Center follow-up study[13] were longitudinally followed to make inferences concerning the behavioral and intellectual influences of intrauterine exposure to diabetes. Direct correlations between mild maternal ketonemia in the second and third trimester and poorer performances on Mental Development Index of the Bayley Scales of Infant Development at age 2, on the Stanford-Binet Intelligence Scales at ages 3–5 years,[61] and on the Bruininks–Oseretsky Test of Motor Proficiency at 6–9 years[67] were found. The associations between exposure to maternal diabetes in utero and psychomotor and cognitive functions in childhood were independent of socioeconomic status and ethnicity, and were similar regardless of gestational or pregestational maternal diabetes status. Moreover, they were not explained by perinatal morbidities occurring more frequently in newborns born to mothers with diabetes.

Blood glucose control throughout gestation may prevent neurological problems in the offspring of diabetic women.[57,65] Sells and associates[68] compared neurodevelopment through 36 months of age in offspring of women with Type 1 diabetes and control infants. Infants of mothers with tight glycemic control during pregnancy had neurological test results similar to those of the control infants, while offspring of mothers with poorer glycemic control during pregnancy scored less well on tests of language development.

Implications for future research

The effects of maternal diabetes during childhood and over the life-course may be viewed as a vicious cycle.[3] Children whose mothers had diabetes during pregnancy are at increased risk of becoming obese and developing diabetes at young ages. Many of these female offspring already have diabetes or abnormal glucose tolerance by the time they reach their childbearing years, thereby perpetuating the cycle. Whether the vicious cycle of the diabetic pregnancy is operating in racial/ethnic groups other than American Indians is possible, but has not yet been adequately investigated. An important research need is to derive risk estimates for childhood obesity, impaired glucose tolerance and Type 2 diabetes that are attributable to maternal diabetes in utero, in populations other than American Indians.

There is recent debate over whether exposure to maternal obesity during pregnancy, in the absence of frank GDM, is also associated with long-term effects on the offspring above and beyond genetic susceptibility. If the hypothesis that maternal obesity during pregnancy drives fuel-mediated teratogenesis is correct, the public health consequences are enormous, since obesity is widespread and increasing. Studies are needed to disentangle the relative contribution of various altered fuels, in addition to glucose, in pregnancies complicated by obesity, to the long-term effects on childhood risks for obesity and impaired glucose metabolism.

Finally, future research is needed to determine whether better glucose control can be achieved throughout pregnancy that would prevent the long-term consequences on the offspring described here. If this is achievable, it will in turn probably reduce the prevalence of diabetes in the next generation of pregnancies and, therefore, be beneficial for future generations as well as for the immediate offspring.

REFERENCES

1. Dabelea D, Hanson RL, Lindsay RS, et al. Intrauterine exposure to diabetes conveys risks for type 2 diabetes and obesity: a study of discordant sibships. Diabetes 2000; 49: 2208–11.
2. Pettitt DJ, Bennett PH, Saad MF, et al. Abnormal glucose tolerance during pregnancy in Pima Indian women. Long-term effects on offspring. Diabetes 1991; 40(suppl. 2): 126–30.
3. Pettitt DJ, Knowler WC. Diabetes and obesity in the Pima Indians: a cross-generational vicious cycle. J Obesity Weight Regl 1988; 7: 61–5.
4. Pettitt DJ, Baird HR, Aleck KA, Bennett PH, Knowler WC. Excessive obesity in offspring of Pima Indian women with diabetes during pregnancy. New Engl J Med 1983; 308: 242–5.
5. Pettitt DJ, Bennett PH, Knowler WC, Baird HR, Aleck KA. Gestational diabetes mellitus and impaired glucose tolerance during pregnancy. Long-term effects on obesity and glucose tolerance in the offspring. Diabetes 1985; 34(suppl. 2): 119–22.
6. Pettitt DJ, Knowler WC, Bennett PH, Aleck KA, Baird HR. Obesity in offspring of diabetic Pima Indian women despite normal birth weight. Diabetes Care 1987; 10: 76–80.
7. Dabelea D, Knowler WC, Pettitt DJ. Effect of diabetes in pregnancy on offspring: follow-up research in the Pima Indians. J Matern Fetal Med 2000; 9: 83–8.
8. Price RA, Charles MA, Pettitt DJ, Knowler WC. Obesity in Pima Indians: large increases among post-World War II birth cohorts. Am J Phys Anthropol 1993; 92: 473–9.
9. Everhart JE, Pettitt DJ, Bennett PH, Knowler WC. Duration of obesity increases the incidence of NIDDM. Diabetes 1992; 41: 235–40.
10. Odeleye OE, Decourten M, Pettitt DJ, Ravussin E. Fasting hyperinsulinemia is a predictor of increased body weight gain and obesity in Pima Indian children. Diabetes 1997; 46: 1341–5.
11. Metzger BE, Silverman BL, Freinkel N, et al. Amniotic fluid insulin concentration as a predictor of obesity. Arch Dis Child 1990; 65: 1050–2.
12. Silverman BL, Rizzo T, Green OC, et al. Long-term prospective evaluation of offspring of diabetic mothers. Diabetes 1991; 40(suppl. 2): 121–5.
13. Silverman BL, Rizzo TA, Cho NH, Metzger BE. Long-term effects of the intrauterine environment. The Northwestern University Diabetes in Pregnancy Center. Diabetes Care 1998; 21(suppl. 2): B142–9.
14. Pettitt DJ. Summary and Comment of: Silverman BL, Rizzo T, Green OC, et al. Long-term prospective evaluation of offspring of diabetic mothers. Diabetes 1991; 40(suppl. 2): 121–5. Diabetes Spect 1992; 5: 39–40.

15. Freinkel N. Banting Lecture 1980. Of Pregnancy and Progeny. Diabetes 1980; 29: 1023–35.
16. Hagbard L, Olow I, Reinand T. A follow up study of 514 children of diabetic mothers. Acta Paediatr 1959; 48: 184–97.
17. Cummins M, Norrish M. Follow up of children of diabetic mothers. Arch Dis Child 1980; 55: 264.
18. Vohr BR, Lipsitt LP, Oh W. Somatic growth of children of diabetic mothers with reference to birth size. J Pediatr 1980; 97: 196–9.
19. Gerlini G, Arachi S, Gori MG, et al. Developmental aspects of the offspring of diabetic mothers. Acta Endocrinol 1986; 277(suppl.): 150–5.
20. Weiss PA, Scholz HS, Haas J, et al. Long-term follow-up of infants of mothers with type 1 diabetes: evidence for hereditary and nonhereditary transmission of diabetes and precursors. Diabetes Care 2000; 23: 905–11.
21. Catalano PM, Thomas A, Huston-Presley L, Amini SB. Increased fetal adiposity: a very sensitive marker of abnormal in utero development. Am J Obstet Gynecol 2003; 189: 1698–704.
22. Gillman MW, Rifas-Shiman S, Berkey CS, Field AE, Colditz GA. Maternal gestational diabetes, birth weight, and adolescent obesity. Pediatrics 2003; 111: e221–6.
23. Whitaker RC, Pepe MS, Seidel KD, Wright JA, Knopp RH. Gestational diabetes and the risk of offspring obesity. Pediatrics 1998; 101: E 91–7.
24. Hanson RL, Elston RC, Pettitt DJ, Bennett PH, Knowler WC. Segregation analysis of non-insulin-dependent diabetes mellitus in Pima Indians: evidence for a major-gene effect. Am J Hum Genet 1995; 57: 160–70.
25. Pettitt DJ, Aleck KA, Baird HR, et al. Congenital susceptibility to NIDDM: role of intrauterine environment. Diabetes 1988; 37: 622–8.
26. Dabelea D, Hanson RL, Bennett PH, et al. Increasing prevalence of Type II diabetes in American Indian children. Diabetologia 1998; 41: 904–10.
27. Franks PW, Looker HC, Kobes S, et al. Gestational glucose tolerance and risk of type 2 diabetes in young Pima Indian offspring. Diabetes 2006; 55: 460–5.
28. Silverman BL, Metzger BE, Cho NH, Loeb CA. Impaired glucose tolerance in adolescent offspring of diabetic mothers: Relationship to fetal hyperinsulinism. Diabetes Care 1995; 18: 611–7.
29. Dorner G, Plagemann A. Perinatal hyperinsulinism as possible predisposing factor for diabetes mellitus, obesity and enhanced cardiovascular risk in later life. Horm Metab Res 1994; 26: 213–21.
30. Alcolado JC, Alcolado R. Importance of maternal history of non-insulin dependent diabetic patients. BMJ 1991; 302: 1178–80.
31. Thomas F, Balkau B, Vauzelle-Kervroedan F, Papoz L. Maternal effect and familial aggregation in NIDDM. The CODIAB Study. CODIAB-INSERM-ZENECA Study Group. Diabetes 1994; 43: 63–7.
32. Young CA, Kumar S, Young MJ, Boulton AJ. Excess maternal history of diabetes in Caucasian and Afro-origin non-insulin-dependent diabetic patients suggests dominant maternal factors in disease transmission. Diabetes Res Clin Pract 1995; 28: 47–9.
33. Groop L, Forsblom C, Lehtovirta M, et al. Metabolic consequences of a family history of niddm (the botnia study) – evidence for sex-specific parental effects. Diabetes 1996; 45: 1585–93.
34. Karter AJ, Rowell SE, Ackerson LM, et al. Excess maternal transmission of type 2 diabetes. The Northern California Kaiser Permanente Diabetes Registry. Diabetes Care 1999; 22: 938–43.
35. Mitchell BD, Kammerer CM, Reinhart LJ, Stern MP, MacCluer JW. Is there an excess in maternal transmission of NIDDM? Diabetoogia 1995; 38: 314–7.
36. Viswanathan M, McCarthy MI, Snehalatha C, Hitman GA, Ramachandran A. Familial aggregation of type 2 (non-insulin-dependent) diabetes mellitus in south India; absence of excess maternal transmission. Diabet Med 1996; 13: 232–7.
37. McCarthy M, Cassell P, Tran T, et al. Evaluation of the importance of maternal history of diabetes and of mitochondrial variation in the development of NIDDM. Diabet Med 1996; 13: 420–8.
38. Gauguier D, Nelson I, Bernard C, et al. Higher maternal than paternal inheritance of diabetes in GK rats. Diabetes 1994; 43: 220–4.
39. Bihoreau MT, Ktorza A, Kinebanyan MF, Picon L. Impaired glucose homeostasis in adult rats from hyperglycemic mothers. Diabetes 1986; 35: 979–84.
40. Gauguier D, Bihoreau MT, Ktorza A, Berthault MF, Picon L. Inheritance of diabetes mellitus as consequence of gestational hyperglycemia in rats. Diabetes 1990; 39: 734–9.
41. Aerts L, Sodoyez-Goffaux F, Sodoyez JC, Malaisse WJ, Van Assche FA. The diabetic intrauterine milieu has a long-lasting effect on insulin secretion by beta cells and on insulin uptake by target tissues. Am J Obstet Gynecol 1988; 159: 1287–92.
42. Pildes RS, Hart RJ, Warrner R, Cornblath M. Plasma insulin response during oral glucose tolerance tests in newborns of normal and gestational diabetic mothers. Pediatrics 1969; 44: 76–83.
43. Van Assche FA, Gepts W. The cytological composition of the foetal endocrine pancreas in normal and pathological conditions. Diabetologia 1971; 7: 434–44.
44. Heding LG, Persson B, Stangenberg M. Beta-cell function in newborn infants of diabetic mothers. Diabetologia 1980; 19: 427–32.
45. Isles TE, Dickson M, Farquhar JW. Glucose tolerance and plasma insulin in newborn infants of normal and diabetic mothers. Pediatr Res 1968; 2: 198–208.
46. Hultquist GT, Olding LB. Pancreatic-islet fibrosis in young infants of diabetic mothers. Lancet 1975; 2: 1015–6.
47. Gautier JF, Wilson C, Weyer C, et al. Low acute insulin secretory responses in adult offspring of people with early onset type 2 diabetes. Diabetes 2001; 50: 1828–33.
48. Warram JH, Krolewski AS, Gottlieb MS, Kahn CR. Differences in risk of insulin-dependent diabetes in offspring of diabetic mothers and diabetic fathers. N Engl J Med 1984; 311: 149–52.
49. Pettitt DJ. Diabetes in Subsequent Generations. In: Dornhorst A, Hadden DR, eds. Diabetes and Pregnancy: an International Approach to Diagnosis and Management. Chichester: John Wiley; 1996, pp. 367–76.
50. Plagemann A, Harder T, Kohlhoff R, Rohde W, Dorner G. Glucose tolerance and insulin secretion in children of mothers with pregestational IDDM or gestational diabetes. Diabetologia 1997; 40: 1094–100.
51. Meigs JB, Cupples LA, Wilson PW. Parental transmission of type 2 diabetes: the Framingham Offspring Study. Diabetes 2000; 49: 2201–7.
52. Lindsay RS, Dabelea D, Roumain J, et al. Type 2 diabetes and low birth weight: the role of paternal inheritance in the association of low birth weight and diabetes. Diabetes 2000; 49: 445–9.
53. Huxtable SJ, Saker PJ, Haddad L, et al. Analysis of parent-offspring trios provides evidence for linkage and association between the insulin gene and type 2 diabetes mediated exclusively through paternally transmitted class III variable number tandem repeat alleles. Diabetes 2000; 49: 126–30.
54. Holemans K, Gerber RT, Meurrens K, et al. Streptozotocin diabetes in the pregnant rat induces cardiovascular dysfunction in adult offspring. Diabetologia 1999; 42: 81–9.
55. Manderson JG, Mullan B, Patterson CC, et al. Cardiovascular and metabolic abnormalities in the offspring of diabetic pregnancy. Diabetologia 2002; 45: 991–6.
56. Bunt JC, Tataranni PA, Salbe AD. Intrauterine exposure to diabetes is a determinant of hemoglobin A(1)c and systolic blood pressure in pima Indian children. J Clin Endocrinol Metab 2005; 90: 3225–9.
57. Cowett RM, Schwartz R. The infant of the diabetic mother. Pediatr Clin North Am 1982; 29: 1213–31.
58. Stehbens JA, Baker GL, Kitchell M. Outcome at ages 1, 3, and 5 years of children born to diabetic women. Am J Obstet Gynecol 1977; 127: 408–13.
59. Persson B, Hanson U, Hartling SG, Binder C. Follow-up of women with previous GDM. Insulin, C-peptide, and proinsulin responses to oral glucose load. Diabetes 1991; 40(suppl. 2): 136–41.
60. Hadden DR, Byrne E, Trotter I, et al. Physical and psychological health of children of Type 1 (insulin-dependent) diabetic mothers. Diabetologia 1984; 26: 250–4.
61. Rizzo T, Metzger BE, Burns WJ, Burns K. Correlations between antepartum maternal metabolism and child intelligence. N Engl J Med 1991; 325: 911–6.
62. Rizzo T, Freinkel N, Metzger BE, et al. Correlations between antepartum maternal metabolism and newborn behavior. Am J Obstet Gynecol 1990; 163: 1458–64.
63. Naeye RL, Chez RA. Effects of maternal acetonuria and low pregnancy weight gain on children's psychomotor development. Am J Obstet Gynecol 1981; 139: 189–93.
64. Dor N, Mosberg H, Stern W, Jagani N, Schulman H. Complications in fetal macrosomia. NY State J Med 1984; 84: 302–5.
65. Pildes RS. Infants of diabetic mothers. N Engl J Med 1973; 289: 902–4.

66. Churchill JA, Berendes HW, Nemore J. Neuropsychological deficits in children of diabetic mothers. A report from the Collaborative Study of Cerebral Palsy. Am J Obstet Gynecol 1969; 105: 257–68.

67. Rizzo TA, Dooley SL, Metzger BE, et al. Prenatal and perinatal influences on long-term psychomotor development in offspring of diabetic mothers. Am J Obstet Gynecol 1995; 173: 1753–8.

68. Sells CJ, Robinson NM, Brown Z, Knopp RH. Long-term developmental follow-up of infants of diabetic mothers. J Pediatr 1994; 125: S9–17.

69. Dabelea D, Pettitt DJ. Intrauterine diabetic environment confers risks for type 2 diabetes mellitus and obesity in the offspring, in addition to genetic susceptibility. J Pediatr Endocrinol Metab 2001; 14: 1085–91.

49 Growth and neuro-development of children born to diabetic mothers and to mothers with gestational diabetes

Asher Ornoy

Introduction

It is well known that diabetes during pregnancy may be associated with an increased rate of spontaneous abortions, intrauterine death and congenital anomalies among the offspring.[1–5] This increase is directly related to the severity of the disease, especially to the blood levels of glycosylated hemoglobin (HbA1c).[3,4,6] The reduction in the prevalence of congenital anomalies among offspring of mothers with pre-gestational diabetes (PGD) observed in the last years is related to the marked improvement of glycemic control in early pregnancy. However, even in well-treated diabetic pregnant women, the rate of congenital anomalies is still significantly higher than in the general population. Generally, no increase in congenital anomalies was observed among children born to mothers with gestational diabetes (GD).[3,5] However, more recent reports have shown that children born to mothers with GD with fasting hyperglycemia or with increased pre-gestational maternal obesity or increased body mass index (BMI), have an increased rate of congenital anomalies, especially of the CNS and are prone to develop at childhood the metabolic syndrome X.[6,7] It is also proposed that the studies demonstrating increased rate of congenital anomalies in offspring of women with GD also include women whose diabetes was first diagnosed in pregnancy, but apparently started before gestation.

In addition, growth disturbances are relatively common among offspring of diabetic mothers. In severe and uncontrolled PGD, intrauterine growth retardation is often found, especially in mothers with diabetic nephropathy.[4,5] In well-controlled PGD or in GD, macrosomia is the more common fetal growth disturbance.[1,5] Growth disturbances have also been encountered in follow up studies on children born to diabetic women.[8]

Many studies have evaluated the postnatal cognitive and neurological development of children born to diabetic mothers. The investigators used a variety of age-appropriate psychometric tests and correlated their findings with the degree of glycemic control and the onset of diabetes (whether PGD or GD). In the present review we will address these issues and also report results of our developmental follow up studies.

The effects of diabetes on intrauterine growth

Growth disturbances in infants of diabetic mothers: General comments

A variety of prenatal and postnatal factors may influence the growth of the offspring of diabetic mothers. Some are attributed to the specific intrauterine milieu imposed by diabetes, which include the severity and onset of diabetes, the degree of diabetic control and the mode of treatment, and others are attributed to postnatal factors, mainly nutrition.

Pedersen, in his monograph,[5] summarized the literature on birthweight, length, organ size and body composition as well as the state of maturity of newborn children. He described the well-known macrosomia (large for gestational age, LGA) in most infants. The fetus responds to maternal hyperglycemia by hyperinsulinemia that reduces his blood glucose levels but may lead to enhanced growth. He also pointed out that in PGD women with nephropathy, there is a high rate of intrauterine growth restriction (IUGR). Farquar[9] described in detail, as early as 1959, the appearance of macrosomic infants born to diabetic mothers and their prognosis. They were described as 'plump, sleek, liberally coated with vernix caseosa, full faced and phletoric.' 'They commonly exceed the mean body weight and crown heel length, and resemble each other.' Farquar also described a variety of perinatal complications, increased neonatal mortality as well as placental enlargement and insufficiency.[9]

Greco et al.[10] studied the gestational age when macrosomia can first be diagnosed ultrasonographically, by repeated measurements of abdominal circumference between 20 and 36 weeks of pregnancy. He found that at week 24, a significant difference in abdominal circumference between macrosomic offspring and offspring of normal birthweight could be observed. The fetuses then maintained their growth profile throughout pregnancy.

Factors related to intrauterine growth

Several substances and hormones are thought to be involved in the imbalanced growth of the fetus in diabetes; amongst them are insulin, glucose, leptin, adiponectin, ghrelin and several growth factors.

Insulin and fetal growth

Maternal hyperglycemia induces fetal hyperglycemia and, in response, fetal hyperinsulinemia. Although the outcome of children of diabetic mothers significantly improved since the 1960s, even in well-controlled diabetic mothers, 15–45% of the newborns are overweight, depending on the degree of diabetic control.

In women with Type 1 diabetes, fetal weight at term was found to correlate with maternal serum levels of IGF1, IGF2 and IGF binding protein,[11] thus pointing to a major role of maternal and/or fetal insulin in the etiology of diabetic macrosomia. In that line, Silverman et al.[8] found when evaluating the amniotic fluid insulin levels, that mean amniotic fluid insulin concentrations were more than twice the control levels in fetuses of mothers with PGD or GD, and that hyperinsulinemic fetuses are often macrosomic. Similarly, high amniotic-fluid insulin levels were observed in obese children by Mezger et al.[12] Hyperinsulinemia would affect the size of insulin responsive tissues such as adipose tissue, which is indeed increased in infants of diabetic mothers. Carpenter et al.[13] examined second trimester amniotic fluid insulin levels in 247 pregnancies at 14–20 weeks of pregnancy. Women with abnormal oral glucose challenge tests and high amniotic-fluid insulin levels often delivered macrosomic infants. They deduced from their findings that maternal glucose intolerance during pregnancy might affect fetal insulin production already in the second trimester of pregnancy.

Glucose and fetal growth

Mello et al.[14] found that infants born to mothers with PGD with glucose blood levels below 95 mg% throughout pregnancy, have children with normal birthweight, while mothers with higher blood glucose levels in the second and third trimester of pregnancy have a high proportion of macrosomic infants. Langer et al.,[15] found that women with GD and average blood glucose levels above 105 mg% had 24% of macrosomic infants, as opposed to 12% in controls. Most recent studies indeed agree that maternal hyperglycemia and high plasma amino acid concentrations have been associated with fetal macrosomia. Lampl and Jeanty[16] examined the

intrauterine growth of 37 fetuses of diabetic mothers in comparison to that of 29 fetuses of nondiabetic nonsmoking mothers. They found that there were asymmetric growth patterns in the fetuses of diabetic mothers with different growth patterns in the head, limbs and abdomen at different stages of pregnancy. The clinical White's class of the diabetic women and the degree of diabetes control as manifested by Hb A1c levels affected these growth patterns.

To further study the role of maternal blood glucose levels during pregnancy on fetal growth, Scholl et al.[17] studied the influence of maternal blood glucose levels in nondiabetic women on the birthweight of their offspring. They found that mean weight of newborns increased by 50 g with maternal blood levels of 99–130 mg% and by 200 g if blood levels were above 130 mg%. However, higher maternal blood glucose levels were associated with a higher rate of pregnancy complications. On the other hand, maternal hypoglycemia was associated with reduced birthweight of term infants. All these studies show that hyperglycemia increases fetal weight and emphasize repeatedly the importance of good glycemic control during diabetic pregnancy.

Blood leptin levels and fetal growth

Leptin, the product of the obesity gene ob/ob is a 167-amino acid protein produced and released by adipose tissue.[18] Leptin is also secreted by various tissues as well as the placenta and is highly correlated with body fat mass and adipocyte size.[19,20] Circulating leptin levels are increased in obese children and adults. As leptin is known to interact with insulin and insulin growth factors, several investigators have studied the relation between leptin, insulin and weight at birth. They found a direct correlation between cord blood levels of leptin and insulin with birthweight. High leptin levels, C peptide and insulin were found in cord blood of macrosomic infants and leptin levels were higher in macrosomic infants of diabetic mothers in comparison to adequate for gestational age (AGA) infants.[20–22]

Hytinantti et al.,[21] found that the increased blood leptin levels observed in newborn infants of PGD mothers were reduced in the third day of life to resemble control values, implying that the high fetal leptin levels in maternal PGD and GD are apparently a result of the influence of disturbed glucose metabolism on fetoplacental leptin metabolism. Leptin concentrations were higher in umbilical vein blood as compared to arterial blood, and were higher in the venous blood of infants of GD mothers compared to controls.[22] These studies show a possible connection of leptin, in the etiology of diabetes-induced fetal macrosomia in both PGD and GD, but the exact role is still unknown.

Blood adiponectin level and fetal growth

Adiponectin, a 30 kDa protein composed of 244-amino acids derived from adipocytes, and in adults it is inversely related to leptin concentrations and reduced in obesity.[19,23] Adiponectin is secreted by the human placenta and fetal tissues.[23,24] It seems to play a role in the regulation of glucose and lipid metabolism as it decreases hepatic glucose production, upregulates fatty acid oxidation and hence decreases insulin resistance. Adiponectin blood levels are reduced in Type 2 diabetes, and apparently in GD but this is still in debate.[19,25]

There are several studies correlating maternal or fetal adiponectin levels in pregnancy and fetal weight at term. Mantzoros et al.[26] found in a study of 304 healthy newborns higher blood levels compared to adults and a positive correlation between their adiponectin serum levels and birth length. Sivan et al.[27] studied adiponectin levels in the cord blood of 51 newborns and found high levels that positively correlated with birthweight. Similarly, Pardo et al.[28] observed a positive correlation between adiponectin levels in the cord blood and birthweight, birth length, gestational age and leptin levels.

Blood levels of ghrelin and fetal growth

Ghrelin is a 28-amino acid peptide primarily secreted by the stomach, hypothalamus and placenta.[29–31] It stimulates the secretion of growth hormone and apparently decreases fat utilization and hence increases adiposity. As it is found in the umbilical cord plasma in full term infants, it was considered that it may play a role in fetal energy balance and growth. In a recent study Farquar et al.[30] found that the umbilical cord levels of ghrelin were inversely related to birthweight z-score and to cord blood glucose. They also found a positive correlation between grelin plasma levels and gestational age in AGA or LGA infants, but a negative correlation in SGA infants. Ghrelin concentrations were higher in the SGA than in AGA and LGA infants, but were independent of maternal diabetes. In a recent study Ng et al.[31] found reduced plasma ghrelin levels in 38 newborns of mothers with Type 1 PGD treated with insulin, in comparison to 40 infants of control nondiabetic mothers and to 42 infants born to mothers with GD treated only by low energy diet. There was no difference in serum leptin levels between the groups, but it correlated with anthropometric parameters: birthweight, body length and subscapular skinfold thickness. Insulin levels were higher in the offspring of the PGD mothers.

It can be concluded that maternal and fetal blood levels of various substances that control normal fetal growth, often deviate in diabetes from the normal and hence affect fetal growth. In addition, the growth hormone – IGF-I–IGF-II axis seems also to be deranged, especially in poorly controlled diabetic pregnancies. The exact relative role that each one of these factors plays in the disturbance of fetal growth, and how it correlates with the severity of diabetes, remains to be elucidated.

Follow-up studies of weight and height in children of diabetic mothers

In developed countries where malnutrition at childhood is very rare and nutrition is optimal, postnatal growth is largely attributed to genetic and prenatal factors. Therefore, the factors affecting fetal growth in diabetic pregnancies also have a major influence on their postnatal growth. Hence, perinatal and/or postnatal factors, such as nutrition and chronic diseases are of secondary importance. The postnatal growth in offspring of diabetic mothers, due to different prenatal factors are to a large extent dependent on birthweight, whether the infant was born SGA, AGA or LGA.

Growth of SGA infants

In the pre-insulin era, most infants of diabetic mothers were of low birthweight due to maternal starvation that was then the way to reduce serum glucose levels and avoid intrauterine fetal death.[5] Since the introduction of insulin, low birthweight in infants of mothers with PGD is usually a sign of severe diabetic vascular complications and is observed in increasing frequencies in women with PGD and hypertension, renal disease or with malformed infants.[5,9,32] It is interesting to note that in studies assessing the in utero early embryonic and fetal growth of diabetic mothers, early fetal growth retardation was accompanied by an increased rate of congenital anomalies.[32] However, overzeallous treatment of diabetes causing periods of reduced blood glucose levels may cause low birthweight. Langer et al.[15] have found that the rate of LBW in women with GD and mean gestational blood glucose levels below 87 mg% was 20%, significantly lower, than in controls that had only 11% of LBW infants.

Low birthweight is a risk factor for a variety of diseases including hypertension, cardiovascular diseases and diabetes. Hence, it is important to reduce the rate of SGA among offspring of diabetic mothers. Indeed, with better treatment of PGD and of GD, more infants are born to such mothers with normal birthweight, thus reducing these specific complications of SGA. As pregnant diabetic women tend to develop thiamine deficiency and thiamine is important for glucose oxidation and for insulin production and cell growth, it may be important to advice dietary supplementation of thiamine to diabetic women during pregnancy as this may at least improve fetal growth in growth-retarded fetuses.[33]

There are few studies describing the growth of low birthweight infants of diabetic mothers. In a relatively recent study published by Biesenbach et al.,[34] 10 children of mothers with PGD and nephropathy were compared to 30 children of mothers with PGD without nephropathy. In the first group, birthweight was significantly reduced (2250 vs. 3554 g). In addition, prematurity was increased to 60% in the mothers with nephropathy with no premature infants in the second group. Reduced growth persisted and at follow-up at 3 years of age, six of the 10 children from the first group had body weight below the 50th percentile and five had height below the 50th percentile, with none in the second group. Language development in the children of the first group was also delayed and they had more infectious diseases.[34]

Growth of AGA or LGA infants

In a follow-up study on infants of diabetic mothers, Silverman et al.[8] found that the higher birthweight of infants born to the mothers with GD and PGD, which was observed in more than 50% of the newborns in his series, gradually disappeared. At 1 year, body weight was similar to that known for the general population of children at that age. Overweight then reappeared after the age of 5 years, and at 8 years, over 50% of the boys had body weight at or above the 90th percentile. A similar trend was observed in girls as almost half of them were at 8 years of age with weight above the 90th percentile. The height of boys and girls at that age was also significantly higher than in the comparison control group. Similar results were reported by Rizzo et al.[35,36] in their studies on children born to diabetic mothers. Vohr et al.[37] found that overweight newborns of mothers with GD have increased fatness at one year of age. Later, at 4–7 years, they had higher body mass index (BMI) and increased skinfold measurement. Other investigators reported[38] that children with high birthweight tended to be overweight and taller as adolescents and as adults. This holds true even in macrosomic infants born to nondiabetic mothers.

Touger et al.[39] studied the growth pattern of Pima Indian children born to diabetic women from birth to 7.7 years of age, in comparison to the growth pattern of children born to nondiabetic mothers at similar ages. They found that the children born to diabetic mothers were heavier at birth than the controls. At 1.5 years they were shorter than the controls but their weight was similar, meaning that they had a higher BMI. At 7.7 years they had the same height as the controls but were heavier. The results of this study are in line with studies on *in utero* growth patterns of fetuses of diabetic mothers, inasmuch as the patterns are strikingly different from the growth patterns of fetuses and infants of nondiabetic mothers.

In a recent study, Schaefer-Graf et al.[40] studied the correlation between birthweight, parental BMI and overweight in childhood in a cohort of 324 pregnancies complicated with GD. They found that the children of mothers with GD have a high rate of overweight, which is positively associated with birthweight and parental obesity with high BMI. Interestingly, breast fed infants of diabetic mothers, while fed in the first week of life, had a higher tendency to develop overweight in later childhood, but breastfeeding after the first week does not seem to have any additional effect.

We have studied the weight and height of 6–12 years old children born to women with well-controlled PGD or GD.[41–43] The children weighed more than age and SES matched control children. There was no correlation between birthweight and the weight at examination, and most children were of normal birthweight. There was no significant difference between the diabetic groups of children and the controls in the head circumference or height. Overweight became more pronounced in the elder, 9–12 years old children. The number of elder children born to mothers with PGD that had a body weight of 90th percentile or above was 4 times higher than in the age appropriate controls.

It can be concluded that prenatal growth and the degree of diabetic control in infants of diabetic mothers influences, to a large extent, their postnatal growth. In infants born SGA, decreased postnatal growth is common, while infants born LGA or even AGA tend to be larger and heavier at childhood and as adults.

The effects of diabetes on postnatal intellectual and neurological development

Studies describing the growth and development of children born to diabetic mothers often report normal physical growth and no significant neurological damage. Children born to diabetic mothers may be able to compensate for slight motor impairment, and their daily function may be normal. However, when coping with complex motor tasks, they may have difficulty in performing adequately. This may be true also for higher intellectual function such as attention span or learning abilities.

The development of children born to diabetic mothers was studied for almost 40 years. Churchill et al.[44] were apparently the first to describe the finding of lower IQ scores in children born to diabetic mothers with acetonuria while children born to diabetic mothers without acetonuria, functioned normally. No effect of insulin treatment on the IQ of the offspring was noted, and there was no correlation of the IQ with the duration of maternal diabetes. Schulte et al.,[45] in their study on the neurological development of newborn infants born to diabetic mothers found longer rapid eye movement (REM) sleep time, seemingly as a sign of reduced brain maturation, in these newborns in comparison to controls. Stehbens et al.[46] examined children born to diabetic mothers at 1, 3 and 5 years of age. The SGA children born to diabetic mothers had lower cognitive scores in comparison to controls. Similarly, Petersen et al.[47] found that SGA children of diabetic mothers had lower verbal performance at 5 years, but the children that did not suffer *in utero* from growth retardation were normal. In contrast, Cummins and Norrish[48] did not find differences in cognitive scores of children born to diabetic mothers at 4.25–13.5 years of age as compared to controls, and Person and Gent[49] found no differences on these measures at 5 years of age. Rizzo et al.[35] also found no developmental delay in children born to mothers with PGD or GD, but found an inverse correlation between maternal blood β-hydroxybutyrate levels and scores on IQ tests for these children. In a later study Rizzo et al.[36] evaluated psychomotor development of children at ages 6–9 years and found a significant negative correlation between maternal second and third trimester β-hydroxybutyrate level and performance on the Bruininks-Oseretzki test that measures fine and gross motor abilities. Yamashita et al.[50] prospectively evaluated the development of 33 children born to diabetic mothers in comparison to 34 control children. They found in these children significantly lower scores on the Tanaka–Binet intelligence test. These investigators did not find any correlation between the IQ of the child and the HbA1c blood levels during pregnancy. This was in contrast to the findings by Sells et al.[51] who reported on an inverse correlation between maternal HbA1c levels during pregnancy of diabetic women and the development of their offspring. Similarly, Hod et al.[52] prospectively evaluated the development of 1-year-old infants of 31 women with PGD in comparison to 41 nondiabetic controls. The authors found lower scores on the Bayley developmental scales in the infants born to the diabetic mothers, in spite of good metabolic control in pregnancy. Kowalczyk et al.[53] also found abnormalities in the development of infants born to diabetic mothers, especially those with poor glycemic control in pregnancy. Nelson et al.,[54] in a series of electrophysiologic studies on infants of diabetic mothers in comparison to controls, found deficit in auditory and visual recognition, the infants having difficulty in visually recognizing objects they had palpated. They also had at 1 year of age slightly lower scores on Bayley mental scales. The authors concluded that infants of diabetic mothers have 'neurophysiologic evidence of persistent slight impairment in hyppocampally-based recognition memory.'

In contrast to these developmental studies performed on children born to mothers with PGD that show developmental delay in various areas, the data on children born to mothers with GD are less conclusive. This issue has important clinical implications since GD is relatively common, and develops exclusively in the second half of pregnancy, often causing significant metabolic dysfunction. This may still lead to an increase in the rate of developmental disorders since the major developmental events of the cerebral cortex occur during the second half of pregnancy.[55]

Children born after high-risk pregnancies tend to show developmental delay, learning difficulties at school and a high rate of attention deficit hyperactivity disorder (ADHD), although predictors of individual outcome are difficult. The Diagnostic and Statistical Manual-IV (DSM-IV) indicates[56] that ADHD is associated with a variety of behavioral problems and is more often diagnosed at school age. Intellectual ability in children with ADHD as well as with learning difficulties is usually within the normal range.

As most developmental studies performed on children born to diabetic mothers were carried out at preschool age, the issue whether diabetes may have some effect on the prevalence of ADHD and learning difficulties was rarely discussed. We therefore performed a series of follow up studies on school-age children to specifically address this issue.

Studies performed by us

The purpose of our studies was to assess the development of early school age children born to mothers with PGD or GD in comparison to pair matched controls, using a number of cognitive, sensory, motor, behavioral and neurological tests. We also intended to correlate the neurological function of these children to the degree of metabolic dysfunction observed in the diabetic mothers.

Subjects and study method

Subjects

The sample consisted of: (a) 57 children (49% girls), born to 48 Type 1 and Type 2 diabetic mothers; (b) 32 children (41% girls) born to 32 women with GD; and (c) 57 control children (44% girls) born to 57 nondiabetic healthy mothers. They were pair matched on age, socio-economic status (SES, based on parental education and occupation), gestational age, birth order, and family size. All children were born between 1982 and 1987 at the Sheba Medical Center, Tel Hashomer, near Tel-Aviv, where the mothers with PGD or GD were also followed up and cared for their diabetes with the goal of achieving optimum glycemic control. All children studied in regular schools. Parental education was similar in the diabetic mothers and controls. Only children born after 34 weeks of gestation participated in the study. Details of the study were described by us elsewhere.[41–43]

The following tests were administered to each participating child:

1. A complete physical examination.
2. The Touwen & Prechtl neurological examination for the child with minor neurological dysfunction.
3. Evaluation of the cognitive score using the Wechsler Intelligence Scales for Children Revised (WISC-R, 1974), and the Bender Visual Gestalt test.
4. The Pollack Taper Test, which is designed to assess attention deficits. The child is asked to repeat a specific sequence of light blinks and auditory taps presented by the tester. The number, sequence and duration of these stimuli is adapted to the child's age. Children with attention deficit tend to obtain lower scores than children with normal attention span. The higher the score, the better is the child's attention to rhythmic stimuli.
5. Bruininks–Oseretsky Motor Development test. This test examines fine and gross motor development of children aged 4.5–14.5 years.
6. Southern California Integration Test, for the evaluation of children's sensory functioning. This test includes three sub tests: manual form perception (MFP), finger identification (FI) and localization of tactile stimuli (LTS).
7. The Conner's abbreviated Parent–Teacher's Questionnaire for the study of hyperactivity and inattention was administered to the parents. The higher the score is, the more hyperactivity and attention problems (ADHD) in the child.

Maternal state of diabetes control in the diabetic women

We examined the medical files of all mothers with PGD for the evaluation of the clinical status, diabetic complications and degree of diabetes control. The laboratory examinations performed included pre and postprandial glucose blood levels which was performed up to 6 times/day by the pregnant women using a glucometer. The clinical details of the women with GD were incomplete and were therefore not considered.

For each woman with PGD we calculated: (1) average blood glucose levels and counted the number of cases of hypoglycemia (<60 mg/dL) or hyperglycemia; (2) the complications of diabetes according to White's classification; and (3) average percent of glycosylated hemoglobin (HbA1c) that was available for only 19 women with PGD. These variables were correlated with the results of the developmental assessments of the children.

Statistical evaluation

We compared research and control groups by paired t-tests for each dependent variable. For comparison of the groups on the Touwen and Prechtl neurological examinations we used the Wilcoxon matched-pair signed-ranks test. Pearson correlations were calculated between the metabolic findings of the diabetic mothers and the scores on the neurodevelopmental tests of their children. The correlation was calculated for each trimester of pregnancy and then for the entire period of pregnancy.

Table 49.1   Comparison of parameters of growth and cognitive scores between control children and children born to mothers with PGD or GD

	Control, Mean (SD)	Mothers with PGD, Mean (SD)	Mothers with GD, Mean (SD)
Birthweight (g)	3381 (582)	3528 (645)	3348 (676)
Head circumference, percentile	48 (24)	47 (24)	47 (22)
Height, percentile	44 (30)	45 (23)	49 (25)
Weight, percentile	44 (30)*	57 (32)	68 (27)
IQ, WISC-R.	118.5 (11)	117.7 (12)	113.5 (14.3)
Verbal WISC-R	114.4 (12)	112.4 (12)	108.0 (11.5)
Performance	119.7 (11.5)	120.4 (19)	116.0 (16.0)
Bender (%)	48.6 (26.5)	48.0 (24)	32.0 (27.0)*

*Significantly different from diabetic or gestational diabetic mothers.

Results

Birthweight, perinatal complications and physical parameters at examination

The average birthweight of the children born to diabetic mothers (PGD and GD) was not significantly different from controls (Table 49.1). Children born to diabetic mothers were heavier than controls in body weight at examination. There was no correlation between birthweight and the weight at examination. There was no significant difference between those born to diabetic mothers and the controls in the average height and head circumference at examination.

Cognitive and neurological development

Table 49.1 also shows the results of the WISC-R and Bender tests for the diabetic and control groups. No differences were found between the groups of children in the WISC-R scores, but the Bender scores of the children born to mothers with GD were slightly lower than controls.

Results of the neurological and the motor assessments of the children are given in Table 49.2. Children born to diabetic mothers had significantly lower scores on the Bruininks–Oseretsky fine and gross motor scores as compared to controls.

No differences between the children of diabetic mothers and the controls were observed in any of the three sub-tests of the Southern California Integration test (NFP, FI and LTS) that were designed to reflect sensory–motor functioning. Children born to mothers with PGD, but not with GD, had a significantly higher number of soft neurological signs in the Touwen & Prechtl examination (Table 49.2). A higher score is indicative of a larger number of soft neurological deficiencies.

Attentional functioning

There was a marked difference on the Pollack Taper test between the control group children and the children born to diabetic mothers, the average score of these children being lower than in controls, meaning lower attention span (Table 49.2). Similarly, children born to mothers with PGD obtained higher scores on the Conner's abbreviated Parent–Teacher's Questionnaire in comparison to controls, indicating more hyperactivity and inattention. However, the differences in the scores were not statistically significant. When the number of children having 15 or more failure points was compared among the groups, it was significantly higher in the children born to diabetic mothers in comparison to controls.

Correlation between neurodevelopmental assessment and severity of PGD

We present the correlation between the results of the neurodevelopmental assessments and the severity of PGD, as indicated by glucose blood levels, urinary acetone, and percent of HbA1c.

Table 49.2   Comparison of motor development (Bruininks–Oseretzki) and of neurological and behavioral evaluation (Touwen & Prechtl, Pollack and Conners) in control children and those born to mothers with PGD or GD

Test	Controls, Mean (SD)	Mothers with PGD, Mean (SD)	Mothers with GD, Mean (SD)
Bruininks total	138 (21)*	129 (20)	121 (27)
Bruininks gross motor	60.8 (12)*	57 (11)	57 (15)
Bruininks fine motor	62.5 (9)*	58 (10)	49 (11)
Touwen & Prechtl (number of failure signs)	4.00**	8.45	4.8
Pollack	28.9 (5.7)*	24.3 (11.2)	24.3 (11)
Conners	7.7 (4.3)	9.1 (4.8)	7.4 (6.3)

*Significantly higher than in children born to mothers with PGD or GD.
**Significantly lower than children born to mothers with PGD.

A negative correlation was found between the percent of HbA1c and the scores on the Bender Gestalt test, as well as the total motor scores on the Bruininks–Oseretzki test, indicating that sensory-motor function of children born to mothers with PGD tends to be lower with higher glycosylated hemoglobin levels. A similar negative correlation was found between positive urinary acetone and the motor ability of the children: the higher the acetonuria, the lower were the total motor scores on the Bruininks test.

A negative but non-significant correlation (−0.25) was found between the percent of HbA1c, and the Pollack Taper test, indicating that a high percent of HbA1c was related to poorer attention ability.

Surprisingly there was a positive correlation between the glucose blood levels and the results of the Bender test and of the IQ on the WISC-R test. The correlation between maternal hyperglycemia and maternal education was found to be positive, indicating that maternal education, rather than high blood glucose, may be the factor responsible for the high WISC-R and Bender–Gestalt scores in these children.

No correlation was found between the medical status of the newborn infants (i.e. hypoglycemia, increased or decreased birthweight) and outcome of any of the associated variables in the children born to diabetic mothers. This emphasizes the importance of the environment of the child in the development of its intellectual capacity, as observed in several other studies of 'high risk' infants.

Conclusions

It is obvious from many studies that in well-controlled diabetes in pregnancy, the intellectual function of the offspring is usually within normal limits. However, fine and gross motor abilities, attention span and activity level are worse among children born to mothers with PGD and GD when compared to matched controls. In some studies the differences from controls is larger in younger than in elder children. It is possible that the metabolic derangement during diabetic pregnancy delays brain maturation and therefore fine neurological functions are impaired at a young age. Advancement in age will enable functional recovery, providing that the child is raised in an environment that is optimal for growth and development. The effects of GD on development may also result from the adverse effects of metabolic diabetic factors (i.e. hyperglycemia and hyperketonemia) during the second half of pregnancy, when higher functions of the brain develop. These results emphasize the importance of good glycemic control throughout pregnancy both in PGD and GD and not only in the first trimester, which is the commonly advised practice.

REFERENCES

1. Macintosh MCM, Fleming KM, Bailey JA, et al. Perinatal mortality and congenital anomalies in babies of women with type 1 or type 2 diabetes in England, Wales and Northern Ireland: population based study. BMJ 2006; 333: 177–80.
2. Clausen TD, Mathiesen E, Ekbom P, et al. Poor pregnancy outcome in women with type 2 diabetes. Diabetes Care 2005; 28: 323–8.
3. Hod M, Diamant YZ. The offspring of a diabetic mother-short and long range implications. Isr J Med Sci 1992; 28: 81–6.
4. Miodovnik M, Mimouni F, St. John Dignan P. Major malformations in infants of IDDM women: Vasculopathy and early first-trimester poor glycemic control. Diabetes Care 1988; 11: 713–8.
5. Pedersen J. The Pregnant Diabetic and Her Newborn: Problems and Management. Baltimore: Williams and Wilkins;1967, pp. 60–74.
6. Sheffield JS, Butler-Koster EL, Casey BM, et al. Maternal diabetes Mellitus and infant malformations. Obstet Gynecol 2002; 100: 925–30.
7. Boney CM, Verma A, Tucker R, et al. Metabolic syndrome in childhood: Association with birth weight, maternal obesity and gestational diabetes mellitus. Pediatrics 2005; 115: e2290–6.
8. Silverman BL, Landsberg L, Metzger BE. Fetal hyperinsulinism in offspring of diabetic mothers. Ann NY Acad Sci 1993; 699: 36–45. J. 1996; 20: 385–96.[R1]
9. Farquhar JW. Prognosis for babies born to diabetic mothers in Edinburgh. Arch Dis Child 1969; 45: 259–63.
10. Greco P, Vimercati A, Scioscia M, et al. Timing of fetal growth acceleration in women with insulin dependent diabetes. Fetal Diagn Ther 2003; 18: 437–41.
11. Lauszus FF, Klebe JG, Flyvbjerc AA. Macrosomia associated with maternal serum insulin-like growth factor –I and –II in diiabetic pregnancy. Obstet Gynecol 2001; 97: 734–41.
12. Metzger BE, Silverman B, Freinkel N, et al. Amniotic fluid insulin as a predictor of obesity. Arch Dis Child 1990; 65: 1050–2.
13. Carpenter MW, Canick JA, Farine D, et al. Amniotic fluid insulin at 14-20 weeks gestation: Association with later maternal glucose intolerance and birth macrosomia. Diabetes Care 2001; 24: 1259–63.
14. Mello G, Parretti E, Mecacci F, et al. What degree of maternal control in women with type I diabetes is associated with normal body size and proportions in full-term infants? Diabetes Care 2000; 23: 1494–8.
15. Langer O, Levy J, Brustman L, et al. Glycemic control in gestational diabetes mellitus—how tight is tight enough: small for gestational age versus large for gestational age. Am J Obstet Gynecol 1989; 161: 646–53.
16. Lampl M, Jeanty P. Exposure to maternal diabetes is associated with altered fetal growth patterns: A hypothesis regarding metabolic allocation to growth under hyperglycemic-hypoxemic conditions. Am J Hum Biol 2004; 16: 237–63.
17. Scholl TO, Sowers MF, Chen X, et al. Maternal glucose concentration influences fetal growth, gestation, and pregnancy complications. Am J Epidemiol 2001; 154: 514–20.
18. Wiznitzer A, Furman B, Zuili I, et al. Cord leptin levels and fetal macrosomia. Obstet Gynecol 2000; 96: 707–13.
19. Lappas M, Yee K, Prmezel M, et al. Release and regulation of leptin, resistin and adiponectin from human placenta, fetal membranes and maternal adipose tissue and skeletal muscle from normal and gestational diabetes mellitus-complicated pregnancies. J Endocrinol 2005; 186: 457–65.
20. Haguel-de mouzon S, Lepercq J, Catalano P. The known and unknown of leptin in pregnancy. Am J Obstet Gynecol 2006; 194: 1537–45.
21. Hytinantti TK, Juntunen M, Kiostinen HA, et al. Postnatal changes in concentrations of free and bound leptin. Arch Dis Child Fetal Neonatal Ed. 2001; 85: F123–6.
22. Vitoratos N, Christodoulacos G, Salamalekis E, et al. Fetoplacental leptin levels and their relation to birth weight and insulin in gestational diabetic pregnant women. J. Obstet Gynecol 2002; 22: 29–33.
23. Chen J, Tan B, Karteris E, et al. Secretion of adiponectin by human placenta: Differential modulation of adiponectin and its receptors by cytokines. Diabetologia 2006; 49: 1292–302.
24. Corbetta S, Bulfamante G, Cortelazzi D, et al. Adiponectin expression in human fetal tissues during mid and late gestation. J Clin Endocrinol Metab 2005; 90: 2397–402.

25. Worda C, Leipold H, Gruber C, et al. Decreased plasma adiponectin concentrations in women with gestational diabetes mellitus. Am J Obstet Gynecol 2004; 191: 2120–4.
26. Mantzoros C, Petridou E, Alexe DM, et al. Serum adiponectin concentrations in relation to maternal and perinatal characteristics in newborns. Eur J Endocrinol 2004; 151: 741–6.
27. Sivan E, Mazak-Tovi S, Pariente C, et al. Adiponectin in human cord blood: Relation to fetal birth weight and gender. J Clin Endocrinol Metab 2003; 88: 5656–60.
28. Pardo IMCG, Geloneze B, Tambascia MA, et al. Hyperadiponectinemia in newborns: Relationship with leptin levels and birth weight. Obesity Res 2004; 12: 521–4.
29. Gualillo O, Caminos E, Blanco M, et al. Ghrelin, a novel placental-derived hormone. Endocrinology 2001; 124: 788–94.
30. Farquar J, Heman M, Wong ACK, et al. Elevated umbilical cord ghrelin concentrations in small for gestational age neonates. J Clin Endocrin Metab 2003; 88: 4324–7.
31. Ng PC, Lee CH, Lam CWK, et al. Plasma ghrelin and resistin concentrations are suppressed in infants of insulin-dependent diabetic mothers. J Clin Endocrinol Metab 2004; 89: 5563–8.
32. Pedersen JF, Molsted-Pedersen L. Early fetal growth delay detected by ultrasound marks increased risk of congenital malformations in diabetic pregnancy. BMJ 1981; 283: 269–71.
33. Bakker SJ, ter Maaten JC, Gans RO. Thiamine supplementation to prevent induction of low birth weight by conventional therapy for gestational diabetes mellitus. Med Hypotheses 2000; 55: 88–90.
34. Biesenbach G, Grafinger P, Zazgornik J, et al. Perinatal complications and three year follow up of infants of diabetic mothers with diabetic nephropathy stage IV. Renal Failure 2000; 22: 573–80.
35. Rizzo TA, Metzger BE, Burns WJ, et al. Correlations between antepartum maternal metabolism and intelligence of offspring. N Engl J Med 1991; 325: 911–6.
36. Rizzo TA, Dooley SL, Metzger BE, et al. Prenatal and perinatal influences on long-term psychomotor development in offspring of diabetic mothers. Am J Obstet Gynecol 1995; 173: 1753–8.
37. Vohr BR, McGarvey ST, Tucker R. Effects of maternal gestational diabetes on offspring adiposity at 4-7 years of age. Diabetes Care 1999; 22: 1284–9.
38. Touger L, Looker HC, Krakoff J, et al. Early growth in offspring of diabetic mothers. Diabetes Care 2005; 28: 585–9.
39. Mikulandra F, Gryuric J, Banovic I, et al. The effect of high birth weight (4000 g or more) on the weight and height of adult men and women. Coll Antropol 2000; 24: 133–6.
40. Schaffer-Graf UM, Pawliczak J, Passow D, et al. Birth weight and parental BMI predict overweight in children from mothers with gestational diabetes. Diabetes Care 2005; 28: 1745–50.
41. Ornoy A, Ratzon N, Greenbaum C, et al. Neurobehaviour of school age children born to diabetic mothers. Arch Dis Child 1998; 79: F94–9.
42. Ornoy A, Wolf A, Ratzon N, et al. Neurodevelopmental outcome at early school age of children born to mothers with gestational diabetes. Arch Dis Child 1999; 81: F10–4.
43. Ornoy A, Ratzon N, Greenbaum C, et al. School-age children born to mothers with pregestational or gestational diabetes exhibit a high rate of inattention and fine and gross motor impairment. J Ped Endocrinol Metab 2001; 14: 681–90.
44. Churchill, JA, Berendes HW, Nemore J. Neuropsychological deficits in children of diabetic mothers: A report from the collaborative study of cerebral palsy. Am J Obstet Gynecol 1969; 105: 257–68.
45. Shulte FJ, Michalis R, Nolte R, et al. Brain and behavioral maturation in newborn infants of diabetic mothers. Neuropediatrics 1969; 1: 24–55.
46. Stehbens JA, Baker GL, Kitchell M. Outcome at age 1,3 and 5 years of children born to diabetic women. Am J Obstet Gynecol 1977; 127: 408–15.
47. Petersen BM, Pedersen SA, Greisen G, et al. Early growth delay in diabetic pregnancy: relation to psychomotor development at age 4. BMJ 1988; 296: 598–600.
48. Cummins M, Norrish M. Follow-up of children of diabetic mothers. Arch Dis Child 1980; 55: 259–64.
49. Person B, Gentz J. Follow-up of children of insulin-dependent and gestational diabetes mothers. Acta Pediatr Scand 1984; 73: 349–58.
50. Yamashita Y, Kawano Y, Kuriya N, et al. Intellectual development of offspring of diabetic mothers. Acta Paediatr 1996: 85: 1192–6.
51. Sells CJ, Robinson NM, Brown Z, et al. Long-term developmental follow-up of infants of diabetic mothers. J Pediatr 1994: 125: S9–17.
52. Hod M, Levy-Shiff R, Lerman M, et al. Developmental outcome of offspring of pregestational diabetic mothers. J Ped Endocrinol Metab 1999; 12: 867–72.
53. Kowaczyk M, Ircha G, Zawodniak-Szalapska M, et al. Psychomotor development in the children of mothers with type 1 diabetes mellitus or gestational diabetes mellitus. J Pediatr Endocrinol Metab 2002; 15: 277–81.
54. Nelson CA, Wewerka SS, Borscheid AJ, et al. Electrophysiologic evidence of impaired cross-modal recognition memory in 8-months – old infants of diabetic mothers. J Pediatr 2003; 142: 575–82.
55. Ornoy A. The impact of intrauterine exposure versus postnatal environment in neurodevelopment toxicity: long term neurobehavioral studies in children at risk for developmental disorders. Toxicol Lett 2003; 140/141: 171–81.
56. American Psychiatric Association. Diagnostic and statistical manual of mental disorders, 4th edn. Washington, DC: American Psychiatric Association; 1994.

50 Diabetes mellitus and the metabolic syndrome after gestational diabetes

Jeannet Lauenborg, Elisabeth R. Mathiesen, Lars Mølsted-Pedersen and Peter Damm

Diabetes mellitus and impaired glucose tolerance in women with previous GDM

Although glucose tolerance returns to normal in the majority of women with GDM shortly after delivery, there is substantial evidence that these women have an increased risk of developing overt diabetes later in life.[1] In the classical studies by O'Sullivan, diabetes was diagnosed in 36% of women 22–28 years after a pregnancy with GDM.[2] A significantly increased risk for diabetes has later been confirmed in other populations, some of which are presented in Table 50.1. However, large variations exist among the different published studies. The trend has been that the reported risk for diabetes is higher in studies from the US compared to European studies. This has been ascribed to many factors where differences in ethnicity, degrees of obesity and diagnostic and screening criteria are the most important.

Methodological considerations

Differences in diagnostic tests and criteria for GDM plays an important role when evaluating and comparing the risk for developing diabetes after a pregnancy with GDM. The higher the blood glucose level needed to fulfil the criteria for the diagnosis of GDM, the higher risk of subsequent development of diabetes is to be expected.

At follow-up the majority of the studies applied a 75-g oral glucose tolerance test (OGTT) evaluated by World Health Organization (WHO 1985 or 1999), National Diabetes Data Group (NDDG) and recently also American Diabetes Association (ADA) criteria.[3–6] The WHO 1999 criteria identified a similar number of cases with diabetes and impaired glucose tolerance (IGT) as WHO 1985, and a similar rate of diabetes but a much higher rate of IGT than the ADA criteria which only uses fasting glucose levels.[7–9] The NDDG criteria probably give a slightly lower incidence rate of IGT.[10]

Women with insulin treated GDM have a significantly higher risk of developing overt diabetes later in life than women treated with diet only.[11,12] However, it should be considered that the plasma glucose level at which insulin therapy is initiated varies between studies. According to the definition of GDM a subset of the women with insulin treated GDM would have Type 1 diabetes with accidental onset during pregnancy. In a Danish population, the majority of these women could be discharged from hospital after delivery without insulin treatment, but a nearly 100% incidence of subsequent development of diabetes was reported.[13] The current GDM definition also allows women with undiagnosed Type 2 diabetes antedating pregnancy to be categorized as having GDM. Thus in populations with a high incidence of these women a relatively high rate of abnormal glucose tolerance in the postpartum period might be expected. The background incidence of both Type 1 and Type 2 diabetes varies considerably among different populations. It has generally been assumed that GDM is associated with an increased risk for later development of Type 2 diabetes and not Type 1 diabetes, but very few studies have addressed this question specifically.

The incidence of overt diabetes in the general population is increasing with age. Hence the time span between index pregnancy and follow-up examination should be considered when comparing the various studies. Accordingly, some studies performing life-table analysis found much higher estimates of the cumulative incidence rate of diabetes than the crude incidence rates.[11,14,15]

The above-mentioned methodological problems underline the significance of an appropriate control group of women. In the relatively few follow-up studies including a control group, women with previous GDM had an excess diabetes risk between 3 and 30%.[2,16–19] For obvious reasons not all women with GDM during a specific period will be available for follow-up several years later, but it is crucial that the women investigated at follow-up constitute a representative and large subset of the initial GDM population to ensure that the study material is not biased.

Table 50.1 Follow-up studies on the incidence of abnormal glucose tolerance after pregnancy in women with previous gestational diabetes

Origin/OGTT	GDM	Control	Length of follow-up	GDM	Control
				Prevalence of glucose intolerance	
Boston, USA, 1979 (2,14)/**	615	328	22–28 years	DM 36%	DM 6%
Melbourne, Australia, 1991 (57)[†]	881		1–19 years	DM 12%; IGT 16%	
Stockholm, Sweden, 1991 (16)/[†]	145	41	3–4 years	DM 3%; IGT 22%	DM 0%; IGT 2%
Copenhagen, Denmark*, 1992 (17)/[†]	241	57	2–11 years	DM 17%; IGT 17%	DM 0%; IGT 5%
Providence, USA, 1993 (29)/[††]	350		<10 years	DM 7%; IGT 4 %	
Chicago, USA, 1993 (11)/**	274		<5 years	DM 41%; IGT 16%	
Los Angeles, USA, 1995 (15)/[††]	671		5 years	T2DM 47%	
Madrid, Spain, 1999 (7)/[†]	788		3–6 months	DM 5%	
London, England, 1999 (8)/[††]	192		<7 years	DM 25%; IGT 29%	
Barcelona, Spain, 2000 (9)/[†]	120		<1 year	DM 2%; IGT 12%; IFG 3%	
Lund, Sweden, 2002 (18)/[†]	229	60	1 year	DM 9%; IGT 22%	DM 0%; IGT 2%
Barcelona, Spain, 2003 (19)/[††]	696	70	0–14 years	DM 6%; IGT 12%	DM 0%
Copenhagen, Denmark*, 2004 (20)/[††]	481		4–23 years	DM 40%; IGT/IFG 27%	
Germany, 2006 (12)/[††]	302		8 years	DM 53%	

Studies presented are those applying an OGTT at follow-up (excl. postpartum follow-up) and with more than 100 subjects with prior GDM. *Only women with previous diet-treated GDM. † 75-g OGTT (WHO 1985), †† 75-g OGTT (WHO 1999), ‡ 75-g OGTT (NDDG), ** 100-g OGTT (NDDG). NGT: normal glucose tolerance. IGT: impaired fasting glucose. DM: diabetes.

Copenhagen series

The participation rates in our two follow-up studies[17,20] were high (81 and 67%), and the participants representative for the total GDM population. All women with GDM were diagnosed by uniform criteria in the same laboratory and treated with diet only. A clear distinction between Type 1 and Type 2 diabetes was made.[21] Ethnically, the material was homogeneous with 90% Scandinavian Caucasians in the first and 75% in the most recent study.

At the first follow-up study[17] glucose tolerance was evaluated according to the WHO 1985 criteria.[3] With a 6-year median observation time since index pregnancy, 34.4% of the 241 women with previous GDM had developed abnormal glucose tolerance; 3.7% had Type 1 diabetes, 13.7% Type 2 diabetes and 17.0% IGT. An OGTT around 2 months postpartum is routinely offered to all our women with GDM, and diabetes was diagnosed at this examination in four women (three Type 1 and one Type 2 diabetes). At follow-up some women were already diagnosed with overt diabetes, but more than half of the women with Type 2 diabetes were diagnosed for the first time at the follow-up study.[17,22,23] In the control group none had diabetes but IGT was found in 5.3%. Women who developed Type 1 diabetes were younger and leaner than the GDM women who did not, with a high prevalence of the Type 1 diabetes typical HLA-DR types DR3 and DR4 and of the autoimmune markers ICA[22] and GAD.[24] Thus it is very likely that women developing Type 1 diabetes after pregnancy have an already ongoing beta-cell destruction during pregnancy which is unmasked by the pregnancy induced insulin resistance as also indicated by others (for review see Mauricio[25]). Type 1 diabetes tended to be diagnosed earlier after pregnancy than Type 2 diabetes. Finally it is likely that some of the GDM women developing diabetes have maturity onset diabetes in

the young (MODY). This is supported by the fact that MODY typical gene mutations have been found in around 5% of women with GDM.[26]

In our latest follow-up study[20] glucose tolerance was evaluated according to the WHO-1999 criteria.[4] The cohort of 481 GDM women included 151 women from the first follow-up resulting in a follow-up length of up to 23 years (median 10 years). Two thirds had abnormal glucose tolerance, 3.9% with known Type 1 diabetes, 17.3% with known Type 2 and 19.3% were diagnosed with diabetes at follow-up while another 26.4% had IGT, impaired fasting glucose (IFG) or both. Even among women with BMI <25 kg/m^2 the incidence of abnormal glucose tolerance was as high as 50%.[27]

In conclusion, women with GDM have a considerably increased risk of developing diabetes (both Type 1 and Type 2 diabetes), IGT or IFG in the years following pregnancy. The incidence of abnormal glucose tolerance increases with increasing follow-up time since pregnancy.[15] Some of the women with previous GDM who develop overt diabetes will, at least in some populations, develop Type 1 diabetes, a fact that might have been underestimated in some studies.

Predictive factors for development of overt diabetes in women with previous GDM

Having confirmed that women with GDM are at risk for subsequent development of overt diabetes it could be relevant, at least in populations with a low prevalence of diabetes, to be able to predict which women among the women with previous GDM who have the highest risk. Yet, the high proportion with diabetes among women with a history of GDM, even in populations previously considered as low risk populations, insinuate that these women comprise a group of potential diabetics decades after delivery.

Many potential predictive factors like, e.g. plasma glucose, plasma insulin, relative weight and age are closely related and hence it is necessary to control for covariance and confounding factors in the analysis of predictive factors for diabetes development, a fact not always taken into consideration.

Table 50.2 summarizes the pregnancy related predictive factors for future diabetes, both Type 1 and Type 2 diabetes, identified by multivariate analysis. Other obvious factors predictive for diabetes are the characteristics also predictive for diabetes in the background population such as age and weight at follow-up.

Predictor variables differ naturally among the different populations studied. Some common features are nevertheless present. The majority of women with GDM who in the postpartum period still have an abnormal OGTT (although not overt diabetic) will normalize their glucose tolerance within one year.[28] However, these women do, a priori, have a more disturbed glucose metabolism compared with women with normal glucose tolerance postpartum and are therefore expected to have an increased risk for diabetes development later in life. In agreement with this the best predictor for later development of diabetes is elevated glucose levels during an OGTT in the postpartum period. The significance of this finding is underlined by the fact that it was found in two ethnically very different populations namely Hispanic Americans[15] and Scandinavian Caucasians[17] with relative risks as high as 11 and 5, respectively. Several studies have shown that the more significant the maternal glucose tolerance during pregnancy is affected, the higher is the risk for future development of abnormal glucose tolerance.[14,15,17,20,28–30] Not surprisingly maternal overweight, a well known risk factor for development of Type 2 diabetes, was also a risk factor in some studies.[9,11,14,20,29] An additional pregnancy or weight gain after the GDM pregnancy has also been related to increased risk of subsequent overt diabetes.[31,32]

Interestingly a low and relatively insufficient insulin secretion during pregnancy predicted development of diabetes in several studies[9,11,17] in accordance with studies in non-GDM populations where a low insulin response to intra venous and oral glucose has been found to predict development of Type 2 diabetes.[33,34]

Although women with GDM as a group have a low prevalence of autoimmune markers of Type 1 diabetes (ICA, GAD) it has been shown that the presence of one or more of these is highly predictive for the later development of Type 1 diabetes.[12,22,35]

In the latest Copenhagen study[20] we found that women diagnosed with GDM in the years 1985–1996 had a 3-fold increased risk of having diabetes compared with women with

Table 50.2 Pregnancy-related independent predictors of subsequent diabetes identified in our latest study in the Copenhagen series[20] and evaluated in previously published studies as either confirming or not confirming that the factors are predictors for subsequent diabetes

Possible predictive factors[a]	OR[b]	Confirming studies	Non-confirming studies
For diabetes			
Pre-pregnancy BMI	1.0/2.2/3.0c	(7,11,19,29)	
Early diagnosis of GDM	3.6	(19)	(7,17)
High fasting BG at GDM diagnosis	2.3	(17)	(7)
IGT postpartum	4.4	(7,17)	
GDM 1987–1996 vs. 1978–1985	3.1		
For Type 2 diabetes			
Pre-pregnancy BMI	1.0/2.6/4.2c	(15,19), (17)d	
Family history of diabetes	1.9		(7,12,14,15,17,19)
Early diagnosis of GDM	2.9	(15)	
High fasting BG at GDM diagnosis	2.1	(15)	
IGT postpartum	3.5	(15)	
For Type 1 diabetes			
IGT postpartum	2.8		
Preterm delivery	3.2	(17)	(14)
Not predictive			
Parity		(12)	(7,14,15,17)
Maternal age at index pregnancy		(14,18)	(7,12,15,17)
Ethnicity		(1)	(17)
LGA infant			(7,14,17,19)

[a]Factors examined by multiple logistic regression analyses in our latest follow-up (20). [b]The results from the multiple logistic regression analyses presented as odds ratio (OR) for diabetes vs. not diabetes adjusted for other predictive factors with length of follow-up as a covariate. [c]Normal weight (BMI <25 kg/m²)/overweight (BMI 25–30 kg/m²)/obesity (BMI >30 kg/m²). [d]Excl. Type 1 diabetic women. Early diagnosis of GDM: GDM diagnosis before 24 weeks of gestation.
High fasting blood glucose (BG): BG > 5.6 mmol/L. IGT: impaired glucose tolerance. Preterm delivery: Delivery before 37 weeks of gestation. LGA: large for gestational age.

GDM in 1978–1985. The 1985–1996 cohort was more over-weight and obese but controlling for this and other known confounders did not change the increased risk. One could speculate if this could be due to inappropriate behavior at work and leisure time, such as e.g. decreased physical activity and increased use of television and computers, fast food etc, all factors we were not able to control for in the analyses. This theory is supported by a study by Hu et al. including a large cohort of female nurses, where physical activity, both at work and leisure time, correlated with a lower incidence of diabetes.[36]

Insulin resistance and the metabolic syndrome

Type 2 diabetes is characterized by insulin resistance/decreased insulin sensitivity primarily in skeletal muscle and decreased insulin secretion,[37] but the primary defect in the pathogenesis of Type 2 diabetes is still unknown. In normoglycemic individuals insulin secretory dysfunction as well as decreased insulin sensitivity have been found to be precursors of diabetes.[33]

Several studies have documented decreased insulin sensitivity in lean as well as obese glucose tolerant women with previous GDM.[38,39] The decreased insulin sensitivity is mainly caused by a reduced non-oxidative glucose metabolism in skeletal muscle tissue.[38] The cellular background for this is not known. A relatively decreased insulin secretion in lean and obese glucose tolerant women with previous GDM has also been found.[9,38,39] Thus women with previous GDM exhibit the metabolic profile of Type 2 diabetes several years after the GDM pregnancy despite a normal glucose tolerance.

The presence of insulin resistance can lead to impaired glucose regulation and overweight, characteristics often accompanied by hypertension or dyslipidemia. The presence of several of these pathophysiological features comprises the metabolic syndrome (X) or the insulin resistance syndrome.[4] As glucose intolerance and overweight are frequent characteristics of women with prior GDM they should theoretically be at risk of the metabolic syndrome. The definitions of the metabolic syndrome[4,40,41] differ at several points. Overweight can be evaluated by either BMI or waist circumference, and there are different cutoff values for hypertension, glucose intolerance, and dyslipidemia. Insulin resistance is evaluated by either the intravenous glucose tolerance test or fasting serum insulin.[40] Recently the International Diabetes Federation (IDF) proposed a new set of criteria for the metabolic syndrome[42] combining two of the previous definitions.[4,41]

The presence of the metabolic syndrome predicts a significantly increased risk of cardiovascular disease[43] and it is mandatory for health care providers to evaluate all the elements of the metabolic syndrome in all subjects with a significantly increased risk of diabetes, such as women with prior GDM. Yet, only few studies have evaluated the prevalence of the metabolic syndrome in women with previous GDM. Although the studies differ regarding design and definitions applied, the risk of the metabolic syndrome is 2- to 3-fold increased in women with prior GDM compared to women without a history of GDM.[27,44,45] In the Copenhagen studies the prevalence of the syndrome was evaluated by

three different definitions.[4,41,42] Up to 40% of the women with previous diet-treated GDM had the metabolic syndrome and this was three times higher than in the control group, even after adjusting for age and BMI, and independent of the definition used.[27] Among glucose tolerant women with prior GDM, the prevalence of the syndrome was more than 2-fold increased compared to the control group, and for normal weight women the risk was 5-fold increased.

Concluding remarks

The increasing prevalence of Type 1 and 2 diabetes world-wide[46] impose the need for early diagnosis of diabetes and prevention. It is well known that Type 2 diabetes often is asymptomatic during the first years, and it has been estimated that the onset of the disease occurs at least 4–7 years before the clinical diagnosis since more than 20% of newly diagnosed Type 2 diabetic patients have micro- or macrovascular diabetic complications.[47,48]

Up to one-third of women with diabetes may have had GDM previously.[49] Substantial evidence indicates that an OGTT should be performed around 2 months postpartum in all women with GDM. First, a high frequency of abnormal glucose tolerance is found at this time,[11,15,17,28,30,50] and second, the result of the OGTT is highly predictive for the development of later overt diabetes.[15,17] Furthermore women with previous GDM should have an OGTT with regular intervals beginning one year after pregnancy. Markers of the metabolic syndrome as abdominal circumference, blood pressure and lipid profile may be investigated in addition to the OGTT.

It is now well described in different populations of subjects with prediabetes that lifestyle changes with increased physical activity, weight loss and a healthy diet can reduce the risk of progressing to Type 2 diabetes.[51–54] Also pharmacological intervention e.g. with metformin has been found to reduce the progression to diabetes.[54] A common characteristic of these studies is that the subjects were seen intensively over a long period of time. In women with prior GDM and IGT after pregnancy, Buchanan et al.[55] found an improvement of insulin sensitivity by prophylactic treatment during 30 months with an insulin-sensitising drug, troglitazone. The effect persisted 8 months after study medication stopped. This was thought to be due to preservation of the pancreatic beta cell. Unfortunately, troglitazone has later been withdrawn from the marked due to side effects but similar products, such as pioglitazone, seems to have similar beneficial effects.[56]

The prevalence of ICA and GAD autoantibodies in GDM pregnancy is low, but the predictive value for later Type 1 diabetes is high. However, routine screening of women with GDM for ICA and/or GAD does not seem indicated before a safe and effective intervention therapy of antibody positive women is available.

Perspectives

Intervention studies in women with prior GDM are few, but due to the substantial evidence for the benefit of intervention in subjects with IGT, women with GDM should be advised to lose weight after pregnancy if they are obese, to eat a healthy diet and to have an active lifestyle including physical activity. Lifestyle changes are probably more effective than pharmacological intervention in preventing diabetes,[54] but further studies are needed.

All women with previous GDM should be offered a regular check of their glucose tolerance, lipid profile, weight, and blood pressure. To implement these measures it is necessary to offer a long-term, continuous program to women with previous GDM including education and stimulation to improve lifestyle. Presently, only very few clinics are able to offer this. However, based on the available evidence a major aim during the next decade will be to implement such programs to the daily clinical life, for the benefit of women with previous GDM.

REFERENCES

1. Kim C, Newton KM, Knopp RH. Gestational diabetes and the incidence of Type 2 diabetes: A systematic review. Diabetes Care 2002; 25: 1862–8.
2. O'Sullivan JB. The Boston Gestational Diabetes Studies: Review and Perspectives. In: Sutherland HW, Stowers JM, eds. Carbohydrate Metabolism in Pregnancy and the Newborn IV. Chapter 26; 1989, pp. 287–94.
3. World Health Organization. World Health Organization Study Group on Diabetes Mellitus. 727 edn. Geneva: World Health Organization; 1985.
4. World Health Organization. Definition, diagnosis and classification of diabetes mellitus and its complications, Report of a WHO consultation, Part 1: Diagnosis and classification of diabetes mellitus. WHO/NCD/NCS/99, 2nd edn. Geneva: World Health Organization; 1999.
5. National Diabetes Data Group. Classification and diagnosis of diabetes mellitus and other categories of glucose intolerance. Diabetes 1979; 28: 1039–57.
6. Report of the Expert Committee on the Diagnosis and Classification of Diabetes Mellitus. Diabetes Care 1997; 20: 1183–97.
7. Pallardo F, Herranz L, Garcia-Ingelmo T, et al. Early postpartum metabolic assessment in women with prior gestational diabetes. Diabetes Care 1999; 22: 1053–8.
8. Kousta E, Lawrence NJ, Penny A, et al. Implications of new diagnostic criteria for abnormal glucose homeostasis in women with previous gestational diabetes. Diabetes Care 1999; 22: 933–7.
9. Costa A, Carmona F, Martinez-Roman S, et al. Post-partum reclassification of glucose tolerance in women previously diagnosed with gestational diabetes mellitus. Diabet Med 2000; 17: 595–8.
10. Motala AA, Omar MA. Evaluation of WHO and NDDG criteria for impaired glucose tolerance. Diabetes Res Clin Pract 1994; 23: 103–9.
11. Metzger BE, Cho NH, Roston SM, Radvany R. Prepregnancy weight and antepartum insulin secretion predict glucose tolerance five years after gestational diabetes mellitus. Diabetes Care 1993; 16: 1598–605.
12. Lobner K, Knopff A, Baumgarten A, et al. Predictors of postpartum diabetes in women with gestational diabetes mellitus. Diabetes 2006; 55: 792–7.
13. Buschard K, Hougaard P, Mølsted-Pedersen L, Kühl C. Type 1 (insulin-dependent) diabetes mellitus diagnosed during pregnancy: a clinical and prognostic study. Diabetologia 1990; 33: 31–5.
14. O'Sullivan JB. Gestational diabetes: factors influencing the rates of subsequent diabetes. In: Sutherland HW, Stowers JM, eds. Carbohydrate metabolism in pregnancy and the newborn. New York: Springer-Verlag; 1979, pp. 425–35.
15. Kjos SL, Peters RK, Xiang A, et al. Predicting future diabetes in Latino women with gestational diabetes. Utility of early postpartum glucose tolerance testing. Diabetes 1995; 44: 586–91.
16. Persson B, Hanson U, Hartling SG, Binder C. Follow-up of women with previous GDM. Insulin, C-peptide, and proinsulin responses to oral glucose load. Diabetes 1991; 40(suppl. 2): 136–41.
17. Damm P, Kühl C, Bertelsen A, Mølsted-Pedersen L. Predictive factors for the development of diabetes in women with previous gestational diabetes mellitus. Am J Obstet Gynecol 1992; 167: 607–16.
18. Aberg AE, Jonsson EK, Eskilsson I, Landin-Olsson M, Frid AH. Predictive factors of developing diabetes mellitus in women with gestational diabetes. Acta Obstet Gynecol Scand 2002; 81: 11–6.
19. Albareda M, Caballero A, Badell G, et al. Diabetes and abnormal glucose tolerance in women with previous gestational diabetes. Diabetes Care 2003; 26: 1199–205.
20. Lauenborg J, Hansen T, Jensen DM, et al. Increasing incidence of diabetes after gestational diabetes mellitus – A long-term follow-up in a Danish population. Diabetes Care 2004; 27: 1194–9.
21. Faber OK, Binder C. C-peptide response to glucagon. A test for the residual beta-cell function in diabetes mellitus. Diabetes 1977; 26: 605–10.
22. Damm P, Kühl C, Buschard K, et al. Prevalence and predictive value of islet cell antibodies and insulin autoantibodies in women with gestational diabetes. Diabet Med 1994; 11: 558–63.
23. Damm P, Kühl C, Hornnes P, Mølsted-Pedersen L. A longitudinal study of plasma insulin and glucagon in women with previous gestational diabetes. Diabetes Care 1995; 18: 654–65.
24. Petersen JS, Dyrberg T, Damm P, et al. GAD65 autoantibodies in women with gestational or insulin dependent diabetes mellitus diagnosed during pregnancy. Diabetologia 1996; 39: 1329–33.
25. Mauricio D, de Leiva A. Autoimmune gestational diabetes mellitus: a distinct clinical entity? Diabetes Metab Res Rev 2001; 17: 422–8.
26. Weng J, Ekelund M, Lehto M, et al. Screening for MODY mutations, GAD antibodies, and Type 1 diabetes-associated HLA genotypes in women with gestational diabetes mellitus. Diabetes Care 2002; 25: 68–71.
27. Lauenborg J, Mathiesen E, Hansen T, et al. The prevalence of the metabolic syndrome in a danish population of women with previous gestational diabetes mellitus is three-fold higher than in the general population. J Clin Endocrinol Metab 2005; 90: 4004–10.
28. Lam KS, Li DF, Lauder IJ, et al. Prediction of persistent carbohydrate intolerance in patients with gestational diabetes. Diabetes Res Clin Pract 1991; 12: 181–6.
29. Coustan DR, Carpenter MW, O'Sullivan PS, Carr SR. Gestational diabetes: predictors of subsequent disordered glucose metabolism. Am J Obstet Gynecol 1993; 168: 1139–44.
30. Catalano PM, Vargo KM, Bernstein IM, Amini SB. Incidence and risk factors associated with abnormal postpartum glucose tolerance in women with gestational diabetes. Am J Obstet Gynecol 1991; 165(4, pt 1): 914–9.
31. Linne Y, Barkeling B, Rossner S. Natural course of gestational diabetes mellitus: long term follow up of women in the SPAWN study. BJOG 2002; 109: 1227–31.
32. Peters RK, Kjos SL, Xiang A, Buchanan TA. Long-term diabetogenic effect of single pregnancy in women with previous gestational diabetes mellitus. Lancet 1996; 347: 227–30.
33. Lillioja S, Mott DM, Spraul M, et al. Insulin resistance and insulin secretory dysfunction as precursors of non-insulin-dependent diabetes mellitus. Prospective studies of Pima Indians. New Engl J Med 1993; 329: 1988–92.
34. Zethelius B, Byberg L, Hales CN, Lithell H, Berne C. Proinsulin and acute insulin response independently predict Type 2 diabetes mellitus in men – report from 27 years of follow-up study. Diabetologia 2003; 46: 20–6.
35. Catalano PM, Tyzbir ED, Sims EA. Incidence and significance of islet cell antibodies in women with previous gestational diabetes. Diabetes Care 1990; 13: 478–82.
36. Hu G, Qiao Q, Silventoinen K, et al. Occupational, commuting, and leisure-time physical activity in relation to risk for Type 2 diabetes in middle-aged Finnish men and women. Diabetologia 2003; 46: 322–9.
37. DeFronzo RA, Bonadonna RC, Ferrannini E. Pathogenesis of NIDDM. A balanced overview. Diabetes Care 1992; 15: 318–68.
38. Damm P, Vestergaard H, Kühl C, Pedersen O. Impaired insulin-stimulated nonoxidative glucose metabolism in glucose-tolerant women with previous gestational diabetes. Am J Obstet Gynecol 1996; 174: 722–9.
39. Kautzky-Willer A, Prager R, Waldhausl W, et al. Pronounced insulin resistance and inadequate beta-cell secretion characterize lean gestational diabetes during and after pregnancy. Diabetes Care 1997; 20: 1717–23.

40. Balkau B, Charles MA, Drivsholm T, et al. Frequency of the WHO metabolic syndrome in European cohorts, and an alternative definition of an insulin resistance syndrome. Diabetes Metab 2002; 28: 364–76.

41. National Institutes of Health. Executive Summary of The Third Report of The National Cholesterol Education Program (NCEP) Expert Panel on Detection, Evaluation, and Treatment of High Blood Cholesterol In Adults (Adult Treatment Panel III). JAMA 2001; 285: 2486–97.

42. Alberti KG, Zimmet P, Shaw J. Metabolic syndrome – a new world-wide definition. A Consensus Statement from the International Diabetes Federation. Diabet Med 2006; 23: 469–80.

43. Lakka HM, Laaksonen DE, Lakka TA, et al. The metabolic syndrome and total and cardiovascular disease mortality in middle-aged men. JAMA 2002; 288: 2709–16.

44. Verma A, Boney CM, Tucker R, Vohr BR. Insulin resistance syndrome in women with prior history of gestational diabetes mellitus. J Clin Endocrinol Metab 2002; 87: 3227–35.

45. Kousta E, Efstathiadou Z, Lawrence NJ, et al. The impact of ethnicity on glucose regulation and the metabolic syndrome following gestational diabetes. Diabetologia 2006; 49: 36–40.

46. Amos AF, McCarty DJ, Zimmet P. The rising global burden of diabetes and its complications: estimates and projections to the year 2010. Diabet Med 1997; 14(suppl. 5): S1–85.

47. Beck-Nielsen H, Groop LC. Metabolic and genetic characterization of prediabetic states. Sequence of events leading to non-insulin-dependent diabetes mellitus. J Clin Invest 1994; 94: 1714–21.

48. Harris MI, Klein R, Welborn TA, Knuiman MW. Onset of NIDDM occurs at least 4–7 yr before clinical diagnosis. Diabetes Care 1992; 15: 815–9.

49. Cheung NW, Byth K. Population health significance of gestational diabetes. Diabetes Care 2003; 26: 2005–9.

50. Kjos SL, Buchanan TA, Greenspoon JS, et al. Gestational diabetes mellitus: the prevalence of glucose intolerance and diabetes mellitus in the first two months post partum. Am J Obstet Gynecol 1990; 163(1, pt 1): 93–8.

51. Eriksson KF, Lindgärde F. Prevention of type 2 (non-insulin-dependent) diabetes mellitus by diet and physical exercise. The 6-year Malmo feasibility study. Diabetologia 1991; 34: 891–8.

52. Pan XR, Li GW, Hu YH, et al. Effects of diet and exercise in preventing NIDDM in people with impaired glucose tolerance. The Da Qing IGT and Diabetes Study. Diabetes Care 1997; 20: 537–44.

53. Qiao Q, Tuomilehto J, Borch-Johnsen K. Post-challenge hyperglycaemia is associated with premature death and macrovascular complications. Diabetologia 2003; 46(suppl. 1): M17–21.

54. Knowler WC, Barrett-Connor E, Fowler SE, et al. Reduction in the incidence of type 2 diabetes with lifestyle intervention or metformin. N Engl J Med 2002; 346: 393–403.

55. Buchanan TA, Xiang AH, Peters RK, et al. Preservation of pancreatic beta-cell function and prevention of type 2 diabetes by pharmacological treatment of insulin resistance in high-risk hispanic women. Diabetes 2002; 51: 2796–803.

56. Xiang AH, Peters RK, Kjos SL, et al. Effect of pioglitazone on pancreatic beta-cell function and diabetes risk in Hispanic women with prior gestational diabetes. Diabetes 2006; 55: 517–22.

57. Henry OA, Beischer NA. Long-term implications of gestational diabetes for the mother. Baillieres Clin Obstet Gynaecol 1991; 5: 461–83.

51 Evidence-based medicine and diabetic pregnancy

Pauline Green and Zarko Alfirevic

Introduction

It seems that increasing number of clinicians are joining one of two very vocal camps. There are the 'evangelists' of evidence-based medicine, who believe that grading of evidence and guidelines based on clinical trials and meta-analyses are the panacea for all clinical mishaps, versus clinicians, who believe that medicine is an art and that so-called evidence has no meaning for doctors who want to provide holistic, individualized patient care. Of course, the truth is somewhere in between. The challenge for tomorrow's doctors is to combine the best of both worlds. It is important to be able to critically appraise the evidence quickly and accurately, and then to apply the knowledge at the bedside, taking into account both the individual needs of the patient and the population perspective.

Critical appraisal of the evidence is only the first step on this journey and not the end of it. Unfortunately, most attempts to start the journey of evidence-informed medicine have failed because the evidence is inadequate or non-existent. This has been a source of frustration for doctors from both camps and also for users of health care.

The public has been increasingly frustrated by the fact that most interventions currently used by health care professionals have not been evaluated according to standards demanded from the pharmaceutical industry. In principle, an evaluation of effectiveness and safety of a 'new' policy of elective Cesarean section to prevent birth trauma or a 'new' diet in diabetic pregnancy should not be less stringent than the evaluation of a new drug. The arguments that clinicians have used successfully to impose strict regulatory mechanisms on the pharmaceutical industry are also relevant when clinicians evaluate new ideas.

Rather than lament on the lack of evidence to guide the management of diabetes in pregnancy, this chapter will try to explain the reasons for it. It is suggested that most of the research related to the management of the diabetic pregnancy follows the pattern seen in other areas of medicine. Published research has concentrated on the clinical questions that have been possible to answer rather than the questions that need to be answered. In order to prove this 'hypothesis', in Table 51.1 the types of diabetic pregnant women and the interventions that may be offered to them in everyday clinical practice are summarized.

The contents of Table 51.1 are only the first part of the clinical question, for example is dietary advice of value for women with pre-existing insulin diabetes or should insulin be given to women with impaired glucose tolerance? The other important part of the question is what is hoped to be achieved by the proposed interventions. Table 51.2 gives the clinical outcomes

---

Table 51.1 Types of diabetic pregnant women and health care interventions suitable for inclusion in clinical trials

Pregnant women*	Interventions
Pre-gestational IDDM	Blood sugar control
Pre-gestational IDDM with complications	Dietary advice
Pre-gestational diet-controlled IDDM	Exercise
Pre-gestational drug-controlled IDDM	Insulin
Gestational diabetes requiring insulin	Oral hypoglycemics
Gestational diabetes, diet controlled	Alternative medicine (e.g. herbs, acupuncture)
Impaired glucose tolerance test	Optimizing fetal and maternal outcome, pre-pregnancy counseling, vitamins/antioxidants, fetal assessment by ultrasound (e.g. fetal growth velocity, Doppler), cardiotocography, antenatal steroids, induction of labor before or at term, Cesarean section before labor, tight glycemic control

*IDDM, insulin-dependent diabetes mellitus.

Table 51.2   Complications that should be used as main outcomes in clinical trials: Clinically relevant adverse outcomes; How many participants are required in a two-arm trial to prove that an intervention can reduce an adverse outcome by 25%?*

Complication	Likely incidence in the control		
	Untreated group (%)	25% reduction (%)	Anticipated total sample size (both groups)
Fetal/neonatal			
Miscarriages/early Pregnancy loss	17[80]	12.75	2292
Fetal anomalies	9.7[80]	7.3	8720
Perinatal mortality	3.6[80]	2.7	12,262
Shoulder dystocia	2.8[68]	2.1	15,878
Erb's palsy	1 0.7 in neonates <4.5 kg,	0.75	45,157
	5 in neonates >4.5 kg	3.75	
Serious neonatal morbidity (seizures, intracranial hemorrhage, encephalo-pathy cerebral palsy)	1	0.75	45,157
Maternal			
Maternal death	0.11[82]	0.08	344,284
Maternal ketoacidosis	1.73[83]	1.3	26,254
Maternal hypoglycemic coma	36[84]	27	878

*Power 80%, alpha 0.05.

that should guide the choice of intervention(s) in the diabetic pregnancy. When reading clinical trial data, it is apparent that many different outcomes have been measured, e.g. fetal or neonatal macrosomia is often used as an outcome measure. This is not included in the present list of important clinical outcomes, as the macrosomia *per se* is not the end point one would wish to judge interventions by. The important end points are those subsequent upon the macrosomia, i.e. birth trauma, shoulder dystocia and Erb's palsy, cerebral hemorrhage due to difficult delivery, seizures due to birth asphyxia or metabolic disturbance in the newborn, and perinatal mortality. Macrosomia would not necessarily lead to any of these problems, therefore the measured outcome needs to be set at a clinically meaningful level. It must be asked whether an intervention being proposed to a patient is capable of reducing the adverse outcomes listed in Table 51.2. The present authors suggest that if an intervention has no impact on these outcomes then it is unlikely to be of clinical value. So, what sort of impact is being sought? Often one finds that researchers are completely unrealistic in their expectations, anticipating reductions in adverse pregnancy outcomes of ≥50%. Very few interventions can achieve this. If they do, the impact is so obvious that clinical trials are at best unnecessary, if not unethical (e.g. Cesarean section for prolonged fetal bradycardia, glucagon for severe maternal hypoglycemia). The vast majority of proposed interventions and management policies can only achieve modest benefits, e.g. ≤25% reduction in important adverse outcomes. With this in mind, the number of women who would be needed to prove that an intervention is capable of achieving its intended aim has been

calculated. (Table 51.2) As a rule, studies with <1000 participants will not be able to give much information about the impact of an intervention on the outcomes that are important to pregnant women with diabetes. The studies will often claim that 'there is no difference in perinatal mortality or birth trauma', but this does not mean that an important clinical difference does not exist. 'No evidence of a difference', which is almost a rule in small studies, should not be confused with 'evidence of no difference'.

The aim of the next section of this chapter is to identify published clinical trials that have set out to answer the questions posed in Tables 51.1 and 51.2. For example, whether elective delivery of a pregnant diabetic woman is better than allowing her to await spontaneous labour or whether the elective use of insulin in mild glucose intolerance will have any advantages over diet alone.

Current evidence from clinical trials

One hundred and three publications of randomized trials from the Cochrane Register of Clinical Trials that may have contained relevant information for the management of diabetes in pregnancy were identified. Of these, 28 publications were excluded: one trial was still recruiting, there was insufficient data collected from a number of other trials, several trials were excluded as they did not contain information relevant to pregnancy and diabetes, and, finally, there were a number of publications which reported on the same randomized trial.

Fetal assessment by ultrasound

Two trials were identified which sought to answer the question as to whether ultrasound could help to identify pregnant women with diabetes who were likely to benefit from an intervention. Buchanon et al.[1] used the third trimester ultrasound to measure the fetal abdominal circumference in women with mild gestational diabetes mellitus (GDM). If the fetal abdominal circumference was large (≥75th centile), women were randomized either to continue with their diet or to start insulin in addition to their dietary therapy: 59 women completed the study but no serious clinically important adverse outcomes were reported (Table 51.2). Rossi et al.[2] also started insulin therapy when ultrasound measurements of the fetal abdominal circumference exceeded the 75th centile in women with mild, diet-controlled GDM: 73 women had an ultrasound fetal abdominal circumference measurement at 28 and 32 weeks gestation, and 68 women had a single measurement at 32 weeks. There were no maternal hypoglycemic episodes in 73 women who took part in the study, but other important adverse outcomes were not reported. For a clinically significant difference in the rate of serious maternal hypoglycemia to be assessed, a sample size of over 800 women would have been required.

Intrapartum glucose control

One study from the USA[3] compared intravenous infusion of 10% invert sugar with lactated Ringer's solution and 5% dextrose in 32 insulin-requiring diabetics prior to labour induction or elective Cesarean section. No serious adverse outcomes were reported. This trial therefore failed to inform of a management strategy which would be of important clinical relevance.

Diet

A Cochrane review by Walkinshaw,[4] included four trials where GDM was managed either by dietary manipulation or with no specific treatment[5,6] (also Ford FA, unpublished work and Okum N, unpublished work). The reviewer concluded that the results were inconclusive, with only one trial of 158 women[6] reporting 'corrected' perinatal mortality of 0% (one baby died with multiple congenital malformations). In this same study there were no reported cases of birth trauma in either group and there were five babies with congenital abnormalities, three in the control group (including the baby with multiple abnormalities that died) and two in the treatment group. Okum reported the reduced incidence of birth trauma with diet [zero of 234 versus four of 223; odds ratio (OR) 0.13, 95% confidence interval (CI) 0.02–0.96].

A study by Bevier et al.,[7] not included in the Cochrane review, also compared diet and home monitoring with routine care in 103 women with a positive glucose challenge test. There were two cases of shoulder dystocia in the control group and one case in the experimental group. However, only 83 of the 103 randomized women were reported on, 48 in the control group and 35 in the experimental group. These numbers are inadequate for assessing any clinically useful difference in the incidence of shoulder dystocia with the chosen intervention.

Seven small trials, with the number of participants ranging from five to 125, compared different types of diet.[8–14] Only trials by Ney et al.[8] and Rae et al.[10] reported substantive outcomes. Ney et al.[8] reported no congenital malformations in 20 diabetic pregnancies, while Rae et al.[10] reported three cases of shoulder dystocia in 124 women.

Insulin

A Cochrane review by Walkinshaw[15] included two trials[16,17] with 182 pre-existing insulin-dependent diabetics. He concluded that there was no clear evidence favouring very tight glycemic control in these women. However, out of the nine clinically important outcomes (as listed in Table 51.2), only the perinatal mortality was reported by Farrag (0%).[17]

A preliminary report by Snyder et al.[18] also described a trial of tight versus very tight diabetic control and reported no difference in the birth trauma between the two groups.

The present authors have identified a further 26 trials focusing on the use of insulin, either comparing its use with diet alone or with no treatment, or in trials comparing different types of insulin, different regimes of delivery of insulin or comparing insulin with oral hypoglycemics.[5,19–43] The population of pregnant women in these studies were either gestational or pregestational diabetics.

Serious maternal morbidity was explicitly reported in nine trials.[27–36] Ketoacidosis was found in one of 10 women in Botta et al.'s[22] study, one of 89 women in Burkhart et al.'s[29] study, three of 23 women in Nosari et al.'s[31] study and no cases in 22 patients in Coustan et al.'s[35] study. The ketoacidosis rate reported in these trials was c. 3.5%, which is higher than in observational studies (Table 51.2). Nevertheless, thousands rather than tens of women are needed to show that an intervention does not affect the incidence of ketoacidosis. Seven studies have also reported severe maternal hypoglycemia.[22,30–33,35,36] The incidence ranged from zero to a high rate of hypoglycemia, with 0% in four studies,[22,30,32,36] 7% in Nachum et al.'s[33] study, 12.5% in Nosari et al.'s[31] study and the high rate of 36.4% in Coustan et al.'s[35] study. It is most likely that these large differences reflect the varying definitions of severe hypoglycemia rather than any true differences in quality of care. This is the reason why severe hypoglycemia is defined by the authors as one that causes unconsciousness. In the three studies with cases of severe hypoglycemia, Coustan et al.[35] defined it as an episode of hypoglycemia requiring hospital treatment with intravenous glucose or glucagon, Nosari et al.[31] characterized it as coma, seizure or a situation requiring hospitalization, intravenous glucose or glucagon, and Nachum et al.[33] defined it as an episode requiring the help of another person.

Perinatal deaths were reported in 14 of the trials.[28–33,36–43] The rates ranged from 0 to 14.5%,[42] but the majority of trials reported a perinatal death rate <5%. Given the low number of patients in these studies and the relatively low perinatal mortality rates it is not surprising that no firm conclusions can be drawn regarding the safety of the various insulin regimens.

No trials reported serious neonatal morbidity as an outcome and only one trial reported Erb's palsy.[43]

Different screening practices

Bebbington et al.'s[44] randomized trial compared routine universal screening of low-risk pregnant women for GDM with selective screening when clinical indications (risk factors) were present: no clinically important outcomes were reported for the 2401 randomized women. A similar trial with 3152 women showed a higher rate of diagnosis of GDM in the universal screening group.[45] Two intrauterine deaths occurred in the routinely screened group after a positive glucose challenge test. Three further randomized trials were identified related to screening for GDM but none referred to clinically important outcomes.[46–48]

Induction versus expectant management

A Cochrane review by Boulvain et al.[49] assessed the effectiveness and safety of elective delivery compared with expectant management in term diabetic pregnant women: only the trial by Kjos et al.[50] was included in the review. This study randomized 200 insulin-requiring diabetic pregnant women to either active induction of labour or expectant management up to 42 weeks gestation. Spontaneous labour occurred in 44% of the expectant management group. Of the clinically significant outcomes that were detailed in the study, only shoulder dystocia actually occurred. All three documented cases occurred in the expectant management group and all were described as mild. There were no cases of birth trauma (including Erb's palsy), no perinatal deaths and no major congenital abnormalities. No maternal outcomes were reported. Again, one is unable to ascertain from this study whether elective delivery in the gestational diabetic confers any benefit as the numbers required to show a 25% improvement in the clinically important outcomes measured would require many more women (Table 51.2).

Vaginal delivery versus Cesarean section

Only one randomized trial compared vaginal delivery and Cesarean section as the mode of delivery at term in pregnant women diagnosed with GDM.[51] All women had been monitored during pregnancy and been given dietary advice, there was no indication that any women required insulin. Out of 84 randomized women with GDM, 44 were allocated to Cesarean section at term. It is reassuring that there were no reported cases of perinatal deaths or congenital malformations. However, >10,000 women would have had be to randomized to exclude the possibility that one of these interventions increases perinatal mortality by 25%.

Exercise

Four studies were identified that assessed the effect of exercise on pregnant women with diabetes.[52–55] Only two of them reported on the present authors' pre-specified outcomes.[52,53] In the randomized trial comparing diet versus diet plus an exercise program in the management of GDM, Jovanovic-Peterson et al.[52] reported that there were no cases of maternal hypoglycemia and no neonatal morbidity in 19 gestational

diabetics. The authors concluded that a cardiovascular-conditioning program might obviate the need for insulin treatment in many women with GDM, but the observations in their study required further testing. Referring to Table 51.2, c. 900 women would be required to assess a difference of 25% in the rate of severe maternal hypoglycemia. Similarly, in the trial by Bung et al.[53] 41 patients with failed diet therapy who would have been treated with insulin were randomized to either receive diet plus exercise or diet plus insulin. There were no reported episodes of hypoglycemia in either group.

Glucose monitoring

Twelve clinical trials studying the various methods of monitoring glucose levels were identified.[56–67] Two studies based the clinical decision to commence insulin therapy on either amniotic fluid insulin levels or mean blood glucose monitoring.[57,67] In both of these studies the present authors' pre-specified outcomes were not reported, although Hopp et al.[67] commented that there were no statistically significant differences in the rates of miscarriage, stillbirth or neonatal death in their two groups. Langer et al.[62] randomized 2461 women with GDM into either conventional (weekly clinic visits) or intensified (home blood glucose monitoring) management groups. A 3-fold higher rate of shoulder dystocia was found in the conventional management group compared with the intensified management group (1.4 vs. 0.4%, $P < 0.0001$). Langer et al.[62] also reported on the percentages of other neonatal trauma events and the number of perinatal deaths. In the following list the conventional management group results come first and the intensified management group results second: seizures, 0.3 versus 0.2%; fracture, 0.7 versus 0.3%; Erb's palsy, 0.1 versus 0%; stillbirths, five versus one; neonatal deaths, three versus three. Langer et al.[62] commented that two neonatal deaths were related to anomalies (anencephaly and holoprosencephaly) and one stillbirth had a cardiac anomaly, but they did not report whether other anomalies had occurred nor which group the anomalies occurred in.

Varner,[59] Rey,[60] and Stubbs et al.[63] all compared clinic visits with the more intensive home blood glucose monitoring in women with either GDM or insulin-dependent diabetes mellitus (IDDM). Varner[59] reported on miscarriage and perinatal death, but only 30 insulin-dependent diabetics were recruited. Rey[60] reported that a significant increase in shoulder dystocia occurred in the clinic visit group (one case in the home-monitoring group versus four cases in the clinic visits group), but on small numbers (347 randomized women). There was one fetal death in the home-monitoring group associated with a true knot of the cord. Stubbs et al.[63] reported one perinatal loss (cot death) in 13 randomized women, but no other clinically important outcomes.

De Veciana et al.[64] recruited 66 gestational diabetics on insulin to monitor blood glucose either pre- or postprandially. Shoulder dystocia (defined as requiring one or more maneuvers) was reported to occur in 18% (six of 33) of the prepandial monitoring group and in 3% (one of 33) of the postprandial monitoring group. Overall, the rate of shoulder dystocia in the 66 gestational diabetics (10.6%) was much higher than in observational studies (2.8%).[68] Such a high incidence of shoulder dystocia probably reflects the definition that was used. As expected, the incidence of Erb's palsy was lower (6 and 3%, respectively) but in all cases the palsy resolved before discharge. One infant in each group had a fracture (one of the clavicle and one of the humerus). There was one unexplained stillbirth in the preprandial monitoring group.

Reller et al.[56] randomized 63 women to either early or late careful diabetic management, but the study design precluded any of the present authors' stated important outcomes. Di Biase et al.[58] randomized 20 IDDM patients to either a telemedicine computerized device, enabling 24-h communication of data, or conventional home blood glucose monitoring. Again, no significant outcome data was reported.

Two trials compared the effect of glycemic control and routine antenatal care in GDM.[61,66] Both trials were in fact pilot studies and too small to draw any conclusions, but both authors concluded that a large randomized trial was feasible.

Hanson et al.[65] studied the effect of hospitalization from 32 weeks gestation compared with a policy of home blood glucose monitoring in 100 pregnant diabetic women. Major congenital abnormalities were reported in three of 46 infants (hospital management) and one of 56 infants (home glucose monitoring). There was one perinatal death in each group. It must be emphasized again that the numbers were too small to draw any meaningful conclusions regarding effectiveness and safety of these interventions.

Diagnosis of gestational diabetes mellitus

Proving that a diagnostic test is reproducible and accurate is only the beginning, and not the end, of its evaluation. Introduction of an effective new screening policy, or a diagnostic test, into clinical practice should be expected to have a major impact on the outcome of diabetic pregnancies. One expects that a test with a better performance (sensitivity, specificity) would restrict interventions, such as blood glucose monitoring and treatment (diet, insulin), to those women who are likely to benefit from such interventions. However,

an excellent diagnostic test may be followed by an ineffective or dangerous treatment package, or vice versa, with the net result of harm rather than benefit. At present, the randomized clinical trial is the only research method that allows an unbiased comparison of various management policies (diagnosis plus treatment) for diabetic pregnant women.

Ten studies were identified that sought to compare different diagnostic tests for GDM,[69–78] but only Court et al.[70] reported the impact of these tests on clinically important outcomes, i.e. perinatal deaths. There were six perinatal deaths in the group of 230 women who used glucose polymer as the test beverage compared with zero deaths in the group of 48 women who were given glucose: two of six deaths were due to congenital abnormality. As far as the present authors could ascertain, no other important clinical outcomes were reported in any of the other studies of diagnostic tests in diabetic pregnancies.

Other

In 1955, Reid[79] evaluated the use of stilboestrol and progesterone in 147 pregnant women with either pre-existing diabetes or GDM. Women were randomized (after stratification by age and parity) to receive (76 women) or not to receive (71 women) hormones from 16 weeks to term. One mother died in each group after Cesarean section. There were four congenital abnormalities in the hormone-treated group and seven in the control group. There were six miscarriages in each group and 17 perinatal deaths in each group.

Summary

In this chapter, the present authors have deliberately set out to be controversial in their approach to evidence-based care of the diabetic pregnancy. It has been attempted to show, by using examples of published clinical trials in this field, that an enormous amount of research time and energy, and patient good will, has produced remarkably little evidence. It is suggested that the way forward is multicentre collaboration rather than intercenter competition. The research agenda should be driven by questions relevant to pregnant diabetic women and their families, rather than the present 'publish or perish' policy.

REFERENCES

1. Buchanon TA, Kjos SL, Montoro MN, et al. Use of fetal ultrasound to select metabolic therapy for pregnancies complicated by mild gestational diabetes. Diabetes Care 1994; 17: 275–83.
2. Rossi G, Somigliana E, Moschetta M, et al. Adequate timing of fetal ultrasound to guide metabolic therapy in mild gestational diabetes mellitus. Results from a randomised study. Acta Obstet Gynecol Scand 2000; 79: 649–54.
3. Wright TE, Martin D, Qualls C, Curet LB. Effects of intrapartum administration of invert sugar and D5LR on neonatal blood glucose levels. J Perinatol 2000; 20: 217–8.
4. Walkinshaw SA. Dietary regulation for 'gestational diabetes' (Cochrane review). In: The Cochrane Library, Issue 1. (Oxford: Update Software, 2002).
5. Langer O, Anyaegbunam A, Brustman L, Divon M. Management of women with one abnormal oral glucose tolerance test value reduces

adverse outcome in pregnancy. Am J Obstet Gynecol 1989; 161: 593–9.
6. Li DFH, Wong VCW, O'Hoy KMKY, et al. Is treatment needed for mild impairment of glucose tolerance in pregnancy? A randomised controlled trial. Br J Obstet Gynaecol 1987; 94: 851–4.
7. Bevier WC, Fischer R, Jovanovic L. Treatment of women with an abnormal glucose challenge test (but a normal oral glucose tolerance test) decreases the prevalence of macrosomia. Am J Perinatol 1999; 16: 269–75.
8. Ney D, Hollingsworth DR, Cousins L. Decreased insulin requirement and improved control of diabetes in pregnant women given a high-carbohydrate, high-fiber, low-fat diet. Diabetes Care 1982; 5: 529–33.
9. Reece EA, Hagay Z, Gay LJ, et al. A randomised clinical trial of a fiber-enriched diabetic diet vs. the standard American Diabetes

Association recommended diet in the management of diabetes mellitus in pregnancy. J Matern Fetal Invest 1995; 5: 8–12.

10. Rae A, Bond D, Evans S, et al. A randomised controlled trial of dietary energy restriction in the management of obese women with gestational diabetes. Aust NZ J Obstet Gynaecol 2000; 40: 416–22.

11. Nolan CJ. Improved glucose tolerance in gestational diabetic women on a low fat, high unrefined carbohydrate diet. Aust NZ J Obstet Gynaecol 1984; 24: 174–7.

12. Magee MS, Knopp RH, Benedetti TJ. Metabolic effects of 1200-kcal diet in obese pregnant women with gestational diabetes. Diabetes 1990; 39: 234–40.

13. Lauszus FF, Rasmussen OW, Henriksen JE, et al. Effect of a high monounsaturated fatty acid diet on blood pressure and glucose metabolism in women with gestational diabetes mellitus. Eur J Clin Nutr 2001; 55: 436–43.

14. Ilic S, Jovanovic L, Pettitt DJ. Comparison of the effect of saturated and monounsaturated fat on postprandial plasma glucose and insulin concentration in women with gestational diabetes mellitus. Am J Perinatol 1999; 16: 489–95.

15. Walkinshaw SA. Very tight versus tight control for diabetes in pregnancy (Cochrane review). In: The Cochrane Library, Issue 1. (Oxford: Update Software, 2002).

16. Demarini S, Mimouni F, Tsang RC, et al. Impact of metabolic control of diabetes during pregnancy on neonatal hypoglycemia: a randomised study. Obstet Gynecol 1994; 83: 918–22.

17. Farrag OAM. Prospective study of 3 metabolic regimens in pregnant diabetics. Aust NZ J Obstet Gynaecol 1987; 27: 6–9.

18. Snyder J, Morin L, Meltzer S, Nadeau J. Gestational diabetes and glycemic control: a randomised clinical trial. Am J Obstet Gynecol 1998; 178: 55.

19. Pardi G, Buscaglia M, Kustermann A, et al. Foetal pulmonary maturation in pregnancies complicated by diabetes and Rh immunization. Eur Respir J 1989; 2(suppl. 3): 50S–52S.

20. Gillmer MDG, Maresh M, Beard RW, et al. Low energy diets in the treatment of gestational diabetes. Acta Endocrinol 1986; 277: 44–9.

21. Schuster MW, Chauhan SP, McLaughlin BN, et al. Comparison of insulin regimens and administration modalities in pregnancies complicated by diabetes. J Mississippi State Med Assoc 1998; 39: 51–5.

22. Maresh M, Alderson C, Beard RW, et al. Comparison of insulin against diet treatment in the management of abnormal carbohydrate tolerance in pregnancy. In: Campbell DM, Gillmer MDG, eds. Nutrition in Pregnancy, Proceedings of the 10th Study Group of the RCOG. London: RCOG; 1983, pp. 255–67.

23. Li P, Yang H, Dong Y. Treating women with gestational impaired glucose tolerance reduces adverse outcome of pregnancy. Chin J Obstet Gynecol 1999; 34: 462–4.

24. Laatikainen L, Teramo K, Hieta-Heikurainen H, et al. A controlled study of the influence of continuous subcutaneous insulin infusion treatment on diabetic retinopathy during pregnancy. Acta Med Scand 1987; 221: 367–76.

25. Jovanovic-Peterson L, Palmer JP, Sparks S, Peterson CM. Jet-injected insulin is associated with decreased antibody production and postprandial glucose variability when compared with needle-injected insulin in gestational diabetic women. Diabetes Care 1993; 16: 1479–83.

26. Jovanovic-Peterson L, Kitzmiller JL, Peterson CM. Randomised trial of human versus animal species insulin in diabetic pregnant women: improved glycemic control, not fewer antibodies to insulin, influences birth weight. Am J Obstet Gynecol 1992; 167: 1325–30.

27. Jovanovic L, Ilic S, Pettitt DJ, et al. Metabolic and immunologic effects of insulin lispro in gestational diabetes. Diabetes Care 1999; 22: 1422–7.

28. Botta RM, Sinagra D, Angelico MC, Bompiani GD. Intensified conventional insulin therapy as compared to micropump therapy in pregnant women affected by type 1 diabetes mellitus. Minerva Med 1986; 77: 657–61.

29. Burkart W, Hanker JP, Schneider HPG. Complications and fetal outcome in diabetic pregnancy. Intensified conventional versus insulin pump therapy. Gynecol Obstet Invest 1988; 26: 104–12.

30. Langer O, Conway DL, Berkus MD, et al. A comparison of glyburide and insulin in women with gestational diabetes mellitus. N Engl J Med 2000; 343: 1134–8.

31. Nosari I, Maglio ML, Lepore G, et al. Is continuous subcutaneous insulin infusion more effective than intensive conventional insulin therapy in the treatment of pregnant diabetic women? Diabet Nutr Metab 1993; 6: 33–7.

32. Thompson DJ, Porter KB, Gunnells DJ, et al. Prophylactic insulin in the management of gestational diabetes. Obstet Gynecol 1990; 75: 960–4.

33. Nachum Z, Ben-Shlomo I, Weiner E, Shalev E. Twice daily versus four times daily insulin dose regimens for diabetes in pregnancy: randomised controlled trial. Br Med J 1999; 319: 1223–7.

34. Maresh M, Gillmer MDG, Beard RW, et al. The effect of diet and insulin on metabolic profiles of women with gestational diabetes mellitus. Diabetes 1985; 34(suppl. 2): 88–93.

35. Coustan DR, Reece EA, Sherwin RS, et al. A randomised clinical trial of the insulin pump vs intensive conventional therapy in diabetic pregnancies. J Am Med Assoc 1986; 255: 631–6.

36. Carta Q, Meriggi E, Trossarelli GF, et al. Continuous subcutaneous insulin infusion versus intensive conventional insulin therapy in Type I and Type II diabetic pregnancy. Diabete Metab (Paris) 1986; 12: 121–9.

37. Persson B, Stangenberg M, Hansson, Nordlander E. Gestational diabetes mellitus (GDM): comparative evaluation of two treatment regimens, diet vs insulin and diet. Diabetes 1985; 34: 101–5.

38. O'Sullivan JB. Prospective study of gestational diabetes and its treatment. In: Stowers JB, Sutherland HW, eds. Carbohydrate Metabolism in Pregnancy and the Newborn. Churchill Livingstone: 1975; pp. 195–204.

39. O'Sullivan JB, Charles D, Dandrow RV. Treatment of verified prediabetes in pregnancy. J Reprod Med 1971; 7: 21–4.

40. O'Sullivan JB, Gellis SS, Dandrow RV, Tenney BO. The potential diabetic and her treatment in pregnancy. Obstet Gynecol 1966; 27: 683–9.

41. O'Sullivan JB, Mahan CM, Charles D, Dandrow RV. Medical treatment of the gestational diabetic. Obstet Gynecol 1974; 43: 817–21.

42. Notelovitz M. Sulphonylurea therapy in the treatment of the pregnant diabetic. S Afr Med J 1971; 45: 226–9.

43. Coustan DR, Lewis SB. Insulin therapy for gestational diabetes. Obstet Gynecol 1978; 51: 306–10.

44. Bebbington M, Milner R, Wilson R, Harris S. A RCT comparing routine screening vs selected screening for GDM in low risk population. Am J Obstet Gynecol 1999; 180: S36.

45. Griffin ME, Coffey M, Johnson H, et al. Universal vs risk factor-based screening for gestational diabetes mellitus: detection rates, gestation at diagnosis and outcome. Diabet Med 2000; 17: 26–32.

46. Hidar S, Chaieb A, Baccouche S, et al. Post-prandial plasma glucose test as screening tool for gestational diabetes: a prospective randomised trial. J Gynecol Obstet Biol Reprod 2001; 30: 344–7.

47. Murphy NJ, Meyer BA, O'Kell RT, Hogard ME. Carbohydrate sources for gestational diabetes mellitus screening. A comparison. J Reprod Med 1994; 39: 977–81.

48. Lamar ME, Kuehl TJ, Cooney AT, et al. Jelly beans as an alternative to a fifty-gram glucose beverage for gestational diabetes screening. Am J Obstet Gynecol 1999; 181: 1154–7.

49. Boulvain M, Stan C, Irion O. Elective delivery in diabetic pregnant women (Cochrane review). In: The Cochrane Library, Issue 1. (Oxford: Update Software, 2002).

50. Kjos SL, Henry OA, Montoro M, et al. Insulin-requiring diabetes in pregnancy: a randomised trial of active induction of labor and expectant management. Am J Obstet Gynecol 1993; 169: 611–5.

51. Khojandi M, Tsai AY/M, Tyson JE. Gestational diabetes: the dilemma of delivery. Obstet Gynecol 1974; 43: 1–6.

52. Jovanovic-Peterson L, Durak EP, Peterson CM. Randomised trial of diet versus diet plus cardiovascular conditioning on glucose levels in gestational diabetes. Am J Obstet Gynecol 1989; 161: 415–9.

53. Bung P, Artal R, Khodiguian N, Kjos S. Exercise in gestational diabetes. An optional therapeutic approach? Diabetes 1991; 40: 182–5.

54. Avery M, Leon AS, Kopher RA. Effects of a partially home-based exercise program for women with gestational diabetes. Obstet Gynecol 1997; 89: 10–5.

55. Lesser KB, Gruppuso PA, Terry RB, Carpenter MW. Exercise fails to improve postprandial glycemic excursion in women with gestational diabetes. J Matern Fetal Med 1996; 5: 211–7.

56. Reller MD, Tsang RC, Meyer RA, Braun CP. Relationship of prospective diabetes control in pregnancy to neonatal cardiorespiratory function. J Pediatr 1985; 106: 86–90.

57. Novak A, Hopp H, Vollert W, et al. Fetal indication for insulin therapy in gestational diabetes. Proceedings of the 14th European Congress of Perinatal Medicine, Helsinki, Finland, 1994, 318.

58. Di Biase N, Napoli A, Sabbatini A, et al. Telemedicine in the treatment of diabetic pregnancy. Annali dell Istituto Superiore di Sanita 1997; 33: 347–51.

59. Varner MW. Efficacy of home glucose monitoring in diabetic pregnancy. Am J Med 1983; 75: 592–6.
60. Rey E. Usefulness of a breakfast test in the management of women with gestational diabetes. Obstet Gynecol 1997; 89: 981–8.
61. Garner P, Okun N, Keely E, et al. A randomised controlled trial of strict glycemic control and tertiary level obstetric care versus routine obstetric care in the management of gestational diabetes: a pilot study. Am J Obstet Gynecol 1997; 177: 190–5.
62. Langer O, Rodriguez DA, Xenakis EMJ, et al. Intensified versus conventional management of gestational diabetes. Am J Obstet Gynecol 1994; 170: 1036–47.
63. Stubbs SM, Brudenell JM, Pyke DA, et al. Management of the pregnant diabetic: home or hospital, with or without glucose meters? Lancet 1980; 1: 1122–4.
64. De Veciana M, Major CA, Morgan MA, et al. Postprandial versus preprandial blood glucose monitoring in women with gestational diabetes mellitus requiring insulin therapy. N Engl J Med 1995; 333: 1237–41.
65. Hanson U, Persson B, Enochsson E, et al. Self-monitoring of blood glucose by diabetic women during the third trimester of pregnancy. Am J Obstet Gynecol 1984; 150: 817–21.
66. Bancroft K, Tuffnell DJ, Mason GC, et al. A randomised controlled pilot study of the management of gestational impaired glucose tolerance. Br J Obstet Gynaecol 2000; 107: 959–63.
67. Hopp H, Vollert W, Ragosch V, et al. Indication and results of insulin therapy for gestational diabetes mellitus. J Perinat Med 1996; 24: 521–30.
68. Conway DL, Langer O. Elective delivery of infants with macrosomia in diabetic women: reduced shoulder dystocia versus increased cesarean deliveries. Am J Obstet Gynecol 1998; 178: 922–5.
69. Sammarco MJ, Mundy DC, Riojas JE. Glucose tolerance in pregnancy. Proceedings of the 41st Annual Clinical Meeting of the American College of Obstetricians and Gynecologists, USA, 1993, 10–11.
70. Court DJ, Mann SL, Stone PR, et al. Comparison of glucose polymer and glucose for screening and tolerance tests in pregnancy. Obstet Gynecol 1985; 66: 491–9.
71. Court DJ, Stone PR, Killip M. Comparison of glucose and glucose polymer for testing oral carbohydrate tolerance in pregnancy. Obstet Gynecol 1984; 64: 251–5.
72. Cheng LC, Salmon YM, Chen C. A double-blind, randomised, crossover study comparing the 50g OGTT and the 75g OGTT for pregnant women in the 3rd trimester. Ann Acad Med 1992; 21: 769–72.
73. Harlass FE, McClure GB, Read JA, Brady K. Use of a standard preparatory diet for the oral gl tol test. Is it necessary? J Reprod Med 1991; 36: 147–50.
74. Helton DG, Martin RW, Martin JN, et al. Detection of glucose intolerance in pregnancy. J Perinatol 1989; 9: 259–61.
75. Berkus MD, Langer O. Glucose tolerance test periodicity: the effect of glucose loading. Obstet Gynecol 1995; 85: 423–7.
76. Bergus GR, Murphy NJ. Screening for gestational diabetes mellitus: comparison of a glucose polymer and a glucose monomer test beverage. J Am Board Fam Plan 1992; 5: 241–7.
77. Jones JS, Horger E. A comparative study of the standard oral and intravenous glucose tolerance tests in pregnancy. Am J Obstet Gynecol 1993; 168: 407.
78. Weiss PAM, Haeusler M, Kainer F, et al. Toward universal criteria for gestational diabetes: relationships between seventy-five and one hundred gram glucose loads and capillary and venous glucose concentrations. Am J Obstet Gynecol 1998; 178: 830–5.
79. Reid DD. Report to the medical research council. The use of hormones in the management of pregnancy in diabetics. Lancet 1955; 2: 833–6.
80. Casson IF, Clarke CA, Howard CV, et al. Outcomes of pregnancy in insulin dependent diabetic women: results of a five year population cohort study. Br Med J 1997; 315: 275–8.
81. Persson B, Hanson U. Neonatal morbidities in gestational diabetes mellitus. Diabetes Care 1998; 21(suppl. 2B): 79–84.
82. Reece EA, Hobbins JC, Mahony MJ, Petrie RH. Handbook of Medicine of the Fetus and Mother. Philiadelphia: JB Lippincott; 1995.
83. Kilvert JA, Nicholson HO, Wright AD. Ketoacidosis in diabetic pregnancy. Diabet Med 1993; 10: 278–81.
84. Rayburn W, Piehl E, Jacober S, et al. Severe hypoglycaemia during pregnancy: its frequency and predisposing factors in diabetic women. Int J Gynaecol Obstet 1986; 24: 263–8.

52 Cost analysis of diabetes and pregnancy

Michael Brandle and William H. Herman

Costs of pregnancy care and adverse outcomes of pregnancy

During the adult reproductive years, women have higher medical expenditures than men.[1] The difference in medical expenditures between women and men is related in large part to pregnancy care, childbirth and its complications. The costs of pregnancy and childbirth include the cost of outpatient prenatal care, hospitalizations, and care of the newborn. Costs increase with higher frequencies of hospitalization,[2] alternative modes of delivery[3,4] and longer stays in hospital.[5] Costs also increase with multiple gestations[6] and with maternal obesity.[7]

Median hospital costs for preterm labor without delivery have been estimated to be US $2200; median hospital costs for preterm labor with early delivery are US $6600. The total annual expenditures for preterm-labor hospitalization in the United States (US) are in excess of $820 million.[2] A recent systematic review of the literature revealed that the range of costs are £600–1300 (US $1000–2200) for an uncomplicated vaginal delivery and £1200–3600 (US $2100–5900) for a Cesarean delivery.[3] In a large Scottish observational study, the health care costs of alternative modes of delivery were estimated to be £1700 for a spontaneous vaginal delivery, £2300 for an instrumental vaginal delivery and £3200 for a Cesarean delivery ($P < 0.001$).[4]

In 1991, the predicted charges for the family (mother and neonate) for a singleton pregnancy was $9800, as compared to $38,000 for twins ($19,000 per baby) and $110,000 for triplets ($36,600 per baby). Hospital charges for a 29-year-old white mother with a singleton pregnancy were $4800, as compared with $8000 for a mother of twins and $15,400 for a mother with a higher order multiple-gestation pregnancy. Daily charges increased from $600 for a singleton neonate to $1000 for each twin and to $1700 for each infant born of a higher order multiple pregnancy.[6]

The average costs of hospital prenatal care are approximately five times higher for mothers who are overweight before pregnancy than for normal-weight mothers.[7] In addition, obesity leads to significantly longer postpartum hospital stays as a result of more frequent Cesarean deliveries and endometritis. The percentage of infants of obese mothers requiring care in a neonatal intensive care unit is c. 3.5 times higher than that of infants of non-obese mothers.[8,9]

Adverse outcomes of pregnancy also contribute to substantially higher costs.[10,11] The inpatient and outpatient treatment costs for very-low-birthweight (VLBW) (birthweight <1500 g) infants during the first year of life was $59,700 (1987 US dollars).[12] Because of the greater mortality in the smallest infants, the average cost was lowest for infants with birthweights <750 g ($49,900) and highest among infants between 750 and 999 g ($79,200).[12] The lifetime costs of major congenital anomalies are also high (Figure 52.1): $393,000 for an infant with a major cardiac defect, $294,000 for spina bifida, $250,000 for diaphragmatic hernia, renal agenesis or dysgenesis, $199,000 for lower limb reduction, $176,000 for omphalocele, $108,000 for gastroschisis, $101,000 for cleft lip or palate, and $84,000 for urinary obstruction. The lifetime cost for one infant with cerebral palsy is estimated to be c. $503,000.

Cost-effectiveness of interventions in pregnancy

Cost-effectiveness analyses (CEA) explicitly compare the costs and outcomes of new treatments with alternative treatments so that the treatments can be ordered on the basis of how much benefit is gained relative to the expense.[13] CEA are being reported more frequently in medicine and specifically in obstetrics.[14] Recent CEA in obstetrics have studied the value of fortifying grain with folic acid to prevent neural tube defects (NTD), prenatal HIV screening, smoking cessation programs and vaginal birth after Cesarean delivery. In general, these interventions have proven to be cost-effective or even cost saving because the treatments are effective and often inexpensive, the risk of adverse outcomes is high, the time to the outcomes is short and the cost of the outcomes is large.

In one study, the economic benefit of fortifying grain with folic acid was assessed as the cost savings from NTD averted minus the costs of folic acid supplementation. In the US, the annual cost savings were estimated to be $94 million with low-level fortification (140 mg/100 gram grain) and $252 million with high-level fortification (350 mg/100 gram grain). The cost–benefit ratio was 4.3 for low-level and 6.1 for

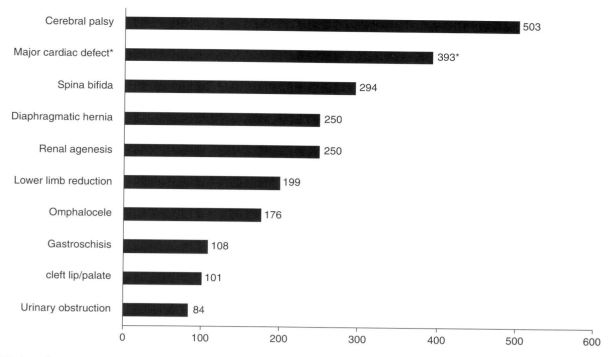

Figure 52.1   Lifetime costs per new case of major congenital anomalies and cerebral palsy in thousands of US dollars (1992 US $). *Weighted average of the lifetime costs of truncus arteriosus, single ventricle, transposition, and tetralogy of Fallot. Adapted from[10].

high-level fortification, suggesting that $4–6 would be saved for each $1 spent on folic acid fortification.[15] Separate CEA performed in the US and the United Kingdom (UK) demonstrated that voluntary HIV screening would cost c. $10,600 per life-year gained in the US,[16] and less than £4000 for each life-year gained in high-HIV-prevalence areas and less than £20,000 for each life-year gained in low-HIV-prevalence areas of the UK.[17] Another CEA demonstrated that if a smoking cessation program decreased the prevalence of cigarette smoking by 1% per year in the US population, it would prevent 1300 low birthweight live births and save $21 million in direct medical costs in the first year and $473 million during the 7 years of the program.[18] Two recent CEA compared elective repeat Cesarean delivery with a trial of labor (vaginal delivery).[19,20] One study found that follow-up routine elective Cesarean delivery cost c. $179 million during the reproductive life of 100,000 women.[19] The prevention of one major adverse neonatal outcome would require c. 1600 Cesarean deliveries and would cost $2.4 million. Another study found that if the

probability of successful vaginal delivery exceeded 0.74, a trial of labor was cost-effective.[20]

Cost-effectiveness of preconception care for women with pre-gestational diabetes

Preconception care for women with established diabetes reduces the incidence of fetal malformations and spontaneous abortions.[21] Three groups have assessed the costs of preconception care relative to the savings resulting from adverse maternal and neonatal outcomes averted. All demonstrated that preconception care for women with established diabetes is cost saving (Table 52.1).[22–24]

A case–control study of women with Type 1 diabetes mellitus was conducted by Scheffler et al to assess the cost–benefit of preconception care.[22] The study estimated the costs of a

Table 52.1   Net savings per pregnancy and cost–benefit ratios of preconception care

Authors (reference)	Net savings (US $)	Savings on early versus no intervention (US $)	Savings on late versus no intervention (US $)	Cost–benefit
Scheffler et al. (22)	6000	7300	5700	5.19
Elixhauser et. al (23)	1700	–	–	1.86
Herman et al. (24)	34,000	–	–	NR

NR, Not reported.

preconception care program using a time–motion methodology, and analyzed actual hospital charges and length of stay for women enrolled in the California Diabetes and Pregnancy Program (CDAPP). These included 102 women with Type 1 diabetes who participated in the preconception care program and subsequently received standard prenatal care: a group of 218 women with Type 1 diabetes who did not participate in the program but who received standard prenatal care served as controls. Each CDAPP participant was randomly matched with an individual from the control group. The matching criteria were the mother's age, race, and severity and duration of diabetes according the White classification system. This procedure yielded 90 cases from the CDAPP group and 90 controls drawn from hospitals outside the program's catchment area. The researchers examined two groups of cases – those enrolled before 8 weeks of gestation and those enrolled after 8 weeks of gestation – and compared them with women who did not enroll in the program. The analysis adopted the perspective of a third-party payer and considered only direct medical costs. For each mother, charges were included through to delivery; for each infant, charges were included from birth through to discharge. Longer term medical costs due to adverse birth outcomes, which are potential savings of the CDAPP, and any potential health benefits to the mother were not included. Costs were expressed in 1988 US dollars; an 8% discount rate was applied to costs but not benefits. Not unexpectedly, the costs of preconception care were greatest for early enrollees ($1300), lower for late enrollees ($800) and lowest for non-enrollees ($0). In contrast, both maternal and neonatal charges increased from early enrollees to late enrollees to non-enrollees: the charges for maternal care increased from $8900 for early enrollees to $9500 for late enrollees to $11,000 for non-enrollees. The charges for neonatal care increased dramatically from $2300 for infants of early enrollees to $6600 for infants of late enrollees to $10,700 for infants of non-enrollees. Compared to non-enrollees, early enrollees experienced savings of $7300 per enrollee and late enrollees experienced savings of $5700 per enrollee. The cost–benefit ratio of the CDAPP was 5.19; thus, for every $1 spent on the program, $5.19 was recovered in charges averted.

A second cost–benefit study by Elixhauser et al.[23] used consensus development, surveys of medical care personnel and a literature review to develop a model to determine whether the additional costs of preconception care are offset by the savings from complications averted. The analyses adopted the perspective of a third-party payer and considered direct medical costs. Costs were calculated in 1989 US dollars; discounting was not performed. Preconception care cost $2600 per enrollee and $4900 per delivery (recognizing that more women receive preconception care than go on to deliver.) The additional cost associated with preconception care was offset by the cost savings associated with adverse maternal outcomes averted ($2000 for women who received preconception care vs. $3200 for those who received prenatal care only, a cost saving of $1200) and adverse neonatal outcomes averted ($7700 for infants of mothers who received preconception care vs. $10,200 for infants of mothers who received prenatal care only, a cost saving of $2500). When the costs of care for the child were recalculated to include medical care for

3 years after discharge from the neonatal intensive care unit, lifetime medical care, residential care, and community services associated with severe congenital malformations, the benefits of preconception care for women with established diabetes were $1700 per enrollee. The cost–benefit ratio was 1.86; thus, for every $1 spent on the preconception care program, $1.86 was gained. When the costs associated with postneonatal intensive care and long-term care were excluded, preconception care saved $480 per enrollee, and the cost–benefit ratio was 1.24.[25]

A third study by Herman et al.[24] assessed pregnancy outcomes, resource utilization and costs among women with Type 1 diabetes who received preconception care (PC) and women who did not receive preconception care [prenatal care only (PN)]. The study found a small increase in outpatient visits (two visits) and a substantial, 20-day decrease in inpatient utilization for women and infants who received PC compared to PN. This consistent and substantial reduction in resource utilization among PC women and their infants as compared to PN women and their infants translated into substantial cost savings. The net cost saving was c. $34,000 per patient (direct medical costs, undiscounted, 1992 US dollars), suggesting that the savings, measured as direct medical costs, may be several times greater than reported by the first two studies.

Cost-effectiveness of interventions in gestational diabetes mellitus

Investigators have studied both the costs of alternative approaches to diagnosing GDM, and the cost-effectiveness of alternative approaches to diagnosing and treating GDM.[26]

Costs of alternative approaches to diagnosing GDM

Over the past two decades, screening for GDM in the US has been performed according to the recommendations of the National Diabetes Data Group (NDDG), the American Diabetes Association (ADA), and the American College of Obstetricians and Gynecologists. Screening has been recommended for all pregnant women and has involved a two-tiered approach: a 1-h 50-g glucose challenge test (GCT) and for women with plasma glucose levels ≥140 mg/dL (7.8 mmol/L) on the GCT a 3-h 100-g oral glucose tolerance test (OGTT).[27]

Many studies have investigated alternative approaches to increase the efficiency and reduce the cost of screening for GDM. Lavin et al.[28] estimated the costs incurred by the hospital laboratory in screening and diagnosing GDM in pregnant women with and without historical and clinical risk factors. They estimated that it cost $5 per patient screened with the 1-h GCT and $329 per case of GDM diagnosed (1980 US dollars). Reed[29] estimated that the laboratory charges per patient screened and per case of GDM detected were $14 and $684, respectively (1984 US dollars) (Table 52.2). Performing a GCT in pregnant women >25 years of age decreased the cost per patient screened to $7 and the cost per case of GDM detected to $386, but missed 24% of women with GDM.

Table 52.2   Cost per case of gestational diabetes mellitus (GDM) diagnosed using various screening protocols

Screening protocol	Cost per GDM case diagnosed (1984 US $)	Cases missed (%)
GCT in all women, if positive OGTT	684	20
GCT in women >25 years of age, if positive OGTT	386	24
GCT only in women with risk factors, if positive OGTT	683	60
OGTT in all women with risk factors	938	48
OGTT in all women	976	0

GCT, 1-h 50-g glucose challenge test.
OGTT, 3-h 100-g oral glucose tolerance test.
Risk factors: birth of a baby weighing ≥4000 g (c.) (≥9lb); a history of two or more pregnancies of fetal death, neonatal death, congenital anomaly, prematurity, excessive weight gain, hypertension or proteinuria; family history of diabetes mellitus.
(Adapted from Reed.[29])

Coustan et al.[30] performed a cost analysis of a population-based study in 6214 universally screened pregnant women using Lavin et al's[29] unit costs for the GCT and OGTT (Table 52.3). A GCT screening threshold of 140 mg/dL (7.8 mmol/L) and NDDG criteria for the OGTT were used. If women <30 years of age with risk factors and all pregnant women ≥30 years of age were screened, the cost per case of GDM diagnosed was $190. However, nearly one-third of women were missed with this protocol because many women with GDM <30 years of age had no other risk factors or had GCT results between 130 and 139 mg/dL. Sensitivity of detection of GDM increased to 95% by screening women <25 years of age with risk factors and all women ≥25 years of age, and by using a threshold of 130 mg/dL (7.2 mmol/L) for the GCT. The cost per case of GDM diagnosed increased from $195 to $215. If universal screening was performed and a GCT threshold of 130 mg/dL was used, the sensitivity was 100% but the cost per case of GDM increased to $249. Coustan et al.[30] noted that if a protocol uses universal screening at ≥25 years of age,

78% of individuals will require screening: the small (22%) decrement in cost that accrues as a result of selective screening must be weighed against the more complex logistics and increased probability of failing to screen high-risk women.

The Fourth International Workshop–Conference on Gestational Diabetes Mellitus[31] suggested that two techniques – the two-tiered protocol with Carpenter–Coustan modifications and the one-tiered protocol (2-h 75-g OGTT) – are both acceptable methods to screen for GDM. Lavin et al.[32] compared the costs and the patient time associated with the two-tiered protocol and the one-tiered modification employing the 2-h OGTT. The two-tiered protocol had lower costs than the one-tiered protocol: low-range and high-range costs for the two-tiered protocol were $3 and $8 per woman; low-range and high-range costs for the one-tiered protocol were $6 and $11 per woman. Test times were 1.4–1.5 h for the two-tiered protocol and 2 h for the one-tiered protocol. Travel time was lower in the one-tiered protocol than in the two-tiered

Table 52.3   Cost per case of gestational diabetes mellitus (GDM) diagnosed using various screening protocols

Screening protocol	Cost per GDM case diagnosed (1980 US $)	Cases missed (%)
GCT in women >30 years of age or if risk factors present, if positive (threshold >140 mg/dL) OGTT	190	35
GCT in all women ≥25 years of age or if risk factors present, if positive (threshold >140 mg/dL) OGTT	192	15
GCT in all women ≥25 years of age or if risk factors present, if positive (threshold >130 mg/dL) OGTT	215	5
GCT in all women, if positive (threshold >140 mg/dL) OGTT	222	10
GCT in all women, if positive (threshold >130mg/dL) OGTT	249	0

GCT, 1-h 50-g glucose challenge test.
Risk factors: pevious GDM; previous macrosomic infant [baby weighing ≥4000 g (c. ≥9lb)]; obesity; previous stillborn or neonatal death; family history of diabetes mellitus.
GTT, 3-h 100-g oral glucose tolerance test.
(Adapted from Coustan et al.[30])

protocol (2 vs. 2.3 h). The authors concluded that the two-tiered protocol appears to be associated with lower costs and less patient time than the one-tiered protocol.

Cost-effectiveness of alternative approaches to diagnosing and treating GDM

CEA are predicated on the demonstration of clinical effectiveness. If an intervention is not effective then it cannot be cost-effective. Ultimately, to determine if the costs of diagnosing GDM are worth paying, studies of cost-effectiveness must include the costs of diagnosing GDM, the costs of providing treatment for GDM, and the costs of the outcomes for the mothers and babies.[26]

Kitzmiller et al.[33] performed a cost-identification analysis of a GDM program in Northern California (Santa Clara Valley). Program costs were defined as the cost of all health resources required to diagnose GDM, monitor blood glucose, maintain blood glucose levels within the target range, and monitor the pregnant women and their fetuses to ensure good outcome. Outcome costs included the costs of all health care resources used for inpatient antepartum care, delivery, postdelivery care, and newborn care. Average reimbursed charges were used to establish direct medical costs (1996 US dollars). The analysis was performed from the perspective of managed care. The average total program costs per case of GDM were $1100. Program costs were higher for women requiring insulin treatment ($1800) than for women with diet therapy only ($800). The total costs of outcomes per case of GDM were $6000: outcome costs per patient were slightly higher in insulin-requiring GDM cases ($6500) than in those treated with diet therapy alone ($5800).

The costs from the Northern California program were also applied to prospectively collected data from a diabetes and pregnancy program at a large teaching hospital in New England.[33] The diagnostic strategy was the same as in the Northern California program, but more patients required insulin therapy in the New England program. Total program costs per case of GDM were $1800. In spite of good program outcomes, the outcome costs per case of GDM were $8900, substantially higher than in the Northern California program ($6000). The authors concluded that the analyses were potentially biased by the selection of complicated cases of GDM referred to the New England program.

Three studies have assessed the cost-effectiveness or cost–benefit of interventions in GDM. In one, the Northern California program, reimbursed charges were applied to the clinical outcomes of a prospective randomized trial of preprandial or postprandial blood glucose monitoring in GDM.[33,34] GDM was treated with insulin in all 66 women. Although mean gestational ages at delivery were similar, the postprandial monitoring group had lower glycohemoglobin levels, significantly lower birthweights, less macrosomia, less neonatal hypoglycemia and fewer Cesarean deliveries.[34] The program costs per case of GDM were slightly higher in the postprandial blood glucose monitoring group ($3800) than in the preprandial blood glucose monitoring group ($3600), but outcome costs per case of GDM were lower in the postprandial monitoring group ($7500) compared to the

preprandial monitoring group ($8000).[33] The incremental cost-effectiveness of the postprandial blood glucose monitoring was $35 per Cesarean delivery averted and $25 per neonatal intensive care unit day prevented. Comparing input and outcome costs for the two blood glucose monitoring groups, the cost–benefit ratio was 2.98 in favor of postprandial blood glucose monitoring; thus, for every $1 spent on postprandial blood glucose monitoring, c. $3 would be saved in averted adverse outcome costs.[33]

Langer et al.[35] performed a prospective population-based study of conventional versus intensified therapy in women with GDM and conducted a cost-benefit analysis. Intensified therapy was defined as self-blood glucose monitoring (SBGM) seven times daily with early institution of insulin therapy. Conventional therapy was defined as four times daily SBGM and weekly assessment of fasting and 2-h postprandial venous plasma glucose.[36] Program costs included the costs of diagnosis, blood glucose evaluation, medication and supplies, and physician, nursing, social worker and dietitian care, and the costs of fetal surveillance. Outcome costs included antepartum and postpartum hospital stay, hospital and physician fees for vaginal or Cesarean deliveries, and neonatal intensive care unit and nursery admissions. Total program costs for the conventional therapy group were $1900 per woman with GDM compared to $2100 per woman with GDM in the intensified therapy group. The total outcome costs for the conventional therapy group were $4600 per woman versus $3900 per woman in the intensified therapy group. There was a 4.37 cost–benefit ratio in favor of the intensified therapy.[35]

Bienstock et al.[37] conducted a retrospective cohort study to compare the costs of prenatal care and subsequent maternal and neonatal outcomes in women with GDM cared for in an inner-city university hospital house-staff clinic versus an inner-city managed-care organization. GDM was defined according to NDDG criteria. There were no differences between groups with respect to baseline maternal demographic factors. The cost of providing care to a patient with GDM by the managed-care organization was $10,000 versus $11,000 for the house-staff fee-for-service clinic setting ($P = 0.20$). A larger percentage of women had >12 visits with their physician and more sonograms were performed in the house-staff clinic compared to the managed-care organization. In contrast, more fetal surveillance tests were performed in the managed-care organization group. The groups had similar rates of insulin treatment, antepartum admissions, Cesarean delivery, and maternal and infant lengths of stay. In the house-staff clinic group, there was a trend toward a lower frequency of preterm delivery (8.9 vs. 13.3%) and significantly less macrosomia (15 vs. 29%). The authors concluded that managed care does not decrease the cost of caring for patients with GDM but does lead to a greater rate of neonatal macrosomia, which may reflect poorer glucose control.

Conclusions

During the adult reproductive years, women have higher medical expenditures than men. The difference in medical expenditures between women and men is largely related to pregnancy care, childbirth, and its complications. The costs of preterm and postpartum maternal hospitalization and the costs of hospital care for infants with adverse outcomes are major sources of increased cost. Because the cost of outcomes is large and the time to outcomes is short, treatments that are effective in preventing adverse outcomes of pregnancy are often cost-effective or even cost saving. Such interventions include folic acid fortification of grain to prevent NTD and smoking cessation programs to prevent low birthweight infants.

Preconception care for women with established diabetes reduces the incidence of fetal malformations and spontaneous abortions. Three groups have assessed the costs of preconception care relative to the savings resulting from adverse maternal and neonatal outcomes averted. All demonstrated that preconception care for women with established diabetes is cost saving. A number of investigators have also assessed the costs of alternative approaches to diagnosing GDM. Although selective screening for GDM is marginally less expensive than universal screening per case of GDM detected, most women require screening and the more complex logistics and increased probability of failing to screen high-risk women may offset any potential cost savings. It appears that a two-tiered approach to screening for GDM (involving a 1-h 50-g GCT followed by a 3-h 100-g OGTT) is more cost-effective than a one-tiered modification (employing a 2-h 75-g OGTT), with respect to both cost of laboratory testing and patient time.

Studies of the cost-effectiveness of alternative approaches to the treatment of GDM have been hampered by the lack of data demonstrating the clinical effectiveness of diagnosis and intervention. To date, cost-effectiveness and cost–benefit analyses of selected interventions have suggested that postprandial blood glucose monitoring is more cost-effective that preprandial monitoring, and that intensified monitoring and insulin treatment is more cost-effective than conventional monitoring.

Because of the high cost of hospitalization for mothers and infants, and the relatively short time course of pregnancy, many prenatal interventions, and particularly those that are relatively inexpensive, are cost-effective or even cost saving from the perspective of a health system. These interventions, like preconception care for women with established diabetes, should be rigorously implemented, as they both improve health outcomes and reduce costs of care. In the area of GDM, either universal screening or selective screening would appear to be cost-effective, depending upon the health system's ability to risk stratify and track pregnant women. Although perhaps counter-intuitive, two-tiered screening appears to be more cost-effective than one-tiered screening, particularly in populations of low diabetes prevalence. Definitive analyses of the cost-effectiveness of alternative approaches to the treatment of GDM will ultimately require more clear-cut demonstration of the clinical effectiveness of those interventions.

REFERENCES

1. Mustard CA, Kaufert P, Kozyrskyj A, Mayer T. Sex differences in the use of health care services. N Engl J Med 1998; 338: 1678–83.
2. Nicholson WK, Frick KD, Powe NR. Economic burden of hospitalizations for preterm labor in the United States. Obstet Gynecol 2000; 96: 95–101.
3. Henderson J, McCandlish R, Kumiega L, Petrou S. Systematic review of economic aspects of alternative modes of delivery. Br J Obstet Gynecol 2001; 108: 149–57.
4. Petrou S, Glazener C. The economic costs of alternative modes of delivery during the first two months postpartum: results from a Scottish observational study. Br J Obstet Gynecol 2002; 109: 214–7.
5. Johnson TR, Zettelmaier MA, Warner PA, et al. A competency based approach to comprehensive pregnancy care. Womens Health Issues 2000; 10: 240–7.
6. Callahan TL, Hall JE, Ettner SL, et al. The economic impact of multiple-gestation pregnancies and the contribution of assisted reproduction techniques to their incidence. N Engl J Med 1994; 331: 244–9.
7. Galtier-Dereure F, Boegner C, Bringer J. Obesity and pregnancy: complications and cost. Am J Clin Nutr 2000; 71(suppl. 5): S1242–8.
8. Galtier-Dereure F, Montpeyroux F, Boulot P et al. Weight excess before pregnancy: complications and cost. Int J Obes Relat Metab Disord 1995; 19: 443–8.
9. Isaacs JD, Magann EF, Martin RW. Obstetric challenges of massive obesity complicating pregnancy. J Perinatol 1994; 14: 10–4.
10. Waitzman NJ, Romano PS, Scheffler RM, Harris JA. Economic costs of birth defects and cerebral palsy – United States, 1992. MMWR Morb Mortal Wkly Rep 1995; 44: 694–9.
11. Vintzileos AM, Ananth CV, Smulian JC, et al. Routine second-trimester ultrasonography in the United States: a cost–benefit analysis. Am J Obstet Gynecol 2000; 182: 655–60.
12. Rogowski J. Cost-effectiveness of care for very low birth weight infants. Pediatrics 1998; 102: 35–43.
13. Weinstein MC, Siegel JE, Gold MR, et al. Recommendations of the Panel on Cost-effectiveness in Health and Medicine. J Am Med Assoc 1996; 276: 1253–8.
14. November MT. Cost analysis of vaginal birth after cesarean. Clin Obstet Gynecol 2001; 44: 571–87.
15. Romano PS, Waitzman NJ, Scheffler RM, Pi RD. Folic acid fortification of grain: an economic analysis. Am J Public Health 1995; 85: 667–76.
16. Zaric GS, Bayoumi AM, Brandeau ML, Owens DK. The cost effectiveness of voluntary prenatal and routine newborn HIV screening in the United States. J Acquir Immune Defic Syndr 2000; 25: 403–16.
17. Postma MJ, Beck EJ, Mandalia S, et al. Universal HIV screening of pregnant women in England: cost effectiveness analysis. Br Med J 1999; 318: 1656–60.
18. Lightwood JM, Phibbs CS, Glantz SA. Short-term health and economic benefits of smoking cessation: low birth weight. Pediatrics 1999; 104: 1312–20.
19. Grobman WA, Peaceman AM, Socol ML. Cost- effectiveness of elective cesarean delivery after one prior low transverse cesarean. Obstet Gynecol 2000; 95: 745–51
20. Chung A, Macario A, El-Sayed YY, et al. Cost effectiveness of a trial of labor after previous cesarean. Obstet Gynecol 2001; 97: 932–41.
21. Kitzmiller JL, Buchanan TA, Kjos S, et al. Pre-conception care of diabetes, congenital malformations, and spontaneous abortions. Diabetes Care 1996; 19: 514–41.
22. Scheffler RM, Feuchtbaum LB, Phibbs CS. Prevention: the cost-effectiveness of the California Diabetes and Pregnancy Program. Am J Public Health 1992; 82: 168–75.
23. Elixhauser A, Weschler JM, Kitzmiller JL, et al. Cost–benefit analysis of preconception care for women with established diabetes mellitus. Diabetes Care 1993; 16: 1146–57.
24. Herman WH, Janz NK, Becker MP, Charron-Prochownik D. Diabetes and pregnancy. Preconception care, pregnancy outcomes, resource utilization and costs. J Reprod Med 1999; 44: 33–8.
25. Elixhauser A, Kitzmiller JL, Weschler JM. Short-term cost benefit of pre-conception care for diabetes. Diabetes Care 1996; 19: 384.

26. Kitzmiller JL. Cost analysis of diagnosis and treatment of gestational diabetes mellitus. Clin Obstet Gynecol 2000; 43: 140–53.
27. National Diabetes Data Group (NDDG). Classification and diagnosis of diabetes mellitus and other categories of glucose intolerance. Diabetes 1979; 28: 1039–57.
28. Lavin JP, Barden TP, Miodovnik M. Clinical experience with a screening program for gestational diabetes. Am J Obstet Gynecol 1981; 141: 491–4.
29. Reed BD. Screening for gestational diabetes – analysis by screening criteria. J Fam Pract 1984; 19: 751–5.
30. Coustan DR, Nelson C, Carpenter MW, et al. Maternal age and screening for gestational diabetes: a population-based study. Obstet Gynecol 1989; 73: 557–61.
31. Metzger BE, Coustan DR. Summary and recommendations of the Fourth International Workshop–Conference on Gestational Diabetes Mellitus. The Organizing Committee. Diabetes Care 1998; 21(suppl. 2): B161–7.
32. Lavin Jr JP, Lavin B, O'Donnell N. A comparison of costs associated with screening for gestational diabetes with two-tiered and one-tiered testing protocols. Am J Obstet Gynecol 2001; 184: 363–7.
33. Kitzmiller JL, Elixhauser A, Carr S et al. Assessment of costs and benefits of management of gestational diabetes mellitus. Diabetes Care 1998; 21(suppl. 2): B123–30.
34. de Veciana M, Major CA, Morgan MA, et al. Postprandial versus preprandial blood glucose monitoring in women with gestational diabetes mellitus requiring insulin therapy. N Engl J Med 1995; 333: 1237–41.
35. Langer O, Conway D, Berkus MD, Xenakis EM. Conventional versus intensified management: cost/benefit analysis. Am J Obstet Gynecol 1998; 178(suppl. 1): S58.
36. Langer O, Rodriguez DA, Xenakis EM, et al. Intensified versus conventional management of gestational diabetes. Am J Obstet Gynecol 1994; 170: 1036–46.
37. Bienstock JL, Blakemore KJ, Wang E, et al. Managed care does not lower costs but may result in poorer outcomes for patients with gestational diabetes. Am J Obstet Gynecol 1997; 177: 1035–7.

53 Quality of care for the woman with diabetes in pregnancy

Alberto de Leiva, Rosa Corcoy and Eulàlia Brugués

Quality assessment and improvement in diabetes care

The aim of health care is to achieve the best health outcomes in the most efficient manner, and the challenge for today's health delivery systems is to increase productivity and quality of care without increasing the economic costs.

Assessment of the quality of health care needs complex measures of the structure (staff, equipment, organization), the process (technical quality) and the outcomes (effectiveness, satisfaction, functional status, quality of life).

Health care delivery depends on efficient communication and cooperation amongst patients, health care services and professionals; this matter is particularly critical regarding chronic disorders in which effective shared-care is pursued by multiple health care providers and professionals, enabling the patient to become actively involved in the process of their care. The effective share of related information is highly facilitated by the operation of an electronic patient record and a telematic infrastructure.

Health care delivery is moving towards disease management, focused on a patient-oriented approach, illness prevention promoting good health and managing long-term care, all of which require integrated activities from generalists, specialists and other health care professionals. This type of care requires effective coordination and an interrelated, multidisciplinary approach.

In addition, the implementation of effective strategies for continuous quality improvement takes advantage of four main areas: (1) efficient use of health care resources (e.g. eliminating practices that are clearly harmful, or without known benefits); (2) linking clinical research to clinical practice (evidence-based care); (3) application of new concepts for improvement of care (the process of care must comply with the 'best practice', including solid methods to monitor and assess the outcomes); and (4) changing clinical practice (design of appropriate models for the management of health care services, based in valid, scientific information).

At a meeting held in St Vincent, Italy, in October 1989, representatives of government health departments and patients' organizations from all European countries met diabetes experts to discuss a set of recommendations – the St Vincent Declaration,[1] a joint initiative of the World Health Organization–Europe and the International Diabetes Federation–Europe (WHO/IDF) – with the intention of creating conditions allowing major reductions in deaths and the burden caused by diabetes mellitus. The declaration meant an important step forward in the general improvement in the quality of delivery of diabetes health care.

One of the main targets of the declaration was to establish monitoring and control systems using state-of-the-art information technology (IT) for quality assurance of diabetes health care provision. A European group of experts was established to design and implement mechanisms for the continuous improvement of the quality of diabetes care in Europe. The term 'continuous quality improvement' was accepted to emphasize the progressive nature of the never-ending process after reaching a determined standard. The assessment requires the comparison of care with standards that are derived from scientific evidence, consensus, good practice and clinical experience.

The St Vincent Declaration pointed out that self-monitoring results in very effective control of treatment. Later in this chapter, the quality assessment of the procedures for self-monitoring glycemic control will be reviewed in some detail.

European DiabCare quality network

A subgroup of the St Vincent Declaration Steering Committee was established to develop instruments and mechanisms for quality assurance in diabetes care. The first initiative of the DiabCare Program was the development of the St Vincent Diabetes Dataset from three main sources: (1) EuroDiabeta, a research project on modeling health care and the implementation of IT in diabetes;[2] (2) the specific recommendations provided by the different working groups of the St Vincent Declaration Steering Committee;[3] (3) the advice provided by more than 130 expert diabetologists from 21 European countries.

DiabCare Basic Information Sheet (BIS) contains 141 fields that include all the necessary data for the analysis of the quality of diabetes care (Figure 53.1). The pertinent analysis provides the performance of care in both aspects of process and outcomes (intermediate and final). Demographic data (age, sex, etc.) are required for a number of purposes. True patient outcomes include the burden of the medical end points of the St Vincent Declaration (such as amputation, blindness, etc.). Symptoms of diabetes-related problems (e.g. painful neuropathy, angina pectoris, etc.) are also recorded. Specific outcomes regarding pregnancies are also included. For the measurement of quality of life, the DiabCare data sets only include information related to duration of hospital admissions and the number of days without the ability to perform normal activities. Assessment of diabetic complications (retinopathy, nephropathy, neuropathy), cardiovascular risk factors, pharmacological treatment and metabolic outcomes [glycated hemoglobin (HbA1c), lipid profile] were considered essential.[4] The computer database (Figure 53.2) contains all the data items of the BIS and additional information with easy access by a single key stroke.

Once a year, at least, the data of all patients under care must be collected in the DiabCare BIS. The performance of the diabetes team is compared with the gold standards of the St Vincent Declaration program. The evaluation of the level of quality should cover the structure (housing, human resources, equipment, logistics), the process (the way the care is organized – from the first call to treatment plan; the annual measurements of indicators – HbA1c, blood pressure, etc; the way the treatment is initiated – use of antihypertensive drugs, cholesterol lowering agents, etc).

The DiabCare Program was designed for those services not having a computer database but having access to computers. In 1991, the feasibility phase, integrating the information from 4000 patients of 29 centers in 19 European countries, was completed. After some minor modifications it gained widespread adoption by centers, and local, regional and national diabetes task forces all over Europe.[5–7]

The DiabCare Feasibility Study[5] demonstrated the achievements obtained by the implementation of local documentation compatible to the DiabCare Diabetes Data Set. It made possible the assessment of the quality of care and to install regional/national quality networks, along with establishing a standard documentation to be used in various health care settings in different countries.

A quality circle is a group of motivated and committed people acting as a structured forum to solve on-the-job problems affecting the quality of their work. Prerequisites for the constitution of the circle are the political awareness and the

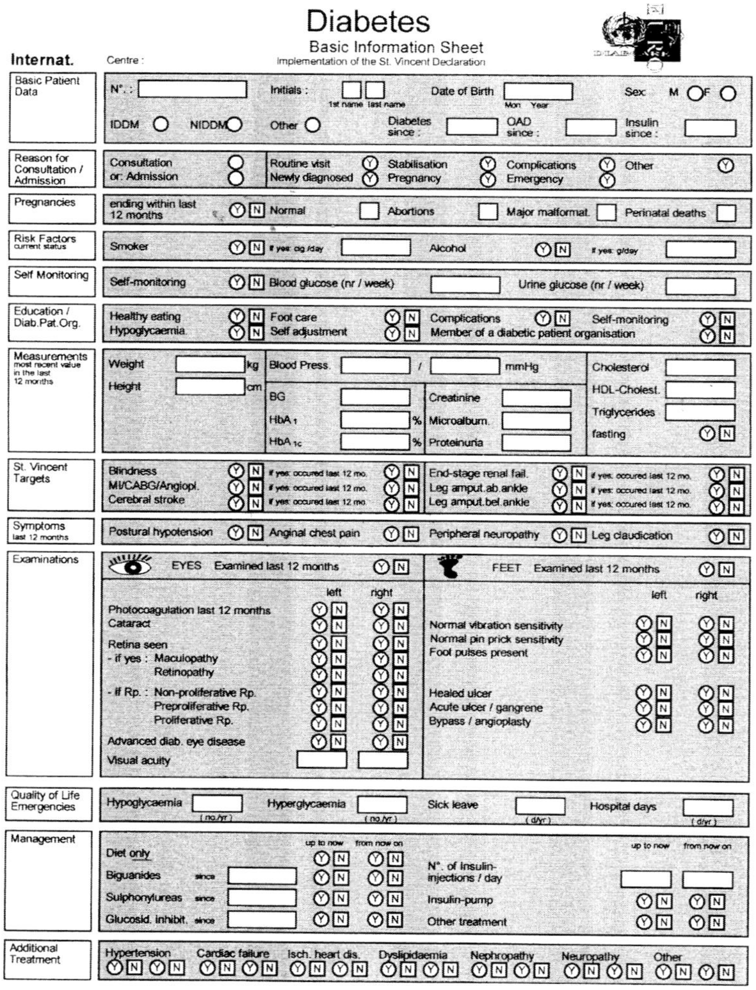
Diabetes
Basic Information Sheet
Implementation of the St. Vincent Declaration
Internat. Centre :
Basic Patient Data: N°. : Initials : 1st name last name; Date of Birth Mon Year; Sex M F; IDDM NIDDM Other; Diabetes since :; OAD since :; Insulin since :
Reason for Consultation / Admission: Consultation or: Admission; Routine visit; Newly diagnosed; Stabilisation; Pregnancy; Complications; Emergency; Other
Pregnancies: ending within last 12 months Y N; Normal; Abortions; Major malformat.; Perinatal deaths
Risk Factors current status: Smoker Y N if yes: cig /day; Alcohol Y N if yes: g/day
Self Monitoring: Self-monitoring Y N; Blood glucose (nr / week); Urine glucose (nr / week)
Education / Diab.Pat.Org.: Healthy eating; Hypoglycaemia; Foot care; Self adjustment; Complications; Self-monitoring; Member of a diabetic patient organisation
Measurements most recent value in the last 12 months: Weight kg; Height cm; Blood Press. / mmHg; BG; HbA_1; HbA_{1c} %; Creatinine; Microalbum.; Proteinuria; Cholesterol; HDL-Cholest.; Triglycerides; fasting Y N
St. Vincent Targets: Blindness; MI/CABG/Angiopl.; Cerebral stroke; if yes: occured last 12 mo.; End-stage renal fail.; Leg amput.ab.ankle; Leg amput.bel.ankle; if yes: occured last 12 mo.
Symptoms last 12 months: Postural hypotension; Anginal chest pain; Peripheral neuropathy; Leg claudication
Examinations: EYES Examined last 12 months Y N; left right; Photocoagulation last 12 months; Cataract; Retina seen; - if yes : Maculopathy; Retinopathy; - if Rp. : Non-proliferative Rp.; Preproliferative Rp.; Proliferative Rp.; Advanced diab. eye disease; Visual acuity; FEET Examined last 12 months Y N; left right; Normal vibration sensitivity; Normal pin prick sensitivity; Foot pulses present; Healed ulcer; Acute ulcer / gangrene; Bypass / angioplasty
Quality of Life Emergencies: Hypoglycaemia (no./yr); Hyperglycaemia (no./yr); Sick leave (d/yr); Hospital days (d/yr)
Management: up to now; from now on; Diet only; Biguanides since; Sulphonylureas since; Glucosid. inhibit. since; N°. of Insulin-injections / day; Insulin-pump; Other treatment
Additional Treatment: Hypertension; Cardiac failure; Isch. heart dis.; Dyslipidaemia; Nephropathy; Neuropathy; Other

Figure 53.1 Basic Information Sheet, DiabCare.

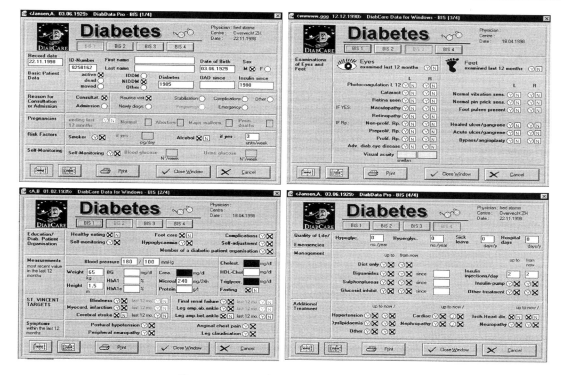

Figure 53.2   DiabCare data for Windows.

involvement of the decision-makers to get things going. The implementation of pilots or demonstration projects make clear what the benefits are and the economic cost.

The quality circle must select targets according to the local health requirements. The information gathered after data collection, data aggregation and analysis (Figure 53.3) of proper indicators (clinical, analytical, etc.), allows a local evaluation (internal comparison); then, sending the aggregated data in anonymous fashion to a server, the comparison with all the other teams sharing the network is possible (external comparison). After all of this, the members of the local quality circle are in the situation to propose and debate measures for quality improvement. These measures are implemented in the following period and the evaluation of their effects will be then

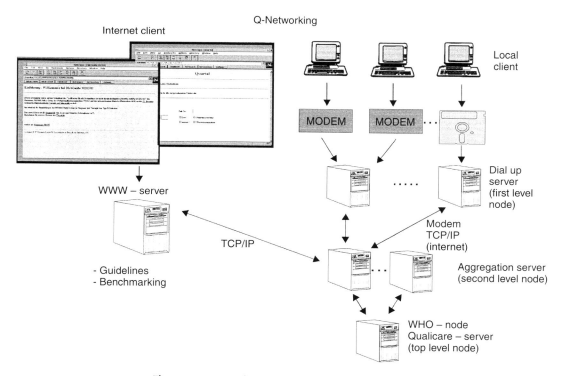

Figure 53.3   DiabCare Q-Net, system architecture.

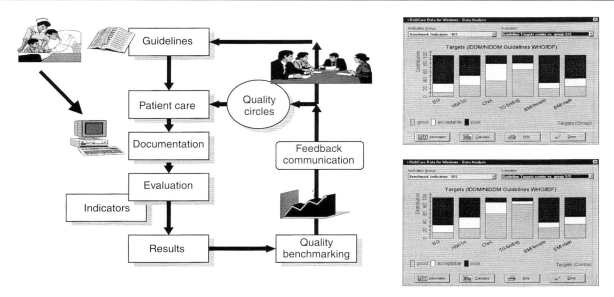

Figure 53.4   Operation of the DiabCare quality circle.

analyzed, following the scheme of continuous assurance and improvement (Figure 53.4).[7]

The present authors' use of DiabCare program, adapted to a net environment in a hospital-based outpatient consultation, has provided a variety of benefits, including Diabetes Data Set exploitation as a registry, diabetes-type characterization, assessment of self blood glucose monitoring (SBGM) status, St Vincent Declaration targets, treatment characterization, outcome for diabetic pregnancies, completeness assessment of medical records, cardiovascular risk factors, identification of groups of patients at risk, etc.[8] On the basis of this information, a quality assurance circle on diabetes care has been operating in the present authors' center since then, following the protocol proposed by the EU Consortium DiabCare Quality Network, integrated in a comprehensive disease management program (the Optidiab System). A recent report about the information provided by the annual evaluation (the 141 parameters of the DiabCare BIS) of >1000 subjects confirmed the burden of Type 2 diabetes patients compared to Type 1 diabetes patients undergoing intensive and specialized care on regular basis.[9]

Interestingly, aggregated and compared data from the central server, integrating national centers from the European DiabCare Quality Network (22,000 patients), lead to the conclusion that the long-term metabolic outcome of patients under intensive management in European specialized centers are far short of achieving their desired goal [HbA1c < mean + four standard deviations (4 SD) of the nondiabetic population]; aggregated HbA1c levels [Diabetes Control and Complication Trial (DCCT) adjusted] recorded at the annual evaluation were optimal for only 26.9% of cases, acceptable for 23.2% and poor in the remaining 49.9% of subjects.[10]

The DiabCare program allows a simple registration procedure for collecting basic data from diabetic pregnant women; the system has also been demonstrated to be useful for limited evaluation of quality assurance in the broad field of diabetes and pregnancy.[11–13]

DiabCare BIS for diabetes and pregnancy

One of the main recommendations of the St Vincent Declaration was the following: 'Achieve pregnancy outcome in diabetic women that approximates to that of nondiabetic women'. In consequence, WHO/IDF guidelines for care and management of pregnant diabetic women have been proposed by an invited group of international experts in the field.[14] The document brought attention to the important differences in the provision of diabetes and obstetrical care in different European countries. Specifically, the relevance of intensive metabolic care before conception, during pregnancy and parturition, as well as the needs of special training and education of the diabetic women contemplating pregnancy, were addressed. For the purpose of developing the quality assurance program, a DiabCare BIS for diabetes and pregnancy was proposed by members of the WHO/IDF Working Group on Pregnancy Outcomes in the Diabetic Woman (Figure 53.5), with data fields addressing diabetes diagnosis, past obstetrical history, prepregnancy counseling, status at entering the specialized interdisciplinary clinic, maternal and newborn outcomes, and reclassification after pregnancy. The OBSQID (OBStetrical Quality Indicators and Data) Perinatal Aggregated Data (PAD) protocol, mainly focused on outcomes, represents a valid alternative proposed by the Quality of Care and Technologies Program, WHO–Europe being exploited for epidemiologic studies.

DiabCard as an instrument for quality assurance

The DiabCard project (EU-AIM 2051) developed the specifications for a chip-card-based medical information system and the requirements for Europewide collection of data about diabetes for clinical and managerial purposes. A common diabetes

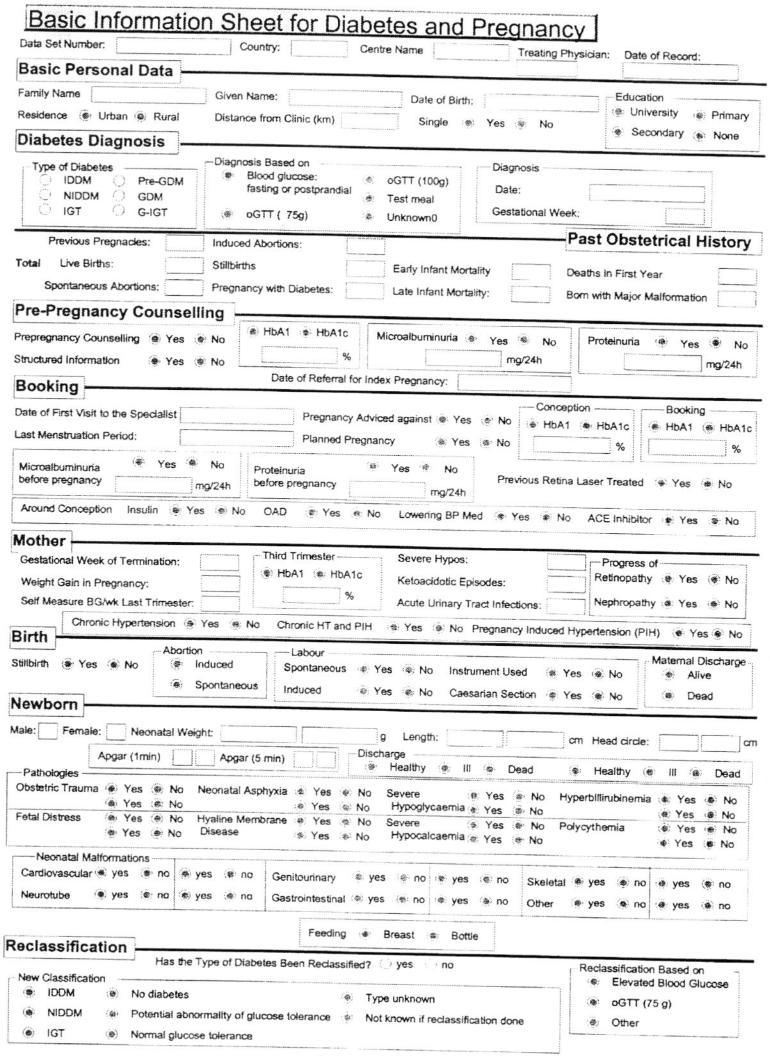

Basic Information Sheet for Diabetes and Pregnancy

Data Set Number: ___ Country: ___ Centre Name ___ Treating Physician: ___ Date of Record: ___

Basic Personal Data

Family Name ___ Given Name: ___ Date of Birth: ___ Education ○ University ○ Primary

Residence ○ Urban ○ Rural Distance from Clinic (km) ___ Single ○ Yes ○ No ○ Secondary ○ None

Diabetes Diagnosis

Type of Diabetes: ○ IDDM ○ Pre-GDM ○ NIDDM ○ GDM ○ IGT ○ G-IGT

Diagnosis Based on ○ Blood glucose: fasting or postprandial ○ oGTT (75g) ○ oGTT (100g) ○ Test meal ○ Unknown0

Diagnosis Date: ___ Gestational Week: ___

Past Obstetrical History

Previous Pregnancies: ___ Induced Abortions: ___

Total Live Births: ___ Stillbirths ___ Early Infant Mortality ___ Deaths in First Year ___

Spontaneous Abortions: ___ Pregnancy with Diabetes: ___ Late Infant Mortality: ___ Born with Major Malformation ___

Pre-Pregnancy Counselling

Prepregnancy Counselling ○ Yes ○ No ○ HbA1 ○ HbA1c ___ % Microalbuminuria ○ Yes ○ No ___ mg/24h Proteinuria ○ Yes ○ No ___ mg/24h

Structured Information ○ Yes ○ No

Date of Referral for Index Pregnancy: ___

Booking

Date of First Visit to the Specialist ___ Pregnancy Adviced against ○ Yes ○ No

Last Menstruation Period: ___ Planned Pregnancy ○ Yes ○ No

Conception ○ HbA1 ○ HbA1c ___ % Booking ○ HbA1 ○ HbA1c ___ %

Microalbuminuria before pregnancy ○ Yes ○ No ___ mg/24h Proteinuria before pregnancy ○ Yes ○ No ___ mg/24h Previous Retina Laser Treated ○ Yes ○ No

Around Conception Insulin ○ Yes ○ No OAD ○ Yes ○ No Lowering BP Med ○ Yes ○ No ACE inhibitor ○ Yes ○ No

Mother

Gestational Week of Termination: ___

Weight Gain in Pregnancy: ___

Self Measure BG/wk Last Trimester: ___

Third Trimester ○ HbA1 ○ HbA1c ___ %

Severe Hypos: ___ Ketoacidotic Episodes: ___ Acute Urinary Tract Infections: ___

Progress of Retinopathy ○ Yes ○ No Nephropathy ○ Yes ○ No

Chronic Hypertension ○ Yes ○ No Chronic HT and PIH ○ Yes ○ No Pregnancy Induced Hypertension (PIH) ○ Yes ○ No

Birth

Stillbirth ○ Yes ○ No

Abortion ○ Induced ○ Spontaneous

Labour Spontaneous ○ Yes ○ No Induced ○ Yes ○ No Instrument Used ○ Yes ○ No Caesarian Section ○ Yes ○ No

Maternal Discharge ○ Alive ○ Dead

Newborn

Male: ___ Female: ___ Neonatal Weight: ___ g Length: ___ cm Head circle: ___ cm

Apgar (1min) ___ Apgar (5 min) ___

Discharge ○ Healthy ○ Ill ○ Dead ○ Healthy ○ Ill ○ Dead

Pathologies:

Obstetric Trauma ○ Yes ○ No / ○ Yes ○ No

Neonatal Asphyxia ○ Yes ○ No / ○ Yes ○ No

Severe Hypoglycaemia ○ Yes ○ No / ○ Yes ○ No

Hyperbilirubinemia ○ Yes ○ No / ○ Yes ○ No

Fetal Distress ○ Yes ○ No / ○ Yes ○ No

Hyaline Membrane Disease ○ Yes ○ No / ○ Yes ○ No

Severe Hypocalcaemia ○ Yes ○ No / ○ Yes ○ No

Polycythemia ○ Yes ○ No / ○ Yes ○ No

Neonatal Malformations:

Cardiovascular ○ yes ○ no / ○ yes ○ no Genitourinary ○ yes ○ no / ○ yes ○ no Skeletal ○ yes ○ no / ○ yes ○ no

Neurotube ○ yes ○ no / ○ yes ○ no Gastrointestinal ○ yes ○ no / ○ yes ○ no Other ○ yes ○ no / ○ yes ○ no

Feeding ○ Breast ○ Bottle

Reclassification

Has the Type of Diabetes Been Reclassified? ○ yes ○ no

New Classification: ○ IDDM ○ NIDDM ○ IGT

○ No diabetes ○ Potential abnormality of glucose tolerance ○ Normal glucose tolerance

○ Type unknown ○ Not known if reclassification done

Reclassification Based on: ○ Elevated Blood Glucose ○ oGTT (75 g) ○ Other

Figure 53.5 Basic Information Sheet for Diabetes and Pregnancy (DiabCare).

data set based on EuroDiabeta was produced and validated in ambulatory and hospital care. An open architecture allowed a bandwidth of different security levels, covered by standards defined by the International Standard Organization (ISO) and the European Telecommunications Standards Institute (ETSI). Security and privacy of the information was provided with the addition of the health professional card for identification and access to the system; the patient card contains most clinically relevant data.[15]

The randomized trial performed in the clinical scenario demonstrated the functionality of DiabCard as a patient record, and the main consequences in facilitating the effective communication between the patient and all levels of health care, and among health care providers as well. DiabCard was equally useful, as DiabCare, for quality assessment, and deserved its high acceptance by patients, promoting their empowerment and active involvement in the health care process (Figure 53.6).[16]

Monitoring glycemic control in diabetes mellitus and during pregnancy in the woman with pregestational or gestational diabetes mellitus.

The primary metabolic abnormality in diabetes mellitus (DM) is hyperglycemia, which is mainly responsible for acute and chronic complications of the disease, including feto-maternal mortality and morbidity.

The results of the DCCT showed that in Type 1 DM strict glycemic control resulted in a significant reduction in the rate of onset and progression of retinopathy, nephropathy and neuropathy.[17] In the United Kingdom Prospective Diabetes Study (UKPDS), the difference of 0.9% in HbA1c between the intensively treated group and the control group was associated with a 25% reduction in risk of microvascular end points;[18] intensive blood glucose control did not reduce the risk of myocardial infarction or stroke, but the control of hypertension was very important in this respect.[19]

Diabetes in pregnancy carries multiple risks to the mother and the fetus/newborn. For this reason, it is recommended to maintain blood glucose levels of 3.5–5.5 mmol/L at fasting and 5.0–8.0 mmol/L postprandially.[20] Although there is still some controversy concerning the implications of a mild degree of glucose intolerance for GDM, the same targets have been recommended

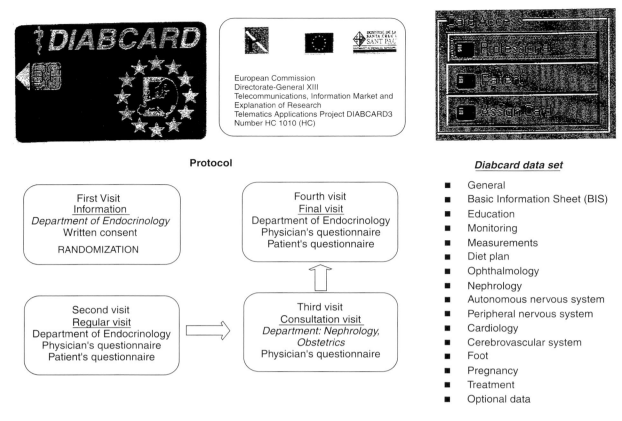

Protocol

First Visit
Information
Department of Endocrinology
Written consent

RANDOMIZATION

Second visit
Regular visit
Department of Endocrinology
Physician's questionnaire
Patient's questionnaire

Third visit
Consultation visit
Department: Nephrology,
Obstetrics
Physician's questionnaire

Fourth visit
Final visit
Department of Endocrinology
Physician's questionnaire
Patient's questionnaire

European Commission
Directorate-General XIII
Telecommunications, Information Market and
Explanation of Research
Telematics Applications Project DIABCARD3
Number HC 1010 (HC)

Diabcard data set

- General
- Basic Information Sheet (BIS)
- Education
- Monitoring
- Measurements
- Diet plan
- Ophthalmology
- Nephrology
- Autonomous nervous system
- Peripheral nervous system
- Cardiology
- Cerebrovascular system
- Foot
- Pregnancy
- Treatment
- Optional data

Figure 53.6   DiabCard system and the clinical scenario.

in these pregnancies, in spite of arguments of insufficient evidence for therapeutic interventions in this condition.[21]

Blood glucose monitoring devices

Portable meters are used for health care workers and by patients. Because of their imprecision and variability, they should not be used for diagnosing diabetes and their value in screening must be limited.

SBGM is recommended for all insulin-treated patients. Glucose can be measured in whole blood, serum or plasma, but plasma is recommended for diagnosis. Although red blood cells are freely permeable to glucose, the concentration of water in plasma is *c.* 11% higher than that of whole blood; as a consequence, the glucose concentration in plasma is higher than in whole blood (being the hematocrit normal). The glucose concentration decreases with time in the assay tube because of *in vitro* glycolysis (on average by 5–7%, or 0.6 mmol/L or 10 mg/dL/h), which can be attenuated by inhibition of enolase with sodium fluoride used in combination with anticoagulants. Therefore, when plasma glucose is going to be analyzed, plasma should be separated from cells within 1 h. Glucose is almost exclusively measured by enzymatic methods (hexokinase, glucose oxidase). For plasma glucose, a coefficient of variation <2.2% is recommended as a target for imprecision.

There is no standard protocol available for the evaluation of blood glucose meters. The evaluation of a single device may be misleading; in general, several units should be tested to explore interdevice variability. The evaluation should include the analysis of the mean difference of the device reading, with respect to a reference procedure at low, medium and high blood glucose concentrations. Other items of the evaluation will include customer acceptability (size, weight, portability, calibration, duration of a test performance, economic cost). Then, a validation protocol using an adequate sample size of recruited patients will follow, covering a wide range of blood glucose levels from the hypoglycemic range to extreme hyperglycemia.

The utilization of memory meters have shown that patients often make incomplete recordings of their daily blood glucose profiles (inaccurate readings, omission of outliers, false reports not recorded in the memory of the meter), usually depicting a trend towards correcting results of readings.[22,23] Of course, adequate training, visual acuity, hypoxia, altitude, hemolysis, hematocrit, hypertriglyceridemia, adequate sample volume,[24] and other technical elements, can influence the results. Reinforcing patient education at regular clinic visits, evaluating his/her technique and frequent comparison of SBGM profiles with concurrent laboratory blood glucose analysis, will assess the reliability of patient reports.

About 30 different brands of meters are commercially available. They use strips containing glucose oxidase or hexokinase; some meters contain a porous membrane that separates erythrocytes, the analysis being carried out in plasma. The meters provide a digital read-out, using reflectance photometry or electrochemistry for the measurements of glucose concentration. There is a wide variability in the performance of the different meters and the level of imprecision remains high. No published reports of glucose meters have achieved the American Diabetes Association (ADA) goal of analytical deviation <5% from reference values.[25,26]

SBGM should be performed at least four times per day in patients with Type 1 DM. It has been demonstrated that monitoring with lower frequency than this is associated with deterioration of glycemic control.[27–29]

Non-invasive or minimally invasive continuous monitoring of blood glucose is a high priority (both to detect unsuspected hypoglycemia and as a further step in the development of an artificial pancreas), allowing automatic measurement of blood glucose and adjustment of insulin administration (Figure 53.7). Transcutaneous sensors and implanted sensors use multiple detection systems [enzymatic (e.g. glucose oxidase), electrode, fluorescence]. The method for sampling in minimally invasive systems takes advantage of the correlation between the concentration of glucose in the interstitial fluid and in blood.[30,31]

Whereas microdialysis systems are inserted subcutaneously, reverse iontophoresis uses a low-level electrical current, which by electro-osmosis moves glucose across the skin, being the glucose concentration measured with a glucose-oxidase detector.[32,33]

Total non-invasive technology for glucose sensing, including techniques of near-infrared spectroscopy, light scattering and photoacoustic spectroscopy, are in progress. The Gluco Watch Biographer and the Continuous Monitoring System (CMS) received a Food and Drug Administration (FDA) license. The Gluco Watch System can analyze glucose three times per hour for up 12 h, and it is best indicated for detection of hypoglycemia. It has provided excellent correlation with SBGM. The CMS includes a subcutaneous glucose sensor connected to an external monitor; it allows glucose measurements every 5 min for 72 h; values are not displayed until being downloaded into a computer at the end of the recorded interval.

It is anticipated that important progress in these methods for non-invasive or minimally invasive glucose monitoring will be made in the near future.

Glycated hemoglobin (HbA1c)

More than 40 years ago, it was observed that normal adult hemoglobin could be separated by chromatographic procedures into a major and various minor components. In one of the minor components – HbA1c – glucose was attached, non-enzymatically, to the terminal N-valine of the beta chain of HbA0. In the following years, numerous assays were developed to measure HbA1c levels.

The average lifespan of erythrocytes is 100–120 days. Measuring HbA1c offers an accurate estimation of the average

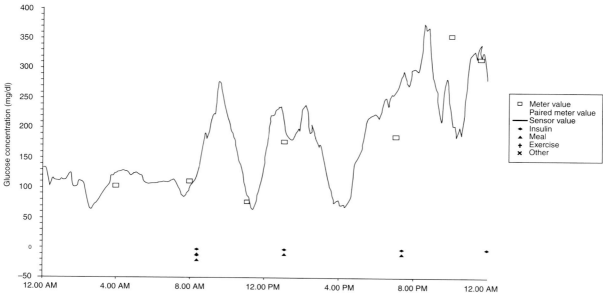

Figure 53.7   Registry of continuous glucose monitoring in interstitial subcutaneous tissue.

blood glucose concentration of the past 2–3 months. HbA1c is used as an integrated estimation of mean glycemia and as a marker of risk for the development of diabetes complications. At present, there are >30 HbA1c assay methods available. Certain methods quantify HbA1c based on charge differences of the glycated components (cation exchange chromatography, agar gel electrophoresis). Other methods analyze structural differences between glycated and non-glycated components (affinity chromatography, immunoassay). Certain methods quantify total glycated hemoglobin, including HbA1c and other hemoglobin–glucose adducts.

In 1996, the American Association of Clinical Chemists (AACC), in collaboration with the ADA established the National Glycohemoglobin Standardization Program. It was decided to adopt the high-performance liquid chromotography (HPLC) reference method used in the DCCT (Bio-Rex 70; between run CV <3%), as the designated comparison method. The UKPDS incorporated the same standardization method; therefore, its HbA1c reports were compatible with those of DCCT. More than 90% of USA laboratories, and many others worldwide, are using this standardization program.[34]

Any condition that shortens erythrocyte survival (hemolytic anemia, acute blood loss) falsely lowers HbA1c test results; in contrast, iron-deficiency anemia increases the value.[35] Glycation may also vary between patients with similar capillary blood glucose levels, and glycation appears to be lower in subjects with a higher body mass index (BMI).[36]

Several hemoglobinopathies interfere with some assay methods; the results can be falsely increased or decreased; non-hemoglobin-based methods for assessing long-term glycemic control may represent useful alternatives in these circumstances.

European guidelines have recommended the classification of blood glucose control by the number of SD the experimental value is from the nondiabetic mean for the particular assay.[37]

The International Federation of Clinical Chemistry (IFCC) has organized a working party to develop a scientifically based method of the production of a primary reference. Electrospray ionization mass spectrometry (ESIMS) has been demonstrated to be a precise measurement of HbA1c, in particular glycation of the beta chain, which has been proposed as a robust procedure for calibration purposes. In a protocol performed with 1022 patients, the comparison of the ESIMS with the ion-exchange chromatographic procedure showed excellent agreement, with values, on average, 0.7% lower with ESIMS. The comparison with DCCT-corrected ion-exchange values gave good agreement, with ESIMS showing an overall lower value of mean 0.4%.[38]

There is a general agreement that the new mass-spectroscopy-based method appears to be more accurate and to reflect 'true' HbA1c. It yields normal (nondiabetic) values that are significantly lower than those used by the National Glycohemoglobin Standardization Program, DCCT and UKPDS (3–5 vs. 4–6%).

The Ames DCA 2000 Analyzer measures HbA1c by an agglutination inhibition immunoassay, allowing results in 6 min with 1 mL of blood. The Ames DCA 2000 analyzer offers reliable results, although showing a trend to lightly underestimate the results in comparison with HPLC.[39] This analyzer gave valid and reliable results when operated by non-medical personnel.

The Primus CLC330 provides an HPLC near-patient HbA1c method, comparable in precision and accuracy to the Ames DCA 2000 Analyzer.[40] Near-patient testing for HbA1c has practical clinical use in the diabetes clinic, avoiding the need for a second appointment and allowing immediate changes in therapy.

Glycated serum proteins

Mostly albumin, and other serum proteins, undergo the process of glycation. The turnover of serum albumin depicts a half-life of 25 days; it provides an index of a mean glycemic level of a shorter interval than HbA1c. The fructosamine assay is the most widely method being used for estimating glycated serum proteins. Nevertheless, although fructosamine levels correlate with HbA1c levels within a population, transference cannot apply for individual values.[41] Also, changes in serum proteins affect the readings of fructosamine;[42] the technique is unreliable in diabetic patients with renal failure,[43] liver cirrhosis and nephrotic syndrome.[44]

Assessment of the effectiveness of self blood glucose monitoring in diabetes in pregnancy

Various randomized controlled trials (RCT)[45–49] and case series studies,[50–55] carried out either in diabetes or obstetrics departments of university hospitals, have evaluated the clinical effectiveness of SBGM in women with GDM or diabetic pregnancies. Blood glucose and HbA1c determinations, as well as maternal and fetal outcomes, were recorded. Some studies examined the costs of hospital care and home monitoring, and the compared costs for a control group receiving standard care.[47,48] The largest of all protocols included a population of 153 women with GDM in the experimental group and 2153 nondiabetics in the control group. The main goal of the case series studies was to assess the feasibility of managing pregnant women with Type 1 DM/GDM at home using SBGM. There was general agreement that women were able to achieve satisfactory blood glucose profiles at home using SBGM; hospital utilization was lower, and infant birthweights and indicators of macrosomia were also more favorable in those women.

Main findings from the RCT demonstrated that patients with Type 1 DM managed by SBGM at home obtained similar results regarding glycemic control to those patients under intensive control in the hospital. Maternal and fetal outcomes were also similar in both groups. Women preferred lower use of the hospital and home management with SBGM. Particularly for GDM, monitoring blood glucose after meals, rather than before, contributed to better metabolic control and better fetal outcomes (there were fewer Cesarean sections for cephalopelvic disproportion, fewer cases of macrosomia and large-for-gestational-age infants, and fewer episodes of neonatal hypoglycemia).[49] In addition, women who utilized SBGM were less likely to require hospital admission, leading to a substantial cost saving.

REFERENCES

1. World Health Organization (Europe) and International Diabetes Federation (Europe). Diabetes care and research in Europe: the St Vincent Declaration. Diabet Med 1990; 7: 360.
2. Eurodiabeta. Information Technology for Diabetes Care in Europe: the Eurodiabeta initiative. Diabet Med 1990; 7: 639–50.
3. Krans HMJ, Porta M, Kee H. Diabetes care and research in Europe. The St Vincent Declaration action programme. G Ital Diabetologia 1992; 12(suppl. 2): 1–56.
4. Piwernetz K, Home PD, Snorgaard O, et al., for the DiabCare Monitoring Group of the St Vincent Declaration Steering Committee. Monitoring the targets of the St Vincent Declaration and the implementation of Quality Managemant in Diabetes Care: the DiabCare Initiative. Diabet Med 1993; 10: 371–7.
5. World Health Organization (WHO). Diabetes care and research in Europe: implementation of the St Vincent Declaration. Report on a joint WHO/IDF Meeting, Budapest 9-11 March 1992. (WHO Regional Office for Europe: Copenhagen, 1992) 1–25, (EUR/ICP/CLR0550235g).
6. World Health Organization (WHO). Recommendations to facili-tate the implementation of the St Vincent Declaration initiatives by national, regional, and local diabetes task forces. Report on the Consensus Workshop, Oslo, 26–27 June 1992. (WHO Regional Office for Europe: Copenhagen, 1992) EUR/ICPCLR0550279g.
7. Piwernetz K, Massi Benedetti M, Vermeij D, et al. DiabCare Thinkshop, 'Quality Network Diabetes'. Diabetes Nutr Metab 1993; 6: 107–22.
8. Corcoy R, Muntaner F, Pou JM, et al. DiabCare data set collection: benefits and warnings. Diabetes Nutr Metab 1993; 6: 389–92.
9. Gallo G, Cermeño J, Brugués E, et al. The burden of type 2 diabetes compared to the burden of type 1 diabetes in patients undergoing intensive and specialized care. Diabetologia 2001; 44(suppl. 1): 16-A.
10. Cubero JM, Hernández M, Brugués E, et al. Metabolic outcome achieved by intensive management in European Diabetes Center are far from desirable targets. Diabetologia 2001; 44(suppl. 1): 17-A.
11. Kerényi Zs, Tamás Gy, Piwernetz K. Pregnancy complicated by diabetes: baseline data. Diabetes Nutr Metab 1993; 6: 365–8.
12. Jówicka E, Krzymierí J, Tracz M, et al. Implementation of the DiabCare program in registration of pregnant diabetic women. Diabetes Nutr Metab 1993; 6: 369–71.
13. Thaisz E, Rappai A, Fövényi J, Závodi E. Screening and care of gestational and insulin-dependent diabtic pregnancies: the first four years experience. Diabetes Nutr Metab 1993; 6: 373–5.
14. Tamás Gy, Hadden DR, Molsted-Pedersen L, et al. WHO/IDF Guidelines for care and management of the pregnant diabetic women. Av Diabetologia 1992; 5: 137–40.
15. Engelbrecht R, Hildebrand C, Kühnel E, et al. A chip card for patients with diabetes. Comput Meth Prog Biomed 1994; 45: 33–5.
16. Engelbrecht R, Hildebrand C, Brugués E, et al. DIABCARD – an application of a portable medical record for persons with diabetes. Med Inform 1996; 21: 273–82.
17. The Diabetes Control and Complications Trial Research Group. The effect of intensive treatment of diabetes on the development and progression of retinopathy in the Diabetes Control and Complications. New Engl J Med 1993; 329: 977–86.
18. UK Prospective Diabetes Study (UKPDS) Group. Intensive blood glucose control with sulphonylureas or insulin compared with conventional treatment and risk of complications in patients with type 2 diabetes (UKPDS 33). Lancet 1998; 352: 837–53.
19. UK Prospective Diabetes Study Group. Tight blood pressure control and risk of macrovascular and microvascular complications in type 2 diabetes: UKPDS 38. Br Med J 1998; 317: 703–13.
20. European Diabetes Policy Group 1998. A desktop guide to type 1 (insulin-dependent) diabetes mellitus. Diabet Med 1999; 16: 253–66.
21. Walkinshaw SA. Dietary regulation for 'gestational diabetes' (Cochrane Review). The Cochrane Library, Issue 2. (Update Software: Oxford, 1999).
22. Ziegler O, Kolopp M, Got I, et al. Reliability of self-monitoring of blood glucose by CSII treated patients with type 1 diabetes. Diabetes Care 1989; 12: 184–8.
23. Strowig SM, Raskin P. Improved glycaemic control in intensively treated type 1 diabetic patients using blood glucose meters with storage capability and computer assisted analysis. Diabetes Care 1998; 21: 1694–9.
24. Devreese K, Leroux-Roels G. Laboratory assessment of five blood glucose meters designed for self-monitoring of blood glucose concentration. Eur J Clin Chem Clin Biochem 1993; 31: 829–37.
25. Weitgasser R, Gappmayer B, Pichler M. Newer portable glucose meters – analytical improvement compared with previous generation devices? Clin Chem 1999; 45: 1821–5.
26. Brunner GA, Ellmere M, Sendlfofer G, et al. Validation of home blood glucose meters with respect to clinical and analytical approaches. Diabetes Care 1998; 122: 495–502.
27. American Diabetes Association. Self-monitoring of blood glucose. Diabetes Care 1996; 19(suppl. 1): S62–6.
28. Schiffrin A, Belmonte M. Multiple daily self-glucose monitoring: it is essential role in long-term glucose control in insulin-dependent diabetic patients treated with pump and multiple subcutaneous injections. Diabetes Care 1982; 5: 479–84.
29. Nathan DS. The importance of intensive supervision in determining the efficacy of insulin pump therapy. Diabetes Care 1983; 6: 295–7.
30. Bolinder J, Ungerstedt U, Arner P. Microdialysis measurement of the absolute glucose concentration in subcutaneous adipose tissue allowing glucose monitoring in diabetic patients. Diabetologia 1992; 35: 1177–80.
31. Hashiguchi Y, Sakakida M, Nishida K, et al. Development of a miniaturized glucose monitoring system by combining a needle-type glucose sensor with microdialysis sampling method. Long-term subcutaneous tissue glucose monitoring in ambulatory diabetic patients. Diabetes Care 1994; 17: 387–96.
32. Tamada JA, Garg J, Jovanovic L, et al. Noninvasive glucose monitoring: comprehensive clinical results. Cygnus Research Team. J Am Med Assoc 1999; 282: 1839–44.
33. Garg SK, Potts RO, Ackerman NR, et al. Correlation of fingerstick blood glucose measurements with Gluco Watch Biographer glucose results in young subjects with type 1 diabetes. Diabetes Care 1999; 22: 1708–14.
34. Little RR, Rohlfing CL, Wiedmayer H-M, et al. The National Glycohemoglobin Standardization Program (NGSP): a five-year progress report. Clin Chem 2001; 47: 1985–92.
35. Guerci B, Durain D, Leblanc H. Multicentre evaluation of the DCA 2000 system for measuring glycated haemoglobin. DCA 2000 Study Group. Diabetes Metab 1997; 23: 195–201.
36. Courturier M, Anman H, Des Rosiers C, Comtois R. Variable glycation of serum proteins in patiens with diabetes mellitus. Clin Invest Med 1997; 20: 103–9.
37. European IDDM Policy Group. Consensus guidelines for the management of insulin-dependent (type 1) diabetes. Diabet Med 1999; 10: 990–1005.
38. Roberts NB, Amara AB, Morris M, Green BN. Long-term evaluation of electrospray ionization mass spectrometric analysis of glycated hemoglobin. Clin Chem 2001; 47: 316–21.
39. Tarim O, Kucukerdogan A, Gunay U, et al. Effects of iron deficiency anemia on hemoglobin A1c in type 1 diabetes mellitus. Pediatr Int 1999; 41: 357–62.
40. Phillipov G, Charles P, Beng C, Philips PJ. Alternate site testing for HbA1c using Primus CLC330 GHb analyzer. Diabetes Care 1997; 20: 607–9.
41. Braadvedt GD, Drury PL, Cundy T. Assessing glycaemic control in disbetes: relationships between fructosamine and HbA1c. NZ Med J 1997; 110: 459–62.
42. Kruseman AC, Mercelina L, Degenaar CP. Value of fasting blood glucose and serum fructosamine as a measure of diabetic control in non-insulin-dependent diabetes mellitus. Horm Metab Res 1992; 26(suppl.): 59–62.
43. Morgan LJ, Marenah CB, Morgan AG, et al. Glycated haemoglobin and fructosamine in non-diabetic subjects with chronic renal failure. Nephrol Dial Transplant 1990; 5: 868–73.
44. Kilpatrick ES. Problems in the assessment of glycaemic control in dibetes mellitus. Diabet Med 1997; 14: 819–31.
45. Stubbs SM, Brudenell JM, Pyke DA, et al. Management of the pregnant diabetic: home or hospital, with or without glucose meters? Lancet 1980; i: 1122–4.
46. Goldstein A, Elliot J, Lederman S. Economic effects of self-monitoring of blood glucose concentrations by women with insulin dependent diabetes during pregnancy. J Reprod Med 1982; 27: 449–50.

47. Varner NW. Efficacy of home glucose monitoring in diabetic pregnancy. Am J Med 1983; 75: 592–6.

48. Hanson U, Person B, Enochsson E, et al. Self-monitoring of blood glucose by diabetic women during the third trimester of pregnancy. Am J Obset Gynecol 1984; 150: 817–21.

49. De Veciana M, Major CA, Morgan M, et al. Postprandial versus prepandial blood glucose monitoring in women with gestational diabetes mellitus requiring insulin therapy. N Engl J Med 1995; 19: 1237–41.

50. Peacock M, Chunter JC, Walford S. Self-monitoring of blood glucose in diabetic pregnancy. Br Med J 1979; ii: 1333–6.

51. Jovanovic L, Peterson CM, Saxena BB, et al. Feasibility of maintaining normal glucose profiles in insulin-dependent pregnant diabetic women. Am J Med 1980; 68: 105–12.

52. Jovanovic L, Druzin ML, Peterson CM. Impact of euglycaemia on the outcome of pregnancy in insulin-dependent diabetic women compared with normal control subjects. Am J Med 1981; 71: 921–8.

53. Espersen T, Klebe JG. Self-monitoring of blood glucose in pregnant diabetics. A comparative study of the blood glucose level and course of pregnancy in pregnant diabetics on an out-patient regime before and after the introduction of methods for home analysis of blood glucose. Acta Obstet Gynecol Scand 1985; 64: 11–4.

54. Goldberg JD, Franklin B, Lasser D, et al. Gestational diabetes: impact of home glucose monitoring on neonatal birth weight. Am J Obstet Gynecol 1986; 154: 546–50.

55. Wecher DJ, Kaufmann RC, Amankwah KS, et al. Prevention of neonatal macrosomia in gestational diabetes by the use of intensive dietary therapy and home glucose monitoring. Am J Perinatol 1991; 8: 131–4.

54 Ethical issues in management of pregnancy complicated by diabetes

Frank A. Chervenak and Laurence B. McCullough

Introduction

Physicians caring for pregnant women with diabetes can confront ethical concerns and issues that arise when the physician's judgments about what is in her clinical interest and/or the fetus's interests differs from her judgment about what is in her or her fetus's interest.[1–6] One way to manage such differences would be to assert the primacy of the physician's judgment. This strategy has been discredited because it leads to paternalism in the care of patients.[7] Paternalism occurs when the physician's clinical judgments fail to take account of the patient's values and beliefs regarding her own health and medical care.[8] To avoid paternalism the physician could opt for the alternative of the primacy of the patient's judgment.[9] This approach, however, can reduce the physician's role to that of mere technician and may also require the physician to act in ways that contradict reasonable medical judgment.

In this chapter the methods of ethics are applied to the problem of differences between the obstetrician and the diabetic pregnant woman about what is in her interest and the fetal patient's interest in a way that avoids these two extremes. Our goal is to identify a framework for clinical judgment and decision-making about the ethical dimensions of the obstetrician–patient relationship. To achieve this goal ethics, medical ethics, and the fundamental ethical principles of medical ethics, beneficence and respect for autonomy will be defined. Secondly, the concept of the fetus as a patient will be identified, emphasizing counseling for a pregnancy complicated by a fetal anomaly. Thirdly, the implications of this concept for the role of Cesarean delivery in the care of pregnant women with diabetes will be discussed. A preventive ethics approach that appreciates the potential for ethical conflict and adopts ethically justified strategies to prevent those conflicts from occurring will be emphasized.[5,10] Preventive ethics helps to build and sustain a strong physician–patient relationship.

A framework for obstetric ethics

Ethics and medical ethics

Ethics can be usefully defined as the disciplined study of morality and draws on the disciplines of the humanities, especially philosophy. Medical ethics can therefore be defined as the disciplined study of morality in medicine and concerns the mutual obligations of physicians and their patients to health care organizations and society. Medical ethics is as old as medicine itself, dating in Western medicine from the Hippocratic Oath and texts. Since the eighteenth century medical ethics has been understood to be secular. By this we mean that medical ethics does not appeal to religious or theological sources of moral authority but to what people can and should agree upon based on careful analysis of concept and rational argument.

Ethics should not be confused with the many sources of morality in a pluralistic society.[11] In most countries, these include law, American political heritage as a free people, the world's religions (most of which now exist in the USA), ethnic and cultural traditions, families, the traditions and practices of medicine (including medical education and training), and personal experience. These sources of morality can be useful reference points for ethical inquiry.

The traditions and practices of medicine, including education and training, constitute an influential, and therefore important, source of morality for physicians. A basic obligation that has emerged from medical traditions and practices is the obligation to protect and promote the interests of the patient.[5,12] This obligation tells physicians what morality in medicine ought to be in very general abstract terms. Providing a more concrete, clinically applicable account of that obligation is the central task of medical ethics.

To undertake this task, medical ethics focuses on the question of: how *ought* the physician to conduct himself or herself with patients? Major tools of ethics for answering this question include ethical principles, because they help the physician to interpret and implement his or her general moral obligation to protect and promote the interests of the patient.[5,12]

Ethical principles

Principle of beneficence

The principle of beneficence requires each of us to act in a way that is expected reliably to produce the greater balance of goods over harms in the lives of others.[5,8,12] To put this principle into clinical practice requires a reliable account of the goods and harms pertinent to the care of the patient, and of how those goods and harms should be reasonably balanced against each other when not all of them can be achieved in a particular situation. In medical ethics, the principle of beneficence requires the physician to act in ways that are reliably expected to produce the greater balance of clinical goods over harms for the patient. The scope of beneficence is limited to clinical goods and harms, because the evidence-based expertise of physicians is clinical and does not extend to other aspects of patient's lives.

Beneficence-based clinical judgment possesses an ancient pedigree: its first expression is found in the Hippocratic Oath and accompanying texts.[5,8] Beneficence-based clinical judgment makes an important claim: to interpret reliably the interests of the patient from medicine's perspective.[5,12] This perspective is provided by accumulated scientific research, clinical experience and reasoned responses to uncertainty. Beneficence-based clinical judgment is therefore a function of evidence-based clinical reasoning and judgment. As such, it is not the function of the individual clinical perspective of a particular physician and therefore should not be based merely on clinical impression or intuition of an individual physician. On the basis of this rigorous, clinical perspective, beneficence-based clinical judgment identifies the clinical goods that can be achieved for the patient in clinical practice based on the competencies of medicine. The clinical goods that medicine is competent to seek for patients are the prevention and management of disease, injury, handicap, unnecessary pain and suffering, and the prevention of premature or unnecessary death.[5] Pain and suffering become unnecessary when they do not result in achieving the other goods of medical care.

It is important to note that there is an inherent risk of paternalism in beneficence-based clinical judgment. This means that beneficence-based clinical judgment, if it is, mistakenly, considered to be the sole source of moral responsibility, and therefore moral authority in medical care, invites the unwary physician to conclude that beneficence-based judgments can be imposed on the patient in violation of her autonomy.[5,8,12] Paternalism can be a dehumanizing response to the patient and therefore should be avoided in the practice of obstetrics.

The preventive ethics response to this inherent paternalism is for the physician to explain the diagnostic, therapeutic, and prognostic reasoning that leads to his or her clinical judgment about what is in the interest of the patient, so that the patient can assess that judgment for herself. This strategy becomes important in the management of pregnancy in diabetic patients as a means to educating the pregnant woman about the implications of diabetes for pregnancy. These include informing her that meticulous outpatient care and even hospitalization may be necessary to optimize outcome. This process of explaining beneficence-based clinical judgment should enhance the patient's ability to understand and deal effectively with the technical aspects of managing a pregnancy complicated by diabetes, and help prepare her for decisions that may need to be made during the course of her pregnancy, e.g. ultrasound examination to detect diabetes-related fetal anomalies or Cesarean delivery to avoid the birth trauma associated with macrosomia.

A major advantage of sharing such beneficence-based clinical judgment for the physician in carrying out this approach is that it promotes compliance with the obstetrician's recommendations, especially those intended to prevent or minimize the complications of pregnancy. Another advantage would be to provide the patient with a better-informed opportunity to make a decision about whether to seek a second opinion. The approach outlined above should make such a decision less threatening to her physician, who has already shared with the patient the limitations on clinical judgment. A final advantage may be a reduction of the percentage (20%) of physicians who reportedly dismiss patients who disagree with them and the high percentage (36%) of patients who report that they have changed physicians who disagree with them.[13]

Principle of respect for autonomy

There has been increasing emphasis in the literature of medical ethics on the principle of respect for autonomy.[8,11] This principle requires one always to acknowledge and carry out the value-based preferences of others, irrespective of what one might think the consequences for them of so doing might be.

The pregnant patient, including the pregnant diabetic patient, increasingly brings to her medical care her own perspective on what is in her interests. The principle of respect for autonomy translates this fact into autonomy-based clinical judgment. Autonomy-based clinical judgment has roots both in the clinical practice of obstetrics and gynecology in the nineteenth century when informed consent practices were developed in the United States,[14] in the twentieth-century law of malpractice that probably codified these emerging best practices, and then in ethics, dating from four decades ago.[8,15] Because each patient's perspective on her interests is a function of her values and beliefs, it is impossible to specify the goods and harms of autonomy-based clinical judgment in advance. Indeed, it would be inappropriate to do so, because the definition of her goods and harms, and their balancing, are the prerogative of the pregnant patient. Not surprisingly, autonomy-based clinical judgment is strongly antipaternalistic in nature.

To understand the moral demands of this principle, an operationalized concept of autonomy is needed, to make it relevant to clinical practice. To do so, three sequential autonomy-related behaviors on the part of the patient are identified: (1) absorbing and retaining information about her condition, and alternative diagnostic and therapeutic responses to it; (2) understanding that information, cognitively, i.e. identifying consequences that can follow from actions; (3) appreciating that information, i.e. believing that it applies to oneself; (4) understanding information evaluatively, i.e. evaluating and rank-ordering those responses; and (5) expressing a value-based preference for a particular response.[16] The physician has a role to play in each of these. They are, respectively: (1) to recognize (and not underestimate) the capacity of each patient to deal with medical information about pregnancy, especially diabetes and pregnancy, to provide information, i.e. disclosure and explanations of all alternatives supported in beneficence-based clinical judgment, and to recognize the validity of the values and beliefs of the patient; (2) not to interfere with but, when necessary, to assist the diabetic pregnant patient in her evaluation and ranking of diagnostic and therapeutic alternative responses to her condition; and (3) to elicit and implement the patient's value-based preference.[5]

Interaction of beneficence and respect for autonomy in obstetric clinical judgment and practice

The ethical principles of beneficence and respect for autonomy play a complex role in obstetric clinical judgment and practice (Box 54.1). There are obviously beneficence-based and autonomy-based obligations to the diabetic pregnant patient.[5] The physician's evidence-based perspective on the pregnant woman's health-related interests provides the basis for the physician's beneficence-based obligations to her. Her own perspective on her health-related and other interests provides the basis for the physician's autonomy-based obligations to her. Because of an insufficiently developed central nervous system, the fetus cannot meaningfully be said to possess values and beliefs. Thus, there is no basis for saying that a fetus has a perspective on its interests. There can therefore be no autonomy-based obligations to any fetus.[5] Hence, the language of fetal rights has no meaning and therefore no application to the fetus in obstetric clinical judgment and practice, despite its popularity in public and political discourse in the United States and other countries. Obviously, the physician has a perspective on the fetus's health-related interests and the physician can have beneficence-based obligations to the fetus, but only when the fetus is a patient. Because of its importance for obstetric clinical judgment and practice, the topic of the fetus as a patient requires detailed consideration.

The concept of the fetus as a patient

The concept of the fetus as a patient is essential to obstetric clinical judgment and practice. This concept has considerable clinical significance because, when the fetus is a patient, directive counseling, i.e. recommending a form of management, for fetal benefit is appropriate and, when the fetus is not a patient, nondirective counseling, i.e. offering but not recommending a form of management, is appropriate. However,

these apparently straightforward roles for directive and nondirective counseling are often challenging to apply in actual perinatal practice because of uncertainty about when the fetus is a patient.

Independent moral status of the fetus

One approach to resolving this uncertainty would be to argue that the fetus is or is not a patient in virtue of personhood, or some other form of independent moral status.[6,9,11,17–19] It will now be shown that this approach fails to resolve the uncertainty and we therefore defend an alternative approach that does resolve the uncertainty.[5]

Independent moral status for the fetus means that one or more characteristics that the fetus possesses in and of itself, and, therefore, independently of the pregnant woman or any other factor, generate and therefore ground obligations to the fetus on the part of the pregnant woman and her physician. Many characteristics have been nominated for this role.[17–19] Given the variability of proposed characteristics, there is considerable variation among ethical arguments about when the fetus acquires independent moral status. Some take the view that the fetus has independent moral status from the moment of conception or implantation.[17–19] Others believe that independent moral status is acquired in degrees, thus resulting in 'graded' moral status.[6,20] Still others hold, at least by implication, that the fetus never has independent moral status so long as it is *in utero*.[9]

Despite an ever-expanding theological and philosophical literature on this subject, there has been no closure on a single authoritative account of the independent moral status of the fetus.[5,19,21] This is an unsurprising outcome because, given the absence of a single method that would be authoritative for all of the markedly diverse theological and philosophical schools of thought involved in this endless debate, closure is impossible. For closure ever to be possible, debates about such a final authority within and between theological and philosophical traditions would have to be resolved in a way satisfactory to all, an inconceivable intellectual and cultural outcome that secular medical ethics does not have the intellectual authority to produce. Therefore, it is proposed that these futile attempts to understand the fetus as a patient in terms of its independent moral status are abandoned and turn instead to an alternative approach that makes it possible to identify ethically distinct senses of the fetus as a patient, and their clinical implications for directive and nondirective counseling.

Dependent moral status of the fetus

Analysis of the dependent moral status of the fetus as a patient begins with the recognition that being a patient does not require that one possesses independent moral status.[22] Rather, being a patient means that one can benefit from the applications of the clinical skills of the physician. Put more precisely, a human being without independent moral status is properly regarded as a patient when two conditions are met: (1) a human being is presented to the physician and (2) there exist clinical interventions that are reliably expected to be efficacious, in that they are reliably expected to result in a greater balance of goods over harms for the human being in question.[23] This is the second sense of the concept of the fetus as a patient, termed the dependent moral status of the fetus.[5]

The present authors have argued elsewhere that beneficence-based obligations to the fetus exist when the fetus is reliably presented for medical interventions, whether diagnostic or therapeutic, that can reasonably be expected to result in a greater balance of goods over harms for the child or person the fetus can later become during early childhood. Whether the fetus is a patient depends on links that can be established between the fetus and its later achieving independent moral status.[5]

Viable fetal patient

One such link is viability. Viability is not, however, an intrinsic property of the fetus because viability must be understood in terms of both biological and technological factors.[21,24] These two factors do not exist as a function of the autonomy of the pregnant woman. When a fetus is viable, i.e. when it is of sufficient maturity so that it can survive into the neonatal period and achieve independent moral status given the availability of the requisite technological support, and when it is presented to the physician, the fetus is a patient.

Viability exists as a function of biomedical and technological capacities, which are different in different parts of the world. As a consequence there is, at the present time, no worldwide, uniform gestational age to define viability. In the United States, the present authors believe, viability presently occurs at c. 24 weeks of gestational age.[25–28]

When the fetus is a patient, directive counseling for fetal benefit is ethically justified. In clinical practice, directive counseling for fetal benefit involves one or more of the following: recommending against termination of pregnancy; recommending for or against aggressive management. Aggressive obstetric management includes interventions such as fetal surveillance, tocolysis, Cesarean delivery or delivery in a tertiary care center when indicated. Non-aggressive obstetric management excludes such interventions. Directive counseling for fetal benefit, however, must take account of the presence and severity of fetal anomalies, extreme prematurity and obligations to the pregnant woman.[5]

It is important to appreciate in obstetric clinical judgment and practice that the strength of directive counseling for fetal benefit varies according to the presence and severity of anomalies. As a rule, the more severe the fetal anomaly, the less directive counseling should be for fetal benefit.[5,29–32] In particular, when there is a very high probability of a correct diagnosis and either a very high probability of death as an outcome of the anomaly diagnosed or a very high probability of severe irreversible deficit of cognitive developmental capacity as a result of the anomaly diagnosed, counseling should be nondirective in recommending between aggressive and non-aggressive management as options.[33] In contrast, when lethal anomalies can be diagnosed with certainty then there are no beneficence-based obligations to provide aggressive management.[5,34] Such fetuses are not patients; they are appropriately regarded as dying fetuses and the counseling should be nondirective in recommending between non-aggressive management

and termination of pregnancy, but directive in recommending against aggressive management for the sake of maternal benefit.[29]

The strength of directive counseling for fetal benefit in cases of extreme prematurity of viable fetuses does not vary. In particular, this is the case for what are termed just-viable fetuses,[5] i.e. those with a gestational age of 24–26 weeks for which there are significant rates of survival but high rates of mortality and morbidity.[25–28] These rates of morbidity and mortality can be increased by non-aggressive obstetric management, while aggressive obstetric management may favorably influence outcome. Thus, it would appear that there are substantial beneficence-based obligations to just-viable fetuses to provide aggressive obstetric management. This is all the more the case in pregnancies beyond 26 weeks gestational age.[25–28] Therefore, directive counseling for fetal benefit is justified in cases of extreme prematurity of viable fetuses considered by itself. Of course, such directive counseling is only appropriate when it is based on documented efficacy of aggressive obstetric management for each fetal indication.

Any directive counseling for fetal benefit must occur in the context of balancing beneficence-based obligations to the fetus against beneficence- and autonomy-based obligations to the pregnant woman (Box 54.1).[5,35] Any such balancing must recognize that a pregnant woman is obligated only to take reasonable risks of medical interventions that are reliably expected to benefit the viable fetus or child later. The unique feature of obstetric ethics is that whether, in a particular case, the viable fetus ought to be regarded as presented to the physician is, in part, a function of the pregnant woman's autonomy.

Obviously, any strategy for directive counseling for fetal benefit that takes account of obligations to the pregnant woman must be open to the possibility of conflict between the physician's recommendation and a pregnant woman's autonomous decision to the contrary. Such conflict is best managed preventively through informed consent as an ongoing dialog throughout the pregnancy, augmented as necessary by negotiation and respectful persuasion.[5,10]

Previable fetal patient

The only possible link between the previable fetus and the child it can become is the pregnant woman's autonomy. This is because technological factors cannot result in the previable fetus becoming a child. This is simply what previable means. The link, therefore, between a fetus and the child it can become, when the fetus is previable, can be established only by the pregnant woman's decision to confer the status of being a patient on her previable fetus. The previable fetus, therefore, has no claim to the status of being a patient independently of the pregnant woman's autonomy. The pregnant woman is free to withhold, confer or, having once conferred, withdraw the status of being a patient on or from her previable fetus according to her own values and beliefs. The previable fetus is presented to the physician solely as a function of the pregnant woman's autonomy.[5]

Counseling the pregnant woman regarding the management of her pregnancy when the fetus is previable should be nondirective in terms of continuing the pregnancy or having an abortion, if she refuses to confer the status of being a patient on her fetus. If she does confer such status in a settled way, at that point beneficence-based obligations to her fetus come into existence and directive counseling for fetal benefit becomes appropriate for these previable fetuses. Just as for viable fetuses, such counseling must take account of the presence and severity of fetal anomalies, extreme prematurity and obligations owed to the pregnant woman.

For pregnancies in which the woman is uncertain about whether to confer such status, the present authors propose that the fetus be provisionally regarded as a patient.[5] This justifies directive counseling against behavior that can harm a fetus in significant and irreversible ways, e.g. poorly controlled hyperglycemia, until the woman settles on whether to confer the status of being a patient on the fetus. This also justifies directive counseling about diagnostic surveillance, e.g. ultrasound examination to detect anomalies. When anomalies are detected, counseling about the disposition of the woman's pregnancy should be nondirective, as explained above.

Nondirective counseling is appropriate in cases of what is termed near-viable fetuses,[5] i.e. those which are 22–23 weeks gestational age for which there are anecdotal reports of survival.[27,28] In the present authors' view, aggressive obstetric and neonatal management should be regarded as clinical investigation, i.e. a form of medical experimentation, and not standard of care.[27,28] There is no obligation on the part of a pregnant woman to confer the status of being a patient on a near-viable fetus, because the efficacy of aggressive obstetric and neonatal management has yet to be proven.

When to offer, recommend and perform a Cesarean section

When to offer, recommend and perform Cesarean delivery is a clinical ethical challenge in the management of a pregnancy complicated by diabetes. In this section an ethically justified approach to offering and recommending Cesarean delivery is provided, based on the ethical principles of beneficence and respect for autonomy, and the concept of a fiduciary.[36] This approach is designed to prevent conflict between the physician and the pregnant woman about intrapartum management.

This approach begins by asking: Is Cesarean delivery substantively supported and vaginal delivery not supported in beneficence-based clinical judgment? Such cases occur with diabetic pregnancies based on clinical factors such as estimation of fetal weight, the maternal pelvis, the degree of control of diabetes in the pregnancy and previous obstetric history (these clinical factors are discussed in detail elsewhere in this book). When evidence or reliable clinical judgment support the view that the fetus' interests are best protected by Cesarean delivery, and there are no maternal contraindications, then such a delivery should be offered and recommended.

In some clinical circumstances, there is scientific controversy as to whether Cesarean delivery is the better alternative. Competing well-founded beneficence-based clinical judgments regarding how to balance the fetal benefit of preventing harm of Cesarean delivery generate these controversies, which are discussed elsewhere in this book. Whenever there is legitimate scientific disagreement about the benefits and risks of Cesarean versus vaginal delivery, both options should be offered to the pregnant woman and discussed with her so that she can exercise her autonomy meaningfully. Such disclosure empowers the woman to emphasize her own perspective in balancing maternal and fetal risks. It is appropriate for the physician to assist the woman's decision-making about both options in the form of a recommendation

In clinical circumstances when Cesarean delivery is substantively supported in beneficence-based clinical judgment but vaginal delivery is more substantively supported, vaginal delivery is the better alternative, but not the only one, e.g. a pregnant diabetic patient whose sugars have been well-controlled during pregnancy and in whom there is no macrosomia. Although Cesarean delivery is supported in beneficence-based clinical judgment, trial of labor is more substantively supported, and therefore should be offered and recommended.

Conclusions

Ethics is an essential dimension of obstetric practice, especially in the care of pregnant diabetic patients. In this chapter a framework for obstetric ethics based on ethical principles and the concept of the fetus as a patient are described. On this basis, two dimensions of the care of diabetes in pregnancy with important clinical dimensions are presented: counseling about fetal anomalies; when to offer and recommend Cesarean delivery. The present authors believe that the clinical application of ethical concepts will strengthen the doctor–patient relationship and therefore enhance the quality of care for pregnant diabetic patients.

REFERENCES

1. Cain J, Stacy L, Jusenius K, Figge D. The quality of dying: financial, psychological, and ethical dilemmas. Obstet Gynecol 1990; 76: 149–52.
2. Park RC. Old bedfellows: ethics and obstetrics and gynecology. Obstet Gynecol 1989; 73: 1–3.
3. Jennings JC. Ethics in obstetrics and gynecology: a practitioner's review and opinion. Obstet Gynecol Surv 1989; 44: 656–61.
4. Skrzydelwski WB. Gynecology and ethics. Eur J Obstet Gynecol Reprod Biol 1990; 36: 274–82.
5. McCullough LB, Chervenak FA. Ethics in Obstetrics and Gynecology. New York: Oxford University Press; 1994.
6. Strong C. Ethics in Reproductive Medicine: A New Framework. New Haven: Yale University Press; 1997.
7. Veatch R. A Theory of Medical Ethics. New York: Basic Books; 1981.
8. Beauchamp TL, Childress JF. Principles of Biomedical Ethics, 4th edn. New York: Oxford University Press; 1994.
9. Annas GJ. Protecting the liberty of pregnant patient. N Engl J Med 1988; 316: 1213–4.

10. Chervenak FA, McCullough LB. Clinical guides to preventing ethical conflicts between pregnant women and their physicians. Am J Obstet Gynecol 1990; 162: 303–7.
11. Engelhardt Jr HT. The Foundations of Bioethics, 2nd edn. New York: Oxford University Press; 1996.
12. Beauchamp TL, McCullough LB. Medical Ethics: The Moral Responsibilities of Physicians. Englewood Cliffs: Prentice-Hall; 1984.
13. Louis Harris and Associates. Views on informed consent and decision making: parallel surveys of physicians and the public. In: President's Commission for the Study of Ethical Problems in Medicine and Biomedical and Behavior Research, Making Health Care Decisions, Volume 2, Appendices: Empirical Studies of Informed Consent. Washington, DC: US Government Printing Office; 1982.
14. Powdely K. Patient consent and negotiation in the Brooklyn gynecological practice of Alexander J.C. Skene: 1863–1900. J Med Philos 2000; 25: 12–27.
15. Faden RR, Beauchamp TL. A History and Theory of Informed Consent. New York: Oxford University Press; 1986.
16. McCullough LB, Coverdale JH, Chervenak FA. Ethical challenges of decision making with pregnant patients who have schizophrenia. Am J Obstet Gynecol 2002; 187: 696–702.
17. Noonan JT, ed. The Morality of Abortion. Cambridge: Harvard University Press; Cambridge, 1970.
18. Noonan JT. A Private Choice. Abortion in America in the Seventies. New York: The Free Press; 1979.
19. Callahan S, Callahan D, eds. Abortion: Understanding Differences. New York: Plenum Press; 1984.
20. Evans MI, Fletcher JC, Zador IE, et al. Selective first-trimester termination in octuplet and quadruplet pregnancies: clinical and ethical issues. Obstet Gynecol 1988; 71: 289–96.
21. Roe versus Wade, 410 US 113 1973.
22. Ruddick W, Wilcox W. Operating on the fetus. Hastings Cent Rep 1982; 12: 10–4.
23. Chervenak FA, McCullough LB. What is obstetric ethics? J Perinat Med 1996; 23: 331–41.
24. Mahowald M. Beyond abortion: refusal of cesarean section. Bioethics 1989; 3: 106–21.
25. Hack M, Fanaroff AA. Outcomes of extremely-low-birth-weight infants between 1982 and 1988. N Engl J Med 1989; 321: 1642–7.
26. Whyte HE, Fitzhardinge PM, et al. External immaturity: outline of 568 pregnancies of 23–26 weeks' gestation. Obstet Gynecol 1993; 82: 1–7.
27. Chervenak FA, McCullough LB. The limits of viability. J Perinat Med 1997; 25: 418–20.
28. Chervenak FA, McCullough LB, Levene ML. An ethically justified, clinically comprehensive approach to periviability: gynaecologic, obstetric, perinatal, and neonatal dimensions. J Obstete Gynecol 2007; 27: 3–7.
29. Chervenak FA, McCullough LB. An ethically justified, clinically comprehensive management strategy for third-trimester pregnancies complicated by fetal anomalies. Obstet Gynecol 1990; 75: 311–6.
30. Chervenak FA, McCullough LB. Does obstetric ethics have any role in the obstetrician's response to the abortion controversy? Am J Obstet Gynecol 1990; 163: 1425–9.
31. Chervenak FA, McCullough LB. Is third trimester abortion justified? Br J Obstet Gynaecol 1995; 102: 434–5.
32. Chervenak FA, McCullough LB. Third trimester abortion: is compassion enough? Br J Obstet Gynaecol 1999; 106: 293–6.
33. Chervenak FA, McCullough LB. Non-aggressive obstetric management: an option for some fetal anomalies during the third trimester. J Am Med Assoc 1989; 261: 3429–30.
34. Chervenak FA, Farley MA, Walters L, et al. When is termination of pregnancy during the third trimester morally justifiable? N Engl J Med 1984; 310: 501–4.
35. Chervenak FA, McCullough LB. Perinatal ethics: a practical method of analysis of obligations to mother and fetus. Obstet Gynecol 1985; 66: 442–6.
36. Chervenak FA, McCullough LB. An ethically justified algorithm for offering, recommending, and performing cesarean delivery and its application in managed care practice. Obstet Gynecol 1996; 87: 302–5.

55 Legal aspects of diabetic pregnancy

Kevin J. Dalton

Introduction: The law and medicine

Legal problems relating to diabetic pregnancy may be considered from three aspects:

1. Legal problems specific to pregnancy in a woman who is diabetic
2. Legal problems specific to diabetes in a woman who is pregnant
3. Legal problems specific to diabetic pregnancy

When an obstetrician or diabetologist hears that the law may be relevant to medicine, immediately he/she will think of medical malpractice and of litigation for alleged negligence. But the law applies to medicine in many other ways. Thus, when considering the legal aspects of diabetic pregnancy, one must look not only at matters arising under civil law, but also those arising under criminal law, administrative law and forensic medicine.

Few obstetricians or diabetologists are trained in medical law, and so concepts that are considered mainstream in law may appear utterly alien to them. A few of these concepts will be explained very briefly here because unless they are understood then the law set out relating to diabetic pregnancy may not be fully understood. For doctors, difficulties often arise with the following legal concepts: the doctrine of precedent, standard of proof, case and statute law, and law in different jurisdictions.

Doctrine of legal precedent

When considering the law relating to any field of medicine, it is essential to recognize that the doctrine of binding precedent is of prime importance in the common-law environment that covers most of the English-speaking world. Briefly, the doctrine of binding precedent states that whenever: (1) a legal case is being tried and (2) a higher court (i.e. an appellate court) has already decided a case that is similar to the present case, then the lower court must follow (i.e. uphold) the previous decision of the higher court. By extension, a court should usually follow the decisions of courts of equal standing within the same jurisdiction. They may even follow decisions made by courts in foreign jurisdictions if they find their decisions helpful.

Sometimes the previous decision of relevance may have been made many decades or even centuries previously.

For example, whenever English courts consider the question of consent to surgery, even today, they will frequently cite a New York court's decision made in 1914.[1]

It is also important to recognize that, in the common-law environment, court decisions that are made in one field of human activity may be readily applicable to other fields. For example, a decision made regarding the liability of an engineer may be highly relevant in deciding a case involving the liability of an architect or a medical doctor. Similarly, a decision made on a case involving only the single disease of hypertension may be relevant to a case involving only diabetes.

It follows from this that when an individual obstetrician or diabetologist discusses a medical case with his/her lawyer, the lawyer has no professional choice other than to accept and follow previous rulings of courts in the same jurisdiction, unless he/she can somehow distinguish the instant case from a related case that the court has already decided.

Standard of proof

In medicine, the level of proof is expected to be c. 95–99% before stating belief in a proposition. This high level of proof, i.e. that one is sure beyond reasonable doubt, is almost identical to the level which the court uses to decide criminal matters that are in dispute.

However, in legal disputes on civil matters, the court requires a level of proof of only 51%. In other words, the court will make its decision on the balance of probability, i.e. when it believes that the proposition in dispute is more likely than not. In medical negligence cases, only this lower level of proof is needed for a decision to be made.

This distinction between making medical decisions or legal decisions is most important.

Case law

From the above, it follows that, in deciding legal cases that arise under point (1) (i.e. problems specific to pregnancy), then previously decided cases relating to any pregnancy, even in nondiabetics, may be highly relevant. Similarly, in deciding cases that arise under point (2) (i.e. problems specific to diabetes), previously decided cases relating to diabetes, even if the diabetic is a man, may be highly relevant. In deciding cases under points (1)–(3), even cases from quite different fields of human activity may be relevant. Thus, in any given jurisdiction in the common-law world, there is a very wide range of case law that may be relevant when considering diabetic pregnancies.

In the common-law jurisdictions there have been many cases litigated that refer to diabetic pregnancy,[2] but in this chapter only the briefest details of just a few of them can be given. For a fuller understanding of each case, and of the rationale for each individual decision that was made, clearly it will be necessary to read the full text of the decision that was handed down by the court – nowadays, such full texts are often available on the World Wide Web.

Statute law

As with case law, in any given jurisdiction there is a considerable amount of statute law that may be relevant when considering diabetic pregnancies.

The law in different jurisdictions

The law relating to health care, and so the law relating to diabetic pregnancy, will differ from one jurisdiction to another. Within the United States the 56 (*sic*) separate jurisdictions have a different body of law, one from another. Even within the British Isles, the four separate jurisdictions each have a different body (and system) of law.

Covering all aspects of the law that relate to diabetic pregnancy in all jurisdictions is beyond the scope of this chapter. Instead, a limited series of topics from different jurisdictions will be considered to illustrate the diversity of the law that may apply to diabetic pregnancy.

Antenatal care

Menopause or pregnancy?

A 47-year-old insulin-dependent diabetic mentioned to her doctor that she had missed her last period and was having hot flushes. He offered no advice on this, nor did he take any action. When he saw her on later occasions, he did not ask about her periods. Subsequently, and unexpectedly, she delivered a 28-week stillborn fetus. She had not realized that she was pregnant. She took legal action against her doctor and claimed for wrongful death of her fetus, who might have survived with better medical care. She also sought damages for 'physical pain, mental anguish, medical expenses, and lost wages'. Even though the Virginia court[3] held (on appeal) that no cause of action lies for the wrongful death of a stillborn child, as it is part of its mother until birth, nevertheless it awarded damages to the mother for her emotional distress.

Fetal macrosomia

In 1988, the Supreme Court of Alabama tried a case[4] in which a diabetic mother who weighed 143 kg delivered a fetus of 5.2 kg. There was shoulder dystocia and the child suffered Erb's palsy. Expert evidence was given relating to two schools of thought on whether a Cesarean section should have been performed. Although the court acknowledged the two schools, it gave greater weight to the breach of a guideline previously issued by the American College of Obstetricians and Gynecologists, which said that there should be an elective Cesarean section when a fetus is believed to weigh >4 kg particularly in a diabetic pregnancy. The court therefore ruled that it was open to the jury to find the obstetrician negligent, despite the two schools of thought.

Other cases where there was fetal macrosomia will be referred to below.

Screening for diabetes in pregnancy

In 1994, a court in Alberta tried a 1988 case[5] in which a macrosomic baby suffered Erb's palsy after shoulder dystocia. During pregnancy the family doctor had failed to implement the universal screening policy for gestational diabetes that had been recommended by the Alberta Medical Association and the Society of Obstetricians of Canada. He also overlooked maternal glycosuria and significant maternal weight gain. He then failed to recognize fetal macrosomia on manual palpation and failed to request an ultrasound scan. The court found that his care was negligent in that he failed to follow guideline recommendations and that he failed to recognize clinical signs.

This Canadian case contrasts with a similar English case decided shortly afterwards. In 1998 the English Court of Appeal decided a 1990 case[6] relating to the screening for diabetes in pregnancy. At 30 weeks gestation a woman exhibited glycosuria ++. Her family doctor carried out a random blood glucose test, which was normal at 4.6 mmol/L. [A glucose tolerance test (GTT) at 30 weeks in her previous pregnancy had also been normal.] Nevertheless, the family doctor referred her to an obstetrician, at a hospital whose policy was to screen selectively rather than universally. The obstetrician saw her at 34 weeks, on which occasion she exhibited no glycosuria. She was considered to be at a low risk of diabetes and was told that no GTT was needed. This followed the screening policy set out in the leading English obstetrical textbook of the time (*Dewhurst's Obstetrics*).[7] The baby delivered at 39 weeks and weighed 5.8 kg. There was insuperable shoulder dystocia and so an emergency Cesarean section had to be carried out. The baby suffered both hypoxic damage to his brain (cerebral palsy) and traction damage to his brachial plexus (Erb's palsy). A claim for clinical negligence was made on the grounds that: (1) a GTT should have been organized at 34 weeks; (2) this would have revealed gestational diabetes; (3) she would then have been delivered by Cesarean section; and (4) the baby would have had no serious injury.

The case was first heard in the High Court, but then it went to appeal. The Court of Appeal held that the obstetrician was entitled to be reassured by the random blood glucose at 30 weeks, i.e. the single episode of glycosuria did not put her in a high-risk group that needed a GTT. When she saw her at 34 weeks there was now no glycosuria and so there was no reason for a GTT. The claim for negligence (along the lines that had been argued) was therefore dismissed, on the grounds that it was both reasonable and not negligent to decide not to carry out a GTT.

These two cases illustrate the fact that different courts in different jurisdictions, when trying similar cases relating to the screening for, and the management of, diabetic pregnancy, may arrive at decisions that on the face of it seem contradictory. Such a situation is by no means unusual in comparative international law.

In English law, the importance of this case is that the Court of Appeal has recognized that universal screening for gestational diabetes is not a legal requirement and that selective screening is sufficient. Furthermore, it accepts that a policy of selective screening may fail to recognize complicated cases. American readers will note that the American Diabetic Association has only recently moved away from recommending universal screening for gestational diabetes and now recommends selective screening.[8]

Hypoglycemic attacks

In pregnancy, diabetic women become more liable to hypoglycemic attacks than before pregnancy. If they are under tighter glycemic control than before pregnancy, then they may even become less aware of their hypoglycemic attacks than they were previously. It may therefore be thought reasonable to discriminate against such women in terms of the activities in which they are allowed to participate. However, an English court has recently ruled as illegal, under the Disability Discrimination Act 1995, a high school's attempt to ban a diabetic student from a watersports holiday in France, on the grounds that there had been hypoglycemic attacks when the student was on an earlier skiing trip.[9]

In England, if a pregnant woman commits a crime when she is hypoglycemic, this fact may provide a valid and sufficient defence in law, although not for all offences (see later). In the case of *R v. Padmore*,[10] a diabetic committed the crime of homicide when in a state of hypoglycemic automatism. The jury cleared him on the grounds that he was unaware of his condition and therefore had no control over his actions.

Dietary control

In gestational diabetes, there is no unambiguous scientific literature to demonstrate that good dietary control, or a special diet, will result in the birth of a smaller infant. Nevertheless, legal cases are often argued on the basis that better diabetic control would have resulted in a smaller baby and in fewer problems at the time of delivery.

One such case was heard in Ontario in 1982.[11] The mother claimed that her doctor's failure to test for, and to diagnose, gestational diabetes led to birth injuries. She had had three vaginal deliveries. Her first child weighed 3.65 kg, and he did well. Her second child weighed 4.4 kg; his delivery was complicated by shoulder dystocia, and he suffered numerous bruises and a fractured clavicle. She requested a Cesarean section for the delivery of her third child, but she was told that this was not necessary, and so again she delivered vaginally. This third child weighed 5.26 kg. His delivery was complicated

by shoulder dystocia, and he suffered brachial plexus palsy and a skull fracture.

The mother brought a legal action, on the grounds that she should have been tested for gestational diabetes and a special diet should have been started in order to minimize the risk of fetal macrosomia.

The court held that the diagnosis of gestational diabetes had never been established during her pregnancy and that it could not be determined retrospectively. Moreover, even if she did have gestational diabetes, there was no convincing evidence that dietary management or insulin would have affected the size of the baby. The expert medical evidence in this case was contradictory, but the judge said that:

> The evidence of Dr Allen [the defence expert] is preferable because his opinion was carefully documented by an assessment of forty studies done by learned researchers. There is no strong body of medical opinion to support the proposition that controlled diet of the mother would have produced a smaller baby.

The case was dismissed.

Although this case was heard in 1982, many would argue that scientific evidence on the benefits of dietary control in gestational diabetes has changed little since then.

Bank robbery

A bank teller who was 28 weeks pregnant came face to face with an armed robber. He pointed a sawn-off shotgun at her and demanded money. She was terrified and feared for her life. Eventually, the robber was arrested and convicted. Later in the pregnancy the woman went on to develop gestational diabetes. She also developed depression and a profound fear of returning to the work at the counter, and needed psychological counseling. She claimed that stress from the robbery had caused her gestational diabetes and that this increased her chance of developing diabetes in later life. At trial, the court took her allegations into account, and so it enhanced the severity of the custodial sentence that was passed.[12]

Labor and delivery

Amniocentesis and delivery

Until recently, it was common to plan the timing of delivery on the basis of testing the amniotic fluid for evidence of fetal lung maturity. In a diabetic pregnancy in South Carolina, the expected date of delivery was only 4 days away. The mother noticed a reduction in fetal movements. A fetal heart rate recording was made, which suggested an active and healthy fetus. Nevertheless, the obstetrician decided upon an amniocentesis with a view to delivery. She admitted that several times during the procedure she stuck the fetus with the amniocentesis needle. Blood was aspirated but no amniotic fluid was obtained. At birth the child had puncture sites on the left and right sides of his face. Right-sided facial paralysis was immediately apparent. As he has grown, his facial appearance has become distorted and his speech is impaired. He cannot close his right eye, and has had several operations on it. His right visual field is restricted. When the case came to trial, evidence was presented of an emotional impact, and of an increased risk of depression and of suicide as he grows older.[13]

Dead or alive?

In New Jersey, an insulin-dependent diabetic became pregnant for the third time. During the pregnancy her diabetes proved difficult to control. At 26 weeks gestation she developed both ketoacidosis and intermittent contractions. She was admitted to hospital but no fetal heart beat could be detected. Fetal death was diagnosed, and the patient and her husband were told the sad news. Labor started spontaneously and so no attempt was made to prevent delivery. Intermittent auscultation during the labor failed to reveal a fetal heart beat: no more accurate a method of detection of fetal heart beat was used. Eventually the baby delivered by the breech, with no one assisting in the birth. Quickly, the baby was taken away and placed in another room. There it became apparent that the baby was in fact alive and pink. He gasped for air and a heart beat was detected. He was rushed to the intensive care nursery. A nurse met the husband on the corridor. She told him the baby was alive, but would soon die, and so it would be best if he did not tell his wife that the baby was still alive. Eventually, a pediatrician arrived and he told everyone that the baby was still alive.

Unfortunately, the baby died 10 days later. With a better quality of medical care, the child may have survived and been born healthy. Not surprisingly, a successful legal action followed, brought on behalf of the parents and the (estate of the) child.[14]

Stillbirth

In obstetrical cases, it is unusual for three of the four principal actors to die before a legal action comes to trial. But fetus, father, and obstetrician all died in a recent (2002) Ontario case; only the mother survived.[15]

She had a stillbirth at 33 weeks gestation. The fetus was normal in weight and in structure. Autopsy failed to reveal a cause of death. Gestational diabetes was never proven medically in this case, but its possibility was contended in argument, and the case revolved around this point. The mother and her partner (who died during the case) brought a legal action on the grounds that the obstetrician (who died a year after the stillbirth) had been negligent in his care. At trial (where the obstetrician's estate and the hospital were co-defendants), the issues in dispute were as follows: (1) gestational diabetes should have been diagnosed; (2) it had not been treated appropriately; (3) it contributed to the stillbirth; and (4) appropriate treatment would have avoided stillbirth.

The expert evidence given to the judge by eminent physicians was contradictory. It well illustrated the considerable confusion and disagreement that abound in the literature concerning screening, diagnosis, and management of gestational diabetes.

After hearing the evidence, the judge decided that on the balance of probabilities: (1) the mother did not have gestational diabetes; (2) even if she did have it, then it did not contribute to the stillbirth; (3) even if she did have it, and even if

it did contribute to the stillbirth, appropriate treatment of the gestational diabetes would not have prevented the stillbirth; and (4) she was treated appropriately. The case was therefore dismissed.

However, it illustrates the complexity of medical issues where a judge sitting alone may be required to reach a decision that is potentially worth many millions of dollars. It also demonstrates how an obstetrician may be sued even when he/she is in his/her grave, on grounds that might seem implausible, as gestational diabetes was never diagnosed.

The baby

Congenital disability

In British Columbia, a mother developed gestational diabetes during her pregnancy, but this was not diagnosed until late. She developed polyhydramnios. Eventually, labor was induced, but it was prolonged and so a Cesarean section was performed. The child was born with numerous defects (these were not specified in the judgment).

The mother started a legal action. She alleged poor medical care, both during the antenatal period and in labor, and so she claimed damages. Her claim on behalf of the child was dismissed because there was no causative link between the standard of care and the child's congenital abnormalities. Only part of the mother's claim for damages was upheld: that for pain and suffering. However, the court held that there was no basis in tort law for her claim of emotional distress for the delivery of a disabled child.[16] Furthermore, it would be wrong in principle to award the mother compensation for lost earnings for devoting herself to the care of her disabled child.

Respiratory distress syndrome

In a South Carolina case from 2000,[17] a woman in her third pregnancy developed gestational diabetes for the first time. Her obstetrician consulted with a diabetologist and her condition was managed by diet alone. Her due date of delivery was known. However, at 36 weeks of gestation the obstetrician attempted an amniocentesis under ultrasound control in order to determine fetal lung maturity. The attempt failed owing to the position of the placenta. However, he told her that the baby was 'big enough' and he delivered her by Cesarean section the next day: the birthweight was 3.75 kg. The parents recollect that the obstetrician was 'enormously happy' during the Cesarean operation, but the baby developed respiratory distress syndrome and was admitted to the neonatal intensive care. In the longer term he went on to have breathing difficulties.

The parents started a legal action against the obstetrician. They alleged that he was negligent in delivering the baby 4 weeks early without medical justification and in violation of accepted medical standards. They also asserted that the doctor was

addicted to the use of drugs and narcotics to the extent that he was not mentally, emotionally or physically able to have provided competent medical care and attention.

They had discovered that the doctor had been treated for alcohol dependency and that he had returned for inpatient treatment <1 month after the Cesarean section: a few days later his partners ousted him from the partnership. At trial the parents asked the court to order release of the doctor's alcohol treatment records, but their motion was refused because it would violate federal and state confidentiality statutes. However, the court rejected the doctor's motion that all reference to his alcohol addiction should be excluded as this could not establish his alcohol status at the time in question and it would only serve to prejudice him in the eyes of the jury. The court took the view that 'the probative value is not substantially outweighed by any prejudicial effect'.

Forensic matters

Detainees

Occasionally, a diabetic pregnant woman may be held in custody, either in jail, or in police detention pending investigations or awaiting trial. Under Britain's Police and Criminal Evidence Act 1984 (PACE), a forensic medical examiner must be called to attend each prisoner who is taking medication for a chronic illness, such as diabetes, and so he/she must therefore be called to attend any diabetic pregnant prisoner. He/she must take an appropriate medical and social history, paying particular attention to whether other drugs (prescribed or not) have been taken recently. Then he/she will carry out an appropriate general and antenatal examination. He/she must then check the patient's blood glucose level at least once during a brief period of custody. Following this, he/she must (at least) discuss the case with a specialist in the management of diabetic pregnancy. If the patient is to remain in brief custody, it is important for him/her to ensure that an appropriate regime of feeding and insulin therapy is in place. However, a diabetic pregnant woman destined for a longer episode of custody will need personal attention and careful ongoing management by a specialist.

In any episode of custody, if a pregnant diabetic becomes unstable, with either hypoglycemia or hyperglycemia, she must be transferred immediately to hospital for appropriate assessment and stabilization. (Clearly, hypoglycemia should be managed by giving glucose or sugar before transfer, if this is possible.) After she has been stabilized in hospital, a decision can then be taken as to when, or whether, she may safely be returned to custody. Clearly, the prison cell is not the safest of places to manage a diabetic pregnancy.

It is important to remember that a pregnant woman will be unfit for interview by the police if her diabetes is in any way unstable at the time of the proposed interview. If an interview takes place when she is (or should be) considered as medically unfit, then any information or confession she gives will be considered unreliable, and so the circumstances of the interview may provide legal grounds for appeal.

Post-mortem examination

Occasionally, a diabetic pregnant woman may die unexpectedly, e.g. in a road traffic accident or suddenly whilst alone.

Hypoglycemia may be the root cause of death. However, at autopsy it is generally not possible to make a firm diagnosis of either hypoglycemia or hyperglycemia. The pathologist will therefore need to take circumstantial evidence into account in determining whether unstable diabetes has played a part in the death.

Administrative and related issues

Public assistance grants

The US Federal Aid for Families with Dependent Children (AFDC) programme is a cash-assistance programme designed to provide ongoing aid to poor families where at least one minor child has been deprived of parental support by reason (inter alia) of a parent's physical incapacity. A number of disadvantaged people started a class action against the Mayor of New York (et al.) in regard to alleged misadministration of AFDC.

One of them was a 30-year-old woman who had developed gestational diabetes. She needed a 2200 calorie-a-day diet, which she could not afford without the monthly special-needs grant of $50 that should have been made available to her. She had first requested the grant when she was at 13 weeks gestation, but she did not receive it until 36 weeks. Although her money was then paid retrospectively, she claimed that she had suffered irreparable injury to herself and her child through deprivation of funds necessary to buy medically required nutrition during a substantial part of her pregnancy.

The District Court agreed to her claim and it certified her as a member of the class action.[18] It also granted (to all the class members) the preliminary injunction that they had requested against the Mayor of New York, relating to the future administration of AFDC.

Employment

Sometimes employers are not sympathetic to women's requests for time off work to attend medical appointments relating to pregnancy. This problem may be worse for pregnant diabetics, as they need more frequent appointments than most women.

There have been many cases where legal action has been taken against an employer, with allegations of discrimination, but the claimants rarely win. The reason for this may be that most cases turn on the intent of one party or the other, and this is difficult to prove after the event, particularly as there is usually no direct evidence of discriminatory intent on the part of the employer. Sometimes claims are brought under the Americans with Disabilities Act. However, temporary, non-chronic impairments of short duration, with little or no long-term impact, are not usually considered in law as disabilities.[19]

Driving

Most countries impose driving regulations on diabetics. Under British regulations, diabetics on treatment with insulin (including gestational diabetics on insulin) are barred from driving heavy goods vehicles and public services vehicles, no matter how good their diabetic control.[20] However, they may drive private cars, provided that they can recognize the symptoms of hypoglycemia. If they cannot recognize hypoglycemia, then they must stop driving. Diabetics on long-term insulin must also meet required visual standards. For those taking insulin, any licence to drive will be limited to 1, 2 or 3 years. Gestational diabetics who are not taking insulin have no driving restrictions. However, if they start insulin therapy in pregnancy, then they must report this fact to the Driver and Vehicle Licensing Authority in Swansea if they wish to continue driving.

Insulin-dependent diabetics who become pregnant often find that their diabetes becomes more difficult to control. Hypoglycemic attacks become more frequent and are more difficult to recognize. Clearly, this presents a danger in terms of driving a car.

In an English case,[21] an insulin-dependent diabetic became pregnant. Her diabetic control had been good but it deteriorated in pregnancy, although she had taken specialist advice about this. One day she drove her car at high speed round a bend, on the wrong side of the road, where she collided with a tractor. She was charged with dangerous driving. Although she pleaded guilty, she claimed that she was unexpectedly hypoglycemic at the time of the accident and so had committed the offence through no fault of her own. The magistrates rejected her claim. They fined her, and they disqualified her from driving for 12 months and until she had passed an extended driving test. She appealed on the grounds that her diabetes provided a special reason entitling the court not to impose a mandatory disqualification for the minimum period under s34 (1) of the Road Traffic Offenders Act (RTA) 1988. At appeal, the court recognized that she was not personally culpable for her offence. Nevertheless, it held that the test to establish the offence of dangerous driving is an objective test, in that the offence lies in the mode of driving, whatever the reason for it. In her case, her temporary condition (of hypoglycemia) was special to her personally and it formed no part of the content of the offence. Thus, these circumstances did not amount to a special reason to avoid an automatic penalty of disqualification, as laid down in s34 of RTA 1988. Her appeal against disqualification was therefore dismissed. Although this decision may seem unfair to the woman, there are clear grounds of public policy as to why she should be disqualified, i.e. the protection of the public and of herself.

Note how the legal consideration of hypoglycemia in this driving case contrasts with that in the case of that of *R v. Padmore*[10] mentioned above. In *R v. Padmore* the initial charge of murder was dismissed, as a conviction for murder requires proof of intention to kill and this was not present during that episode of hypoglycemia. By contrast, a conviction for dangerous driving does not require any specific intention to drive dangerously.

Certification of diabetics

In England, diabetics who wish to drive must ask their doctor to complete a certificate to confirm that they have not had evidence of blackouts or loss of consciousness within the past 5 years, and have not had any significant episodes of hypo-

glycemia. The present author has recently been involved in one such case. A family doctor had signed this certificate for a diabetic patient, but he signed negative answers to these two questions. He failed to mention that 5 years previously the patient had caused a motoring accident in which a heavy truck was driven through the central reservation of a major motorway, and that the episode was attributed to hypoglycemia. Thus, the doctor had signed false entries on the driving licence application, which misled the Driving and Vehicle Licensing Authority into issuing another heavy goods vehicle licence. A few months later the driver had a more serious trucking accident in which three people were killed: two adults and one child. Again, this accident was attributed to hypoglycemia. On this occasion the driver was imprisoned for causing death by dangerous driving.

The family doctor was called before the Professional Conduct Committee of the General Medical Council to face charges that included making false and misleading entries on a patient's driving licence application form. He was found guilty of serious professional misconduct and the General Medical Council reprimanded him.[22]

The cost of diabetes care

Looking after diabetic women in pregnancy is expensive and so those who are ineligible for care provided by the state or by their insurance may be tempted to run their pregnancies without appropriate diabetic care. Sometimes insurers will deny funding to their insurees. But this will bring increased morbidity for mother and fetus.

For these reasons, and for longer term reasons of cost reduction, most American states have now enacted measures to require comprehensive insurance reimbursement for diabetes care, e.g. Massachusetts has its Diabetes Cost Reduction Act 2000.

The Americans with Disability Act may also be invoked in such cases. Under the Americans with Disabilities Act, in 2000 a Maine court awarded $60,000 in both compensatory and discriminatorial damages against a health maintenance organization HMO that had refused to fund a sign-language interpreter for the antenatal visits of a pregnant diabetic who was deaf, and whose husband was deaf too.[23] The couple were unable fully to communicate with their physician about dietary concerns or about complications that arose in the pregnancy.

Examination fraud

Two lawyers were married. She was an insulin-dependent diabetic; he had a history of professional setbacks, including loss of employment and bar exam failures in both Texas and California. She then became pregnant: he reacted with violent rage and depression, and the marriage deteriorated. Her diabetic pregnancy suffered a series of complications. In an attempt to save her own health, the marriage and also the future for their unborn baby, she agreed to her husband's request that she should take the state bar examination in his place. She did so, and she obtained the ninth highest mark in the state. She then went on to deliver a healthy child. However, the examination fraud was later discovered, and they were both prosecuted and disbarred.[24] They lost their jobs and now they are now divorced.

Excuse for non-performance

A diabetic solicitor was pregnant, but she continued in her law practice throughout the pregnancy, which ended in a Cesarean section. In the final few days of her pregnancy, when she was preparing for her imminent delivery, she missed an important court deadline for submission of certain papers relating to the case of a client. The court therefore struck out her client's case. She did not become aware of this problem until a few days after delivery. She therefore apologized to the court and to her client, and she made an application to court for a reversal of its decision, on the grounds that she was unable to conduct her affairs properly under the circumstances of her health. The court rejected her submission on the grounds that she knew she was to deliver soon and should have submitted the papers earlier, or made alternative arrangements by handing the case over to a colleague.[25] Her client's case therefore remained struck out.

Related medical matters

Involvement of other specialists in the care

Nowadays, reputable doctors would agree that diabetic pregnancy must be managed by an obstetrician with significant experience of such cases, but it has not always been so. In an Ontario case from 1982,[26] a pregnant woman at 37 weeks gestation was found to have glucose and ketones in her urine. Her family doctor admitted her to hospital for investigation of suspected diabetes. This diagnosis was confirmed the following day, but she was not referred to a diabetologist or an obstetrician, and no special treatment was started. Instead, she was allowed home. A few days later she went into diabetic ketoacidosis and fetal death occurred: her stillborn child was delivered 2 days later. She brought a legal action. The court held that the family doctor's failure to start insulin therapy on the evening she was first admitted to hospital was 'merely error in judgement'. However, the doctor's failure to act positively once the diagnosis of diabetes was confirmed constituted professional negligence, as also did his decision to discharge her from hospital at a time when her diabetes was not under control. The court held that damages could not be awarded for loss of the fetus or grief. However, it did award general damages to the mother for her physical pain and suffering.

By contrast, another pregnant diabetic (who also had epilepsy) sued her obstetrician because he *did* refer her on to another specialist for ongoing care. Her obstetrician had looked after her in two previous pregnancies, but early in her third pregnancy he discovered that she was HIV positive and so he referred to another hospital for care. She took legal action against him on the grounds that he had denied her treatment solely because she was HIV positive, in violation of various disability discrimination laws. In his defence, the obstetrician explained to the court that he had never used AZT, which is recommended for such patients, and that this is

why he referred her to another hospital. The court accepted his explanation, and the case was dismissed.[27]

In a Californian case from 1992,[28] Dr Klvana (a licensed doctor who practised obstetrics) was convicted of: nine counts of second degree murder, five counts of aiding and abetting the practice of medicine without a licence, one count of conspiracy to practise medicine without a licence, 19 counts of preparing a fraudulent insurance claim, 10 counts of presenting a false insurance claim, two counts of grand theft, and two counts of perjury. One of these cases involved a diabetic pregnancy. The patient concerned was an insulin-dependent diabetic, and he saw her throughout the pregnancy. At 30 weeks gestation she found glucose in her urine and so she consulted a diabetologist. He advised her that her diabetes was out of control and so she increased her insulin dosage. She told Dr Klvana about this consultation and about the increase of insulin dosage. At 34 weeks she experienced uterine contractions. Dr Klvana examined her in his office (i.e. not at the hospital) and he found that her cervix was already 3 cm dilated. He told her she would deliver that afternoon. Later he found that her cervix was 5 cm dilated and so he ruptured the membranes. At his next examination he found the cervix to be 9 cm dilated; she had not yet been transferred to hospital. Soon, the premature infant was delivered in the office. The baby was bluish purple in color and wheezing, and he would not cry. Dr Klvana advised the mother that the baby would be all right within 24 h. He sent them both home, with instructions for her to give the baby sugar water, and to return within 1–2 days. He did not consult or refer to a pediatrician. The mother went home and slept, but when she awoke her baby was dead. At autopsy the baby's cause of death was given as perinatal complications associated with a diabetic mother and prematurity.

The case came to trial. At trial, the following further facts emerged:

> Klvana visited [the patient] later that morning. He told her that the police would accuse them both of killing the baby if she told them that she had planned a hospital delivery but did not know the name of the hospital. Klvana indicated that he would insert the name of a hospital in her medical records. Klvana stated that the baby would have died anyway even if hospitalized immediately.

Mental illness

Sometimes a diabetic woman may be mentally ill. She may then become pregnant. If so, she may not receive the care necessary for her health and safety, nor for that of her fetus. In Oregon, a 25-year-old woman of 32 weeks gestation had a schizoaffective disorder and severe social problems. Management of her diabetic pregnancy proved problematic, as she was a regular defaulter from health care. An application to commit her to the care of the Mental Health Division was made, but she opposed it. At the civil commitment hearing, no expert testimony was presented on the dangers generally posed by diabetes in pregnancy, nor about the specific risks to the patient or her fetus. Moreover, her attorney argued that she was not a danger to herself or others. The commitment hearing agreed that she was not a danger to herself, but it considered that her mental illness (through her diabetes being incorrectly managed) presented a danger to the fetus, and so a committal order was made. She appealed the decision. Although the Court of Appeals heard general evidence about diabetes and pregnancy, it did not hear any evidence relating to the patient's specific circumstances, which would have needed expert medical testimony. The court therefore reversed the committal order, on the ground that insufficient evidence had been presented to prove that her diabetes presented a specific threat to herself and her fetus.[29]

This case illustrates the importance of thorough preparation before a medical case is taken to court, as otherwise a decision that is medically undesirable, even though legally sound, may be handed down.

Consent to sterilization

In Colorado in 1976, a schizophrenic woman had badly controlled diabetes and she defaulted from care. Her mother wanted this diabetic daughter to be sterilized, on the grounds that any future pregnancy would be dangerous to both mother and baby. Moreover, the daughter had already had a preterm delivery at 34 weeks gestation. The mother argued that her daughter did not have the capacity to understand the risks of pregnancy in the face of unstable diabetes and she had a history of preterm delivery. However, the daughter refused to be sterilized and so the matter was taken to court. The Supreme Court ruled in favor of the mentally ill daughter, on the basis that the legal case turned on her understanding of the concept of sterilization, and not on her understanding of the risks of diabetic pregnancy and preterm delivery.[30] Thus, the mentally ill daughter could not be sterilized unless she herself consented to surgery.

Congenital abnormality following failed sterilization

It is well known that cardiac defects are more common in children born of diabetic mothers. A Missouri case involved a woman who had a previous history of difficult pregnancy complicated by gestational diabetes. Her husband had a vasectomy and this was followed by negative semen analysis. But she fell pregnant again, this time with twins. A repeat semen analysis was positive, and so the vasectomy had failed. Eventually the babies delivered, but one had a severely defective heart condition. Despite multiple operations and a prolonged period of hospitalization, he died at 7 months of age.

A legal action followed, on the grounds that the vasectomy must have been performed incorrectly. At that time in Missouri, claims for damages arising from birth defects were not in themselves actionable. Nevertheless, the claim was for medical expenses associated with the birth defects, lost income and emotional distress.

The Court of Appeals[31] held that, as a matter of law, a negligent vasectomy alone will not normally be the cause of a child's birth defects; it is too far removed from the damage and it is not the cause of the damage. Furthermore, it follows that negligent performance of a vasectomy was not the proximate cause of the medical expense resulting from the child's birth defects. Thus, the claim for damages was dismissed.

Involuntary participation in research

In 1976 an insulin-dependent diabetic was delivered by Cesarean section at the Boston Hospital for Women. She became infected afterwards and then she became sterile. Later she discovered that her obstetrician had curetted her uterus after the operation. She claimed that she was thus unknowingly the subject of an experiment, in that her obstetrician wanted to obtain tissue for a research study on maternal infant health problems in diabetic pregnancy, which was being funded at the hospital by the National Institute for Neurological Disease and Blindness.

The obstetrician denied this. He claimed that performing curettage was part of his standard treatment of diabetic women in childbirth, so that he could study the uterine decidua to determine the effect of diabetes on the vascular system, and to determine if future pregnancies were desirable.

She brought a legal action against the hospital. However, the court determined that the hospital could not be held liable, as she was the obstetrician's private patient.[32]

Expert witnesses

A diabetic woman from Michigan died in early pregnancy due to the complications of undiagnosed diabetes (these were not detailed in the judgment). The (husband and estate of the) plaintiff took legal action and they brought a claim against the specialist in internal medicine who had last treated her. They also put forward supportive evidence from a doctor whose principal work was that of a pathologist and a coroner. However, under cross-examination he had to acknowledge that he only practised internal medicine on a limited 'moonlight basis'. Following a review by the Court of Appeals,[32] his evidence was not admitted, on the grounds that he was not an appropriate expert to comment on the actions of a specialist in internal medicine. The case was therefore dismissed.

This case illustrates that if the management of a medical case is to be criticized, this can only reasonably be done by a doctor who is expert in the relevant area of medicine.

Conclusions

From the legal point of view, the topic of diabetic pregnancy is a very wide one. But most legal issues or disputes that arise in relation to diabetic pregnancy will already have arisen in health fields outside of diabetic pregnancy, or even in fields well outside of medicine, and a court will take such external references into account. Very few cases will arise in diabetic pregnancies that have not already been addressed previously, at least in a related fashion, by one jurisdiction or another.

Finally, it is important to remember that, just like medicine, the field of medical law is changing continuously and more rapidly than hitherto. What a court may have decided last year may not be valid next year, if the law or our medical understanding changes in the interim. An example here lies in the American Diabetic Association's recent change in the guidelines relating to universal or selective screening for gestational diabetes.[8]

These are but two of the reasons why it is so important in the field of legal medicine to keep up to date, not only with changes in medical understanding but also with changes in medical law, both locally and in other jurisdictions.

REFERENCES

1. Schloendorff v. Society of New York Hospital [1914] 105 NE 92 MLC 0678.
2. In researching this paper, >100 decided legal cases relating to diabetic pregnancy were found by the present author.
3. Shoemaker v. Hotchkiss [1984] 4 Va Cir 166: 6684.
4. James v. Wooley [1998] a/a 523 So 2d 110.
5. Pierre v. Marshall [1994] 8 WWR 478.
6. Hallatt v. North West Anglia Health Authority [1998] 4ML 2; [1998] Lloyd's Rep Med 197 (CA).
7. Dewhurst CJ (ed). Integrated Obstetrics and Gynaecology for Postgraduates, 4th edn. Oxford: Blackwell, 1986.
8. American Diabetic Association. Gestational diabetes mellitus: a position statement. Diabetes Care 2002; 25: S94–6.
9. White v. Clitheroe Royal Grammer School [2002], reported on www.diabetes.org.uk/news on 30.04.02.
10. R v. Padmore, reported in The Times, 17 December 1999.
11. Quiroz v. Austrup, Simpson and Kitchener–Waterloo Hospital [1982] ACWSJ 538408; 17 ACWS (2d) 245.
12. USA v. Murray [1999] US Court of Appeals Fourth Circuit: 97–6735.
13. Rush v. Blanchard [1993] 310 SC 375; 426 SE 2d 802: 23794.
14. Careys v. Lovett and others [1993] 132 NJ 44; 622 A.2d 1279: A-8.
15. Wereszczakowski and Darrock v. Swales and St Joseph's Health Centre, [2002] Ont Sup CJ, 98-CV–140516.
16. Oliver v. Ellison, Mitchell and the Salvation Army Grace Hospital [2001] BC CA; 2001 BCD Civ J 2079 – CA 024495.
17. Watson v. Chapman [2000] SC CA Op 3272.
18. Brown, Corredor et al. v. Giuliani et al. [1994] USDC Eastern District of New York, 158 FRD 251; CV-94–2842 (CPS).
19. LaCoparra v. Pargament Home Ctrs Inc [1997] 982 F Supp 213, 228 (SDNY).
20. Drivers' Medical Group, Driver and Vehicle Licensing Authority. For Medical Practitioners: At a Glance Guide to the Current Medical Standards of Fitness to Drive. Swansea: Driver and Vehicle Licensing Authority; 2002.
21. Jarvis v. Director of Public Prosecutions [2000] Queen's Bench Division 164 JP 15.
22. General Medical Council v. Krishnamurthy, Hearing of the GMC's Professional Conduct Committee in Manchester on 29 August 2002. (The present author sat on the panel at this hearing, which was in public and before the national press.)
23. US v. York Women's Care Associates [2000] US District Court for the District of Maine.
24. re Lamb on Disbarment [1989] 49 Cal 3d 239; 776 P.2d 765; 260 Cal Rptr 856–S007499.
25. Florida Municipal Liability Self Insurers Program v. Mead Reinsurance Corporation, and the Town of Pembroke Park [1993] US Dist. LEXIS 7501; 7 Fla. L. Weekly Fed. D. 191.
26. MacRae v. MacKenzie and West Lincoln Memorial Hospital [1984] Ontario High Court of Justice, ACWSJ 446604; 24 ACWS (2d) 514.
27. Lesley v. Chie [2001] 250 F.3d 47 (1st Cir).
28. People v. Klvana [1992] 11 Cal App 4th 1679; 15 Cal Rptr 2d 512.
29. State of Oregon v. Ayala [1999] 164 Ore App 399; 991 P.2d 100; A101430.
30. re Romero (Incapacitated Person) [1990] 790 P.2d 819; 1990 Colo. LEXIS 306; 14 BTR 541.
31. Williams and Williams v. van Biber [1994] 886 SW.2d 10: WD 47567.
32. Schwartz v. Boston Hospital for Women [1976] USDC Southern District of New York, 422 F Supp 53; 71 Civ 1562.
33. McDougall v. Schanz and others [1999] 461 Mich 15; 597 NW.2d 148.

56 Diabetologic education in pregnancy

Lluis Cabero-Roura and Maria Goya Canino

Introduction

All complications of pregnancy in diabetic patients are directly or indirectly related to the degree of metabolic control, as many of these affect the course of gestation, as embryonic or fetal lesions. This is as true for pre-gestational diabetics, insulin-dependent or not, as it is for gestational diabetics. The only way to reduce complications to a minimum, to be close to the numbers encountered in a normal population, is for a pregnant woman to achieve a blood glucose level as near as possible to normoglycemia. To achieve this objective requires a major effort, not only on the part of the therapeutic team, but on the patient herself.

Maybe more than in any other illness, during pregnancy it is true to say that treatment is only possible with the patient's direct and active participation. To treat her, she is not only prescribed a certain medication that she should take several times a day, but she is also asked to change her habits, and from the first visit until childbirth the rhythm of her life and habits revolve around metabolic control. The patient's participation is indispensable, and is only obtained when, firstly, she understands what is requested and why; and, secondly, when she has the necessary knowledge, which she must continuously acquire, so that her effort is effective and results in completion of gestation.

Transmitting sufficient motivation, knowledge and skills to the patient is called diabetologic education. This is a cornerstone in the management of patients with diabetes because they are the ones who actually put it into practice and follow the therapeutic regime recommended by the help group.

The recognition of diabetics' needs to be involved in their own treatment dates back to the discovery of insulin. A drug with a very small therapeutic margin and potentially serious secondary effects, it cannot be taken orally nor can it be administered exclusively in hospitals because the patient needs it every day. The insulin-dependent diabetic needs to know how to administer it, and how to recognize the effects produced by too much or too little, and how to compensate for this. The Joslin Clinic in Boston was one of the first centers to establish formal education for diabetics; this can now be considered the general approach, at least as far as the theoretical definition of overall care for diabetics is concerned. The efficacy of structured diabetologic education in achieving better glycemic profiles and in reducing complications in patients with access to such education has been shown in many studies. However, we are a long way from achieving generalized easy access to diabetologic education programs, and it is true to say that even in highly developed countries there is a notable difference between the recommended standards and everyday reality.[1]

Reaction to the disease

The reaction to the diagnosis of a chronic disease is similar to the process of grieving: in fact, it is a grieving process brought about by the loss of health. It involves a number of phases, from initial denial to final acceptance, which are normal provided that their duration and intensity do not exceed certain limits. In any case, medical staff dealing with the chronically ill should be familiar with these phases in order to understand certain types of behavior or attitudes, and to be able to respond in the most effective way at any given time:

- *Shock phase or initial denial.* The patient rejects the diagnosis, believing that it is due to a laboratory error or interpretation, and that it is not actually happening to her. He/she may request a second opinion, repeat tests or argue about the reliability of the tests.
- *Protest phase.* This involves rebellious or angry reactions. Not complying with medical instructions, or deception and evasiveness in response to compliance may be seen in this phase.
- *Anxiety phase.* Melancholic or inhibited reactions.
- *Negotiation phase.* The disease is accepted, but the patient tries to set limits on the impact that this will have in her life. One characteristic may be a partial acceptance of the proposed instructions: 'Okay, I'll do the controls but only twice a day', or 'I'll follow the diet but I'm not injecting myself with insulin.'
- *Adaptation phase.* 'If there is no way back, I better do as best I can.'

During pregnancy, it is slightly different.[2] Women with Type 1 and Type 2 diabetes already have a known disease at the start of the gestation period, and, therefore, it might be expected that they would be in the adaptation phase. However, this is not always the case. Furthermore, one of the educator's first interventions should be to identify exactly which phase the patient is in. Sometimes, the patient can remain in the anxiety or negotiation phase for years, while at other times the patient can be in a hidden denial phase. Identifying which phase the patient is in is fundamental to be able to focus the situation effectively and to reinforce or begin, if appropriate, the education process efficaciously. Getting over the initial phases, especially if they are prolonged, is more difficult in these patients than in gestating patients, because their experiences are more prolonged and intense, and because sometimes elaborate schemes are created (excessive family or work problems, supposed difficulty in response or negative effects of the disease, etc.) to justify an evasive attitude to diabetes.

Gestational diabetics scarcely have time to progress through the different phases. They could easily stay in the first phase because they do not perceive any inconvenience as a consequence of the disease. However, frequently, this is not the case, because the fetus is presented as being the most affected in the process, this makes them advance quickly to the negotiation or adaptation phase. As the inconvenience is perceived as transitory, and the effect on their lifestyle is of low intensity, this also adds to a quick acceptance. However, in some cases, the initial denial phase is strongly manifested.[3] Continuation of pregnancy without the relief of specific problems or without the detection of fetal anomalies can reinforce this attitude of distrust of the diagnosis or its relevance, and convert it into a definitive attitude. Sometimes, it is difficult to overcome this response which is theoretically reinforced by events, or rather by the absence of events, and the best that can be obtained is to control the patient's evolution and to hope that she is in the percent of patients who do not spontaneously develop complications. Fortunately, this is not a normal response.

In both types of diabetes, the presence of the fetus and the knowledge that it will be the main beneficiary of the correct treatment provide the patient with a stimulus.[4] The concept of the fetus as a patient is a key factor in the transmission of information, and it is undoubtedly helpful in making the pregnant patient's attitude, in most cases, a collaborative one.

Diabetologic education

The objective of medical care for diabetic patients is to normalize glycemia levels and to minimize the complications of the disease. Achieving near normal glycemia levels delays the onset of chronic complications, reduces the number of medical visits and hospital stays, and lowers health costs. During pregnancy, the goal of metabolic management (glycemic monitoring, dietary regulation and insulin therapy) is to prevent or minimize the postnatal sequelae of diabetes – macrosomia, shoulder distocia, birth injury and postnatal metabolic instability – in the newborn (Table 56.1). If this goal is to be achieved, glycemic control must be instituted early and aggressively. Normoglycemia is associated with reduced perinatal mortality and morbidity.[5]

To obtain normal or near normal glycemic controls, it is necessary for the diabetic to become sufficiently skilled in choosing, distributing, and preparing foods conveniently, to be able to self-administer insulin, and to periodically check glycemia levels. The objective of diabetologic education is to give the patient the knowledge and skills to be able to attend to his own daily care. Medical care that does not enable diabetics to gain a good degree of independence in the control of their disease is insufficient care, which will, in the medium- to long-term, struggle to reflect satisfactory results. In the case of pregnant women, medical control without the active participation of the patient creates a serious obstacle to obtaining normal perinatal results. Without an adequate diabetic education and with a minimum of instructions, serious imbalances may be avoided, but it is practically impossible to achieve euglycemia in many cases, especially in previously diagnosed diabetics.[6]

Table 56.1   Objectives of diabetology education in pregnancy

	Gestational diabetes	Pre-gestational diabetes
Short-term	Diabetes awareness Mutual interference between diabetes and gestation Basic management skills	Identification: • Degree of previous training • Degree of independence achieved • Family support Knowledge: • Interrelation between diabetes and gestation Increase: • Level of awareness and skills • Degree of independence
Medium to long-term	Diabetes of healthy habits Prevention /detection of diabetes • Diabetes Type 2 • Gestational diabetes in another pregnancy	Promote healthy attitudes Promote positive and proactive attitudes to the disease Prevention of complications in a new pregnancy

Diabetologic education is a collaborative and interactive process which is established between the diabetic and the educator.[7] The process includes:

- Knowledge of the specific individual educational needs
- Identification of the objectives of specific individual self-controls
- Education and direct follow-up to help the diabetic meet the objectives set
- Evaluation of the achievement of the objectives set

In diabetes, an educator can be defined as a healthcare professional with thorough knowledge and skills in physiology, pathology, social relations, communication and education, and with experience in the care of diabetic patients. This role can be undertaken by nurses, doctors, psychologists, dieticians, etc. since the function is neither specific nor exclusive to any one group. In multidisciplinary teams, all the members should possess knowledge and sufficient training for the role, even although the role is assumed and led by a certain member of the team.[8]

Education in self-management should be aimed at diabetics and, as far as possible, at their family and friends so that they can offer the diabetic the necessary support and so that they are able to act appropriately in a crisis. The content of the information and training given to patients should include topics such as the physiopathology of diabetes mellitus; its short- and long-term consequences; appropriate kinds of food, physical activity, drug therapy, self-control of glycemia, the prevention and management of acute and chronic complications, how to act in situations of conflict, psychosocial adaptation, and the use of the health service.[9] Pregnant women or those of child-bearing age considering pregnancy should also be made aware of how the disease can influence the gestation and the fetal development; how the pregnancy affects the metabolic balance; to what extent the disease could influence the aggravation or appearance of chronic complications; and which are the general treatment principles during this period.[10]

The information and the method of educating should be adapted to the personal characteristics of each individual, taking into account the level of education, knowledge and prior preparation, capacity of understanding and learning, existence of concomitant diseases, social or cultural differences, lifestyle and predisposition or capacity to collaborate.[11]

Although the final objective of getting a healthy newborn baby with the minimum possible interference to health or discomfort to the mother is similar for all patients, individual objectives may vary greatly. With each individual patient, it is necessary to establish learning objectives which are both reasonable and achievable. During the first visit, the educator should identify the needs and the specific objectives of each gestating or nonpregnant patient and, thus, establish a learning calendar which will enable each patient to participate fully. Furthermore, the educator should set down a number of indicators which can be evaluated to determine the success of the process. Depending on the degree of independence that the patient manages to obtain, the rhythm of the gestation follow-up schedule can be established with either more or fewer

visits. The ideal situation is one in which the pregnant patient has sufficient resources to make small adjustments to correct glycemic deviations, and to be able to identify when to go to the hospital or call the doctor when warning signs appear.

Despite the obvious needs to instill diabetic patients with autonomy in the daily control of the disease, the existence of inadequate education programs or the failure to implement such programs is a problem in general. More than half of the diabetic population receives little or no diabetology education. A national survey carried out in the USA in patients with diabetes Type 1, in insulin-dependent diabetes Type 2 patients, and in noninsulin-dependent diabetes Type 2 patients revealed that 41, 51, and 76% of them, respectively, had never taken a class, course or any other diabetology education-related program.[13]

It is not simply an issue of gestational diabetics not having sufficient resources to manage their metabolic changes, because this would be a limited problem moderated by the dysfunction and the short period of duration. A good number of diabetic adults clearly lack the skills associated with management of the disease, such as preparation of an adequate diet, adjusting the insulin dose, or making adequate compensation for occasional glycemic deviations. Hospitalization of patients with poor metabolic control is frequently attributed to their insufficient awareness of self-control. It is also more likely that such patients end up developing complications or requiring emergency services.

Deficits in training are not solely due to lack of awareness and skills; often an incomplete first educational stage has led the patient to make supposed 'deductions' or 'misunderstandings' and, over the passage of time, these have been assumed by the patient to be correct. Detection of these suppositions can be complex: they do not arise during the interview, but rather based on the suspicion that they do exist, the interviewer has to review in great detail all the knowledge that the patient should have. The types of errors that the patient has incorporated into the daily control can be wide-ranging, affecting the diet, such as its distribution and preparation, types of food containing carbohydrates and their approximate proportion, choosing food when eating out, as well as insulin-administering techniques and their effect, dosage errors, effects of exercise, etc. The task of correcting skills and knowledge is as difficult as that of identifying them, given that the patient is usually reluctant to accept that over an often prolonged period of time, he has been forming habits which were not only incorrect but also, at times, counterproductive. The educator should have sufficient communication and educational skills not only to explain the error but also to convince the patient that the analysis being carried out is appropriate and that the resulting change in attitude will have a positive effect on his own control.

An educational model will be effective depending on the extent of independence it gives the patient to participate effectively in the management of his disease. The time required for a complete educational process is usually greater than the gestational period; however, if it is a basic issue for an existing diabetic, then its importance is more relative for gestational diabetics. The specific objective for pregnancy should be clear. *For gestational diabetes*: be aware of the disease, know the basics so that it does not interfere with fetal development, in the medium- to long-term acquire healthy eating and lifestyle habits, and take a preventative and proactive approach towards Type 2 diabetes or gestational diabetes in a new pregnancy. *For existing diabetics*: detection of deficits or errors in the educational process to date, identify patient's degree of independence, evaluate degree of family support, increase their awareness and skills, facilitate the maximum degree of independence possible during pregnancy, in the medium to long term promote healthy attitudes, and adopt a stance of prevention of complications in a new pregnancy.

Guidelines of diabetes care and pregnancy: Hospital Maternal–Infantil Vall D'Hebron

The acquisition of knowledge and abilities on the part of the patient can be subdivided into three stages that are continuous and superimposed:

1. Informative stage
2. Training stage
3. Support stage

Informative stage

All the patients who go to a diabetes and gestation clinic should receive complete, clear and comprehensible information of the basic aspects related their illness. A patient should understand:

- What is happening
- What dangers she and her fetus may encounter
- Why complications can arise
- What treatment we propose and why

This means that the following should be explained:

- What diabetes is and the relationship it has with pregnancy
- The influence of diabetes in the course of the pregnancy:
  ◦ How diabetes influences the development of the fetus and neonates
  ◦ What long-term repercussions it can have for the patient and her baby
- What is the fundamental cause of the complications, and the relationship with the glycemia levels
- Why the diabetes must be treated during pregnancy, how it is treated, and the importance of the diet:
  ◦ What are the carbohydrates and what purpose do they serve
  ◦ What types of HCO there are, and which are forbidden and which are not
  ◦ Which are the fundamental rules that should be continued in a suitable diet: (a) the proportion of carbohydrates; (b) the number of meals/day; and (c) the preparation of the food

- The purpose of exercise
- What is the metabolic autocontrol and why it is important. How glycemia levels can be determined
- What is insulin and when it is used

If the patient is able to answer these sections clearly and concisely after the informative stage, we will have achieved half of the treatment. We will gain a faithful collaborator who will feel an active part of the therapeutic team. But to transmit this knowledge requires special ability. It does not require a great volume of information, rather the opposite. The information that is transmitted should be important, clear, concise, and suffcient.

Important

A patient cannot assimilate the entire importance of diabetes in half an hour, nor in 3 days. Only key points should be chosen for transmission, keeping in mind that the objective is to motivate the patient to follow the treatment. She should receive enough information so that she considers it important to remember it, but not so much as to worry her unnecessarily and magnify the risks, nor to disconcert her with a great number of figures or of secondary details.

Clear

The information must be made accessible for the patient, appropriate to her language and level of education. It serves no purpose to choose the fundamental points of the illness correctly if, later, an excessive amount of scientific language is used, with terms that are not comprehensible for those without any scientific training, or with tortuous rhetorical constructions, so that when concluding a sentence nobody can remember how it began. The chosen level should be the lowest in the group. Nobody is offended when simple words and short sentences are used, nor when they are spoken slowly, stressing those words that need to be highlighted. The opposite can occur where half the patients look bewildered, having lost the thread of the explanations some time beforehand. The educator should never forget that he/she speaks for them and not for a committee of experts.

Concise

The patient is not an expert in perinatology, and her notions of medicine can be very limited. It is very probable that most of what is said is unknown to her, and the amount learned is inversely proportional to the volume of new concepts supplied. It is relatively easy to remember three sentences, but very difficult to retain thirty. The educator should be able to synthesize and extract the basic points that are important for the patient to know.

Sufficient

The information cannot be broken into fragments, as this causes it to lose value. If how to follow a diet is well explained, but the justification is omitted, the most probable thing is that the patient will not follow it. What is the point in changing her routine if she has no clear reason for doing so?

On the other hand, the objective of the information is not its omission but its receipt and assimilation. Thus it may be appropriate to repeat the same arguments, or the same concepts with different arguments, as many times as necessary until the patient understands what is being explained.

Although the information can be transmitted in an individualized way, we prefer the interactive group, in which we include, weekly, all the patients in gestation that go to the clinic for the first time in their present pregnancy, whether diabetic or not. The group offers the advantages of acceptance, participation, and collaboration.

Acceptance

The patient is from the first moment with women in the same situation. This allows her to accept the process better. She does not have the sensation of being alone, or of being a strange case, but rather there is a reference group that shares the same problems. This normalizes the diabetes.

Participation

The group grants a certain degree of freedom and stimulus. A comment from one can suggest a question to another which spontaneously would not have occurred to her. What we would not sometimes think about because it is considered banal or inadequate is verbalized with more freedom if somebody has said something similar. It is easier to request a repetition of an explanation if it is seen that there is another person who has not understood than when the patient is alone in which case there are times she remains silent so as not to appear dumb. Individual 'embarrassment is diluted in the group.

Collaboration

The use of the knowledge and the experience of patients themselves – whether pregestational diabetics or women that have had gestational diabetes in previous pregnancies – allows reinforcement of the information that is given. If one knows how to channel their participation they become of the educator and their previous experience is a 'guarantee' that what is being said is true and what is requested is possible.

On the other hand, the inclusion of the pre-gestational diabetic in the group offers another possibility: to assess, without their having the sensation of being examined, the degree of previous diabetic education and to know which are the areas that need to be reinforced.

The reactions and the difficulties of the patients before the situation are sometimes linked to the diabetes type. The pregestational diabetic already has an idea about what diabetes involves and also regarding what is normal or abnormal as for glycemia, but her concepts do not always correspond to needs of the pregnancy. The fact that, frequently, figures of slightly high glycemia, are tolerated in the general diabetic population, causes certain patients to consider them normal and refuse later to accept the normoglycemia concept.

When gestation begins not only the illness is distorted in a way that frequently surprises the patient herself, but she should also understand that what she had considered as normal has ceased, so that levels of glucose that before were considered good are now unacceptable. That she understands that the euglycemia is fundamental during pregnancy is indispensable in the treatment process. In this sense the concept

of the fetus as patient is basic. The pregnant patient should understand that the increase of attention that is requested, the greater adjustment in the metabolic control, is designed to safeguard her son from feeling any consequences of the illness.

The gestational diabetic patient, on the other hand, is a woman that may not have had any contact with diabetes. She may feel well (she does not have an illness, or pain, or any negative symptom). She may have been told by her doctor that she has a metabolic problem that will last only for some months. The first effort is to ensure that the patients believes what is being said, and later accepts that, in order to treat the illness of which she is unaware, it is necessary for her to change her daily habits. This acceptance requires an effort that the therapeutic team should facilitate and value. Also, the patient receives a great deal of information that needs to be assimilated in a short period of time. Thus, she needs support from the medicine personnel who assist her.

In general, we could say that the gestational diabetic patient needs to receive a greater amount of new information, but that this is easier to transmit, because it is made on a clean base, from zero. Maybe it will entail an effort that she accepts the presence of metabolic dysfunction, but once she has made it she will not offer further resistance. While the pre-gestational diabetic patient can have sufficient knowledge, this should be reassessed and corrected. It is, on occasions, much more difficult to change an erroneous idea and requires greater effort and ability on the part of the educator than to establish a new one.

Training stage

The general ideas that have been expounded in the information stage should be transferred to each patient and adapted to her characteristics. If first it has been explained to a patient how to treat her diabetes, now the necessary instruments should be provided so that she can undertake the task. The key points are diet, metabolic control, and administration of insulin.

Diet

The patient needs to know how to:

- Check the degree of understanding of the written diet
- Calculate the quantity of foods
- Cook the various foods
- Carry out simple substitutions
- Calculate the diet if she eats out
- Adjust the diet if activities different to the habitual ones are carried out (evenings out, holiday periods, etc.)

Metabolic control

The patient needs to know about:

- The technique for obtaining capillary blood
- Reading of reactive ribbons of blood and urine
- How the reflectometer functions
  ○ Management and conservation
  ○ Most usual errors

- Registry of the values obtained in the diabetes notebook
- Other data that should be noted: diet excesses (transgressions), decrease in night rest, infections, etc.
- The situations when she should visit her doctor outside the usual regular appointment

Administration of insulin

The patient needs to know:

- The places for the administration of insulin
- The administration technique
- The types of insulin that will work
- Fundamental differences between them
- Metabolic objectives: which are the glycemic margins taken as normal
- How to proceed if the wrong dosage is administered.
- Precautions to take if insulin is administered (hypoglycemia prevention)
- How to act if faced with hypoglycemia

Instruction

The instruction on each one of these sections should be given as the patient needs it. The first two are general, while the third is reserved for the gestational diabetic patients that require insulin. In the case of the pregestational diabetics, this stage may not be training as much as confirmation that she has acquired the necessary skills.

As well as giving general information the group facilitates understanding and acceptance of the process, and the training should be carried out in a personalized way. Each pregnant patient has her own characteristics: habit schedules, family relations, work type, way of cooking, etc. The diet should adapt to these peculiarities, so that it accomplishes the objective but does not become an uncomfortable straitjacket that distorts the whole daily activity of patient.

The time that each woman requires to incorporate this knowledge is variable, depending on her learning capacity, previous notions, and stress level and, of course, the competence of the person who is training her. The patient always feels at a certain disadvantage with respect to the health personne they speak to her of her illness, they know it, they know more about her than she does herself if the health care provider is not capable of creating a relaxed and pleasant atmosphere, of mutual trust from the beginning, if the patient perceives by means of the language or the educator's attitude that she is too slow, or simply that she is in a hurry or indifferent because other patients need attention, the most probable thing is that she will say she has understood everything perfectly only to please the trainer or for shame that her ineptitude will be discovered. The time that each patient requires does not matter. The fundamental thing is that in the end she has acquired the necessary capacity and that she has progressed.

Also, if possible complications have been dealt with, it must be explained when she can expect them and how identify them at an early stage, so that she can go to the doctor's surgery before the situation becomes serious.

Obstetric self-control

The patient needs to be able to control fetal well-being and to know the usual fetal movements:

- What they mean and how they are controlled
- Why they can diminish
- How to act in this case

The patient should be made aware of the alarm signs:

- How to identify the contractions, and which are those that could be worrying
- What other symptoms should receive attention, when should the patient consult, and in what case should she go to the hospital emergency department

Each one of these informative sections should be given at the time in which it can be used by the patient or when she enters a specific risk situation.

Support stage

The attention has to also be personalized and maintained different intensity, according to the necessities, during the whole gestation.

During each visit the following should be checked:

- Suitability of the diet, solving possible errors
- Correction in the punction technique and in the collection of results
- Correct handling and administration of insulin
- Appropriate control of fetal movements

The patient's instruction is not finished until the moment of delivery. New situations can appear every day (a different food that causes an unexpected glycemic response, changes in the rhythm of fetal movements, etc.) and these may require explanation so that the patient understands what has happened and can act appropriately if the situation arises again. If in the two previous stages a bond has been established with the pregnant patient, the communication will be easy and the patient will not only quickly detect possible risky situations, but will also feel she participates in the treatment.

At this stage we can delegate to the patient herself, according to the degree of autonomy that has been reached:

- Modifications in the diet
- Adjustments in the dosage of insulin

It is an appropriate and effective policy to try to engage the patient to the maximum in her own control, making her perceive the importance of her role as part of the therapeutic team. This will diminish the degree of restlessness concerning the illness, will make her feel useful and in control of the situation, and will reduce the perception of discomfort from the treatment. The degree of delegation degree will depend on each patient, on her previous preparation, on the speed of understanding and learning, on the family and social support that is available to here. The assistance team should be willing to go as far as the patient can and want. For example, for women with good knowledge and appropriate capacity for decision-making, adjusments in the doses of insulin are made at home rather than during clinic visits: confirmation that her decisions have been correct can be made by phone. Changes in dosage or substantial variations in the diet are not the doctor's exclusive decisions but reasoned and shared, allowing greater participation of the patient as her level of autonomy is greater.

The assistance team must have enough preparation to be able to accept a relationship of collaboration and dialogue with the patient, what is much more difficult than to be shielded by the traditional doctor–patient or nurse–patient relationship. They should be able to listen to her and to respond appropriately to her needs. If the patient completes the treatment because she is ordered, she will do it only during the period in which she perceives the doctor's authority, but if she does it because she understands its function and agrees on its utility, she will prolong it. The whole time that is invested in education will be saved later, allowing the metabolic situation to remain stable and diminishing the incidence and the seriousness of the complications.

REFERENCES

1. American Diabetes Association. Third-party reimbursement for diabetes care, self-management education and supplies. Diabetes Care 2002; 25(suppl. 1): S134–5.
2. American Diabetes Association. National standards for diabetes self-management education. Diabetes Care 2002; 25(suppl. 1): S140–7.
3. American Association of Diabetes Educators. The scope of practice for diabetes educators and the standards of practice for diabetes educators. Diabetes Educ 2000; 26: 25–31.
4. Brown SL, Pope JF, Hunt AE, Tolman NM. Motivational strategies used by dietitians to counsel individuals with diabetes. Diabetes Educ 1998; 24: 313–8.
5. Clements S. Diabetes self-management education (technical review). Diabetes Care 1995; 18: 1204–14.
6. Glasgow RE. A practical model of diabetes management and education. Diabetes Care 1995; 18: 117–26.
7. Peyrot M, Rubon RR. Modeling the effect of diabetes education on glycemic control Diabetes Educ 1994; 20: 143–8.
8. Heins JM, Nord WR, Cameron M. Establishing and sustaining state-of the art diabetes education programs: research and recommendations. Diabetes Educ 1992; 18: 501–8.
9. Greene DS, Beaudin BP, Bryan JM. Addressing attitudes during diabetes education: suggestions from adult education. Diabetes Educ 1993; 19: 497–502.
10. Armstrong CL, Brown LP, York R, Robbins D, Swank A. From diagnosis to home management: nutritional considerations for women with gestational diabetes. Diabetes Educ 1991; 17: 455-9.
11. Rubin RR, Peyrot M, Saudek CD. Effect of diabetes education on self-care, metabolic control and emotional well-being. Diabetes Care 1989; 12: 673–9.
12. Padgett D, Mumford E, Hynes M, Carter R. Meta-analysis of the effects of educational and psychosocial interventions on the management of diabetes mellitus. J Clin Epidemiol 1988; 41: 1007–30.
13. Greenfield S, Kaplan SH, Ware Jr JE, Yano EM, Frank HJ. Patients' participation in medical care: effects on blood sugar control and quality of life in diabetes. J Gen Intern Med 1988; 3: 448–57.

57 Databases: A tool for quality management of diabetic pregnancies

Dina Pfeifer, Rony Chen and Moshe Hod

Introduction

Predicting the likelihood that databases will become an important instrument for medical quality improvement is at least as obvious as the prediction that a woman in labor will deliver. Databases are not a novelty. Although used by clinicians for only a century, there are earlier historical examples of simple types of database that served as a major engine of change and progress, displaying a convincing evidence of its usefulness over a respectable period of time.[1]

In most instances, the benefits of clinical databases have long been recognized. Formerly, data were stored in paper form, analysis meant calculation by hand or with a simple calculator, and statistical tables were used for accepting or rejecting hypothesis at defined levels of statistical significance.[2] In practice this has led to a restricted number of comparisons. Today we have databases, statistical and graphical packages, and comparisons between many variables and data sets are done with ease. Meta-analysis is becoming an increasingly popular method of comparing, combining and summarizing the outcomes of published studies, though provoking controversies at the same time. Some authors believe that meta-analysis may be as reliable as randomized controlled trials, whereas others believe that the technique should be used only to generate rather than test hypotheses.[3–5]

Database research is generally considered to be cheaper and faster than trials, but is weaker on research design. Such problems include incomplete data on the case mix, a lack of concurrent controls, and an inability to ascertain important outcomes or to identify the role of association among the multiple outcomes of interest.[6,7] While a lack of progress has partly been a consequence of a lack of interest on the part of clinicians, managers and researchers, it has also reflected the demanding requirements for creating high-quality databases.[8]

Database developments

Developments in computer technology and mass production of computer processors and other components have made computers and data-input devices affordable. The rapid development of newer and better equipment has made cutting-edge technology affordable even for low-income countries. In response to growing demand, the software market has become ultrasophisticated in addressing the vast range of user needs.

Various database architectures are in use. Database structures must be defined prior to data entry and are set as institutional administrative databases, clinical databases or national registries.[9] As a result, users of statistical techniques need no longer be concerned with the arithmetical and algebraic details of various statistical methods, and can concentrate instead on understanding the underlying ideas and basic principles of statistical analyses, and look into outcomes of the analysis.[10,11] The advantages of electronic databases include: minimal storage space, fast and accurate searches, ease of updating data, easy data management, merge of data from various sources, multiuser access, interactivity, networking, internet access, data presentation and reporting, and simple back-up.

When making a decision concerning which database software to use, care must be taken not to be unduly influenced by price and availability, but primarily by hardware capacity, software compatibility, programming requirements and technical expertise required. The analysis process frequently requires the simultaneous use of a number of complementary software packages. Therefore, the decision for software purchase should be established on the ability for the interface of various applications, the format in which the data are stored and simplicity of use.

Evidence-based medicine and databases

Evidence-based medicine integrates the best available data from clinical research into clinical practice to enhance the quality of decisions made, so achieving the best possible outcomes.[12–14] The precise role of evidence-based medicine is being widely debated in view of its applicability to individual patients. Continuous collation of data at the level of provision of medical services, though not being pure clinical research, as an alternative approach is considered closer to reality.[8] The advantages include high generalizability through the participation of a wider scale of health care providers, the ability to rapidly generate large samples, and the opportunity to study conditions and interventions.[8,15] However, practitioners have difficulty in finding, assessing, interpreting and applying current best evidence.

The importance of data comparison of institutional data is invaluable for increasing excellence through the Hawthorne effect. An example of this approach is the Obstetrical Quality Indicators and Datacollection (OBSQID) database of the World Health Organization's (WHO) Regional Office for Europe, which includes aggregated data on more than 14 million births in 43 countries and offers a forum for comparing obstetrical quality data at its internet site for either aggregated or case-based data (Figure 57.1).[16] In coordination with representatives of most participating institutions, the OBSQID project variables and coding were standardized, nevertheless mostly reflecting uniformity with clinical data already available. Thus, comparison of data was made possible and so increased the ability to effectively reuse data to produce further information of evidence-based medicine.

Despite of the wealth of available data, the issue of data quality should also be assessed. The incomplete data, limited detection of outcomes (e.g. maternal mortality 42 days after delivery, congenital malformations diagnosed after discharge), interrupted time series, coding accuracy and methods of data verification applied, are some of the problems encountered in the endeavor to maintain such regional databases. A substantial challenge of maintaining or improving obstetrical outcomes spins the process of comparing the data on more than initially agreed basic information. An increase of active participation of clinicians and researchers in designing other databases is increasingly emphasized and is applied to ensure meaningfulness and usefulness for the quality measurement.

Evidence or lack of it?

The St Vincent Declaration integrates a commitment to continuous quality improvement through routine measure of outcomes, benchmarking and consolidation of processes in diabetic care.[17,18] Since its proclamation in 1989, different types of diabetes databases, national registries, subregional and regional databases or other types of information systems, have been developed to meet objectives set in the declaration.[19–22] The process of continuous quality improvement demands not only the gathering of reliable and validated data, but also acting upon this data. Many standardization, logistical and legal problems have been encountered, and have subsequently led to a better understanding of the successful implementation of these databases.[23–25]

Diabetes in pregnancy is not a rare condition and represents a specific area of diabetes population management. When a decision has to be made about measures or treatments in women or neonates from such pregnancies, physicians face a dearth of comparative evidence. However, reproducibility of results is often limited and most risk estimates are based on uncontrolled observational studies. According to the St Vincent Declaration, the ultimate goal for the management of pregnancies complicated by diabetes should be a maternal or neonatal outcome approaching that of the nondiabetic population. Some of previously set databases (e.g. DIABCARE) and national registries collected data on diabetes in pregnancy, primarily Type 1 diabetes.[21] Yet there seems to be an appreciable gap between the obstetrical and perinatal information collected, and maternal diabetes-related data sets, preventing the necessary outcome of monitoring, benchmarking, and clinical auditing to monitor changes. The situation is particularly complex with respect to gestational diabetes.

Several multicenter studies have been undertaken in recent years to provide baseline data on the outcomes of diabetic pregnancies with respect to obstetrical interventions, dietary and treatment alternatives, subsequent short- and long-term effects on offsprings' morbidity and mortality, as well as development and progression of long-term diabetes complications during the course of pregnancy. Systematic review of the literature in order to find evidence of best practice reveals a scarcity of adequate information on obstetrical outcomes, decision-making, guidelines and protocols in relation to diabetes in pregnancy. To implement changes in the clinical practice an audit mech-anism should be initiated to continuously re-evaluate outcomes and practices. Strengthening epidemiological assessment has become an imperative strategy of diabetes surveillance and it is considered essential for quality management of diabetes in pregnancy too. The annual rate of pregnancies complicated by diabetes at an average maternity hospital is usually too small to be informative, making average data from several years necessary for analysis. Therefore, adverse effects may reflect performance in the past rather than the present.[14] Variations may be substantial to such a degree that it is impossible to assess its influence on real differences of an intervention or outcome. Because of small numbers or rare outcomes, the sample size is inadequate for statistical analysis, usually making comparisons between subgroups impossible.

Large patient samples and a broad origin of data is a clear benefit of multicenter study, however, great care should be taken in harmonization of methodology. Examples of national and international data collection tools of WHO Pan European Database on Diabetes in Pregnancy are presented in Figure 57.2 (aggregated data) and Figure 57.3 (case-based data). Case-based data can be merged with basic information related to obstetrical history, diagnoses and interventions (Figure 57.1) for detailed analysis of perinatal outcomes or with other databases containing data on metabolic control, dietary measures, diabetic complications, etc. Data and conclusions derived in such a way should be of a quality relevant for the institutions and applicable to the patients.[26]

Some cautions and concerns

Administrative and clinical databases are valuable assets which should be considered as evidence. However, the challenge

Draft

OBSQID Basic Information Sheet
SAMPLE - DO NOT USE

Mother

Case Identification Code

Residence Urban ○ Rural ○

Time to clinic (hours:minutes) [ ][ ] : [ ][ ]

Mother's Year of Birth 1 9 [ ][ ]

Single Yes ○ No ○

Education
University ○
Secondary ○
Primary ○
None ○

Reproductive History

Abortions
Spontaneous [ ]
Induced [ ]
Ectopic [ ]

Deliveries
Vaginal [ ]
Caesarean sections (CS) [ ]

Outcome
Number of live born [ ]
Number of stillborn [ ]
Number of preterm deliveries (<37 weeks) [ ]
Number of early neonatal deaths [ ]
Number of late neonatal deaths [ ]

Well-Being
Score on the WHO/EURO well-being scale
5 weeks before expected delivery [ ]
4 to 6 weeks after delivery [ ]
Violence during pregnancy   No ○ Yes ○

Present Pregnancy

Pregnancy
Height (cm) [ ][ ][ ]
First pre-natal visit (week) [ ][ ]
Weight (kg) at delivery [ ][ ][ ]
Weight gain (kg) [ ][ ]
Smoke No ○ 1-3 ○ >3 ○ Cigs. per day
Alcohol No ○ <=15 ○ >15 ○ g/day (15g =1 unit)
Drug abuse Yes ○ No ○

Ultrasound
Number of scannings [ ]
First scan (week) [ ]
Last scan (week) [ ]
Scan for malformations Yes ○ No ○
Multiple gestation detected (week) [ ]

Pathology
If "Yes", please specify   No ○ Yes ○

Threatened abortion [ ]
Threat premature labour [ ]
Antepartum haemorrhage (APH) [ ]
Gestational hypertension [ ]
Pre-eclampsia [ ]
Eclampsia [ ]
Placenta praevia [ ]
Placenta abruption [ ]

Yes
Suspected IUGR [ ]
IVF (ART) [ ]
Blood group immunization [ ]
Infection [ ]
Cardiovascular disease [ ]
Other (give ICD-10 Code) [ ][ ][ ].[ ]

IDDM before pregnancy [ ] } ⟹ { Preconceptional treatment [ ]
NIDDM before pregnancy [ ]   Vascular complications [ ]
Gestational diabetes [ ] If yes → Insulin treatment [ ]

Delivery

Onset
Induced ○
Spontaneous ○
Planned CS ○

Calculated date of delivery (dd-mm-yy) [ ][ ] - [ ][ ] - [ ][ ]
Based on LMP ○ US ○
Certain Yes ○ No ○

Birth
Spontaneous ○
Forceps ○
Vacuum extraction ○
Assisted breech ○
CS before labour
 Elective ○
 Acute ○
CS during labour
 Elective ○
 Acute ○

Attended by
Physician ○
Nurse/Midwife ○
Other ○
Unattended ○

Analgesics
None ○
Opioid [ ]
Inhalation [ ]
Regional [ ]
Other [ ]

Blood Transfusion
No Yes Units
Hb level ○ ○
HCT level ○ ○ [ ][ ]
Symptoms ○ ○

Anaesthesia
General [ ]
Epidural/Spinal [ ]
Pudendal [ ]
Other [ ]

Maternal Discharge
Home ○
Transferred ○
Dead ○
Days after delivery [ ]

Date of delivery (dd-mm-yy) [ ][ ] - [ ][ ] - [ ][ ]

Special Condition
If "Yes", please specify   No ○ Yes ○
Rupture of membrane > 24h [ ]
Episiotomy [ ]
Lacerations [ ]
Hysterectomy < 48h [ ]
Retained placenta [ ]
Bleeding > 1000 ml [ ]
Shoulder dystocia [ ]
Other (give ICD-10 code) O [ ][ ].[ ]

Infant

General
Infant number (multiple gestation) [ ] of [ ]
Sex Male ○ Female ○
Birthweight [ ][ ][ ][ ] g
Length [ ][ ] cm
Head circum. [ ][ ] cm
Cord-blood pH at delivery [ ].[ ][ ]
Artery ○ Vein ○ Unknown ○

Apgar
at 1 minute [ ]
at 5 minutes [ ]

Feeding
No Yes
Breastfeeding in delivery room ○ ○
Breast milk only ○
Infant formula ○
Formula and breast milk ○

Pathology
If "Yes", please specify   No ○ Yes ○
RDS/Hyaline membrane [ ]
Other respiratory conditions [ ]
Seizure within 7 days [ ]
Congenital malformations (ICD-10 Code) Q [ ][ ]
Breech presentation at delivery [ ]
Transverse lie at delivery [ ]
Hyperbilirubinaemia [ ]
Sepsis [ ]
Other (including infections) (ICD-10 Code) P [ ][ ].[ ]

Cause of Death
Congenital malformations [ ]
Pregnancy-related disorders [ ]
Birth asphyxia/trauma [ ]
Immaturity-related disorder [ ]
Infection [ ]
Other [ ]

Discharge
Home ○
Transferred ○

Death Prenatal ○ Intranatal ○ Postnatal ○
Days after delivery [ ]

Filled in by [   ]   Revision 1 Apr 1998

Figure 57.1   OBSQID Basic information sheet.

OBSQID Perinatal Aggregated Data - Diabetes (DPAD)

Draft

WHO ID number or country acronym

Year
- ○ 1999
- ○ 2000
- ○ 2001

Data Level
- ○ National   ○ Regional   ○ Local

Location (if regional/local)

Women who gave birth (all deliveries)

Infants born (all births)

A

Women with pre-gestational diabetes mellitus

IDDM   NIDDM

IGT   MODY

Women with vascular complications

Retinopathy   Nephropathy

Deterioration

Retinopathy   Nephropathy

Pre-pregnancy counselling/care

HbA1C >8%
1 trimester

3 trimester

B **Women with**

... GDM

... persisting DM post delivery

... persisting IGT post delivery

Treated with insulin

Post partum evaluation

		Induced	Spontaneous	Total	**A: Pre-GDM**	**B: GDM**
1. *Abortions						
2. Intrauterine deaths (22–27 completed weeks)						
3. Antenatal deaths (>27 completed weeks)						
Total antenatal deaths if 2/3 not available						
4. Fetal deaths during delivery						

Figure 57.2 OBSQID Aggregated data sheet for pregnancies complicated by diabetes.

Draft

	A: Pre-GDM	**B: GDM**
5. Preterm births (<32 completed weeks)		
6. Preterm birth (32–36 completed weeks)		
7. Labour induced		
8. Caesarean sections		
9. Forceps/vacuum extractions		
11. Early neonatal death (0–6 days)		
12. Late neonatal death (7–27 days)		
Total neonatal deaths if 11/12 not available		
13. Maternal PIH/PET		
14. Eclampsia (during pregnancy – 10 days after delivery)		
15. Macrosomia (>4000 g)		
16. Shoulder dystocia		
17. Apgar <=6 @ 5 minutes (>31 completed weeks)		
18. Major congenital malformations		
19. Infants with RDS		
22. Neonatal admissions to NICU		

Enter all data as absolute numbers.
Avoid leading zeros.
Where data are unavailable please leave
the field blank.

Filled in by

Date

Name

Address

Revision 17 Sep 1999

Figure 57.2   cont'd

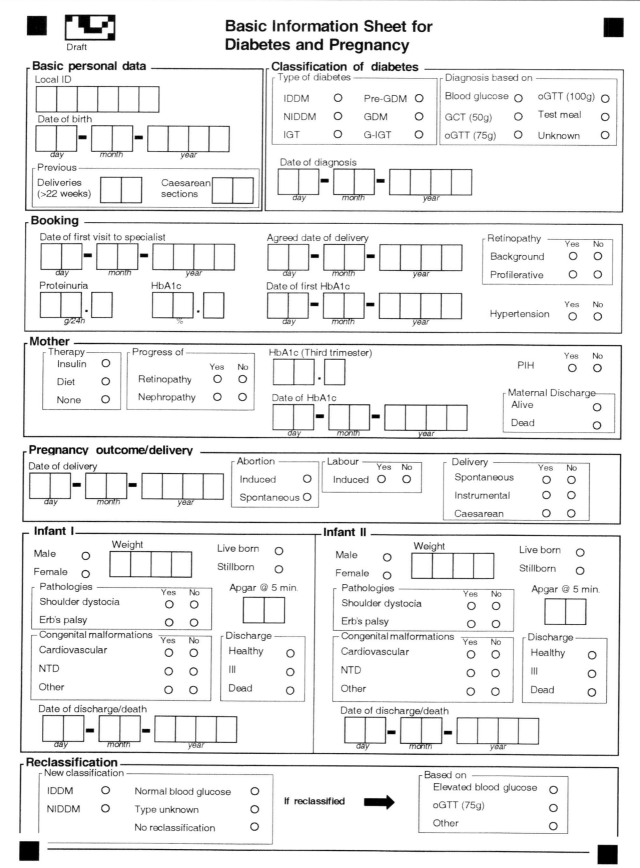

Figure 57.3   OBSQID Case based data collection sheet for pregnancies complicated by diabetes.

remains to identify means by which various data can be collated from disparate sources into a single structure and used effectively. Frequently, diabetes- and pregnancy-related data are stored in several databases of unequal design. Attempts to successfully merge data sets, avoiding unrealistic assumptions and oversimplifications, should be done in a systematic fashion, with special consideration to consistency and validity of underlying data.

Databases are technologically sophisticated, complex, and fascinating objects. When creating a database the objective of establishing it should be clear and not affected by architecture or functional characteristics. Limitations and potentially negative consequences of database use for quality improvement should be questioned early in the process. Dealing with these challenges will probably turn out to be at least as important to the implementation and full effectiveness of databases as the technical side of the effort.[1] New statistical methods are required to analyse raw data from large databases, as traditional statistical methods using models that adjust for covariates do not eliminate biases. In fact, inherent biases are magnified, not minimized, by large databases.[10,27] Furthermore, an overlooked problem is that an overwhelming number of feasible comparisons show some results to be statistically significantly simply by chance.[2,28]

Databases will not help directly any individual patient with the management of his or her condition. Rather, they will be tools in the development of new or improved methods of achieving better health, prediction, diagnoses and treatment of disease, and in establishing more cost-efficient ways of operating health services.[29] However, the results are often of uncertain generalizability, as they tend to be carried out in atypical settings. It is difficult to make adjustments in complex case-mix conditions, as databases usually contain minimal set of variables.

Once a database is established it should be run for an extended period of time to provide an overview of the epidemiological situation. Although some flexibility is beneficial, a basic variable set should be kept fixed to allow for comparisons and a minimal data set should be defined. Funding to run the service should be secured, feedback to the contributors must occur at regular intervals and, if on-line access is granted, the database should be updated regularly. Contributions to the database should be seen as part of ongoing work and so considered as highly beneficial.

Due to dangers inherent in modern technology, every care should be taken to improve the security of data, control of its dissemination and the potential for abuse minimized.

Legal and ethical issues are clearly important, and are relevant to international conventions and policies concerned with human rights.[30,31] European legislation is not entirely clear on the issues of keeping case-based data in registers, the need for consent and how to consider aggregated databases.[23]

According to European Directive 95/46,[32] informed consent is necessary if personal data are to be used for purposes other than those for which they were originally gathered, but consent is not required if the data are not personal.[31] The public is sensitized to the potential for breaches of privacy. Many acknowledge the fundamental need for privacy, but only a few recognize that there may be circumstances under which the benefits to the public outweigh the cost of some limited loss of privacy. To get a pertinent snapshot of an epidemiological situation, data collection needs to be universal, i.e. population based. If patients refuse consent to their details being stored in registries then the epidemiological picture of the disease would be distorted.

Conclusions

It may seem difficult and cumbersome to establish an epidemiological surveillance system for diabetes in pregnancy. In fact, it is a matter of organizing available data rather than searching for new data-collection mechanisms, and extending use of the database to the epidemiological dimension. An epidemiological surveillance system could be attained by provision of routinely collected and aggregated data by centers providing obstetrical and neonatal care for pregnant diabetics and their infants. If diabetes and pregnancy is considered a public health issue, it is strongly recommended that epidemiological models should be further developed and implemented at various levels of services to provide data for the dimensioning of the current and future diabetes care systems.[33] Benefits of the surveillance system should be clearly articulated: (1) utilization of perinatal performance indicators related to a subset of diabetic pregnancies in situation analysis, and for comparison with the general population; (2) benchmarking to aid target setting; (3) identification of areas of particular concern in terms of the need for improved management; (4) forecasting of trends in gestational diabetes prevalence; and (5) implementation of the St Vincent Declaration. Critical attention should be given to database design, data sources and their validity, methodologies and interpretation of findings, and the implications for clinical practice.

REFERENCES

1. Davidoff F. Databases in the next millennium. Ann Intern Med 1997; 127: 770–4.
2. Egberts J. Databases and the statistical usage of (perinatal) results. Am J Obstet Gynecol 1998; 178: 192.
3. Moher D, Cook DJ, Eastwood S, et al. Improving the quality of reports of meta-analyses of randomised controlled trials: the QUOROM statement. QUOROM Group. Br J Surg 2000; 87: 1448–54.
4. Stroup DF, Berlin JA, Morton SC, et al. Meta-analysis of observational studies in epidemiology: a proposal for reporting. Meta-analysis of observational studies in epidemiology (MOOSE) group. J Am Med Assoc 2000; 283: 2008–12.
5. Olkin I. Meta-analysis: reconciling the results of independent studies. Stat Med 1995; 14: 457–72.
6. Smith DM. Database research: is happiness a humongous database? Ann Intern Med 1997; 127: 725.
7. Imamura K, McKinnon M, Middleton R, Black N. Reliability of a comorbidity measure: the Index of Co-Existent Disease (ICED). J Clin Epidemiol 1997; 50: 1011–6.
8. Black N. Developing high quality clinical databases. Br Med J 1997; 315: 381–2.
9. Iezzoni LI. Assessing quality using administrative data. Ann Intern Med 1997; 127: 666–74.

10. Katz BP. Biostatistics to improve the power of large databases. Ann Intern Med 1997; 127: 769.
11. Beck JS, Brown RA. Medical Statistics on Personal Computers, 2nd edn. London: BMJ Publishing Group; 1995.
12. Knottnerus JA, Dinant GJ. Medicine based evidence, a prerequisite for evidence based medicine. Br Med J 1997; 315: 1109–10.
13. Olatunbosun OA, Edouard L. The teaching of evidence-based reproductive health in developing countries. Int J Gynaecol Obstet 1997; 56: 171–6.
14. Sheldon T. Promoting health care quality: what role performance indicators? Qual Assur Health Care 1998; 7 (suppl.): S456–50.
15. Black N. A regional computerised surgical audit project. Qual Assur Health Care 1990; 2: 263–70.
16. World Health Organization, Regional Office for Europe, Quality of Care and Technologies. Copenhagen: WHO; 2000. http://qct.who.dk
17. World Health Organization and International Diabetes Federation. Diabetes care and research in Europe: the Saint Vincent declaration. Diabet Med 1990; 7: 360.
18. Dunne F, Brydon P, Proffitt M, et al. Approaching St Vincent. Working toward the St Vincent targets. Diabet Med 2001; 18: 333–4.
19. Piwernetz K, Benedetti MM, Johansen KS. Advanced health care initiatives in Europe on quality development, epidemiology and medical documentation. Diabete Metab 1993; 19: 213–7.
20. Palmer AJ, Brandt A, Gozzoli V, et al. Outline of a diabetes disease management model: principles and applications. Diabetes Res Clin Pract 2000; 50(suppl. 3): S47–S56.
21. Alexander W, Bradshaw C, Gadsby R, et al. An approach to manageable datasets in diabetes care. Br Diabetic Assoc Diabet Med 1994; 11: 806–10.
22. Henrichs HR, Piwernetz K, Sonksen PH, et al. The feedback between monitoring and improvement of quality of diabetes care. Diabete Metab 1993; 19: 70–3.
23. Vaughan NJ, Massi Benedetti M. A review of European experience with aggregated diabetes databases in the delivery of quality care to establish a future vision of their structure and role. Diabetes Nutr Metab–Clin Exp 2001; 14: 86–7.
24. Bloomgarden ZT. Computers in diabetes. Diabetes Care 1997; 20: 457–9.
25. Buxton C, Gibby O, Hall M, et al. Diabetes information systems: a key to improving the quality of diabetes care. Diabet Med 1996; 13(suppl. 4): S122–8.
26. Johansen KS, Hod M. Quality development in perinatal care – the OBSQID project. Int J Obstet Gynecol 1999; 64: 167–72.
27. Byar DP. Problems with using observational databases to compare treatments. Stat Med 1991; 10: 663–6.
28. Bland JM, Altman DG. Multiple significance tests: the Bonferroni method. Br Med J 1995; 310: 170.
29. Council of Europe Steering Committee on Bioethics. The Icelandic Act on a Health Sector Database and Council of Europe Conventions. Strasbourg: Ministry of Health and Social Security; 1999.
30. Lazaridis EN. Database standardization, linkage, and the protection of privacy. Ann Intern Med 1997; 127: 696.
31. Morrow JI. Data protection and patients' consent. Informed consent should be sought before data are used by registries. Br Med J 2001; 322: 549–50.
32. European Parliament. Directive on the Protection of Individuals with Regard to the Processing of Personal Data. European Parliament: Brussels; 1995.
33. Glasgow RE, Wagner EH, Kaplan RM, et al. If diabetes is a public health problem, why not treat it as one? A population-based approach to chronic illness. Ann Behav Med 1999; 21: 159–70.

58 Introduction to technological disease-management tools and eHealth networks: The future of better care delivery in diabetes and pregnancy

Moshe Hod, Linda Harnevo and Yossef Bahagon

Introduction

Technologies are now playing an increasing role in presenting physicians with new information on which to base their diagnosis and treatment. The EuHealthNet project aims at building a technology platform to enable integration of healthcare knowledge, patient specific clinical data and data from monitoring devices both at the individual patient level and at the public health level.

Objectives are:

(i) Integrating *vertical data* of an individual patient into a *comprehensive*-personal health record;

(ii) *Anytime, anywhere access* to full patient health records

(iii) Improving *quality of care*, through Decision Support Systems

(iv) *Optimizing clinical workflow efficiency* – in particular, the day-to-day quality of life of patients with chronic diseases.

The St Vincent Declaration integrates a commitment to continuous quality improvement through routine measure of outcomes, benchmarking and consolidation of processes in diabetic care. Since its proclamation in 1989, different types of diabetes databases, national registries, subregional and regional databases or other types of information systems, have been developed to meet objectives set in the declaration. Diabetes in pregnancy is not a rare condition and represents a specific area of diabetes population management. When a decision has to be made about measures or treatments in women or neonates from such pregnancies, physicians face dearth of comparative evidence, reproducibility of results is often limited and most risk estimates are based on uncontrolled observational studies.

Recent national audits demonstrate that the goal of the St Vincent Declaration is far from being met in nonselected, geographically based populations, without uniform management guidelines of diabetic pregnancies. Infants of women with pregestational diabetes still have a 4- to 6-fold increased risk of PNM and higher risk for major congenital anomalies. It should be said that these large-scale national population based studies performed over the past years in England, France, Denmark, Scotland, and the Netherlands include in their statistics nonspecialist units inexperienced and ill-equipped in treating diabetic pregnancies.

There is no doubt that specialist centers with substantial skills in the care of diabetic pregnancies may achieve outcomes that come within reach of the St Vincent Declaration. As today, while no more than 30–50% of the pre-GDM pregnancies are planned or undergoing pre-pregnancy counselling, and achievement of desired level of glycemic control is achieved in no more than 50% of the patients, the aim of the St Vincent declaration seems remote from accomplishment. We must be honest and ask ourselves, is the aim of the St Vincent declaration unapproachable? It may be, that establishing national/international-based registry programs for all women with pre-gestational diabetes will identify those who want to conceive, thus, enabling the foundation of pre-pregnancy consultation programs. Desired level of glycemic control can be achieved by the use of technologies such as combination of glucose sensors and insulin pumps ('closing the loop') and the use of personal health record (PHR) with integrated clinical decision support (CDS) systems. These in turn could lead to improved perinatal outcome.

The following chapter has two aims: to introduce recent innovations in the field of medical informatics and its potential application to the management of diabetic pregnancy and to present the 'EuHealthNet' Pan European project implemented in diabetes and pregnancy.

Introduction to health care informatics

In order to appreciate the impact that eHealth networks and the implementation of disease management tools have in improving the outcome and treatment of any particular medical situation (especially in this chapter, in diabetes and pregnancy) it is essential to have a solid background in medical informatics and its evolution in the recent years. Thus, we introduce the reader to these recent innovations and their application to the management of diabetic pregnancy. This introduction will review the following subjects:

- Introduction to medical informatics
- A future scenario
- The patient health record (PHR)
- Health care communication informatics
- Evidence-based medicine(EBM)
- Clinical decision support systems (CDSS)
- IT and database developments, including the EuHealthNet

Health care is an information-based science. Much of clinical practice involves gathering, synthesizing, and acting on information. Biomedical informatics is the scientific field dealing with biomedical information, data and knowledge – their storage, retrieval, and optimal use for problem solving and decision-making. It accordingly touches on all basic and applied fields in biomedical science and is closely tied to modern information technologies, notably in the areas of computing and communication.[1] The field emerged in the last few years as a merger of several distinct scientific disciplines, among them structural biology, statistical genetics, genomics-oriented computer science, biochemical kinetics analysis and medical informatics. The ability to creatively integrate and expand results from a variety of highly complex, multidisciplinary and information resources, holds a great challenge with a true benefit in means of quality of decision making. It is all about sculpturing medical information in a way that floods an insight not seen otherwise.

In an article by Kukafka et al. Shortliffe describes four categories of biomedical informatics and their respective foci from the cell to the population: bioinformatics, imaging informatics, clinical informatics and public health informatics. Clinical informatics is the scientific discipline that aims to enhance human health by developing novel information technology, computer science and knowledge management methodologies to prevent disease, deliver more efficient and safer patient care, increase the effectiveness of translational research, improve knowledge access and facilitate technology-enhanced education.[2]

One of the most studied and developed domains in the field of clinical informatics are applications directed at improving patient safety and preventing medical error. The growing sophistication of computers and software allows information technology to play a vital part in reducing that risk – by streamlining care, improving communication, increasing access to knowledge, assisting with decisions, catching and correcting errors and providing feedback on performance.[3]

From the financial point of view, a 2005 RAND research highlight, which summarized several health research publications, concluded that, properly implemented and widely adopted, health information technology (HIT) would save money and significantly improve health care quality. HIT includes a variety of integrated data sources, including electronic medical records, decision support systems, computerized physician order entry for medications etc. Large overall savings were found compared with costs. Annual savings in US from efficiency alone could be $77 billion or more. Health and safety benefits could double the savings while reducing illness and prolonging life. The study proposed a range of policy options that could be used to speed the development of HIT benefits: 'Our findings strongly suggest that it is time for government and other payers to aggressively promote the adoption of effective Health Information Technology.'[4]

In the last few years the field of medical informatics has gained significant governmental, institutional and initiators attention both in the US and Europe.

Office of the National Coordinator for Health IT

The Office of the National Coordinator (ONC) for Health IT in the US was founded in 2004. The ONC's task is to coordinate the development and integration of IT in the health care sector. Quotes from the ONC's Statement of Principles:

> The Benefits Health IT Can Bring to Our Nation – Fewer Mistakes, Lower Costs, Less Hassle, Better Care ... Health care IT investment is critical to US economy. Investment in IT should be a top priority ... Federal government should use its purchasing power to spur health care IT adoption, and the private sector should collaborate with the government to encourage technology use in health care since the benefits of health care IT clearly outweigh the costs.

Agency for Health care Research and Quality

The Agency for Health care Research and Quality (AHRQ) is the main federal agency charged with the improvement of the quality, safety and efficiency of Health care services. As the AHRQ stated in its 2007 budget request:

> Emerging information about ambulatory care suggests that the patient safety crisis in hospitals is only the tip of the iceberg ... There is a desperate need for better information sharing availability at the point-of-care

European Commission eHealth Action plan for Europe 2004–2010

The 2004 EPSCO Health Council issued a report that comprises the European Commission eHealth Action plan for Europe 2004–2010. The action plan includes a sequential set of actions to be taken by EU member states and the Commission over the period 2004–2010 in three target areas:

- Common challenges, including setting national roadmaps for e-Health, deploying e-Health systems and health information network, setting targets for interoperability, the use of electronic health records and clarification of legal framework
- Pilot actions accelerating implementation of e-Health e.g. tele-consultation, e-prescription, e-referral, tele monitoring and tele-care
- Evaluation, confirmation of benefits and dissemination of best practices: 'The main objectives of the action plan are to improve access and boost quality and effectiveness of eHealth services offered in Europe, and enhance the European eHealth industry by making eHealth systems and services more interoperable and integrated.'

Individual e-Health sites

A recently published public report by Stroetmann et al. evaluated ten individual e-Health sites using methods developed by the EU eHealth Impact project. The study showed that across a wide range of eHealth applications clear evidence can be found of the benefits of information and communication technologies in routine health care settings. These benefits range from improvements in quality, safety, costs, efficiency and better access to care: 'The eHealth Impact project conclusively demonstrated that there is over a 2:1 ratio between economic benefits and costs.'[5]

The lack of current or comprehensive information on the legal implications of using many types of eHealth applications is well known. The EU 2004 e-Health Action Plan states that by 2009 the 'legally eHealth' European Commission will have defined a 'framework for greater legal certainty of e-Health products and services liability within the context of existing product liability legislation.' The lack of such a framework is not confined to the EU. The main aims of the project, which reports in 2007, are to analyze the existing EU eHealth legal framework, develop an accessible knowledge base on legal and regulatory aspects of eHealth, develop a series of case studies to explore and elucidate the practical implications of the identified legislative issues in the use of eHealth, and to make recommendations to meet any legislative and regulatory needs.

One major impediment to adoption is the fear that e-health technology will only add to physicians already demanding workload. Usability factors will determine implementation since many physicians find that the time commitment involved in learning and using computers is too great, resulting in additional stress.[6] A concern also exists that e-health may also exacerbate inequities in health care due to socioeconomic inequities in Internet access.[7,8]

A future scenario

BA is a 53-year old woman. Upon her weekly log in to her personal health record (PHR) she notices that the 'health maintenance' label, in the lower corner of the screen, is flashing. BA clicks on it and sees a message that 2 years have passed since her last mammogram and the system recommends her to get a mammogram. BA thinks she has recently had one and is not sure she needs it. She clicks on the message and it changes to a view of all of her mammograms over the past 5 years. It appears the system is correct; she does indeed need a mammogram. By clicking on the message for the new mammogram she is able to send an electronic message to the radiology department at her local hospital and confirm an appointment for her mammogram next week. Using her PHRs built-in Google search engine, with its pre-defined medical search algorithm, BA 'Googles' pre-appraised high quality information regarding new methods of diagnosing breast cancer. She is particularly impressed with a short video that shows a world-renowned breast cancer specialist discussing the importance of mammogram and the overall great outcomes for patients with early stage disease. Armed with this information she feels much more a part of her health care experience and she arrives right on time for her mammogram appointment.

On her last visit at her primary care physician's office, BA had given him a passkey to log in to her PHR. Back at his office, BA's primary care provider, Doctor Smith is reviewing results in his electronic health record system. Doctor Smith's office houses no books or patient charts. Patient specific evidence-based medical information and best practices are delivered instantaneously, on request from leading web resources directly to the electronic health record (EHR). Patient medical information, such as records from emergency department visits and hospitalizations appears on Doctor Smith's e-mail inbox and are transferred to the EHR transparently. Doctor Smith gets a quick note from the PHR indicating that BA has accepted a recommendation to get a mammogram and scheduled the test. A week later, Doctor Smith gets a note in the EHR from radiology indicating that BA's study has come back positive. He is able to click on the message and review the latest treatment guidelines and prognosis information for breast cancer and prepare himself for the difficult phone call with BA. Doctor Smith schedules BA for a needle localization biopsy and 2 weeks later, he reviews the results on the phone with a surgeon. BA has cancer, but it is early stage and the prognosis should be very good. Doctor Smith has another difficult phone call with BA, but BA is grateful that the cancer has been diagnosed early and that she stands a very good chance of cure. Doctor Smith suggests that video recordings of patients with a similar diagnosis that can be accessed through the PHR might be helpful for BA. At the end of the phone call, BA has an appointment with an oncologist and scheduling information has been conveyed over the phone and sent to her PHR. Prior to her visit with the oncologist, BA logs onto her PHR and fills out several forms with personal questions about her treatment. She is pleased to see that she is being asked sensitively about her religious beliefs and practices including her approach to blood products and her desire to seek aggressive treatments for her cancer should that be necessary. She submits all of the responses and arrives at the oncologist's office prepared for the discussion that will ensue. She has already read on the PHR about some of the treatments that she will discuss with the oncologist and the visit goes very well. The oncologist and BA decide on a treatment plan that involves radiation, chemotherapy, and surgery. It is an aggressive strategy, but the oncologist explains that this is in part due to a risky genetic profile uncovered in the many blood tests that BA has had so far. He is able to pull up the genetic profile via the EHR in the office, display it and show BA how her risk changes based on the profile. Given the fact that BA has expressed a desire to be very aggressive about her treatment in the electronic forms, the oncologist is able to further support this approach. He even recommends that BA's three sisters have genetic screening and more frequent mammograms. Since two of them are already signed up for the PHR, the oncologist is able to transmit summary recommendations to their profiles based on this information. The oncologist finishes his day by submitting a treatment plan to the inpatient system via the EHR. At one point, he accidentally orders chemotherapy mixed in saline when it should be mixed in dextrose solution. The EHR quickly fires a pop-up window pointing out the error and then goes on to assist him in calculating the best doses of chemotherapy to treat BA's cancer given her genetic risk profile, weight and kidney function. BA is admitted to the hospital exactly five weeks from the moment that she first clicked on the link describing the need to get a mammogram. BA's world is the future. The high quality, rich information and common-sense efficiency inherent in BA's care are all within our grasp. In fact, we have seen similar and even greater transformations in equally complex sectors.[9]

Personal health record (PHR)

'The focus of the 21st-century health care system must be the patient.'[10] In 1998, an international group of lay people and health professionals met to envision a more patient friendly health care system, one created 'through the patient's eyes.' They agreed quickly on a guiding principle: 'Nothing about me without me.'[11] Over the past several years, there has been a remarkable upsurge in activity promoting the adoption of electronic health records (EHRs). By contrast, personal health record (PHR) systems have not received the same level of attention. Most consumers and patients receive care from many health care providers, and consequently their health data are dispersed over many facilities' paper- and EHR-based record systems.[12] A fragmented system of storing and retrieving essential patient data impedes optimal care. PHRs are:

> electronic application(s) through which individuals can maintain and manage their health information (and that of others for whom they are authorized) in a private, secure, and confidential environment.[13]

The essence of PHRs is being consumer-patient focused hence empowering patients by allowing them to be involved and responsible for their own health status and health care decisions, i.e. promote preventive and chronic diseases self-care. PHR core benefits include improving patient satisfaction, improving patient health data validity and quality control,

supporting patient safety initiatives, supporting patient and health services mobility, cooperation and shared care and providing ready access to emergency patient data. Figure 58.1 shows an example of a PHR.

PHRs have been under development since the mid to late 1990s. The Markle Foundation Connecting for Health Initiative, a public–private endeavor working toward an interoperable health information infrastructure, provides the following PHR definition:

> The Personal Health Record (PHR) is an Internet-based set of tools that allows people to access and coordinate their lifelong health information and make appropriate parts of it available to those who need it. PHRs offer an integrated and comprehensive view of health information, including information people generate themselves such as symptoms and medication use, information from doctors such as diagnoses and test results, and information from their pharmacies and insurance companies. Individuals access their PHRs via the Internet, using state-of-the-art security and privacy controls, at any time and from any location. Family members, doctors or school nurses can see portions of a PHR when necessary and emergency room staff can retrieve vital information from it in a crisis. People can use their PHR as a communications hub: to send e-mail to doctors, transfer information to specialists; receive test results and access online self-help tools. PHR connects each of us to the incredible potential of modern health care and gives us control over our own information.[14]

Online PHRs are seen as offering portability, interoperability and security, and help meet many Western governments' aims of personalizing care and increasing patient participation in the way decisions are made regarding their care. Equally important, they can be a substrate for anonymous population-based research based upon grouping of patients by diagnoses and clinical risk strata. Clinical data collection targeting implementation of quality indicators, such as the Pan-European Obstetrical Quality Indicators (OBSQID) project, that aims at continuous promotion of best perinatal practices, could be greatly facilitated by information gathered anonymously from PHRs of specific patient populations.

PHRs are coming close to the top of the health care technology agenda in many countries. In the US they form a significant part of the government's national health IT strategy and have been implemented by various regional and local health care systems and providers. In July 2006 the American Health Information Management Association (AHIMA) demonstrated its advocacy for the empowerment of individuals to manage their health care by issuing a joint Position Statement for Consumers of Health Care on the Value of Personal Health Records with the American Medical Informatics Association (AMIA).

> Using a PHR will help people make better health decisions and improves quality of care by allowing them to access and use information needed to communicate effectively with others about their health care.

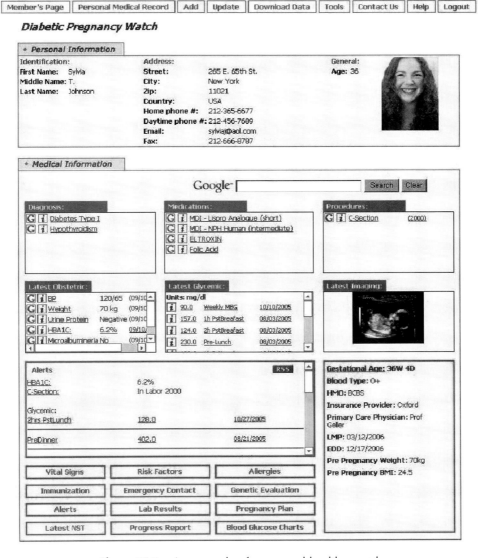

Figure 58.1   An example of a personal health record.

In Europe, PHRs are being developed by various national health information technology programmes e.g. in France and England.

Endsley et al. have identified three types of PHR that have been developed in recent years: a provider-owned and provider-maintained digital summary of clinically relevant health information made available to patients, a patient-owned software program that lets individuals enter, organize and retrieve their own health information and that captures the patient's concerns, problems, symptoms, emergency contact information, etc. and a portable, interoperable digital file in which selected, clinically relevant health data can be managed, secured and transferred. Platforms for portable PHRs include smart cards, personal digital assistants, cellular phones and USB-compatible devices that can be plugged into almost any computer.[15]

One of the most evident scenarios in which PHR can play a vital role is the case of the obstetrical follow-up. Obstetrics is an ideal speciality for implantation and evaluation of a PHR.

It is a well-defined field with a relatively standard course of care for a common condition, and it focuses on events that occur over a set interval of time lasting approximately 10 months (including postpartum care). Communication among patients and providers is a key element in ensuring quality of care, because all patients have their care transferred from outpatient to inpatient settings and back being cared for by different providers. PHR can improve communication among an antepartum unit, the outpatient office and the labor floor, i.e. the availability of important data such as the most recent blood pressures measured in the primary physician clinic is vital to the care of a patient suspected of having pre-eclampsia. Another example is the crucial roll of the tight follow-up needed for pregnant women with diabetes. 2004 marks the 15th anniversary of the St Vincent declaration and cumulative data indicate that pregnancy outcome remains poor among women with diabetes, even in top-rated medical centers throughout western Europe. Several published European studies revealed an undesirably high rate of both perinatal mortality and malformations. PHR has the potential to play major role in intensifying management in diabetic pregnancies. A tight follow-up and care could lead to a significant reduction of prenatal morbidity and mortality in pregnancies complicated by diabetes, by preventing both the excessive congenital anomaly rate and the reducing metabolic complications.

Beyond improving the quality of care for prenatal patients, given that obstetrics is a large contributor to the current malpractice crisis, PHR and its accompanying decision support tools could potentially mitigate medicolegal risks. It is quite possible that the costs of implementing such a system might be offset by reduced malpractice claims. Consider a patient who had an ultrasound examination the day before presenting in labor that suggests that her fetus may be macrosomic. The provider who does not have access to this report runs a greater risk of encountering a bad newborn outcome than a provider who has immediate access to that ultrasound report.

Personal health record systems are more than just static repositories for patient data; they combine data, knowledge, and software tools, which help patients to become active participants in their own care. When PHRs are integrated with electronic health record systems, they provide greater benefits than would stand-alone systems for consumers.[16]

While PHRs have many potential benefits to patients, caregivers, and institutions, the supporting evidence of specific benefits and the business case for PHR adoption are limited. Furthermore, the technology supporting PHRs is still evolving. As with EHR adoption, the impediments to PHR adoption are not limited to technical ones. Issues regarding PHRs concept and adoption include: security and confidentiality, accuracy of data, integration with other electronic patient data systems used by health professionals, ownership of data, extent of shareability of data across systems and across borders, back-up issues in case of loss of data stored on USB devices, and funding issues.

Widespread adoption and use of PHRs will not occur unless they provide perceptible value to users, easy to learn and use, and have associated costs (both financial and effort) that are easily justified related to the PHRs perceived value.

Health care communication informatics

Informatics is poised to have a major impact in patient–clinician communication. Electronic communication has the potential of moving medicine inexorably toward such transparency, enabling doctors and patients to share knowledge, responsibility, and decision making more equally. As e-mail communication becomes more widespread, interactions between patients and physicians, such as follow-up inquiries, receiving data from home monitoring (e.g. blood glucose levels) and adjusting of medication accordingly, will be facilitated. E-mail communications creates the potential for improved continuity of care because patients can interact with their personal physician asynchronously via e-mail. E-mail

may also promote communications between providers e.g. physician–physician and physician–pharmacist. Speciality consultations could include an e-mail message with an electronic attachment of a patients test results, a digital radiograph or a scanned photo of a skin lesion. In a clinical crossroads article, Slack demonstrates the value that patient–physician e-mail can have in improving patient care, and also catalogues the incomplete but encouraging underlying evidence. The article emphasizes that informatics can help physicians better incorporate into clinical practice one of the most underused resources in medicine, the patient, whose help is greatly enhanced through this new technology.[17] Despite the benefits of electronic communication, potential disadvantages do exist. Patient advocacy groups have expressed their concern about the confidentiality of e-mail communication and the delay in receiving a response. Physicians are also concerned about communication through electronic technology because it may deteriorate the patient–physician relationship. Furthermore, e-mail bypasses the conventional administrative screening and consequently can overload a clinician with unnecessary electronic mail.[18] Physician resistance to e-mail communication was apparent in a 2002 study showing that only 6% of respondents reported using e-mail to contact a physician or other health care professional.[19] The American Medical Association (AMA) has released guidelines for doctors using e-mail in an attempt to standardize electronic communication. These suggestions advise establishing timely responses, discouraging e-mail communication for insistent matters, explaining electronic mail procedures to patients, and making the patients informed that e-mails can be printed or copied and inserted into standard patient records.[20] Urged on by the AMA and the American College of Physicians, insurers and health plans are exploring ways of paying doctors for using e-mail.[21]

Handheld memory devices such as smart cards and USB memory devices are another advantage of electronic communication. They are small sized devices that transmit electronic information to a computer system and contain a patient's electronic health record. They can provide physicians with a patient's complete medical history, immunizations, allergies, blood type, prostheses, measurements, laboratory results, and so on.[22]

One of the most concerning issues are the confidentiality and security issues. The Health Insurance Portability and Accountability Act of 1996 (HIPAA) regulations require that comprehensive policies and procedures be established to safeguard electronic health records and patient confidentiality.[23] E-mail and handheld memory devices communication can be protected through encryption using public key cryptography.[24]

Evidence-based medicine and health information access

The practice of evidence-based medicine (EBM) is the integration of current best research evidence with clinical expertise, and patient values to achieve the best possible patient management.[25] In the modern world of rapidly expanding scientific knowledge, increased patient self-advocacy, and limited health care resources, EBM defines a way to optimize medical decision-making. There is a rich literature about the frequency of questions occurring in clinical practice (0.7–1.5 per patient).[26] The vast majority are 'foreground questions' concerning management of a specific patient. 'Background questions' that seek more general medical information are fewer, especially among more experienced clinicians. Nonetheless, current information sources, such as electronic textbooks, focus on providing answers to background questions. In fact, questions about therapy consist above than 50% of clinical questions, while diagnostic issues account for less than 30% of questions.[27] Green et al. demonstrated that a group of residents believed that 70% of evidence-based answers to their questions would have changed the management of patients and that 34% of questions might involve harm for the patient if not answered.[28] Marshall reported that 80% of participating physicians changed their care as a result of evidence. He also calculated that these changes reduced mortality risk in 19% of patients, avoided hospitalization in 12% of cases, changed diagnostic tests in 51% and drug choice in 45%. Overall length of stay in hospital was reduced in 19% of patients.[29] Searching for health information was one of the most common uses of the web.[30] Internet use by physicians has grown from 89% in 2001 to 96% in 2002, and 90% of physicians use the Internet to research clinical issues, making it the most common professional Internet activity for physicians. Additionally, 70% of doctors claim that the web influences treatment and diagnosis of patients.[31] Search engines allow quick access to an ever-increasing knowledge base.[32] The Google search engine, for example, gives users ready access to more than three billion articles on the web and has far exceeded PubMed as the search engine of choice for retrieving medical articles.[33] A recently published article suggests that in difficult diagnostic cases, it is often useful to 'Google for a diagnosis.'[34]

From the patients point of view, an 2002 Cochrane review concluded that trials indicates decision aids improve knowledge and realistic expectations; enhance active participation in decision making; lower decisional conflict; decrease the proportion of people remaining undecided, and improve agreement between values and choice. The effects on persistence with chosen therapies and cost-effectiveness require further evaluation.[35] About 20% of adults in the US use the Internet to access health information.[36] Eighty percent of patients are online, and 90% of online patients claim that web access has increased their understanding of health conditions.[37] Growing numbers of patients bring online search results into their physician's offices, expecting their physicians to interpret the information.

Nevertheless, a significant proportion of consumer web sites are not peer reviewed, are influenced by sponsorships and advertisements, and are not continuously updated.[38] The American Medical Association (AMA) guidelines stress clear indications of content, site ownership and sponsorship, privacy procedures, payment information (if applicable), recent updates, qualified peer review, off-site links, and navigational ease.[39] Thus far, these principals have nor been endorsed by the Internet health care world, and no regulatory process currently exists to guarantee Internet health care quality.[40] MEDLINE plus (http://medlineplus.gov) is an example of a regulated health care information web site that can provide useful medical information to both physicians and patients.[41]

Clinical decision support systems (CDSS)

In part, PHRs represent a repository for patient data, but PHR systems can also include decision-support capabilities that can assist patients in managing their health. Today's clinicians face significant challenges with an information explosion that is taxing their time, demanding more accountability from them and increasing pressure to contain costs. The top priority is the quality of patient care; yet due to growing complexity of health care, it becomes increasingly more difficult achieve this goal, despite the many advances achieved in health care during the last 50 years. The highly publicized Institute of Medicine report 2000, *To Err Is Human: Building a Safer Health System*, outlined the pervasiveness of medical errors in routine health care and the potential danger those errors pose for patients on a daily basis.[42] Between 6.6 and 13.6% of medical errors which occur in hospitalized patients lead to death, which equates to between 44,000 and 98,000 patient deaths every year. What would be the global response if 110 jumbo jets, each carrying 400 passengers crashed each year, killing all on board? In fact, medical errors are the 5th to 8th most common cause of death in the US.[43] Emerging information about ambulatory care suggests that the patient safety crisis in hospitals is only the tip of the iceberg. Similar follow-on studies concerning the British National Health System came to similar conclusions.[44] In 2001, the IOM catalogued studies of under use, overuse, and misuse of care and concluded the performance of the US health system 'has floundered in its ability to provide consistently high quality care to all Americans' and noted that the system 'frequently falls short in its ability to translate knowledge into practice.' Thus, the IOM described the US health system as facing 'a large chasm between today's system and the possibilities of tomorrow.' The report ties the problems and potential solutions together in a vision for a health care system that is safe, patient-centered and evidence-based.[45] In 2003, the RAND Corporation found that on average patients receive recommended care only 54.9% of the time.[46]

One of the main causes of the above-mentioned chasm is the gap between the most current and evidence-based clinical and health knowledge, and the information that is typically applied in making health and care decisions at the very moment they are made; the point of care. Where answers to clinical questions are provided by the literature, they are buried in textbooks or in one or more journal articles. Unfortunately, only few clinicians have ready access or the time required to search medical databases, read articles, and synthesizes their findings in the busy clinical setting. As a result, the focus has changed toward approaches that provide highly concise information in the context of the specific patient and clinical problem.[47] Rapid access to answers, which are provided in a synthesized and succinct patient-specific, actionable knowledge, manner, embedded within an electronic clinical tool, remains the key to solving this dilemma.[48] Clinical decision support systems (CDSS) are typically designed to integrate a medical knowledge base, patient data and an inference engine to generate case specific advice. The first CDSS used in clinical practice were developed in the 1970s. The electronic integration of patient information, evidence-based reference material and clinical decision support results in knowledge driven care. For example, CDSS interventions can detect potential medical errors, suggest optimal clinical strategies, organize the details of a plan of care, help gather and present data needed to execute this plan, and ensure that the best clinical knowledge and recommendations are utilized to improve health management decisions. Patient context in terms of age, gender, current problems, current drugs, co-morbidities etc. and workflow context, such as stage in treatment, location of care, determined resources etc., are essential for delivering actionable knowledge. The potential benefits of using electronic decision support systems in clinical practice fall into three broad categories:[49]

- *Improved patient safety*, e.g. through reduced medication errors and adverse events and improved medication and test ordering
- *Improved quality of care*, e.g. by increasing clinicians' available time for direct patient care, increased application of clinical pathways and guidelines, facilitating the use of up-to-date clinical evidence, improved clinical documentation and patient satisfaction
- *Improved efficiency in health care delivery*, e.g. by reducing costs through faster order processing, reductions in test duplication, decreased adverse events, and changed patterns of drug prescribing favoring cheaper but equally effective generic brands

Multiple studies demonstrated CDSS beneficial in improving outcomes at some health care institutions and practice sites by making needed medical knowledge readily available to knowledge users.[50–55]

A recently published systematic review of literature on the effect of health information technology on quality, efficiency, and costs of care found that three major benefits on quality were demonstrated – increased adherence to guideline-based care, enhanced surveillance and monitoring, and decreased medication errors.[56]

Yet, at many other sites, CDS has been problematic, stalled in the planning stages, or never even attempted due to significant barriers to its use. These include cost, technical issues; system interoperability, concerns about privacy and confidentiality, and lack of a well-trained clinician informatics workforce to lead the process.[3,57]

On June 2006 a special American Medical Informatics Association (AMIA) committee issued by the US Office of the National Coordinator for Health Information Technology (ONC) presented its conclusions in a white paper titled 'The Roadmap for National Action on Clinical Decision Support.' The roadmap recommended a series of federal and private activities to improve CDS development, implementation and use throughout the United States health sector:

The immediate goal of these activities is to ensure that optimal, usable and effective clinical decision support is widely available to providers, patients, and individuals where and when they need it to make health care decisions. The ultimate goal of these activities is to improve the quality of health care services and to improve health in the United States.

IT and database developments

Developments in computer technology and mass production of computer processors and other components have made computers and data input devices affordable. The rapid development of newer and better equipment has made cutting edge technology affordable even for low-income countries. In response to growing demand, the software market has become ultra sophisticated in addressing the vast range of user needs.

The integration of IT and networking, imaging, data at the level of the individual and data from monitoring products should create solutions that will help hospitals, and clinics address four important issues:

- Be able to *integrate vertical data* of the individual into the personal medical files.
- *Access* of full patient medical records *anytime, anywhere* (from within health care institutions or any other patient's choice of health care provider) with built-in knowledge-based elements allowing for minimization of risk of errors.
- *Improve quality of care*, through effective storage of the information, to be used by the same doctors again, or by other health providers of the same patient, or anonymously be used for local, regional, nationwide and international comprehensive research, in order to reach conclusions and hence improve treatments.
- *Critical time-savings* through improving workflow efficiency and, on the other hand, the day-to-day life of patients with chronic diseases can be dramatically improved if the level of awareness is elevated to a level that will make an impact on their responsiveness to their medical customized treatments. Moreover, their daily routine and check-ups (e.g., in diabetes patients check their sugar levels various times a day) directly integrated into their personalized chart can be continuously monitored, and alerts and disasters can be taken into account immediately using a cell phone and/or the Internet.

The 'EuHealthNet': Scientific and technological objectives

The 'EuHealthNet' is an eHealth network implemented to measure outcome in diabetes and pregnancy.

Vertical integration

IT aspects/solutions (which can be transferred)

- *Interoperability* of information-medical systems by building agents that self configure themselves to collect information (genetic data from bio-bank, blood analysis, information collected from external devices, etc.) from existing databases in the different institutions, on pre-defined common parameters

- Enable *transfer of information between systems* via a network using same agents in the opposite direction
- Enable extraction of data from external devices, into the same unified system, seamlessly
- Enable extraction of data from external devices, into same unified system, via the Internet
- *Interconnect external devices* using blue-tooth technology, or other, through the unified system (i.e. glucometers, pumps and sensors)

Medical aspects

The system will download of data from personal medical devices (glucometers, insulin pumps, sensors, fetal monitors, ultra sound, etc.) directly into the personal medical file on a unified system, using the Internet (from an ASP application).

Medical–IT combined

- *Interconnect external medical devices* using blue-tooth technology, or other, through the unified system (i.e. glucometers, pumps and sensors, fetal monitors, etc.)
- *Build a feedback mechanism* between the medical files, the individual and the medical devices using blue-tooth technology and cell phones. Consequently, send messages and feedback alerts from a network through a cellular phone as feedback from data downloaded from medical devices (especially wearable ones)
- Integrate genetic data from bio-banks into the integrated personal medical file; unification of formats
- Automatically create an electronic birth certificate to include parts of the mother's medical file, and use the genetic information of parents to automatically update the origin of the new born (medical file of new bon starts from the pre-natal information from conception time)

Horizontal integration
IT aspects/solutions (which can be transferred)

- Build the system in a way so that the information is stored in 'virtual saves' – using two digital keys to open – a network key and an authorized person (the patient, and authorized health care provider)
- Build the system in a way to link the following services: Authentication, Authorization and Control (to every piece of information)
- Design the data base agents (see vertical integration) to seamlessly integrate the information from all kinds and format

The information is displayed in the different languages, allowing automatic translation of main medical terms achieved, using common standards.

Medical aspects–IT combined
Development of standards
- Standards for electronic birth certification: the medical file of newborn is automatically generated by the system, using the mother medical file (and father's if in the system), to include genetic information, bio-bank information, fetal status information, and labor information
- Standards for unification of medical data, using interoperability to convert data into a web-display for textual data and support of medical imaging (web viewer DIACOM-compatible)

Connecting information Connect the information in a medical file (diagnosis, medications, allergies, medical procedures, treatments etc.) to a search engine which will identify related information directly to the items in the file, enable smart questions and deliver an 'evidence-based' search result per demand.

Horizontal and vertical
Medical–IT combined

Anonymous accessibility Build the database in a way that the textual and medical information are accessible anonymously using the authentication/authorization modules. The information of a person resides in different sets of servers. One is specifically designed for the individual private data for authentication, and serves to authenticate, and the other to set the authenticated party the right authorization. Then the authenticated person receives a digital key to open the medical information which is then transferred with no names (allowing a maximum security), as during transmission, only medical data is transmitted without names, or names without any medical data attach to it. Images are stored in a third server to allow transmission of large digital pictures (only when and if broadband is available).

One-to-one identifier Develop a one-to-one identifier for patients (clients) to be used by the authentication server as well as by the connector–integration module to be identified by the system as a single identity to integrate data for patients

Information labelled by tags Build the database in such a way so that information labelled by tags which will be interpreted by an authorization server (so that only authenticated authorized people will have rights to the information). Integrate these tags with the authorization server to be able to build partial authorization of the information. The patients and the health care providers can see some of the information. Some of the information can be seen either only by the patient and/or only by health care providers (such as psychiatric information in some countries).

Medical

Goal 1: Inform clinical practice To bring information tools to the point of care, by creating a full network for retrieval of medical data, for data entry (the traditional replacement of EHR systems) for use in hospitals, as well as in physicians' offices and public and private clinics – either a new web-system or integration of the existing systems to be able to 'push' the information when needed by a centralized index system.

Goal 2: Interconnect clinicians To build an inter-operational health information infrastructure, allowing the patient's clinicians complete access to critical health care information when treatment decisions need to be made. Moreover, the information is kept in a common very secure database system, which enables the building of local, regional, national and international registries.

Goal 3: Personalize care To utilize health information technology in a way that will give consumers more access and involvement in their health care decisions. To enable patients to have their medical information available at all times: by Internet, phone, smart cards, and GSM SIM cards, PDAs, and Disk On Keys. To enable patients to download their data from the personal medical devices directly into their personal records online, or transfer it using a phone.

Goal 4: Improve health care by creating local, regional, national and international registries on diseases To expand capacity for research by building registries to be used by local hospitals that will be able to share and collect anonymous data from other health institutions for quality of care measurement, by adopting new technologies, using a network to monitor patients (such as diabetics, cancer, AIDS, etc.) and bring research advances and improvements faster into local medical practice.

Goal 5: Improve population health To expand public health monitoring capacity, quality of care measurement, research findings to allow for faster effective implementation into medical practice – using local, regional, national and international registries, and a common research center to identified crucial parameters.

'EuHealthNet': The project

EuHealthNet is about a pan-European effort of commercial companies and network of researchers, health care providers, and professional institutions (centers of excellence throughout Europe) to build a comprehensive eHealth network, integrated with medical devices from different types (sensors, glucometers, tension meters, insulin pumps, scales, fetal monitors, etc.) as well as with phones, PDAs, Smart Cards, etc. (Figure 58.2).

The researcher specialists of the centers of excellence - are working together to design the application that is implemented into the system, for specialist-dependent data entry system and/or the integration into the medical devices, and software packages used in each of the sub-specialties. In addition, the companies are working with researchers from the different hospitals to build the prototype of the devices to be integrated into the system. At this stage the participating centers are from Denmark, Holland, Sweden, Spain, Italy, Germany, France, UK, Ireland, Poland, Slovenia, and Israel.

During the second step, the number of hospitals in each country will increase, and additional countries will be added. All the hospitals involved in the project will share a very secure database. Each hospital will have an allocated designated partition in the database, and will have full access to its own data. However, the participants of the project can only retrieve and review the comprehensive data (coming from all the centers) anonymously, under definite restrictions imposed by the steering committee of the project, and by the ethics committees of each hospital.

The technical outputs of the project

A full eHealth network, with a sophisticated secure DB solution, modules for retrieval of data (in multiple ways including cellular communication), modules for data entry (general medicine, diabetes, pregnancy and paediatrics), synchronization with multiple devices, and more.

The Online Research Centre that is supported by the common very secure anonymous database, will allow each of the networks (and within each of the centers) to perform its own analysis and combine and compare results with each of the other institutes participating in the project, to reach the most comprehensive conclusions and enable development of new treatments on behalf of the patients, as well as local, regional, national and international registries.

The Online Information Centre, integrated within the patients' personal medical files, will allow various facilities.

The EuHealthNet Information Centre

The Centre, integrated within the patients' personal medical files, will be able to expose new drugs, new technologies, and new medical devices to both the health care provider and the patient, whenever the file is reviewed.

- With the help of the anonymous data, centers involved in the project will be able to improve the quality and efficiency of specific drugs (e.g. manufacturers of types of drugs, tension meter, glycemic meters and other meters, sensors, ultra sound monitors, etc.) and have a unique opportunity to build an anonymous registry of users.
- The Information Centre will enable the patients and their health care providers complete awareness and involvement in the patient's medical condition.

The Physician Decision Support Tool

This tool, integrated within the patient's medical file, when viewed by a physician (regulated by the authentication–authorization

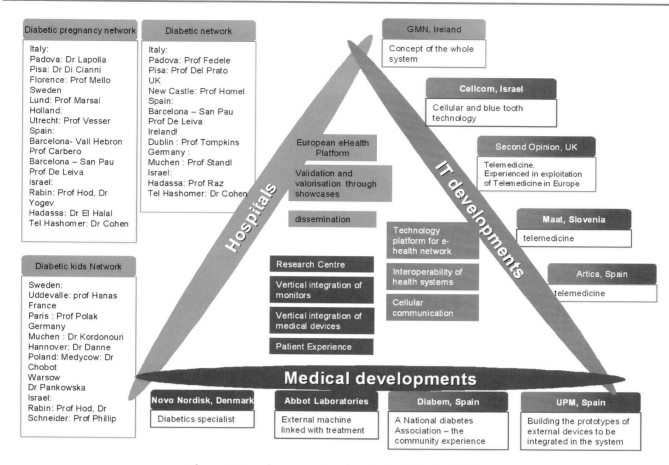

Figure 58.2   The consortium involved with EuHealthNet.

servers) will enable the physician to receive support for decision making from several levels:

- Pre-designed recommendations based on the specific parameters within the personal medical file (taking into account all the data: levels of blood sugar, complications, status (child, pregnant woman, adult), etc).
- Linked to medical based medicine existing sites
- Linked to journals

A patient's portal is developed, for each of the networks, and of course will be enriched by every step along the roadmap. An immediate step to improve consumer access to personal and customized health information, providing secure health information via the Internet, the phone, PDAs, smart card, GSM SIM cards, etc. The portal enables authorized beneficiaries to have access to information about the health care services they have received under the project, as well as have full access to information related to their physical condition, through the Information Centre capabilities, which are developed as part of the project. The portal includes online training for illiterate computer users.

As a showcase of the validation and valorization of the EuHealthNet, the researcher in charge of each center of excellence – for each of the key applications of this project (gynaecology, diabetes and paediatrics) – work together to design the application that is implemented into the system, for specialist-dependent data entry system and/or the integration into the medical devices, and software packages used in each of the subspecialities.

The showcase for validation and valorisation of the EuHealthNet project, all through the project, is diabetes, implemented in different sectors to further enhance the complexity of the system: (1) Diabetic Pregnancy Network, (2) Diabetic Kids Network, and (3) Diabetic Network.

Main innovations claimed by EuHealthNet

The EuHealthNet technology has a differentiated solution that delivers a full eHealth Network, around the patient, which includes modules for all the participants in the health care community: patients, hospitals, clinics community level and private), other health care providers. Within this solution we integrated two major centers of information and research: the Online Research Centre and the Online Information Centre.

Online Research Centre

The Online Research Centre, supported by the common very secure anonymous database, allows hospitals and physicians to perform their own analysis and combine and compare results with each of the other institutes participating in the local network, to reach the most comprehensive conclusions and enable development of new treatments on behalf of the patients.

Online Information Centre

The Online Information Centre, integrated within the patients personal medical files, allows:

- Patients and their health care providers complete awareness and involvement in the patient's medical condition
- The commercial companies to directly expose their drugs, new technologies, and new medical devices to the patient, whenever the file is reviewed (only with the patient's permission)
- In the future when the product is commercialized, with the help of the anonymous data base, commercial companies using the network, of course anonymous use (ONLY supervised by ethics committees), the ability to improve the quality and efficiency of their specific products (e.g., manufacturers of types of drugs, pumps, meters, sensors, ultra sound monitors, etc.), and have a unique opportunity to build an anonymous registry of users, and address them in the commercialisation phase with the patients' permission) in targeted advertising

A patient's portal is used to improve consumer access to personal and customized health information, providing secure health information via the Internet, the phone, PDAs, smart card, GSM SIM cards, etc. The portal enables authorized beneficiaries to have access to information about the health care services they receive, as well as have full access to, information related to their physical condition, through the Information Centre capabilities, which makes part of the network. The portal includes online training for illiterate computer users.

Challenges and expectations facing countries' health sectors and the role of e-Health

- Health care systems have to face major challenges.
- There are increasing expectations of citizens who want the best care available, and at the same time to experience a reduction in inequalities in access to good health care.
- Increasing mobility of patients and health professionals within a better functioning internal market.
- There is a need to reduce the so-called 'disease burden', and to respond to emerging disease risks (for example, new communicable diseases like SARS).
- The difficulties experienced by public authorities in matching investment in technology with investment in the complex organizational changes needed to exploit its potential.
- The need to limit occupational accidents and diseases, to reinforce well-being at work and to address new forms of work-related diseases.

- Management of huge amounts of health information that need to be available securely, accessibly, and in a timely manner at the point of need, processed efficiently for administrative purposes,
- The need to provide the best possible health care under limited budgetary conditions.

eHealth: systems and services that benefit the health sector

eHealth systems and services combined with organisational changes and the development of new skills are key tools to face these major challenges. They can deliver significant improvements for access to care, quality of care, and the efficiency and productivity of the health sector.

The amount and complexity of health-related information and knowledge has increased to such a degree that a major component of any health organization is information processing. The health sector is clearly an information intensive sector that increasingly depends on information and communication technologies. These technologies are supporting progress in medical research, better management and diffusion of medical knowledge, and a shift towards evidence-based medicine. e-Health tools support the aggregation, analysis and storage of clinical data in all its forms; information tools provide access to the latest findings; while communication tools enable collaboration among many different organizations and health professionals.

Empowering health consumer: patients and healthy citizens

Both as patients and as healthy citizens, people can benefit from better personal health education and disease prevention. They need support in managing their own diseases, risks – including work-related diseases – and lifestyles. A growing number of people are looking proactively for information on their medical conditions. They want to be involved actively in decisions related to their own health, rather than simply accepting the considerable discrepancy ('asymmetry') in knowledge between themselves and health professionals. e-Health services provide timely information tailored to individuals in need.

Personalized systems for monitoring and supporting patients are also currently available; examples include wearable or implantable communication systems for continuous monitoring of patients' heart conditions. These systems can help shorten or completely avoid patient stay in hospitals, while ensuring monitoring of their health status.

Having access to comprehensive and secure electronic health records has been shown to improve quality of care and patient safety. This will facilitate appropriate treatment of patients in providing health professionals with a better knowledge of the patient's history and of previous interventions by other colleagues. If interoperable, given patient mobility, electronic health records will also improve conditions for treatment in other countries.

Assisting health professionals

e-Health tools and applications can provide fast and easy access to electronic health records at the point of need. They can support diagnosis by non-invasive imaging-based systems. They support surgeons in planning clinical interventions using digital patient specific data, provide access to specialized resources for education and training, and allow radiologists the possibility to access images anywhere. Thus, the workplace is being redefined and extended. Digital data transfer enables more effective networking among clinical institutions across Europe, and the creation of a European network of centers of reference. Electronic health records also enable the extraction of information for research, management, public health or other related statistics of benefit to health professionals.

Supporting health authorities and health managers

Health authorities and managers are responsible for the proper organization and running of health systems. They do this against the background of increasing budgetary pressures and rising patient expectations. e-Health systems can play a major part in meeting those pressures by making the health sector more productive, and delivering better results with fewer resources. Unfortunately, the currently available paper-based information aggregation and processing has major limitations.

Integrated and comprehensive data can be provided in good time using e-Health tools; such as electronic health records and support for care flow management. Automatic data extraction from electronic health systems that operate according to standards and countries' legal requirements on data protection and privacy could provide missing data that facilitates proper evaluation of much needed resources and eradicates the huge administrative burden of filling in separate forms for reimbursement, a clear example of a productivity gain to be achieved through e-Health systems and services.

e-Health systems can empower managers by spreading best practices and helping to limit inefficient and inappropriate treatment. This is the single most important step in releasing resources and ensuring broad access for everyone to quality care. In addition, e-Health opens new opportunities for people who live in remote areas with only limited health care

services, as well as marginalized groups (such as persons with different degrees of disability, whether minor or more severe). e-Health is already proving in the Western and developing world that it can provide a platform for telemedicine services such as tele-consultations (second medical opinion); tele-monitoring; and tele-care, either in the home or the hospital.

Conclusions

It is no exaggeration to declare that the years to come portend the 'decade of health information technology'.[58] Health care IT in not a panacea for all that ails medicine, but it has the potential to improve the quality of care as well as the personal experience for patients.

It may seem difficult and cumbersome to establish an epidemiological surveillance system for diabetes in pregnancy. Rather it is a matter of organizing available data than searching for new data collection mechanisms, and extending its use to the epidemiological dimension. An epidemiological surveillance system could be attained by provision of routinely collected and aggregated data by centers providing obstetrical and neonatal care for pregnant diabetics and their infants. If diabetes and pregnancies are considered public health issues, it is strongly recommended that epidemiological models should be further developed and implemented at various levels of services to provide data for the dimensioning of the current and future diabetes care systems. Benefits of the surveillance system should be clearly articulated: (1) utilization of perinatal performance indicators related to subset of diabetic pregnancies in situation analysis, and for comparison with general population; (2) benchmarking and aid to target setting; (3) identification of areas of particular concern in terms of need for improved management; (4) forecasting of trends in gestational diabetes prevalence; (5) implementation of St Vincent Declaration. Critical attention should be given to database design, data sources and its validity, methodologies and interpretation of findings, its implication for clinical practice.

When combined with organizational changes and the development of new skills, eHealth can help to deliver better care for less money within citizen-centered health delivery systems. It thus responds to the major challenges that the health sector is currently facing.

REFERENCES

1. Definition adapted from Stanford's Medical Informatics department. Available at www.openclinical.org [Accessed 11 January 2007].
2. Kukafka R, O'Carroll PW, Gerberding JL, et al. Issues and opportunities in public health informatics: a panel discussion. J Public Health Manag Prac 2001; 7: 31–42.
3. Bates DW, Gawande AA. Improving safety with information technology. N Eng J Med 2003; 348: 2526–34.
4. Health Information Technology: Can HIT Lower Costs and Improve Quality? Available at http://www.rand.org/pubs/research_briefs/RB9136/RAND_RB9136.pdf [Accessed 29 November 2006].
5. Stroetmann KA, Jones T, Dobrev A, Stroetmann VN. eHealth is it worth it? The economic benefits of implemented eHealth solutions at ten European sites.
6. Mitchell E, Sullivan F. A descriptive feast but an evaluative famine BMJ 2001; 322: 279–82.
7. Kassirer J. Patients, physicians and the internet. Health Aff (Millwood) 2000; 19: 115–23.
8. Brodie M, Flournoy RE, Altman DE, et al. Health information, the Internet and the digital divide. Health Aff (Millwood) 2000; 19: 255–65.
9. Adapted from Osheroff et al. A roadmap for national action on clinical decision support. 2006. Available at http://amia.org/inside/initiatives/cds/ [Accessed 28 November 2006].
10. Frist WH. N Engl J Med 2005; 352: 267–72.
11. Delbanco TL, Berwick DM, Boufford JI, et al. Healthcare in a land called People Power: nothing about me without me. Health Expect 2001; 4: 144–50.

12. McDonald CJ, Overhage JM, Dexter PR, et al. Canopy computing: using the Web in clinical practice. JAMA 1998; 280: 1325–9.
13. US HHS http: //www.hhs.gov/healthit/glossary.html [Accessed 28 November 2006].
14. Markle Foundation, Connecting for Health. The Personal Health Working Group Final Report, 1 July 2003.
15. Endsley S, Kibbe DC, Linares A, Colorafi K. An introduction to personal health records. Fam Pract Manag 2006; 13: 57–62.
16. Tang PC, Ash JS, Bates DW, Overhage JM, Sands DZ. Personal health records: definitions, benefits, and strategies for overcoming barriers to adoption. J Am Med Inform Assoc 2006; 13: 121–6.
17. Slack WV. A 67-year-old man who e-mails his physician. JAMA 2004; 292: 2255–61.
18. Moyer CA, Stern DT, Katz SJ, et al. We got mail. Am J Manag Care 1999; 5: 1513–22.
19. Baker L, Wagner T, Singer S, et al. Use of the Internet and e-mail for health care information. JAMA 2003; 289: 2400–6.
20. Bovi AM, for the Council on Ethical and Judicial Affairs of the American Medical Association – Ethical guidelines for use of electronic mail between patients and physicians. Am J Bioeth 2003; 3: W–IF2.
21. Gottlieb S. US doctors want to be paid for email communication with patients. BMJ 2004; 328; 1155.
22. Ward SR. Health smart cards: merging technology and medical information. Med Req Serv Q 2003; 22: 57–65.
23. US department of Health and Human Services, Office for civil rights. Health Insurance Portability and Accountability Act. Available at http:/hhs.gov/ocr/hipaa. [Accessed 1 December 2006].
24. Pangalos G, Mavridis I, Ilioudis C, et al. Developing a public key infrastructure for a secure regional e-health environment. Methods Inf 2002; 41: 414–8.
25. Sackett DL, Rosenberg WM, Gray JA, et al. Evidence-based medicine, what it is and what it isn't. BMJ 1996; 312: 71–2.
26. Smith, R. What clinical information do doctors need? BMJ 1996; 313: 1062–8.
27. Ebell M. Information at the point of care: Answering clinical questions. J Am Board Fam Pract 1999; 12: 225–35.
28. Green ML, Ciampi MA, Ellis PJ. Residents' medical information needs in clinic: Are they being met? Am J Med 2000; 109; 218–23.
29. Marshall JG. The impact of the hospital library on clinical decision-making: The Rochester Study. Bull Med Lib Assoc 1992; 80: 169–78.
30. Powell J, Clarke A. The www of the World Wide Web: who, what, and why? J Med Internet Res 2002; 4: e4.
31. Knoop CA, Lovich D, Silverstein MB, et al. Vital signs: e-health in the United States. Boston, MA: The Boston Consulting Group; 2003, pp. 9–39.
32. Giustini D. How Google is changing medicine. BMJ 2005; 331: 1487–8.
33. Steinbrook R. Searching for the right search-reaching the medical literature. N Engl J Med 2006; 354: 4–7.
34. Tang H, Kwoon JH. Googling for a diagnosis-use of Google as a diagnostic aid: Internet based study. BMJ, oi: 10.1136/bmj.39003.640567. AE [Published 10 November 2006].
35. O'Connor AM, Stacey D, Entwistle V, et al. Decision aids for people facing health treatment or screening decisions. Cochrane Database System Rev 2003; Issue 1. [Art. No.: CD001431. DOI: 10.1002/14651858.CD001431].
36. Baker L, Wagner TH, Singer S, Bundorf MK. Use of the internet and e-mail for healthcare information. JAMA 2003; 289: 2400–6.
37. Knoop CA, Lovich D, Silverstein MB, et al. Vital signs: e-health in the United States. Boston, MA: The Boston Consulting Group; 2003, pp. 9–39.
38. Eysenbach G, Powell J, Kuss O, et al. Empirical studies assessing the quality of health information for consumers on the World Wide Web. JAMA 2002; 287: 2691–700.
39. Winker MA, Flanagin A, Chi-Lum B, et al. Guidelines for medical and health information sites on the Internet. JAMA. 2000; 283: 1600–6.
40. Bodenheimer T, Grumbach K. Electronic technology. JAMA 2003; 290: 259–64.
41. Ullrich P, Vaccaro A. Patient education on the Internet. Spine 2002; 26: E185–8.
42. Institute of Medicine. To Err is Human: Building a Safer health System. Washington, D.C.: National Academy Press; 2000.
43. American Hospital Association. Hospital Statistics. Chicago, IL. 1999.
44. National Patient Safety Agency. 2003. Seven Steps to Patient Safety: A Guide for NHS Staff.
45. Institute of Medicine. Crossing the Quality Chasm: A New Health System for the 21st Century. Washington, D.C.: National Academy Press; 2001.
46. McGlynn EA, Asch SM, Adams J, et al. The quality of health care delivered to adults in the United States. N Engl J Med 2003; 348: 2635–45.
47. Chueh H, Barnett GO. 'Just-in-time' clinical information. Acad Med 1997; 72: 512–7.
48. Haynes RB. Of studies, syntheses, synopses and systems: the '4S' evolution of services for finding current best evidence. ACP J Club 2001; 134: A11–3.
49. E. Coiera. The Guide to Health Informatics, 2nd edn. London: Arnold; 2003.
50. Johnston ME, Langton KB, Haynes RB, Mathieu A. Effects of computer-based clinical decision support systems on clinician performance and patient outcome: a critical appraisal of research. Ann Intern Med 1994; 120: 135–42.
51. Hunt DL, Haynes RB, Hanna SE, Smith K. Effects of computer-based clinical decision support systems on physician performance and patient outcomes. JAMA 1998; 280: 1339–46.
52. Chertow GM, Lee J, Kuperman GJ, et al. Guided medication dosing for inpatients with renal insufficiency. JAMA 2001; 286: 2839–44.
53. Gandhi TK, Bates DW. Computer adverse drug event (ADE) detection and alerts. In: Shojania K, Duncan B, McDonald K, Wachter R, eds. Making Health Care Safer: A Critical Analysis of Patient Safety Practices. AHRQ Publication No. 01-E058. Rockville, MD: Agency for Healthcare Research and Quality; 2001, pp. 79–85.
54. Raschke RA, Gollihare B, Wunderlich TA, et al. A computer alert system to prevent injury from adverse drug events: development and evaluation in a community teaching hospital. JAMA 1998; 280: 1317–20. [Erratum, JAMA 1999; 281: 420].
55. Kaushal R, Bates DW. Computerized physician order entry (CPOE) with clinical decision support systems (CDSSs). In: Shojania K, Duncan B, McDonald K, Wachter R, eds. Making Health Care Safer: A Critical Analysis of Patient Safety Practices. AHRQ Publication No. 01-E058. Rockville, MD: Agency for Healthcare Research and Quality; 2001; pp. 59–69.
56. Chaudry B, Wang J, Wu S, et al. Systematic review: impact of health information technology on quality, efficiency, and costs of medical care. Ann Int Med 2006; 144: 742–52.
57. Hersh W. Health care information technology progress and barriers. JAMA 2004; 292 2273–4.
58. Department of Health & Human Services Web site. The decade of health information technology: delivering consumer-centric and information-rich health care. Available at: http://www.hhs.gov/healthit/documents/hitframework.pdf [Accessed 28 November 2006].

59 Optimal contraception for the diabetic woman

Siri L. Kjos

Introduction

For a woman with diabetes to decide whether and when she desires to become pregnant is not simply a question of choice. A planned or unplanned pregnancy can have lifelong implications for her own health and most importantly for the health of her future child. Whether she has Type 1, Type 2 or prior gestational diabetes mellitus (GDM), optimizing her health prior to pregnancy should be a primary educational and medical goal promoted by her health care providers. Pregnancy planning can reduce her risk for elective abortion by offering her reliable methods to prevent conception or for spontaneous abortion by enabling her to plan a pregnancy in good glycemic control. Her own risk of developing serious medical complications such as ketoacidosis, accelerated retinopathy or proteinuria can similarly be reduced by controlling her medical problems prior to conception. Lastly, her risk of giving birth to an anomalous infant can be reduced by achieving euglycemia at conception and during embryogenesis. The risk of major congenital anomalies in offspring of women with Type 1[1] and Type 2[2] diabetes has been shown to be increased by up to 20–25%, and to be more than doubled (>5.5%) in GDM[3] when initial fasting glucose levels were >120 mg/dL. Achieving euglyemic control prior to and early in pregnancy has been shown to normalize rates of congenital malformations in women with Type 1 diabetes.[4] In the woman with GDM, there may be an additional long-term health benefit in avoiding pregnancy: a subsequent pregnancy has been shown to increase their risk of subsequent diabetes c. 3-fold.[5] Periodic testing for diabetes, regardless of the contraceptive method used, is recommended in all women with prior GDM,[6] especially prior to a subsequent pregnancy.

This chapter will discuss methods with a low failure rate, specifically combination oral contraceptives, progestin-only oral contraceptives, longer acting (injectable and implantable) hormonal methods and the intrauterine devices (IUD), in women with diabetes. Barrier methods will not be addressed, as they are metabolically neutral and have no medical contraindication to their use except for their significantly higher failure rates.

Hormonal contraceptives

The formulation, dosage and route of delivery all influence the various metabolic and endocrine effects of hormonal contraceptive methods in diabetic women. The first question to consider is whether estrogen-containing oral contraceptives should be prescribed. Estrogen is always prescribed in combination with pro-gestins and most commonly as a combination oral contraceptive. More recently, it has become available in combination with progestins delivered via intramuscular or transvaginal routes. Estrogen beneficially decreases the rate of breakthrough bleeding, thus increasing patient continuation of oral contraceptives. However, estrogen stimulates hepatic globulin production in a dose-dependent fashion. It produces an increase in angiotensinogen II levels, which in turn produces a slight but significant increase in mean arterial blood pressure,[7] and an increase in coagulation factors which thereby increases thromboembolic risk.[8] Estrogen also increases high-density lipoprotein and triglyceride levels, while decreasing low-density lipoprotein levels.[9] Important for the care of diabetic women, estrogen does not have any significant effect on carbohydrate metabolism.[10] In the general population these metabolic effects of combination oral contraceptives are subclinical and have been minimized by a steady decrease in ethinyl estradiol dosage in pill preparations. Currently, the lowest combination oral contraceptive preparations contain 20 mg of ethinyl estradiol. In women with medical conditions, generally the lowest dose preparations should be prescribed to minimize metabolic side effects, unless other medical conditions dictate otherwise. Estrogen- containing oral contraceptives should be avoided in women with hypertension or a history of thromboembolic disease.

If estrogen prescription is contraindicated, a progestin-only method should be selected. Progestin-only methods can be delivered via the oral, intramuscular, subcutaneous or intrauterine route, each with advantages and disadvantages. While progestins have a neutral effect on blood pressure[7] and coagulation factors,[8] they adversely decrease glucose tolerance, increase insulin resistance and increase low-density lipoprotein levels parallel to the dose and potency of the progestin formulation.[11] Thus, similar to estrogen, the lowest dose and least 'androgenic' progestin formulation should be selected in diabetic women.

Combination and progestin-only oral contraception

Type 1 and Type 2 diabetes

In diabetic women, formulations which contain the lowest dose and potency of progestin should be selected to minimize deterioration in glucose tolerance[11,12] and lipid metabolism.[9] These include the newer, less androgenic progestins or lower dose preparations containing the older progestins. Prospective studies with 1-year follow-up have shown combination preparations with low doses of older progestins, either norethindrone (≤0.75 mg mean daily dose) or triphasic levonorgestrel preparations, or newer progestins (gestodene, desogestrel) to have minimal effect on diabetic control, lipid metabolism[13–15] and cardiovascular risk factors.[16,17] All preparations examined in these studies also contained a low estrogen dosage (≤35 mg). The progestin-only oral contraceptive, containing 0.35 mg of norethindrone, has also been similarly studied in diabetic women and found to have no significant effect on carbohydrate or lipid metabolism.[15]

While recent short-term studies have shown oral contraceptive use to be safe in women with Type 1 diabetes, no long-term, prospective studies have been done which evaluate their effect on diabetic sequelae. While one older retrospective study suggested that thromboembolic disease may be accelerated by combination oral contraceptive use,[18] newer studies, which control for underlying risk factors, have not. Studies have not found any increased risk of or progression of diabetic sequelae (retinopathy, renal disease or hypertension) with past or current use of oral contraceptives.[19,20] In a case–control study, young women with Type 1 diabetes who either used or had never used oral contraception were followed for up to 7 years. There was no difference in the mean glycosylated hemoglobin levels (HbA1c), the mean albumin excretion rates or retinopathy scores.[20] Similarly, in a cross-sectional study of 384 women with Type 1 diabetes, no association was found between the use of oral contraceptives, either current, past or present, and the severity of retinopathy, hypertension or HbA1c levels when the known risk factors for diabetic sequelae were controlled for.[19]

The reluctance to prescribe oral contraceptives in diabetic women stems from the increase in cardiovascular complications and hypertension associated with both diabetes and older preparations of combination oral contraceptives. Current evidence from short-term trials in healthy women[9,21–24] have failed to find an association between cardiovascular risk markers and low-dose combination oral contraceptives. Furthermore, large, prospective cohort trials of healthy women have found no evidence for any excess risk of myocardial infarction with the use of low-dose oral contraceptives.[25–29] The increased risk for cardiovascular events appears to be related to their diabetes and not to oral contraceptive use. A recent multicenter, case–control study, examining acute myocardial infarction in women between the ages of 20 and 44, found that the use of combined oral contraceptives was associated with an increased risk of acute myocardial infarction in women with known cardiovascular risk factors, especially in those with hypertension.[29] Similarly, the risk of cerebral thromboembolism in young women has been related to known risk factors for stroke and not to combination oral contraceptive exposure. In a case–control study examining almost 500 women, aged 15–44, with documented cerebral thromboembolism, diabetes, prior thromboembolic disease, hypertension and migraine headaches were significantly associated with cerebral thromboembolism, but not the use of combination oral contraceptives.[30]

In summary, of the current available data, low-dose combination oral contraceptives can be used in diabetic women. The lowest dose/potency of both estrogen and progestins should be selected. In diabetic women with coexisting vascular disease, progestin-only oral contraceptives are preferred, because of the lack of effect of progestin on coagulation or blood pressure.

Currently, there are no studies examining either the retrospective use or the short-term prospective use of oral contraceptives in women with Type 2 diabetes. In the absence of studies, and given the generally safety of low-dose oral contraceptives, the guidelines suggested for prescription in women with Type 1 diabetes should be followed.

Women with Type 1 or Type 2 diabetes using oral contraceptives should be monitored more frequently than others for changes in blood pressure and weight. A baseline evaluation of weight, blood pressure, and fasting lipids are recommended. Consultation between the woman's internist/primary care physician and her gynecologist should occur to establish a monitoring program which involves both specialists. Her gynecologist should be aware of her diabetic therapy, home glucose monitoring regimen and any vascular sequelae, while the internist should be aware of the type of birth control and specific metabolic side effects. Blood pressure, weight, and glycemic parameters should be established. After 1 month and every 4–6 months thereafter the patient should return for blood pressure and weight measurements, as well as for evaluation of glycemic control. Lipids should be reassessed annually in diabetic women and more frequently if abnormal values are detected, following standard guidelines.[31]

Prior history of GDM

Over half of women with a history of GDM will develop diabetes, primarily Type 2, in their lifetime.[6,32] Their risk for subsequent diabetes varies and parallels the background rates for Type 2 diabetes for their ethnic group.[33,34] Periodic testing every 1–3 years for diabetes is recommended in women with prior GDM.[6] Testing should be done after delivery and prior to a subsequent pregnancy, as undiagnosed diabetes and untreated hyperglycemia,[2] which is often asymptomatic, has been associated with an increased risk for major congenital malformations. Additionally, recent evidence suggests that a subsequent pregnancy after a pregnancy complicated by GDM may be diabetogenic. In a cohort of Latino women, a second pregnancy following GDM was shown to triple the risk of subsequent diabetes.[35] Thus, women with prior GDM need effective contraception that does not accelerate their already increased risk of developing diabetes.

For the same reasons as in women with Type 1 and Type 2 diabetes, the lowest dose and potency progestin and estrogen combination oral contraceptive should be selected, in order to minimize adverse deterioration in glucose tolerance, lipid metabolism, and blood pressure effects. Combination oral contraceptives with low-dose/potency progestins have been shown, in short-term studies, to have no adverse effect of on glucose and lipid metabolism.[36–38] Recently, in a longer retrospective follow-up of 904 women with prior GDM, the long-term use of low-dose/potency progestin combination oral contraceptives had no effect on cumulative incidence rates of diabetes. After 3 years of uninterrupted use of the combination oral contraceptive, the diabetes rate (25.4%) was almost identical to non-hormonal forms of contraception (26.5%).[39] However, breastfeeding women who were using the progestin-only oral contraceptive had an almost a threefold increase in the risk of development of diabetes, which was further increased with the duration of uninterrupted use.[29] Thus, the progestin-only oral contraceptive should not be given to women with prior GDM who are breastfeeding. In breastfeeding women either a non-hormonal method or a low-dose combination oral contraceptive can be initiated 6–8 weeks postpartum, after the establishment of lactation. It is not clear whether the use of progestin-only oral contraceptives in non-breastfeeding women with prior GDM has any adverse effect.

Evidence supports the use of low-dose/ potency progestin combination oral contraceptive use in women with prior GDM. As these preparations do not accelerate the development of diabetes, routine testing for diabetes using fasting plasma glucose levels should be performed every 1–3 years, regardless of the contraceptive method used.[6] A confirmed fasting plasma glucose level ≥126 mg/dL is diagnostic of diabetes, and a fasting plasma glucose level ≥110 mg/dL and <126 mg/dL is diagnostic of impaired fasting glucose.[40]

Long-acting hormonal methods

The two long-acting preparations that have been in use for some time contain progestational agents only; one, depomedroxyprorgesterone acetate (DMPA), is delivered via injection and the other as a subdermal implant containing levonorgestrel (Norplant; recently withdrawn from the US market). Currently, no studies address the use of either DMPA or levonorgestrel implants (Norplant) in women with diabetes or prior GDM. However, data regarding thier effect on carbohydrate metabolism in healthy women are available. Norplant has been shown to have no significant effect on carbohydrate metabolism during its 5-year insertion period in healthy women.[41] In contrast, DMPA injections significantly increase fasting and post-glucose challenge levels of both insulin and glucose.[42,43] Recently, in Navajo women, who as an ethnic group are at high risk for diabetes, the use of DMPA contraception for ≥1 year was associated with an 8-fold increased risk in the development of Type 2 diabetes compared to combination or progestin-only oral contraceptives.[44] DMPA contraception has also been associated with increased weight

gain,[45] which is undesirable in women with Type 2 diabetes or with prior GDM. Thus, if contraindications to estrogens exist, a progestin-only oral contraceptive would be preferable, based on their demonstrated safety in women with Type 1 diabetes.[15] In select patients where compliance is a problem, strong consideration should be given to the IUD.

New progestin-only implant products, one containing levonorgestrel (Norplant II)[46] and another containing 3-ketodesogestrel (Implanon),[47] may provide alternative choices as studies become available. Also, long-acting combination hormonal methods will offer new alternatives. A monthly combination contraceptive injection containing estradiol cypionate and MPA has recently become available, but information regarding its effect on carbohydrate metabolism is lacking.[48] Similarly, hormone-releasing vaginal rings deliver sustained release of etonogestrel and ethinyl estradiol in lower dosage and serum concentrations than when taken orally.[49] Again, in the absence of data, these methods remain second-line choices. They should only be prescibed if similar guidelines for periodic monitoring of glycemia and lipids are followed.

Intrauterine devices

The legacy of the Dalkon Shield intrauterine device (IUD) was to associate IUD use with pelvic inflammatory disease (PID), a complication that in diabetic women could precipitate life-threatening ketoacidosis. Physicians caring for diabetic women have since been reluctant to prescribe the IUD. This misconception is being slowly reversed. Studies have shown that the development of pelvic inflammatory disease and subsequent tubal infertility were not related to the use of the IUD, *per se*, but the exposure risk for sexually transmitted disease.[50–52] Newer copper-medicated IUD, currently on the market, have not been associated with any increase in risk of PID after the post-insertion period. In a large meta-analysis involving almost 60,000 women-years of copper-medicated IUD use, the overall incidence of PID associated with IUD use was 1.6/1000 women-years of IUD use.[53]

Similarly, none of the studies examining copper-medicated IUD use in diabetic women with either Type 1[54,55] or Type 2[56] diabetes have found any support for an increased risk of PID. In two controlled trials examining copper-medicated IUD use in healthy and Type 1 diabetic women, followed for 1[54] or 3[55] years, there were no cases of PID. The rates of perforations, failure, expulsion, pain, and discontinuation were not different between diabetic and healthy control women. Similarly, in a 3-year uncontrolled study in women with Type 2 diabetes, no cases of PID were found.[56] In fact, no study which has examined IUD use in diabetic women,[54–59] has found any demonstrable increase in PID. However, caution must be exercised. The risk of PID is extremely low with use of medicated IUDs in the general population, making it highly unlikely that large enough studies can ever be conducted in diabetic women to demonstrate the absence of any increase in risk.[60]

In addition to the copper-medicated IUD, a levonorgestrel-releasing IUD provides an excellent alternative. It can be considered a hybrid of a long-acting hormonal method and an

IUD. The levonorgestrel-releasing IUD has been extensively used during the past decade and provides extremely effective contraception with a 5-year cumulative failure rate of 0.71/100 women.[61] The IUD provides sustained low-dose (20 mg daily) release of levonorgestrel, which inhibits pregnancy by thickening the cervical mucus,[62] and by inhibiting motility and function of sperm,[63] rather than by inhibiting ovulation. The high levels of levonorgestrel released into the endometrium decreases menstrual bleeding and atrophies the uterine lining.[64,65] This effect would be a desirable benefit in obese, Type 2 diabetic women, who tend to be parous, older and at higher risk of endometrial cancer.

In summary, either the copper-medicated or levonorgestrel-releasing IUD provide excellent long-term pregnancy protection, and their use should be encouraged in women with overt diabetes and prior GDM. General gynecological principles should be followed for proper patient selection, insertion, and monitoring of IUD use. Ideal candidates are parous, without a history of PID and at low risk for sexually transmitted disease. General prophylaxis with insertion or removal has not been shown to provide any benefit and is not indicated.

Conclusions

Women with either Type 1 or Type 2 diabetes or prior GDM can be offered several contraceptive options, which when properly selected and closely monitored do not accelerate their disease process or affect their medical therapy. Their contraceptive choice should address their individual lifestyle preferences as well as their state of health and possible pregnancy plans. Consultation and coordinated medical care between their internists and gynecologists should occur. Most importantly, each diabetic or potentially diabetic woman needs to be educated and be an active participant in her pregnancy planning, which allows her to choose either to avoid conceiving or to time her pregnancy to meet personal and health reasons. This can only happen when she is provided with an effective contraceptive method.

REFERENCES

1. Mills JL, Baker L, Goldman AS. Malformations in infants of diabetic mothers occur before the seventh gestational week. Diabetes 1979; 28: 292–3.
2. Towner D, Kjos SL, Leung B, et al. Congenital malformations in pregnancies complicated by NIDDM. Diabetes Care 1995; 18: 1446–51.
3. Schaefer UM, Songster G, Xiang A, et al. Congenital malformations in offspring of women with hyperglycemia first detected during pregnancy. Am J Obstet Gynecol 1997; 177: 1165–71.
4. Fuhrmann K, Reiher H, Seemler K, et al. The effect of intensified conventional insulin therapy before and during pregnancy on malformation rate in offspring of diabetic mothers. Exp Clin Endocrinol 1984; 83: 173–7.
5. Peters RK, Kjos SL, Xiang A, Buchanan TA. Long-term diabetogenic effect of a single pregnancy in women with prior gestational diabetes mellitus. Lancet 1996; 347: 227–30.
6. Metzger BE, Coustan DM and the Organizing Committee. Summary and recommendations of the Fourth International Workshop–Conference on Gestational Diabetes Mellitus. Diabetes Care 1998; 21(suppl. 2): B161–7.
7. Wilson ES, Cruickshank J, McMaster M, et al. A prospective controlled study of the effect on blood pressure of contraceptive preparations containing different types of dosages and progestogen. Br J Obstet Gynaecol 1984; 91:1254–60.
8. Meade TW. Oral contraceptives, clotting factors and thrombosis. Am J Obstet Gynecol 1982; 142: 758–61.
9. Godsland IF, Crook D, Simpson R, et al. The effects of different formulations of oral contraceptive agents on lipid and carbohydrate metabolism. N Engl J Med 1990; 323: 1375–81.
10. Spellacy WN, Buhi WC, Birk SA. The effect of estrogens on carbohydrate metabolism: glucose, insulin and growth hormone studies on one hundred seventy-one women ingesting premarin, mestranol and ethinyl estradiol for six months. Am J Obstet Gynecol 1971; 114: 388–92.
11. Perlman JA, Russell-Briefel R, Ezzati T, et al. Oral glucose tolerance and the potency of contraceptive progestins. J Chronic Dis 1985; 338: 857.
12. Spellacy W. Carbohydrate metabolism during treatment with estrogen, progestogen and low-dose oral contraceptive preparations on carbohydrate metabolism. Am J Obstet Gynecol 1982; 142: 732.
13. Skouby SO, Jensen BM, Kuhl C, et al. Hormonal contraception in diabetic women: acceptability and influence on diabetes control of a nonalkylated estrogen/progestogen compound. Contraception 1985; 32: 23.
14. Skouby SO, Molsted-Pedersen L, Kuhl C, et al. Oral contraceptives in diabetic women: metabolic effects of four compounds with different estrogen/progestogen profiles. Fertil Steril 1986; 46: 858.
15. Radberg T, Gustafson A, Skryten A, et al. Oral contraception in diabetic women. Diabetes control, serum and high density lipoprotein lipids during low-dose progestogen, combined oestrogen/progestogen and non-hormonal contraception. Acta Endocrinol 1981; 98: 246.
16. Peterson KR, Skouby SO, Sidelmann J, et al. Effects of contraceptive steroids on cardiovascular risk factors in women with insulin-dependent diabetes mellitus. Am J Obstet Gynecol 1994; 171: 400–5.
17. Peterson KR, Skouby SO, Vedel P, Haaber AB. Hormonal contraception in women with IDDM. Diabetes Care 1995; 18: 800–6.
18. Steel JM, Duncan LJP. Serious complications of oral contraception in insulin-dependent diabetics. Contraception 1978; 17: 291.
19. Klein BEK, Moss SE, Klein R. Oral contraceptives in women with diabetes. Diabetes Care 1990; 13: 895.
20. Garg SK, Chase HP, Marshal G, et al. Oral contraceptives and renal and retinal complications in young women with insulin-dependent diabetes mellitus. J Am Med Assoc 1994; 271: 1099–102.
21. Loke DFM, Ng CSA, Samsioe G, et al. A comparative study of the effects of a monophasic and a triphasic oral contraceptive containing ethinyl estradiol and levonorgestrel on lipid and lipoprotein metabolism. Contraception 1990; 42: 535–54.
22. Petersen KR, SKouby SO, Pederson RG. Desogestrel and gestodene in oral contraceptives: 12 months' assessment of carbohydrate and lipoprotein metabolism. Obstet Gynecol 1991; 78: 666–72.
23. Runnebaum B, Grunwald K, Rabe T. The efficacy and tolerability of norgestimate/ethinyl estradiol (250mg of norgestimate/35mg of ethinyl estradiol): results of a open, multicenter study of 59,701 women. Am J Obstet Gynecol 1992; 166: 1963–8.
24. van der Vange N, Kloosterboer HJ, Haspels AA. Effect of seven low-dose combined oral contraceptive preparations on carbohydrate metabolism. Am J Obstet Gynecol 1987; 156: 918–22.
25. Stampfer MJ, Willet WC, Colditz GA, et al. A prospective study of past use of oral contraceptive agents and risk of cardiovascular disease. N Engl J Med 1988; 319: 1313.
26. Porter JB, Hunter JR, Jick H, et al. Oral contraceptives and nonfatal vascular disease. Obstet Gynecol 1985; 66: 1.
27. Porter JB, Jick H, Walker AM. Mortality among oral contraceptive users. Obstet Gynecol 1987; 70: 29.
28. Rosenberg L, Palmer JR, Lesko SM, et al. Oral contraceptive use and the risk of myocardial infarction. Am J Epidemiol 1990; 131: 1009.
29. WHO Collaborative Study of Cardiovascular Disease and Steroid Hormone Contraception. Acute myocardial infarction and combined oral contraceptives; Results of an international multicenter case-control study. Lancet 1997; 349: 1202–9.

30. Lidegaard Ø. Oral contraceptives, pregnancy and the risk of cerebral thromboembolism: the influence of diabetes, hypertension, migraine and previous thrombotic disease. Br J Obstet Gynaecol 1995; 102: 153–9.

31. National Cholesterol Education Project. Second Report of the Expert Panel on Detection, Evaluation and Treatment of High Blood Cholesterol in Adults.

32. O'Sullivan JB. Diabetes after GDM. Diabetes 1991; 40(suppl. 2): 131–5.

33. Kjos SL, Peters RK, Xiang A, et al. Predicting future diabetes in Latino women with gestational diabetes: utility of early postpartum glucose tolerance. Diabetes 1995; 44: 586–91.

34. Pettitt DJ, Knowler WC, Baird HR, Bennet PH. Gestational diabetes: infant and maternal complications of pregnancy in relation to third-trimester glucose tolerance in Pima Indians. Diabetes Care 1979; 3: 458–64.

35. Peters RK, Kjos SL, Xiang A, Buchanan TA. Long-term diabetogenic effect of a single pregnancy in women with prior gestational diabetes mellitus. Lancet 1996; 347: 227–30.

36. Skouby SO, Kuhl C, Molsted-Pedersen L, et al. Triphasic oral contraception: metabolic effects in normal women and those with previous gestational diabetes. Am J Obstet Gynecol 1985; 153: 495.

37. Skouby SO, Anderson O, Saurbrey N, et al. Oral contraception and insulin sensitivity: in vivo assessment in normal women and women with previous gestational diabetes. J Clin Endocrinol Metab 1987; 64: 519.

38. Kjos SL, Shoupe D, Douyan S, et al. Effect of low-dose oral contraceptives on carbohydrate and lipid metabolism in women with recent gestational diabetes: results of a controlled, randomized, prospective study. Am J Obstet Gynecol 1990; 163: 1822.

39. Kjos SL, Peters RK, Xiang A, et al. Contraception and the risk of type 2 diabetes mellitus in Latina women with prior gestational diabetes mellitus. J Am Med Assoc 1998; 280: 533–8.

40. The Expert Committee on the Diagnosis and Classification of Diabetes Mellitus. Report of the Expert Committee on the Diagnosis and Classification of Diabetes Mellitus. Diabetes Care 1997; 20: 1183–97.

41. Konje JC, Otolorin EO, Ladipo AO. The effect of continuous subdermal levonorgestrel (Norplant) on carbohydrate metabolism. Am J Obstet Gynecol 1992; 166: 15–9.

42. Liew DFM, Ng CSA, Yong YM, et al. Long term effects of depo-provera on carbohydrate and lipid metabolism. Contraception 1985; 31: 51.

43. Fahmy K, Abdel-Razik, Shaaraway M, et al. Effect of long-acting progestaten-only injectable contraceptives on carbohydrate metabolism and its hormonal profile. Contraception 1991; 44: 419–29.

44. Kim C, Seidel KW, Degier EA, Kwok YS. Diabetes and depot medroxyprogesterone contraception in Navajo women. Arch Intern Med 2001; 1616: 1766–71.

45. World Health Organization. Special programme of research, development, and research training in human reprodcution: a multi-centered phase III comparative clinical trial of depot medroxyprogesterone acetate given 3-monthly at doses of 100mg, or 150mg. Contraception 1986; 34: 223–35.

46. Sivin I, Viegas O, Campodonico I, et al. Clinical performance of a new two-rod levonorgestrel contraceptive implant: a three-year randomized study with Norplant implants as controls. Contraception 1997; 55: 73–80.

47. Zheng SR, Zheng HM, Qian SZ, et al. A long-term study of the efficacy and accetability of a single-rod hormonal contraceptive implant (Implanon) in healthy women in China. Eur J Contracept Reprod Health Care 1999; 4: 85–93.

48. Kaunitz AM, Garceau RJ, Cromie MA. Comparative safety, efficacy and cycle control of Lunelle monthly contraceptive injection (medroxyprogesterone acetate and estradiol cypionate injectable suspension) and Ortho-Novum 7/7/7 oral contraceptive (norethindrone/ethinyl estradiol triphasic). Lunelle Study Group. Contraception 1999; 60: 179.

49. Timmer CJ, Mulders TM. Pharmacokinetics of etonogestrel and ethinylestradiol released from a combined contraceptive vaginal ring. Clin Pharmacokinet 2000; 39: 233.

50. Cramer DW, Schiff I, Schoenbaum SC, et al. Tubal infertility and the intrauterine device. N Engl J Med 1985; 312: 941.

51. Lee NC, Rubin GL, Ory HW, et al. Type of intrauterine device and the risk of pelvic inflammatory disease. Obstet Gynecol 1983; 62: 1.

52. Lee NC, Rubin GL. The intrauterine device and pelvic inflammatory disease revisited: new results form the Women's Health Study. Obstet Gynecol 1988; 72: 1.

53. Farley TMM, Rosenberg MJ, Rowe PJ, et al. Intrauterine devices and pelvic inflammatory disease: an international perspective. Lancet 1992; 339: 785–8.

54. Skouby SO, Molsted-Pedersen L, Kosonen A. Consequences of intrauterine contraception in diabetic women. Fertil Steril 1984; 42: 568.

55. Kimmerle R, Weiss R, Berger M, Kurz K-H. Effectiveness, safety and acceptablilty of a copper intrauterine device (CU Safe 300) in type I diabetic women. Diabetes Care 1993; 16: 1227–30.

56. Kjos SL, Ballagh SA, La Cour M, et al. The copper T380A intrauterine device in women with type II diabetes mellitus. Obstet Gynecol 1994; 84: 1006–9.

57. Gosen C, Steel J, Ross A, et al. Intrauterine contraception in diabetic women. Lancet 1982; 1: 530–5.

58. Lawless M, Vessey MP. Intrauterine device use by diabetic women. Br J Fam Plan 1982; 7: 110–1.

59. Wiese J. Intrauterine contraception in diabetic women. Fertil Steril 1977; 28: 422.

60. Kjos SL. Contraception in diabetic women. Obstet Gynecol Clin N Am 1996; 23: 243.

61. Andersson K, Odlind V, Rybo G. Levonorgestrel-releasing and copper-releasing (Nova T) IUDs during five years of use: a randomized comparative trial. Contraception 1994; 49: 56.

62. Jonsson B, Landgren B-M, Eneroth O. Effects of various IUDs on the composition of cervical mucus. Contraception 1991; 43: 447.

63. Rivera R, Yacobson I, Grimes D. The mechanism of action of hormonal contraceptives and intrauterine contraceptive devices. Am J Obstet Gynecol 1999; 181: 1263.

64. Andersson K. Levonorgestrel releasing IUD – more than a contraceptive. Acta Obstet Gynecol Scand 1994; 73(suppl. 161): 55.

65. Lahteenmake P, Haukkamaa M, Puolakka J, et al. Open randomized study of the use of levonorgestrel releasing intrauterine system as an alternative to hysterectomy. Br Med J 1998; 316: 1122.

60 Hormone replacement therapy and diabetes

Bari Kaplan, Michael Hirsch and Dov Feldberg

Introduction

After the onset of menopause, the average woman in developed countries lives for nearly 30 years in an estrogen-deficient state. Both estrogen and progesterone affect cells response to insulin. This response, in turn, affects the level of blood glucose. Unfortunately, less than 20% of these women receive any form of treatment.[1]

The use of postmenopausal hormone replacement therapy (HRT) poses one of the most difficult health care decisions women face today. HRT offers well-established benefits, including alleviation of vasomotor symptoms, management of urogenital atrophy and libido decline, and prevention of osteoporosis and fractures. It may also provide a cardiovascular protective effect, reduce the risk of colorectal cancer[2] and lower overall mortality rates.[3,4] However, concerns regarding the safety of HRT have recently been raised.[5]

HRT is prescribed less often for women with diabetes than for nondiabetic women.[6–10] The reasons for this is unclear, although fear of adverse effects among both patients and physicians may play an important role. Many cautions are included in the product literature and, until recently, both diabetes and hypertension were listed as contraindications in the *British National Formulary*.[11] In addition, studies have shown that women 65 years of age or older with chronic medical disease tend to be under treated for other, unrelated, disorders.[12]

Carbohydrate metabolism and aging

The prevalence of Type 2, or noninsulin-dependent, diabetes increases with age,[12–14] affecting *c.* 20% of individuals more than 65 years old. Older individuals with Type 2 diabetes tend to be leaner than younger ones. Most studies demonstrate an age-related increase per decade of 10–20 mg/L in fasting glucose concentrations and *c.* 150 mg/L in postprandial glucose concentrations.[12–15] This is accompanied, on average, by a small increase in fasting hepatic glucose output, impaired noninsulin-dependent glucose disposal,[12,13] and less insulin release in the early and late phase after glucose challenge.[16] The distribution of insulin moieties also appear to shift with age.[17] Other endocrine changes, particularly in adrenal function, may contribute to this process.[12]

Obesity, fat distribution, and body composition also alter with age. Generally, fat mass increases until about the age of 65 and then it begins to decrease.[18] Lean body mass decreases steadily from the fifth or sixth decade onward. In women, adiposity tends to concentrate in the abdomen (central obesity). Obesity itself increases insulin resistance, and the emerging dyslipidemia and disturbances in the coagulation system.

The weight gain and altered body composition are, in turn, affected by changing habits in dietary intake and physical activity with aging, which alone may play a role in increasing insulin resistance. Individuals with leaner body mass have lower skeletal muscle volume, the main target tissue that lowers plasma glucose concentrations in reaction to insulin.

Effects of menopause on carbohydrate metabolism

Type 2 diabetes occurs more often in women than men in the older age group. Whether menopause contributes to this difference remains unclear because the discrimination of changes associated with menopause from those due to aging is difficult. Any changes observed in individual women followed through menopause will be influenced by aging and, given the extended duration of the perimenopause, such studies are extremely difficult to undertake.

No effect of menopause on fasting plasma glucose levels was found in women who became postmenopausal during the course of the Framingham Study.[19] Similarly, there was no effect of menopause on fasting or on the 2-h oral glucose tolerance test (OGTT) glucose, or insulin levels, in the prospective study of Matthews et al.[20]

Nevertheless, menopause is associated with many characteristics of the insulin resistance syndrome, including increased cardiovascular morbidity and mortality, and accretion of generalized and visceral adiposity. Reduced lean body mass, sedentary lifestyle and, possibly, reduced estrogen-dependent blood flow to skeletal muscles, may result in decreased peripheral glucose uptake, impaired insulin secretion and increased insulin resistance.

Some insight into whether menopause affects insulin and glucose metabolism may be gained from experimental studies of the effects of estrogen and progesterone. Early studies consistently demonstrated increased pancreatic insulin secretion in response to glucose in animals treated with estrogens,[21–23] similar observations were subsequently made in islet cells isolated from estrogen-treated animals.[24–26]

Estrogen and progesterone may augment the pancreatic insulin response to glucose. However, estrogen apparently increases the sensitivity of insulin-dependent metabolic processes, such as tissue glucose uptake and lipid synthesis, to insulin,[27–29] whereas progesterone has the opposite effect.[30–32] Therefore, menopause might be expected to result in some reduction in pancreatic insulin output and deterioration in glucose tolerance, but the effects on insulin sensitivity are likely to depend on the relative contributions of the two hormones. It is conceivable that insulin sensitivity might increase with the reduction in progesterone concentrations at menopause.

Effects of diabetes mellitus on postmenopausal women

Women with Type 1 diabetes frequently go through menopause at an earlier age, in average age of 41.6 years than nondiabetic women with an average age of 49.9 years.[33]

Diabetes mellitus (DM) was found to be associated with an increase in uterine size in postmenopausal women.[34] In addition, the relative risk of endometrial cancer in diabetic women is 4-fold higher than in nondiabetic women.[27,35] The risk of endometrial cancer also increases with the use of unopposed estrogen in non-hysterectomized women[36] and is reduced with the use of cyclical or continuous progestins.[37–39]

Women become more prone to urinary and vaginal infections during and after menopause, this problem is greater in women with diabetes.[40] Over the course of 2 years, women with diabetes were 1.5 times as likely to have a urinary tract infection with symptoms and twice as likely to have one without symptoms as women without diabetes were. Both risks were higher in women who took insulin and women who had had diabetes for at least 10 years.

According to most studies, Type 2 diabetes is associated with high bone mineral densities (BMD)[41,42] and Type 1, or insulin-dependent diabetes, with decreased BMD. The prospective Iowa Women's Health Study of >30,000 women revealed that women with Type 1 diabetes were 12.25 times more likely to have an incident hip fracture than nondiabetic women; the relative rate for women with Type 2 diabetes was only 1.7.[43] Most studies have reported no consistent relationship between metabolic control of diabetes and BMD.

Possible mediators of the osteopenia are microangiopathy at the bone tissue, and changes in insulin, insulin-related growth factors (IGF) and other cytokines involved in bone metabolism.[44] Recent studies have also tentatively attributed the higher incidence of hip fractures in Type 1 diabetics to the absence of amylin, a 37-amino-acid polypeptide normally secreted by the pancreatic beta cells. Amylin binds to calcitonin receptors, lowers plasma calcium concentrations, inhibits osteoclasts and stimulates osteoblasts.[45] Leptin may play a role in bone regulation in Type 2 diabetes.

Effect of HRT on carbohydrate metabolism

In nondiabetic postmenopausal women, HRT seems to have no increased effect on future diabetic risk. Gabal et al.[46] reported no change in the age-adjusted relative risk of developing Type 2 diabetes in postmenopausal women followed for 11.5 years. Similarly, in a prospective follow-up study of 12 years, Manson et al.[47] noted no increase in the incidence of Type 2 diabetes among past users of HRT; the relative risk (RR) in current users was 0.8 (RR 0.67–0.96). These findings did not change significantly after multivariate adjustment for age, body mass index (BMI), family history of diabetes and coronary risk factors. Accordingly, one 10-year literature review found no compelling evidence for a reduced risk of diabetes in women treated by HRT.[48]

HRT reportedly contributes to the control of glucose levels. The Women Health Initiative (WHI) study, have shown that healthy postmenopausal women who took combined conjugated equine estrogen (CEE)/ medroxyprogesterone acetate (MPA)[49] or CEE alone,[50] develop diabetes at a lower rate than women who did not take hormones. Hazard ratio was 0.79 (95% CI 0.67–0.93, $P = 0.004$) for the combined treatment and 0.88 (95% CI 0.77–1.01, $P = 0.072$) in the only estrogen treated women. These data suggests that combined therapy with estrogen and progestin reduces the incidence of diabetes, possibly mediated by a decrease in insulin resistance unrelated to body size.[49] Postmenopausal therapy with estrogen alone may reduce the incidence of treated diabetes. However, the effect was smaller than that seen with estrogen plus progestin.[50] Similar results were also obtained in several other well controlled studies. In the Heart and Estrogen/progestin Replacement (HERS) study data,[51] a randomized double blind placebo controlled HRT trial in women with coronary heart disease, treatment by combined continuous CEE/MPA in non DM women, fasting glucose remained unchanged in the treatment group but increased significantly in the placebo treated women. Likewise, Incidence of DM was 6.2% in the treated group versus 9.5% in the placebo. The calculated relative hazard to develop DM was 0.65 (95% CI 0.480–0.89, $P = 0.006$) and the number needed to treat to prevent a single case of DM was 30 (95% CI 18–103).

Calculated insulin resistance (HOMA-IR) was reduced by 12.9% for HRT compared to controls, fasting glucose by 2.5%, and fasting insulin by 9.3%, in nondiabetic postmenopausal women.[52] Os et al.[53] investigated 99 women treated by transdermal beta-estradiol for 1 year combined by 14 days of MPA every 3 months. Insulin sensitivity increased during the only estrogen treatment period but this effect was negated by the adding of MPA. In another study,[54] in 30 women treated by sequential E2/NETA compared to placebo during 6 months, a steady decline in insulin sensitivity was observed, however, in parallel to that observed in the placebo group. The reduced insulin sensitivity may be explained by doing all measurements during the only estrogen treatment phase. In a cross sectional study of 427 postmenopausal women, only CEE/MPA treatment did show a reduction in insulin resistance if compared to placebo.[55] No such effect was seen in the E2/NETA, raloxifene or tibolone treated women. Contrarily, in a prospective randomized control trial (RCT) on 71 non-obese women treated with either CEE/MPA combined treatment or placebo for one year, HRT was associated with significantly worsening of insulin sensitivity.[56]

In diabetic postmenopausal women, HRT confers too, a better control of carbohydrate metabolism. One study reported lower glycosylated hemoglobin (HbA1c) levels (i.e. greater glycemic control) in 14 overweight diabetic women treated by HRT [2 months of CEE 0.625 mg, followed by combined CEE/MPA 5mg than in an equal number of age- and weight-matched untreated women.[57] The treated women also showed a reduction in total cholesterol, but no change in triglyceride (TG), fasting glucose or insulin concentrations. These findings were confirmed in another study wherein short-term (6 weeks) oral estradiol was administered to women with Type 2 diabetes.[58] In a retrospective study of c. 15,000 women with Type 2 diabetes in northern California, glycemic control improved to an equal degree with either estrogen or estrogen–progestin replacement therapy.[59]

Somewhat different conclusion was derived from studies conducted with HRT in American Indians, who have a particularly high prevalence and incidence of the disease. The Strong Heart Study (SHS), which investigated 13 tribes in three geographic areas, noted a 40–70% prevalence of Type 2 diabetes in women aged 45–74.[60] Postmenopausal estrogen therapy led to a reduction in fasting glucose but was associated with deterioration in glucose tolerance. The authors concluded that long-term use of estrogen use may increase the risk of Type 2 diabetes.

It may be concluded that although most of the data support a positive effect of HRT on glucose metabolism in both diabetic and nondiabetic postmenopausal women, the ultimate results depends on the population being studied and characteristics of the HRT.

Hormone replacement therapy in the diabetic patient

Traditionally, the prevention of severe renal disease and retinopathy has been the primary target in the long-term management of diabetes. It seems that HRT carries neutral effect toward these goals. In a 10-year follow-up of women with late-onset diabetes, HRT use was found to be unrelated to the severity of retinopathy or the incidence of macular edema.[61] In another study, 6 months of CEE/MPA treatment failed to reverse micro-albuminuria in postmenopausal diabetic patients.[62]

Effect of HRT on cardiovascular risk

Diabetes is a major risk factor for coronary heart disease (CHD) in women and event rates increase substantially after menopause. Older individuals with diabetes are more prone to cardiovascular and peripheral vascular complications than

older individuals without diabetes, and they have a poorer prognosis in the presence of these complications.[13]

This risk is greater in women than in men. Many observational studies have shown that HRT reduces mortality due to coronary heart disease (CHD) by c. 50%; however, this has not been confirmed in RCT. Two long-term prospective randomized studies, the HERS[63] and the WHI,[64] suggested that HRT may actually increase the risk of coronary vascular disease. This was particularly true during the first year after the initiation of hormonal treatment. Therefore, HRT is not currently indicated for the primary or secondary prevention of CHD. However, it is important to note, that, among younger healthy postmenopausal women, aged 50–59 years at baseline, a tendency for reduced CHD was observed during a 7-year period of CEE only treatment.[65] In diabetic women specifically, there are, at present, no long-term studies. The many short-term studies infer that HRT may have beneficial effects on glucose homeostasis, the lipid profile and fibrinolytic activity, all compatible with the prevention of CHD. A recent study suggested that women with Type 2 diabetes may stand to benefit more from any HRT cardioprotection than their nondiabetic counterparts because of their higher absolute baseline risk.[66] Nevertheless, the unknown effect of HRT on endometrial cancer and venous thromboembolism, which occur more often in diabetic women than in the general population, need to be considered.

Some of the inflammatory biomarkers should also be considered in regard to HRT in diabetics. C-reactive protein (CRP), a marker of inflammation, is associated with increased cardiovascular risk; its levels are increased in diabetes. Both combined and estrogen only HRT, regardless of specific type of preparation, cause a significant increase in the CRP concentration.[67] This has been also verified in Type 2 diabetic women.[68] However, levels of IL-6, another inflammatory biomarker of increased CHD, remained unchanged in nondiabetics[69] as well as in DM women during HRT.[70]

Effect of HRT on atherosclerosis

One case–control study reported an absence of adverse effects of HRT on the risk of fatal and non-fatal myocardial infarctions in diabetic women,[71] and another 27 month observational follow-up study reported a positive impact of HRT, with fewer myocardial infarctions in estrogen-treated compared to untreated patients after percutaneous transluminal coronary balloon angioplasty (PTCA).[72] A larger cross-sectional study on 623 postmenopausal women with diabetes showed that atherosclerosis, as determined by the intimal–medial wall thickness of the common and internal carotid arteries, was reduced in the internal carotid in both current and former users of HRT.[73]

Effect of HRT on vascular reactivity

Menopause and diabetes have independent and adverse impacts on microvascular reactivity, as measured by forearm cutaneous vasodilation in response to acetylcholine and nitroprusside. HRT was found to improve this relaxation response in both healthy and diabetic subjects.[74] Another in vitro study conducted in patients with Type 2 diabetes given

HRT for 6 months yielded similar results, demonstrating an effect of HRT on both endothelium-dependent and -independent mechanisms of vascular relaxation.[75] Other studies on vascular function failed to confirm beneficial effect of HRT. In short term controlled study no significant effect of HRT was shown during performance of isometric exercises or intra-venous infusion of vasoactive substances. However, mental stress induced blood pressure elevation, was moderated by estrogen only treatment in the diabetic patients but not in the nondiabetics.[76] HRT also failed to reduce elevated levels of endothelin-1, a natural vasoconstrictor, which is characteristic of Type 2 diabetes.[77] In a small prospective study, low dose E2/NETA, failed to improve endothelial function in postmenopausal diabetics.[78] Finally, there was no effect on clinic or ambulatory blood pressure, arterial load indexes or circadian blood pressure variations in the diabetic group, as was anticipated according to such improvements noted in nondiabetic women treated by HRT.[79]

Effect of HRT on the coagulation system

Short-term (3 month) treatment with oral estradiol in diabetic women led to a significant increase in tissue plasminogen activator activity and, thereby, an improvement in fibrinolytic activity.[28] As observed by others, the increase in tissue plasminogen activator activity was noted only when TG levels were within the normal range.[13] Other effects on the coagulation system included a small reduction in antithrombin level. There was no change in the levels of fibrinogen, the von Willebrand factor, prothrombin, protein S or protein C, or in resistance to activated protein C.[80]

Effect of HRT on blood lipids

Many studies show beneficial effect of HRT on lipid profile in postmenopausal diabetic women. Data from a large survey conducted between 1988 and 1994, presented a better lipoprotein profile and glycemic control among current HRT users postmenopausal diabetic women if compared to never users or previous users of HRT.[81] Overall, HRT increased HDL cholesterol and reduced LDL cholesterol, LDL/HDL ratio and lipoprotein-A compared to placebo or no treatment. Combined HRT had no effect on triglycerides.[52] Recent data from the Diabetes Heart Study,[68] related HRT use to a significant reduction of LDL cholesterol levels in Type 2 DM patients. Apolipoprotein A1 levels are increased by c. 20% in diabetic subjects and can be reduced by HRT.[82] In one study, short-term oral estradiol treatment of postmenopausal diabetic women increased high-density lipoprotein (HDL) cholesterol and its subfraction HDL2 and apolipoprotein A1, whereas low-density lipoprotein (LDL) cholesterol and apolipoprotein B levels decreased.[58,83] Andersson et al.,[83] using a double-blind crossover placebo-controlled design, investigated 25 postmenopausal women with Type 2 diabetes treated with oral estradiol. Blood tests performed after 68 days yielded a decrease in blood glucose, HbA1c, total cholesterol and LDL cholesterol and an increase of HDL cholesterol.[83] A study on combined continuous HRT compared to placebo

for 6 months[84] revealed somewhat different results compared to estradiol only treatment. Apo-lipoprotein A and B, total cholesterol, LDL cholesterol, fibrinogen and fructosamin were reduced whereas; TG and HDL cholesterol remained unchanged.

Usually, the effect of HRT in diabetic is milder, compared to nondiabetic population. This was shown, in a large cross-sectional population study, where HRT use was associated with lower increase of HDL cholesterol and higher rise of triglycerides (TG).[64] No significant difference was observed in other lipemic variables as LDL cholesterol and apolipoprotein A or B. Similarly, data from the Strong Heart Study (SHS),[85] a cross-sectional analysis of diabetic and nondiabetic American Indian population characterized by high prevalence of DM, showed that HRT in the diabetics resulted in relative smaller changes if compared to the effect on nondiabetics. HDL cholesterol was increased and plasminogen activator inhibitor (PAI) was reduced by the hormonal treatment. No significant changes were noted in CRP, LDL cholesterol and fibrinogen levels. Another cross-sectional study of 694 diabetic patients also showed that HRT (type and length of treatment not specified) caused an increase in HDL cholesterol, but to a lesser degree than in the nondiabetic control women, resulting in proportionally lower levels of HDL, HDL2, and HDL3 cholesterol. TG increased to a greater extent than in controls. LDL cholesterol and apolipoprotein B decreased, and apolipoprotein A increased to a similar degree in both groups.[86]

Effect of type and mode of delivery of HRT

Evaluating type and mode of delivery of HRT is quite cumbersome. Whereas, some large RCT exists for postmenopausal women in general, only relatively small studies were conducted in diabetics. These too, are heterogeneous in the number of women included in the study, duration of treatment and type of risk factors being assessed. Timing of blood sampling during the study also carries a significant effect, especially in cyclical combined estrogen/progestin regime, where differences may ensue between the only estrogen and the combined estrogen/progestin phases of treatment. As for the nondiabetic population, effect may be changed by nature of the hormonal constituents and route of administration. Since the variability of the estrogenic component is limited, CEE or E2, most of the expected diversity will depend on the wide selection of progestins available. Transdermal hormonal treatment differs mainly by avoiding hepatic first pass of highly concentrated blood hormones characteristic to the oral route. Whereas, hysterectomized women are generally treated by estrogen only regimen, combined estrogen/progestin treatment in non-hysterectomized women can be administered as continuous, cyclic or long cycle regime. Absolute dose and proportions of each of the hormonal constituents also vary significantly among HRT formulations. Nevertheless, an effort is made to summarize existing data in the diabetic menopausal population.

In diabetics, oral CEE only treatment reduced total and LDL cholesterol and increased HDL cholesterol. There was some increase in triglycerides and reduction of fasting glucose and HBA1c. There was an increase in coagulation factors along with some augmentation of the fibrinolytic activity.[87–89] No data was found for either oral or transdermal E2 only treatments.

Adding continuous progestins to oral estrogens, mostly CEE/MPA[57,89] or E2/NETA[90–92] usually resulted in a reduction of total cholesterol and LDL cholesterol. Though, HDL cholesterol remained unchanged instead of increasing as in estrogen only treatment. No significant change was observed for triglycerides, fasting glucose, inflammatory biomarkers, and blood pressure measurements. Continuous combined E2/NETA formulations reduced total cholesterol, triglycerides and coagulation factors II, VIII and XI, while keeping LDL and HDL cholesterol, fasting glucose, and plasminogen activity unchanged.[92,93] It was therefore hypothesized that the impact of combined oral E2/NETA treatment on cardiovascular risk factors in diabetic women is probably neutral.[91]

Cyclic combined oral HRT revealed variable effect depending probably on its progestin content. E2/NETA formulation[94] was characterized by a decrease of total, HDL, LDL cholesterols, triglycerides, factor VII, elastin, and HBA1c. Adding micronized progesterone (MP) to E2[95] kept HDL cholesterol and triglycerides still elevated like in the only estrogen treated women.

In transdermal estrogen treatment combined with either cyclic transdermal NETA[94] or oral MP[95] neutralize effect was seen for glycemic, lipemic, and coagulation variables. Adding oral dedrygeston to trans-dermal E2 further reduced total cholesterol, LDL cholesterol, and HBA1c values.[96] Adding continuous oral norethisterone acetate (NETA) to transdermal estradiol in diabetics, significantly reduced CRP concentrations.[97]

Most studies report that oral estradiol and transdermal estrogen have no adverse effect on insulin resistance.[98] A few trials have actually shown a positive effect of oral estrogen, which the authors suggested was mediated by a reduction in fasting glucose and insulin levels, and an increase in the glucose metabolism rate. Luotola et al.[99] examined the effects of orally administered cyclical NETA given with continuous 17β-estradiol in 30 postmenopausal women followed over 6 months. The combination had little effect, although in women who commenced the study with impaired glucose tolerance, there was some improvement in glucose response. This is in agreement with another study showing that the addition of a progestin does not appear to reverse the observed benefit of estrogen[100] DeCleyn et al.[101] studied 20 postmenopausal women before and 2 months after taking conjugated equine estrogens, and then after 6 months of cyclically administered dydrogesterone (20 mg for 12 days). The lack of change in glucose and the reduction in insulin concentrations suggested that combined therapy improves insulin sensitivity and elimination in postmenopausal women. It was reported that medroxyprogesterone acetate given together with oral estrogen may abolish any beneficial effect on carbohydrate metabolism.[98]

Comparison of oral and transdermal combined hormonal treatment yielded no effect of transdermal treatment on glucose tolerance or insulin concentrations. Neither treatment caused significant insulin resistance compared with baseline levels, but with the oral treatment insulin resistance was significantly greater during the combined phase than the estrogen-only phase.[102]

Longer period of HRT may reverse the effect gained in short term treatments. Short-term treatment with unopposed transdermal estradiol caused a decrease in insulin resistance, but long-term treatment after intermittent MPA was introduced had no effect on either insulin secretion or insulin resistance.[53]

It can be concluded that HRT probably does not impair metabolic balance in postmenopausal diabetics and can even improve insulin sensitivity. Considering various type of treatment regimen, it seems likely, that transdermal route probably carries lesser changes in most glycemic, lipemic and coagulation variables. A similar conclusion emerges from a large cross sectional study on postmenopausal women in the Lund area,[103] detecting lower incidence of impaired glucose tolerance and higher levels of HDL among users of cyclic transdermal E2/NETA treatment. The use of progestins like dydrogesterone and MP, may interfere even less, with the advantageous metabolic effect induced by estrogens.

Effects of hormone replacement therapy on obesity and body composition

Central abdominal fat is associated with increased insulin resistance.[104] The effect of HRT on accretion of visceral adiposity remains unclear. While short-term studies have shown that it is preventive, longer term studies fail to support this finding.[98] HRT reduces lean body mass and waist to hip ratio. However, this effect was rather small although statistically significant.[105] In a study of young postmenopausal women of normal range body weights, previous use of HRT was associated with reduced intra-abdominal fat, but not reduced abdominal subcutaneous fat, sagital diameter, fat-free mass, total fat, insulin sensitivity or body weight.[106] In a small RCT conducted on 57 postmenopausal women, adding growth hormone to HRT increased significantly lean body weight and reduced fat mass further more than that achieved by HRT alone.[107] In overweight postmenopausal women with Type 2 diabetes, HRT reduced the waist-to-hip ratio but not the total fat mass.[57]

Conclusions

Diabetes is apparently not a contraindication for HRT. HRT does not have adverse effects on glycemic control in women with diabetes and certain preparations may even have a positive effect. Some forms also improve the lipid profile in this population. It seems that transdermal hormonal therapy, containing estrogens combined with natural progesterone or NETA, may be the preferable regimen recommended for the diabetic patient, interfering less with an already deranged metabolism.

At present, the use of HRT for the prevention or treatment of cardiovascular disease is unclear, and women should be informed about these data before starting therapy for other reasons. This should not prevent clinicians from prescribing HRT in diabetic women mainly for menopausal symptom control and maybe for the prevention of osteoporosis. However, since there are no long-term studies in women with diabetes who have received HRT, definitive conclusions cannot be reached. On the basis of the data collected so far, however, it is suggested that the risk–benefit ratio is similar to that for the nondiabetic population. Both the decision to prescribe HRT and the specific preparation used should always be tailored to the individual. Individual assessment of the potential benefits and risks of long-term HRT should be performed in women with diabetes as it is for all women when HRT is considered.

REFERENCES

1. Ravnikar VA. Barriers for taking long-term hormone replacement therapy: why do women not adhere to therapy? Eur Menopause J 1996; 3: 90–3.
2. Lester S, Moore V. Oral oestrogen replacement therapy versus placebo for hot flushes (Cochrane Review). The Cochrane Library 1, 2002.
3. Cauley JA, Seeley DG, Browner WS, et al. Estrogen replacement therapy and mortality among older women: the study of osteoporotic fractures. Arch Intern Med 1997; 157: 2181–7.
4. Henderson BE, Paganini-Hill A, Ross RK. Decreased mortality in users of estrogen replacement therapy. Arch Intern Med 1991; 151: 75–8.
5. WHI, Database of Systematic Reviews 2006 Issue 3 of Long term hormone therapy for perimenopausal and postmenopausal women. Cochrane Database of Systematic Reviews 2006 Issue 3.
6. Feher MD, Issacs AJ. Is hormone replacement therapy prescribed for post-menopausal diabetic women? Br J Clin Pract 1996; 50: 431–2.
7. Moorhead T, Hannaford P, Warskyj M. Prevalence and characteristics associated with use of hormone replacement therapy in Britain. Br J Obstet Gynaecol 1997; 104: 290–7.
8. Lawrenson RA, Newson RB, Feher MD. Do women with diabetes receive hormone replacement therapy? Pract Diabetes Int 1998; 15: 71–2.
9. Keating NL, Cleary PD, Rossi AS, et al. Use of hormone replacement therapy by post-menopausal women in the United States. Ann Intern Med 1999; 130: 545–53.
10. Troici RJ, Cowie CC, Harris MI. Hormone replacement therapy and glucose metabolism. Obstet Gynecol 2000; 96: 665–70.
11. British Medical Association (BMA) and Royal Pharmaceutical Society of Great Britain. British National Formulary. London: BMA/Royal Pharmaceutical Society of Great Britain; 1999, pp. 38.
12. Carey VJ, Walters EE, Colditz G, et al. Body fat distribution and risk of non-insulin-dependent diabetes mellitus in women. The Nurses' Health Study. Am J Epidemiol 1997; 145: 614–9.
13. Morrow LA, Halter JB. Treatment of the elderly with diabetes. In: Kahn CR, Weir GC, eds. Joslin's Diabetes Mellitus, 13th edn. Malvern, PA: Lea & Febiger; 1994, pp. 552–9.
14. Meneilly GS, Tessier D. Diabetes in the elderly. Diabet Med 1995; 12: 949–60.
15. Meneilly GS, Dawson K, Tessier D. Alterations in glucose metabolism in the elderly patient with diabetes. Diabetes Care 1993; 16: 1241–7.
16. Shimizu M, Kawazu S, et al. Age-related alteration of pancreatic b-cell function: increased proinsulin and proinsulin-to-insulin molar ratio in elderly, but not in obese, subjects without glucose intolerance. Diabetes Care 1996; 19: 8–11.
17. Perry III HM, Morley JE, Horowitz M, et al. Body composition and age in African-American and Caucasian women: relationship to plasma leptin levels. Metabolism 1997; 46: 1399–405.
18. Silver AJ, Guillen CP, Kahl MJ, et al. Effect of aging on body fat. J Am Geriatr Soc 1995; 41: 211–3.
19. Hjortland MC, McNamara PM, Kannel WB. Some atherogenic concomitants of the menopause: the Framingham Study. Am J Epidemiol 1976; 103: 304–11.
20. Matthews KA, Meilahn E, Kuller LH, et al. Menopause and risk factors for coronary heart disease. N Engl J Med 1989; 321: 641–6.
21. Barnes B, Regan J, Nelson W. Improvement in experimental diabetes following the administration of Amniotin. Am Med Assoc 1933; 101: 926–7.
22. Nelson W, Overholser M. The effect of oestrogenic hormone on experimental pancreatic diabetes in the monkey. Endocrinology 1936; 20: 473–80.
23. Griffiths M, Young F. Does the hypophysis secrete a pancreotropic hormone? Nature 1940; 146: 266–7.
24. Costrini N, Kalkhoff R. Relative effects of pregnancy, estradiol and progesterone on plasma insulin and pancreatic islet insulin secretion. Clin Invest 1971; 50: 992–9.
25. Howell S, Tyhurst M, Green I. Direct effects of progesterone on rat islets of Langerhans in vivo and in tissue culture. Diabetologia 1977; 13: 579–83.
26. Faure A, Sutter-Dub M-T. Insulin secretion from isolated pancreatic islets in the female rat. Short and long term estradiol influence. J Physiol 1979; 75: 289–95.
27. Hager D, Georg J, Leitner J, Beck P. Insulin secretion and content in isolated rat pancreatic islets following treatment with gestational hormones. Endocrinology 1972; 91: 977–81.
28. Ashby J, Shirling D, Baird J. Effects of progesterone on insulin secretion in the rat. J Endocrinol 1978; 76: 479–86.
29. Bailey C, Ahmed-Sorour H. Role of ovarian hormones in the long-term control of glucose homeostasis. Diabetologia 1980; 19: 475–81.
30. Neilsen J. Direct effect of gonadal and contraceptive steroids on insulin release from mouse pancreatic islets in organ culture. Acta Endocrinol 1984; 105: 245–50.
31. McKerns K, Coulomb B, Kaleita E, DeRenzo E. Some effects of in vivo administered oestrogens on glucose metabolism and adrenal cortical secretion in vitro. Endocrinology 1958; 63: 709–22.
32. Samos LF, Roos BA. Diabetes mellitus in older persons. Med Clin N Am 1998; 82: 791–803.
33. Diabetes 2001.
34. Gull B, Karlsson B, Milsom I, Granberg S. Factors associated with endometrial thickness and uterine size in a random sample of post-menopausal women. Am J Obstet Gynecol 2001; 185: 386.
35. Purdie DM, Green AC. Epidemiology of endometrial cancer. Best Pract Res Clin Obstet Gynaecol 2001; 15: 341–54.
36. Grady D, Gebretsadik J, Kerlikowske K, et al. Hormone replacement therapy and endometrial cancer risk: a meta-analysis. Obstet Gynecol 1995; 85: 304–13.
37. Sturdee DW, Wade-Evans T, Paterson ME, et al. Relations between bleeding pattern, endometrial biopsy and oestrogen treatment in post-menopausal women. Br Med J 1978; 1: 1575–7.
38. The Writing Group for the PEPI Trial. Effects of hormone replacement therapy on endometrial histology in post-menopausal women. J Am Med Assoc 1996; 275: 370–5.
39. Sturdee DW, Ulrich LG, Barlow DH, et al. The endometrial response to sequential and continuous combined oestrogen progestogen replacement therapy. Br J Obstet Gynaecol 2000; 107: 1392–400.
40. Am J Epidemiol 2005.
41. Barrett-Connor E, Holbrook TL. Sex differences in osteoporosis in older adults with non-insulin-dependent diabetes mellitus. J Am Med Assoc 1992; 268: 3333–7.
42. Lunt M, Masaryk P, Scheidt-Nave C, et al. The effect of lifestyle, dietary dairy intake and diabetes on bone density and vertebral deformity prevalance: The EVOS Study. Osteoporos Int 2001; 12: 688–98.
43. Nicodemus KK, Folsom AR, Iowa Women's Health Study. Type 1 and type 2 diabetes and incident hip fractures in postmenopausal women. Diabetes Care 2001; 24: 1192–7.
44. Leidig-Bruckner G, Ziegler R. Diabetes mellitus a risk for osteoporosis? Exp Clin Endocrinol Diabetes 2001; 109(suppl. 2): S493–S514.
45. Horcajada-Molteni MN, Chanteranne JB, Lebecque P, et al. Amylin and bone metabolism in streptozotocin-induced diabetic rats. Bone Miner Res 2001; 16: 958–65.
46. Gabal LL, Goodman-Gruen D, Barrett-Connor E. The effect of post-menopausal estrogen therapy on the risk of non-insulin-dependent diabetes mellitus. Am J Public Health 1997; 87: 443–5.
47. Manson JE, Rimm EB, Colditz GA, et al. A prospective study of postmenopausal estrogen therapy and subsequent incidence of non-insulin-dependent diabetes mellirus. Ann Epidemiol 1992; 2: 665–73.

48. Barrett-Connor E. Postmenopausal estrogen therapy and selected (less-often-considered) disease outcomes. Menopause 1999; 6: 14–20.

49. Effect of oestrogen plus progestin on the incidence of diabetes in postmenopausal women: results from the Women's Health Initiative Hormone Trial. Diabetologia 2004; 47.

50. The effect of conjugated equine oestrogen on diabetes incidence: the Women's Health Initiative randomised trial. Diabetologia 2006; 49.

51. Kanaya AM, Herrington D, Vittinghoff E, et al. Glycemic effects of postmenopausal hormone therapy: the Heart and Estrogen/progestin Replacement Study. A randomized, double-blind, placebo-controlled trial. Ann Intern Med 2003; 138: 1–9.

52. Salpeter SR, Walsh JME, Ormiston TM, et al. Meta-analysis: effect of hormone-replacement therapy on components of the metabolic syndrome in postmenopausal women. Diabetes Obes Metab 2006; 8: 538.

53. Os I, Os A, Abdelnoor M, et al. Insulin sensitivity in women with coronary heart disease during hormone replacement therapy. J Womens Health (Larchmt). 2005; 14: 137–45.

54. Walker RJ, Lewis-Barned NJ, Sutherland WH, et al. The effects of sequential combined oral 17beta-estradiol norethisterone acetate on insulin sensitivity and body composition in healthy postmenopausal women: a randomized single blind placebo-controlled study. Menopause 2001; 8: 27–32.

55. Christodoulakos G, Lambrinoudaki I, Panoulis C, et al. Serum androgen levels and insulin resistance in postmenopausal women: association with hormone therapy, tibolone and raloxifene. Maturitas 2005; 50: 321–30.

56. Goodrow GJ, L'Hommedieu GD, Gannon B, Sites CK. Related Articles, Links Predictors of worsening insulin sensitivity in postmenopausal women. Am J Obstet Gynecol 2006; 194: 355–61.

57. Samaras K, Hayward CS, Sullivan D, et al. Effects of postmenopausal hormone replacement therapy on central abdominal fat, glycemic control, lipid metabolism and vascular factors in type 2 diabetes: a prospective study. Diabetes Care 1999; 22: 1401–7.

58. Brussaard HE, Gevers LJ, Frolich M, et al. Short-term oestrogen replacement therapy improves insulin resistance, lipids and fibrinolysis in postmenopausal women with NIDDM. Diabetologia 1997; 40: 843–9.

59. Ferrara A, Karter AJ, Ackerson LM, et al. Hormone replacement therapy is associated with better glycemic control in women with type 2 diabetes: The Northern California Kaiser Permanente Diabetes Registry. Diabetes Care 2001; 24: 1144–50.

60. Zhang Y, Howard BV, Cowan LD, et al. The effect of estrogen use on levels of glucose and insulin and the risk of type 2 diabetes in American Indian postmenopausal women: the strong Heart Study. Diabetes Care.

61. Klein BE, Klein R, Moss SE. Exogenous estrogen exposures and changes in diabetic retinopathy. The Wisconsin Epidemiologic Study of Diabetic Retinopathy. Diabetes Care 1999; 22: 1984–7.

62. Manning PJ, Sutherland WH, Allum AR, de Jong SA, Jones SD. HRT does not improve urinary albumin excretion in postmenopausal diabetic women. Diabetes Res Clin Pract. 2003; 60: 33–9.

63. Hulley SB, Grady D, Bush TL, et al. Randomized trial of estrogen plus progestin for secondary prevention of coronary heart disease in postmenopausal women. Heart and Estrogen/Progestin Replacement Study (HERS) Research Group. J Am Med Assoc 1998; 280: 605–13.

64. Manson JE, et al., Women's Health Initiative Investigators. Estrogen plus progestin and the risk of coronary heart disease. N Engl J Med 2003; 349: 523–34.

65. Hsia J, Langer RD, Manson JE et al., for the Women's Health Initiative Investigators. Conjugated Equine Estrogens and Coronary Heart Disease: The Women's Health Initiative. Arch Intern Med 2006; 166: 357–65.

66. Sattar N, McKenzie J, MacCuish AC, Jaap AJ. Hormone replacement therapy in type 2 diabetes mellitus: a cardiovascular perspective. Diabet Med 1998; 15: 631–3.

67. Ridker PM, Hennekens CH, Rifai N, et al. Hormone replacement therapy and increased plasma concentration of C-reactive protein. Circulation 1999; 100: 713–6.

68. Bowden DW, Lohman K, Hsu FC, et al. Hormone replacement therapy is associated with increased C-reactive protein in women with Type 2 diabetes in the diabetes heart study. Diabet Med 2006; 23: 763–7.

69. Pradhan AD, Manson JE, Rossouw JE, et al. Inflammatory biomarkers, hormone replacement therapy, and incident coronary heart disease: prospective analysis from the Women's Health Initiative observational study. JAMA 2002; 288: 980–7.

70. Manning PJ, Sutherland WH, Allum AR, de Jong SA, Jones SD. Effect of hormone replacement therapy on inflammation-sensitive proteins in post-menopausal women with Type 2 diabetes. Diabet Med 2002; 19: 847–52.

71. Abu-Halawa SA, Thompson K, Kirkeeide RL, et al. Estrogen replacement therapy and outcome of coronary balloon angioplasty in post-menopausal women. Am J Cardiol 1998; 82: 475.

72. Kaplan RC, Heckbert SR, Weiss NS, et al. Postmenopausal estrogens and risk of myocardial infraction in diabetic women. Diabetes Care 1998; 21: 1117–21.

73. Dubuisson JT, Wagenknecht LE, D'Agostino Jr RB, et al. Association of hormone replacement therapy and carotid wall thickness in women with and without diabetes. Diabetes Care 1998; 21: 1790–6.

74. Lim SC, Caballero AE, Arora S, et al. The effect of hormonal replacement therapy on the vascular reactivity and endothelial function of healthy individuals and individuals with type 2 diabetes. J Clin Endocrinol Metab 1999; 84: 4159–64.

75. Perera M, Petrie JR, Hillier C, et al. Hormone replacement therapy can augment vascular relaxation in post-menopausal women with type 2 diabetes. Hum Reprod 2000; 17: 497–502.

76. Manwaring P, Phoon S, Diamond T, Howes LG. Effects of hormone replacement therapy on cardiovascular responses in post-menopausal women with and without type 2 diabetes. Maturitas 2002; 43: 157–64.

77. Saltervo J, Puolakka J, Ylikorkala O. Plasma endothelin in post-menopausal women with type 2 diabetes mellitus and metabolic syndrome: a comparison of oral combined and transdermal oestrogen-only replacement therapy. Diabetes Obes Metab 2000; 2: 293–8.

78. Kernohan AF, Spiers A, Sattar N, et al. Effects of low-dose continuous combined HRT on vascular function in women with type 2 diabetes. Diab Vasc Dis Res. 2004; 1: 82–8.

79. Hayward CS, Samaras K, Campbell L, Kelly RP. Effect of combination hormone replacement therapy on ambulatory blood pressure and arterial stiffness in diabetic postmenopausal women. Am J Hypertens 2000; 14: 699–703.

80. Hahn L, Mattsson LA, Andersson B, Tengborn L. The effects of oestrogen replacement therapy on haemostatic variables in post-menopausal women with non-insulin-dependent diabetes mellitus. Blood Coagul Fibrinolysis 1999; 10: 81–6.

81. Crespo CJ, Smit E, Snelling A, Sempos CT, Andersen RE. NHANES III. Hormone replacement therapy and its relationship to lipid and glucose metabolism in diabetic and nondiabetic postmenopausal women: results from the Third National Health and Nutrition Examination Survey (NHANES III). Diabetes Care. 2002; 25: 1675–80.

82. Sun Z, Larson IA, Ordovas JM, et al. Effects of age, gender and lifestyle factors on plasma apolipoprotein A-IV concentrations. Atherosclerosis 2000; 15: 381–8.

83. Andersson B, Mattsson LA, Hahn L, et al. Estrogen replacement therapy decreases hyperandrogenicity and improves glucose homeostasis and plasma lipids in postmenopausal women with noninsulin-dependent diabetes mellitus. J Clin Endocrinol Metab 1997; 82: 638–43.

84. Manning PJ, Allum A, Jones S, Sutherland WH, Williams SM. The effect of hormone replacement therapy on cardiovascular risk factors in type 2 diabetes: a randomized controlled trial. Arch Intern Med 2001; 161: 1772–6.

85. Zhang Y, Howard BV, Cowan LD, et al. Associations of postmenopausal hormone therapy with markers of hemostasis and inflammation and lipid profiles in diabetic and nondiabetic american Indian women: the strong heart study. J Womens Health (Larchmt). 2004; 13: 155–63.

86. Robinson JC, Folsom AR, Nabulsi AA, et al. Can postmenopausal hormone replacement improve plasma lipids in women with diabetes? The Atherosclerosis Risk in Communities Study Investigators. Diabetes Care 1996; 19: 480–5.

87. Friday KE, Dong C, Fontenot RU. Conjugated equine estrogen improves glycemic control and blood lipoproteins in post-menopausal women with type 2 diabetes. J Clin Endocrinol Metab 2001; 86: 48–52.

88. Sztejnsznajd C, Silva ME, Nussbacher A, et al. Estrogen treatment improves arterial distensibility, fibrinolysis, and metabolic profile in postmenopausal women with type 2 diabetes mellitus. Metabolism 2006; 55: 953–9.

89. Manwaring P, Morfis L, Diamond T, Howes LG. The effects of hormone replacement therapy on plasma lipids in type II diabetes. Maturitas 2000; 34: 239–47.

90. McKenzie J, Jaap AJ, Gallacher S, et al. Metabolic, inflammatory and haemostatic effects of a low-dose continuous combined HRT in women with type 2 diabetes: potentially safer with respect to vascular risk? Clin Endocrinol (Oxf) 2003; 59: 682–9.

91. Scott AR, Dhindsa P, Forsyth J, Mansell P, Kliofem Study Collaborative Group. Effect of hormone replacement therapy on cardiovascular risk factors in postmenopausal women with diabetes. Diabetes Obes Metab 2004; 6: 16–22.

92. Cornu C, Mercier C, Ffrench P, et al. Postmenopause hormone treatment in women with NIDDM or impaired glucose tolerance: the MEDIA randomized clinical trial. Maturitas 2000; 37: 95–104.

93. Perera M, Sattar N, Petrie JR, et al. The effects of transdermal estradiol in combination with oral norethisterone on lipoproteins, coagulation, and endothelial markers in postmenopausal women with type 2 diabetes: a randomized, placebo-controlled study. J Clin Endocrinol Metab 2001; 86: 1140–3.

94. Darko DA, Dornhorst A, Kennedy G, Mandeno RC, Seed M. Glycaemic control and plasma lipoproteins in menopausal women with Type 2 diabetes treated with oral and transdermal combined hormone replacement therapy. Diabetes Res Clin Pract 2001; 54: 157–64.

95. Araujo DA, Farias ML, Andrade AT. Effects of transdermal and oral estrogen replacement on lipids and glucose metabolism in postmenopausal women with type 2 diabetes mellitus. Climacteric 2002; 5: 286–92.

96. Stojanovic ND, Kwong P, Byrne DJ, et al. The effects of transdermal estradiol alone or with cyclical dydrogesterone on markers of cardiovascular disease risk in postmenopausal women with type 2 diabetes: a pilot study. Angiology 2003; 54: 391–9.

97. Sattar N, Perera M, Small M, Lumsden MA. Hormone replacement therapy and sensitive C-reactive protein concentrations in women with type-2 diabetes. Lancet 1999; 354: 1908.

98. Fineberg SE. Glycaemic control and hormone replacement therapy: implications of the Postmenopausal Estrogen Progestogen Intervention (PEPI) study. Drugs Aging 2000; 17: 453–61.

99. Luotola H, Pyorala T, Loikkanen M. Effects of natural oestrogen/progestogen substitution therapy on carbohydrate and lipid metabolism in post-menopausal women. Maturitas 1986; 8: 245–53.

100. Grodstein F, Stampfer MJ, Manson JE, et al. Postmenopausal estrogen use and progestin use and the risk of cardiovascular disease. N Engl J Med 1996; 335: 453–61.

101. DeCleyn K, Buytaert P, Coppens M. Carbohydrate metabolism during hormonal substitution therapy. Maturitas 1989; 11: 235–42.

102. Spencer CP, Godsland IF, Cooper AJ, et al. Effects of oral and transdermal 17beta-estradiol with cyclical oral norethindrone acetate on insulin sensitivity, secretion, and elimination in postmenopausal women. Metabolism 2000; 49: 742–7.

103. Shakir YA, Samsioe G, Nerbrand C, Lidfeldt J, Women's Health in the Lund Area study. Combined hormone therapy in postmenopausal women with features of metabolic syndrome. Results from a population-based study of Swedish women: Women's Health in the Lund Area study. Menopause 2004; 11: 549–55.

104. Sites CK, Calles-Escandon J, Brochu M, et al. Relation of regional fat distribution to insulin sensitivity in postmenopausal women. Fertil Steril 2000; 73: 61–5.

105. Chen Z, Bassford T, Green SB, et al. Postmenopausal hormone therapy and body composition–a substudy of the estrogen plus progestin trial of the Women's Health Initiative. Am J Clin Nutr 2005; 82: 651–6.

106. Sites CK, L'Hommediew GD, Brochu M, Poehlman ET. Previous exposure to hormone replacement therapy and confounders in metabolic studies. Menopause 2000; 8: 281–5.

107. Blackman MR, Sorkin JD, Munzer T, et al. Growth hormone and sex steroid administration in healthy aged women and men: a randomized controlled trial. JAMA 2002; 288: 2282–92.

61 The genetics of diabetic pregnancy

Mark Forbes and Andrew T. Hattersley

Introduction

Genetic factors play a critical role in diabetic pregnancy; they are important in the etiology of maternal hyperglycaemia and also the fetal response to hyperglycaemia. This chapter reviews these two areas. The understanding of the genetics of common, polygenic diabetes is still incomplete especially for Type 2 diabetes. In contrast, the molecular genetics of monogenic diabetes has been almost completely defined. Studying pregnancy in monogenic diabetes, can give insights into normal physiology and the more common forms of gestational diabetes and diabetic pregnancy.

Genes in the etiology of maternal diabetes

Genetic predisposition plays an important role in determining whether a mother has diabetes before she is pregnant or whether she develops diabetes during pregnancy. In most cases in addition to this genetic susceptibility, there is also a considerable environmental component in both Type 1 diabetes or Type 2 diabetes. It is only in monogenic diabetes that the diabetes or hyperglycemia occurs almost exclusively as a result of genes. There are very different issues in the polygenic, complex forms of diabetic pregnancy and the rarer monogenic forms. These are therefore dealt with separately.

Polygenic diabetes

Pre-pregnancy Type 1 diabetes

In most European, Caucasian diabetic pregnancy clinics Type 1 diabetes is the commonest cause of diabetes diagnosed before pregnancy. This is not the case in patients from high prevalence Type 2 populations from the Asian and African continents, where Type 2 diabetes is often as common, or more common, than Type 1. Genetic factors are very important in Type 1 diabetes, even though it is rarely familial. The risk of diabetes before the age of 18 is approximately 6% in siblings of Type 1 diabetic patients, 2% in the offspring of diabetic mothers and 4% in the offspring of diabetic fathers. Although these familial risks are low, the relative risk is greatly increased

compared to a population risk of Type 1 diabetes of 0.4%. The critical role of non-genetic factors is made clear in observations in identical twins: if one twin has Type 1 diabetes the risks of the second twin developing diabetes is in the region of 40%. The nature of the environmental component is uncertain: and might possibly be antigens such as cows' milk and specific viruses or alternatively, reduced exposure to infection resulting in a failure of the immune system to differentiate self and non-self antigens (the hygiene hypothesis).[1]

In contrast to our poor understanding of the environmental factors of Type 1 diabetes, there have been considerable advances in the molecular genetics. There is strong evidence for genetic variation in key components of the autoimmune pathway playing a role in the susceptibility to Type 1 diabetes which are reviewed in detail elsewhere.[2] By far the strongest genetic determinant discovered is the HLA complex.[3] This explains approximately 40–50% of the genetic susceptibility. However, there has been five other definite susceptibility genes defined: insulin,[4] CTLA4,[5] lymphoid tyrosine phospatase,[6] and the interferon-induced helicase (IFIH1) region.[7] Further progress will be made in the coming years by using large patient resources (thousands of patients and matched controls) and whole genome association studies (studying 500,000 markers). It is unlikely, however, that defining the genetic susceptibility in Type 1 patients will alter our management of diabetic pregnancy. Type 1 diabetes usually results in a complete loss of beta-cell function, especially by the time women desire pregnancy, and hence etiological genetic studies play no role in determining the management of the pregnant Type 1 mother that have no endogenous insulin secretion.

Pre-pregnancy Type 2 diabetes

Pre-pregnancy Type 2 diabetes is increasingly common. To have Type 2 diabetes prior to becoming pregnant, onset would have to be early compared to the typical late middle or old age. A key component of subjects diagnosed when young is that they are very likely to have a considerable genetic predisposition, coupled with increased environmental factors such as increased obesity and reduced physical exercise. Table 61.1 includes a comparison of the likely characteristics of early-onset and compares it with late-onset Type 2 diabetes and gestational diabetes. Evidence for the genetic susceptibility includes the increased prevalence of Type 2 diabetes among

Table 61.1 Comparison of the relative role of genetic factors and obesity in young-onset Type 2 diabetes, gestational diabetes and late-onset Type 2 diabetes

	Early-onset Type 2 diabetes	Gestational diabetes	Late-onset Type 2 diabetes
Age of diagnosis	25–45 years	18–40 years	>45 years
Parental history of Type 2 diabetes	+++	++	+
High prevalence racial origin	+++	++	+
Obesity	+++	+++	+

parents and siblings of patients and the fact that families usually come from high prevalence races. This is in keeping with the hypothesis that the greater the genetic predisposition, the earlier the age of diagnosis and supported by linkage studies, in which it has been easier to define genetic susceptibility loci in young-onset diabetic patients compared to patients diagnosed latter.[8]

Although there is clear evidence for genetic susceptibility in Type 2 diabetes, the molecular genetics is considerably less well define than Type 1 diabetes. It is hoped that defining the molecular genetics of Type 2 diabetes will help define the pathogenesis of this complex condition. To date, studies claiming to have found susceptibility genes have rarely been replicated, usually due to the fact that the sample sizes used are too small to reliably detect the small relative risk associated with individual polymorphisms. Any of the initial studies with strongly positive results and relative risks in the region of >1.5 have always overestimated the strength of the association. Hence studies of similar size attempting to replicate the initial result have failed to find any association. As large studies, in the order of 2000–8000 subjects in total are used, it has been shown that genuine predisposing polymorphisms the relative risk is between 1.1 and 1.4. Polymorphisms with this small relative risk will only be detected with large studies and meta-analysis so small studies can be ignored until they are replicated. There are few genes that have shown consistent analysis in large studies and meta-analyses and are now considered to be established these are: TCF7L2,[9] PPAR,[10] Kir6.2,[11] and Calpain 10.[12] Further studies using thousands of patients and controls and examining over 500,000 variants are likely to define new Type 2 diabetes susceptibility polymorphisms in the near future, at least in European Whites. As the majority of studies to date have been performed in European subjects, it is uncertain whether they will define important genes or polymorphisms in the high prevalence populations, where pre-pregnancy Type 2 diabetes is more common.

Gestational diabetes

Gestational diabetes and the relationship to Type 1 diabetes

Type 1 diabetes may be diagnosed for the first time in pregnancy but this is relatively rare. There is an increase in the presence of islet antibodies in gestational diabetes especially in Scandinavian populations suggesting a proportion of patients with gestational diabetes have a slow autoimmune destruction of the beta cell.[13,14] It might be expected that the molecular genetics are similar to latent-autoimmune diabetes in adults (LADA). In keeping with this here is some evidence that HLA associations are present, in patients with gestational diabetes and pancreatic autoantibodies.[13]

Gestational diabetes and the relationship to Type 2 diabetes

Patients who are diagnosed with diabetes or glucose intolerance in pregnancy, and who then return to normal glucose tolerance after pregnancy are known to be at high risk of developing Type 2 diabetes. Estimates of the risk vary between 10 and 50% within 5 years of the pregnancy, depending on the racial group and diagnostic criteria used for gestational diabetes. This would suggest that there is likely to be a similar etiology in gestational diabetes and Type 2 diabetes, with the pregnancy associated insulin resistance precipitating hyperglycemia during pregnancy. It also suggests that the molecular genetics for gestational diabetes will considerably overlap with Type 2 diabetes in the same population.

To date, studies into defining the genetic predisposition to gestational diabetes have had limited success, with no genes showing reproducible association across studies. The main problem has been achieving sufficiently large cohorts for these studies. This has proved considerably more difficult than collecting large collections of Type 2 subjects, partly because one is limited only to women, and also that they need to be diagnosed during pregnancy. It now seems more likely that genetic susceptibility variants will be defined in Type 2 diabetes and then tested in large cohorts of patients with gestational diabetes, using national collaborations and combining cohorts to achieve sufficient power to see the small relative risks.

The published studies thus far have been limited to a few key candidate genes. Early insulin response was reduced in a small study in pregnant women who were homozygous for the −30 polymorphism in the glucokinase gene.[15] This common variation glucokinase mutation was not associated with gestational diabetes in a second small study.[16] However the same variant has been shown in large studies to be associated with both a small increase in fasting glucose (0.1 mmol/L per allele) in pregnancy and also an associated increase in offspring birthweight.[17]

The Trp64Arg polymorphism of the β_3-adrenergic receptor gene was more common in subjects with gestational diabetes in a small study[18] However, this was not replicated in a larger Greek study.[19] We know from studies in Type 2 diabetes that studies of this size (200–500 subjects) usually result in false positives and false negative results.

The largest studies have been in Swedish patients with over 500 cases and over 1100 controls and these have shown some evidence of association with the Type 2 diabetes susceptibility polymorphism E23K in the KCNJ11 gene encoding the Kir6.2 unit of the potassium ATP (K^{ATP}) channel.[20] Other studies in the ABCC8 gene encoding the SUR1 subunit of the K^{ATP} channel have been variable reflecting their small size,[21,22] 2000 #2531}

Until larger cohorts are collected it is unlikely that significant progress will be made in defining the genetic susceptibility to gestational diabetes.

Monogenic diabetes

In marked contrast to the limited progress made in defining polygenic influences in pre-pregnancy gestational diabetes, there have been considerable advances in our understanding of causal monogenic mutations in diabetic pregnancy.

Maturity-onset diabetes of the young

Maturity-onset diabetes of the young (MODY) was initially a clinical classification defined on the basis of dominantly inherited, familial, early-onset (usually before 25 years), noninsulin-dependent diabetes resulting from beta-cell dysfunction.[23] Considerable advances in defining the molecular genetics of this condition mean that there are at least six genetic sub-types recognized, with the majority of these having discreet phenotypes allowing them to be recognized clinically.[23,24] These are outlined in Table 61.2. By far the most common subtypes are hepatic nuclear factor-1 alpha; (HNP-1α) and glucokinase. Within gestational diabetes and diabetic pregnancy clinics glucokinase is probably the most common, although frequently it is not recognized as being MODY as the mild hyperglycemia associated with this dominant condition may not be diagnosed in the parents.

Glucokinase. Glucokinase is the critical enzyme for phosphorylating glucose to glucose-6-phosphate in the pancreas and liver. It is the rate-determining step in both of these tissues and has been called 'the pancreatic glucose sensor'. Mutations throughout the gene encoding glucokinase result in mild fasting hyperglycemia which is present from birth and deteriorates only slightly with age.[25] Typically, the fasting blood glucose will be between 5.5 and 8.0 mmol/L.[25] Consistent with a glucose sensing disorder, the glucose remains regulated at this higher level. In keeping with this, subjects with glucokinase mutations have been shown to have a relatively small increment in response to a glucose load in an oral glucose tolerance test (OGTT).[25] As the level of hyperglycemia is mild, it is rare for patients to be symptomatic or develop diabetic complications. This means that most patients are detected by

screening. Pregnancy is one time when asymptomatic women are screened for hyperglycemia and therefore many glucokinase patients present with gestational diabetes. Many studies have looked at the prevalence of glucokinase mutations in gestational diabetes, which has ranged between 0 and 6% in predominantly European Caucasian groups.[26] As there are no common mutations, these patients can only be detected by full sequencing of the gene. This is both labor intensive and expensive. Ellard and colleagues chose to try and define the phenotype of glucokinase patients in an attempt improve the specificity of the subjects screened. They used the following criteria that had been found in glucokinase MODY families:

1. Fasting blood glucose, both before, during and after pregnancy was consistently >5.5 mmol/L but did not exceed 8.5 mmol/L.
2. In at least one oral glucose tolerance test there was a glucose increment during the OGTT (2-h glucose – a fasting glucose) of <3.5 mmol/L.
3. Either a parent or child also had fasting hyperglycemia consistent with a dominant family history.
4. Subjects were treated with insulin during pregnancy but were managed with diet outside pregnancy.

With these strict criteria they found that 75% (15/20) had a glucokinase mutation.[26] This is clear evidence that selection of phenotype is appropriate prior to screening for the glucokinase mutation. These criteria may have been over-prescriptive, particularly as treating with is a characteristic of the doctor as much as of the characteristic of the pregnancy. Furthermore, family history may be difficult to accurately ascertain as fasting blood glucose needs to be measured in other family members which is not practical within the normal clinical setting. Less strict criteria also increased the detection rate, but they were less specific when they were applied to patients from high prevalence populations.[27] The considerable variation in diabetic pregnancy outcome with differing fetal genotype (Figure 61.1) means that the recognition of glucokinase pregnancies is important.

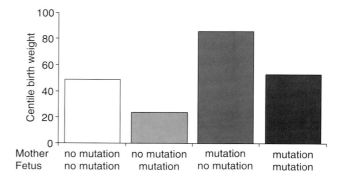

Figure 61.1   The impact of glucokinase mutations in mother and fetus on birth weight centile. (Adapted from Hattersley et al.[40])

Table 61.2   Comparison of the different sub-types of monogenic diabetes that may present in the diabetic pregnancy clinic

	GDM/pre-pregnancy diabetes	Prevalence in diabetic pregnancy clinic	Onset of hyperglycemia Median age diagnosis (range) years	Severity of hyperglycemia	Other features
Glucokinase (MODY2)	Most GDM	3%	From birth14 (0 –85)	Fasting glucose 5.5–8 mmol/L mild deterioration with age	Low renal threshold for glucose
HNF-1α (MODY 3)	Most pre-pregnancy	1%	Adolescence Young adults 22 (6–70)	Progressive May become severe	Sensitive to the glucose lowering effects of sulfonylureas
HNF-4α (MODY 1)	GDM/pre-pregnancy	0.5%	Adolescence, Young to middle aged adults, 32 (12–72)	Progressive May be severe	Sensitive to the glucose lowering effects of sulfonylureas
HNF-1β (MODY5)	GDM/pre-pregnancy	0.3%	Adolescence young adults 24 (6–45)	Progressive May be severe. Rapidly need insulin treatment	Renal cysts Developmental renal disease Renal failure Uterine abnormalities Short
Maternally inherited diabetes and deafness (3243 mutation)	GDM/pre-pregnancy	0.5%	Young to middle aged adults 32 (11–72)	Progressive	Bilateral neural deafness onset as young adult Renal tract abnormalities Pigmented retinopathy Short
Kir6.2/SUR1 diabetes	Pre-pregnancy	0.05%	First 6 months 0.1 (0–0.5)	Insulin dependent if not on sulfonylureas	20% have developmental delay

Hepatic nuclear factor 1 alpha. In most MODY families, patients with HNF-1α mutations diagnosed in the last two decades have been diagnosed before the age of 20. The majority will therefore have pre-pregnancy diabetes. These patients have a strong autosomal dominant family history with a single parent affected and often a grandparent or aunt or uncle on the same side as their affected parent. Typically they are not overweight and present with symptomatic diabetes. As shown in Table 61.2, specific features which characterize HNF-1α MODY include a low renal threshold, meaning that detection by glycosuria is frequent. These patients are very sensitive to sulfonylureas and can be successfully treated with low doses.[28,29] In a randomized control trial sulfonylureas have been shown to be four times more effective than they are in patients with Type 2 diabetes.[29]

The prevalence of HNF-1α mutations in diabetic pregnancy clinics has not been extensively studied. Weng et al. sequenced 66 subjects with gestational diabetes and a family history of diabetes (excluding known MODY families) and found on subject with an HNF-1α mutation and one subject with a HNF-4α mutation.[14] When a diagnosis of HNF-1α MODY has been made, patients can typically be treated with diet or low-dose sulfonylureas. In many cases transferring such patients from sulfonylurea to insulin prior to conception will result in a deterioration of glycemic control. Sulfonylureas have been safely and effectively used in gestational diabetes.[30] It is likely that patients with known HNF-1α mutations and excellent glycemic control on sulfonylurea treatment prior to pregnancy should remain on this treatment during pregnancy. The improved pregnancy outcome, as a result of improved glycemic control, outweighs the uncertainty about sulfonylurea safety in pregnancy. If there is any question of suboptimal glycemic control on sulfonylureas then clearly rapid transfer to insulin would be appropriate.

Other subtypes of MODY. HNF-4α mutations will often present in women before pregnancy. Characteristics may be similar to HNF-1α as shown in Table 61.2: of note they are responsive to sulfonylureas.[31]

HNF-1β mutations usually result in diabetes in the early twenties but the age of diagnosis is very variable and hence can occur before, during or after pregnancy.[32] There is one report of woman presenting with gestational diabetes who had two pregnancies complicated by severe fetal cystic renal disease: one fetus had severe renal failure *in utero* but the second pregnancy resulted in a live child with only moderate renal impairment.[33] Generally, HNF-1β diabetes is not responsive to sulfonylureas and most of these patients will require insulin treatment both during and after pregnancy.[34] Some patients may have uterine and other genital abnormalities which interfere with normal pregnancy.[32]

MODY due to mutations in IPF1 and NEUROD1 are too rare to have any information on pregnancy in these families. It is likely they are similar to other transcription factor mutations.

Other monogenic forms of diabetes

Patients with many other monogenic forms of diabetes may occur in pregnant women (Table 61.3). In some patients the likelihood of pregnancy is reduced: patients with severe insulin resistance may have reduced fertility as a result of the associated polycystic ovarian syndrome and some of the multi-system syndromes that include diabetes suffer from severe neurological defects. The commonest form of monogenic diabetes in the diabetic pregnancy clinic outside the MODY genes is maternally inherited diabetes and deafness due to the mitochondrial 3243tRNA leucine mutation. Permanent neonatal diabetes has recently been shown to frequently result from mutations in the Kir6.2 gene. These are dealt with in more detail below.

Mitochondrial tRNA leucine 3243 mutation. The 3243mtDNA was common is a large Japanese study of the patients attending a diabetic pregnancy clinic. The mutation was present in 6–8% of pre-gestational Type 2 diabetes and gestational diabetes but it was not found in Type 1 diabetes.[35] Interestingly, the subjects with the mutation were more likely to have spontaneous abortions. The prevalence of 3243 mutations is higher

Table 61.3   Impact of monogenic diabetes mutations on birth weight and other clinical features in the neonatal period

	Birthweight	Other features at birth
Glucokinase (MODY2)	Reduced by 500 g	Mild hyperglycemia detectable from first day
HNF-1α (MODY 3)	No effect	–
HNF-4α (MODY 1)	Increased by 800 g	Moderate hypoglycaemia in neonatal period lasts >48 h but <6 months
HNF-1β (MODY5)	Reduced by 700 g	Renal cysts often detected able on antenatal ultrasound. Rare cases of transient neonatal hyperglycemia
Maternally inherited diabetes and deafness (3243 mutation)	Reduced but no formal studies	–
Kir6.2/SUR1 permanent neonatal diabetes	Reduced by 1000 g	Marked hyperglycemia within 24 h but may not be detected
6q imprinted anomalies transient neonatal diabetes	Reduced by 1500 g	Very marked hyperglycemia within 24 h usually detected

in Oriental then European populations[36] and so is likely to be less common in the diabetic pregnancy clinic in European countries.

Permanent neonatal diabetes due to mutations in Kir6.2. Neonatal diabetes arises in about 1 in 100,000–200,000 births. Approximately half have permanent neonatal diabetes, which will persist throughout life, and therefore present in the diabetic pregnancy clinic. The commonest cause of permanent neonatal diabetes are mutations in the *KCNJ11* gene which encode the Kir6.2 gene.[37] These patients are usually diagnosed in the first 3 months of life, but may present any time within 6 months. They present with marked hyperglycemia and/or ketoacidosis and are insulin dependent, shown by having absent or very low levels of C-peptide but, unlike Type 1 diabetes, they do not have auto-antibodies.[37] Traditionally, they will have been treated with insulin throughout life.

Although these activating mutations in Kir6.2 reduce the closing of the K^{ATP} channel in responses to ATP generated through metabolism, they may still secrete insulin in response to sulfonylureas, which bind to the SUR1 subunit of the K^{ATP} channel binding to the SUR1 subunit.[38] Recently, it was shown that 90% of patients with mutation in Kir6.2 could transfer from insulin to sulfonylureas and all achieved better glycemic control.[39]

Most patients described to date have been spontaneous mutations but it likely that with improved diabetes care, more of these patients will reach reproductive age and will be seen in diabetic pregnancy clinics. This may be another group that are best managed through pregnancy on sulfonylureas rather than insulin as glycemic control will be considerably better.

Fetal genetics altering fetal growth

Diabetes genes may result in a variation in fetal growth during diabetic pregnancy. Fetal growth in a diabetic pregnancy clearly reflects many aspects of the maternal environment, particularly the glycemic control of the mother. By achieving tight glycemic control throughout the pregnancy, considerable improvements in outcome have been possible. However, for a given level of maternal glycemia there remains considerable variation in fetal outcome. This could reflect other aspects of maternal environment such as placental function, maternal lipids, other nutrient supplies and environmental factors such as smoking. It is also possible that genetic factors inherited by the fetus determine the fetal response to the maternal environment. This could explain a lot of variation seen in the outcome of diabetic pregnancy which is not explicable by measured maternal factors.

Diabetes genes in fetal growth

The idea that diabetes genes were important in the predisposition of mothers to hyperglycemia in pregnancy is not unexpected, given their role in the predisposition to Type 2 diabetes. A novel concept which has been developed since 1998 is that the genes that cause monogenic diabetes or

predisposed to Type 2 diabetes may result in reduced fetal growth.[40,41] This is an interesting area where further study is required and may help to explain at least part of the association between low birthweight babies and the predisposition to Type 2 diabetes as adults. The initial observations were made in monogenic diabetes, but there is increasing evidence that these same observations apply to Type 2 diabetes and the general population.

Fetal genetic effects in glucokinase pregnancy

Glucokinase mutation effects on glycemia are present from birth. This means therefore, that any mutation carrier, whenever diagnosed, will have had relative fasting hyperglycemia during pregnancy. Therefore their children will have been exposed to hyperglycemia *in utero* regardless of whether the mother was diagnosed with gestational diabetes or not. It is therefore possible to study the outcome of mothers with glucokinase mutations retrospectively. These studies have resulted in some fascinating insights.

A mother with a heterozygous glucokinase mutation is the perfect scenario for studying the impact of a fetal glucokinase mutation, as she will transmit this mutation to 50% of her offspring. As anticipated, the presence of maternal fasting hyperglycemia meant that mothers with a mutation have children which are, on average, greater than 600 g heavier than those of mothers without the mutation.[40] However, it is clear from the studies that there is a marked dichotomy of fetal response, depending on whether the fetus has an inherited mutation or not. Offspring who inherited the mutation were over 500 g lighter than offspring who had not inherited the mutation.[40] This means that in the mothers with the glucokinase mutation the macrosomia was almost completely confined to foetuses who did not inherit the mutation. Those who inherited the mutation had a normal distribution of birthweight (see Figure 61.1). This result is strong evidence that the sensing of glucose by the fetus is through glucokinase. As glucokinase is involved in the phosphorylation of glucose to glucose-6-phosphate, this effect is specific to maternal glycemia, and is not a result of a fetal response to lipids or other fuels. It is interesting that even the relatively mild hyperglycemia of a heterozygous mutation could have a large impact on birthweight.

Fetal insulin hypothesis

The most important impact of these results in glucokinase mutations is that it establishes that a gene involved in glucose metabolism can also have a considerable impact on birthweight. This led to the fetal insulin hypothesis which proposes that the association of low birthweight, with subsequent Type 2 diabetes and insulin resistance could have a genetic explanation.[41] On the basis of the glucokinase observations it was proposed that altered insulin sensing, insulin secretion or insulin action could result in reduced fetal growth by reducing insulin mediated growth *in utero* as well as predisposing to Type 2 diabetes by altering glucose metabolism. This hypothesis has been tested in a wide variety of situations. There is increasing evidence to support that at least part of the explanation of the association between low birthweight and later diabetes may be due to a genetic mechanism.

Support for the fetal insulin hypothesis from monogenic diabetes studies

There has been strong evidence for the principle that genes resulting in monogenic diabetes have a large impact on fetal growth. In addition to the observation of glucokinase, which acts on glucose sensing (see above), there is also greatly reduced birthweight in mutations that reduce insulin secretion or action. The impact n fetal growth on monogenic diabetes mutations are outlined in Table 61.3. When hyperglycemia is detectable soon after birth due to reduced insulin secretion (e.g. Kir6.2 neonatal diabetes) it is not surprising that there is also reduced insulin secretion *in utero* and hence low birthweight.[42] More striking is that mutations in HNF-1β are associated with a 800g reduction in birthweight despite diabetes not usually developing until early adult life (Edghill and Hattersley, personal communication). This observation is compatible with the role of HNF-1β in pancreatic stem cells[43] which is supported by loss of function mutations resulting in reduced pancreatic size and mild exocrine failure as well as beta-cell dysfunction.[32] The only exception to diabetes mutations reducing birthweight are mutation in HNF-4α that result in an increase of birthweight of 800 g (Pearson, Steele and Hattersley, personal communication). This greatly increases the risk of macrosomia especially when the mothers are diabetic and babies greater than 4.5 kg are common. As 13% of mutation carriers are detected to have neonatal hypoglycemia related to sustained hyperinsulinism it is likely that the increased birthweight reflects increased insulin secretion *in utero*. All the monogenic examples identify the considerable impact of insulin mediated growth on the human fetus and highlight the fact that it can be altered as a result of genetic mutations.

Although observations in monogenic diabetes establish the principle of this pathway being important and alterable by fetal genetics, any association between low birthweight and diabetes cannot be explained by rare mutations, as they are too infrequent. In order to establish genes as playing a role in this association, studies of the general population are required.

Support for the fetal insulin hypothesis from studies of the population and susceptibility genes

In an article outlining the fetal insulin hypothesis, Hattersley and Tooke proposed two predictions that could be tested in the general population:

- That paternal insulin resistance or Type 2 diabetes should be associated with reduced birthweight of offspring. This represented the concept that the genetic predisposition inherited by the father would be, at least in part, transmitted to his offspring and result in reduced insulin mediated growth.
- Polymorphisms associated with the predisposition to Type 2 diabetes would also be associated with reduced fetal birthweight.

The evidence for these two proposals will be considered separately.

Paternal associations with birthweight of offspring. There is increasing evidence that whilst the subsequent development of maternal diabetes results in increased offspring birthweights, particularly when the mother develops early onset diabetes, paternal Type 2 diabetes/insulin resistance results in reduced offspring birthweight. This has now been found in a wide variety of populations.

The most comprehensive study was performed in the Pima Indians by Lindsay and colleagues and showed clear evidence of a dichotomy between the offspring of fathers and mothers who went on to develop Type 2 diabetes. It appears that the small babies that went on to develop diabetes usually had a diabetic father, whilst the large babies who went on to develop diabetes had a diabetic mother.[44] The reduced birthweight of offspring has also been seen in fathers who go on to develop Type 2 diabetes in a UK population.[45,46] In a large UK male cohort, a weak inverse relationship was seen between insulin resistance, as measured by HOMA, and fetal birthweight in offspring after correction for BMI and other potential covariables.[46] However no relationship was seen between paternal insulin resistance and offspring birthweight in a prospective study of 1000 UK families.[47]

Molecular genetic studies. Slow progress in defining the Type 2 diabetes susceptibility genes has meant that testing the fetal insulin hypothesis by molecular genetic techniques has been limited and to date disappointing. The main problem is that the association of low birthweight with a predisposition to Type 2 diabetes is weak. Also, the contribution of any individual polymorphism is very weak. This means that the vast majority of studies are not powered to see an association. Further confounding factors are that if the fetus has a predisposing polymorphism which the mother also has, this polymorphism this tends to increase the birthweight due to the predisposition to gestational diabetes. The impact on fetal birthweight may not be seen without allowing for maternal genotype. Very few studies have looked at this. There are 2 studies which have shown that the association of polymorphisms, within the same population, with Type 2 diabetes and also low birthweight. In a large Dutch cohort a polymorphism 5′ to the IDF1 gene was associated with Type 2 diabetes and subsequently with low birthweight.[48,49] However, the association of this polymorphism with diabetes and low birthweight of offspring has not been replicated in other studies.[50] In the Pima Indian, Lindsay and colleagues found that the polymorphism 5′ to the insulin gene (INS VNTR) was associated with low birthweight and Type 2 diabetes (at least in association studies).[51] This would clearly fit with the fetal insulin hypothesis; however, it has proved difficult to replicate the association of INS VNTR with Type 2 diabetes or low birthweight and the INS VNTR, apart from being associated with low birthweight, has also been associated with increased birth size[52] and no change in birth size.[53]

We can conclude from these studies that there is no strong molecular genetic evidence in support of the fetal insulin hypothesis. The paternal studies do suggest a moderate influence of Type 2 diabetes genes on reducing birthweight. It is likely that the resolution will be that there are some genes that alter birthweight but not predispose to Type 2 diabetes, other genes will predispose to Type 2 diabetes but not alter birthweight and a third group of genes predispose to Type 2 diabetes and to low birthweight. The resolution of the genes involved in fetal growth will take a considerable additional study.

Conclusion

In this chapter we have outlined the important role of genes in causing (monogenic) and predisposing to (polygeic) maternal diabetes in pregnancy. We have also outlined the strong monogenic evidence that the same genes can alter the fetal response to the hyperglycemic environment and shown that the inheritance of a susceptibility to Type 2 diabetes from a diabetic father results in reduced fetal growth. Molecular genetic studies are still in their infancy and it is clear that large studies are required in order to improve our understanding of the role of individual genetic variants in diabetic pregnancy. This area will be of increasing importance in the future.

REFERENCES

1. Filippi C, von Herrath M. How viral infections affect the autoimmune process leading to type 1 diabetes. Cell Immunol 2005; 233: 125–32.
2. Maier LM, Wicker LS. Genetic susceptibility to type 1 diabetes. Curr Opin Immunol 2005; 17: 601–8.
3. Cucca F, Lampis R, Congia M, et al. A correlation between the relative predisposition of MHC class II alleles to type 1 diabetes and the structure of their proteins. Hum Mol Genet 2001; 10: 2025–37.
4. Bell GI, Horita S, Karam JH. A polymorphic locus near the human insulin gene is associated with insulin-dependent diabetes mellitus. Diabetes 1984; 33: 176–83.
5. Ueda H, Howson JM, Esposito L, et al. Association of the T-cell regulatory gene CTLA4 with susceptibility to autoimmune disease. Nature 2003; 423: 506–11.
6. Bottini N, Musumeci L, Alonso A, et al. A functional variant of lymphoid tyrosine phosphatase is associated with type I diabetes. Nat Genet 2004; 36: 337–8.
7. Smyth DJ, Cooper JD, Bailey R, et al. A genome-wide association study of nonsynonymous SNPs identifies a type 1 diabetes locus in the interferon-induced helicase (IFIH1) region. Nat Genet 2006; 38: 617–9.
8. Frayling TM, Wiltshire S, Hitman GA, et al. Young-onset type 2 diabetes families are the major contributors to genetic loci in the Diabetes UK Warren 2 genome scan and identify putative novel loci on chromosomes 8q21, 21q22, and 22q11. Diabetes 2003; 52: 1857–63.
9. Grant SF, Thorleifsson G, Reynisdottir I, et al. Variant of transcription factor 7-like 2 (TCF7L2) gene confers risk of type 2 diabetes. Nat Genet 2006; 38: 320–3.
10. Altshuler D, Hirschhorn JN, Klannemark M, et al. The common PPARgamma Pro12Ala polymorphism is associated with decreased risk of type 2 diabetes. Nat Genet 2000; 26: 76–80.
11. Gloyn AL, Weedon MN, Owen K, et al. Large-scale association studies of variants in genes encoding the pancreatic beta-cell K-ATP channel subunits Kir6.2 (KCNJ11) and SUR1 ABCC8) confirm that the KCNJ11 E23K variant is associated with Type 2 diabetes. Diabetes 2003; 52: 568–72.
12. Weedon MN, Schwarz PE, Horikawa Y, et al. Meta-analysis and a large association study confirm a role for calpain-10 variation in type 2 diabetes susceptibility. Am J Hum Genet 2003; 73: 1208–12.
13. Ferber KM, Keller E, Albert ED, Ziegler AG. Predictive value of human leukocyte antigen class II typing for the development of islet autoantibodies and insulin-dependent diabetes postpartum in women with gestational diabetes. J Clin Endocrinol Metab 1999; 84: 2342–8.
14. Weng J, Ekelund M, Lehto M, et al. Screening for MODY mutations, GAD antibodies, and type 1 diabetes–associated HLA genotypes in women with gestational diabetes mellitus. Diabetes Care 2002; 25: 68–71.
15. Zaidi FK, Wareham NJ, McCarthy MI, et al. Homozygosity for a common polymorphism in the islet-specific promoter of the glucokinase gene is associated with a reduced early insulin response to oral glucose in pregnant women. Diabet Med 1997; 14: 228–34.
16. Allan CJ, Argyropoulos G, Bowker M, et al. Gestational diabetes mellitus and gene mutations which affect insulin secretion. Diabetes Res Clin Pract 1997; 36: 135–41.
17. Weedon MN, Frayling TM, Shields B, et al. Genetic regulation of birth weight and fasting glucose by a common polymorphism in the islet cell promoter of the glucokinase gene. Diabetes 2005; 54: 576–81.
18. Festa A, Krugluger W, Shnawa N, et al. Trp64Arg polymorphism of the beta3-adrenergic receptor gene in pregnancy: association with mild gestational diabetes mellitus. J Clin Endocrinol Metab 1999; 84: 1695–9.
19. Alevizaki M, Thalassinou L, Grigorakis SI, et al. Study of the Trp64Arg polymorphism of the beta3-adrenergic receptor in Greek women with gestational diabetes. Diabetes Care 2000; 23: 1079–83.
20. Shaat N, Ekelund M, Lernmark A, et al. Association of the E23K polymorphism in the KCNJ11 gene with gestational diabetes mellitus. Diabetologia 2005; 48: 2544–51.
21. Rissanen J, Markkanen A, Karkkainen P, et al. Sulfonylurea receptor 1 gene variants are associated with gestational diabetes and type 2 diabetes but not with altered secretion of insulin. Diabetes Care 2000; 23: 70–3.
22. Krugluger W, Festa A, Shnawa N, et al. A serine/alanine polymorphism in the nucleotide-binding fold-2 of the sulphonylurea receptor-1 (S1369A) is associated with enhanced glucose-induced insulin secretion during pregnancy. J Inherit Metab Dis 2000; 23: 705–12.
23. Stride A, Hattersley AT. Different genes, different diabetes: lessons from maturity-onset diabetes of the young. Ann Med 2002; 34: 207–16.
24. Fajans SS, Bell GI, Polonsky KS. Molecular mechanisms and clinical pathophysiology of maturity-onset diabetes of the young. N Engl J Med 2001; 345: 971–80.
25. Stride A, Vaxillaire M, Tuomi T, et al. The genetic abnormality in the beta cell determines the response to an oral glucose load. Diabetologia 2002; 45: 427–35.
26. Ellard S, Beards F, Allen LIS, et al. A high prevalence of glucokinase mutations in gestational diabetic subjects selected by clinical criteria. Diabetologia 2000; 43: 250–3.
27. Kousta E, Ellard S, Allen LI, et al. Glucokinase mutations in a phenotypically selected multiethnic group of women with a history of gestational diabetes. Diabet Med 2001; 18: 683–4.
28. Pearson ER, Liddell WG, Shepherd M, Corrall RJ, Hattersley AT. Sensitivity to sulphonylureas in patients with hepatocyte nuclear factor 1 alpha gene mutations: evidence for pharmacogenetics in diabetes. Diab Med 2000; 17: 543–5.
29. Pearson ER, Starkey BJ, Powell RJ, et al. Genetic aetiology of hyperglycaemia determines response to treatment in diabetes. Lancet 2003; 362: 1275–81.
30. Langer O, Conway DL, Berkus MD, Xenakis EM, Gonzales O. A comparison of glyburide and insulin in women with gestational diabetes mellitus. N Engl J Med 2000; 343: 1134–8.
31. Pearson ER, Pruhova S, Tack CJ, et al. Molecular genetics and phenotypic characteristics of MODY caused by hepatocyte nuclear factor 4alpha mutations in a large European collection. Diabetologia 2005; 48: 878–85.
32. Bingham C, Hattersley AT. Renal cysts and diabetes syndrome resulting from mutations in hepatocyte nuclear factor-1β. Nephrol Dial Transplant 2004; 19: 2703–8.
33. Bingham C, Ellard S, Allen L, et al. Abnormal nephron development associated with a frameshift mutation in the transcription factor hepatocyte nuclear factor-1 beta. Kidney Int 2000; 57: 898–907.

34. Pearson ER, Badman MK, Lockwood CR, et al. Contrasting diabetes phenotypes associated with hepatocyte nuclear factor-1alpha and -1beta mutations. Diabetes Care 2004; 27: 1102–7.
35. Yanagisawa K, Uchigata Y, Sanaka M, et al. Mutation in the mitochondrial tRNA(leu) at position 3243 and spontaneous abortions in Japanese women attending a clinic for diabetic pregnancies. Diabetologia 1995; 38: 809–15.
36. Maassen JA, Kadowaki T. Maternally inherited diabetes and deafness: a new diabetes subtype. Diabetologia 1996; 39: 375–82.
37. Gloyn AL, Pearson ER, Antcliff JF, et al. Activating mutations in the gene encoding the ATP-sensitive potassium-channel subunit Kir6.2 and permanent neonatal diabetes. N Engl J Med 2004; 350: 1838–49.
38. Hattersley AT, Ashcroft FM. Activating mutations in Kir6.2 and neonatal diabetes: new clinical syndromes, new scientific insights, and new therapy. Diabetes 2005; 54: 2503–13.
39. Pearson ER, Flechtner I, Njolstad PR, et al. Switching from insulin to oral sulfonylureas in patients with diabetes due to Kir6.2 mutations. N Engl J Med 2006; 355: 467–77.
40. Hattersley AT, Beards F, Ballantyne E, et al. Mutations in the glucokinase gene of the fetus result in reduced birth weight. Nat Genet 1998; 19: 268–70.
41. Hattersley AT, Tooke JE. The fetal insulin hypothesis: an alternative explanation of the association of low birth weight with diabetes and vascular disease. Lancet 1999.
42. Slingerland AS, Hattersley AT. Activating mutations in the gene encoding Kir6.2 alter fetal and postnatal growth and also cause neonatal diabetes. J Clin Endocrinol Metab 2006; 91: 2782–8.
43. Maestro MA, Boj SF, Luco RF, et al. Hnf6 and Tcf2 (MODY5) are linked in a gene network operating in a precursor cell domain of the embryonic pancreas. Hum Mol Genet 2003; 12: 3307–14.
44. Lindsay RS, Dabelea D, Roumain J, et al. Type 2 Diabetes and Low Birth Weight. Diabetes 2000; 49: 445–9.
45. Hypponen E, Smith GD, Power C. Parental diabetes and birth weight of offspring: intergenerational cohort study. BMJ 2003; 326: 19–20.
46. Wannamethee SG, Lawlor DA, Whincup PH, et al. Birthweight of offspring and paternal insulin resistance and paternal diabetes in late adulthood: cross sectional survey. Diabetologia 2004; 47: 12–8.
47. Knight B, Shields BM, Hill A, et al. Offspring birthweight is not associated with paternal insulin resistance. Diabetologia 2006; 49: 2675–8.
48. Vaessen N, Heutink P, Janssen JA, et al. A polymorphism in the gene for IGF-I: functional properties and risk for type 2 diabetes and myocardial infarction. Diabetes 2001; 50: 637–42.
49. Vaessen N, Janssen JA, Heutink P, et al. Association between genetic variation in the gene for insulin-like growth factor-I and low birthweight. Lancet 2002; 359: 1036–7.
50. Frayling TM, Hattersley AT, McCarthy A, et al. A putative functional polymorphism in the IGF-I gene: association studies with type 2 diabetes, adult height, glucose tolerance, and fetal growth in U.K. populations. Diabetes 2002; 51: 2313–6.
51. Lindsay RS, Hanson RL, Wiedrich C, et al. The insulin gene variable number tandem repeat class I/III polymorphism is in linkage disequilibrium with birth weight but not Type 2 diabetes in the Pima population. Diabetes 2003; 52: 187–93.
52. Dunger DB, Ong KK, Huxtable SJ, et al. Association of the INS VNTR with size at birth. ALSPAC Study Team. Avon Longitudinal Study of Pregnancy and Childhood. Nat Genet 1998; 19: 98–100.
53. Mitchell SM, Hattersley AT, Knight B, et al. Lack of support for a role of the insulin gene variable number of tandem repeats minisatellite (INS-VNTR) locus in fetal growth or type 2 diabetes-related intermediate traits in United Kingdom populations. J Clin Endocrinol Metab 2004; 89: 310–7.

62 The integration of compliance, communication and culture to enhance health care delivery

Nieli Langer

Introduction

Health communication is the singularly most important tool health professionals have to provide health care to their patients. Health care providers depend upon their ability to communicate in order to gather pertinent information, explain procedures and regimens, respond to patients' queries, give the patient directions about self-care and establish a therapeutic humane relationship. The clarity, timeliness, and cultural sensitivity of human communication in health care are often critical to the physical and emotional well-being of all concerned.

Kreps and Thornton[1] addressed several problem areas in health care linked to communication deficiencies:

- Low levels of patient compliance/cooperation
- Miscommunication and misinformation
- Culturally incompetent awareness and behavior

Noncompliance (non-adherence)

Perhaps no aspect of diabetes care seems as frustrating to care providers as the problems that result from noncompliance. Multiple issues contribute to whether a diabetic patient adheres to the prescribed treatment. These influences are similar to those for other chronic diseases such as hypertension, asthma and mental health disorders. On average, one-quarter of patients do not adhere to treatment recommendations.[2] The prevalence of non-adherence suggests that as many as 188.3 million medical visits result in patients not following a prescribed health regimen. The results of meta-analysis indicate that across the spectrum of chronic disease and outcome assessments, adherence (compared to non-adherence) may reduce the risk of a poor treatment outcome by 26%.[3]

How patients perceive the relevance of suggested therapies often explains how the treatments conform to their 'health beliefs model.'[4] This model is the patient's belief in his/her own susceptibility to a disease or illness. It is the belief regarding the degree of severity of the illness and the consequences for health and daily functioning; belief in the efficacy of the treatment for the illness; belief about the barriers and costs related to treatment; and, cues to action. Each of these contributing factors has been shown to influence the degree to which a patient will/will not adhere to a treatment protocol.[5] The frequency or complexity of prescribed medical therapies is an important determinant of compliance as is the presence of side effects.[6]

The quality of the provider–patient relationship also influences compliance. However, as cooperative and diligent as the care provider–patient partnership is in monitoring and reassessing care, we must not dismiss the data that demonstrates that only about 30% of pregnant and nonpregnant Type 1 and 2 diabetic women in both the United States and Europe are able to achieve the recommended levels of glycemic control (Figure 62.1). It begs the question: can glycemic control be sustained in the long run by chronically ill diabetic women? In addition, one must consider other factors: is the ability of GDM women to achieve established levels of glycemic control the result of a milder form of the disease, the relatively short duration of adherence to a diabetic protocol (often less than 9 months) or the inherent motivational factor to deliver a healthy fetus? Studies have shown (Figure 62.2) that the level of compliance in blood glucose testing was relatively low for pregnant and nonpregnant diabetic women when unaware of the existence of a computer chip to record an accurate reading. They would also alter test results.

In addition to all the diverse influences that may contribute to noncompliance, we need to also recognize that patients and care providers rely on different variables when weighing the concept of 'willing and able' relative to compliance. Care providers value compliance as a necessary component to treatment since they believe that the benefits of compliance outweigh the impact of social, psychological, and economic

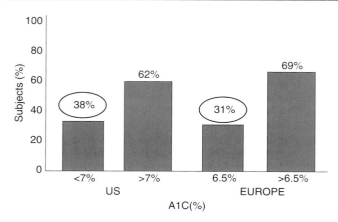

Figure 62.1 Patients who achieved established levels of HbA1c. (Modified from Harris et al. Diabetes Care 1999; 22: 403–8; and Liebl. Diabetologia 2002; 45: S23–8.)

factors on the patient's life. For the physician, patients' noncompliance is synonymous with disobedience. Patients value convenience, money, cultural beliefs, habits, body image, etc. Patients use their judgment when presented with a medical protocol and decide *if* to adhere to the protocol and/or which components of the protocol they will adhere to from their subjective, cultural, autonomous life view. Noncompliant or non-adherent patient behaviors:

- **No-show** to an appointment
- **Not** having the prescription filled
- **Not** taking the correct dose or forgetting to take the requisite doses
- **Not** taking the medication in a timely manner
- **Discontinuing** the medication without medical consultation

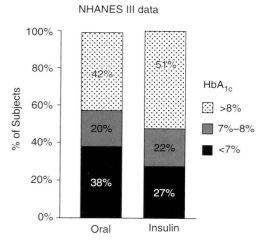

- 62% *of patients* on oral are not *at ADA goal of HbA1c <7%*
- 73% *of patients* on insulin are not *at ADA goal (HbA1c <7%)*

Figure 62.2 Patient distribution by level of glycemic control in insulin and oral anti-diabetic therapies. Sixty-two percent of patient on oral are not at ADA goal of HbA1c <7%. Seventy-three percent of patient on insulin are not at ADA goal of HbA1c <7%. (Modified from Harris et al. Diabetes Care 1999; 22: 403–8.)

Medical paternalism (physician-directed practice) at one end of the care continuum and patient self-determination at the opposite end cannot obscure the valid underlying concerns about relationships between noncompliance and poor clinical outcomes; these are well documented. Compliance influences glycemic control. Patients who fail to adhere to the diabetic protocol prescribed by their clinician suffer very poor outcomes. Recurrent diabetic crises are, in part, attributable to noncompliance. Noncompliance may represent an important component of unnecessary health care costs[7–10] yet for some noncompliant patients, any factor that can improve aspects of adherence to the diabetic protocol becomes a 'necessary' health care cost.

Many of the problems and crises of diabetes management in pregnancy have emotional and psychosocial sources in addition to medical ones. Many studies have shown a correlation between glucose control and psychological factors such as mood disturbances.[11–13] In 1998, we[12] reported that chronically ill pregnant diabetic women display significantly greater anxiety and hostility in comparison to nondiabetic women. However, regardless of the level of glycemic control or the severity of the disease, the mood profiles of these women were not affected. Although near-normal glycemic control with a strict management approach using either insulin or glyburide therapy is achievable for GDM women, chronically ill patients are often unable or unwilling to achieve established levels of glycemic control.

Although historically the blame and burden of failing to follow a medical regimen have been shouldered by the patient, a more realistic and empowering interactive perspective defines compliance in terms of cooperation between the patient and practitioner, where responsibility for health care outcomes are shared jointly. Instead of viewing patient noncompliance as a maladaptive characteristic, it is more productive to view the problem as related to the kind of communication relationship established between the patient and practitioner.

Patient–practitioner communication

The most basic and powerful way to connect to another person is to listen; probably, the most important thing we ever give each other is our attention. When we are listened to, it makes us unfold and expand. Relating to other people is both therapeutic and growth-enhancing. 'Man becomes man with the other self. He would not be man at all without the I–thou relationship.' (Martin Buber). Effective communication is the core of every helping relationship and listening is the foundation of every medical and social service interaction.

Human communication occurs when a person responds to a message and assigns meaning to it. Relationships in the health care setting developed through interpersonal communication can elicit cooperation and thus compliance. In human communication we simultaneously send and receive many messages on many different levels. Once you have communicated something to someone via spoken words, facial expressions, environmental cues or feelings, you cannot retract it. By restating or changing the messages sent, you do not remove previous messages; you merely add on to them. The irreversible nature of human communication underscores the importance of careful communication in health care. Whatever the health care professional says, it will always be remembered to some extent by the patient.

For patients, professional competence and communication are equally important. Researchers have linked poor communication to misdiagnoses, the ordering of unnecessary tests, and the failure of patients to follow treatment plans. Patients do not always understand what their care providers tell them, and they often leave their offices uncertain of how they are supposed to maximize self care. An article appeared in the science section of the *New York Times* (June 2004) in which a series of studies reported that good doctor–patient communication resulted in lower blood sugar levels in diabetic patients and lower blood pressure in hypertensive patients. The message conveyed that if patients believe they are in a good relationship with their doctors, there may be a strong chance their health will benefit, too.

Active listening implies the active participation of both the care provider in his capacity in the health care environment as well as that of the patient who, too, has a responsibility to participate in his/her own health care. Active listening refers to nonverbal communication such as eye contact; look at clients when they speak. It involves verbal behavior such as responding by reflecting: using comments such as 'I see what you mean' signaling that you are listening and encourages the patient to continue. It also involves avoidance of sending discouraging messages by interrupting, changing the subject or not acknowledging what the patient says. As a result, patients are empowered because they feel worthwhile as human beings; feel accepted by the care provider, and are, therefore, comfortable to explore their presenting problem.

Unhelpful communication behaviors may include: interrupting the patient's explanation, preaching, blaming, extensive probing and questioning, especially with 'why' questions and adapting a patronizing attitude. These behaviors are hindrances to the interaction because they place patients on the defensive and make them feel worthless. These behaviors may also encourage avoidance so that debilitating issues remain unexplored. Empowerment is not just abstract social service jargon; a practical attitude and environment is attainable when conditions of genuineness, respect, and empathy are generated and used to facilitate the dialogue and produce several options for care.

When the pregnant diabetic patient seeks health services, the interview is more than an exchange of information or filling out a standardized form. The patient and the care provider send and interpret verbal and nonverbal stimuli. The changing medical environment is increasing its insistence on a more cooperative relationship between care provider and patient, with the patient taking a more active and informed role than ever before. For the patient diagnosed with gestational diabetes, the care provider is faced with a patient who does not complain of any disease symptoms yet is tagged 'sick.' The practitioner's role is to explain to a pregnant patient who 'feels well' what is the nature of her disease, why adherence to a diabetic protocol (diet management, injection/oral medication,

exercise) can positively influence the pregnancy outcome while allaying anxiety and fear.

In the patient–provider relationship, the care provider and patient each brings his/her own expertise to the medical encounter and each respects the ideas of the other. In the case of a chronic disease, this means the recognition that while health professionals are experts on the specific illness, patients are experts on their own lives. Patients are the best sources of information about the attitudes, beliefs, and lifestyle issues that affect their acceptance of medical treatments. Miscommunication often leads patients to incorrectly interpret the health care instructions explained to them by providers, making it difficult for a patient to adhere to a medical protocol. Likewise, care providers can misinterpret information given them by patients resulting in incorrect diagnoses and in inappropriate treatment plans. Part of establishing an effective provider–patient relationship is being able to communicate clearly and accurately. Listening for patients' meanings and values becomes the starting point for gaining patients' confidence and establishing two-way communication. Satisfaction, communication and consultation style are all factors in the care provider-patient relationship.

Strengths perspective communication fits well with patient empowerment. The strengths perspective focuses on capabilities, assets, and positive attributes rather than problems and pathologies. This generative model enhances patients' resources for problem solving, coping, and healing. It appears to add an element of control which is very important to a sense of well being. Listening and attending behaviors that communicate empathy, encouragement, support, respect, and nonjudgmental acceptance are the most effective to implementing an environment of empowerment and potential adherence to a medical protocol.

Displaying empathy, the sharing of another's perceptual field and world of meaning, can improve the quality of information exchange. An empathetic care provider can help troubled patients express their own fears, problems, needs, anger and expectations. Basic to an empathic exchange is respect. A distressed person needs to believe that the listener really wants to understand and will maintain privacy, withhold judgment, and reserve advice for the appropriate time. The comments of the care provider should be brief, concrete, and jargon-free. Tone and inflections should promote sharing and be fully congruent with body language. Asking the patient for clarification and checking perceptions are appropriate counseling skills. A concise rephrasing of the patient's current emotions, perceptions, and plans is often the best response. We, as care providers, need to recognize and remember that people are often able to direct their lives more than they realize; they have some freedom to choose even if their options are restricted by environmental variables or inherent biological or personality dispositions.

One of the biggest hindrances to change in the patient–care provider dialogue is the continued emphasis on changing doctors' behaviors even though it takes two to generate a relationship. Studies suggest that the more equal the relationship between doctors and patients, the more likely it will translate into health benefits. Physicians need to develop sensitivity that will help them identify those aspects of patients' behavior that are determined by their socio-cultural backgrounds, i.e., 'inflated' respect for authority that discourages communication. Patient passivity may be a risk factor in the treatment of diabetes. In addition, patients often experience embarrassment with limited health literacy when they do not understand what the doctor has said. And, of course, asking for clarification is seriously impeded by the imbalance in power between the white-coated physician and the patient in the paper-wrapped gown.

Patients need the opportunity to practice asking questions and interpreting answers. A doctor needs to assess the patient's baseline understanding before providing extensive information: 'Before we go on, could you tell me what you already know about diabetes?' Physicians should use plain language, not medical terminology, vague terms and words that may have different meanings to a lay person. In addition, physicians need to facilitate the patient's understanding by saying, 'I always ask my patients to repeat things back to me to make sure I have explained them clearly.' Or, if a new skill like using a self-monitoring blood glucose machine is taught, the doctor should have the patient demonstrate the action. The doctor might also consider providing the patient and the family with written instructions and educational material to review at home. Tailoring information to a patient's individual needs and limiting it to the most important points can save time in the long run and result in better control of chronic illness that may lead to shorter and less frequent office visits.

In order to manage diabetes successfully, patients must be able to set goals and make decisions that are both effective and fit their values and lifestyles while addressing physiological and psychosocial factors. The role of the pregnant diabetic woman is to be a well-informed active partner in her care, i.e. adherence to the diabetic protocol with the use of self-monitoring blood glucose, maintenance of a healthy diet and exercise and frequent fetal testing. The role of the practitioner is to help these women achieve goals and overcome barriers through education, appropriate care recommendations and support.

In health care, stories are the means by which people make sense of their personal health conditions. By listening to the stories a patient tells about her pregnancy, the care provider can learn about that woman's cultural orientation, health belief system and psychological orientation towards her condition. Some care providers are reluctant to ask women to tell their stories, preferring not to get too 'personal' with their patients. Some providers would rather just perform diagnostic tests and keep the interpersonal communication with their patients to a minimum. However, by failing to encourage patients to tell their stories, these providers are potentially losing a wealth of health information that would help them be more effective at providing health care to their patients.

Patients need to be encouraged to share their stories since their own interpretations of their health conditions are legitimate and important. By legitimizing consumers' personal narratives about their health, health care providers can validate the worth of individual consumers, encourage them to participate in their own health care, establish good working relationships with them and learn a great deal about physical and symbolic health conditions.

Narratives can easily be used by health care providers, too. They enable them to humanize communication with clients/patients. Stories are also a means to emphasize components of the health care regimen that the provider wishes the patients to pay attention to, remember and, therefore, to co-manage in the form of compliance.

Culture and health communication

The cultural impact of beliefs, values and attitudes strongly influence health care for both the practitioner and the client. Anthropology teaches us that disease, health and illness are culturally defined. A person's beliefs influence their perceptions of health and illness. Beliefs dictate which symptoms will be considered appropriate to take to a doctor, how patients will understand the cause and treatment of their illness, what patients expect of physicians, what personal and moral meanings patients will ascribe to their illness and how they will answer the recurrent questions 'Why me? Why now? What did I do to deserve this?' Practitioners' failure to address these beliefs may result in the loss of a powerful source of information and a potent tool for healing since this knowledge can often improve outcomes.[14]

Before you continue reading the chapter, take the time to respond to the following modified *Cultural Competence in Health Care Quiz*.[15] It will provide you with a baseline about your current knowledge, skills and attitudes about culture as a significant factor in health care communication.

Cultural competence in health care quiz

1. Cross-cultural misunderstandings between obstetricians and pregnant diabetic women can lead to mistrust and frustration. These misunderstandings will probably ***not have*** an impact on objectively measured clinical outcomes.
   A. True
   B. False
2. When the patient and provider come from different cultural backgrounds, the medical history obtained ***may not*** be accurate.
   A. True
   B. False
3. When a provider expects that a pregnant diabetic woman will understand her condition and follow the diabetic protocol, she is ***more likely*** to do so than if the provider has doubts about the patient's willingness or ability to adhere to the protocol and expresses these doubts with either verbal or body language.
   A. True
   B. False

4. When taking a medical history from the patient with a limited ability to speak the language, which of the following is the *least* useful?
   A. Asking questions that require the patient to give a simple 'yes' or 'no' answer, such as 'Have you been able to modify your diet?' Have you been able to include exercise in your lifestyle?'
   B. Encouraging the patient to give a description of her medical situation and beliefs about health and illness.
   C. Asking the patient whether she would like to have a qualified interpreter for the medical visit.
   D. Asking the patient questions such as 'How has your condition changed since the last office visit?' 'What makes your condition get better or worse?'

5. When a patient is not adhering to the diabetic protocol after several visits, which of the following approaches is *not likely* to lead to adherence?
   A. Involving family members
   B. Repeating the instructions very loudly and several times to emphasize the importance of the protocol
   C. Agreeing to a compromise in the protocol components
   D. Spending time listening to the patient's explanation of her culture's folk or alternative remedies.

6. When a patient who has not adhered to the diabetic protocol states that she cannot afford the medications prescribed, *it is* appropriate to assume that financial factors are indeed the real reasons and not explore the situation further.
   A. True
   B. False

7. If a family member speaks the language of the medical consultation as well as the patient's native language and is willing to act as interpreter, this is *the best* possible solution to the problem of interpreting.
   A. True
   B. False

8. Which statement is *true*?
   A. People who speak the same language have the same culture.
   B. Cultural background, diet, religious, and health practices, as well as language, can differ widely within a given country or part of a country.
   C. An alert provider can usually predict a patient's health behaviors by knowing what country or culture she comes from.

9. Minority and immigrant patients in the United States who go to traditional healers and use traditional medicines *generally avoid* conventional Western treatments.
   A. True
   B. False

10. Which of the following is *good advice* for a provider attempting to use and interpret non-verbal communication?
    A. The provider should recognize that a smile may express unhappiness or dissatisfaction in some cultures.
    B. To express sympathy, a health care provider can lightly touch a patient's arm or pat the patient on the back.
    C. If the patient will not make eye contact with a health care provider, it is likely that the patient is hiding the truth.
    D. When there is a language barrier, the provider can use hand gestures to bridge the gap.

11. Some symbols – a positive nod of the head, a pointing finger, or a 'thumbs-up' sign – are universal and *can help* bridge the language gap.
    A. True
    B. False

12. Out of respect for a patient's privacy, the provider *should always* begin a relationship by seeing an adult patient alone and drawing the family in as needed.
    A. True
    B. False

The correct answers are to be found at the end of the chapter in Appendix 1.

Cultural assessment

Cultural assessment is the process of obtaining an overview of the patient's characteristics in order to identify needs. By shifting the questioning from a medical to a patient-oriented focus, the practitioner may begin to learn and understand the world view and social organization of the patient. This can be accomplished by the use of some/all of these questions:

1. What do you call your problem? What name does it have?
2. What do you think caused it?
3. When do you think it started?
4. What does your sickness do to you?
5. How severe is it? Will it have a long or short course?
6. What do you fear most about your sickness?
7. What are the chief problems your sickness has caused for you?
8. What treatment should you receive? What are the most important results you hope to receive?[16]

Alternatively, the care provider can use some form of the following Patient Cultural Status Exam[17] to illicit medical information that is also socially and culturally less stressful to the patient than a customary medical interview:

1. How would you describe the problem that has brought you here?
2. Who in the community and your family helps you with your problem?
3. How long have you had this problem?
4. Do you know anyone else with it?
5. Tell me what happened to them when dealing with this problem.
6. What do you think is wrong with you?
7. What might other people think is wrong with you?
8. Tell me about people who **don't** get this problem.
9. Why has this happened to you, and why now?
10. What do you think will help clear up this problem?
11. If specific tests, and/or medications are listed, ask what they are and what they do.
12. Apart from me, who else do you think can make you feel better?
13. Are there therapies that make you feel better that I don't know about?

The awareness of the dynamics that result from cultural differences such as value preferences, perception of illness, health beliefs, and communication style will help practitioners adapt treatment plans that meet culturally unique needs. The lack of awareness of cultural issues increases social distance, and breaks down communication. It is an ethical obligation for physicians to develop sensitivity to cultural and educational differences if they hope to make interventions that are consistent with the values of their patients.

In diabetes, pregnant patients are expected to follow a complex set of behavioral actions to care for their diabetes on a daily basis. Self-care in diabetes often involves a complex regimen that varies across patients and situations. It is rarely a standard prescription but rather a regimen that resembles a series of 'if–then' statements. Improvements in medical care such as intensive insulin regimens require more patient counseling, education and support than simpler regimens, such as 'take one shot a day and watch the sweets.' Diabetes treatment is predominantly behavioral (involving daily medication, glucose testing, exercise and dietary actions). While most patients may take their medication, they are far less compliant with timing or adjusting medication administration.

Working with the patient to reach agreement on a treatment plan that makes sense in the context of her life will facilitate her adherence to self-management when she leaves the physician's office and resumes her day-to-day life. The GDM patient faces a temporary illness unless she develops Type 1 or Type 2 diabetes. In order to mitigate the onset of Type 2 diabetes and/or metabolic syndrome, the postpartum patient needs to consider a lifestyle change that would include a healthy diet and exercise.

The patient with pre-gestational diabetes is wrestling with a life-long illness in which failure to maximize glucose control may seriously compromise both her and her fetus. The physician is obliged to use understandable language, provide constructive, culturally appropriate advice and create a humane environment conducive to adherence to a medical protocol. Satisfaction, communication and cultural competence are all factors in the doctor–patient relationship. Practitioners and patients need to pool their expertise to pattern customized treatment plans that are suitable to the patient and her disease. It is incumbent upon all health care practitioners and health care consumers to recognize the importance of communication in health care, to understand the many ways effective, culturally sensitive communication can be used to promote health.

The doctor–patient relationship is more than a commercial transaction between retailers and consumers. It is a hallowed relationship in which both parties are interdependent and, therefore, allies. Much has happened in the medical profession and in society to distort that relationship, i.e. medical technology and the imposition of managed care into the equation has led to a certain estrangement between doctor and patient. These factors have contributed to the almost adversarial relationship that sometimes evolves between doctors and patients instead of as allies in pursuit of a common goal. It is time we begin to refocus on the purpose inherent in the patient–physician bond: souls rendering service to one another.

Appendix 1: Answers to culture quiz

1. **False:** Low levels of cultural competence can obstruct the process of making an accurate diagnosis and may cause the provider to order contraindicated medication.

2. **True:** Patient may not understand the questions or be reluctant to disclose symptoms because of language and cultural barriers. The care provider may also misunderstand the patient's explanation of her symptoms.

3. **True:** People (students, patients, etc.) generally rise to the challenge or fail in response to their perception of the physician's (teacher's, etc.) level of expectation [Pygmalion theory].

4. **The correct answer is 'A.'** While it may seem easier to ask questions that require a simple 'yes' or 'no' answer, this format seriously limits the ability of the patient to communicate information necessary for diagnosis and/or assessment. The most effective way to proceed under these circumstances is to combine an open-ended question such as 'Tell me about your difficulties altering your diet plan' and using a more directed question such as 'Which of the meals is easiest for you to anticipate and prepare?' A qualified interpreter is also a valuable asset.

5. **The correct answer is 'B.'** Non-adherence can be the result of many factors. Simply repeating the same instructions may not be addressing the real issues that are preventing adherence. Repetition may also be demeaning and offensive if the patient cannot communicate. Family members can provide valuable support. It may also be possible to set small, realistic goals in order to achieve long-term behavioral change. Making an effort to understand the patient's beliefs in alternative remedies may offer valuable clues to her resistance to compliance.

6. **False:** You can explore payment options with the patient but you also need to explore cultural and psychological factors that may preclude adherence to the diabetic protocol.

7. **False:** This is an inappropriate responsibility for families to take on. They lack objectivity and the technical knowledge to convey the provider's message accurately. Professional interpreters have been trained to provide accurate, sensitive two-way communication and uncover areas of uncertainty or discomfort.

8. **The correct answer is 'B.'** People from the same continent, country, same part of the country and even the same city may have major differences in cultural heritage, traditions and language, as well as differences in socioeconomic status, education, etc. It is the aggregate of all of these that make up a person's 'culture.'

9. **False:** In the United States, some minority and immigrant groups first use their traditional medications before turning to conventional Western medicine, or use both concurrently.

10. **The correct answer is 'A.'** In most cultures smiling is an expression of joy while in others, e.g. Chinese, may smile when they are discussing uncomfortable issues. The other responses are incorrect: body language is not

universal; interpersonal greetings vary widely from one culture to another; beliefs about touching vary widely; some cultures perceive eye contact as a sign of respect yet direct eye contact may be interpreted as an invasion of privacy; a hand gesture in one culture may create a social bond while the same gesture in another culture may represent an offense.

11. **False:** see answer to # 10

12. **False:** In many of the world's cultures, a patient's health problem is also considered the family's problem and it is offensive to exclude family members from any medical interaction. The care provider needs to assess the patient's preference for inclusion/exclusion of family members during a medical visit. The provider might ease any tension around this issue by assuring family members that they will be asked to return to the examining room shortly.

REFERENCES

1. Kreps GL, Thornton BC. Health Communication: Theory and Practice. Illinois: Waveland Press; 1992.
2. DiMatteo MR. Variations in patients' adherence view of 50 years of research. Med Care 2004; 42: 200–9.
3. DiMatteo MR, Giordani PJ, Lepper HS, Croghan TW. Patients adherence and medical treatment outcomes: a meta-analysis. Med Care 2002; 40: 794–811.
4. Pham DT, Fabienne F, Thibaudeau MF. The role of the health belief model in amputees' self-evaluation of adherence to diabetes self-care behaviors. Diabetes Educ 1996; 22: 126–32.
5. Rosenstock IM. Historical origins of the health belief model. Health Educ Monog 1974; 2: 328.
6. Ley P. Communicating with patients: Improving communication, satisfaction and compliance. London: Croom Helm; 1988.
7. Kuo YF, Raji MA, Markedes KS, et al. Inconsistent use of diabetes medications, diabetes complications, and mortality in older Mexican Americans over a 7-year period. Diabetes Care 2003; 26: 3054–60.
8. Chen HS, Jap TS, Chen RL, Lin HD. A prospective study of glycemic control during holiday time in type 2 diabetic patients. Diabetes Care 2004; 27: 326–30.
9. Skinner TC. Recurrent diabetic ketoacidosis: Causes, prevention and management. Horm Res 2002; 57: 78–80.
10. American Diabetes Association: Hyperglycemic crisis in diabetes [Position Statement]. Diabetes Care 2004; 27: S94–S102.
11. Langer N, Langer O. Emotional adjustment to diagnosis and intensified treatment of gestational diabetes. Obstet Gynecol 1994; 84: 329–34.
12. Langer N, Langer O. Pre-existing diabetes: Relationship between glycemic control and emotional status in pregnancy. J Matern–Fetal Med 1998; 7: 257–63.
13. Langer N, Langer O. Comparison of pregnancy mood profiles in gestational diabetes and preexisting diabetes. Diabetes Educ 2000; 26: 667–72.
14. Weston WW, Brown JB. The importance of patients' beliefs. 1989. In: Stewart M, Roter D eds. Communication with Medical Patients. Newbury Park, CA: Sage; 1989, pp. 77–85.
15. Manager's Electronic Resource Center; Management Sciences for Health. erc.msh.org [16 October 2006].
16. Kleinman A. Patients and Healers in the Context of Culture: An Exploration of the Borderland Between Anthropology, Medicine, and Psychiatry. Berkley: University of California Press; 1980.
17. Pfeifferling JH. A cultural prescription for medicine. In: Eisenberg L, Kleinman A, eds. The Relevance of Social Science for Medicine. Boston: Reidel; 1981.

63 Diabetes and infertility

Avi Ben-Haroush and Benjamin Fisch

Introduction

Patients with diabetes mellitus often have reproductive disturbances. For women these include delayed menarche, menstrual irregularities, subfertility, early onset of menopause, and increased incidence of spontaneous abortions, and for men impotence, hypospermia, and impaired spermatogenesis. The exact mechanisms underlying diabetes-related infertility remain unknown. Studies have implicated a central effect on the pituitary–gonadal axis, abnormal antral follicle development, as in polycystic ovary syndrome (PCOS), and microangiopathy or other tissue-damaging factors.

This chapter reviews the known data on the association between diabetes and infertility, including the cumulative information on the pivotal role of insulin resistance in the pathogenesis of prediabetic states such as PCOS, and the effect of insulin-sensitizing drugs, such as metformin. The risks of spontaneous abortion and male infertility are discussed as well.

Type 1 diabetes and reproductive disturbances

Delayed menarche and menstrual irregularities

Prior to the identification and isolation of insulin in 1921, diabetic women rarely underwent secondary sexual development.[1] Today, menarche is usually delayed if the disease develops in the prepubertal years, and early if it precedes the onset of the disease.[2,3] Almost one-third of diabetic women of reproductive age have some form of menstrual dysfunction.[4] In a study of 337 women with Type 1 diabetes, Burkart et al.[5] noted an inverse correlation between age at menarche and patient age, with age at menarche being 0.8–2 years higher in diabetic patients than in the patients in whom diabetes developed after menarche, and 0.4–1.3 years higher than in nondiabetics. The increase was most pronounced if the diabetes was diagnosed between 3 and 8 years of age. A delay in menarche was also noted in a later retrospective study of 100 diabetic women when the disease was diagnosed before the age of menarche and before 10 years of age:[6] the average age at menarche in this series was 13.5. In addition, there was a significant correlation between menstrual disturbances and both late menarche and diabetic complications.[6] The authors suggested that one possible explanation for the delayed menarche

in Type 1 diabetes is the characteristic weight loss that occurs at the time of diagnosis.

Burkart et al.[5] found that the prevalence of primary amenorrhea was 3.6% in women with Type 1 diabetes, compared to 1.5% in healthy controls and in women with late-onset diabetes. The rates of oligomenorrhea and secondary amenorrhea were 14 and 7%, compared to 12% in the patients with late-onset diabetes. Menstrual irregularities were more frequent at the time of diabetes onset, although 76% of the patients had not complained of any change in menstrual bleeding and it normalized with time. Over 70% of patients <35 years of age had spontaneous conceptions and only 2.1% were infertile; both these rates are similar to those in the control group.

Yeshaya et al.[6] also noted a 32% rate of oligomenorrhea, amenorrhea, and polymenorrhea, which was in agreement with the study of Bergquist[7] but higher than the 21.6% reported by Kjaer et al.[8]

Infertility

A questionnaire survey of an unselected population of 18- to 49-year-old diabetic women (*n* = 245) and a comparable control group (*n* = 253) failed to yield differences in the cumulative rates of pregnancies and involuntary infertility (17%).[9,10] However, the diabetic women had significantly fewer pregnancies (1.4 vs. 1.7) and fewer births per pregnancy than controls, and more were nulliparous (48 vs. 38%). Half of all the diabetic pregnancies were planned. The women reported that their diabetes had a negative influence on their attitude toward having children.

Briese and Muller,[11] in a study of 672 diabetic women between the ages of 17 and 42, of whom 72% were taking insulin, found that one third had successful pregnancies, but only one in 10 delivered more than once after the diabetes became manifest. At the time of the study, 126 patients (19.1%) were attempting pregnancy, about one-fifth of them for >2 years. Manifestations of diabetes occurred significantly earlier in the patients who did not achieve pregnancy. Infertility was correlated with daily insulin dose but was unrelated to duration of diabetes.

Euglycemia at the time of conception is crucial for the success of the pregnancy. Considering the difficulties in achieving and maintaining tight glycemic control for long periods, clomiphene citrate (CC) may be used to enhance fecundability in diabetic patients with good glycemic control.[12] This new 'sweet' indication for the use of CC is probably debatable. Nevertheless, fertility, like all other health issues in diabetic patients, depends on good metabolic control.

It may be concluded that although diabetic patients tend to have a negative attitude towards pregnancy and motherhood, their fertility potential is usually not substantially impaired when in good glycemic control.

Mechanisms for infertility

Hypothalamic–pituitary–gonadal dysfunction

Uncontrolled Type 1 diabetes is thought to disrupt normal hypothalamic–pituitary–gonadal function, and animal studies have suggested that poorly controlled Type 1 diabetes may adversely affect the uterovaginal outflow tract and/or ovarian function. However, clinical studies do not relate this factor to menstrual dysfunction.[4] Similarly, pituitary function, as assessed by basal gonadotropins and gonadotropin-releasing hormone (GnRH)-stimulated gonadotropin release, appears to be normal in young women with Type 1 diabetes. Although there is some evidence that pituitary function declines with increasing duration of diabetes, this issue has not been thoroughly investigated. Therefore, the oligo/amenorrhea in Type 1 diabetes appears to be principally hypothalamic in origin and may represent intermittent (and perhaps reversible) failure of the GnRH pulse generator. This is similar to the mechanism in anorexia nervosa or in women who engage in endurance training.[4] The exact pathophysiology of the GnRH neuronal system dysfunction is still not well understood, but attention is currently focused on increased central opioidergic activity, increased central dopaminergic activity and central glucose deprivation.

Role of insulin

The role of insulin in folliculogenesis has been studied extensively. Insulin receptors have been localized in the ovary, within the stromal cells, granulose and theca cells of developing follicles.[13] Studies that specifically examined primordial follicles localized insulin receptors primarily to the oocyte.[14] Some growth factors promote the primordial to primary follicle transition to a greater degree in the presence of insulin.[15] Direct ovarian organ culture studies have demonstrated that high concentrations of insulin stimulate primordial follicle development in the hamster.[16] Insulin also stimulates androgen production by cultured theca cells,[17] as well as estrogen and progesterone production by cultured granulosa cells.[18]

Kezele et al.[19] suggested that insulin's site of action is likely the oocyte and that its activity is mediated via the insulin receptor, not the insulin-like growth factor (IGF)-I receptor. Thus, insulin helps to coordinate the primordial to primary follicle transition at the level of the oocyte. Abnormal insulin levels may alter or inhibit early follicular development.

Role of catecholamines

Impaired hypothalamic regulation of gonadotropin secretion may be caused by disrupted noradrenergic feedback.

Monoamines and opioids are involved in the regulation of luteinizing hormone (LH) secretion.[20] Substances that block hypothalamic adrenergic receptors or activate opioid receptors suppress the release of GnRH and the preovulatory LH surge. The actions of opioids appear to involve noradrenergic mechanisms.[21] Thus, increased norepinephrine turnover in the preoptic areas may be a prerequisite for the LH surge, and the noradrenergic control of LH secretion is regulated by an opioid pathway.[22] Bitar[23] suggested that the endocrine abnormalities in diabetes are due, at least in part, to a functional deficit in noradrenergic neurons within the hypothalamus. Therefore, diabetes could suppress the cyclic reproduction function by disrupting these regulatory mechanisms.

Microangiopathy and decreased ovarian superoxide dismutase activity

Microangiopathy is the major cause of tissue damage in Type 1 diabetes[24] and may therefore be a mechanism for ovulatory dysfunction as well. The risk of microangiopathic abnormalities does not appear to increase linearly with the duration of diabetes, nor can it be prevented by good glycemic control.[24] Nitric oxide (NO), an important mediator in the regulation of the blood–follicle barrier and ovulation, is inactivated in the presence of clinical and experimental diabetes, leading to impaired endothelial-dependent vascular activity.[25] This state can be reversed by administration of insulin or free-radical scavengers, such as superoxide dismutase (SOD).[26] Powers et al.[27] localized endothelial NO synthase (NOS), inducible NOS, SOD and the LH receptor to the same population of endothelial cells surrounding the preovulatory follicle. They suggested that short periods of hyperglycemia may cause a decrease in activity of ovarian SOD, thereby increasing the production of superoxide anion and disrupting the homeostatic vascular activity of NO. Specifically, the loss of the protective activity of SOD in diabetes may compromise the signaling of NO within the ovarian microvasculature at the time of ovulation.

Insulin resistance and polycystic ovary syndrome

PCOS is a heterogeneous disorder affecting 5–10% of women of reproductive age.[28] It is characterized by chronic anovulation with oligo/amenorrhea, infertility, typical sonographic appearance of the ovaries, i.e. multiple small follicles distributed around the ovarian periphery or throughout the echodense stroma[29] and clinical or biochemical hyperandrogenism. As anovulation accounts for an estimated 40% of all cases of female infertility, PCOS, being the most common cause of anovulation, is the most important cause of this type of infertility.[30]

Insulin resistance is present in 40–50% of patients, especially in obese women,[31] making PCOS a prediabetic state. The prevalence of impaired glucose tolerance (IGT) in PCOS is 31–35%, and the prevalence of Type 2 diabetes mellitus is 7.5–10%.[32] The conversion rate from IGT to overt Type 2 diabetes is increased 5- to 10-fold in women with PCOS.[33]

Women with PCOS are at increased risk of pregnancy and neonatal complications; a recent meta-analysis[34] demonstrated that these women are at higher risk of developing gestational diabetes [odds ratio (OR) 2.94; 95% confidence interval (CI): 1.70–5.08], pregnancy-induced hypertension (OR 3.67; 95% CI: 1.98–6.81), pre-eclampsia (OR 3.47; 95% CI: 1.95–6.17) and preterm birth (OR 1.75; 95% CI: 1.16–2.62). Their babies had a significantly higher risk of admission to a neonatal intensive care unit (OR 2.31; 95% CI: 1.25–4.26) and a higher perinatal mortality (OR 3.07; 95% CI: 1.03–9.21), unrelated to multiple births.

Hyperinsulinemic insulin resistance

Insulin resistance is defined as the decreased ability of insulin to stimulate glucose disposal into target tissues, or a reduced glucose response to a given amount of insulin. Chronic hyperinsulinemia is a compensatory response to this target tissue resistance. Several mechanisms have been suggested to explain insulin resistance, including peripheral target tissue resistance, decreased hepatic clearance, or increased pancreatic sensitivity. Studies with the euglycemic clamp technique indicate that hyperandrogenic woman with hyperinsulinemia have peripheral insulin resistance and a reduced insulin clearance rate due to decreased hepatic insulin extraction.[35,36]

The peripheral insulin resistance in PCOS is uniquely due to a defect beyond the activation of the receptor kinase, namely, reduced tyrosine autophosphorylation of the insulin receptor.[37,38] The reduced signal transmission caused by excessive phosphorylation of serine residues on the insulin receptor also explains the hyperandrogenism caused by the concomitant serine phosphorylation of P450c17, the key enzyme in ovarian and adrenal androgen biosynthesis, which increases the 17,20-lyase activity and androgen production.[38,39] Thus, insulin resistance may be causally related to overactivity of cytochrome P450c17.[40] Insulin, by acting via its own receptors, appears to promote ovarian and adrenal androgen biosynthesis,[41,42] amplifying LH-induced androgen production by theca cells and resulting in hyperandrogenemia.[43,44] Amelioration of the hyperinsulinemia leads to a dramatic decline in circulating androgens to normal levels.[45] Hyperinsulinemia may also upregulate IGF-I receptors, which are potent stimulators of LH-induced androgen synthesis, and increase the bioavailability of IGF-I secondary to the suppression of IGF binding protein (BP) I (IGF-BPI) production by the liver.[46,47] Additionally, insulin may potentiate the response of adrenal steroidogenesis to adrenocorticotropic hormone (ACTH),[48] and enhance the expression of hyperandrogenism by its inhibitory effect on hepatic sex hormone binding globulin (SHBG) production,[49] thereby increasing the bioavailability of androgens. Figure 63.1 presents the potential mechanisms of insulin resistance in PCOS.

Although some studies indicate that androgens can induce hyperinsulinemia, most of the evidence supports hyperinsulinemia as the primary factor leading to hyperandrogenism.[50,51]

Both lean and obese women with PCOS may be insulin resistant.[52–55] Affected lean women appear to have an intrinsic and still poorly understood form of insulin resistance,[37,38] and

obese women probably have this form in addition to insulin resistance due to overweight.

Clinical findings that suggest the presence of insulin resistance and hyperinsulinemia include body mass index (BMI) >27 kg/m^2, waist-to-hip ratio >0.85, waist >100 cm, acanthosis nigricans and numerous achrochordons (skin tags).[56] However, according to the American Diabetes Association (ADA) Consensus Conference,[57] there is still no satisfactory method for determining insulin resistance in the clinical practice setting. None of the tests, such as fasting insulin, glucose or glucose-to-insulin ratio, has been shown to be a useful predictor of the ovulatory response to insulin-sensitizing drugs. Although the fasting glucose-to-insulin ratio (<4.5) correlates with insulin sensitivity as determined by the insulin–glucose clamp,[58] it has never been tested as a predictor of response to insulin-sensitizing therapy.[33]

Hyperinsulinemia and impaired ovulation

Dale et al.[59] examined the correlation between insulin metabolism and outcome of gonadotropin stimulation in 42 infertile, CC-resistant women with PCOS. Using continuous infusion of glucose with the model assessment test, they identified 17 patients with insulin resistance who required higher doses of gonadotropins and a longer duration of treatment to achieve follicular maturation. In this group, 35% of the cycles were cancelled due to a multifollicular response compared to 2.5% in the noninsulin-resistant PCOS group. Moreover, although the ovulation rate in completed cycles was similar between the groups, the conception rate was significantly better in the women with noninsulin-resistant PCOS.

Hyperinsulinemia and obesity correlate directly with the failure to ovulate in response to CC, or with the need for multiple repeated courses and increasing doses of CC.[60,61] Thus, women with PCOS and severe insulin resistance are more likely to fail to respond to CC.[62] BMI is a major determinant of insulin resistance and hyperinsulinemia. Insulin resistance is unlikely in women with BMI <22 kg/m^2, common in women with BMI >27 kg/m^2 and almost always present in women with BMI >30 kg/m^2.[63] In obese women, weight reduction can reduce circulating androgen, LH and insulin concentrations, and, thereby, may induce ovulation and even improve the pregnancy rate.[64–66] The difficulty obese women have in losing weight, coupled with the fact that 10–30% of women with PCOS are lean, led to the introduction of insulin-sensitizing drugs to improve peripheral insulin sensitivity and reduce plasma insulin concentrations.[33,67,68]

Metformin

Metformin is an oral biguanide, category B drug for pregnant women, which has been approved for the treatment of Type 2 diabetes mellitus. It is thought to affect multiple metabolic pathways, decreasing glucose absorption, and suppressing hepatic glucose output and gluconeogenesis.[69,70] Metformin also improves the action of insulin at the cellular level by enhancing glucose uptake by fat and muscle cells,[71,72] and by increasing insulin receptor binding.[73] The reduction in

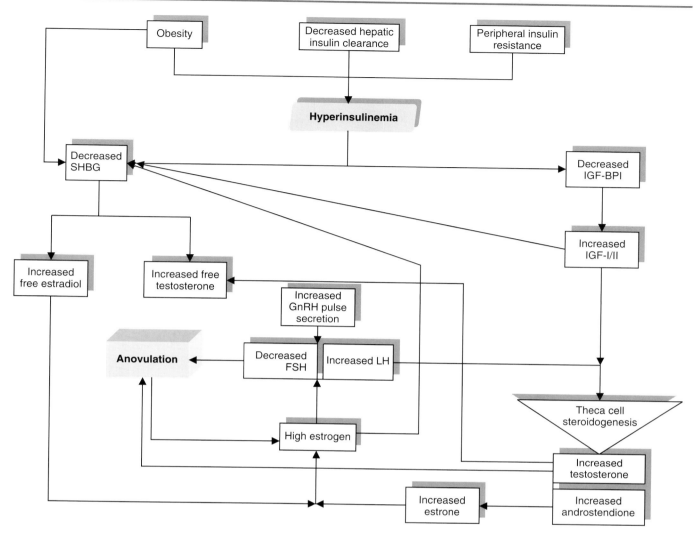

Figure 63.1   Presents the potential mechanisms of insulin resistance in PCOS.

free fatty acid release from adipose tissue further enhances insulin sensitivity.[74] Recently, Attia et al.[75] showed that metformin directly inhibits androgen production in human thecal cells. Importantly, the actions of metformin are not associated with an increase in insulin secretion and, hence, with hypoglycemia. It is possible that the weight loss that often accompanies protracted metformin therapy may account for some of the beneficial effects observed in many studies.[76,77]

Metabolic and endocrine effects of metformin

Women with PCOS and fasting hyperinsulinemia who were treated with metformin showed a significant decrease in fasting insulin and total testosterone levels, and an increase in SHBG, leading to a decrease in the free testosterone index. In addition, there was a significant decline in mean BMI, the waist-to-hip ratio, hirsutism, and acne, as well as an improvement in menstrual cyclicity. No changes in the LH level or in LH-to-follicle-stimulating hormone (FSH) ratio were observed. The greatest decline in testosterone and its free index occurred in the patients with the most pronounced

hyperandrogenemia. Women with high levels of dehydroepiandrosterone sulfate (DHEAS) exhibited less improvement in menstrual cycle regularity, no change in hirsutism, and an increase in levels of IGF-I.[78] In addition, plasma 17-hydroxyprogesterone response to human chorionic gonadotropin (hCG) was significantly lower after treatment,[79] and the adrenal steroidogenesis response to ACTH was reduced, supporting the hypothesis that the high insulin levels associated with PCOS may cause an increase in plasma levels of adrenal androgens.[48] Accordingly, decreasing serum insulin concentrations with metformin also reduce ovarian cytochrome P450c17 alpha activity and ameliorate hyperandrogenism.[80] Thus, metformin apparently affects ovarian steroidogenesis, possibly via decreased insulin action.[81]

Spontaneous ovulation after metformin treatment

Vrbikova et al.[82] showed that a 6-month course of metformin 1000 mg daily significantly improved the menstrual cycle pattern in 58% of the 24 women evaluated. In a study of 50 women with PCOS given metformin 1500 mg daily for

12 months, Baysal et al.[83] found a statistically significant decrease in mean BMI, with no differences in fasting serum insulin and testosterone levels. Metformin improved menstrual patterns in 60% of cases. The authors speculated that the changes in menstrual cyclicity in response to metformin possibly occurred independent of insulin sensitivity or circulating insulin concentrations. A similar effect has also been reported by others.[77,84–86]

Metformin treatment and ovulation induction with CC

CC-resistant and obese women have a high prevalence of insulin resistance. This subgroup may benefit more from treatment with metformin. In a large prospective trial, an oral glucose tolerance test (OGTT) was performed in 61 obese women with PCOS before and after administration of metformin 500 mg or placebo three times daily for 35 days.[87] Those who failed to ovulate spontaneously were given CC 50 mg daily for 5 days, concomitant with metformin or placebo. This regimen was successful in 19 of 21 women (90%) in the metformin group and two of 25 women (8%) in the placebo group. Overall, 31 of the 35 women (89%) treated with metformin ovulated spontaneously or in response to CC, compared with only three of the 26 untreated women (12%). This finding agrees with other studies reporting an increase in pregnancy rate with combined metformin–CC treatment.[88–92] In a comparative study,[93] 154 infertile women with oligomenorrhea and hyperandrogenism were studied. Patients receiving metformin alone had an increased ovulation rate compared with those receiving CC alone (75.4 vs. 50%). Patients on metformin had similar ovulation rates compared with those in the combination group (75.4 vs. 63.4%). Pregnancy rates were equivalent in the three groups. Response to metformin was independent of body weight and dose. Additionally, nonsmoking predicted better ovulatory response overall as well as lower fasting glucose for CC and lower androgens for metformin. By contrast, however, Ng et al.[88] noted no improvement in ovulation rate in CC-resistant women after metformin treatment, despite a significant reduction in BMI and serum testosterone and fasting leptin concentrations. Similarly, Legro et al.[94] randomly assigned 626 infertile women with PCOS to receive CC plus placebo, metformin plus placebo, or a combination of CC and metformin for up to 6 months. The live birth rates were 22.5, 7.2, and 26.8%, respectively. Therefore, CC was superior to metformin in achieving live birth.

In a novel study,[95] the combination of metformin and the aromatase inhibitor, letrozole, was studied in infertile women with PCOS that were randomly divided into metformin–letrozole (29 patients) and metformin–clomiphene groups (30 patients). After an initial 6–8 weeks of metformin, they received either letrozole (2.5 mg) or clomiphene (100 mg) from days 3–7 of their menstrual cycle. Endometrial thickness was significantly higher in letrozole group. The pregnancy rate in letrozole group (10 patients, 34.50%) as compared with clomiphene group (five patients, 16.67%) did not show significant difference, whereas full-term pregnancies were higher in letrozole group [10 patients (34.50%) vs. three patients (10%)].

Metformin treatment and ovulation induction with FSH

De Leo et al.[89] showed that cycles performed with metformin had significantly fewer follicles measuring >15 mm in diameter on the day of hCG administration. In addition, hCG was withheld in a significantly lower percentage because of excessive follicular development. Plasma levels of E2 were significantly higher in cycles treated with FSH alone than in those treated with FSH and metformin. Similarly, Palomba et al.[96] performed a randomized controlled trial and concluded that in insulin-resistant women with PCOS, metformin pre-treatment and co-administration with FSH increases the mono-ovulatory cycles. Yarali et al.[90] concluded that in CC-resistant PCOS patients with normal glucose tolerance, metformin may restore ovulation with no improvement in insulin resistance. However, it has no significant effect on ovarian response during recombinant FSH treatment.

Metformin treatment and *in vitro* fertilization

Stadtmauer et al.[91] hypothesized that metformin may improve the quality of oocytes retrieved from patients with PCOS by reducing hyperinsulinemia and by modulating the local insulin and IGF levels. They retrospectively analyzed 46 women with CC-resistant PCOS who underwent 60 cycles of *in vitro* fertilization (IVF) embryo transfer with intracytoplasmic sperm injection. In half the cycles, patients received metformin 1000–1500 mg daily, starting with the cycle prior to gonadotropin treatment. The authors found that the metformin cycles were associated with a decrease in the total number of follicles on the day of hCG treatment, with no change in mean follicular diameter. There was no effect on mean number of oocytes retrieved, although the mean number of mature oocytes and embryos cleaved was higher. Fertilization rates (64 vs. 43%) and clinical pregnancy rates (70 vs. 30%) were also increased. Metformin led to a modulation of preovulatory follicular fluid IGF levels, with increases in IGF-I and decreases in IGF-BPI. Doldi et al.[97] compared the stimulation characteristics and IVF outcomes of the standard short GnRH antagonist protocol for ovarian stimulation with or without metformin in 40 patients. The metformin group was characterized by a statistically significant decrease in the number of ampoules of rFSH and estradiol levels, fewer cancelled cycles and lower rate of OHSS (5 vs. 15%, $P < 0.05$). The mean number of mature oocytes was increased with metformin treatment. No difference was found in the number of cleaved embryos.

Contrary to these findings, however, Fedorcsak et al.[98] reported that in woman with PCOS who received long-term downregulation and stimulation with recombinant FSH, insulin resistance was not related to either hormone levels or IVF outcome. Obesity was independently associated with relative gonadotropin resistance. The same group of investigators, also reported that co-administration of metformin is likely to increase the number of oocytes collected after ovarian stimulation in insulin-resistant women with PCOS but is unlikely to reduce the requirement for FSH.[99] In recent randomized controlled trials,[100–102] metformin did not lead to any improvement in IVF/ICSI outcomes among patients with PCOS. However, improved pregnancy rates[101] improved pregnancy outcome and reduced risk of OHSS[102] were reported.

Metformin treatment in pregnancy

In addition to poor conception rates, pregnancy loss rates are high (30–50%) in the first trimester in women with PCOS. Hyperinsulinemia may contribute to the early pregnancy loss by adversely affecting endometrial function and environment. Serum glycodelin, a putative biomarker of endometrial function, is decreased in women with early pregnancy loss. IGF-BPI may also play an important role in pregnancy by facilitating adhesion processes at the feto-maternal interface. Jakubowicz et al.[103] studied 48 women with PCOS before and after administration of metformin 500 mg (n = 26) or placebo (n = 22) three times daily for 4 weeks. OGTT were performed, and serum glycodelin and IGF-BPI were measured during the follicular and CC-induced luteal phases of menses. The authors found a decrease in mean area under the serum insulin curve after glucose administration. In the metformin group, follicular and luteal phase serum glycodelin and IGF-BPI concentrations were significantly increased, as was the luteal phase blood flow in the spiral arteries, as indicated by a 20% decrease in resistance index. Thus, metformin-induced changes may reflect an improved endometrial milieu for the establishment and maintenance of pregnancy.

In a later study, the same group studied 96 women with PCOS who became pregnant during a 4.5 year period, of whom 65 had taken metformin during pregnancy and 31 had not.[104] Early pregnancy loss rate was 8.8% in the metformin group compared with 41.9% in the control group. The authors concluded that metformin administration during pregnancy reduces first trimester pregnancy loss in women with PCOS. Similar results were reported others.[105,106]

Glueck et al.[107] prospectively followed 33 nondiabetic women with PCOS who conceived while taking metformin and gave birth to live babies; 28 took metformin through delivery. These findings were compared with the file data of 39 nondiabetic women with PCOS giving birth to live babies who were not given metformin. One of the 33 pregnancies (3%) achieved during metformin therapy was associated with gestational diabetes mellitus (GDM), compared to eight of 12 (67%) previous pregnancies in the same group achieved without metformin and to 14 of 60 pregnancies (23%) in the control group (total non-metformin GDM rate, 31.9%). Thus, metformin was associated with a 10-fold reduction in GDM in women with PCOS. Importantly, these findings emphasize the possible role of metformin in preventing GDM and overt diabetes in these patients.

Metformin does not appear to be teratogenic.[108] In a recent meta-analysis, Gilbert et al.[109] evaluated the rate of major malformations in eight studies of exposure to metformin in the first trimester of pregnancy. In their analysis, after adjustment for publication bias, metformin treatment was associated with a statistically significant 57% protective effect. After pooling the studies, the malformation rate in the disease-matched control group was approximately 7.2%, statistically significantly higher than the rate found in the metformin group. Therefore on the basis of the data available today, there is no evidence of an increased risk for major malformations when metformin is taken during the first trimester of pregnancy.

Type 1 diabetes and spontaneous abortions

Epidemiology

Women with Type 1 diabetes are at increased risk of both first trimester spontaneous abortions and major congenital malformations. The magnitude of the risk depends on the degree of metabolic control in the first trimester.[110] Stricter control is necessary to avoid spontaneous abortions than major malformations. At the same time, the timely institution of intensive therapy yields excellent results with regard to spontaneous abortions, whereas the risk of major malformations remains elevated compared to nondiabetic pregnancy even when control is good.[111]

The multicenter Diabetes in Early Pregnancy (DIEP) study, which was designed to answer questions about causes of spontaneous abortion and malformations, found that the risk of spontaneous abortion increased from 9% with good glucose control to 45% when the glycemic level was markedly elevated.[112] Recently, Temple et al.[113] showed that among 242 diabetic pregnancies, the poor control group [glycosylated hemoglobin (HbA1c) >7.5%] had a 4-fold higher spontaneous abortion rate than the fair-control group [relative risk (RR) 4.0, 1.2–13.1].

Dorman et al.[114] found that improvement in maternal care over the past 30 years in the USA was accompanied by a significant temporal decline in the rates of spontaneous abortion for women with Type 1 diabetes as follows: up to 1969, 26.4%; 1970–1979, 31.0%; 1980–1989, 15.7%; $P < 0.05$. No differences were noted for the nondiabetic partners of Type 1 diabetic men (up to 1969, 4.2%; 1970–1979, 9.5%; 1980–1989, 5.7%; $P > 0.05$). Current rates in Denmark and the UK are about 17.5%.[115,116]

Etiology

Although some authors attribute spontaneous abortions in diabetic pregnancy to early fetal growth delay,[117] others suggest that this finding is probably an artifact of incorrectly estimated ovulation date.[118,119] To clarify this issue, Ivanisevic et al.[120] confirmed the pregnancy duration in their cohort by beta-human chorionic gonadotropin (hCG) measurements within a fortnight of the missed menstrual period. They found that the risk of spontaneous abortion in the Type 1 diabetic pregnancies with delayed embryonal growth was eight times higher than in the diabetic pregnancies with a normal growth pattern, which were matched for gestational age, prepregnancy weight, newborn birthweight and sex. Neither group had fetal malformations. Corresponding HbA1c levels were 9.39 ± 2.37 and 7.3 ± 1.5% ($P = 0.006$), confirming the relationship between embryonal growth, spontaneous abortions and abnormal metabolic control of diabetic pregnancy.

On the basis of in vitro findings of an association of high levels of β-hydroxybutyrate (beta-HOB) and malformations and growth retardation, Jovanovic et al.[121] studied these factors in diabetic and nondiabetic women. Although the first trimester beta-HOB levels were significantly higher in the diabetic group, they tended to be lower, not higher, in mothers in both groups who had a malformed infant or pregnancy loss. The biological significance of this trend remains unclear.

There is considerable amount of clinical and experimental evidence suggesting the involvement of free-radical-mediated oxidative processes in the pathogenesis of diabetic complications. These might be contributory factors to conceptus damage, leading to embryonic death and abortion or the appearance of fetal malformations.[122] Another hypothesis claims that the diabetic milieu causes a reduction in phosphatidylinositol turnover, leading to a disruption in the arachidonic acid cascade and resulting in a deficiency of prostaglandins, particularly prostaglandin E2 (PGE2). Accordingly, it was found that yolk sac prostaglandin levels were undetectable in diabetic women prior to elective abortion but high in normal controls.[123]

Other researchers introduced a mouse model of premature programmed cell death to explain adverse pregnancy outcomes in diabetes. In this model, raised glucose concentrations altered gene expression in developing tissues, leading to apoptosis in key progenitor cells of the mouse blastocyst or mouse postimplantation embryos, resulting in abnormal morphogenesis or miscarriage.[124] Although these findings are still preliminary and limited to mouse, the paradigm is supported by examples in other cell systems including human-derived cell lines.[124]

Diabetes and male infertility

Erectile dysfunction

Diabetic men have a higher prevalence of erectile dysfunction (ED) than nondiabetic men. Erectile function is primarily a vascular phenomenon, triggered by neurologic controls and facilitated by appropriate hormonal and psychological components. All of these factors are affected by diabetes. Recent advances in the understanding of the physiology of penile vasculature and its role in male sexual performance have influenced the clinical approach to ED. A thorough history and physical examination are an important aspect of ED management. It is also important to rule out secondary causes such as hypogonadism and thyroid abnormalities.[125]

A large cohort study of 31,027 men between the ages of 53 and 90[126] showed that the age-adjusted RR of ED was 1.32 [95% confidence interval (CI) 1.3–1.4) in those who had diabetes compared to those who did not. These findings remained significant in multivariate regression analyses (Type 1 diabetes: RR = 3.0, 95% CI 1.5–5.9; Type 2 diabetes: RR = 1.3, 1.1–1.5). In men with Type 2 diabetes, the risk of ED increases with increased duration of disease. Another study reported ED in 86.1% of diabetic males, varying in degree from mild in 7.7%, to moderate in 29.4%, to severe in 49.1%.[127] The prevalence of ED was three times higher in the group over 50 years of age compared those under 50 years of age, and was also higher in the group with a long (>10 years) history of disease compared to those with a history of <5 years. Men with poor metabolic control were 12.2 times more likely to report ED than men with good metabolic control. Over half the diabetic patients with ED had one or more

diabetes-related complication compared with 20.5% of those without ED.

Various treatment modalities have been suggested for ED in diabetic patients. The development of oral medications that inhibit the action of phosphodiesterase in the penile vasculature has revolutionized the treatment of impotence in diabetic men. These drugs are currently the treatment of choice for most patients.[126,128] However, some authors claim that self-intracavernous injection of vasoactive substances is still the sole effective therapeutic modality when ED is severe, and that younger men with Type 2 diabetes treated with low doses of PGE1 are more likely to respond to oral sildenafil (Viagra) than men with Type 1 diabetes or men treated with mixtures of vasoactive drugs.[129]

Retrograde ejaculation

Retrograde ejaculation causes <2% of all cases of male infertility but it is the leading cause of aspermia,[130] the incidence of which is increased in patients with diabetes because of the presence of diabetic neuropathy. Treatment approaches include drugs such as imipramine or ephedrine,[131] insemination with sperm-rich urine obtained after masturbation, bladder washing after masturbation for sperm retrieval and assisted reproduction technology using the intracytoplasmic sperm injection.

Impaired semen production

In adult rats, long-term diabetes with sustained hyperglycemia leads to significant testicular dysfunction associated with decreased fertility potential,[132] and this may also be true for humans. Garcia-Diez et al.,[133] in a study of 80 patients with Type 1 diabetes, found significant alterations in semen parameters and levels of prolactin and testosterone. In all patients, seminal insulin concentrations were higher than serum concentrations. The authors speculated that the hormone freely crosses the blood–testis barrier. The levels of insulin in serum and seminal plasma did not correlate with semen parameters and were not suitable markers of seminal quality.

Padron et al.[134] studied 32 adolescents with Type 1 diabetes and aged-matched controls. The Type 1 diabetes group had significantly lower semen volume, motility and morphology, non-significantly lower sperm count, and significantly higher seminal fructose and glucose levels. There were no differences in plasma testosterone levels. No correlation was detected between clinical parameters (age at onset and duration of diabetes and time since first ejaculation), semen parameters, plasma testosterone level, glycemia or glycosuria.

In another study, subjects with Type 1 or Type 2 neuropathic diabetes showed a highly significant increase in total sperm output and sperm concentration compared to age-matched nondiabetic controls.[135] Sperm motility and semen volume were reduced by about 30 and 60%, respectively. Sperm morphology and quality of sperm motility remained unaffected. The authors suggested that the significant decrease in semen volume could be the result of Leydig cell hyperplasia, which in turn may stimulate spermatogenesis and atonia of the bladder and urethra, resulting in retrograde ejaculation.

Conclusions

Type 1 diabetes is associated with delayed menarche if diabetes is diagnosed prior to 11 or 12 years of age. Menstrual disturbances, such as oligomenorrhea, amenorrhea, and polymenorrhea, occurr in 16–30% of women. Diabetes apparently does not affect the ability to conceive, but affected women have fewer pregnancies and fewer births per pregnancy than controls. Suggested mechanisms for infertility in diabetes are hypothalamic–pituitary dysfunction, impaired folliculogenesis, functional deficit in noradrenergic neurons within the hypothalamus, microangiopathy, and decreased ovarian SOD activity.

PCOS is a metabolic disorder with widespread systemic effects. The accompanying insulin resistance and hyperinsulinemia mark this syndrome as a prediabetic state, with high incidence of IGT, GDM, and overt diabetes. Fertility may also be impaired due to anovulation, impaired implantation and higher rates of spontaneous abortions. All of these effects may be related to the hyperinsulinemia. Lifestyle interventions, such as weight loss and exercise, should be the first line of treatment in women with PCOS. Those who cannot maintain weight loss and those who are not overweight but nevertheless hyperinsulinemic should be considered candidates for metformin treatment. Metformin, an insulin-sensitizing drug, is being evaluated for its potential long-term disease-modifying effect, such as prevention of GDM and diabetes. Its use may also help restore spontaneous ovulation and improve menstrual cyclicity, improve the success rate of induction of and decrease early pregnancy loss. Though not all of these benefits have been proven by evidence-based medicine, given the drug's relatively low rate of side effects and the growing experience with metformin in the treatment of women with PCOS receiving fertility treatment and even those in early pregnancy, we believe, in agreement with others, that metformin should be considered in women with PCOS and insulin resistance.

Although the risk of major malformations remains elevated, despite good to excellent metabolic control, the risk of spontaneous abortions is substantially lower in well-treated women and is comparable to that seen in nondiabetic women. Male diabetic patients may suffer from impotence, retrograde ejaculation and sexual dysfunction, as well as from impaired semen production.

REFERENCES

1. Drash A. Diabetes mellitus in childhood. J Pediatr 1971; 78: 919–41.
2. Post RH. Early menarchial age of diabetic women. Diabetes 1962; 11: 287–90.
3. Tattersal RB, Pyke DA. Growth in diabetic children. Lancet 1973; 2: 1105–9.
4. Griffin ML, South SA, Yankov VI, et al. Insulin-dependent diabetes mellitus and menstrual dysfunction. Ann Med 1994; 26: 331–40.
5. Burkart W, Fischer-Guntenhoner E, Standl E, Schneider HP. Menarche, menstrual cycle and fertility in diabetic patients. Geburtshilfe Frauenheilkd 1989; 49: 149–54.
6. Yeshaya E, Orvieto R, Dicker D, et al. Menstrual characteristics of women suffering from insulin-dependent diabetes mellitus. Int J Fert Menopausal Stud 1995; 40: 269–73.
7. Bergquist N. The gonadal function in female diabetics. Acta Endocrinol 1954; 15: 3–20.
8. Kjaer K, Hagen C, Sando SH. Epidemiology of menarche and menstrual disturbances in an unselected group of women with insulin-dependent diabetes mellitus compared to controls. J Clin Endocrinol Metab 1992; 75: 524–9.
9. Kjaer K, Hagen C, Sando SH, Eshoj O. Infertility and pregnancy outcome in an unselected group of women with insulin-dependent diabetes mellitus. Am J Obstet Gynecol 1992; 166: 1412–8.
10. Pedersen KK, Hagen C, Sando-Pedersen SH, Eshoj O. Infertility and pregnancy outcome in women with insulin-dependent diabetes. An epidemiological study. Ugeskr Laeger 1994; 156: 6196–200.
11. Briese V, Muller H. Diabetes mellitus – an epidemiologic study of fertility, contraception and sterility. Geburtshilfe Frauenheilkd 1995; 55: 270–4.
12. Peled Y, Rabinerson D, Kaplan B, et al. A 'sweet' indication for ovulation induction. Hum Reprod 1996; 11: 1403–4.
13. El-Roeiy A, Chen X, Roberts VJ, et al. Expression of the genes encoding the insulin-like growth factors (IGF-I and II), the IGF and insulin receptors, and IGF binding proteins 1–6 and the localization of their gene products in normal and polycystic ovary syndrome ovaries. J Clin Endocrinol Metab 1994; 78: 1488–96.
14. Samoto T, Maruo T, Ladines-llave C, et al. Insulin receptor expression in the follicular and stromal compartments of the human ovary over the course of follicular growth, regression, and artesia. Endocr J 1993; 40: 715–26.
15. Nilsson E, Skinner MK. Cellular interactions that control primordial follicle development and folliculogenesis. J Soc Gynecol Invest 2001; 8: S17–20.
16. Yu N, Roy S. Development of primordial and prenatal follicles from undifferentiated somatic cells in oocytes in the hamster prenatal ovary in vitro: effect of insulin. Biol Reprod 1999; 61: 1558–67.
17. McGee EA, Sawetawan C, Bird I, et al. The effect of insulin and insulin-like growth factors on the expression of steroidogenic enzymes in a human ovarian thecallike tumor cell model. Fert Steril 1996; 65: 87–93.
18. Willis D, Mason H, Gilling-Smith C, Franks S. Modulation by insulin of follicle stimulating hormone and luteinizing hormone actions in human granulosa cells of normal and polycystic ovaries. J Clin Endocrinol Metab 1996; 81: 302–9.
19. Kezele PR, Nilsson EE, Skinner MK. Insulin but not insulin-like growth factor-1 promotes the primordial to primary follicle transition. Mol Cell Endocrinol 2002; 192: 37–43.
20. Kalra SP. Mandatory neuropeptide-steroid signaling for the preovulatory luteinizing hormone-releasing hormone discharge. Endocrinol Rev 1993; 14: 507–38.
21. Nishihara M, Hiruma H, Kimura F. Interactions between the noradrenergic and opioid peptidergic systems in controlling the electrical activity of luteinizing hormone-releasing hormone pulse generator in ovariectomized rats. Neuroendocrinology 1991; 54: 321–6.
22. Dyer RG, Grossmann R, Mansfield S, et al. Opioid peptides inhibit noradrenergic transmission in the preoptic area to block LH secretion: evidence from neonatally androgenised rats. Brain Res Bull 1988; 20: 721–7.
23. Bitar MS. The role of catecholamines in the etiology of infertility in diabetes mellitus. Life Sci 1997; 61: 65–73.
24. Chittenden SJ, Shami SK. Microangiopathy in diabetes mellitus. Causes and prevention and treatment. Diabetes Res 1991; 17: 105–14.
25. Mayhan WG. Impairment of endothelium dependent dilatation of the basilary artery during diabetes mellitus. Brain Res 1992; 580: 297–302.
26. Hattori Y, Kawasaki H, Kazuhiro A, Kanno M. Superoxide dismutase recovers altered endothelium-dependent relaxation in diabetic rat aorta. Am J Physiol 1991; 261: H1086–94.
27. Powers RW, Chambers C, Larsen WJ. Diabetes-mediated decreases in ovarian superoxide dismutase activity are related to blood–follicle barrier and ovulation defects. Endocrinology 1996; 137: 3101–10.
28. Franks S. Polycystic ovary syndrome. N Engl J Med 1995; 333: 853–61.

29. Adams J, Polson DW, Franks S. Prevalence of polycystic ovaries in women with anovulation and idiopathic hirsutism. Br Med J Clin Res Ed 1986; 293: 355–9.
30. Nestler JE, Stovall D, Akhter N, et al. Strategies for the use of insulin-sensitizing drugs to treat infertility in women with polycystic ovary syndrome. Fert Steril 2002; 77: 209–15.
31. Franks S, Gilling-Smith C, Waston H. Insulin action in the normal and polycystic ovary. Metab Clin N Am 1999; 28: 361–78.
32. Ehrmann DA, Barnes RB, Rosenfield RL, et al. Prevalence of impaired glucose tolerance and diabetes in women with polycystic ovary syndrome. Diabetes Care 1999; 22: 141–6.
33. Nestler JE. Should patients with polycystic ovarian syndrome be treated with metformin? Hum Reprod 2002; 17: 1950–3.
34. Boomsma CM, Eijkemans MJ, Hughes EG, et al. A meta-analysis of pregnancy outcomes in women with polycystic ovary syndrome. Hum Reprod Update 2006; 12: 673–83.
35. Poretsky L. On the paradox of insulin-induced hyperandrogenism in insulin-resistant states. Endocrinol Rev 1991; 12: 3–13.
36. O'Meara NM, Blackman JD, Ehrman DA, et al. Defects in beta-cell function in functional ovarian hyperandrogenism. J Clin Endocrinol Metab 1993; 76: 1241–7.
37. Ciaraldi TP, el Roeiy A, Madar Z, et al. Cellular mechanisms of insulin resistance in polycystic ovarian syndrome. J Clin Endocrinol Metab 1992; 75: 577–83.
38. Dunaif A, Xia J, Book CB, et al. Excessive insulin receptor serine phosphorylation in cultured fibroblasts and in skeletal muscle. A potential mechanism for insulin resistance in the polycystic ovary syndrome. J Clin Invest 1995; 96: 801–10.
39. Zhang L, Rodriguez H, Ohno S, Miller WL. Serine phosphorylation of human P450c17 increases 17,20-lyase activity: implications for adrenarche and the polycystic ovary syndrome. Proc Natl Acad Sci USA 1995; 92: 106–19.
40. Ehrmann DA, Rosenfield RL, Barnes RB. Detection of functional ovarian hyperandrogenism in women with androgen excess. N Engl J Med 1992; 327: 157–62.
41. Barbieri RL, Makris A, Randall RW. Insulin stimulates androgen accumulation in incubations of ovarian stroma obtained from women with hyperandrogenism. J Clin Endocrinol Metab 1986; 62: 904–10.
42. Barbieri RL, Smith S, Ryan KJ. The role of hyperinsulinemia in the pathogenesis of ovarian hyperandrogenism. Fert Steril 1988; 50: 197–212.
43. Nahum R, Thong KJ, Hillier SG. Metabolic regulation of androgen production by human thecal cells in vitro. Hum Reprod 1995; 10: 75–81.
44. Willis DS, Watson H, Mason HD, et al. Premature response to luteinizing hormone of granulosa cells from anovulatory women with polycystic ovary syndrome: relevance to mechanism of anovulation. J Clin Endocrinol Metab 1998; 83: 3984–91.
45. Murray RD, Davison RM, Russell RC. Clinical presentation of PCOS following development of an insulinoma: case report. Hum Reprod 2000; 15: 86–8.
46. Suikkari AM, Koivisto VA, Rutanen EM. Insulin regulates the serum levels of low molecular weight insulin-like growth factor-binding protein. J Clin Endocrinol Metab 1988; 66: 266–72.
47. Suikkari AM, Koivisto VA, Koistinen R. Dose–response characteristics for suppression of low molecular weight plasma insulin-like growth factor-binding protein by insulin. J Clin Endocrinol Metab 1989; 68: 135–40.
48. La Marca A, Morgante G, Paglia T, et al. Effects of metformin on adrenal steroidogenesis in women with polycystic ovary syndrome. Fert Steril 1999; 72: 985–9.
49. Botwood N, Hamilton-Fairley D, Kiddy D. Sex hormone-binding globulin and female reproductive function. J Steroid Biochem Mol Biol 1995; 53: 529–31.
50. Geffner ME, Kaplan SA, Bersch N, et al. Persistence of insulin resistance in polycystic ovarian disease after inhibition of ovarian steroid secretion. Fert Steril 1986; 45: 327–33.
51. Dunaif A, Green G, Futterweit W, Dobrjansky A. Suppression of hyperandrogenism does not improve peripheral or hepatic insulin resistance in the polycystic ovary syndrome. J Clin Endocrinol Metab 1990; 70: 699–704.
52. Chang RJ, Nakamura RM, Judd HL, Kaplan SA. Insulin resistance in nonobese patients with polycystic ovarian disease. J Clin Endocrinol Metab 1983 57: 356–9.
53. Dunaif A, Graf M, Mandeli J, et al. Characterization of groups of hyperandrogenemic women with acanthosis nigricans, impaired glucose tolerance, and/or hyperinsulinemia. J Clin Endocrinol Metab 1987; 65: 499–507.
54. Dunaif A, Segal KR, Futterweit W, Dobrjansky A. Profound peripheral insulin resistance, independent of obesity, in polycystic ovary syndrome. Diabetes 1989; 38: 1165–74.
55. Dunaif A, Segal KR, Shelley DR, et al. Evidence for distinctive and intrinsic defects in insulin action in polycystic ovary syndrome. Diabetes 1992; 41: 1257–66.
56. Barbieri RL. Induction of ovulation in infertile women with hyperandrogenism and insulin resistance. Am J Obstet Gynecol 2000; 183: 1412–8.
57. American Diabetes Association (ADA). Consensus Development Conference on Insulin Resistance. Diabetes Care 1998; 21: 310–4.
58. Legro RS, Finegood D, Dunaif A. A fasting glucose to insulin ratio is a useful measure of insulin sensitivity in women with polycystic ovary syndrome. J Clin Endocrinol Metab 1998; 83: 2694–8.
59. Dale PO, Tanbo T, Haug E, Abyholm T. The impact of insulin resistance on the outcome of ovulation induction with low-dose follicle stimulating hormone in women with polycystic ovary syndrome. Hum Reprod 1998; 13: 567–70.
60. Shepard MK, Balmaceda JP, Leija CG. Relationship of weight to successful induction of ovulation with clomiphene citrate. Fert Steril 1979; 32: 641–5.
61. Lobo RA, Gysler M, March CM, et al. Clinical and laboratory predictors of clomiphene response. Fert Steril 1982; 37: 168–74.
62. Murakawa H, Hasegawa I, Kurabayashi T, Tanaka K. Polycystic ovary syndrome. Insulin resistance and ovulatory responses to clomiphene citrate. J Reprod Med 1999; 44: 23–7.
63. Weyer C, Bogardus C, Mott DM, Pratley RE. The natural history of insulin secretory dysfunction and insulin resistance in the pathogenesis of type 2 diabetes mellitus. J Clin Invest 1999; 104: 787–94.
64. Bates GW, Whitworth NS. Effects of obesity on sex steroid metabolism. J Chronic Dis 1982; 35: 893–6.
65. Pasquali R, Antenucci D, Casimirri F, et al. Clinical and hormonal characteristics of obese amenorrheic hyperandrogenic women before and after weight loss. J Clin Endocrinol Metab 1989; 68: 173–9.
66. Clark AM, Thornley B, Tomlinson L, et al. Weight loss in obese infertile women results in improvement in reproductive outcome for all forms of fertility treatment. Hum Reprod 1998; 13: 1502–5.
67. Homburg R. Should patients with polycystic ovarian syndrome be treated with metformin? Hum Reprod 2002; 17: 853–6.
68. Seli E, Duleba AJ. Should patients with polycystic ovarian syndrome be treated with metformin? Hum Reprod 2002; 17: 2230–6.
69. Meyer F, Ipaktchi M, Clauser H. Specific inhibition of gluconeogenesis by biguanides. Nature 1967; 213: 203–4.
70. Wollen N, Bailey CJ. Inhibition of hepatic gluconeogenesis by metformin. Synergism with insulin. Biochem Pharmacol 1988; 37: 4353–8.
71. Jacobs DB, Hayes GR, Truglia JA. Effects of metformin on insulin receptor tyrosine kinase activity in rat adipocytes. Diabetologia 1986; 29: 798–801.
72. Matthaei S, Hamann A, Klein HH. Association of metformin's effect to increase insulin-stimulated glucose transport with potentiation of insulin-induced translocation of glucose transporters from intracellular pool to plasma membrane in rat adipocytes. Diabetes 1991; 40: 850–7.
73. Bailey CJ. Metformin: an update. Gen Pharmacol 1993; 24: 1299–309.
74. Abbasi F, Kamath V, Rizvi AA. Results of a placebo-controlled study of the metabolic effects of the addition of metformin to sulfonylurea-treated patients. Evidence for a central role of adipose tissue. Diabetes Care 1997; 20: 1863–9.
75. Attia GR, Rainey WE, Carr BR. Metformin directly inhibits androgen production in human thecal cells. Fert Steril 2001; 76: 517–24.
76. Crave C, Fimbel S, Lejeune H, et al. Effects of diet and metformin administration on sex hormone-binding globulin, androgens, and insulin in hirsute and obese women. J Clin Endocrinol Metab 1995; 80: 2057–62.
77. Glueck CJ, Wang P, Fontaine R, et al. Metformin-induced resumption of normal menses in 39 of 43 (91%) previously amenorrheic women with the polycystic ovary syndrome. Metabolism 1999; 48: 511–9.
78. Kolodziejczyk B, Duleba AJ, Spaczynski RZ, Pawelczyk L. Metformin therapy decreases hyperandrogenism and hyperinsulinemia in women with polycystic ovary syndrome. Fert Steril 2000; 73: 1149–54.
79. La Marca A, Egbe TO, Morgante G, et al. Metformin treatment reduces ovarian cytochrome P-450c17alpha response to human chorionic gonadotrophin in women with insulin resistance-related polycystic ovary syndrome. Hum Reprod 2000; 15: 21–3.

80. Nestler JE, Jakubowicz DJ. Decreases in ovarian cytochrome P450c17 alpha activity and serum free testosterone after reduction of insulin secretion in polycystic ovary syndrome. N Engl J Med 1996; 335: 617–23.

81. Koivunen RM, Morin-Papunen LC, Ruokonen A, et al. Ovarian steroidogenic response to human chorionic gonadotrophin in obese women with polycystic ovary syndrome: effect of metformin. Hum Reprod 2001; 16: 2546–51.

82. Vrbikova J, Hill M, Starka L, Vondra K. Prediction of the effect of metformin treatment in patients with polycystic ovary syndrome. Gynecol Obstet Invest 2002; 53: 100–4.

83. Baysal B, Batukan M, Batukan C. Biochemical and body weight changes with metformin in polycystic ovary syndrome. Clin Exp Obstet Gynecol 2001; 28: 212–4.

84. Fleming R, Hopkinson ZE, Wallace AM, et al. Ovarian function and metabolic factors in women with oligomenorrhea treated with metformin in a randomized double blind placebo-controlled trial. J Clin Endocrinol Metab 2002; 87: 569–74.

85. Glueck CJ, Wang P, Fontaine R, et al. Metformin to restore normal menses in oligo-amenorrheic teenage girls with polycystic ovary syndrome (PCOS). J Adolesc Health 2001; 29: 160–9.

86. Velazquez E, Acosta A, Mendoza SG. Menstrual cyclicity after metformin therapy in polycystic ovary syndrome. Obstet Gynecol 1997; 90: 392–5.

87. Nestler JE, Jakubowicz DJ, Evans WS, Pasquali R. Effects of metformin on spontaneous and clomiphene-induced ovulation in the polycystic ovary syndrome. N Engl J Med 1998; 338: 1876–80.

88. Ng EH, Wat NM, Ho PC. Effects of metformin on ovulation rate, hormonal and metabolic profiles in women with clomiphene-resistant polycystic ovaries: a randomized, double-blinded placebo-controlled trial. Hum Reprod 2001; 16: 1625–31.

89. De Leo V, la Marca A, Ditto A, et al. Effects of metformin on gonadotropin-induced ovulation in women with polycystic ovary syndrome. Fert Steril 1999; 72: 282–5.

90. Yarali H, Yildiz BO, Demirol A, et al. Co-administration of metformin during rFSH treatment in patients with clomiphene citrate-resistant polycystic ovarian syndrome: a prospective randomized trial. Hum Reprod 2002; 17: 289–94.

91. Stadtmauer LA, Toma SK, Riehl RM, Talbert LM. Metformin treatment of patients with polycystic ovary syndrome undergoing in vitro fertilization improves outcomes and is associated with modulation of the insulin-like growth factors. Fert Steril 2001; 75: 505–9.

92. Khorram O, Helliwell JP, Katz S, Bonpane CM, Jaramillo L. Two weeks of metformin improves clomiphene citrate-induced ovulation and metabolic profiles in women with polycystic ovary syndrome. Fertil Steril 2006; 85: 1448–51.

93. Neveu N, Granger L, St-Michel P, Lavoie HB. Comparison of clomiphene citrate, metformin, or the combination of both for first-line ovulation induction and achievement of pregnancy in 154 women with polycystic ovary syndrome. Fertil Steril 2007; 87: 113–20.

94. Lergo RS, Barnhart HX, Schlaff ??, et al. Clomiphene, metformin, or both for infertility in the polycystic ovary syndrome. N Engl J Med 2007; 356: 551–66.

95. Sohrabvand F, Ansari Sh, Bagheri M. Efficacy of combined metformin-letrozole in comparison with metformin-clomiphene citrate in clomiphene-resistant infertile women with polycystic ovarian disease. Hum Reprod 2006; 21: 1432–5.

96. Palomba S, Falbo A, Orio Jr F, et al. A randomized controlled trial evaluating metformin pre-treatment and co-administration in non-obese insulin-resistant women with polycystic ovary syndrome treated with controlled ovarian stimulation plus timed intercourse or intrauterine insemination. Hum Reprod 2005; 20: 2879–86.

97. Doldi N, Persico P, Di Sebastiano F, Marsiglio E, Ferrari A. Gonadotropin-releasing hormone antagonist and metformin for treatment of polycystic ovary syndrome patients undergoing in vitro fertilization-embryo transfer. Gynecol Endocrinol 2006; 22: 235–8.

98. Fedorcsak P, Dale PO, Storeng R, et al. The impact of obesity and insulin resistance on the outcome of IVF or ICSI in women with polycystic ovarian syndrome. Hum Reprod 2001; 16: 1086–91.

99. Fedorcsak P, Dale PO, Storeng R, Abyholm T, Tanbo T. The effect of metformin on ovarian stimulation and in vitro fertilization in insulin-resistant women with polycystic ovary syndrome: an open-label randomized cross-over trial. Gynecol Endocrinol 2003; 17: 207–14.

100. Onalan G, Pabuccu R, Goktolga U, et al. Metformin treatment in patients with polycystic ovary syndrome undergoing in vitro fertilization: a prospective randomized trial. Fertil Steril 2005; 84: 798–801.

101. Kjotrod SB, von During V, Carlsen SM. Metformin treatment before IVF/ICSI in women with polycystic ovary syndrome; a prospective, randomized, double blind study. Hum Reprod 2004; 19: 1315–22.

102. Tang T, Glanville J, Orsi N, Barth JH, Balen AH. The use of metformin for women with PCOS undergoing IVF treatment. Hum Reprod 2006; 21: 1416–25.

103. Jakubowicz DJ, Seppala M, Jakubowicz S, et al. Insulin reduction with metformin increases luteal phase serum glycodelin and insulin-like growth factor-binding protein 1 concentrations and enhances uterine vascularity and blood flow in the polycystic ovary syndrome. J Clin Endocrinol Metab 2001; 86: 1126–33.

104. Jakubowicz DJ, Iuorno MJ, Jakubowicz S, et al. Effects of metformin on early pregnancy loss in the polycystic ovary syndrome. J Clin Endocrinol Metab 2002; 87: 524–9.

105. Thatcher SS, Jackson EM. Pregnancy outcome in infertile patients with polycystic ovary syndrome who were treated with metformin. Fertil Steril 2006; 85: 1002–9.

106. Khattab S, Mohsen IA, Foutouh IA, et al. Metformin reduces abortion in pregnant women with polycystic ovary syndrome. Gynecol Endocrinol 2006; 22: 680–4.

107. Glueck CJ, Wang P, Kobayashi S, et al. Metformin therapy throughout pregnancy reduces the development of gestational diabetes in women with polycystic ovary syndrome. Fert Steril 2002; 77: 520–5.

108. Glueck CJ, Phillips H, Cameron D, et al. Continuing metformin throughout pregnancy in women with polycystic ovary syndrome appears to safely reduce first-trimester spontaneous abortion: a pilot study. Fert Steril 2001; 75: 46–52.

109. Gilbert C, Valois M, Koren G. Pregnancy outcome after first-trimester exposure to metformin: a meta-analysis. Fertil Steril. 2006; 86: 658–63.

110. Greene MF. Spontaneous abortions and major malformations in women with diabetes mellitus. Semin Reprod Endocrinol 1999; 17: 127–36.

111. Pregnancy outcomes in the Diabetes Control and Complications Trial. Am J Obstet Gynecol 1996; 174: 1343–53.

112. Mills JL, Simpson JL, Driscoll SG, et al., the National Institutes of Child Health and Human Development – Diabetes in Early Pregnancy Study: incidence of spontaneous abortion among normal and insulin-dependent diabetic women whose pregnancies were identified within 21 days of conception. N Engl J Med 1988; 319: 1617–23.

113. Temple R, Aldridge V, Greenwood R, et al. Association between outcome of pregnancy and glycaemic control in early pregnancy in type 1 diabetes: population based study. Br Med J 2002; 325: 1275–6.

114. Dorman JS, Burke JP, McCarthy BJ, et al. Temporal trends in spontaneous abortion associated with type 1 diabetes. Diabetes Res Clin Pract 1999; 43: 41–7.

115. Lorenzen T, Pociot F, Johannesen J, et al. A population-based survey of frequencies of self-reported spontaneous and induced abortions in Danish women with type 1 diabetes mellitus. Danish IDDM Epidemiology and Genetics Group. Diabet Med 1999 16: 472–6.

116. Casson IF, Clarke CA, Howard CV, et al. Outcomes of pregnancy in insulin dependent diabetic women: results of a five-year population cohort study. Br Med J 1997; 315: 275–8.

117. Pedersen JF, Molsted-Pedersen L, Lebech PE. Is the early growth delay in the diabetic pregnancy accompanied by a delay in placental development? Acta Obstet Gynecol Scand 1986; 65: 675–7.

118. Steel JM, Wu PS, Johnstone FD, et al. Does early growth delay occur in diabetic pregnancy? Br J Obstet Gynaecol 1995; 102: 224–7.

119. Hieta-Heikurainen H, Teramo K. Comparison of menstrual history and basal body temperature with early fetal growth by ultrasound in diabetic pregnancy. Acta Obstet Gynecol Scand 1989; 68: 457–9.

120. Ivanisevic M, Bukovic D, Starcevic V, et al. Influence of hyperglycemia on early embryonal growth in IDDM pregnant women. Coll Antropol 1999; 23: 183–8.

121. Jovanovic L, Metzger BE, Knopp RH, et al. The Diabetes in Early Pregnancy Study: beta-hydroxybutyrate levels in type 1 diabetic pregnancy compared with normal pregnancy. NICHD – Diabetes in Early Pregnancy Study Group (DIEP). National Institute of Child Health and Development. Diabetes Care 1998; 21: 1978–84.

122. Damasceno DC, Volpato GT, de Mattos Paranhos Calderon I, Cunha Rudge MV. Oxidative stress and diabetes in pregnant rats. Anim Reprod Sci 2002; 72: 235–44.

123. Schoenfeld A, Erman A, Warchaizer S, et al. Yolk sac concentration of prostaglandin E2 in diabetic pregnancy: further clues to the etiology of diabetic embryopathy. Prostaglandins 1995; 50: 121–6.

124. Moley KH. Hyperglycemia and apoptosis: mechanisms for congenital malformations and pregnancy loss in diabetic women. Trends Endocr Metab 2001; 12: 78–82.

125. Dey J, Shepherd MD. Evaluation and treatment of erectile dysfunction in men with diabetes mellitus. Mayo Clin Proc 2002; 77: 276–82.

126. Bacon CG, Hu FB, Giovannucci E, et al. Association of type and duration of diabetes with erectile dysfunction in a large cohort of men. Diabetes Care 2002; 25: 1458–63.

127. el-Sakka AI, Tayeb KA. Erectile dysfunction risk factors in noninsulin dependent diabetic Saudi patients. J Urol 2003; 169: 1043–7.

128. Boulton AJ, Selam JL, Sweeney M, Ziegler D. Sildenafil citrate for the treatment of erectile dysfunction in men with type II diabetes mellitus. Diabetologia 2001; 44: 1296–301.

129. Perimenis P, Markou S, Gyftopoulos K, et al. Switching from long-term treatment with self-injections to oral sildenafil in diabetic patients with severe erectile dysfunction. Eur Urol 2002; 41: 387–91.

130. Silva PD, Larson KM, Van Every MJ, Silva DE. Successful treatment of retrograde ejaculation with sperm recovered from bladder washings. A report of two cases. J Reprod Med 2000; 45: 957–60.

131. Gilja I, Parazajder J, Radej M, et al. Retrograde ejaculation and loss of emission: possibilities of conservative treatment. Eur Urol 1994; 25: 226–8.

132. Cameron DF, Rountree J, Schultz RE, et al. Sustained hyperglycemia results in testicular dysfunction and reduced fertility potential in BBWOR diabetic rats. Am J Physiol 1990; 259: E881–9.

133. Garcia-Diez LC, Corrales Hernandez JJ, Hernandez-Diaz J, et al. Semen characteristics and diabetes mellitus: significance of insulin in male infertility. Arch Androl 1991; 26: 119–28.

134. Padron RS, Dambay A, Suarez R, Mas J. Semen analyses in adolescent diabetic patients. Acta Diabetol Lat 1984; 21: 115–21.

135. Ali ST, Shaikh RN, Siddiqi NA, Siddiqi PQ. Semen analysis in insulin-dependent/non-insulin-dependent diabetic men with/without neuropathy. Arch Androl 1993; 30: 47–54.

64 Early pregnancy loss and perinatal mortality

Kinneret Tenenbaum-Gavish, Galia Oron and Rony Chen

Introduction

Diabetes is one of the most prominent medical disorders complicating pregnancy, probably affecting 1 out of 250 pregnant women.[1–3] Gestational diabetes occurs in up to 15% of all pregnancies[4,5] and it is estimated that approximately 10% of diabetic pregnancies are due to pre-gestational diabetes.[6] Furthermore, diabetes is considered a major risk factor for congenital malformations, stillbirth, and neonatal death, all constituting increased perinatal mortality (PNM).[2,5,7] Achieving desired level of glycemic control prior to and during pregnancy is crucial in order to reduce the PNM.[8–13]

Definitions

Perinatal mortality

Perinatal mortality (PNM) still remains the standard measure to evaluate adverse pregnancy outcome. There is a considerable difficulty in estimating PNM due to numerous systems used and substantial differences in definitions of PNM. Even the World Health Organization's (WHO) reports do not all follow the same definitions.[14–16] The American National Vital Statistics System and the British CEMACH (Confidential Enquiry into Maternal and Child Health) both use gestational age as the basis for calculation of stillbirth and neonatal death but differ in the referred gestational age (20 vs. 24 weeks of gestation).[2] In the Netherlands, gestational age >24 weeks and/or birth weight >500 g were used and a French survey used either 22 weeks of gestation or 500 g at birth for their study.[13,15] This variance between reports makes international comparisons somewhat more difficult and may hinder identification of temporal or geographic trends. Furthermore, little can be said about the standard of care which is reflected by these adverse pregnancy outcome measures.

The following definition of PNM has been adapted internationally:

$$\frac{\text{still births} + \text{deaths from 0 to 6 days of age}}{\text{all live births} + \text{still births}} \times 100.$$

Live birth was defined by the WHO as:

The complete expulsion or extraction of a product of conception, irrespective of the duration of pregnancy, which after such separation breathes or shows any evidence of life, such as beating of the heart, pulsation of the umbilical cord, or definite movement of voluntary muscles, whether or not the umbilical cord has been cut, or the placenta is attached, each product of such a birth is considered live born.[14]

Common causes of perinatal mortality

The cause of death can be identified in 65–75% of cases, depending on expertise of the multi-disciplinary team involved.[17]

Stillbirth or fetal death is defined as an involuntary loss in which the fetus (>20 weeks' gestation) showed no evidence of life (i.e. no heartbeat or respiration) on delivery.[18] In other studies stillbirth is the death of a fetus >24 or 28 weeks of gestation.[4] There are considerable variations regarding the rates of stillbirth in different countries. The WHO's report on the topic of stillbirths (defined there at >28 weeks of gestation and >1000 g and excluding 'lethal' congenital anomalies) reported an almost 50-fold difference in stillbirth rates between high and low income countries.[16] Stillbirth may account for up to 50% of cases of PNM and the underlying cause may remain obscure depending on resources applied.[19] Causes for stillbirth are generally grouped into three categories: fetal, placental, and maternal (Table 64.1).[17]

Neonatal death is the death of a live born infant before the age of 28 days. Neonatal death can be divided into early and late neonatal deaths. Early neonatal death is defined as the death of a live-born infant during the first 7 days after birth. Late neonatal death is the death of a live-born infant after 7 days but before 29 days of birth.[2,20,21] Neonatal death is largely attributed to four factors: preterm delivery, infections (mainly sepsis and pneumonia), birth asphyxia, and fetal anomalies affecting the neonatal period.[20]

Early pregnancy loss

Early pregnancy loss is an indirect measure related to quality of care before and during early pregnancy. Early pregnancy loss or spontaneous abortion refers to pregnancy loss at less than 20 weeks gestation in the absence of elective medical or surgical measures to terminate the pregnancy.[20]

Table 64.1   Percentage occurrence and causes of stillbirth

Category	Percent occurrence	Causes
Fetal	25–40	Chromosomal anomalies, congenital malformations, infections, hydrops
Pacental	Up to 25	Placental abruption, cord accidents, infections, feto-maternal hemorrhage, placenta previa
Maternal	5–10	Hypertension, vascular disease, thrombophilia, trauma, substance abuse
Other	–	Combined causes, e.g. maternal illness causing placental abruption or insufficiency, or cause unknown

Etiology of perinatal mortality

Diabetes affects the metabolism of all nutrients (carbohydrates, fatty acids and proteins), glucose being the most prominent. Glucose and those other metabolic fuels operating at the different stages of pregnancy may account for the multitude of pathologies inflicted upon the offspring of the diabetic mother. These pathologic conditions range from congenital malformations and intrauterine fetal death to macrosomia, respiratory distress and hyperbilirubinemia. Poor metabolic control may also induce alternations in levels of fatty acids and amino acids. This provides an altered environment in which the embryo and fetus of the diabetic mother may be exposed to changes in gene expression and increased teratogensis.[22,23]

Hyperglycemia by itself, is involved in the pathogenesis of factors contributing to PNM throughout the entire length of pregnancy.[24] *In vitro*, high glucose levels generate free oxygen radicals which are linked to mechanisms of cellular damage.[22–25] Not surprisingly, the congenital malformation rate (which largely contributes to higher rate of PNM in pregnancies complicated by diabetes) was found to be inversely related to maternal age and directly related to the level of glycemic control during early pregnancy.[26,27] Good glycemic control brings about adequate levels of glucose and insulin and is therefore associated with lower levels of ketones. It was suggested that maternal ketosis plays an important part in the occurrence of congenital malformations in the fetus.[28]

Later in pregnancy, maternal hyperglycemia is translated into fetal hyperplasia of pancreatic islet cells and hyperinsulinemia. Pedersen and colleagues[29,30] linked this to early neonatal hypoglycemia. A series of studies by Salvesen et al.[31,32] demonstrated that hyperinsulinemia is related to cord blood acidemia and hypoxemia. It is suggested that hypoxemia and academia are related to increased rates of stillbirth and neonatal death observed in the diabetic population. Furthermore, insulin has an anabolic effect on muscle and adipose tissue linked to fetal macrosomia.[32,33] Macrosomia in its turn is related to increased risk of PNM and shoulder dystocia.[34]

Perinatal mortality in the diabetic population

Although steps forward in modern obstetrics allow early detection of congenital malformation and assessment of fetal well-being, PNM rates in the diabetic population still remain up to five times higher than those of the general population.[3,24]

In order to try to achieve further reduction in PNM rates of diabetic women, focus should be put on the various components constituting overall perinatal outcome in the different stages of the diabetic pregnancy. A closer examination of the various components comprising PNM rate may help elucidate specific points at which intervention might assist in the overall reduction of PNM in the diabetic population.

Numerous studies have demonstrated that there is an inverse relationship between maternal blood glucose levels and adverse pregnancy outcome. Pioneer work done during the 1960s and 1970s allowed the inverse relationship between mean blood glucose levels and perinatal mortality to be plotted. These studies suggest that normalization of blood glucose levels might equal the PNM in the diabetic population to that of nondiabetic population.[35] Karllson and Kjellmer divided their diabetic gravid patients into three groups according to White's classification and mean blood glucose levels. MBG <100, 100–150, >150 were related to PNM of 3.8, 16, and 24% respectively, but no association was found between White's classification and PNM.[35] The established inverse relationship between maternal metabolic control in patients with pre-gestational diabetes and the risk for PNM[36] was also demonstrated in patients with gestational diabetes (also related to maternal age and obesity).[37,38]

Early pregnancy loss

The altered intrauterine conditions in women with diabetes are probably associated with increase in early pregnancy loss rate. However, the exact quantification of the added risk in the diabetic population is difficult to assess due to the indefinable incidence of miscarriages in the general population.[44,45]

Pre-gestational diabetes

The incidence of pregnancy loss in the diabetic population has declined substantially since the introduction of insulin in the early twentieth century. During the 1940s and 1950s the reported pregnancy loss rate ('sudden fetal death') was approximately 20%.[46] This might reflect the association between enhanced glycemic control (both pre-conceptionl and during the first weeks of organogenesis) and the decreased rate of malformations.[47] Most of the studied reporting outcome of miscarriage included patients with pre-gestational diabetes, without a specific distinction between Type 1 and Type 2 diabetes. The reported rate of spontaneous abortions in women with Type 1 diabetes is approximately 17%.[48] The pooled estimate risk for early pregnancy loss in patients with Type 1 and Type 2 diabetes was calculated to be 3.23 RR (95% CI, 1.64–6.36).[3]

Good glycemic control around the period of conception reduces the risk of early pregnancy loss to that observed in nondiabetic population. High levels of HbA1c above normal range showed progressively high pregnancy-loss rates. Lower levels of HbA1c were associated with lower early pregnancy-loss rates among women with Type 1 DM.[18,49,50] Therefore HbA1c can be regarded as an indirect measure of adverse outcome and be used for quality control.

A threshold level of HbA1c of 10–12% correlating with mean blood glucose (MBG) of 150–170 mg/dL, is suggested as the upper limit for reducing the risk of spontaneous abortions.[51]

Gestational diabetes mellitus

Only few studies investigating GDM and pregnancy outcome have included *early* pregnancy loss as one of the outcome measures examined. Therefore, there is a scarcity of data concerning the exact proportion of spontaneous pregnancy loss in this specific sub-group of diabetic patients.

Rudge et al.[52] described pregnancy results in women with abnormal glucose tolerance including women diagnosed with GDM. They reported an abortion rate of 0.8% in the group of patients with altered diurnal glycemic profile without frank diabetes (as opposed to no abortions in the control group). There is evidence to support the theory that some metabolic abnormalities such as insulin resistance and high levels of fasting blood glucose may be apparent at early stages of pregnancy in women who are subsequently diagnosed with gestational diabetes.[53] An alternative explanation is that this constitutes a group of women with undiagnosed Type 2 diabetes.

These studies and others offer circumferential support that GDM represents a metabolic disorder that interferes with the outcome of pregnancy from conception to delivery even though it is generally diagnosed throughout the third trimester.

Stillbirth (late fetal loss)

Stillbirth is a major component of PNM in the diabetic population (see Tables 64.2 and 64.3). Congenital malformations are thought to be the most established causes of stillbirth in the diabetic population. The most common malformations are cardiovascular, and neural tube defects,[2] but diabetes was not found to be predictive of any specific malformations.[19,54,55]

Fetal metabolic acidosis with and without hypoxemia (as discussed above) are more prevalent in the diabetic population.[31,32,56] Their presence may offer an additional explanation for late fetal demise in the diabetic population. Most studies investigating the pathophysiological basis for fetal death unrelated to congenital anomalies were done in women with PGDM[29,56] but it is reasonable to assume that women with GDM may share the same pathophysiological events as they also present the same high stillbirth rates.

The higher prevalence of other recognized risk factors for stillbirth such as maternal obesity, hypertension, and advanced maternal age in the diabetic population may all contribute to higher stillbirth rates.[2,57] Late fetal death occurs more often in women with poor metabolic control, ketoacidosis and vascular complications probably as a result of fetal metabolic acidemia and hypoxemia.[58] Landon et al.[58] found that women with Type 1 diabetes with vascular complications were at greater risk for abnormal fetal surveillance tests and subjected to more obstetric interventions such as induction of labor. In the group of patients who needed intervention, fetal cord pH was significantly lower then the non-intervention group. This may also serve as an indirect measure of fetal academia (in diabetic women as a possible cause of fetal compromise which may lead to intrauterine fetal death).

Pre-gestational diabetes

The reported rate of congenital malformation in patients with Type 1 diabetes in some population based studies is 3- to 5-fold higher than that of the general population.[15,48] Congenital anomalies in women with Type 2 diabetes are also significantly higher than that of the general population and contribute to the increased PNM rate reported in this sub-group of patients.[12,13] The congenital malformation rate in patients with Type 2 diabetes is equal, or even exceeds that of Type 1 diabetes.[12,13,59]

Stillbirth rate in women with pre-gestational diabetes may reach 28–46 per 1000 live births, a rate three to five times higher than that of the general population.[2,12,38] Lauenborg et al.,[19] in an audit on 25 cases of stillbirth in Type 1 diabetes patients found a direct relationship between poor glycemic control both before and during pregnancy (measured by HbA1c levels) and higher incidence of stillbirth. The relative risk for stillbirth in patients with Type 2 diabetes was found to be 4.7 (95% CI, 3.7–6.0).[12] Cundy et al.[38] reported a 7-fold increase in the risk for late fetal death in women with Type 2 diabetes which contributed to a high PNM rate of 46 per 1000 in that study. This was attributed to maternal factors such as obesity and advanced maternal age more prevalent in his study group. Furthermore, patients with Type 2 diabetes tend to be of lower socio-economic class and part of an ethnic minority group, demographic differences that are interrelated to lack of preconception care and may be confounding in interpretation of results.[2,12,38]

Gestational diabetes mellitus

The stillbirth rate in patients with GDM is greater than that of general population. The exact extent of increase in stillbirth rates is dependant upon the severity of glucose intolerance and degree of glycemic control. Stillbirth rate are only slightly increased when good glycemic control is achieved (stillbirth rate of 4.8 vs. 4.2 per 1000).[11] Pettitte et al.[57] reported increased risk of stillbirth mainly related to excessive fetal growth, which is also a measure of increased hyperglycemia and hyperinsulinemia. The threshold for this pregnancy complication seems to be between 105 and 110 mean blood glucose (MBG), patients who achieve glycemic control below these values have stillbirth rate comparable to those of general population.[51]

Table 64.2 Perinatal mortality in pre-gestational diabetes mellitus

Author	Number of participants	Total PNM	Stillbirth	Neonatal death	Preterm Ω	Macrosomia LGA	Birth trauma	Congenital anomalies
CEMACH[2] 2005	3808 (2767 Type 1; 1041 Type 2)	NA	26.8/1000 (Type 1 25.8/1000; Type 2 29.2/1000)	9.3/1000 (Type 1 9.3/1000; Type 2 9.2/1000)	36%	Macrosomia 21% (*); LGAA 51.7%	Shoulder dystocia 7.9%; Erb's palsy 4.5/1000	41.8/1000
French multicentric[13]	435 (289 Type 1; 146 Type 2)	44/1000	34.5/1000	Type 1 3/1000; Type 2 21/1000	38.2%	Macrosomia 17.3%	Shoulder dystocia 7.6%	41/1000
Machintosh et al.[12]	2359 (1707 Type 1; 652 Type 2)	31.8/1000	26.8/1000	9.3/1000	NA	NA	NA	46/1000
Jensen et al.[34]	1215 (Type 1)	31/1000	21/1000	NA	41.7%	LGA 62.5%	NA	50/1000
Clausen et al.[39]	301 (240 Type 1; 61 Type 2)	66/1000 (Type 2)	NA	NA	38% Type 1, 31% Type 2	LGA 51% Type 1; 56% Type 2; Macrosomia 5% Type 1; 8% Type 2	NA	29/1000 (Type 1); 67/1000 (Type 2)
Evers et al.[40]	323 Type 1	28/1000	18.5/1000	9.25/1000	32.2%	LGA 45.1%	Shoulder dystocia 14%	88/1000

*No significant difference in macrosomia rate between Type 1 and Type 2.

Table 63.3   Perinatal mortality in gestational diabetes mellitus

Author	Number of participants	Total PNM	Stillbirth	Neonatal death	Preterm Ω	Macrosomia LGA	Birth trauma	Metabolic
Crowther et al.[41]	1000 (490 intervention, 510 routine care)	NA	0/506 vs. 3/524	0/506; 2/524	NA	Macrosomia 10% vs. 21%; LGA 13% vs. 22%	Shoulder dystocia 1%; vs. 3% RR 0.46 (95% CI 0.19–1.10)	Jaundice 9% (both)
O'Sullivan et al.[37]	187 GDM	64/1000	NA	NA	22.5%	NA	NA	NA
Dunne et al.[42]	216 (*)	NA	0	0	NA	LGA 25–37%	NA	NA
Ramtoola et al.[43]	294	116/1000	81/1000	38/1000	22%	Macrosomia 16%	NA	Hypoglycemia 14%; Hyperbilirubinemia 39%
Ray et al.[10]	428	NA	NA	NA	19.2%	LGA 15.9%	Shoulder dystocia 3%	NA

*GDM + IGT.

Neonatal death

Preterm delivery

Pre-gestational diabetes. Preterm delivery is strongly related to adverse neonatal outcome.[2,4,13] Over one-third of infants of pre-gestational diabetic mothers were born prematurely.[2] The rate of preterm delivery (both spontaneous and induced) in Type 1 diabetic population is as high as 45%.[13] Poor glycemic control (elevated HbA1c) levels and vascular complications (pre-eclampsia and nephropathy) are predictive factors for preterm labor.[60–62]

The CEMACH enquiry reported the risk for preterm delivery in the diabetic population (Type 1 and Type 2 diabetes) to be nearly 5-fold higher in comparison to the general population. Up to two-thirds of preterm deliveries were induced ('medically indicated'), and nearly 37% of them were due to presumed fetal compromise.[2] Some studies indicate that the proportion of induced preterm delivery due to presumed fetal compromise is greater in the diabetic population than that of general population.[2]

Diabetes complicated by nephropathy or vascular disease causes an overall higher preterm delivery even when compared to a group of women with chronic hypertension, which might suggest there are other pathophysiological factors contributing to the adverse outcome.[60]

Gestational diabetes mellitus. There is an association between increased incidence of preterm delivery and gestational diabetes. Hedderson et al.[63] found that the risk for preterm delivery increased with increasing levels of glycemia (ranging from abnormal screening, but normal diagnostic glucose tolerance test to GDM). The relative risk for preterm labor was 1.42 (95% CI, 1.15–1.77) for the GDM group compared to normal controls. This association was also present for both induced and spontaneous preterm labor.[63–65]

The degree of glucose intolerance or 'early onset' of GDM is linked to a higher incidence of preterm labor. This may suggest an inverse relation between length of pregnancy and poor glycemic control, and identify poor glycemic control as a marker of increased risk for preterm delivery.[9]

Macrosomia

Pre-gestational diabetes. Macrosomia is associated with increased PNM and increased birth trauma. Birth related trauma in women with pre-gestational diabetes are much higher than those in the general population: shoulder dystocia (more then 2-fold), birth related fractures, and Erb's palsy (more than 10-fold).[2,10,53] Higher rates of shoulder dystocia carry an increased risk of PNM. Sheiner et al. found PNM rates of 3.7% in infants suffering from shoulder dystocia versus 0.5% in those without (OR 7.4, 95% CI, 3.5–14.9).[66]

Mondestein et al. reported that PNM is increased among diabetic pregnancies at all birth weight categories over 1250 g,[67] but especially when fetal weight exceeded 4000 g, thus doubling the risk of fetal death in the diabetic population reaching 5.9/1000 births (adjusted RR 2; 95% CI, 1.8–2.2).[67]

There was no significant difference between the rates of macrosomia in infants born to women with Type 1 diabetes compared with those born to women with Type 2 diabetes.[2] In unselected diabetic populations of patients with Type 1 and Type 2 diabetes, up to 50% of infants of diabetic mothers are born at weights >90th percentile. These patients were suboptimal in their glycemic control, as reflected by HbA1c levels.[2,53,66] The risk for delivery of a macrosomic child is directly related to glycemic control measures throughout pregnancy.

Gestational diabetes mellitus. A high rate of macrosomia is also reported in infants of mothers diagnosed with GDM (increased risk of 2- to 4-fold).[5,9] Women with GDM who attend an intensive pregnancy surveillance have a 4-fold decrease in the risk birth related complications compared with GDM patients receiving 'standard' prenatal care.[41]

Langer et al.[68] demonstrated the relationship between glycemic control (namely mean blood glucose levels <105) and reduced incidence of macrosomia.

The above is not direct evidence for the relationship between metabolic control, macrosomia, and reduced PNM. However, it is logical to assume that intensive prenatal care results in better glycemic control which contributes to improved outcome.

Respiratory and metabolic complications

Admission to neonatal intensive care units (NICU) or other special care units is more common in infants of diabetic mothers, and reaches up to 50% of neonates.[2,13,33]

The NICU admission rate is an indirect measure of morbidity and of quality of care in the diabetic population (both PGDM and GDM). The majority of admissions are due to a myriad of conditions that may all contribute to early or late PNM in the diabetic population, such as hypoglycemia, hyperbilirubinemia, respiratory distress due to lung immaturity, etc. Premature infants are more prone to episodes of hypoglycemia than term infants;[33] however, even after correction for preterm birth the proportion of infants of diabetic mothers hospitalized in NICU is still significantly higher than general population.[2,33,62,64] For instance, the rate of hypoglycemia in infants born to Type 1 diabetes may reach 50% in premature infants and 23% in term infants.[61] Pulmonary complications ranging from transient tachypnea to respiratory distress are more common in infants of diabetic mothers resulting from abnormal lung maturation caused by hyperinsulinemia.[51] There is a direct relationship between higher rates of respiratory complications and poor glycemic control,[24,33] but there is little information concerning the estimated threshold of glycemia which carries an increased risk for respiratory complications.[51] Another problem is the lack of data relating directly to the relationship between higher rates of these 'metabolic' complication and PNM. These complications may carry an increased risk for morbidity and mortality, but exact quantification of this added risk is difficult due to lack of information. It is believed that with modern resources, the greater part of these complications have a minor influence on actual mortality rates, but may cause increase in morbidity.

What can be done to reduce the rate of perinatal mortality in pregnancies complicated by diabetes?

The St Vincent declaration given in 1989 set a goal to equalize pregnancy outcomes of women with diabetes mellitus to those of nondiabetic women within 5 years. Although there has been considerable advancement in the ability to detect fetal anomalies, establish fetal well-being and maturity, this goal, which was perceived as feasible at the time (especially in light of the conceivable improvement in pregnancy outcomes of insulin-dependant diabetic women), has not been met. The presence of diabetes is thought to increase the risk for congenital malformation by as much as 10-fold, stillbirth (up to 5-fold), and neonatal death (3- to 4-fold).[3]

Furthermore, some reports imply that the trend toward decline in PNM rates in the diabetic population is less than the decline in PNM observed in the general population during the same time period.[4,18]

Good glycemic control is a fundamental part in avoiding adverse pregnancy outcome. In order to elucidate possible causes for this apparent failure to meet goals set at St Vincent, two important issues must be addressed. The first issue is the extent at which the diabetic population meets the health care practitioners' criteria for 'good diabetic control'.

There are very few randomized control trials (RCTs) regarding the relationship between glycemic control and pregnancy outcome.[69] The DCCT (Diabetes Control and Complications Trial) suggested that early and tight glycemic control might reduce pregnancy-loss rates and congenital anomalies rates equal to those of general population.[70] This finding was not repeated in the Cochrane's review on three other RCTs.[69] Conversely, observational studies (which included less selective populations) failed to demonstrate such a substantial reduction.[2,13] Some of the difference can be explained by the fact that different cut-off points for HbA1c levels to distinguish between poor and good glycemic control were used. There were also dissimilarities regarding the time in which the predictive HbA1c measurement was taken (first trimester, first antenatal visit etc.), and the number of measurements used to categorize women in 'poor' versus 'optimal' control. It is clear that a single HbA1c measurement can not be used as an absolute predictor for pregnancy complications.

HbA1c may reflect long-term average glycemic control, but there are many limitations to its use, raising important questions regarding its adequacy as a measure of glycemic control (vs. other methods such as self-monitoring blood glucose levels, MBG or fasting blood glucose). Furthermore the optimal HbA1c level that should be set as a treatment goal is beyond the scope of this chapter. Langer and colleagues[71] provided support for those calling to rely on maternal glucose levels as a measure of glycemic control rather then HbA1c. They showed that strict glycemic control resulting in near normoglycemia leads to perinatal morbidity and mortality rates almost comparable to those of nondiabetic population. Other studies also hold up the hypothesis that intensive care consisting of maternal glucose monitoring and decisions concerning insulin treatment based upon its results are related with enhanced perinatal outcome.[72,73]

The second issue regarding the failure to meet St Vincent goals is related to preconception counseling in the diabetic population. Preconception counseling is significant due to the fact that the crucial phase of organogenesis takes part during early pregnancy, at which timely and adequate metabolic control is important for optimal pregnancy outcome.

A meta-analysis[8] reviewing 14 cohort studies concerning patients with PGDM, calculated a major malformation rate of 2.1% in women attending PCC versus 3.5% in those without PCC (RR 0.36; 95% CI, 0.22–0.59). This connection between preconception care (PCC) and reduction in adverse pregnancy outcome (mainly spontaneous abortions and congenital anomalies) was also demonstrated in other studies.[13,15,34,74] The topic of PCC may need special attention in women with Type 2 DM as they tend to differ in lifestyle, age, and economical background and often require change in treatment regime (oral antiglycemics drugs or insulin).[2,15,39]

The route towards improved PCC attendance remains somewhat obscure. Some of the factors associated with low attendance rates such as education level, socio-economic status, and ethnic background are not in the hands of health care providers. However, diabetic patients should be counseled against PCC failure and unplanned pregnancies, and provided with accessible preconception education and care programs.

Tables 64.2 and 64.3 summarize data regarding PNM and its various components in women with pre-gestational and gestational diabetes, respectively.

REFERENCES

1. Metzger BE, Coustan DR, et al. The Organising Committee. Summary and recommendations of the 4th international Workshop Conference on Gestational Diabetes Mellitus. Diabetes Care 1998; 21(suppl. 2): 161–7.
2. Confidential Enquiry into maternal and child health: Pregnancy of women with type 1 and type 2 diabetes 2002–03 in England, Wales and Northern Ireland. London: CEMACH; 2005.
3. Inkster M, Fahey TP, et al. Poor glycated heamoglubin control and adverse pregnancy outcomes in type1 and type 2 diabetes mellitus: systematic review of observational studied. BMC Pregnancy and Childbirth 2006; 6: 30.
4. American College of Obstetricians and Gynecologists Clinical management guidelines for obstetrician–gynecologists. ACOG practice bulletin no. 30. Washington DC: ACOG; 2001.
5. Jovanovic L, Pettitt DJ. Gestational diabetes mellitus. JAMA 2001; 286: 2516–8.
6. American Diabetes Association. Clinical practice recommendations 2004. Diabetes Care 2004; 27: S88–S90.
7. Wood ST, Sauve R, et al. Prediabetes and perinatal mortality. Diabetic Care 2000; 23: 1752–4.
8. Ray JG, O'Brien TE, et al. Preconception care and the risk of congenital anomalies in the offspring of women with diabetes mellitus: a meta analysis. QJM 2001; 94: 435–44.
9. Langer O, Yogev Y, et al. Gestational diabetes: the consequence of not treating. Am J Obstet Gynecol 2005; 192: 989–97.
10. Ray JG, Vermeulen MJ, et al. Maternal and neonatal outcomes in pregestational and gestational diabetes mellitus, and the influence of

maternal obesity and weight pain: the DEPOSIT study. QJM 2001; 94: 347–56.

11. Yogev Y, Most O, et al. Gestational diabetes mellitus: Is there a risk for perinatal mortality? Am J Obstet Gynecol 2004; 191(suppl.): s51.

12. Machintosh MC, Fleming KM, et al. Perinatal mortality and congenital anomalies in babies of women with type 1 or type 2 diabetes in England, Wales and Northen Ireland: Population based study. BMJ 2006; 333; 177–80.

13. Diabetes and Pregnancy group, France. French multicentric survey of outcome of pregnancy in women with pregestational diabetes. Diab Care 2003, 26: 2990–3.

14. World Health Organization. Manual of the International Statistical Classification of Diseases, Injuries and Causes of Death, 9th revision, vol 1. Geneva: World Heath Organization; 1977.

15. Evers IM, W de Valk H, et al. Risk of complications of pregnancy in women with type 1 diabetes: nationwide prospective study in the Netherlands. BMJ 2004.

16. Lawn J, Shibuya K, Stein C. No cry at birth: global estimates of intrapartum stillbirths and intrapartum-related neonatal deaths. Bull World Health Organ 2005; 83: 409–17.

17. Cunningham FG, Leveno KJ, et al. Fetal death. In: William's Obstetrics, 22nd edn. (suppl. 4). Norwalk, CT: Appleton & Lange; 2005.

18. Barfield W, Martin J, Hoyert D. Racial/ethnic trends in fetal mortality in United States, 1990–2000. MMWR Morbid Mortal Wkly Rep 2004; 53: 529–32.

19. Lauenborg J, Mathiesen E, et al. Audit on stillbirths in women with pregestational type 1 diabetes. Diabetic Care 2003; 26: 1385–9.

20. Canningham FG, Gant NF, Leveno KJ, et al., eds. In: Obstetrics in Broad Perspective. 21st edn. Williams & Williams Obstetrics 2001.

21. American College of Obstetricians and Gynecologists. Perinatal and infant mortality statistics. Committee Opinion No 167. Washington: ACOG; 1995.

22. Lee AT, Plump A, et al. A role for DNA mutations in diabetes-associated teratogenesis in transgenic embryos. Diabetes 1995; 44: 20–4.

23. Eriksson UJ, Borg LA, et al. Diabetic embryopathy. Studies with animal and in vitro models. Diabetes 1991; 40(suppl. 2): 94–8.

24. Carrapato MR, Marcelino F, et al. The infant of the diabetic mother: the critical developmental window. Early pregnancy 2001; 5: 57–8.

25. Fine EL, Horal M, et al. Evidence that elevated glucose causes altered gene expression, apoptosis and neural tube defects in a mouse model of diabetic pregnancy. Diabetes 1999; 48: 2454–62.

26. Towner D, Kojs SL, et al. Congenital malformations in pregnancies complicated by NIDDM. Diabetes Care 1995; 18: 1446–51.

27. Scaefer UM, Songster G, et al. Congenital anomalies in offsprings of women with hyperglycemia first detected during pregnancy. Am J Obstet Gynecol 1997; 177: 1165–71.

28. Jovanovic L, Metzger BE, et al. β-hydroxybutyrate levels in type 1 diabetic pregnancy compared with normal pregnancy. Diabetes Care 1998; 21: 1978–84.

29. Pedersen J, Pedersen LM, et al. Assessors of fetal perinatal mortality in diabetic pregnancy. Analysis of 1,332 pregnances in Cooenhagen series 1946–1972. Diabetes 1974; 23: 302–5.

30. Pedersen J. The pregnant diabetic and her newborn. In: Williamms and Wilkins 2nd edn. Baltimore; 1977.

31. Salvesen DR, Freeman J, et al. Prediction of fetal academia in pregnancies complicated by maternal diabetes mellitus by biophysical profile scoring and fetal heart rate monitoring. Br J Obstet Gynecol 1993; 100: 277–33.

32. Salvesen DR, Brudenell JM, et al. Fetal beta-cell function in pregenancies complicated by maternal diabetes mellitus: relationship to fetal academia and macosomia. Am J Obstet Gynecol 1993; 168: 1363–9.

33. Williams AF. Hypoglycemia of the newborn. Review of the literature. CHD/97.1. Geneva: World Health Organization; 1997. http://www.who.int/child-adolescent-health/publication/NUTRITION/WHO_CHD_97.1htm

34. Jensen DM, Damm P, et al. Outcomes in Type 1 diabetic pregnancies. Diabetes Care 2004, 27: 2819–23.

35. Karllsson K, Kjellmer I. The outcome of diabetic pregnancies in relation to the mother's blood sugar level. Am J Obstet Gynecol 1972; 112: 213.

36. Kitzmiller JL, Cloherty JP, et al. Diabetic pregnancy and perinatal morbidity. Am J Obstet Gynecol 1978; 131: 560–79.

37. O'sullivan JB, Charles D, et al. Gestational diabetes and preinatal mortality rate. Am J Obstet Gynecol 1973; 1: 901–4.

38. Cundy T, Gamble G, et al. Perinatal mortality in Type 2 diabetes mellitus. Diabet Med 2000; 17: 33–9.

39. Clausen TD, Matheisen E. Poor pregnancy outcome in women with type 2 diabetes. Diabetes Care 2005; 28: 323–8.

40. Evers IM, de Valk HW, et al. Risk of complications of pregnancy in women with type 1 diabetes: nationwide prospective study in the Netherlands. BMJ 2004; doi: 10.1136/bmj.38043.583160.EE

41. Crowther CA, Hiller JH, et al. Effect of treatment of gestational diabetes mellitus on pregnancy outcomes. N Engl J Med 2005; 352: 2477–86.

42. Dune F, Brydon P, et al. Pregnancy in women with Type 2 diabetes: 12 years outcome 1990–2002. Diabet Med 2003; 20: 734–8.

43. Ramtoola S, Home P, et al. Gestational impaired glucose tolerance does not increase perinatal mortality in a developing country: cohort study. BMJ 2001; 322: 1025–6.

44. Griebel CP, Halvorsen J, et al. Management of spontaneous abortion. Am Fam Physician 2005: 72: 1243–50.

45. Stovall TG. Early pregnancy loss and ectopic pregnancy. In: Berek JS and Novak's Gynecology, 14th edn; 2007.

46. Miller HC, Hurwitz D, et al. Fetal and neonatal mortality in pregnancies complicated by diabetes mellitus. JAMA 1944; 124: 271.

47. Miodovnik M, Skillman CA, et al. Effect of maternal hyperketonemia in hyperglycemic pregnant ewes and their fetuses. Am J Obstet Gynecol 1986; 154: 394–401.

48. Casson IF, Clarke CA, et al. Outcome of pregnancy in insulin dependent diabetic women: results of a five year population cohort study. BMJ 1997; 315: 275–8.

49. Mills JL, Simpson JL, et al. Incidence of spontaneous abortion among normal women and insulin-dependent diabetic women whose pregnancies were identified within 21 days of conception. New Engl J Med 1988; 319: 1617–23.

50. Jovanovic L, Knopp RH, et al. Elevated pregnancy losses at high and low extremes of maternal glucose in early and normal diabetic pregnancy. Diabetic Care 2005; 28: 1113–7.

51. Langer O. The association between glucose thresholds and perinatal complications. In: Diabetes and pregnancy dilemma: leading change with proven solutions. Langer O ed. University Press of America; 2006; 14:231–5.

52. Rudge MV, Calderon I, et al. Perinatal outcome of pregnancies complicated by diabetes and by maternal daily hyperglycemia not related to diabetes. Gynecol Obstet Invest 2000; 50: 108–12.

53. Smirnakis KV, Martinez A, et al. Early pregnancy insulin resistance and subsequent gestational diabetes mellitus. Diabetes Care 2005; 28: 1207–8.

54. Kuhoury MJ, Becerra JE, et al. Clinical–epidemiologic assessment of pattern of birth defects associated with human teratogenens: application to diabetic embrypathy. Pediatrics 1989; 84: 658–65.

55. Becerra JE, Kuhoury MJ, et al. Diabetes mellitus during pregnancy and the risks for specific birth defects: a population-based case–control study. Pediatrics 1990; 85: 1–9.

56. Bradley RJ, Brundenell JM, et al. Fetal acidosis and hyperlacticemia diagnosed by cordocentesis in pregnancies complicated by maternal diabetes mellitus. Diabet Med 1991; 8: 464–8.

57. Pettitt DJ, Knowles WC, et al. Gestational diabetes: infant and maternal complications of pregnancy in relation to third trimester glucose tolerance in Pima Indians. Diabetes Care 1980; 3: 458–64.

58. Landon MB, Langer O, et al. Fetal surveillance in pregnancies complicated by insulin-dependent diabetes mellitus. Am J Obstet Gynecol 1992; 167: 617–21.

59. Roland JM, Murphy HR, et al. The pregnancies of women with type 2 diabetes: poor outcomes but opportunities for improvement. Diabet Med 2005; 22: 1774–7.

60. Sibai BM, Caritis SN, et al. Preterm delivery in women with pregestational diabetes mellitus or chronic hypertension relative to women with uncomplicated pregnancies. The national institute of child health and human development maternal–fetal medicine units network. Am J Obstet Gynecol 2000; 183: 1520–4.

61. Lepereq J, Coste J, et al. Factors Associated with preterm delivery in women with type 1 diabetes. Diabetes Care 2004; 27: 2824–8.

62. Watson D, Rowan J, et al. Admissions to neonatal intensive care following pregnancies complicated by geastational or type 2 diabetes. Aust N Z Obstet Gynecol 2003; 43: 429–32.

63. Hedderson MM, Ferrara A, et al. Gestational diabetes mellitus and lesser degrees of pregnancy hyperglycemia: association with increased risk of spontaneous preterm delivery. Obstet Gynecol 2003; 102: 850–6.

64. Svare JA, Hansen BB, et al. Perinatal complications in women with gestational diabetes mellitus. Acta Obstet Gynecol Scand 2001; 80: 899–904.

65. Lao TT, Ho LF. Does maternal glucose intolerance affect the length of gestation in singleton pregnancies? J Soc Gynecol Investig 2003; 10: 366–71.

66. Sheiner E, Levy A, et al. Determining factors associated with shoulder dystocia: a population based study. Eur J Obstet Gynecol 2006; 126: 11–5.

67. Mondestin MA, Ananth CV, et al. Birth weight and fetal death in the united states: the effect of maternal diabetes during pregnancy. Am J Obstet Gynecol 2002; 187: 922–6.

68. Langer O, Yogev Y, et al. Gestational diabetes: Does an association exist between deviant fetal growth and glycemic control? Am J Obstet Gynecol 2004; 189: 151.

69. Walkinshaw SA. Very tight versus tight glycemic control for diabetes in pregnancy. Cochrane database Syst Rev 2000; 2: CD00226.

70. The Diabetes Control and Complications Trial Research Group. The effect of intensive treatment for diabetes on development and progression of long-term complications in insulin dependent diabetes mellitus. N Engl J Med 1993; 329: 977–86.

71. Langer O, Rodriguez DA, et al. Intensified versus conventional management of gestational diabetes. Am J Obstet Gynecol 1994; 170: 1036–46.

72. Jovanovic L, Peterson CM, et al. Maternal postprandial glucose levels and infant birth weight: The diabetes in early pregnancy study. Am J Obstet Gynecol 1991; 164: 103–11.

73. de Veciana M, Major CA, et al. Postprandial versus preprandial blood glucose monitoring in women with gestational diabetes mellitus requiring insulin therapy. N Engl J Med 1995; 333: 1237–41.

74. Steel JM, Johnstone FD, et al. Can prepregnancy care of diabetic women reduce the risk of abnormal babies? BMJ 1990; 301: 1070–4.

Index

Note: Page references in *italics* refer to Figures; those in **bold** refer to Tables
GDM = gestational diabetes mellitus